CONTACT —LENS— PRACTICE

Edited by

Montague Ruben FRCS, FRCOphth.

Honorary Consultant Ophthalmologist
Moorfields Eye Hospital
University of London

and

Michel Guillon PhD

Contact Lens Research Consultants
Pimlico
London
UK, and
University of Paris
Orsay
France

CHAPMAN & HALL MEDICAL
London · Glasgow · New York · Tokyo · Melbourne · Madras

Published by Chapman & Hall, 2–6 Boundary Row, London SE1 8HN

Chapman & Hall, 2–6 Boundary Row, London SE1 8HN, UK

Blackie Academic & Professional, Wester Cleddens Road, Bishopbriggs, Glasgow G64 2NZ, UK

Chapman & Hall Inc., One Penn Plaza, 41st Floor, New York NY10019, USA

Chapman & Hall Japan, Thomson Publishing Japan, Hirakawacho Nemoto Building, 6F, 1-7-11 Hirakawa-cho, Chiyoda-ku, Tokyo 102, Japan

Chapman & Hall Australia, Thomas Nelson Australia, 102 Dodds Street, South Melbourne, Victoria 3205, Australia

Chapman & Hall India, R. Seshadri, 32 Second Main Road, CIT East, Madras 600 035, India

First edition 1994

© 1994 Chapman & Hall

Typeset in 10/12 Palatino by Falcon Graphic Art, Wallington, Surrey

Printed and bound in Hong Kong

ISBN 0 412 35120 X

A catalogue record for this book is available from the British Library

Library of Congress Cataloguing-in-Publication data
Contact lens practice/edited by Montague Ruben and Michel Guillon. – – 1st ed.
    p. cm.
  Includes bibliographical references index
  ISBN 0-412-35120-X (alk. paper)
  1. Contact lenses. I. Ruben, Montague. II. Guillon, Michel.
  [DNLM: 1. Contact Lenses. WW 355 C7557 1994]
RE977.C6C5558 1994
617.7'523–dc20
DNLM/DLC
for Library of Congress
                                       93–8749
                                         CIP

Contents

PART FOUR ANATOMICAL AND PHYSIOLOGICAL FACTORS 185

PART FIVE CLINICAL TECHNIQUES 273

PART SIX PRACTICAL ROUTINE 497

Contributors

Christine Astin
Moorfields Eye Hospital
City Road
London EC1V 2PD
UK

W.J. Benjamin
The University of Alabama Birmingham
School of Optometry
The Medical Centre
University Station
Birmingham
Alabama 35294
USA

J.A. Bonanno
School of Optometry
University of California
Berkeley
California 94720
USA

I.M. Borish
College of Optometry
University of Houston
Houston
Texas
USA

N.S.C. Borisuth
The University of Chicago
Visual Sciences Center
939 East 57th Street
Chicago
Illinois 60637
USA

Barbara E. Caffery
60 Bloor Street West
Suite 705
Toronto
Canada M4W 3B8

L.G. Carney
Queensland University of Technology
School of Optometry
2 George Street
Brisbane Queensland 4000
Australia

T. Chan-Ling
Department of Anatomy F13
Sydney University
Sydney
New South Wales 2006
Australia

I. Cox
Bausch and Lomb
Ocular Research Dept
1400 North Goodman Street
PO Box 450
Rochester
New York 14692-0450
USA

C. Ducharme
Boston Eye Associates
1244 Boyleston Street
Suite 202
Chestnut Hill
MA 02167
USA

I. Fatt
406 Boylton Avenue
Berkeley
California 94707
USA

Sharon Fekrat
The University of Chicago
Chicago
Illinois
USA

C. Fowler
Vision Sciences
Aston University
Birmingham B4 7ET
UK

O.-C. Geyer
Institute for Medical Aid
Bahnhofstr. 19a
6330 Wetzler
Germany

W.S. Gibson
24 Murray Road
Wokingham
Berkshire RG11 2TB
UK

T. Grosvenor
College of Optometry
Central Campus
University of Houston
Houston
Texas 77004
USA

J.-P. Guillon
Contact Lens Research Consultants
42 Vauxhall Bridge Road
London SW1V 2RX
UK

M. Guillon
Contact Lens Research Consultants
42 Vauxhall Bridge Road
London SW1V 2RX
UK

R.M. Hill
College of Optometry
Ohio State University
338 West 10th Avenue
Columbus
Ohio 43210
USA

A. Ho
Cornea and Contact Lens Research Unit
School of Optometry
University of New South Wales
PO Box 1
Kensington 2033
New South Wales
Australia

N.F. Burnett Hodd
7 Devonshire Street
London WIN 1FT
UK

T.A. Horbett
Department of Chemical Engineering and
Centre for Bioengineering
BF-10 University of Washington
Seattle
Washington 98195
USA

T. John
Cornea Research Unit
University of Chicago Medical Centre
939 E 57th Street
Chicago
Illinois 60637
USA

J.E.L. Josephson
60 Bloor Street West
Suite 705
Toronto
Ontario
Canada M4W 3BB

K.R. Kenyon
Schepeus Eye Research Institute
20 Staniford Street
Boston
Massachusetts 02114
USA

Y. Kikkawa
613 Koyoen Mansions
6–25 Monjo-cho Koyoen
Nishinomiya 662
Japan

S.L. Kwok
College of Optometry
Central Campus
University of Houston
Houston
Texas 77204-6062
USA

J.G. Lawrenson
Reta Lila Weston Institute of Neurological
    Studies
University College London Medical School
Riding House Stree
London W1P 7PN
UK

G.E. Lowther
School of Optomety
University of Alabama at Birmingham
Birmingham
Alabama 35294
USA

B.R. Masters
Uniformed Services University of
    The Health Sciences
Department of Anatomy and Cell Biology
4301 Jones Bridge Road
Bethesda
Maryland 20814
USA

Nancy B. Mateo
To the Point Writing Service
2515 Parkland No. H
Ann Arbor
Michigan 48104
USA

M. Millodot
Hong Kong Polytechnic
Hung Hom
Kowloon
Hong Kong

Eleanor F. Mobilia
Cornea Service
Massachusetts Eye and Ear Infirmary
Boston
Massachusetts
USA

Judith A. Morris
Contact Lens Department
Moorfields Eye Hospital
City Road
London
UK

S.E.G. Nilsson
Department of Ophthalmology
University of Linköping
S-58185 Linköping
Sweden

M. O'Neal
AL/CFHV
Wright-Patterson AFB
Ohio 45433
USA

R.M. Pearson
City University
Department of Optometry and Visual
   Science
311–21 Goswell Road
London EC1V 7DD
UK

M.J.A. Port
City University
Department of Optometry and Visual
   Science
Dame Alice Owen Building
311–21 Goswell Road
London EC1V 7DD
UK

D.C. Pye
School of Optometry
University of New South Wales
Kensington 2033
New South Wales
Australia

R. Rabbetts
31 Fratton Road
Portsmouth
Hampshire PO1 5AB
UK

B. Ratner
NESAC/BIO, BF-10
University of Washington
Seattle
Washington 98195
USA

M.F. Refojo
Eye Research Institute
Retina Foundation
20 Staniford Street
Boston
Massachusetts 02114
USA

P. Rosenthal
Scleral Lens Clinic
Massachusetts Eye and Ear Infirmary
Boston
Massachusetts
USA

T.J.P. Rouwen
Central Military Hospital
Department of Ophthalmology (poli G)
PO Box 90-000
3500 AA Utrecht
The Netherlands

M. Ruben
20 Seven Stones Drive
Broadstairs
Kent CT10 1TW
UK

G. Ruskell
Department of Optometry and Visual
   Science
City University
Dame Alice Owen Building
311–321 Goswell Rd
London EC1V 7DD
UK

A.G. Sabell
234 Hole Lane,
Northfield
Birmingham
UK

W.A. Sammons
Jigsaw Consultants
11 Stillions Close
Windmill Hill
Alton
Hampshire GU34 2RX
UK

O.D. Schein
Wilmer Ophthalmology Institution
Johns Hopkins Hospital
Baltimore
Maryland 21205
USA

M. Sheridan
30 Simcoe Way
Dunkeswell
Honiton
Devon EX14 0UR
UK

A. Slonovic
Department of Ophthalmology
University of Toronto
Toronto
Canada

Fiona Stapleton
Moorfields Eye Hospital
City Road
London EC1V 2PD
UK

Judith Stechler
Moorfields Eye Hospital
City Road
London EC1V 2PD
UK

R.W.W. Stevenson
Optometry Department
Glasgow Caledonian University
Glasgow
UK

Janet Stone
Optometrist
formerly Lecturer in Contact Lenses
The Institute of Optometry
56–62 Newington Causeway
London SE1 6DS
UK

D. Taylor
Hospital For Sick Children
Great Ormond Street
London WC1
UK

A.A. Thaer
In co-operation with the Institute for Medical
   Vision Aid
and Helmut Hund GmbH
Bahnhofst. 19a
6330 Wetzler
Germany

Brenda J. Tripathi
The University of Chicago
Chicago
Illinois
USA

R.C. Tripathi
Professor of Ophthalmology
   and Visual Science
University of Chicago
5841 South Maryland Avenue
Chicago
Illinois 60637
USA

R.E. Weisbarth
Ciba Vision Corporation
Professional Services
11460 Johns Creek Parkway
Duluth
Georgia 30136
USA

B.A. Weissman
Jules Stein Eye Institute
UCLA School of Medicine
800 Westwood Plaza
Los Angeles
California 90024
USA

S. Zantos
School of Optometry
University of New South Wales
Kensington 2033
New South Wales
Australia

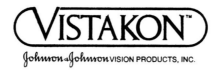

POST OFFICE BOX 10157
JACKSONVILLE, FLORIDA 32247
(904) 443-1000

As the world's leading contact lens company, Vistakon is proud to sponsor the special edition of Contact Lens Practice. Contact lens practice is a multi-disciplinary science, which is in a constant state of change as new materials and developments enable an increasing number of patients to be successfully fitted. In order to keep in touch with these developments it is necessary for contact lens practitioners to have comprehensive sources of information at their fingertips and this book provides such information.

At Vistakon we have achieved our world-wide leadership position with Acuvue® only as a result of the support we have received from the eye care professionals. It is the professional acceptance of the advantages that disposable lenses in general, and Acuvue in particular, have to offer the patient that has made Acuvue the number one selling lens in the world.

We are committed to continuing support of the eye care professional in developing the contact lens business around the world. We see the continuing education of the professions and the education of students as being essential and hope that this book is able to provide a valuable asset in this process.

Bernard W. Walsh
Worldwide Franchise Chairman

ORIGINS OF THE CONTACT LENS   1

A.G. Sabell

1.1 INTRODUCTION

With the exception of contact appliances devised for diagnostic purposes it can be assumed that an important, if not indispensible requirement is that the lens or shell should be capable of being worn on the eye surface for a useful number of hours. In the earlier years of contact lens use, this was frequently not possible. The history of the contact lens is a study of the struggles and achievements of a small number of pioneers whose work has enabled the present day practitioner to satisfy the needs of his patient in a relatively rapid and easy manner. Good comfort and lengthy wearing times can now be regarded as the norm rather than the exception. This is not to imply that 'everything in the garden is rosy'. Each innovation brings with it a new set of problems, many of which may not have existed previously.

The history of any aspect of human achievement, or indeed of human folly, is created around a catalogue of names. It is the lives and work of these individuals which are being celebrated and recorded by the historian so that future generations shall be conscious of their efforts, of their successes and their failures. It is hoped that by paying reference to this aspect, the future generations may avoid some of the errors of their predecessors and make more rapid progress in their own work. In the medical field we have seen the widespread use of eponyms, and some of these are found within the field of contact lens practice. There are those who deplore the use of eponyms but, from the historian's viewpoint, they add colour to the subject and act as a constant memorial to those who created the foundations upon which we build.

Many publications have appeared on historical aspects of contact lenses both in journals and as sections in textbooks. Those who find an interest in the origins of their speciality will find endless entertainment in exploring the agreement and disagreement portrayed therein, as well as in the degree to which errors creep in and often become perpetuated by other authors. One can only recommend exploration of the original source material listed as references so that readers can formulate their own interpretation of the work and opinions of these contact lens pioneers. To the general public, contact lenses are a recent innovation and surprise is usually expressed by patients on being told that we have already passed the centenary of the first practical use of these lenses.

1.2 THE PRECLINICAL CONTRIBUTORS

Disagreement exists as to the point of origin of the contact lens. Many sources today quote Leonardo da Vinci (circa 1508) as exhibiting the earliest material relating to the subject.

Contact Lens Practice. Edited by Montague Ruben and Michel Guillon.
Published in 1994 by Chapman & Hall, London. ISBN 0 412 35120 X

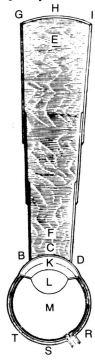

Il ne rɛſte plus qu'vn autre moyen pour augmenter la grandeur des images, qui eſt de faire que les rayons qui viennent de diuers points de l'obiet, ſe croiſent le plus loin qu'il ſe pourra du fonds de l'œil. mais il eſt bien ſans cõparaiſon, le plus important & le plus conſiderable de tous. Car c'eſt l'vnique qui puiſſe ſeruir pour les obiets inacceſſibles, auſſy bien que pour les acceſſibles, & dont l'effet n'a point de bornes: en ſorte qu'on peut en s'en ſeruant augmenter les images de plus en plus iuſques a vne grandeur indefinie. Comme par exemple, d'autãt que la premiere des trois liqueurs dont l'œil eſt rempli, cauſe a peu prés meſme refraction que l'eau commune, ſi on applique tout contre vn tuyau plein d'eau, comme E F, au bout duquel il y ait vn verre G H I, dont la figure ſoit toute ſemblable a celle de la peau B C D qui couure cette liqueur, & ait meſme rapport a la diſtance du fonds de l'œil; il ne ſe fera plus aucune refraction a l'entrée de cet œil; mais celle qui s'y faiſoit auparauant, & qui eſtoit cauſe que tous les rayons qui venoient d'vn meſme point de l'obiet commencoient a ſe courber dés cet endroit-

Figure 1.1 Water in contact with the eye which reduced the power of the cornea, as discussed by Rene Descartes.

Next quoted is the published work of Rene Descartes (1637) who described a water-filled tube to be applied to the surface of the eye having a convex glass at its front end (Fig. 1.1) This, he appreciated, could not be retained in position and in this respect cannot be equated with the concept of a contact lens as we know it. Likewise, the apparatus described by Leonardo was an experiment in optical theory of the eye and not a clinical corrective device. Duke Elder (1970) cites the work of Phillipe de la Hire, a French mathematician as postulating in 1685 the application of a solid glass

lens directly to the cornea. As with Descartes' apparatus, this would appear to be a telescopic or image magnifying device rather than a means of remedying a visual disorder. The extensive experimental work of Thomas Young (1801), on the mechanism of the eye also included the use of a water-filled tube, in this case to investigate the nature of accommodation (Fig. 1.2).

1.2.1 SIR JOHN FREDERICK WILLIAM HERSCHEL

Herschel, writing around 1828, on light and on the structure of the eye and vision, refers to Thomas Young's investigations as well as to the astigmatic correcting spectacle lens devised by George Biddell Airy. This latter work was described by Airy in a lecture to the Cambridge Philosophical Society in 1825 and was published some two years later in their *Transactions*. It is Herschel's chapter in the *Encyclopaedia Metropolitana* that so precisely anticipates the developments in terms of contact lenses which were to begin some 60 years later and which were to occupy the various pioneers for a further period of 60 years. Referring to the effects of corneal astigmatism he says:

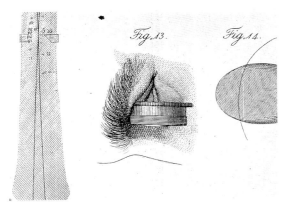

Figure 1.2 The Thomas Young experiment using a water filled tube in contact with the eye.

It is obvious, that the correction of such a defect could never be accomplished by the use of spherical lenses. The strict method, applicable in all such cases would be to adapt a lens to the eye, of nearly the same refractive power, and having its surface next the eye an exact intaglio fac-simile of the irregular cornea, while the external should be exactly spherical of the same general convexity as the cornea itself; for it is clear, that all the distortions of the rays at the posterior surface of such a lens would be exactly counteracted by the equal and opposite distortions at the cornea itself. But the necessity of limiting the correcting lens to such surfaces as can be truly ground in glass, to render it of any real and every day use, and which surfaces are only spheres, planes, and cylinders, suggested to Mr Airy the ingenious idea of a double concave lens, in which one surface should be spherical and the other cylindrical.

This statement by Herschel is followed by the oft-quoted footnote:

Should any very bad cases of irregular cornea be found, it is worthy of consideration, whether at least a temporary distinct vision could not be procured, by applying in contact with the surface of the eye some transparent animal jelly contained in a spherical capsule of glass; or whether an actual mould of the cornea might not be taken, and impressed on some transparent medium.

So much seems to be contained within these lines which over future years was to emerge in terms of practicality. For instance although the triggering factor of Airy's cylindrical spectacle was for the correction of a regular astigmatic error, Herschel uses the term 'cases of irregular cornea', exactly the condition for which the first vision-correcting contact lenses were to be tried. Second, Herschel uses the term

'. . . in contact with. . .' the very title now universally used for this corrective appliance. He foresees the use of eye impressions as a means of arriving at the shape required for the posterior surface of the contact lens, The expression '. . . and impressed on some transparent medium. . .' seems to imply that glass might not constitute that substance: an event which has certainly come to pass. Finally, one might even suggest that his use of the expression '. . . animal jelly. . .' constituted visions of a flexible substance for the appliance bounded by a rigid front surface certainly explored by exponents of the 'piggyback lenses' attempted for some irregular cornea cases.

This publication by Herschel was, for many years quoted as the earliest known reference to the contact lens by authors of historical material. Since the paper by Hofstetter and Graham (1953) it became popular to regard Leonardo da Vinci as the originator of the underlying principle, to the extent that the British Contact Lens Association adopted the drawing by Leonardo of a man with his face immersed in what appears to be a goldfish bowl as their 'logo'. As to whether this work can legitimately be regarded as the origin of the contact lens is best left to the reader, who is recommended to peruse the extensive paper on the ophthalmic work of Leonardo published by Walter Gasson (1976). The paper by Enoch (1956), who clearly rates the contribution by Descartes as having greater relevence to the development of modern contact lenses, nevertheless provides a useful comparative review of the thinking of these three pioneers.

1.3 THE EARLY CLINICAL PIONEERS

1.3.1 ADOLF EUGEN FICK

The statement has been made by several writers on contact lens history that, so far, no discovery has been made of any practical attempt to employ contact appliances therapeutically between the postulation of Herschel and the publications relating to the practical clinical attempts at using contact lenses which took place in the late 1880s. Of these, the first to be published was that of Eugen Fick (1888), who described at some length his attempts to find suitable cases having irregular corneal surfaces with which he might assess the efficacy of some glass 'Contactbrillen' which he had arranged to be made following impressions of rabbits' eyes and of those of human cadavers. The centenary of this publication on the first attempts to use contact lenses for the correction of visual disorders was celebrated by a number of publications among which was a special supplement to *The Optician*, which was entitled '100 Years of the Contact Lens'. This appeared in May 1988 and contained contributions by several authors interested in the history of this subject. Among these may be found a detailed appraisal of Fick's 1888 paper (Sabell, 1988). This contains observations on a number of issues described by Fick and their relevance to present-day contact lens wear. It is unnecessary to elaborate on this first clinical paper as it has been discussed fully in the centenary publications, as well as in the paper by Mann (1938), which marked the 50th anniversary of Fick's work, Graham (1959), in a detailed review of Fick's original paper, seeks to show that the lenses which he made in his first attempts were in fact corneal lenses, albeit probably covering the entire cornea. Fick's later lenses made by Professor Abbe at Jena, clearly had a scleral component and were, from a comfort viewpoint, superior to the earlier forms.

1.3.2   JEAN BAPTISTE EUGENE KALT

Of the other publications of work performed in the late nineteenth century, the announcement of Eugene Kalt's contribution by Panas (1888), took place on 20 March 1888, only days after the publication of Fick's paper.

Kalt's aim appears to have been the remodelling of the corneal curvature in keratoconic patients by the wearing of his 'coques de verre', glass contact shells to act as orthopaedic splints for the deformed cornea. By the time of this announcement he had apparently tried this out on only two patients; not that Fick had completed many more trials. Although de Carle (1988), States that Fick had tried out his contact lenses on 17 patients, the 1888 publication clearly states that he had obtained 17 names of potential patients from the records of the Ophthalmological Poliklinik; of these, only ten could be located and four had to be rejected as unsuitable when seen. Fick had therefore used only six patients; one keratoconic and five with corneal opacity of varying degree. Also, at the time his paper was completed not one of the six had actually been issued with the contact lenses to wear.

Returning to Kalt's work, we find that Dr Panas describes these lenses as '. . . glass shells similar to those which are sometimes used in the treatment of symblepharon and of the size of shells used as ocular prostheses'. He continues, 'The cornea being very thinned, conforms exactly to the concavity, and so becomes straightened out'. Panas emphasizes the visual improvement brought about with the contact lens in place but says that only the future would reveal to what extent the cornea might be permanently reshaped. He announced that their results on the two patients were ready to be published when their attention was drawn to Fick's paper.

One interesting variation which has crept in to historical reviews over the years relates to the status of Kalt. Attention has been drawn to this by Graham (1959) who implies that the first paper in which the description '. . . an optician, E. Kalt,. . .' appears, was that of Joseph Pascal (1941). This was followed shortly after by the first edition of Theodore Obrig's book *Contact Lenses*, published in 1942, in which the same designation is applied, Obrig, in his paper of 1937, in which he reviews the 'Historical Background' to contact lenses, made no mention of Kalt whatever; nor do Kalt and Panas appear in the bibliography of his book. Mann (1938) refers to 'E. Kalt of Paris . . . also wished to treat keratoconus. . .' but made no reference to Panas either in her text or in her bibliography. It seems highly unlikely that two E. Kalts existed, one an optician and the other an ophthalmologist. There is no doubt that Jean Baptiste Eugene Kalt (1861–1941), who trained in ophthalmology under Dr Panas, was the person who attempted to use contact lenses to remodel conical corneas in the 1887–8 period. Whether Kalt himself was present at the meeting of the Academy of Medicine in Paris on 20 March 1888 when Panas presented an account of his early trials is difficult to say. Certainly Kalt was present at the meeting of the Society of Ophthalmology of France in 1893 at which Chevallereau read his paper on contact lenses in the 'Treatment of keratoconus', and took part in the ensuing discussion when something of a confrontation developed between Kalt and Sulzer over precedence in the recommendation of contact lenses for keratoconus therapy (see Chevallereau, 1893). Curiously, while most of the earlier references by writers to the origins of contact lenses mention the roles played by Fick, August Müller and F.A. Müller of Wiesbaden, they fail to bring Kalt into the picture. Perhaps this relative obscurity also accounts for the uncertainty over Kalt's status.

1.3.3 AUGUST MÜLLER

The third member of the early clinical workers, August Müller of Gladbach (1889), published a detailed account in his doctoral thesis of problems which he encountered in attempting to correct his own 14 dioptres of myopia by means of 'hornhautlinsen'. Although not a corneal lens as we know it today, this does appear to be the first usage of the term. Müller, in this inaugural dissertation, compared his results between spectacles and contact lenses for his high myopia. Pearson (1978) published a detailed review of the contents of Müller's thesis. The thesis itself inevitably contains misinterpretation of some factors, only to be expected at such an early stage in the work; it did however contain many very relevant observations and deductions.

1.3.4 THE MÜLLERS OF WIESBADEN

The other major personalities of this introductory phase of contact lenses were the artificial eye makers at Wiesbaden in Germany. Despite the name, they were unrelated to August Müller. The firm of F.A. Müller and Sons had been first established at Lauscha, a centre for the manufacturing of glass, in 1868. The family had moved to Wiesbaden in 1875 and it is reported that in 1887 a particular patient was sent to the Mullers by Dr Theodore Saemisch to be fitted with a protective glass shell. Malignant growth affecting the lids of his right eye had necessitated their partial removal exposing the cornea to inevitable degeneration. The patient's left eye was highly myopic and had a cataract and it was considered essential to conserve the vision of his right eye if possible by means of the protective shell.

Various accounts published over the last 50 years of these events have tended to disagree in certain respects. For the most part they state that Saemisch's patient was sent to the Müllers with a request for the protective shell to be blown for his right eye. An exception, for some reason appears in the account by Dickinson and Hall (1946), in which it is claimed:

> . . . F.E. Müller, artificial-eye maker of Wiesbaden, made a protective contact glass for a patient referred to him by a Dr Saemisch for the fitting of an artificial eye. Müller realised that the sight of the

remaining eye would soon be seriously jeopardised from exposure, as the lids had been removed on account of a cancerous condition. He therefore sought permission from Saemisch to blow a thin shell of glass designed to protect the cornea from exposure. The doctor at once agreed. . .

Was this wishful thinking on the part of these authors or were they privy to some information not available to others? Dickinson and Hall conclude, 'The first contact glass, therefore, was a protective, and not a refractive, device'.

1.3.5   AN EARLIER CONTENDER?

If we accept this contention, that the Saemisch/Wiesbaden device was for protection, and therefore a therapeutic device rather than for correction of refractive error, we must begin to look for earlier evidence of such appliances as constituting the first practical attempts to employ contact appliances. One such reference is made by Duke-Elder and Abrams (1970) and by Duke-Elder and MacFaul (1972) who state that William White Cooper, founder of the ophthalmological department at St Mary's Hospital, London, in his book *Wounds and Injuries of the Eye* (London, 1859), recommended the insertion of a 'glass mask' filling the fornices, in order to prevent formation of symblepharon following lime burns of the eye. These authors go on to say that this technique was successfully applied by Ridley (1963) using his particular 'flush-fitting' moulded scleral lenses. It would appear from these observations that there may well be an earlier contender for the honour of having first used a contact appliance nearly 30 years earlier than the 1887 pioneers.

1.4   THE END OF A CENTURY

Returning to the 1890s we can find several references to papers or discussions in medical meetings relating to the use of contact lenses; these hinge mainly around the subject of keratoconus. They appear to show little progress in contact lens terms. Dr D.E. Sulzer of Geneva (1891, 1892) published an extensive account of his research into the surface contours of the cornea in normal eyes which included regular astigmatism. The paper deals with the effect of these surface variations on vision. While he does not relate these observations directly to contact lenses, we may in looking back say that they did contain material pertinent to much later attempts to fit such lenses. Shortly after, in May 1892, Sulzer had published his paper entitled *On The Optical Treatment of Keratoconus and Irregular Astigmatism and the Astigmatism due to Corneal Scarring*. In this, he refers to the poor visual results published by Fick in the paper of 1888 which he attributed to the use of blown glass lenses. Sulzer described his own results on three patients using ground contact lenses and, while his visual results may have been better, little progress was being made in patient tolerance. Although Sulzer's paper appeared in a French ophthalmological journal, he made no reference to or acknowledgment of the attempts made by Kalt, which were reported in 1888.

Fick, in September 1892, replied to some of Sulzer's observations in his paper *Some Notes on the Contact Lens*. It is in this paper that Fick states that the lenses supplied to him by Professor Abbe of Jena had, unknown to him at the time, been of blown construction and not ground as he had reported.

In November of the same year there appeared a paper by Professor Hont Dor of Lyon, discussing the optical correction of keratoconus and irregular astigmatism for which he had tried the use of conical spectacle lenses in 1876. He then comments on Fick's work of 1888 and mentions Fick's choice of 2% glucose for filling the precorneal space. He expressed his own preference for a physiological solution of sodium chloride – much more familiar to practitioners today. Dor refers to the announcement by Sulzer at the previous meeting of the French Ophthalmological Society that some of his lenses had been ground by an optician named Benzoni in Geneva. As a result, Dor ordered two of these for his own trials; complaining as he did so of the price that he was charged for them (40 francs each). On examining them he was apparently well satisfied with the quality of workmanship. Dor also found that patients' physical reactions to the lenses were disappointing, but observed that the use of cocaine rendered them tolerable. Dor reports the visual results in nine patients with various visual disorders, none being keratoconic. He comments on the difficulties found in inserting the lenses free from air bubbles but regarded the lenses as making a useful contribution to the quick diagnosis of irregular corneas and having good potential for experiments on possible astigmatic contractions of the crystalline lens during accommodation.

In 1893, Dr M.A. Chevallereau discussed various forms of treatment for keratoconus before the French Ophthalmological Society, quoting results from two patients on whom he had employed superficial thermocauterization with apparently effective results. In the discussion which followed this presentation, Dr Abadie referred to a case in which he had used the contact lenses as 'advocated by Dr Sulzer'. This was immediately challenged by **Eugene Kalt**, who informed Dr Abadie that the optical treatment by contact lenses was first used in 1887 by Fick in Switzerland and by himself in France and was thus recommended by them in 1888 and not by Dr Sulzer in 1892. At this, Sulzer replied that the idea of using contact lenses was very old, 'dating back to the previous century' and could not therefore be attributed to Dr Kalt. He went on to suggest that in any case, the lenses used by Kalt had failed to adhere to the cornea adequately. Kalt thereupon retorted that adhesion was a factor resulting from atmospheric pressure as

the clinging together of two wet sheets of glass.

In 1896 A.E. Fick's book entitled *Diseases of the Eye and Ophthalmoscopy* was published. From it we may deduce that little progress had been made with contact lenses and indeed that little enthusiasm had been aroused. In the chapter on 'Diseases of the Cornea', Fick writes:

I have proposed to treat conical cornea with a 'contact glass', that is, with a glass ground so as to have the form of the normal anterior segment of the eye, this glass to be laid directly upon the affected eye, the space between glass and cornea being filled with some aseptic fluid of the same refractive index as that of the cornea. If this were done, the influence of the conical cornea upon the path of the luminous rays would be destroyed. Unfortunately, I have found no case exactly suited for the application of such a contact glass, but the improved visual acuity in proper cases of irregular corneal astigmatism has been surprising.

Not much space devoted to a novel treatment often attributed to the author, and in a textbook of nearly 500 pages! In the section devoted to irregular astigmatism, Fick advocates the use of stenopaic spectacles, not contact lenses, which suggests that he did not have too much faith in their future.

The 1890s ended with a letter by Fick to the correspondence section of the journal in which his first paper had appeared. This letter, published in 1897 was in response to a paper by T. Lohnstein, which had appeared in December 1896 on the optical management of irregular astigmatism by means of the hydrodiascope, Fick's letter, headed 'Hydrodiascope and Contact Lens' appears to end publications on the topic so far as the nineteenth century was concerned – something of a 'damp squib'!

1.5   THE FIRST DECADE OF THE TWENTIETH CENTURY

The next ten years were even worse; very few publications are found which report the use of contact lenses. One, of indirect relevance to our subject was the paper by Drysdale (1900) which laid the way for the radiuscope, now a basic tool of the contact lens practitioner. Another 'peripheral' item was by Benson (1902), giving some of his observations on the use of fluorescein, the introduction of which he attributed to Straub (1888), coinciding therefore with Fick's publication. Benson, of course, does not relate the use of fluorescein to contact lenses; this connection was to come later. Several of the publications over this decade are cited by Much (1932) and appear to deal exclusively with the management of keratoconic patients and often are comparing the use of the hydrodiascope with that of contact lenses.

1.6   1910 TO 1920

After 1910 things began to pick up slightly, and also to diversify in terms of the uses for which contact lenses could be employed. One important publication of 1910 was the book entitled *Das Künstliche Auge* by Friedrich A Müller and Albert C Müller of the firm of F.A. Müller and Sons of Wiesbaden. The authors were sons of the founder of the firm and the book carries the inscription 'dedicated to our father's memory'. While most of the book is devoted to conventional artificial eyes, pages 68 to 72 are devoted to their 'Kontakt-Adhäsionsbrillen', beginning with their description of the case referred to them in 1888 by Dr Saemisch; this apparently being the first published account of this event.

In terms of contact lens manufacturing during these earlier years, the names of several opticians had been mentioned in publications but it would seem that such contact lenses were made on a very small scale to individual requests by the surgeons concerned. Rycroft (1932) suggests that any so-called 'ground' lenses in the early days had been made in two seperate parts – a single, curved, optically ground corneal portion was produced, which was afterwards either fused or cemented to the scleral section. Throughout the last decade of the nineteenth century, however, the firm of Carl Zeiss at Jena was gradually developing what was to become the first one piece fully ground lens the originator of what is today's 'preformed' systems. Their first lenses were launched in 1911, followed a year later by a lens intended for keratoconics. By 1920, Zeiss were offering a four lens fitting set which was described by Dr W Stock of Jena as consisting of four corneal radii: 6.5 mm, 7.1 mm, 8.1 mm and 9.0 mm; the sceral radii were all 12 mm; corneal diameters were all 12 mm and overall size was 20 mm round. There was no displacement of the corneal segment. The apparently curious choice of back optic radii becomes apparent by virtue of the resultant heights of each corneal segment, being: 5.0 mm, 4.5 mm, 4.0 mm and 3.0 mm. Over this decade we find publications such as that by Erggelet (1913) on the use of contact lenses for monocular aphakia and his paper (1914) on their use in assessment of binocular vision, Hanke (1916), discussed their value in the prevention of symblepharon. Nevertheless the correction of keratoconus still occupied the centre of the stage and we find communications on the management of this disorder by both the Zeiss ground lenses as well as the blown Müller type (von Hippel, 1918). The option of the hydrodiascope was still in evidence (Lüdemann, 1917), which illustrates the limitations still exhibited by the two available forms of contact lenses.

1.6.1   DIAGNOSTIC LENSES

The introduction of the slit lamp by Gullstrand (1911) which when suitably mounted in combination with the binocular stereomicroscope as presented by Henker (1916), opened up a new and promising field of application for the contact lens. While Sugar (1941) credits Salzmann with having first employed Fick's keratoconic contact lens to examine the anterior chamber angle by ophthalmoscopy, Koeppe (1918, 20) introduced specialized diagnostic contact lenses for both gonioscopy and for fundus examination by means of the newly developed slit lamp microscope. A review of these and later forms of diagnostic contact lenses was published by the present author some years ago (Sabell, 1970).

1.7 THE THIRD DECADE

Between 1920 and 1930, although Muller's blown lenses were clearly still in use for Keratoconus (von Hippel, 1918; Lauber, 1923; Sitchevska, 1932), we begin to notice much progress in the development of the Zeiss range of lenses. The number of publications on contact lenses also shows a noticeable increase. Dohme (1922) described in at least two journals his use of Zeiss lenses for keratoconus. Some names of authors had become familiar through repeated publications relating to contact lens usage. One example is Professor Erggelet of Jena, whose first report in 1913 on monocular aphakia was followed in 1914 by discussion of binocular vision aspects of contact lenses. His 1916 contributions relate mainly to keratoconus. Erggelet (1920) wrote comparing the contact lens, the hydrodiascope and 'immersion spectacles'. Five years later he explored the relationship between contact lenses and spectacles during accommodation for near objects. This latter topic was taken up by Rugg-Gunn (1931). Erggelet was still expressing views on contact lenses and their modes of fitting into the 1930s. By 1930 the view had been clearly reached of the superiority in comfort of the blown Müller lenses over the regular spherical ground types. In his investigations into contact lens intolerance, Erggelet had employed fluorescein solution to compare tear exchange between the two types, which demonstrated clearly the superiority in this respect of the Müller lenses. Fischer (1929), appears to be the first to raise the question of corneal respiration as a factor in contact lens toleration and had advocated the presence of an air bubble between the lens and the eye to act as a reservoir for exhaled carbon dioxide.

1.7.1 THERAPEUTIC APPLICATIONS

As regards reasons for using contact lenses, we find further expansion of ideas. Ruben (1975) cites Friede (1926) and Müller-Welt (1926) as advocating their use in ptosis, while Comberg is credited by Mann (1938) with having produced 'a lead glass protective lens for X-ray work'. Illig (1929) wrote on the prevention and management of symblepharon, although Mann (1938) claims that he first employed contact lenses for this purpose as early as 1915. Weihmann (1923) advocated the use of 'bandage contact lenses' in the treatment of corneal ulcers, while Meyerbach's paper (1926) describes their use in cases of descemetocele.

Despite this diversification, keratoconus remained the condition of greatest interest for the use of contact lenses. At the beginning of the previous decade, Clausen (1920) had published a paper entitled *Keratoconus and its Treatment*, in which he reported on two patients whom he fitted with Muller lenses which gave a reasonable vision standard whereas spectacles had failed to do this. One of these patients was able to wear his lenses 'all day long without interruption' and with no adverse corneal effects being observed. His other patient tolerated the lenses for periods of 'several hours'. Clausen confirmed the limitations of the Müller lenses 'as decribed by Siegrist', namely the need for a large bank of fitting lenses from which patients could be supplied direct. In addition there was the time consuming, 'hit-and-miss' system for finding a suitable fit combined with satisfactory vision. Clausen did comment, however, that a well fitting Müller lens did not need to be filled with saline for insertion as did the Zeiss lenses, as the tears infiltrated readily to occupy the space between lens and cornea. He also recommended that sustained corneal pressure be avoided, commenting on the corneal lesions and exfoliation which had been observed in patients using ground lenses. This he attributed to the tendency of the ground lens to become sucked on to the eye surface, a trend not only seen regularly in full clearance scleral lenses up to 25 years after his observation, but also seen with some of the steeply fitted corneal lenses of up to 50 years later! Nine years later we find Clausen (1929) still reporting good results with Müller lenses, although he had recently observed one case of heavy corneal infiltration following their use. At this time he reported on his experimental work in conjunction with Professor Wiegand, a physicist, to produce and assess 'plastic contact lenses' made by Carl Zeiss from 'cellon'. These, he found, like their glass counterparts also produced 'conjunctival strangulation'. Obrig (1942, 1957) presents details of the US patent granted to Albert Wigand of Halle in Germany in June 1923 for manufacture of 'Contact Bowls' from cellon and celluloid.

By the late 1920s, the development work on Zeiss lenses had become very apparent largely due to the work of Professor Leopold Heine of Kiel University. Heine (1929) introduced his fitting range of Zeiss lenses which were all afocal in air but which contained a range of corneal radii from 5.00 mm to 11.00 mm. The aim was to correct a very wide range of ametropia by means of the liquid lens. By this time Heine was also advocating a range of haptic radii from 11.00 mm to 13.00 mm in steps of 0.5 mm. Unlike most ophthalmologists of the time, Heine was already thinking of the use of contact lenses

for correcting ametropia in otherwise normal eyes; in other words as a cosmetic alternative to spectacles. This clearly was approved by the firm of Zeiss who saw in it great commercial possibilities. One sees evidence of this from the promotional literature produced by this firm during the next decade.

One new trend seen towards the late 1920s was the appearance of publications in English-speaking journals on the subject of contact lenses. Apart from C .H. May's translation of Fick's original paper in *Archives of Ophthalmology* (1888), all communications during the late nineteenth and early twentieth centuries appear to have been in either German or French journals. O'Rourke (1928), published a paper entitled *The Optical Correction of the Conical Cornea with the Contact Lens*, in which he presents a very large and elaborate apparatus by means of which patients may insert their contact lenses. His illustration also shows what appears to be an old fashioned 'button hook', similar to those used in Victorian times to fasten shoe buttons, which he advocates for the removal of the lenses.

1.8 THE 1930s

Moving into the 1930s we find a very marked increase in the numbers of contact lens publications, including many in the English language. A further change is noticeable in that many authors are beginning to look back at the earlier years of contact lens development and to present either exclusively historical reviews, such as that by Dr Victor Much (1932), who presents a most impressive and useful bibliography relating to the early development of the contact lens field. Several other authors at this period when presenting general reviews of their clinical usage of contact lenses chose to begin their publications with an introductory historical review (Rugg-Gunn, 1931; Sitchevska, 1932; Rycroft, 1932; Obrig, 1937). Possibly this trend was expressing a wish to rethink the past in order to find the way forward and to escape from the limitations imposed by the two forms of contact lens in use at that time. Olga Sitchevska makes clear in her paper of 1932 the clinical limitations of both the Zeiss lenses and those of the Müllers.

Not only was interest in contact lenses spreading to the UK and the USA, but we are now beginning to find publications in many other countries and across many continents. In Italy, Professor Vincenzo Gualdi of Florence in a paper published in 1934, describes his lenses as 'corneal contact lenses' and, although these were ground with a single curve over the entire back surface, of radii between 10.50 mm and 13.00 mm, they were sufficiently large (around 20.00 mm) as to be supported by the sclera at the extreme edges of the lens. It is difficult in terms of present day terminology to equate these with corneal lens design. Nor is it possible to imagine their successful application, indeed Obrig (1942) stated that they 'have not proved satisfactory in the hands of the few men known by the author to have tried them'.

In the UK, one of the earlier users of contact lenses was Andrew Rugg-Gunn (1930, 1931) who describes the processes involved in fitting Zeiss lenses and discusses in some detail contact lens optics. He makes clear the problems experienced at this time over inserting full clearance lenses without trapping air bubbles. This problem was also discussed by Affleck Greeves (1931) and, from today's viewpoint, they all seem to have been making very 'heavy weather' of a relatively simple task. In sharp contrast was the observation of Clausen (1920), speaking of the blown Muller lenses:

It is very easy to put them in, there is no need to fill the shell with a sterile solution of sodium chloride beforehand, . . . the space between cornea and rear wall of the shell will very soon be filled with lachrymal fluid which will also remove any air bubbles present.

Rugg-Gunn, in his concluding section on the usage of contact lenses, expresses the interesting opinion that he felt 'that the psychology of the British people will prove to be on the whole unfavourable' to the future use of contact lenses. Things were however to prove somewhat different!

The 1930s was perhaps the most significant decade in the history of contact lenses. At the beginning there had been little progress to break the deadlock between blown and ground lenses. By the end of the decade we had moulded lenses which combined the comfort and toleration seen with the Müller type and the superior vision correction associated with the Zeiss lens. In addition, we had begun to move into the era of plastic lenses. The route towards deliberate rather than accidental tear exchange had been explored and demonstrated, and the beginning of the change over from the use of glass to acrylic materials was to open up the way to successful corneal lenses, and to further massive exploration of alternative materials. 1939 saw the start of the Second World War, which was to prove the watershed between the contact lens as a predominantly clinical tool and its random use for correction of minor ametropia. Also by 1939, significant advances had been made in eye impression procedures with the introduction of new cold alginate materials and improved designs for impression trays.

1.8.1 EYE IMPRESSIONS

By the end of the 1920s there had been renewed interest in eye impression techniques. Although the concept had been suggested by Herschel in 1828 and practical attempts had been made by Fick and by August Müller in the 1880s, they had both lacked suitable materials for developing the procedure. Von Csapody (1929) had revised interest in the possibilities of eye impressions by trying various materials and by settling on the use of a low melting point paraffin wax which he hardened on the eye surface by irrigating with refrigerated liquid paraffin so as to be able to remove the impression without distortion. Poller's Negocoll, a new alginate material was introduced around 1930 and appeared to offer a useful alternative to wax impressions. Although intended for making anatomical models for museums, Negocoll, and its casting material Hominit, was brought to the attention of a young ophthalmological student who was, over the next 20 years, to have a significant influence on the development of contact lenses. Joseph Dallos received his MD from the University of Budapest in 1928 and joined the staff of the University Eye Clinic. He soon found himself involved in research into the clinical possibilities of the contact lens. Rapidly he became aware of the serious limitations of the two available form of lenses and set about trying to find a solution to these problems. In doing so, he made a very marked contribution to the subject and indeed remained committed to this field of activity right up to his death in 1979. He contributed many papers relating to contact lenses (Dallos, 1933 to 1980). (The present author has written extensively on the work of Dallos – Sabell, 1979, 1980, 1988, 1989.)

1.8.2   FULL CLEARANCE FITTING

In terms of contact lens fitting, there developed, during the 1930s, two distinct schools of thought, The first favoured complete clearance of the cornea and limbal area by the contact lens optic zone, The second advocated a much closer corneal fit; capillary clearance over the central cornea with somewhat greater limbal clearance. The former philosophy was epitomized by the work, in the USA of such practitioners as William Feinbloom, an active and original thinker who was to make several very interesting contributions to contact lens design over the 1930s and 1940s. The other great US name

was that of Theodore Obrig, who, embracing the 'full clearance' philosophy, spent much time attempting to provide a breakthrough in the field of contact lens solutions. It was widely believed, right up to the mid-1940s, that someone might devise a solution for use with full clearance contact lenses which would break the limiting factor which had been first described by Fick (1888) and later, in more detail by Sattler (1938). Sattler's veil would frequently onset after some two to three hours of contact lens wear when using full clearance, unfenestrated lenses. Its cause was, over the years attributed to a number of factors, such as a fall in pH of the fluid behind the lens resulting from corneal emision of carbon dioxide. This led to experimentation with various buffered solutions such as those described by Gifford (1933, 1935) and by Feldman (1937). The 'magic' contact lens solution failed to materialize, however, despite some very exotic options which were explored by Obrig (1957).

The full clearance philosophy was, no doubt derived from two factors. First, a continuing reluctance to have the contact lens resting directly onto the cornea. This was brought about by inability to deal effectively with corneal opacification and also the limitations in the pre-antibiotic days of controlling corneal infection. Second, it was observed that sustained corneal pressure, especially in the limbal region, resulted in marked intolerance as with the earlier Zeiss lenses. Steps to correct this had been taken by the Zeiss researchers Fertsch and Hartinger (1931) who had proposed the blending of the step junction between optic and haptic zones. Joseph Dallos (1975) claimed that it was he who had originally made this suggestion to Hartinger.

1.8.3   CLOSE FITTING LENSES

One of the exponents of the minimum clearance fitting method was A. Müller-Welt (1934), who began work in Stuttgart, Germany, in the mid-1920s using glass lenses blown into female dies. Nelson (1938) gave a fairly detailed review of Müller-Welt's lenses, which he preferred to the ground lenses of Zeiss. Later, Müller-Welt emigrated to Canada and the USA, where he gradually evolved moulded acrylic lenses of a similar design to the blown glass ones he had been making in Germany. Both his glass lenses and his later acrylic ones were fitted to minimum clearance philosophy using preformed fitting sets. After his move to North America, Mueller-Welt as he was now called, described his transition to acrylic scleral lenses (1950) and later (1957) his experiences with corneal lenses.

One appealing aspect of the minimum clearance lens was its lack of insertion difficulties. This was made clear by several authors, originally as early as 1920 by Clausen in respect of the Müller of Wiesbaden blown lenses. The Mueller-Welt lenses as described by Nelson could easily be regarded as a logical development from this earlier form.

The second and major exponent of the minimum clearance technique was, of course Joseph Dallos, and the reader should refer to the various papers by this contact lens pioneer.

By the late 1930s it was widely accepted that contact lenses with regular spherical haptic portions were unsatisfactory for many patients. Although some workers created preformed lenses having aspheric haptic zones (Eggers, 1939; Feinbloom, 1945; Forknall, 1948; Mueller-Welt, 1950), there were always some eyes for which an impression would prove to be the best answer. Nelson (1938) quotes from the paper by Dallos (1933) on this very point, saying:

> However, just as there is a certain percentage of feet which can tolerate only individually made shoes, the same will be the case with contact lenses, and the molding will never be, therefore, entirely unnecessary.

This comment by Dallos reflects his early problems with eye impressions, partly responsible for his abandoning this technique in favour of his 'type shell' approach. This has been discussed in more detail elsewhere (Sabell, 1989).

Dallos left Hungary in 1937, moving to London at the invitation of a small group of British ophthalmologists. Here, along with his technician and erstwhile brother-in-law George Nissel, he took charge of Hamblin's newly created Contact Lens Centre at 18, Cavendish Square, London. The purpose and work of this unit was described by Rugg-Gunn (1938).

1.9 THE YEARS OF CHANGE – THE 1940S

Although in many ways a major World War can exert an adverse effect on progress in some fields by restricting supplies and communication, in other areas it will lead to incredibly rapid advancement. In terms of contact lenses, the reduced communication between Germany, a major centre and originator of contact lens technology, and the rest of the Western world, which was only just beginning to take up this challenge, probably did exert some restrictive effect. That contact lenses were employed in the UK for certain trained personnel whose services may have been lost owing to refractive errors can be seen from some of the case reports presented by Dickinson and Hall (1946). Ruben (1979), in his obituary of Joseph Dallos, refers to his war-time work 'with the RAF ophthalmologist, Wing-Commander Livingstone, on special cases requiring contact lenses'. These instances came to the attention of the general public, and especially of servicemen and women, and were reflected in the immediate post-war period by increasing numbers of requests for contact lenses, mainly for simple refractive errors. Thus the war years formed a turning point from the days when the contact lens would have been tried on medical advice to the beginnings of 'consumer demand' for the product. It is apparent from Zeiss promotional literature of the late 1930s (Fig. 1.3) that this firm at least foresaw the approaching trend, which was probably only delayed by the war years.

1.9.1   POST-WAR DESIGNS

In the post-war years, new designs of preformed haptic lenses were appearing, with a view to improving toleration and to render more easy the processes of fit assessment. In the immediate post-war period, and up to early 1947, impression lenses were not yet available in polymethylmethacrylate (PMMA) in the UK, and any patient who could not be fitted by the preformed Dixey

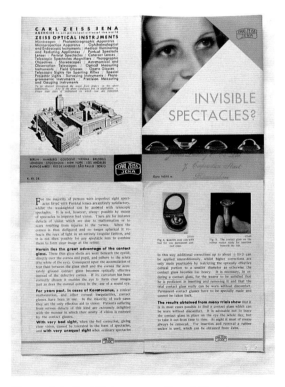

Figure 1.3 Carl Zeiss promotional literature.

lenses* had to be supplied with moulded glass lenses. This situation was remedied by the setting up (by George Nissel) of a manufacturing laboratory, and also by the establishment, in London, of an overseas branch of Obrig Laboratories from the USA. Nevertheless, the post-war period resulted in much interest in preformed haptic lenses. There was, at that time (and inexplicably still is in some quarters), the belief that eye impressions constituted 'an ordeal' for the patient. This author would suggest that, if this is so, it is an attitude transmitted from and reinforced by the practitioner, and needs rarely be the case. Additionally, the fitting of contact lenses from eye impressions was demanding of a certain level of acquired experience on the part of the practitioner, as had been demonstrated by Dallos in the early 1930s; it also called for a level of practical 'workshop involvement'. These factors in themselves were to add to the popularity of the preformed approach of the post-war period, which of course extended into and beyond the 1950s with the advent of the corneal lens. As examples of the post-war preformed haptic era in the UK, we have the 'transcurve lens' of Norman Bier (1948) and the 'wide-angle lens' of George Nissel (Jenkin & Tyler-Jones, 1969). One should also not forget the 'offset lens' of Forknall (1948). There were also several cone haptic lenses introduced, based on the US 'Feincone lenses' (Feinbloom, 1945; McKellen, 1948).

1.9.2   FENESTRATED HAPTIC LENSES

The most significant advance of the immediate post-war period was the introduction of fenestration. For this, the full clearance system of fitting had to be abandoned in favour of the close fitting techniques of Dallos. It has been stated that the techniques associated with fenestration of haptic lenses were

---

* For a description of Dixey contact lenses, see Ridley (1946).

developed independently by both Bier and Dallos; this has been discussed elsewhere (Sabell, 1989). Bier's application for a British patent based on a contact lens having 'a plurality of holes . . . for the purpose of permitting lachrymal fluid to flow through the lens while it is in position on the eye', was submitted in January 1945 and was finally accepted in September 1947, which may explain the delay in published information on this feature by Bier (1948). In the meantime, Dallos had already made reference to his own experiments into contact lens ventilation in his paper *Sattler's Veil* (1946). The evolution of these Dallos lenses was described by the present author (Sabell, 1980).

By the late 1940s, the scleral lens had almost reached its full development. A small number of minor refinements to lens design or to techniques of fitting and manufacture have been introduced since, but to all intents and purposes the fenestrated haptic lens of today is essentially that of the post-war years.

1.9.3 CORNEAL LENSES

The other main development of this period was undoubtedly the introduction of a potentially successful corneal lens by Tuohy (see Nugent, 1950). That corneal lens types had been tried from time to time since the days of Fick and Kalt has been clearly described by Graham (1959), but without success as compared to the scleral lenses of the period. This was essentially due to the material, glass being too heavy, the inability to make lenses to the same thinness as the modern corneal lens without becoming very vulnerable and the surface characteristics of glass lacking the slight adhesive properties essential to create appropriate lens movement during blinks. It was therefore the advent of PMMA which provided the suitable material for the route into smaller and thinner contact lenses.

So much has been published since 1948 on the subject of corneal lens designs, and over more recent years on oxygen-permeable copolymers as alternatives to pure PMMA, that it impossible to review these in detail. We must wait many more years before being able to assess the place in contact lens history of these materials. One thing is clear, that the more successfully contact lenses are tolerated, the more widely they are used and the duration of wearing times become extended. These great improvements in lens comfort and toleration which we have witnessed increasingly make us aware of the adverse consequences of over-use of these appliances. Many of the writers of the 1930s were categorically stating that the wearing of contact lenses had no harmful effects upon the eyes. It would appear that if relatively small numbers of people are wearing the lenses and/or they can be tolerated only for an hour or two and then must be removed for several hours, that little in the way of harmful effects will be seen. It was the increasingly prolonged wearing of the early corneal lenses in the middle to late 1950s that began to focus interest on undesirable corneal changes. Corneal oedema effects had been descibed by Fick in his first paper and had been increasingly understood in terms of contact lens wear by the 1930s, when gas exchange had been discussed by Fischer (1929). Sattler had, with the advantages offered by improving slit-lamp design in the 1930s, been able to further clarify understanding of contact-lens-induced oedema. Interest in corneal physiology and its relationship to contact lens wear may be illustrated by the papers cited by Obrig and Salvatori (1957) – Cogan (1941), Cogan and Kinsey (1942), Kinsey *et al.* (1942), Kinsey (1952), Smelzer (1952), Smelzer and Ozanics (1953) and Smelzer and Chen (1955). With the aid of developing technology, these have led to the spate of literature which began in the late 1960s with Fatt, Hill and many others. These seem to have led to an obsession with oxygen in recent times, which, however, did not totally convince everyone (Dallos, 1980). Clearly, when one examines critically the results of each new contact lens advance, it becomes apparent that there is no such thing as 'pure progress'!

1.9.4 'SOFT' LENSES

The other major change to the contact lens scene which occurred in the 1960s was the introduction of fully flexible contact lenses, beginning with the paper by Wichterle and Lim (1960) and Wichterle *et al.* (1961) and not long after this of the US patent for silicon rubber contact lenses to W.E. Becher in 1962 (cited by Ruben, 1975). It is interesting to recall that the firm of C.W. Dixey, when introducing their lathe-turned PMMA haptic lenses during the Second World War, used in their trade literature the title 'Flexible contact lenses'. The introduction of hydrogel materials into the contact lens world opened the way to many new lines of research and development as well as introducing the contact lens field to a new category of worker – the polymer chemists. Their involvement has been ceaseless over the past 30 years and yet we are still very conscious of being nowhere near to a perfect contact lens material. The volume of contact lens publications over the last three decades has been so vast that the historians of the next century will be faced with a very formidable task.

1.10   CONCLUSION

As with the history of so many fields, that of the contact lens will be subject to variations of opinion and interpretation by different authors; this will always be the case. These individual opinions, which may or may not be accurate, can become reinforced when reproduced without comment by future writers and can become accepted without question by many readers. The various contact lens historical publications exhibit examples of such discrepancies. Some of these may arise in the translation of material from one language to another while others will be created by inflexibility of the viewpoint of some authors. No doubt the reader will identify such examples in this present review! One of the great pleasures to the historian is the identification of such variations in other writings and the attempt to retrace steps from original sources and if possible, to find some explanation as to how the differences in interpretaion could arise. No doubt the question as to who originated the contact lens will be debated far into the future.

REFERENCES

Airy, G.B. (1827) On a peculiar defect in the eye and a mode of correcting it. *Trans. Camb. Philos. Soc.*, **2**, 267–71.

Benson, A.H. (1902) A note on the value of the fluorescein test. *Ophthal. Review*, **21**, 121–30.

Bier, N. (1948a) The tolerance factor and Sattler's veil influenced by a new development of the contact lens. *The Optician*, 2nd January, 557–9.

Bier, N. (1948b) The practice of ventilated contact lenses. *The Optician*, **116**, 497–501.

Bier, N. (1957) Patent specification, in *Contact Lens Routine and Practice*, 2nd edn, Butterworths, London, pp. 243–56.

Bier, N. and Cole, P.J. (1948) The transcurve contact lens fitting shell. *The Optician*, **115**, 605–6.

Chevallereau, M.A. (1893) Traitement du keratocone. *Bull. Mem. Soc. Ophthal.*, **11**, 385–92.

Clausen, B. (1920) Keratokonus und seine Behandlung. Ber. 42 Vers. d. *Deutsch. Ophth. Gesellsch.*, Heidelberg, 288–94.

Clausen, B. (1929) Meeting reports and discussion. *Klin. Mbl Augenheilk.*, **82**, 112–13.

Cogan, D.G. (1941) Some practical considerations pertaining to corneal edema. *Archs. Ophthal.*, **25**(4), 552–6.

Cogan, D.G. and Kinsey, V.E. (1942) Physiologic studies on the cornea. *Science N.Y.*, **95**, 607–8.

Dallos, J. (1933) Ueber Haftglaser und Kontaktschalen. *Klin. Mbl Augenheilk.*, **91**, 640–59.

Dallos, J. (1936) Contact glasses, the invisible spectacles. *Archs. Ophthal.*, **15**, 617–23.

Dallos, J. (1938) The individual fitting of contact glasses. *Trans. Ophthal. Soc. U.K.*, **57**, 509–20.

Dallos, J. (1946) Sattler's veil. *Brit. J. Ophthal.*, **30**, 607–13.

Dallos, J. (1954) Ventilated glass contact lenses. Correspondence: *Brit. J. Ophthal.*, **38**, 319–20.

Dallos, J. (1956) Dallos contact lenses. Correspondence. *Archs. Ophthal.*, **55**, 443–4.

Dallos, J. (1964) Individually fitted corneal lenses made to corneal moulds. *Brit. J. Ophthal.*, **48**, 510–12.

Dallos, J. (1965) Kontaktkamra szaruhartyamosashoz es csarnokdializizishez. *Szemeszet.*, 212–13.

Dallos, J. (1970) In praise of glass. *The Dispensing Optician*, October/November.

Dallos, J. (1980) The myth of oxygen permeability. *J. Brit. Contact Lens Ass.*, **3**, 28–9.

Dallos, J. and Hughes, W.H. (1972) Sterilization of hydrophilic contact lenses. *Brit. J. Ophthal.*, **56**, 114–19.

De Carle, J. (1988) Who fitted the first contact lens?, in *100 Years of the Contact Lens. An Optician Supplement*, May, **4**.

Descartes, R. (1637) Discours de la méthode, Discours No.7, *La Dioptrique*, 74–91.

Dickinson, F. and Hall, K.G.C. (1946) An Introduction to the Prescribing and Fitting of Contact Lenses. Hammond and Hammond, London, chapter 1.

Dohme, B. (1922a) Die Korrektion des Keratokonus mit den Geschliffenen Zeissishen Kontaktglasern. *Ztschr. Augenheilk.*, **48**, 106–12.

Dohme, B. (1922b) Zeissche Kontaktglaser bei Keratokonus. *Deutsche Med. Woch.*, **48**(33), 1121.

Dor, H. (1892) Sur les verres de contact. *Revue Gen. Ophthal.*, **11**, 493–7.

Drysdale, C.V. (1900) On a simple direct method of obtaining the curvature of a small lens. *Trans. Opt. Soc.*, **2**, 1–12.

Duke-Elder, S. and Abrams, D. (1970) Ophthalmic Optics and Refraction P.713, in *A System of Ophthalmology*, **5**, H. Kimpton, London.

Duke-Elder, S. and MacFaul, P.A. (1972) Chemical Injuries, in *A System of Ophthalmology*, **14**(2), 1048–9, H. Kimpton, London.

Eggers, H. (1939) Suggestions for a new design of stock contact lenses. *Archs. Ophthal.*, **22**, 403–5.

Enoch, J.M. (1956) Descartes' contact lens. *Am. J. Optom.*, **33**, 77–85.

Erggelet, H. (1913) Zur Korrektion der einseitigen Aphakie. *Ztschr. Ophthal. Optik.*, **33**.

Erggelet, H. (1914) Diebedeutung der Fickschen kontaktglaser für die Beurteilung des Zweiangigen Sehens durch Brillenglaser. *Klin. Mbl Augenheilk.*, **52**, 240–6.

Erggelet, H. (1916) Zur Korrektion des Keratokonus. *Klin. Mbl Augenheilk.*, **56**, 624.

Erggelet, H. (1920) Haftglaser, Hydrodiaskop, Taucherbrillen. *Zbl. Ges. Ophthalm.*, **3**, 361.

Erggelet, H. (1925) Das Nahglas für das Akkommodierende astigmatische Auge. *Zeitschr. Ophthal. Optik.*, 5–6.

Feinbloom, W. (1945) The tangent cone contact lens series. *Optom. Wkly*, **36**, 1159–61.

Feldman, J.B. (1937) pH and buffers in relation to ophthalmology. *Archs. Ophthal.*, **17**, 797–810.

Fertsch, F. and Hartinger, H. (1931) Patent application cited in *Contact Lenses* 3rd edn (eds T.E. Obrig and P.L. Salvatori), Obrig Laboratories, New York, 444–6.

Fick, A.E. (1888) Eine Kontaktbrille. *Schweiger's Archs Augenheilk.*, **18**, 279–89.

Fick, A.. (1892) Einige Bemerkungen über die Contactbrille. *Klin. Mbl Augenheilk.*, **30**, 306–10.

Fick, A.E. (1896) Diseases of the eye and ophthalmoscopy. Translation by A.B. Hale (1902), King, Manchester, 261.

Fick, A.E. (1897) Hydrodiaskop und Kontaktglas. *Klin. Mbl Augenheilk.*, **35**, 129–32.

Fischer, F.P. (1929) Ueber den Gasaustausch der Hornhaut mit der Luft. *Schweiger's Archs Augenheilk.*, **102**, 146.

Forknall, A.J. (1948) Offset contact lenses. *The Optician*, **116**(3006), 419–21.

Forknall, A.J. (1959) Some notes on haptic lenses. *Brit. J. Physiol. Opt.*, **16**, 96–115.

Friede, R. (1926a) Eine neuartige Vorrichtung zum Anheben von gelahmten Augenlidern. *Dtsch. Opt. Wschr.*, **12**, 240.

Friede, R. (1926b) Eine Ersatz für die Ptosisbrille. *Opt. Rdsch.*, **230**.

Gasson, W. (1976) Leonardo da Vinci – Ophthalmic Scientist. *Ophthal. Optician*, **16**, 393–541.

Gifford, S.R. (1935) Reaction of buffer solution and ophthalmic drugs. *Archs. Ophthal.*, **13**, 78–82.

Gifford, S.R. and Smith, R.D. (1933) Effect of reaction on ophthalmic solutions. *Archs. Ophthal.*, **9**, 227–33.

Graham, R. (1959) The evolution of corneal contact lenses. *Am. J. Optom.*, **36**(2), 55–72.

Greeves, R.A. (1931) A method of inserting contact lenses. *Lancet*, **1**, 752–3.

Gualdi, V. (1934) Neue Hornhaut-haftglaser zur Korrektion aller Ametropien. *Klin. Mbl Augenheilk.*, **92**, 775–9.

Gullstrand, A. (1911) Demonstration der Nernstlampe. *Ber. 37 Versamml. dt Ophth. Ges.*, 374–6.

Hanke, V. (1916) A contact glass for use in symblepharon. *Zeitschr. Augenheilk.*, **36**, 101.

Heine, L. (1929) Die Korrektur saemtlicher Ametropien durch geschliffene Kontaktschalen. *Ber. 13. Congr. Ophthal.*, Amsterdam, **1**, 232–4.

Henker, O. (1916) Ein Trager für die Gullstrandsche Nernstspaltlampe. *Zeitschr. Ophth. Optik.*, **4**, 75–85.

Herschel, J.F.W. (1845) Light in *Encyclopaedia Metropolitana* (Section XII: Of the structure of the eye, and of vision), **4**, 398.

Hoffstetter, H.W. and Graham, R. (1953) Leonardo and contact lenses. *Am. J. Optom.*, **30**(1), 41–4.

Illig (1929) Eine Glasschale zur Verhutung und Behandlung des Symblepharon. *Arch. Augenheilk.*, **82**, 94.

Jenkin, L. and Tyler-Jones, R.A. (1969) *Theory and practice of contact lens fitting*, 2nd edn Hatton Press, London 13–21.

Kinsey, V.E. (1952) An explanation of the corneal haze and halos produced by contact lenses. *Am. J. Ophthal.*, **35**(5), 691–5.

Kinsey, V.E. *et al.* (1942a) Sodium chloride and phosphorus movement and the eye. *Archs. Ophthal.*, **27**(6).

Kinsey, V.E. *et al.* (1942b) Water movement and the eye. *Archs. Ophthal.*, **27**(2).

Koeppe, L. (1918) Die Mikroskopie des lebenden Augenhintergrundes mit starken Vergrosserungen im fokalen Lichte der Gullstandschen Nernstspaltlampe. *Albrecht v Graefes Arch. Ophthal.*, **95**, 282–306.

Koeppe, L. (1920) Die Mikroskopie des lebenden Kammerwinkels im fokalen Lichte der Gullstrandschen Nernstspaltlampe. *Albrecht v Graefes Arch. Ophthal.*, **101**, 238–56.

Lauber, H. (1923) On improvement of vision with Müller's lenses. *Klin. Mbl Augenheilk.* **72**, 239.

Leonardo da Vinci, (1508) *Manuscript Codex D. Codex of the eye.*

Ludemann, (1917) Hydrodiaskop oder Kontaktglas zur Korrektur des Keratokonus. *Zeitschr. Augenheilk.*, **37**, 267.

Mann, I. (1938) The history of contact lenses. *Trans. Ophthal. Soc. U.K.*, **58**, 109–36.

May, C.H. (1888) A contact lens. (Translation of paper by A.E. Fick). *Archs. Ophthal.*, **19**, 215–26.

McKellen, G.D. (1949) Conical contact lenses. *Brit. J. Ophthal.*, **33**, 120–7.

Meyerbach, F. (1926) Descemetocele and its correction with a contact lens. *Klin. Mbl Augenheilk.*, **77**, 507.

Much, V. (1932) Über Haftglaser, geschichtliches. *Arch. Augenheilk.*, **105**, 390–414.

Mueller-Welt, A. (1934) Über Haftglaser. *Klin Mbl Augenheilk.*, **94**, 108.

Mueller-Welt, A. (1950) The Mueller-Welt fluidless contact lens. *Optom. Weekly*, **41**, 831–4.

Mueller-Welt, A. (1957) Trial case fittings. *Contacto*, **1**(2) 28–30.

Müller, A. (1889) *Brillenglaser und Hornhautlinsen.* Inaugural dissertation, University of Kiel.

Müller, F.A. and Müller, A.C. (1910) Das kunstliche Auge. J.F. Bergmann, Wiesbaden.

Nelson, F. (1938) Contact lenses with spheric optic and aspheric haptic part. *Am. J. Ophthal.*, **21**, 775–9.

Nugent, M.W. (1950) The Tuohy corneal lens, a second report. *Archs Ophthal.*, **43**, 232–7.

Obrig, T.E. (1937) Fitting of contact lenses for persons with ametropia. *Archs Ophthal.*, **17**, 1089–120.

Obrig, T.E. (1942) *Contact Lenses*, Chilton Co., Philadelphia.

Obrig, T.E. (1947) Solutions used with contact lenses. *Archs Ophthal.*, **38**, 668–76.

Obrig, T.E. and Salvatori, P.L. (1957) *Contact Lenses*, 3rd edn, Chilton Co., Philadelphia.

O'Rourke, D. (1928) The optical correction of conical cornea with the contact glass. *Trans. Am. Acad. Ophthal. Otolaryng.*, **32**, 260–9.

Panas, P. (1888) Traitement optique du keratocone. *Ann. D'Occulist.*, **99**, 293.

Pascal, J.I. (1941) The origins and development of contact lenses. *Opt. J. and Rev. Optom.*, **78**(2), 57–61.

Pearson, R.M. (1978) August Muller's inaugural dissertation. *J. Brit. Contact Lens Ass.*, **1**(2), 33–6.

Poller, A. (1931) *Das Pollersch Verfahren zum Abformen und lebenden und tote, sowie an gegenstanden.* Urban & Scharzenberg, Berlin.

Ridley, F. (1946) Recent developments in the manufacture, fitting and prescription of contact lenses of regular shape. *Proc. Soc. Med.*, **39**(12), 842–8.

Ridley, F. (1963) Scleral Contact Lenses. *Archs Ophthal.*, **70**, 739–45.

Ruben, M. (1975) *Contact Lens Practice*, Baillière Tindall, London, pp. 23, 312.

Ruben, M. (1979) Obituary of Joseph Dallos. *Brit. Med. J.*, **2**, 217.

Rugg-Gunn, A. (1930) Contact glasses for ametropia. *Lancet*, **2**, 1067–9.

Rugg-Gunn, A. (1931) Contact glasses. *Brit. J. Ophthal.*, **15**, 549–74.

Rugg-Gunn, A. (1938) The contact lens centre, its purpose and policy. *Brit. Med. J.*, **2**, 278–9.

Rycroft, B.W. (1932) Contact glasses. *Brit. J. Ophthal.,* **16**, 461–72.

Sabell, A.G. (1970) Some notes on diagnostic contact lenses. *Ophthalmic Optician,* **10**(22), 1160–78.

Sabell, A.G. (1979) Dr Joseph Dallos: an appreciation. *The Contact Lens J.,* **8**(5) 16–18.

Sabell, A.G. (1980) An ophthalmic museum. *The Contact Lens J.,* **9**(2) 15–19; (3), 16–22; (4), 10–18; (6), 3–18.

Sabell, A.G. (1988) The early years in *100 years of the contact lens,* (Optician Supplement) 6–21.

Sabell, A.G. (1989) The history of contact lenses, in *Contact Lenses* (eds Phillips and Stone) Butterworths, London.

Sattler, C.H. (1938) Erfahrungen mit Haftglasern. *Klin. Mbl Augenheilk.,* **100**(2), 172–7.

Siegrist, A. (1916) Die Behandlung des Keratokonus. *Klin Mbl Augenheilk.,* **56**, 400–21.

Siegrist, A. (1920) Demonstration des Keratokonus. *Ber. d. 42. Versamml. Ophthal. Ges.,* Heidelberg, 339–40.

Sitchevska, O. (1932) Contact glasses in keratoconus and in ametropia. *Am. J. Ophthal.,* **15**, 1028–38.

Smelser, G.K. (1952) Relation of factors involved in maintenance of optical properties of cornea to contact lens wear. *Archs Ophthal.,* **47**(3), 328–43.

Smelser, G.K. and Chen, D.K. (1955) Physiologic changes in the cornea induced by contact lenses. *Archs Ophthal.,* **53**(5), 676–9.

Smelser, G.K. and Ozanics, V. (1953) Structural changes in the corneae of guinea pigs after wearing contact lenses. *Archs Ophthal.,* **49**(3), 335–40.

Sugar, H.S. (1941) Gonioscopy and glaucoma. *Archs Ophthal.,* **25**, 674–717.

Sulzer, D.E. (1891–2) La forme de la cornée humaine et son influence sur la vision. *Archiv. d'Ophthal.,* Part 1, 11, 419–34; Part 2, 12, 32–50.

Sulzer, D.E. (1892) La corréction optique du keratocone, de l'astigmatisme irregulier et de l'astigmatisme cicatriciel. *Bull. Soc. Fr. Ophthal.,* **10**, 113–20.

von Csapody, I. (1929) Abgusse der lebenden Augapfeloberflache für Verordnung von Kontaktglasern. *Klin. Mbl Augenheilk.,* **82**, 818–22.

von Hippel, E. (1918) Über die Behandlung des Keratokonus mit Mullerschen Kontaktglasern. *Klin. Mbl Augenheilk.,* **60**, 320.

Weihmann (1923) Verbandlose Behandlung des Ulcus Corneae mit durchsichtigen Kontaktschalen. *Klin. Mbl Augenheilk.,* **70**, 236.

Wichterle, O. and Lim, D. (1960) Hydrophilic gels for biological use. *Nature,* **185**, 117–18.

Wichterle, O., Lim, D. and Dreifus, M. (1961) A contribution to the problem of contact lenses. *Cesk. Oftal.,* **17**, 70–5.

Young, T. (1801) On the mechanism of the eye. *Phil. Trans. R. Soc.,* **16**, 23–88.

PART TWO

Material Technology

INTRODUCTION

The history of the development of the contact lens (see Chapter 1) has been concerned with the ideology of achieving maximal tolerance and best acuity and for the therapeutic device protection with minimal complications.

There are many secondary issues concerned with tolerance of the device which for example may be metabolic and/or sensory. The history has shown how the inventions of materials have largely influenced the development of the lens. The chemical formulation (see Chapter 2) illustrates how 'needs' control development. Thus the fitters of the 1930s used the then new technology of thermolabile acrylates to replace glass. Later, in the 1950s, the same class of materials was used to develop the corneal rigid lens (see Chapter 27). From the 1950s onwards the rapid advances in contact lens manufacture and the understanding of the criteria for safe contact lens wear gave rise to a different approach. Thus the chemists were able to produce materials that satisfied the criteria demanded by the physiologist, clinician and manufacturer.

But even with present-day sophisticated investigative research it has been impossible to find the ideal material for all clinical needs. Polymethylmethacrylate (PMMA) is thermolabile and therefore mouldable by heat processing. This technology could be applied for all sizes of lenses but with limitations as to thickness. But using lathe generation, very thin, small lenses could be manufactured by automated methods. Coatings and copolymers attempted to resolve the hydrophobic nature of the contact lens surface.

The co-existence of silicone rubbers and resins opened up for the researcher the possibility of having gas permeation materials but restrictions due to manufacturing technology, hydrophobicity of surface and undue flexibility of the lens plus the surface coating problems (see Chapter 47) has to a degree made advances, with such materials difficult.

The compromise has been with silastic acrylate copolymers and cellulose acetate butyrate (CAB) copolymers to provide materials capable of generation and with gas permeable properties (see Chapter 3). To satisfy the gas permeable requirements, fluorocarbon and other new materials have been assessed but an entirely satisfactory rigid material has yet to be found.

The soft hydrophilic materials have been developed from the original polyhema (of low water content) to vinyl and other copolymers of very high water content and commensurate increased gas transmissibility for the lens. There are also ionic polymers of different chemistry that can be formulated to provide better surface tolerances.

Added to this enormous potential of polymers, there are biopolymers of cellulose or collagen made with added acrylics to prevent undue rapid biodegeneration when worn.

In desperation of finding a polymer that will withstand long periods of wear without spoilage the conventional materials can be offered for use on short-term disposable lens systems (see Chapter 47).

Soft materials have the advantage of tolerance and in special instances of irregular corneal shape the combination of hard and soft has been used (see Chapters 28, 29 and 35).

There are methods of identifying the chemistry of a material but the easiest way is to establish the material's physical characteristics. For example, the gas permeability, water content (for hydrophilic), specific gravity and elasticity are sufficient to distinguish one material from another. The finished lens has many other physical properties to consider, such as gas transmissibility, surface finish, flexibility, ionic or non-ionic surface and sorption properties; and there are many others that are pertinent to research on the function of the lens on the eye.

The whole subject of biocompatibility (see Chapter 47) and the problems that arise for each aspect of non-compatibility (see Chapters 25, 26 and 47) is indeed the future for contact lens advancement.

Providing the material satisfies the physiological criteria for corneal cell metabolism and the lens design permits the lens to use such criteria to that optimum, then there is one remaining problem – the ultimate goal must be to have a contact lens surface that maintains a tear film in the same form and function as the precorneal tear film (see Chapter 21).

CHEMICAL COMPOSITION AND PROPERTIES 2

M.F. Refojo

2.1 CHEMISTRY OF CONTACT LENS MATERIALS

2.1.1 MONOMERS, POLYMERS AND COPOLYMERS

Contact lenses are made of plastics, which are synthetic or semi-synthetic macromolecular materials also known as polymers. The semi-synthetic polymers are naturally occurring, chemically modified biopolymers, such as proteins and polysaccharides. Polymers are made by the condensation or addition of monomers, which are the links in the polymeric chains. When all the monomeric units are identical, the material is a homopolymer. When two or more kinds of monomers have been combined in a polymerization reaction, the result is a copolymer. There are several kinds of copolymers. The comonomers can be distributed in the polymer chain either in a random fashion or alternating regularly. In block copolymers, one monomer type can form chains to which chains of another monomer are joined in alternating fashion. In graft copolymers, a monomer of one type is polymerized onto a pre-existing polymer formed from different monomers. The arrangement of the comonomers greatly affects the properties of copolymers. Telechelic polymers are macromolecules that can react at both ends with other monomers to generate new polymers with different properties.

Plasma, or glow discharge, polymerization is a procedure used to chemically bond very thin polymeric surfaces onto other materials. Plasma polymerization has been used to form hydrophilic surfaces on hydrophobic contact lenses. The plasma polymerization reaction is carried out in high vacuum; a gas, such as hydrogen, nitrogen, or water vapour, or a more complex molecule is reacted onto the surface of the lens. The plasma state of the gaseous molecules is generated by means of radiofrequencies or microwaves.

The properties of a polymer depend on the monomer(s) and on the polymerization procedure. A polymerization reaction is triggered by an initiator that activates the monomer molecules to link to each other. The reaction is usually started by heating or by irradiating the monomers which contain a very small amount of an initiator. The polymer is further treated by a curing process that consists of additional heat or irradiation to complete the polymerization. The polymerization can be carried out in a solvent or in bulk, resulting in polymers with different physical and mechanical properties.

Contact Lens Practice. Edited by Montague Ruben and Michel Guillon. Published in 1994 by Chapman & Hall, London. ISBN 0 412 35120 X

2.1.2 THERMOPLASTICS AND THERMOSET POLYMERS

Polymer and plastic are synonyms. The latter term reflects the plasticity that makes some of these materials amenable to moulding under heat and pressure, but not all plastics can be moulded. Plastics can be classified according to their behaviour when heated. If they melt under heat, they are thermoplastics and can be moulded. Thermoplastics may also dissolve in some solvents. Certain molecules, called cross-linking agents, can react with two or more polymeric chains, linking them together by a bridge; the resulting polymer is said to be cross-linked. A cross-linked polymer is a thermosetting plastic that does not melt or dissolve. Glassy plastics, both thermoplastics and thermoset, can be shaped by mechanical means, such as the use of cutting tools in a lathe. Plastic objects can also be formed by a cast moulding technique, a process in which the polymerization is carried out in moulds such that the liquid monomers polymerize and take the form of the mould.

2.1.3 MANUFACTURE TECHNIQUES FOR CONTACT LENSES

Monomers can be polymerized in bulk to form contact lens blanks, rods, or sheets, depending on the shape and size of the container in which the polymerization reaction is carried out. The rods and sheets of plastics can then be cut into lens blanks, which are lathed and polished into finished lenses. Semi-finished lenses can also be obtained by carrying out the polymerization in moulds that have the shape, for example, of the back curvature of a lens.

Spin casting of contact lenses is done by polymerizing the monomer mixture, in a solvent or in bulk, in rotating open moulds. Cast moulding is done by polymerizing the monomer mixture in closed moulds. The casting technique must take into account the shrinkage of the total volume of the prepolymer mixture and the resulting polymer. Shrinkage occurs because the distance between the unreacted monomers is larger than the length of the covalent bonded monomer units formed upon polymerization.

Moulded lenses can be made only from thermoplastic polymers by injection of powder melt or by compression of plastic sheet in the proper moulds. Because the thermal expansion of most plastics is relatively high, shrinkage of the moulded lenses must be taken into account.

Internal stresses can develop when a moulded plastic is cooled and when lenses are lathed and polished. Annealing is the slow cooling of a hot plastic to relieve internal stresses. Annealing can reduce brittleness and the distortions that stressed lenses may suffer with normal use, but any hard plastic lens can retain residual stresses even after annealing.

2.2 CLASSIFICATION OF CONTACT LENSES BY MATERIALS

From a materials point of view, contact lenses can be classified as follows:

1. Rigid (hard) lenses:
    poly (methyl methacrylate);
    oxygen-permeable (RGP) materials:
        cellulose acetate butyrate,
        silicone resins,
        siloxane-methacrylates,
        fluoro-siloxane-methacrylates,
        alkyl styrene copolymers.
2. Flexible fluoropolymer lens.
3. Elastomeric lenses:
        silicone rubber,
        acrylic rubber.
4. Soft hydrophilic (hydrogel) lenses:
        hydrogels of non-ionic polymers:
            low hydration (Group I),
            high hydration (Group II).

hydrogels of ionic polymers:
    low hydration (Group III),
    high hydration (Group IV).
5.   Lenses with rigid permeable optics and soft hydrophilic periphery.
6.   Biopolymer lenses:
    polysaccharides,
    proteins.

2.2.1 RIGID (HARD) LENSES

Poly(methyl methacrylate)

Poly(methyl methacrylate) (PMMA) is the prototype material for all rigid contact lenses. PMMA is a commercial plastic, and some of its trade names (Plexiglas, Lucite, Perspex) are easily recognized by the general public. The excellent tissue tolerance of pure, fully polymerized PMMA, its optical properties, resistance to discoloration, light weight and good manufacturing properties have contributed greatly to the development of the contact lens industry.

Because non-cross-linked PMMA is thermoplastic, many of these contact lenses have been made by moulding. However, to increase the scratch resistance and the physical stability of the lens upon hydration (moisture absorption about 1%), some manufacturers used crosslinked PMMA to make contact lenses by lathing and abrasion-polishing techniques.

The single most important drawback of PMMA as a contact lens material is its extremely low oxygen permeability. However, as a consequence of the fitting of a great number of PMMA contact lenses, much has been learned about corneal physiology, particularly the need for PMMA lens movement to allow corneal oxygenation and minimize corneal swelling.

The realization of the need for corneal oxygenation under a contact lens stimulated the search for new contact lens materials with high oxygen permeability. The objective of this search has been to find materials having the desirable properties of PMMA but with highly enhanced oxygen permeability.

Oxygen-permeable (RGP) materials

Cellulose acetate butyrate

Cellulose acetate butyrate (CAB) is a common transparent commercial plastic. The interest in this plastic for the manufacture of contact lenses derived from its relatively high oxygen permeability compared with PMMA. CAB is a derivative of a very abundant natural polysaccharide – cellulose – in which the three free hydroxyl groups in its monomeric unit, glucose, have been esterified to acetyl and butyryl groups. Cellulose esters can be prepared with varying degrees of substitution. Because the proportion of acetate and butyrate, as well as of free hydroxyl groups, can be varied, CAB is not a single material but rather a family of potentially useful contact lens materials. A commonly used CAB contains about 13% substitute acetyl groups, 37% butyryl groups and 1 to 2% free hydroxyl groups. The physical and chemical properties of CAB vary according to the ratio of acetyl to butyryl in the cellulose molecule; increasing butyryl (decreasing acetyl) content increases the flexibility and decreases the moisture absorption of the plastic. CAB is a non-cross-linked thermoplastic, and CAB contact lenses can be made by moulding. It can absorb up to 2% of moisture by weight, which, together with the lack of cross-links, contributes to the distortion and warping of some CAB lenses.

Commercial CAB may contain additives, such as plasticizers, that improve its physical properties for diverse industrial uses. However, these additives can leach from the plastic, and an additive-free CAB should be used for contact lens manufacture.

Silicone resins

Silicon is a chemical element that must not be confused with silicone, which is the generic name for polymers with a backbone of silicon and oxygen links. The importance of the silicone polymers as contact lens materials is based on the high oxygen permeability that the silicon–oxygen moiety imparts. The most familiar silicone contact lenses are those made of flexible silicone rubber (see page 00), but some rigid silicone resin lenses are also available.

Silicones have a poly(siloxane), $[-Si-O-]_n$, backbone, with two organic radicals such as methyl ($-CH_3$), phenyl ($-C_6-H_5$), or vinyl ($-CH=CH_2$) attached to each silicon atom. A silicone resin has a larger proportion of phenyl to methyl radicals than a silicone rubber, and proportionally more vinyl groups to produce higher cross-linking density. The phenyl groups and the cross-links impart rigidity to the silicone resin. To maintain its rubbery elasticity, a silicone rubber is richer in methyl radicals and poorer in cross-links than a silicone resin. Because the oxygen permeability of poly(methyl-phenyl-siloxane) decreases exponentially with decreasing methyl (increasing phenyl) content, the silicone resin contact lenses have substantially lower oxygen permeability than do the silicone rubber lenses. The phenyl groups, which are bulkier than the methyl groups, hinder the mobility of the siloxane segments in the polymer chain, making it more difficult for the oxygen molecules to pass through the rigid macromolecular network. The higher density of cross-links in the resins also hinders the movement of the oxygen molecules through the polymer mass.

Oxygen permeability For a gas such as oxygen to permeate through a contact lens, the gas must dissolve in the polymer surface and then diffuse, impelled by its own kinetic energy, from a place of higher to a place of lower concentration in the polymer. For poly(siloxanes), the oxygen permeability, $P = D \cdot k$, is high because the diffusivity, D, of the oxygen in silicone is facilitated by the flexibility of the polymer molecules, which allows the small oxygen molecules to move throughout the polymer network with little restraint. The phenyl groups and the vinyl cross-links in the silicone resins lower the flexibility of the silicone network and reduce the oxygen permeability. The solubility of oxygen in silicone (expressed by the Henry's Law solubility coefficient, and given by the factor k in the permeability equation) is of the same order of magnitude as in other polymers, and contributes less to the oxygen permeability of silicones than does its diffusivity factor.

Water wettability When water completely wets a surface, its contact angle is zero, and the surface is said to be hydrophilic. When the water contact angle on a surface is larger than zero, the surface is said to be less hydrophilic, or more hydrophobic, than a perfectly wettable surface. An ideal contact lens material should have hydrophilic surfaces. Silicone materials are by their nature hydrophobic, because the predominant chemical groups that surround the poly(siloxane) backbone are hydrophobic. Nevertheless, the surface of silicone contact lenses can be chemically modified to contain a high proportion of hydrophilic groups, such as hydroxyl ($-OH$) or carboxyl ($-COOH$), attached to the alkyl radical on the poly(siloxane) backbone. These treatments result in more comfortable and useful silicone contact lenses. Unfortunately some of these hydrophilic surfaces are not long lasting. Silicone resin rigid lenses that have hydrophilic surfaces cannot be polished or otherwise mechanically modified for better fit, hence the hydrophilic surface becomes as hydrophobic as the bulk of the lens.

An often-used procedure to render hydrophobic contact lenses hydrophilic is plasma treatment, which consists of subjecting a gas, such as oxygen, nitrogen, or water vapour, to an electric discharge in a vacuum where the gas is ionized. The ionized gas reacts with the contact lens surface, forming a new hydrophilic surface. The disadvantage of this treatment is that the hydrophilic surface may rub off, and the lens again becomes hydrophobic.

Siloxane-methacrylates

The oxygen permeability of rigid contact lenses was improved by copolymerization of methyl methacrylate with certain siloxanyl (–Si–O–Si–) alkyl (–CH_2–CH_2–CH_2–) methacrylate (CH_2=C–COO–) monomers. One typical monomer of this type is methacryloxypropyltris(trimethylsiloxy)silane (TRIS):

$$CH_2=\underset{\underset{O}{\|}}{\overset{\overset{CH_3}{|}}{C}}-C-O-CH_2-CH_2-CH_2-\underset{\underset{\underset{CH_3-\underset{|}{Si}-CH_3}{|}}{\overset{|}{O}}}{\overset{\overset{\overset{CH_3}{|}}{CH_3-\overset{|}{Si}-CH_3}}{\overset{|}{O}}}{Si}-O-\underset{\underset{CH_3}{|}}{\overset{\overset{CH_3}{|}}{Si}}-CH_3$$

(eqn 2.1)

Several monomers of the TRIS type have been used in the manufacture of various proprietary contact lenses. These monomers differ in the amount and configuration of the siloxane radicals attached to the alkyl methacrylate moiety. One of these monomers, methyldi(trimethylsiloxy)silylpropylglycerol methacrylate (SiGMA) (2.2), also includes a hydrophilic radical in the alkyl moiety:

The oxygen permeability coefficient of the siloxanyl alkyl methacrylate polymers depends on the number of siloxane bonds and their distribution through the polymer network. In contrast to the silicone rubbers and resins mentioned above, which are polymers with backbones made entirely of siloxane bonds, the siloxanylalkyl methacrylate copolymers have a backbone of carbon-to-carbon linkages, with branches that are relatively short compared with the length of the polymer backbone and that may contain several siloxane bonds per branch. Therefore, the siloxane–methacrylate (or siloxanylalkyl methacrylate) contact lenses do not contain silicone and should not be called silicone methacrylates; they do contain silicon and could be termed silicon methacrylates.

The pioneer work in developing an oxygen-permeable, silicon-containing rigid methacrylate contact lens was done in the early 1970s and resulted in the first lens of this type, the Polycon lens. Several similar contact lens materials followed, based on the same general idea. Usually these contact lens materials are copolymers of a given siloxanylalkyl methacrylate with methyl methacrylate and some other monomers to contribute rigidity and hydrophilicity. A common ingredient is a cross-linking agent, such as ethylene glycol dimethacrylate, that contributes hardness and lens stability. Methacrylic acid is also commonly used to improve wettability, but other hydrophilic monomers

$$CH_2=\underset{\underset{O}{\|}}{\overset{\overset{CH_3}{|}}{C}}-C-O-CH_2-\underset{\underset{OH}{|}}{CH}-CH_2-O-CH_2-CH_2-CH_2-\underset{\underset{\underset{CH_3-\underset{|}{Si}-CH_3}{|}}{\overset{|}{O}}}{\overset{\overset{\overset{CH_3}{|}}{CH_3-\overset{|}{Si}-CH_3}}{\overset{|}{O}}}{Si}-CH_3$$

(eqn 2.2)

such as hydroxyethyl methacrylate and acrylamide derivatives may be used as well in these contact lens materials.

The original idea behind the development of oxygen-permeable hard contact lenses was to maintain as far as possible the desirable properties of the PMMA contact lenses, but with the highest possible oxygen permeability. Such desirable properties as oxygen permeability, wettability and physical and chemical stability are obtained by the right combination of monomers. However, an ingredient that improves one property, such as oxygen permeability, might contribute to the deterioration of another property, such as wettability. Therefore, the contact lens chemist must find the formulation that maximizes all the desirable properties. Although there are some differences in the chemical composition of the diverse siloxanylalkyl methacrylate contact lenses on the market, sometimes the difference in lenses from the same manufacturer may be only in the proportion of the monomers. Other apparently small differences in composition can result in substantial differences in lens performance. A siloxanylalkyl methacrylate contact lens material was apparently the first material of this type to include dimethyl itaconate (2.3) in its formulation to improve the rigidity and hardness.

$$\begin{array}{c} CH_2-COO-CH_3 \\ | \\ CH_2=C-COO-CH_3 \end{array} \quad \text{(eqn 2.3)}$$

The formula of dimethyl itaconate is similar to that of methyl methacrylate with the $-CH_2-COO-CH_3$ radical replacing a methyl ($-CH_3$) radical.

Fluoro-siloxane-methacrylates

These contact lens materials were derived from the copolymers used to make the siloxanylalkyl methacrylate contact lenses, but in addition to the monomers mentioned above for these materials, they also contain some fluorinated monomers. Different fluorinated methacrylates, such as 2,2,2,-trifluoro-1-(trifluoromethyl)ethyl methacrylate (2.4) and bis-hexafluoroisopropyl itaconate (2.5), can be used in the fluoro-siloxane-methacrylate contact lens materials.

$$\begin{array}{c} CH_3 \\ | \\ CH_2=C-COOCH(CF_3)_2 \end{array} \quad \text{(eqn 2.4)}$$

$$\begin{array}{c} CH_2COOCH(CF_3)_2 \\ | \\ CH_2=C-COOCH(CF_3)_2 \end{array} \quad \text{(eqn 2.5)}$$

In general, the siloxanylalkyl methacrylate moiety imparts oxygen permeability to the polymer, which the fluorinated monomer does also but only to a minor degree. However, addition of the fluorinated monomer to the polymer formulation permits the use of a major proportion of the siloxanylalkyl methacrylate moiety, and hence a higher oxygen permeability, without detriment to the mechanical properties of the lens. The fluorinated moieties are hydrophobic, but they may impart some resistance to mucoprotein adhesion on the contact lenses. The hydrophobicity of the siloxanylalkyl and fluoroalkyl methacrylate moieties must be modified by the addition of methacrylic acid or other hydrophilic monomer in the polymer formulation. Rigidity of the contact lens is due to the presence of methyl methacrylate or dimethyl itaconate, or the cross-linking agent, or both, and in some cases also the fluoro derivative.

Alkyl styrene copolymers

These materials are characterized by their low density, such that they may float on water, and relatively high refractive index

(n_D about 1.59, versus 1.49 for PMMA). The principal idea in developing alkyl styrene contact lenses was, again, the relatively high oxygen permeability of these materials. The alkyl styrenes used in contact lenses are *para*-isopropyl styrene (2.6) and *para*-tertiary butyl styrene (2.7).

$$CH=CH_2$$

CH$_3$–CH–CH$_3$　　　(eqn 2.6)

$$CH=CH_2$$

CH$_3$–C–CH$_3$
　　CH$_3$　　　(eqn 2.7)

The oxygen permeability characteristics of the alkyl styrenes are due to the presence of the bulky alkyl group (isopropyl or tertiary butyl) which hinders the packing of the polymer chains and contributes to void formation in the plastic for the passage of gas molecules. The looseness of the polymer structure is shown in their low density, which is an indication of gas permeability. In contrast to the oxygen permeability coefficient ($D \cdot k$) of polystyrene, which is about 2.5 barrers (1 barrer = 1×10^{-11} cm^3·cm/cm^2·s·mmHg), the oxygen permeabilities of poly(isopropyl styrene) and poly(tertiary butyl styrene) are about 13 and 16 barrers, respectively.

Polystyrene and the poly(alkyl styrenes) are hydrophobic materials; therefore alkyl styrene contact lenses must be made from copolymers with hydrophilic monomers such as vinyl pyrrolidone or hydroxyethyl methacrylate. The copolymers may also contain other comonomers such as methyl methacrylate and a cross-linking agent to impart stability, rigidity and machinability. Some contact lenses of higher oxygen permeability than the alkyl styrene lenses have been made from copolymers of an alkyl styrene with a siloxanylalkyl methacrylate, methyl methacrylate, a hydrophilic monomer, and a cross-linking agent.

2.2.2　FLEXIBLE FLUOROPOLYMER LENS

Organofluorine compounds are distinguished by their inertness, hydrophobicity and lubricity. Fluorocompounds have, in general, a low refractive index and high density. These compounds are of interest in the contact lens field because of their relatively high oxygen permeability and resistance to coating, as well as the potential for reduced friction between the lens and the lid, which would afford better lens tolerance.

The only contact lens material of this kind currently available is made by the copolymerization of a high-molecular-weight telechelic perfluoropolyether (which imparts high oxygen permeability) with methyl methacrylate (which imparts stiffness) and vinyl pyrrolidone (which imparts hydrophilicity). The perfluoro- prefix in an organic compound indicates that all the hydrogen atoms in the molecule have been replaced by fluorine atoms. The telechelic perfluoropolyether used in this lens is α, ω-methylene methacrylate perfluoropoly-(oxyethylene) poly(oxymethylene) (2.8); where m and n determine an average molecular weight between 500 and 15 000 Da.

Like other kinds of contact lens materials, particularly the siloxanyl alkyl methacrylate copolymers, the perfluoropolyether/methyl methacrylate/vinyl pyrrolidone copolymers

$$CH_2=\underset{\underset{O}{\overset{\|}{C}}}{\overset{\overset{CH_3}{|}}{C}}-C-O-CH_2-CF_2-CF_2--(CF_2-CF_2-O-)^m-(CF_2-O)^n-CF_2-CH_2-O-\underset{\underset{O}{\overset{\|}{C}}}{\overset{\overset{CH_3}{|}}{C}}-C=CH_2$$

$$(\text{eqn } 2.8)$$

can be made with different proportions of the components to obtain materials with diverse degrees of oxygen permeability, stiffness and wettability. Not only can the proportion of the comonomers be altered, but also, for example, a hydrophilic monomer other than vinyl pyrrolidone can be used in the formulation. Furthermore, the perfluoropolyether can be of various molecular weights. Because the material is apparently not amenable to mechanical forming, these flexible fluoropolymer lenses are manufactured by a moulding procedure.

2.2.3 ELASTOMERIC LENSES

Silicone rubber

The oxygen permeability of poly(dimethyl siloxane) (2.9), the most common silicone rubber, is unsurpassed at this time by any other material with properties suitable for the manufacture of contact lenses:

but often for silicone rubber contact lenses a certain proportion of the methyl groups are replaced by phenyl and vinyl groups. Some specialized silicone rubbers have other organic radicals as well. The silicone polymers are oils or semi-solid greases. The rubbers and resins are cross-linked polymers forming three-dimensional polymer networks. The cross-links are usually vinyl bridges. Because cross-linked poly(dimethyl siloxane) forms relatively weak materials, inorganic fillers such as silica are often added to these silicone rubbers. However, in the contact lens field the best silicone derivatives are the poly(dimethyl diphenyl vinyl siloxanes), which without a filler are strong enough for contact lenses, and, of course, transparent, and still maintain high oxygen permeability, although lower than that of poly(dimethyl siloxane).

Because silicone rubber contact lenses are not easily amenable to mechanical cutting and polishing, they are made by moulding:

$$\underset{\underset{CH_3}{|}}{\overset{\overset{CH_3}{|}}{CH_3-Si}}-O(-\underset{\underset{CH_3}{|}}{\overset{\overset{CH_3}{|}}{Si}}-O)_n-\underset{\underset{CH_3}{|}}{\overset{\overset{CH_3}{|}}{Si}}-CH_3 \qquad (\text{eqn } 2.9)$$

$$-\underset{\underset{CH_3}{|}}{\overset{\overset{CH_3}{|}}{Si}}-O-\underset{\underset{Ph}{|}}{\overset{\overset{Ph}{|}}{Si}}-O-\underset{\underset{Ph}{|}}{\overset{\overset{CH_3}{|}}{Si}}-O-\underset{\underset{-CH}{|}}{\overset{\overset{CH_3}{|}}{Si}}-O-\underset{\underset{CH_3}{|}}{\overset{\overset{CH_3}{|}}{Si}}-CH_3$$
$$-CH_2 \qquad (\text{eqn } 2.10)$$

The silicone rubbers are organic–inorganic polymers with a backbone of silicon and oxygen linkages (siloxane moiety). In the poly(dimethyl siloxane) formula, the subscript *n* represents a number that determines the molecular weight of the polymer. Two organic radicals are attached to each silicon atom in the backbone. In poly(dimethyl siloxane) these radicals are methyl groups,

Formula (2.10), a poly(methyl phenyl vinyl siloxane), has the following groups (listed here in their order from left to right in the formula): dimethyl siloxy, diphenyl siloxy, methyl phenyl (Ph) siloxy, methyl vinyl siloxy. The silicone chain is terminated by a trimethyl siloxy radical.

Although the high oxygen permeability of

silicone rubbers has made them very attractive for use in contact lenses, their strong hydrophobicity has been a deterrent. The surfaces of silicone rubber contact lenses can be made hydrophilic by chemical and physical treatments. However, if, to increase the hydrophilicity, the alkyl radicals in the silicone polymer are replaced by hydroxyl groups, the resulting hydrophilic surface would be short lasting, because the –Si–OH groups will react with each other, liberating water, or react readily with some components of the tear films, in either case rendering the lens surface hydrophobic. Glow discharge has been the most successful treatment to render silicone lenses hydrophilic. This procedure does not substitute the alkyl radical for the hydroxyl radical, but attaches hydrophilic groups to the alkyl radicals in the polysiloxane chain. Nevertheless, the resulting ultrathin hydrophilic surface can rub off and the lens may again become hydrophobic.

The silicones are lipophilic materials, so the silicone rubber contact lenses tend to absorb lipids such as the cholesterol and cholesterol esters present in the tear film and other lipid contaminants that may come in contact with the lens.

The water vapour permeability of silicone rubber greatly surpasses even its very high oxygen permeability. Therefore, in the absence of a stable tear film on the front surface of a silicone rubber lens, the tear film or the epithelium under the lens may dry. The result can be attachment of the lens to the corneal surface and the complications of epithelium erosion that such an adhesion creates. This phenomenon could also take place with other water-permeable contact lenses, such as the ultrathin, high-hydration hydrogel contact lenses (see pages 00 and 00).

Water vapour permeability Because it might appear paradoxical that such a hydrophobic material as silicone rubber has a high water permeability, it will be worthwhile to comment here on the mechanisms of water permeability across membranes. Water can move across a membrane through two mechanisms, bulk flow and diffusion. Bulk flow of water takes place through porous membranes when there is a hydrostatic pressure difference across the membrane. Essentially, during bulk flow the molecules of water move together through pores in the membrane. This is not the mechanism whereby water permeates through silicone rubber. Thus, one can apply a hydrostatic pressure across a silicone rubber contact lens and water will not pass through the lens in any significant amount. By the diffusion mechanism, the water molecules move through the membrane independent of each other by a transport process called diffusive permeability. Diffusive permeability depends on two factors: the solubility of the permeating substance, in this case water in the silicone contact lens, and the diffusion factor. Water will diffuse through certain membranes, such as silicone rubber contact lenses, when there is a difference in the activity of water across the membrane. Activity is a thermodynamic concept related to concentration. For gases or vapours the activity of the diffusing species is related to its partial pressure. Thus, if the partial pressure of a gas such as oxygen or a vapour such as water is different across a contact lens, the gas or vapour will pass through the lens from the side of high to the side of low partial pressure. If a silicone lens has liquid water under it and air at less than 100% relative humidity in front of it, water from under the lens will pervaporate through the lens (permeate through the lens and evaporate from its surface).

Acrylic rubber

Acrylic rubber contact lenses are made of polymers that have a carbon-to-carbon backbone similar to that of rigid lenses of the methyl methacrylate type. By having acrylic-type rather than methacrylic-type monomers in the polymer, and/or higher alkyl homologues in the ester radical of the methacrylate moiety such as butyl rather than the methyl ester in methyl methacrylate, the resulting polymer is soft and rubbery rather than rigid at room temperature. The property of softness or rigidity at room temperature is related to the glass transition temperature, which is the temperature at which a glassy polymer becomes soft. Thus, acrylic rubber polymers are said to have a low glass transition temperature.

$$\underset{\overset{|}{CH_3}}{CH_2{=}C}\ COOCH_2CH_2CH_2CH_3$$

(eqn 2.11)

$$\underset{\overset{|}{H}}{CH_2{=}C}\ COOH$$

(eqn 2.12)

The original developers of the acrylic rubber contact lenses, who wanted a soft, non-water-absorbing contact lens that could be manufactured by the standard lathing and polishing techniques used for rigid lenses and xerogels (hydrogels in their dry state), took advantage of the glass transition temperature properties of acrylic polymers. They started with a copolymer of *n*-butyl methacrylate (2.11) and acrylic acid (2.12): poly(*n*-butyl methacrylate-co-acrylic acid) (2.13).

The copolymer is slightly cross-linked with ethylene glycol dimethacrylate for stability of the end product. A lens can be cut and polished from this copolymer because it is hard at normal manufacturing temperature. Then the lens is reacted (esterified) with *n*-butanol (2.14), which converts the lens from a hard lens at room temperature to a soft lens: poly(*n*-butyl methacrylate-co-butyl acrylate) (2.15). The lens size increases about 5% after the esterification reaction.

The finished lenses have also been described as PBABMA (poly-butyl acrylate-co-butyl methacrylate) lenses; due to the flexibility of the polymer chains, they have a relatively high oxygen permeability. PBABMA is hydrophobic and, except if some of the acrylic acid remains unreacted, this material should not wet better than PMMA.

2.2.4 SOFT HYDROPHILIC CONTACT LENSES

Soft hydrophilic contact lenses are made of a unique class of materials called hydrogels, which consist of a hydrophilic polymer network that absorbs water to a certain maximum capacity. The hydrophilic network is usually made from slightly cross-linked polymers or copolymers with a carbon-to-carbon backbone, to which are attached the hydrophilic groups. The dry cross-linked polymer is called a xerogel. When the xerogel is placed in water or an aqueous environment, it swells to its equilibrium swelling which depends on, in addition to the hydrophilic character of the polymer and its degree of

$$-(CH_2{-}\underset{\overset{|}{\underset{\overset{|}{\underset{\overset{|}{\underset{|}{CH_3}}{(CH_2)_3}}{O}}{C{=}O}}}{\overset{|}{C}})^m(CH_2{-}\underset{\overset{|}{\underset{|}{OH}}{C{=}O}}{\overset{\overset{|}{H}}{C}})^n{-}\ +\ CH_3(CH_2)_2OH \longrightarrow -(CH_2{-}\underset{\overset{|}{\underset{\overset{|}{\underset{\overset{|}{\underset{|}{CH_3}}{(CH_2)_3}}{O}}{C{=}O}}}{\overset{|}{C}})^m(CH_2{-}\underset{\overset{|}{\underset{\overset{|}{\underset{\overset{|}{\underset{|}{CH_3}}{(CH_2)_3}}{O}}{C{=}O}}}{\overset{\overset{|}{H}}{C}})^n{-}\ +\ H_2O$$

(eqn 2.13)   (eqn 2.14)   (eqn 2.15)

cross-linking, the composition of the aqueous solution, the temperature, and the hydrostatic and osmotic pressures applied to the hydrogel.

The water of hydration in a hydrogel contact lens can evaporate. Thus, the hydration of a hydrogel contact lens is constant only under the constant conditions that may exist in a closed container at a given temperature. When a hydrogel lens is on the eye, however, one can expect some fluctuations in the hydration and hence in the size of the lens.

The polymer network in a hydrogel contains hydrophilic groups, such as hydroxyl (–OH), carboxyl (–COOH), amide (–ONH–), or lactam (–NCO). Ionizable groups, such as carboxyl, are not as desirable in a hydrogel contact lens as the non-ionizable groups, because the hydration of hydrogels with ionizable groups can fluctuate more than those with non-ionizable groups with changes in pH and ionic environment. Furthermore, hydrogels with carboxylic groups are more reactive to the environment and can bind positive-charge components of the tear film.

The original hydrogel contact lenses were made of cross-linked poly(2-hydroxyethyl methacrylate) (PHEMA). Formula (2.16) represents two poly(2-hydroxyethyl methacrylate) chains cross-linked by an ethylene glycol dimethacrylate bridge. Because ethylene glycol dimethacrylate (EGDMA) is always present in small amounts in the HEMA monomer, practically all HEMA contact lenses have cross-links of EGDMA. Other cross-linking agents are also often added to HEMA hydrogels. Without cross-links, most hydrophilic polymers, but not high-molecular-weight PHEMA, would be soluble in water. The cross-links control the degree of swelling and give stability to the polymer. Most hydrogels for contact lenses are cross-linked by about one cross-link per 100 or more monomer units in the polymer.

Another common impurity in HEMA monomer is methacrylic acid, which is not always completely removed from HEMA

$$
\begin{array}{cc}
CH_3 & CH_3 \\
| & | \\
-(CH_2-C-CH_2-C)^m- \\
| & | \\
C=O & C=O \\
| & | \\
O & O-CH_2-CH_2-OH \\
| \\
CH_2 \\
| \\
CH_2 \\
| \\
O & O-CH_2-CH_2-OH \\
| & | \\
C=O & C=O \\
| & | \\
-(CH_2-C-CH_2-C)^n- \\
CH_3 & CH_3
\end{array}
\qquad (eqn\ 2.16)
$$

prior to its polymerization. Methacrylic acid will copolymerize with HEMA, and therefore it cannot leach from the lens. The small amount of methacrylic acid usually present in many types of hydrogel contact lenses will not affect the properties of the lens very much. However, in the presence of increasing amounts of methacrylic acid moieties, which are sometimes added to achieve higher hydration, the lenses will achieve not only higher hydration but also more reactivity and more sensitivity to changes in the pH of the environment.

Glyceryl methacrylate (2.17) is closely related chemically to HEMA. However, because it carries two hydroxyls per molecule versus one in HEMA, its homopolymer is much more hydrophilic than polyHEMA:

$$
\begin{array}{c}
CH_3 \\
| \\
CH_2=C \\
| \\
COOCH_2-CH-CH_2OH \\
| \\
OH
\end{array}
\qquad (eqn\ 2.17)
$$

Like PHEMA, poly(glyceryl methacrylate) is non-ionic and inert. Because glyceryl methacrylate is highly hydrophilic, to obtain hydrogels useful for contact lenses it should be copolymerized with a less hydrophilic monomer such as methyl methacrylate, as in crofilcon lenses.

Another type of hydrophilic monomer, which is used in bufilcon hydrogel contact lenses, is *N*-(1,1 -dimethyl-3-oxobutyl)-acrylamide (2.18) or, for short, diacetone acrylamide. This compound, as its name indicates, is a derivative of acrylamide (2.19). Cross-linked polyacrylamide hydrogels are widely used as a biochemical analytical tool to separate biopolymers, but they have not been useful for the manufacture of contact lenses. Diacetone acrylamide forms neutral polymers that are more resistant to hydrolysis than polyacrylamide because the amide group is shielded by the adjacent methyl groups. However, diacetone acrylamide is more reactive than HEMA and glyceryl methacrylate because its keto group (C=O) and the neighbouring carbon atoms can enter into cross-linking and other types of reactions:

$$
\begin{array}{c}
\overset{\displaystyle H}{\underset{\displaystyle \underset{\displaystyle CONH-\underset{\displaystyle CH_3}{\underset{|}{C}}-CH_2-\overset{O}{\overset{||}{C}}-CH_3}{|}}{CH_2=C}} \qquad CH_3
\end{array}
\tag{eqn 2.18}
$$

$$
\begin{array}{c}
\overset{\displaystyle H}{\underset{|}{CH_2=C}}-CONH_2
\end{array}
\tag{eqn 2.19}
$$

Diacetone acrylamide, as well as HEMA, produces polymers of relatively low hydrophilicity. To obtain hydrogel contact lenses of higher hydration, the most commonly used monomer has been vinyl pyrrolidone (VP) (2.20), which, although it does not belong to the family of acrylics, copolymerizes well with these compounds.

$$
\begin{array}{ccc}
CH_2 & \!\!\!\!\!\!\!\!\!\!\!\!\! & CH_2 \\
| & & | \\
CH_2 & & C=O \\
& \diagdown \quad \diagup & \\
& N & \\
& | & \\
& CH=CH_2 &
\end{array}
\tag{eqn 2.20}
$$

Vinyl pyrrolidone, as a comonomer with HEMA (as in vifilcon and perfilcon contact lenses) or with methyl methacrylate (as in lidofilcon contact lenses), is most commonly found in the high-hydration hydrogels. The hydrophilicity of vinyl pyrrolidone is due to the lactam moiety which forms a dipole between the nitrogen atoms and the carbonyl group. Although the pyrrolidone moiety appears not to be charged, an aqueous solution of poly(vinyl pyrrolidone) is slightly acidic (pH 4–5).

In 1986 the US Food and Drug Administration and the hydrogel contact lens manufacturers in the USA classified hydrogel contact lenses in four groups:

Group I: Non-ionic, low-water-content (38–50% water)
Group II: Non-ionic, high-water-content (51–80% water)
Group III: Ionic, low-water-content (hydration as in Group I)
Group IV: Ionic, high-water-content (hydration as in Group II)

The number of different monomers used in the hydrogel contact lens field is not very large, and only a few are the main ingredients in these materials. HEMA and VP are the most commonly used monomers. EGDMA is a commonly used cross-linking agent, although several others are used in various formulations. Several lenses contain a diversity of monomers, which contribute to their ultimate properties but often seem to be added just to obtain a polymer that is different. In the ionic hydrogels, the most common ingredient imparting this property is methacrylic acid or its sodium salt.

Hydrogels of non-ionic polymers

Low hydration (Group I)

In this group are all the lenses made of cross-linked polyHEMA, such as the polymacon material (Soflens, Hydron) and the tefilcon material (CibaSoft). Also in this group are the tetrafilcon materials (AO Soft, Aquaflex), which are made of terpolymers of HEMA, MMA, and VP, cross-linked with divinyl benzene (2.21):

$$CH=CH_2$$

$$CH=CH_2 \qquad \text{(eqn 2.21)}$$

and crofilcon (CSI), which is a cross-linked copolymer of glyceryl methacrylate with MMA.

Other materials in this group are the hefilcons (Flexlens, Sofsite, Naturvue), which are compounds of cross-linked copolymers of HEMA with VP, and phemfilcon (Durasoft), which is a copolymer of HEMA with 2-ethoxyethyl methacrylate (2.22):

$$CH_2=\overset{\overset{\displaystyle CH_3}{|}}{C}-COO-CH_2-CH_2-O-CH_2-CH_3$$

$$\text{(eqn 2.22)}$$

High hydration (Group II)

In this group are the lidofilcons (Sauflon, CW 79, B&L 70), which are made from copolymers of VP with MMA, and vifilcon (Softcon), which is a cross-linked graft copolymer of HEMA onto PVP.

Another non-ionic hydrogel used as a contact lens material under the generic name of atlafilcon is made of a cross-linked polyvinyl alcohol (PVA) polymer $[-(CH_2-CH(OH))_n-]$. Depending on the amount of cross-linking, PVA hydrogel contact lenses can be of either low or high hydration. Although PVA has been an easily available hydrophilic polymer used in several artificial tear formulations and PVA hydrogels have also long been known, the development of a PVA hydrogel contact lens is very recent, and its characterisitics and performance are not yet well known.

Hydrogels of ionic polymers

Low hydration (Group III)

Contact lens materials in this group are etafilcon (Hydromarc, Vistamarc), which is made of cross-linked copolymers of HEMA with methacrylic acid and sodium methacrylate; bufilcon (Hydrocurve II, Softmate), which is made of copolymers of HEMA with diacetone acrylamide and methacrylic acid; deltafilcon (Amsoft, Aquasoft), which is made from cross-linked copolymers of HEMA, isobutyl methacrylate and methacrylic acid; droxifilcon (Accugel), which contains methacrylic acid in addition to HEMA and PVP; phemifilcon (Durasoft), which is made of HEMA, ethoxyethyl methacrylate and methacrylic acid; and ocufilcon (Tresoft), which contains a cross-linked copolymer of HEMA and methacrylic acid.

High hydration (Group IV)

In this group are perfilcon (Permalens), which is a copolymer of HEMA with VP and methacrylic acid, and etafilcon A (Vistamarc) and ocufilcon C (Ocu-Flex), the latter two of which contain the same components as listed for lenses of low hydration (Group III), but polymerized in different proportions to obtain high hydration.

2.2.5 LENSES WITH RIGID PERMEABLE OPTICS AND SOFT HYDROPHILIC PERIPHERY

These lenses were developed to obtain in one lens the comfort of hydrogel lenses and the optics of rigid lenses. This idea was introduced in the early 1970s, when the original hydrogel contact lenses were gaining in popularity but were not giving as good optical corrections, particularly for astigmatism, as the then popular PMMA lenses. Ideally one would have a PMMA contact lens with a hydrogel marginal edge to reduce the physical discomfort of the hard lenses. In 1971 a contact lens was described with a rigid, gas-permeable, poly(4-methyl-1-pentene) (2.23) optical centre and a hydrophilic edge of poly(acrylic acid). Poly(4-methyl-1-pentene), also called poly(isobutylethylene) or TPX, is an optically clear, hydrophobic polymer with good oxygen permeability. This olefinic polymer has not reached practical application as a contact lens material, probably due to its hydrophobicity, low resistance to ageing, and low glass transition temperature (29 °C), which is lower than the eye temperature (34 °C) and would cause the lens to change from a glassy to a rubbery state.

$$-(CH_2-CH-)_n$$
$$|$$
$$CH_2$$
$$|$$
$$CH_3CHCH_3 \qquad \text{(eqn 2.23)}$$

None of these early patented contact lenses with a rigid centre and a soft hydrophilic skirt reached commercial use. More recently a contact lens of this type (Saturn II®), made of a composite of materials called synergicon, has become available. This lens consists of a rigid, circular central portion with a soft hydrophilic skirt. The rigid portion, which constitutes the optical part of the lens, is made of pentasilcon. Pentasilcon is poly(tertiary butyl styrene-co-methyl methacrylate-co-maleic anhydrideco-pentamethyl disiloxanyl methacrylate-co-1,1,1-trimethyl propane trimethacrylate). Thus, it is an oxygen-permeable rigid material, with two ingredients that contribute to oxygen permeability: the styrene and the siloxanyl methacrylate derivatives. Trimethyl propane trimethacrylate is the cross-linking agent, methyl methacrylate contributes to the rigidity of the material, and the maleic anhydride moiety (2.24), after it hydrolyses in water to maleic acid (2.25), will contribute to the wettability of the lens surface:

$$-CH-CH-$$
$$|\qquad|$$
$$O=C\qquad C=O$$
$$\backslash\quad\diagup$$
$$O \qquad \text{(eqn 2.24)}$$

$$-CH-CH-$$
$$|\qquad|$$
$$O=C\qquad C=O$$
$$|\qquad|$$
$$OH\quad OH \qquad \text{(eqn 2.25)}$$

The hydrophilic portion of the synergicon material, which comprises the soft portion of the lens, is a copolymer of HEMA with methoxyethyl methacrylate, cross-linked with the same agent used in the hard portion of the lens.

2.2.6 BIOPOLYMERS

In this group of contact lens materials are included the lenses made from polymers of natural origin, such as polysaccharides and proteins. The natural polymers used for contact lenses are usually chemically modified to obtain the desired properties of strength and transparency, as well as to optimize their manufacturing properties. These naturally occurring polymers are available in large amounts and are usually inexpensive, but they are biodegradable.

Polysaccharides

The most important polysaccharide in the contact lens field is cellulose, which is used in the form of its derivative, cellulose acetate butyrate (CAB) (see page 00). Another polysaccharide proposed for contact lenses is chitin, which is poly-*N*-acetyl-D-glucosamine; its formula closely resembles cellulose. Chitin is the biopolymer that forms the exoskeleton of insects and crustaceans.

Proteins

Reconstituted proteins and modified collagen have been mentioned as contact lens materials. Collagen lenses have perhaps received the most attention and have been in the experimental stage for several years, but apparently none has reached the commercial stage. The greatest potential advantage of these materials, which are a kind of hydrogel, may be that they can be made of high water content and their mechanical properties are superior to those of most synthetic hydrogels of similar high hydration. On the negative side is the potential for micro-organism proliferation. Proteins are susceptible to micro-organisms, and because contact lenses are normally used in an environment propitious for micro-organism proliferation, protein lenses would require special care and caution.

BIBLIOGRAPHY

Refojo, M.F. (1976) Contact lenses. In *Encyclopedia of Polymer Science and Technology*, Suppl. 1 (ed. R.N. Bikales), Wiley-Interscience, New York, pp. 195–219.

Refojo, M.F. (1978) The chemistry of soft hydrogel lens materials. In *Soft Contact Lenses – Clinical and Applied Technology* (ed. M. Ruben), Wiley Medical, New York, pp. 19–39.

Refojo, M.F. (1979) Contact lenses. In *Kirk-Othmer Encyclopedia of Chemical Technology*, Vol. 6, 3rd ed. John Wiley, New York, pp. 720–42.

Refojo, M.F. (1984) The siloxane bond in contact lens materials: The siloxanyl alkyl methacrylate copolymers. *Ann. Ophthalmol.*, **16**, 1009–13.

Refojo, M.F. (1984) The siloxane bond in contact lens materials: Effect of methyl and phenyl content on oxygen permeability of silicone lenses. *Int. Cont. Lens Clin.*, **11**, 83–5.

Refojo, M.F. and Dabezies, O.H. Jr (1984) Classification of the types of materials used for construction of contact lenses. In *Contact Lenses: The CLAO Guide to Basic Science and Clinical Practice* (ed. O.H. Dabezies Jr), Grune & Stratton, Orlando, FL, pp. 11.1–11.11.

Refojo, M.F. (1988) Rigid contact lens materials and oxygen permeability. In *The Cornea: Transactions of the World Congress on the Cornea III* (ed. H.D. Cavanagh), Raven Press, New York, pp. 267–71.

Tighe, B. (1984) Contact lens materials. In *Contact Lenses: A Textbook for Practitioners and Students* (eds. J. Stone and A.J. Phillips), Butterworths, London, pp. 377–399.

William J. Benjamin

Manufacturers of contact lenses . . . should endeavor to make their lenses of some semi-pervious material to allow for oxygen – carbon-dioxide exchange through it. Or, perhaps they should concentrate their efforts in designing the lenses in such a way as to allow continuous interchange of the lacrimal fluid between lens and the eye. (Edward Goodlaw, 1946)

3.1 INTRODUCTION

It was apparently Goodlaw, in 1946, who concluded that contact lenses impede the oxygen supply to the cornea from the atmosphere, such that contact lenses should be made permeable to oxygen. In the first experiment to investigate this possibility, Smelser (1952) found that the visual effects of corneal swelling were the result of hypoxia induced by wearing oxygen-impermeable haptic contact lenses. Perhaps no single physiological discovery has caused such alteration of material and design of contact lenses, leading to an enhancement of the human eye's ability to tolerate their wear. Subsequent basic and clinical research by many authors has implicated contact-lens-induced hypoxia as a major cause of acute and chronic anatomical, physiological and biochemical changes within the corneal

layers (Lowther & Hill, 1974; Hill, 1977; DeDonato, 1981). Corneal hypoxia has been lessened by the advent of oxygen-permeable contact lenses and the magnitude of hypoxic corneal trauma has also decreased. Duration of contact lens wear was lengthened, as foretold by Goodlaw and Smelser, and other former restrictions on lens wear were loosened. Corneal traumas became more subtle rather than overt, a result of chronic hypoxia rather than acute anoxia. The degree to which wear of contact lenses could approach a mythical 'convenient care-free' optical correction for ametropia became linked to the amount of oxygen allowed to reach the cornea during contact lens wear.

Supply of molecular oxygen (O_2) to a cornea comes from several routes when the eye is not wearing a contact lens. From the posterior surface oxygen diffuses into the cornea from a reservoir of approximately 55 mmHg partial pressure of oxygen, equivalent to 7.4% O_2 as a proportion of atmospheric pressure at sea level, present in the aqueous fluid as a result of oxygenation carried to the eye by blood in the ophthalmic artery. Radially, at the limbus, oxygen diffuses a short distance into the cornea from capillaries also supplied by the ophthalmic artery. Anteriorly, oxygen diffuses across the tear film to most of the open-eye cornea from the atmosphere, being composed of 20.9% O_2 or 159

Contact Lens Practice. Edited by Montague Ruben and Michel Guillon.
Published in 1994 by Chapman & Hall, London. ISBN 0 412 35120 X

mmHg partial pressure at sea level. In the closed-eye state, the anterior corneal surface obtains oxygen from the palpebral conjunctiva, though some oxygen may enter the palpebral fissure from the atmosphere and diffuse into the underlying cornea especially if the lids are not entirely closed (Benjamin, 1982; Benjamin & Hill, 1986a). Excluding oxygen that might make its way between lagophthalmic eyelid margins, the mean oxygen supply to the closed-eye central cornea has been shown to be 7.7% (59 mmHg) for the population (Fatt & Bieber, 1968; Efron & Carney, 1979a; Benjamin, 1982) but varies widely between individuals (Efron & Carney, 1979a; Benjamin & Hill, 1986a, 1988a) and significantly between corneal locations on the same individual (Benjamin, 1982; Benjamin & Hill, 1988a). The closed-eye superior cornea, for instance, receives about 1.1% less oxygen than does the closed-eye central cornea (Benjamin, 1982; Benjamin & Hill, 1988a; Benjamin & Rasmussen, 1988), even though the horizontal strip of cornea underlying the palpebral fissure may receive more than 7.7% oxygen. It is generally assumed that the limbal route may supply oxygen to only the most peripheral 1.0 mm of the cornea, which becomes more significant when contact-lens-induced hypoxia is present.

The status of the palpebral conjunctival vasculature determines the supply of oxygen to the closed-eye cornea. Oxygen supplied by the palpebral vasculature decreases with age (Isenberg & Green, 1985) and can be adversely affected by vasoconstrictors (Isenberg & Green, 1984). Palpebral oxygen supply may be enhanced during the heat of the summer, when peripheral capillary beds are dilated for heat exchange, and reduced in the cold when such heat is best retained (Benjamin & Hill, 1988a). Vascular density may not be uniform over the palpebral surface and, therefore, not all regions of the closed-eye cornea may receive the same amount of oxygen (Benjamin, 1982; Benjamin & Rasmussen, 1988).

On average, about 7% of the corneal area is covered in the open-eye state by the upper eyelid. The vertical extent of superior cornea covered by the upper eyelid averages 2.1 mm with a standard deviation of 0.9 mm in Caucasians (Benjamin, 1982) and is probably increased for patients of oriental ancestry. A smaller portion of the inferior cornea is covered in a few individuals by the lower eyelid. Therefore, oxygen diffuses across the tear film into these limited portions of the anterior cornea from the palpebral conjunctivae even in the open-eye state. Superior corneal oxygenation via the palpebral conjunctiva is probably supplemented in the open-eye state by atmospheric oxygen that may diffuse vertically from the palebral aperture. Mean oxygenation for the superior cornea at a point 1 mm below the superior limbus has been found to be 10.4% (79 mmHg) in the open-eye state (Benjamin, 1982; Benjamin & Hill, 1988a). This represents an average contribution of 2.7% oxygen by the atmosphere above that which might be expected (7.7%) from the palpebral conjunctiva and/or limbal vasculature. In actuality, the supply of oxygen to a particular superior corneal site probably depends on the site's distance from the eyelid margin across which atmospheric oxygen must diffuse. Figure 3.1 shows oxygen distributions across layers of the central and superior cornea in the open-eye and closed-eye states (Fatt, 1968; Fatt & Bieber, 1968; Fatt *et al.*, 1969). Partial pressure of oxygen was assumed to be 55 mmHg at the posterior corneal surface. Partial pressures at the anterior corneal surface were assumed to be 159 mmHg, 79 mmHg, 59 mmHg and 50 mmHg for the open-eye central cornea, open-eye superior cornea, closed-eye central cornea and closed-eye superior cornea, respectively (taken from Table 3.1).

A barrier to the diffusion of oxygen from the anterior oxygen reservoirs (that is, the atmosphere and/or palpebral conjunctiva) to

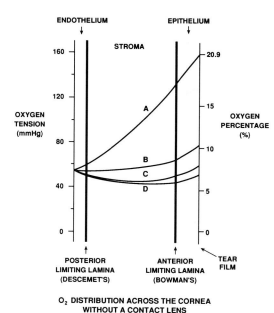

Figure 3.1 Oxygen tension and percentage distributions across the corneal layers, for central (A,C) and superior (B,D) corneal sites under open-eye (A,B) and closed-eye (C,D) conditions. The diagram of the cornea is a representation; thicknesses of the epithelium and endothelium have been emphasized relative to the stroma.

the anterior cornea is posed by the wear of a contact lens, while the posterior (aqueous fluid) and radial (limbus) oxygen supplies are considered intact. Figure 3.2 shows central corneal oxygen profiles for contact lenses allowing 15%, 10%, 5% and 0% oxygen to be present at the anterior corneal surface, respectively (Fatt, 1968; Fatt & Bieber, 1968; Fatt *et al.*, 1969). Note that the corneal epithelium receives oxygen almost exclusively from the anterior supply route, and that minimal oxygen is present at the basal layer of the epithelium when oxygen is not available from the anterior supply route. Investigators differ about the stability of the oxygen concentration at the corneal endothelium when anterior oxygenation is reduced due to contact lens wear (Fatt, 1968; Fatt *et al.*, 1969; Kwok, 1985; Stefansson *et al.*, 1987). Contact-

lens-induced hypoxia, therefore, should primarily and directly influence the metabolism of cells within the corneal epithelium, anterior limiting membrane (Bowman's layer), and anterior stroma (Fatt, 1968; Fatt & Bieber, 1969). Wear of contact lenses decreases the amount of oxygen available to the posterior stroma and perhaps even the endothelium to a small extent.

Oxygenation of the anterior cornea underneath a contact lens is brought about by diffusion of atmospheric oxygen through the contact lens and by influx of oxygenated tear fluid underneath the contact lens as a result of blinking (Fatt & Hill, 1970; Fatt & Liu, 1984). So-called 'tear pumping' supplies oxygenation of the order of 1–3% O_2 (7–22 mmHg) to corneal tissue under the periphery of rigid contact lenses, depending on their design, and is important for rigid lenses having limited ability to pass oxygen

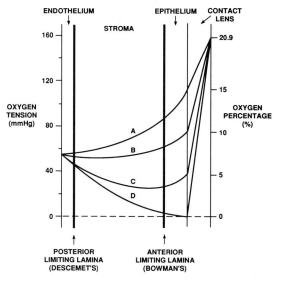

Figure 3.2 Oxygen tension and percentage distributions across the corneal layers, for the central cornea wearing contact lenses allowing 15% (A), 10% (B), 5% (C), and 0% (D) oxygen to be present at the anterior surface.

Table 3.1 Population average oxygen percentages and tensions at the cornea, without contact lens wear

Condition	O$_2$ (%)	O$_2$ Tension (mm Hg)
Open-eye, central cornea	20.9	159
Open-eye, superior cornea	10.4	79
Closed-eye, central cornea	7.7	59
Closed-eye, superior cornea	6.6	50

through the lens matrix. Such oxygenation becomes progressively less available to tissue lying more centrally under a rigid contact lens, because freshly 'pumped' tear fluid does not efficiently reach the central cornea and because the peripheral cornea first consumes oxygen before it can reach the central cornea. Central circular clouding, shown in Figure 3.3, was a physiological result of progressive corneal hypoxia from the periphery to the centre of the open-eye cornea underlying polymethylmethacrylate (PMMA) contact lenses (Berger, 1974; Allaire *et al.*, 1978; Garr-Peters & Ho, 1987). PMMA had a negligible ability to pass atmospheric oxygen through the polymer to the underlying cornea, so that the anterior oxygen supply was entirely the result of tear pumping.

Oxygenation via tear pumping for daily wear of contact lenses became progressively

less important as corneal hypoxia was reduced by oxygen transmitted to the cornea through increasingly permeable rigid and soft contact lens materials (Fatt & St Helen, 1971; Fatt & Lin, 1976). In the case of hydrogel (soft) contact lenses, corneal oxygenation via the open-eye tear pump mechanism was thought to be less than 1% (Polse, 1972, 1979; Efron & Carney, 1979b, 1983), though more significant 'tear pumps' for soft lenses have been postulated (Hill, 1967; Parrish & Larke, 1981). A 'closed-lid' tear pump thought to occur with rapid eye movements (REMs) during overnight wear of rigid (intralimbal) contact lenses (Benjamin & Simons, 1984) was shown not to be effective in supplying oxygen to the central cornea under these lenses (Benjamin & Rasmussen, 1985). Movement of rigid lenses on the closed-eye cornea due to REMs may, however, expose portions of the peripheral cornea to the palpebral conjunctiva at various times and for varying durations during sleep, so that peripheral corneal hypoxia during extended wear of rigid (intralimbal) lenses may not be as severe as peripheral hypoxia induced by overnight wear of hydrogel (paralimbal) lenses (Benjamin 1986; Benjamin & Rasmussen, 1988). Many rigid lenses and even soft lenses become adherent to the cornea during overnight wear, such that they apparently do not move across the cornea even when REMs are present. For these reasons, alleviation of lens-induced corneal hypoxia has been overwhelmingly tied to the ability of corneal contact lenses to transmit atmospheric oxygen through their matrices to the anterior

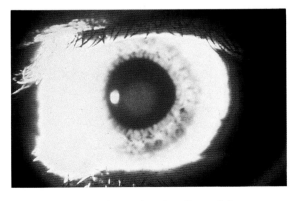

Figure 3.3 Central circular clouding of the cornea following wear of an oxygen-impermeable rigid corneal contact lens.

cornea. Thus, methods of determining the degree to which contact lenses succeed in this endeavour have received considerable interest in the contact lens field.

The Clark-type oxygen electrode (Clark, 1956) was first applied to corneal physiology by Hill and Fatt.(1963a,b) After a brief period of collaboration in the use of the electrode at the University of California at Berkeley, Professor Hill relocated to The Ohio State University and these two original investigators began separately to use their particular talents to tackle the problems of quantifying the ability of contact lenses to allow oxygenation of the cornea. So began two great parallel efforts in corneal science related to contact lenses: Irving Fatt, having a background in engineering, over the years developed and refined a laboratory technique for measuring oxygen permeability of materials and oxygen transmissiblity of contact lenses *in vitro* based on American Society for Testing and Materials standards for measurement of oxygen flow through thin plastic films; and Richard Hill, having a background in neurophysiology, developed a physiological technique for estimating the concentration of oxygen in the tear film underneath a contact lens, in terms of its equivalent percentage at the corneal surface *in vivo*. Both measurement systems entailed the use of a Clark-type polarographic oxygen sensor, a schematic for which is shown in Figure 3.4.

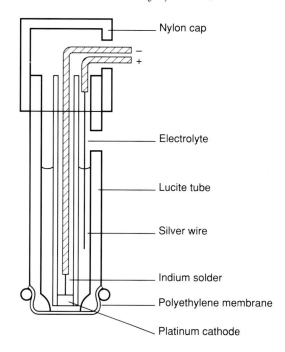

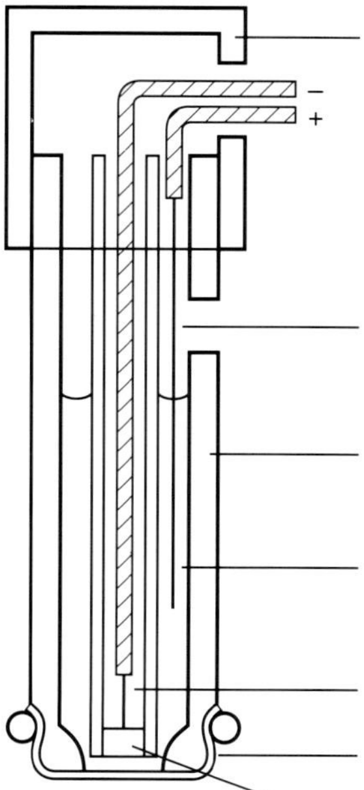
Nylon cap
–
+
Electrolyte
Lucite tube
Silver wire
Indium solder
Polyethylene membrane
Platinum cathode

Figure 3.4 Diagram of the Clark-type oxygen sensor as originally published by Clark (1956). An electrochemical reaction takes place at the platinum cathode and silver anode when an electrical potential is formed between the two electrodes. The current developed by the reaction is proportional to the concentration of molecular oxygen at the sensor cathode.

3.2 PERMEABILITY OF MATERIALS AND TRANSMISSIBILITY OF CONTACT LENSES

Rate of oxygen flow through a contact lens is the essential value determined in any method of deriving oxygen *transmissibility* or *permeability*. Oxygen flow rate is the net volume of oxygen gas passing through the exposed area of test sample (contact lens) per unit time under specified conditions, including temperature, sample thickness, area of sample exposed to oxygen flow and partial pressures of oxygen on both sides of the sample. Oxygen transmissibility and permeability increase with temperature, so that their measurements have been standardized at eye temperature (35 °C). Oxygen permeability values of non-hydrogel materials are about 50% higher at eye temperature than at room temperature, but the difference is only of minor consequence for hydrogel materials. Having measured oxygen flow rate, oxygen transmissibility of the contact lens (Dk/L) and oxygen permeability of its material (Dk) can be calculated using eqn 3.1, knowing the area of the contact lens through which oxygen must have passed (A, in cm^2), the thickness of the lens or sample (L) and the oxygen tension difference between anterior and posterior lens surfaces at equilibrium measurement. This difference, $P_A - P_P$, in mmHg, is usually set so that P_A is approximately 159 mmHg and P_p is zero:

$$Dk = \frac{L \times (\mu l\ O_2/s)}{(P_A - P_P) \times A} \times \frac{ml}{10^3 \mu l} \qquad \text{(Eqn 3.1)}$$

Dk, oxygen permeability of test sample; P_A, (barometric pressure – vapour pressure) (0.209); P_p, zero; L, thickness of test sample (measured); A, exposed area of test sample (measured); $\mu l\ O_2/s$, rate of oxygen flow (measured).

Oxygen transmissibility (Dk/L). This is the oxygen permeability (Dk) divided by the thickness (L), in cm, of the measured sample under specified conditions. Oxygen transmissibility units are (cm/s) (ml O_2/[ml × mmHg]), or equivalently (cm^3[O_2])/(cm^2 × s × mmHg). For Dk/L units in terms of hectopascals instead of mmHg, Dk/L magnitudes using mmHg in the denominator should be multiplied by 0.75. Oxygen transmissibility is a physical property of both lens material and lens thickness; it depends on design of the contact lens. Dk/L is equal to the oxygen flow rate divided by the area of lens exposed to oxygen flow and the difference in oxygen tension (partial pressure of oxygen) between atmospheres at the two exposed surfaces of the sample contact lens. Contact lenses having low oxygen transmissibilities (low-Dk/L lenses) are indicated by Dk/L values below 12 × 10^{-9} units, medium-Dk/L lenses range from 12 to 25 × 10^{-9} units and high-Dk/L lenses have values greater than 25 × 10^{-9} units. Throughout the rest of this chapter, 10^{-9} and the transmissibility unit will be dropped in favour of the term 'Dk/L unit' determined at eye temperature.

While oxygen transmissibility (Dk/L) is theoretically a function of the oxygen permeability (Dk) of the contact lens material and thickness of the contact lens sample, its experimental determination can be practi-

cally performed without actually knowing the Dk of the material or the thickness of the contact lens. Oxygen transmissibility (Dk/L) determinations are usually more important than calculation of permeability (Dk) for finished contact lenses incorporating various powers and designs. This is because Dk/L is the result of permeability of the lens material and lens design. Therefore, Dk/L is more applicable than Dk to individual lenses that are placed on the eye.

Oxygen permeability (Dk). This is the oxygen flow under specified conditions through a unit area of contact lens material of unit thickness when subjected to unit pressure difference. Oxygen permeability is stated in units of (cm^2/s) (ml O_2/[ml × mmHg]), or equivalently, (cm^3[O_2] × cm)/(cm^2 × s × mmHg). For units in terms of hectopascals instead of mmHg, Dk magnitudes using mmHg in the denominator should be multiplied by 0.75. Oxygen permeability is a physical property of the material and is theoretically not a function of the thickness or design of the material sample. Materials having low oxygen permeabilities (low-Dk materials) are indicated by Dk values below 15 × 10^{-11} units, medium-Dk materials range from 15 to 30 × 10^{-11} units and high-Dk materials have values greater than 30 × 10^{-11} units. The Dk of water is 80 × 10^{-11} units at eye temperature. Throughout the rest of this chapter, 10^{-11} and the permeability unit will be dropped in favour of the term 'Dk unit' determined at eye temperature.

Oxygen permeability (Dk) of the lens material is equal to the oxygen transmissibility (Dk/L) of the contact lens sample multiplied by the sample thickness (L). Thus, accuracy and reliability of oxygen permeability values depend practically on accurate and reliable determinations of oxygen transmissibilities (Dk/L) and thicknesses (L) of contact lenses under controlled test conditions. If the aim of an investigation is to determine oxygen permeability (*Dk*) of materials used in the production of contact lenses, oxygen flow through test samples having standardized designs should be measured to eliminate variability resulting from different lens designs. Standardized test samples should have parallel or near-parallel anterior and posterior surfaces, such that sample thickness does not significantly vary over the central area exposed to oxygen flow. In the case of manufactured contact lenses, the near-parallel condition has been interpreted to correspond to dioptric powers within the range +3.00 to –3.00 for the polarographic technique noted later. This large range of values is because the polarographic sensor samples oxygen over a small area corresponding to its cathode diameter. For techniques that sample over a larger area of lens surface, such as the coulometric and gas-to-gas techniques, a more restricted range of +0.50 to –0.50 dioptres may be appropriate. In actuality, however, refractive power of contact lenses with parallel surfaces can vary significantly with lens design and refractive index (Weissman, 1982).

Thickness (*L*) is the radial thickness within the central area of the test sample, or the harmonic mean thickness (Fatt, 1988) of the area of test sample exposed to oxygen flow during measurement. These two definitions are identical for standardized test samples. To be consistent with other definitions and equations in this chapter, (*L*) has been given in centimetres (cm). The harmonic mean thickness of a radially symmetric contact lens (*L*$_{HM}$) could be that thickness calculated from a series of (*h* + 1) radial thickness measurements at intervals from the centre (point 0) to the edge (point *h*) of the circular area exposed to oxygen flow during measurement of oxygen flow. The intervals between thickness measurements should allow each annular ring between measurements to be of the same area:

$$L_{HM} = \frac{h + 1}{1/L_0 + 1/L_1 + 1/L_2 + 1/L_3 + \ldots + 1/L_h}$$

(Eqn 3.2)

L_{HM} harmonic mean thickness of radially symmetric test sample; L_{0-h}, radial thicknesses measured at intervals of equal annular area from the centre (L_0) to the edge (L_h) of the exposed sample area.

3.2.1 THE POLAROGRAPHIC TECHNIQUE

A contact lens test sample is placed in an apparatus, shown in Figure 3.5., with its central front surface area in contact with room air at eye temperature. The back surface of the lens sample is separated from the electrodes of a polarographic oxygen sensor by a thin aqueous layer. The gaseous environment at the anterior lens surface and the oxygen sensor are separated by the contact lens and the aqueous film (and, perhaps, a filter-paper disk), which act as barriers to the net flow of oxygen from the anterior environment to the platinum cathode of the oxygen sensor. When a small electrical potential is created between the cathode and anode of the oxygen sensor, oxygen molecules are reduced to hydroxyl ions at the cathode, consuming four electrons per molecule. At the silver anode, hydroxyl ions are oxidized to water, supplying the electrons for reactions at the cathode. These chemical reactions establish a current across the gap between cathode and anode and bring the concentration of oxygen molecules to nearly zero at the surface of the cathode. After a few minutes an O_2 concentration gradient is established, from approximately 159 mmHg (at sea level) at the anterior surface of the test sample, to zero (assumed) at the surface of the cathode against the thin aqueous film at the back surface of the lens (or, against a filter-paper disk separating the electrode from the posterior lens surface). Oxygen molecules that diffuse down this gradient are immediately eliminated by reduction at the sensor cathode, and the equilibrium current is proportional to the rate of oxygen flow across the test contact lens.

With appropriate instrument calibration, the rate of oxygen flow (μl O_2/s) to the cathode can be calculated from the measured current. Oxygen transmissibility and permeability can then be computed using eqn 3.1, having also measured thickness (L) and knowing the surface area (A) of the platinum cathode exposed to oxygen flow.

Room air is usually allowed to directly contact the anterior surface of the contact lens when oxygen flow is measured through rigid or flexible non-hydrogel test samples. To reduce evaporation from hydrogel lenses, the air can be prehumidified and water saturated. An optional method of measurement

is to place a reservoir of standard saline solution on top of the test sample (against the anterior contact lens surface). The reservoir should be constantly and consistently stirred so as to distribute oxygen as evenly as possible within the solution. Hydrogel lenses require proper hydration during measurement, such that an aqueous reservoir is sometimes used. When an aqueous reservoir is placed at the front surface of the test sample, consideration must be given to the 'boundary layer effect' discussed on page 49.

An aqueous film must be present at the surface of the oxygen sensor for the described electrochemical reactions to take place. This film is present within the lens material when hydrogel lenses are tested but is not present during testing of non-hydrogel lenses. Rigid and flexible non-hydrogel

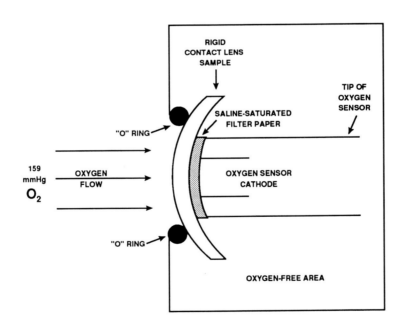

POLAROGRAPHIC TECHNIQUE

Figure 3.5 In the 'polarographic technique', oxygen that diffuses across the lens from the anterior contact lens environment establishes an equilibrium current across the electrodes of the polarographic sensor placed against the back surface of the lens. In the case of a rigid lens, as shown, an 'aqueous bridge' separates the lens surface from the sensor. The aqueous bridge is necessary to allow the electrochemical reaction involving molecular oxygen to occur at the sensor tip.

lenses will not support, by themselves, polarographic measurement of oxygen at their surfaces. Therefore, a filter-paper disk soaked in saline is typically used as an 'aqueous bridge' between a non-hydrogel surface and the oxygen sensor (Fatt & Chaston, 1981), but other forms of aqueous bridges have been used (Refojo *et al.*, 1977; Fatt, 1984). Unfortunately, the filter paper (a type of 'cigarette paper' reported by Fatt and Chaston in 1981) acts as an additional barrier to the flow of oxygen and its influence must be corrected before the actual oxygen transmissibility or permeability of test samples can be properly determined. A procedure for correction of the 'boundary layer effect' is discussed on page 51.

3.2.2 THE COULOMETRIC TECHNIQUE

A contact lens test sample is placed in an apparatus, shown in Figure 3.6, with exposed front and rear lens surface areas in contact with gas mixtures at eye temperature (35 °C). The gaseous environments at the anterior and posterior lens surfaces are separated by the contact lens, which acts as a barrier to the net flow of oxygen from the anterior environment to the posterior environment. The two environments and the contact lens can be purged of all detectable oxygen gas. Once purged, an oxygen-containing humidified gas is allowed to fill the anterior environmental chamber and to diffuse through the contact lens. Humidified inert carrier gas, initially oxygen-free, is allowed to flow across the posterior environmental chamber at the posterior lens surface and to remove oxygen molecules that have crossed the semi-permeable contact lens barrier. The carrier gas, now containing a small concentration of oxygen, is directed to a coulometric sensor, which creates a current proportional to the concentration of oxygen flowing past the detector. With appropriate instrument calibration, such that the concentration of oxygen at the detector is precisely

known, the rate of oxygen flow (μl O_2/s) past the detector can be determined and recorded. As already noted, oxygen transmissibility and permeability can then be calculated using eqn 3.1 (Winterton *et al.*, 1987, 1988).

As with the polarographic technique, gases are usually allowed to directly contact the anterior lens surface when oxygen flows through rigid or flexible non-hydrogel test samples (Winterton *et al.*, 1987, 1988). A reservoir of standard saline solution or, perhaps, a water-saturated gas must contact the test sample (against the anterior contact lens surface) when oxygen flow through hydrogel lenses is measured with the coulometric technique. The reservoir should be constantly and consistently stirred so as to quickly distribute incoming carrier gas during the purge and especially oxygenated test gas during measurement (Winterton *et al.*, 1987, 1988). When using an aqueous reservoir at the front surface of the test sample, consideration must again be given to the 'anterior boundary layer effect', discussed on page 49 (Fatt, 1989).

An important distinction between the coulometric technique and the polarographic technique is the manner in which oxygen is detected at the posterior surface of the contact lens test sample. A free flow of oxygen from the entire exposed posterior lens surface to the oxygen sensor is established using the coulometric oxygen sensor, unhindered by an 'aqueous bridge' or by the necessity for small polarographic electrodes to be positioned against the posterior lens surface. Thus, the coulometric technique does not suffer from the 'posterior boundary layer effect', discussed on page 49 (Winterton *et al.*, 1987, 1988).

3.2.3 THE GAS-TO-GAS TECHNIQUE

A contact lens test sample is placed in an apparatus (Fig. 3.7), with exposed front and rear lens surface areas in contact with room air. The gaseous environments at the anterior

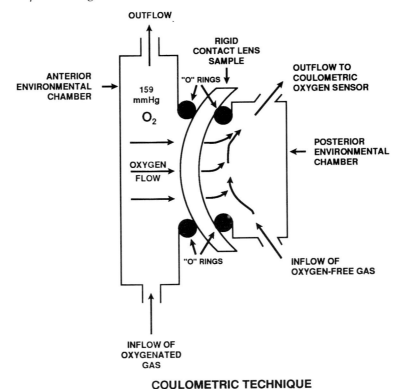

COULOMETRIC TECHNIQUE

Figure 3.6 In the 'coulometric technique', oxygen that diffuses across the lens from the anterior environmental chamber to the posterior environmental chamber is carried by a flow of inert gas to a coulometric oxygen sensor.

and posterior lens surfaces are separated by the contact lens, which will act as a barrier to the net flow of oxygen from the anterior environment to the posterior environment. The two environments and the contact lens can be purged and pressurized with pure oxygen gas (100% O_2), such that pressure in the posterior environment is 1 atmosphere (atm, or 760 mmHg), pressure in the anterior environment is 3 atm (2280 mmHg), and temperatures of the lens and chambers are at eye temperature (35 °C). Pressure transducers allow accurate recording of pressure within the two environmental chambers; the oxygen tensions are equal to the pressures within each chamber (Fatt, 1991a).

Pressure within the anterior environ-ment is maintained at 3 atm and pressure within the closed posterior environment increases as oxygen flows from the volume of higher pressure (in the anterior environ-ment) to the volume of lower pressure (in the posterior environment). The transduc-ers having been previously calibrated, the pressure increase in the closed posterior chamber is recorded from 760 mmHg to 767.6 mmHg (a 1% change in pressure) over a duration of approximately 10 min. Because volume has been held constant in the posterior environment, the rate of oxy-gen flow (in g mol/s) through the contact lens can be calculated (Fatt, 1991a) from the recorded rate of pressure increase using the gas law ($PV = nRT$):

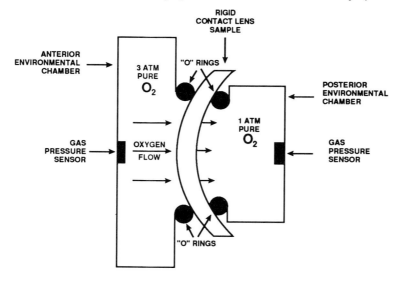

GAS-TO-GAS TECHNIQUE

Figure 3.7 In the 'gas-to-gas technique', both sides of the contact lens are differentially pressurized with pure oxygen gas. Because the anterior environmental chamber has more pressure than the posterior environmental chamber, oxygen flows from the anterior to the posterior environment. Since the posterior environmental chamber is of constant volume, there is a pressure change within the chamber that is sensed by a pressure transducer.

$dP/dt = dn/dt\ (RT/V)$ (Eqn 3.3)

dP/dt, rate of pressure increase, in mmHg/s; dn/dt, rate of oxygen flow, in g mol/s; V, volume of posterior environment, in ml; R, constant = 6.236×10^4 mmHg ml/g mol./°K; T, absolute temperature = 308K.

Knowing the rate of oxygen flow in g mol/s, the rate can be converted to µl/s. Oxygen transmissibility and permeability can then be calculated using eqn 3.1, where $P_A - P_P =$ 1520 mmHg (Fatt, 1991a).

As with the coulometric technique, gas is allowed to contact the anterior and posterior lens surfaces directly when oxygen flows through rigid and non-hydrogel test samples. Thus far, the pressure difference between anterior and posterior environments has made this technique inapplicable to hydrogel lenses.

An important distinction between the gas-to-gas technique and the coulometric and polarographic techniques is the manner in which oxygen is detected after passing through the posterior surface of the non-hydrogel test sample. A free flow of gas from the entire exposed posterior lens surface into the posterior environment is established. Because only oxygen is contained in the gas, the pressure change in the posterior environment is indicative of the flow of oxygen through the test sample. There is no sensor specific for oxygen, nor is there the need for an 'aqueous bridge'. Thus, the 'gas-to-gas technique' does not suffer from the 'boundary layer effect' discussed next. Also, the gas-to-gas method can be used for measurement of Dk and Dk/L for any gas.

3.2.4 ANTERIOR AND POSTERIOR BOUNDARY LAYER EFFECTS

When saline is placed against the surface of a test sample, oxygen does not diffuse freely through the surface. A relatively stagnant layer of saline next to the lens surface, called the 'boundary layer', acts as an additional barrier to the flow of oxygen through the contact lens surface (Fig. 3.8) (Fatt & Chaston, 1981). Boundary layers reduce the flow of oxygen through the test sample (Garr-Peters & Ho, 1987). Transmissibility of the boundary layer is independent of sample thickness and cannot be totally eliminated by stirring of saline at the surface. Rates of oxygen flow determined for samples with a boundary layer lead to an under-estimation of the actual Dk/L or Dk values of contact lenses. Such values must be corrected for the 'boundary layer effect' peculiar to the measurement technique used, to state accurately the transmissibility and permeability of test samples.

The boundary layer effect is insignificant when a gas directly contacts both polymer surfaces (Fatt & Chaston, 1981). Gas molecules are so mobile that they arrive at the front lens surface faster than they can be transported into the material and are carried away faster from the back surface than they can be transported through the lens. Diffusion through the contact lens is then the rate-limiting step for oxygen transport.

A significant boundary layer may be present at the anterior or posterior sample surfaces, or at both surfaces, depending on the measurement technique used and the conditions of the test. When a reservoir of standard saline is in contact with the anterior lens surface of hydrogel lenses during measurement of oxygen flow, an anterior boundary layer is present. This may occur during measurements of hydrogel lenses with the polarographic and coulometric techniques. The gas-to-gas technique, as noted, has not yet been applied to hydrogel lenses. If the investigator wishes to do so, an anterior saline reservoir may be used with all three techniques, even when measurements of non-hydrogel lenses are desired.

A boundary layer is present at the posterior surface of a test sample being measured polarographically, because an aqueous bridge is necessary for the electrochemical

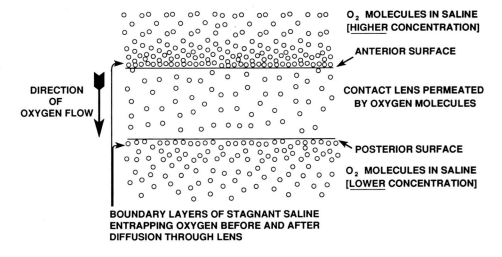

ANTERIOR AND POSTERIOR BOUNDARY LAYER EFFECTS

Figure 3.8 A 'boundary layer effect' occurs when oxygen molecules arrive at the front surface of the contact lens faster than they can be transmitted through the lens, or when oxygen molecules arrive at the back surface faster than they can be carried away.

reaction to take place. For a hydrogel lens, the posterior boundary layer is a thin film that is established between the back surface of the gel lens and the polarographic sensor cathode. For a non-hydrogel lens, the posterior boundary layer is a combination of two thin films on either side of a wet filter paper disk (including the filter-paper disk), separating the back surface of the lens from the cathode. The coulometric and gas-to-gas techniques are free of a posterior boundary layer effect.

To correct for a boundary layer effect, oxygen transmissibility (Dk/L) may be determined for test samples of the same material and design having different thicknesses. A plot of the inverse of these transmissibilities (L/Dk) versus thickness (L) yields a line with slope equal to $1/Dk$ of the test samples and a y-intercept equal to L/Dk of the boundary layer. The line, such as that shown in Figure 3.9, may be derived using the least squares method of statistical computation. Knowing the true oxygen permeability (Dk) of the material (the inverse of the slope) and thick-

ness of any particular test sample, the actual oxygen transmissibility of a test sample (Dk/L) may be computed (Fatt & Chaston, 1982a).

This correction procedure can be used for anterior or posterior boundary layer effects. In fact, should measurements incorporate anterior *and* posterior boundary layers, e.g. when polarographic measurements are made of lenses using an anterior saline reservoir, the outlined correction will simultaneously solve for both effects. The slope of the line in Figure 3.9 should be the same regardless of the magnitude or number of boundary layers, even if the intercept does vary with severity or combination of boundary layers.

The resistance of boundary layers to the flow of oxygen is small in comparison to the resistance of low-Dk or thick contact lenses (< 15 Dk units). While the absolute resistance of boundary layers remains constant as Dk increases, the relative impact of boundary layers on oxygen flow does increase with respect to the resistance of the contact lens. Therefore, the certainty with which the cor-

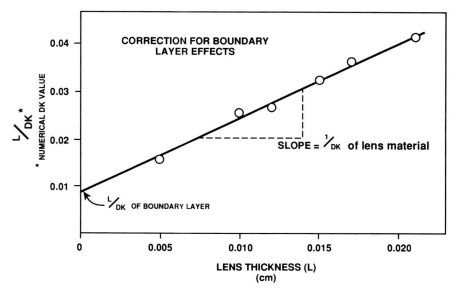

Figure 3.9 Graph showing correction for the boundary layer effect. A plot of L/Dk versus thickness will yield a straight line with a slope of $1/Dk$. Resistance of the boundary layer to passage of oxygen is constant for all thicknesses of contact lens material.

rection for the boundary layer effect can be applied is reduced for contact lenses of higher *Dk*. Above a value of 100 *Dk* units the correction becomes so uncertain, even given measurements of several samples having different thicknesses, that it is best to perform measurements with a method that avoids the boundary layer effect. For rigid and non-hydrogel flexible lenses, this would mean use of the coulometric or gas-to-gas methods. With respect to hydrogel lenses that generally contain less than 80% water, *Dk* is now practically limited to at most 37 *Dk* units. The permeability at eye temperature of a 'mythical' hydrogel lens containing 100% water might be slightly above 90 *Dk* units. When hydrogel materials are devised that have values significantly greater than 100 *Dk* units, a new modification of current *Dk/L* and *Dk* measurement technology will be necessary or the number of measurements made for each of the several thicknesses in Figure 3.9 will need to be increased to enhance the certainty of correction for boundary layers; or, one might choose to use the equivalent oxygen percentage (EOP) technique covered on page 00.

3.2.5 TYPE I AND TYPE II EDGE EFFECTS

When there is a difference between the front surface area exposed to flow of oxygen and the back surface area through which oxygen flow must be detected, a so-called 'edge effect' may influence the measured oxygen transmissibility and permeability of test samples (Garr-Peters & Ho, 1987). A diagram of the type I edge effect for the polarographic technique is shown in Figure 3.10. Oxygen may 'funnel' from a larger area at the front surface than has been placed in the calculation of *Dk/L* and *Dk* from the measured oxygen flow rate. In other words, the area of sample exposed to flow of oxygen ('*A*' in eqn 3.1) has not been properly determined, and is in fact larger than the area calculated from the polarographic cathode diameter (Brennan *et al.*, 1987a; Fatt *et al.*, 1987). The type I edge effect is not present when using the coulometric and gas-to-gas methods.

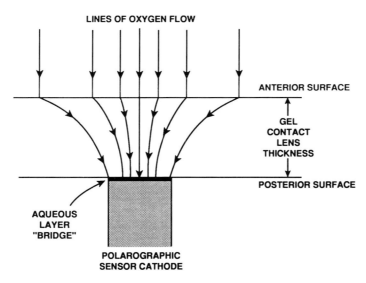

Figure 3.10 The 'type I edge effect' is caused by oxygen flow through a front surface area that is greater than the back surface area. This is often referred to as an oxygen 'funnel'.

Polarographic *Dk/L* and *Dk* values that have not been corrected for the type I edge effect are, therefore, an over-estimation of their actual magnitudes (Brennan *et al.*, 1987a; Fatt *et al.*, 1987). Correction for the type I edge effect (Brennan *et al.*, 1987b; Fatt *et al.*, 1987) is achieved by modification of the area factor (*A*) in eqn 3.1. The area through which oxygen flows to the detector is approximately 25% higher than the cathode diameter for hydrogel lenses and appears to be unrelated to oxygen permeability of gel materials. For high-*Dk* (> 37 *Dk* units) rigid materials the area appears to be 25% larger and for low-*Dk* (< 15 *Dk* units) rigid materials 15% larger. Therefore, polarographic *Dk/L* and *Dk* values for hydrogel and high-*Dk* lenses corrected for the type I edge effect are approximately 25% lower than their uncorrected values. This proportion falls to 15% for low-*Dk* rigid materials (Fatt, 1991b).

A second type of edge effect may be apparent in the coulometric and gas-to-gas methods, but should not be a factor in the polarographic method. Using the former methods, oxygen that has diffused through the anterior lens surface may extend radially into the lens matrix peripheral to the exposed front surface area before exiting the sample through the exposed posterior surface (Garr-Peters & Ho, 1987). A diagram of such an edge effect is shown in Figure 3.11. This type II edge effect should hinder the flow of oxygen through a test sample by less than 3%. The type II edge effect is thickness-dependent, being of slightly higher magnitude for samples with thick peripheries (Barrer *et al.*, 1962; Fatt, 1991a). Therefore, uncorrected *Dk/L* and *Dk* values should under-estimate their actual magnitudes by only a minor amount when the coulometric and gas-to-gas methods have been used. This small discrepancy is less than the repeatability of *Dk* and *Dk/L* measurements (5–10%).

3.3 PERCENTAGE OF OXYGEN AT THE ANTERIOR CORNEAL SURFACE

There has not been a direct measurement technique reported that will adequately measure the concentration of oxygen at the surface of the cornea under a contact lens. To assess this concentration of oxygen indirectly, the corneal response to contact lens wear is evaluated and compared to responses occurring when the cornea has been exposed

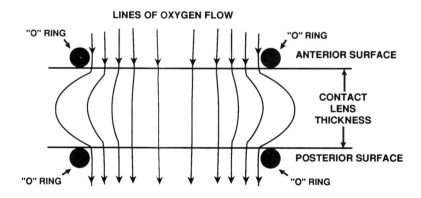

TYPE II EDGE EFFECT

Figure 3.11 The 'type II edge effect' is caused by the expansion of oxygen flow into lens material peripheral to the exposed front and back surface areas of the lens.

to standard environments having graded levels of oxygenation. It is thought that if the corneal response to various concentrations of oxygen is known, then the concentration of oxygen at the surface of the contact-lens-wearing cornea can be predicted. The response that is measured, however, must not be significantly influenced by factors other than corneal oxygen supply for the described relationship to hold.

In the 'equivalent oxygen percentage' (EOP) method, the oxygen uptake rate of the anterior cornea is used as the corneal response that serves as an indirect measure of corneal hypoxia. The uptake rate is a result of placement of a membrane-covered polarographic oxygen sensor against the anterior corneal surface for periods of 4–60 s (Fig. 3.12). The sensor has been previously calibrated and bathed in 20.9% O_2 (159 mmHg). The cornea depletes the oxygen dissolved in the sensor membrane over the period of corneal contact with the membrane. Recording of the oxygen depletion results in an oxygen depletion curve, and the relative depletion rate in mmHg/s over a specified span of time or oxygen concentration is called the corneal 'oxygen uptake rate'. Corneal oxygen uptake rates can be determined for the unstressed cornea and immediately after the cornea has been placed under hypoxic and other stresses.

Application of different anterior gaseous environments to the cornea for periods as short as 5 min, such atmospheres having progressively lower percentages of oxygen (progressively more stressful hypoxias) will result in corneal oxygen uptake rates that are increasingly higher (Roscoe & Wilson, 1984a; Benjamin & Hill, 1988b). Five minutes of exposure to the environmental stress or static contact lens wear is over 2.5 times that period necessary to ensure corneal gaseous equilibrium prior to measurement and has been shown to result in consistent corneal oxygen uptake rates. Five minutes between uptake rate measurement and application of another stressful condition are allowed for the cornea to aerobically stabilize between readings. This period is 2.5 times that duration needed for the cornea to recover from short-term hypoxia (Hill & Fatt, 1964; Hill, 1965; Benjamin & Hill, 1986a). Representative oxygen depletion curves for corneas having been exposed to atmospheres ranging from 0 to 20.9% O_2 are shown in Figure 3.13. Mean

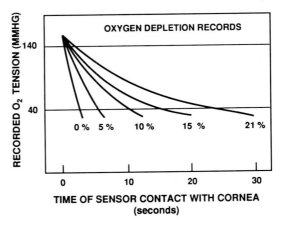

Figure 3.13 Representative oxygen depletion curves for corneas that were exposed to progressively lower percentages of oxygen. Note that as the cornea is deprived of oxygen, the oxygen depletion rate (the 'oxygen uptake rate') progressively increases.

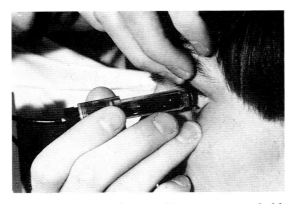

Figure 3.12 A polarographic sensor is held against the cornea while oxygen is depleted from the membrane covering the sensor tip.

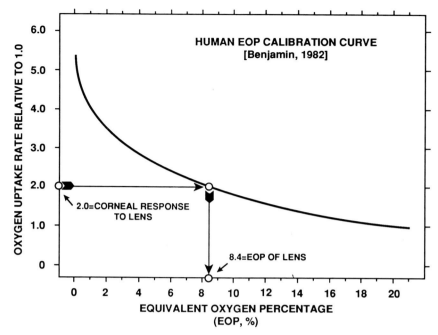

Figure 3.14 The EOP calibration curve, plotting oxygen uptake rate relative to a baseline at 1.0 versus oxygen percentage in the anterior corneal environment (the EOP). A contact lens associated with an uptake rate of 2 times baseline (2.0) has an EOP of 8.4%.

corneal oxygen uptake rates that have been calculated from such depletion curves have been plotted in Figure 3.14 against the percentages of oxygen that were contained in the anterior corneal environments.

Should the corneal oxygen uptake rate be measured immediately after 5 min of open-eye static contact lens wear, then the percentage of oxygen that induces an equivalent corneal oxygen uptake rate can be interpolated from Figure 3.14. Hence, the term 'equivalent' is used in equivalent oxygen percentage (EOP). In the example shown, the

oxygen uptake rate associated with wear of a contact lens was two times (2.0) that of the baseline unstressed cornea (1.0) and the interpolated EOP was 8.4%. Low EOP values are below 6%, medium EOP values fall between 6 and 11%, and high EOP values are greater than 11% (Table 3.2). Because EOP values are determined for contact lenses *in vivo*, eye temperature is automatically achieved.

Though anterior and posterior boundary layers are represented by the pre- and post-lens tear films, correction of EOP values for

Table 3.2 EOP, *Dk/L*, and *Dk*: what is high and what is low?

	EOP (%)	*Dk/L* (DK/L units)	*Dk* (Dk units)
Low values	< 6	< 12	< 15
Medium values	6–11	12–25	15–30
High values	> 11	> 25	> 30

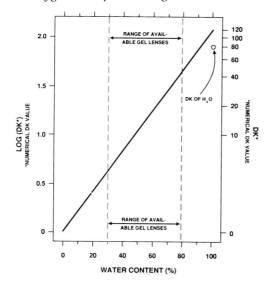

Figure 3.17 The log of *Dk* for hydrogel materials is linearly related to water content. This plot was derived from that of Sarver *et al.* (1981)[1] and of Fatt and Chaston (1982a) after correction for the edge effect. An unexplained phenomenon, the *Dk* of water (80) is not the same as the extrapolated *Dk* of a gel lens having 100% water content (115–120).

keted by Wesley-Jessen and Ciba Vision Corporation constitute barriers to oxygen flow. However, as these materials are non-uniformly distributed across the lens aperture, oxygen may be able to diffuse around any 'opaqued' spots or lines having reduced permeability and through the lens materials. The result may be only subclinical resistance to oxygen transmission due to the 'opaqued' portions of these lenses. So-called 'opaqued' contact lenses need to be tested in order to assess whether the 'opaqued' material significantly reduces oxygen supply to the cornea or not.

The practitioner is most concerned with corneal oxygen availability under the particular contact lens being worn. This amount of oxygen is related to *Dk/L* (transmissibility) and its non-identical twin, EOP, of the contact lens. As we have already noted, these relative estimates of oxygen performance are highly correlated with each other and depend on lens design (that is, thickness of the lens) in addition to material permeability. Unfortunately, there is a critical thickness minimum at some point or points on a lens specific for each contact lens material in order to provide stability of parameters and durability of wear. Thicknesses of hydrogel and non-hydrogel lenses also become greater by incorporation of refractive power, which is a function of refractive index. For these reasons, therefore, required lens thickness is positively related to water content in hydrogel lenses. Low-water content lenses may be suitable in relatively thin designs; high-water content lenses require thick designs in order to function properly. Figure 3.18, shows EOP and *Dk/L* for theoretical critical

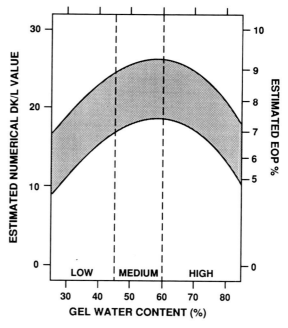

Figure 3.18 When *Dk/L* is calculated from known *Dk* values using estimated minimum thicknesses for hydrogel lenses of various water contents, medium-water content lenses reveal the greatest potential for oxygen transmissibility (*Dk/L*). EOP values have been included for reference.

Table 3.3 Water contents of some common hydrogel materials

Gel material	Water content (%)	
phemfilcon A	30	
dimefilcon A	36	
isofilcon		
polymacon tefilcon phemfilcon A	38	
crofilcon A polymacon	39	Low water
tetrafilcon A hefilcon A etafilcon A deltafilcon A & B	43	
bufilcon A	45	
droxfilcon	47	
ocufilcon B	53	
bufilcon A methafilcon A & B phemfilcon A vifilcon A focofilcon A ocufilcon C	55	Medium water
etafilcon A tetrafilcon B	58	
lidofilcon A	70	
perfilcon A	71	High water
surfilcon A	74	
lidofilcon B	79	

thickness minima of hydrogel materials ranging from 30 to 80% water. The reader will note that medium-water content lenses (45 to 60% water) are better than low-water (< 45% water) and high-water (> 60% water) lenses in terms of oxygen performance.

The necessary designs offset, to a large extent, the 'oxygen advantage' that accompanies an increase of water content from low-water to medium-water content materials.

When comparing medium-water content lenses to high-water content lenses, it appears, the additional material permeability attributed to water content is more than offset by design compromises resulting in additional thickness. Most successful extended-wear hydrogel lenses are of the medium-water content variety, for it is in this range that EOP and *Dk/L* are currently maximized. Daily-wear hydrogel lenses must be more durable, yet the emphasis on oxygen transport is not as great as with extended-wear lenses. Hence, daily-wear hydrogels are often of low water content.

EOP and *Dk/L* are not limited by the oxygen permeability of water for rigid and non-hydrogel flexible materials. The oxygen-permeable component of the lens material is silicone (siloxane) and/or a fluoropolymer. The extent to which these can be incorporated into a rigid material is limited by the increased flexibility of the material and reduced wettability caused by these permeable substances. In general, as the rigid lens material is made more permeable to oxygen, the critical thickness to maintain stability of surface curvature on the eye is correspondingly increased and in-eye wettability (Bourassa & Benjamin, 1989) is decreased. When flexure is an unwanted complication of rigid lens wear, additional lens thickness may be incorporated into the prescription. When wettability is a problem for the patient, low-*Dk* materials may be more bio-compatible. These attributes detract from enhanced oxygen performance derived from materials of progressively higher *Dk*. Even so, it appears that rigid and non-hydrogel flexible contact lenses have the potential to provide greater oxygen to the cornea than do

hydrogel lenses (Table 3.4), for these limitations are not as severe with respect to oxygen permeability as is the water content limitation with hydrogel lenses. When significant flexibility is not a problem, as when fitting spherical (non-toric) corneas, very high EOP and *Dk/L* values (> 11% EOP or > 25 *Dk/L* units) can be achieved with rigid lenses because they can be made thin with high-*Dk* materials. Flexible non-hydrogel 'soft' lenses, such as those made of silicone elastomer, may have incredibly high EOP and *Dk/L* values (> 15% EOP or > 50 *Dk/L* units) because the limitations imposed on oxygen permeability by flexibility and water content are not applicable. Sadly, it was the inherently poor wettability of pure silicone elastomer that has thus far ruined its potential in the contact lens field.

Coatings and deposition on contact lens surfaces have the potential to act as barriers to oxygen flow as lenses age (Benjamin & Hill, 1980; Hill & Goings, 1981). In these quoted studies a protein component of tear fluid was denatured on gel lens surfaces in an amount that ultimately led to coatings that were opaque and up to twice the thickness of the lenses being tested. The EOPs of the coated lenses were correspondingly reduced

Table 3.4 Oxygen permeabilities for some common non-hydrogel materials (Barrer *et al.* 1962; Fatt 1991a) minimum thicknesses, *Dk/L*, and EOP values for –3 D, +3 D lenses

Material	*Dk* (*Dk* units)	Minimal estimated thickness (mm)	Estimated central transmissibility and EOP (*Dk/L* units, %)	
			–3 D Lens	+3 D lens
PMMA	0	0.06	0, 0	0, 0
Polycon II	9	0.08	11, 5	5, 3.5
Boston IV	22	0.10	2, 8	12, 5
Paraperm EW	38	0.12	32, 10	18, 7
Equalens	49	0.14	35, 10.5	21, 8
Fluoroperm	63	0.16	39, 11	25, 9
Silicone elastomer	104*	0.10	104, 16	55, 13

* As produced in the Silsoft and Danker elastomer lenses (Fatt, 1988, 1991a). The bulk permeability of silicone elastomer may be as high as 400 to 600 *Dk* units. Minimal thickness for this soft material is not limited by flexibility on the eye.

by half or more of the value of the EOPs when the gel lenses were new (7%). It would be exceedingly rare, if ever, that patients might allow this much deposition to accumulate on lens surfaces (Fatt & Morris, 1977; Benjamin *et al.*, 1981). Because coatings and deposits are of high oxygen permeability and are very thin, they have a subclinical impact on oxygen flow through contact lenses (Fatt & Morris, 1977; Refojo *et al.*, 1982).

3.5 FOR THE CLINICIAN: AN OXYGEN SUMMARY

Practitioners must keep in mind several aspects of oxygen transport when dealing with their contact-lens-wearing patients. The first aspect is that determinations of *Dk*, *Dk/L* and EOP are not exact sciences as currently performed. Considerable variability in results are shown by different investigators who use different measurement techniques and methods of correction for the various flaws in those techniques described above. The terms, units, and relationships between *Dk*, *Dk/L* and EOP are of sufficient complexity to result in significant confusion for clinicians concerning actual values and interpretation. It is all too easy for a company to advertise the highest *Dk*, *Dk/L*, or EOP value found amongst several different investigators, and considerable 'fog' or 'smoke' seems to surround many attempts to 'clear the air' of any discrepancies. A log change in units indicated by an asterisk in 'fine print' at the bottom of the page, say from 10^{-11} to 10^{-12}, can be enough to position the numerical *Dk* value of a particular material positively compared to other materials for which *Dk* has been stated in conventional units. Simply stated, it is difficult for the practitioner to obtain a straight answer about any particular lens material or lens design. This situation is not unusual when marketing of products is allowed to dominate the science surrounding them.

Second, the practitioner is concerned with the contact lens that will actually go on the patient's eye. *Dk/L* and EOP values are each representative of oxygen transport only at a specific lens thickness. The practitioner must extrapolate this data to the particular lens design and mode of wear that will be used. Aside from a few basic clinical principles, noted in Figure 3.19, this is a difficult task because contact lens prescriptions are unique to individual patients. The material and design that optimizes corneal oxygenation for one patient, balanced against flexibility, wettability, and mode of wear, will not be the same for another. The requisite data to discern the 'oxygen difference' is usually not available for individual cases.

Third, published EOP or *Dk/L* values 'of contact lenses' are actually not derived from the entire distributions of thickness within the lens apertures, but are valid for only a

1. Thin designs are better, but thinness also applies to the periphery of a lens as well as the centre. Use plus and minus lenticular designs or aspheric surfaces when possible.
2. For rigid lenses, high-*Dk* materials are better when flexure and wettability are not significant problems. Rigid extended wear may be an option in these cases.
3. For rigid lenses, low-*Dk* materials are better when flexure and wettability problems are substantial.
4. For rigid lenses, medium-*Dk* materials are better when flexure and wettability problems are significant but manageable with limited design modification.
5. For hydrogel lenses, oxygen transport is maximized with materials having medium water content. Daily wear and extended wear may be options in these cases.
6. For spherical hydrogel lenses, extended wear is contraindicated when refractive power exceeds −8 D or +3 D.
7. For toric hydrogel lenses incorporating prism, extended wear is contraindicated when refractive power exceeds −6 D or +1 D in the most vertical meridian.

Figure 3.19 Some general 'rules of thumb' concerning oxygen transport.

single thickness. Each point on the cornea will respond only to the primary amount of oxygen that it receives through the lens thickness overlying it, or in the case of daily-wear rigid lenses, to that also supplied secondarily by tear pumping and mixing under the lens.

Plus lenses are well known for their lack of capacity to deliver oxygen to the cornea. However, their reputation is based on central EOP and Dk/L measurements relevant only to the thickest portions of these lenses. Plus lenses become thinner at the periphery where EOP and Dk/L are correspondingly higher. Thus, they are not as poor in terms of oxygenation over the entire corneal surface as would seem to be the case. Fortunately, rigid plus corneal lenses are of intralimbal design, have access to the 'tear pump' to reduce hypoxia (though the pump is least effective at the lens centre), and are not generally prescribed for cosmetic extended wear. They can be lenticularized and/or aspheric surfaces can be used to help thin the lens centre. With hydrogel plus lenses, maximum hypoxia is concentrated near the visual axis. Clinical signs of significant central hypoxia are readily noted by the practitioner and visual disturbances are readily noticed by the patient. Hypoxia of lesser magnitude is concentrated in the corneal periphery, nearer the limbus, across which the reduced hypoxic stress has less chance to draw infiltration (Gordon & Kracher, 1985) and vascularization (De Donato, 1981). This is particularly important at the superior cornea. Plus hydrogel lenses can be worn in daily wear with special attention given to monitoring the central cornea for hypoxic stress. Up to +3 D may be attempted in cosmetic extended wear with high-Dk gel materials in thin designs.

Minus contact lenses have the reputation of being excellent oxygen transmitters. Again, this is based on central EOP and Dk/L values at the thinnest portion of minus lenses. EOP and Dk/L become progressively diminished toward the peripheries of these lenses. Hence, minus lenses

are not as good in terms of oxygenation over the entire corneal surface as would seem to be the case. Like plus lenses, rigid high-minus corneal lenses are of intralimbal design, can be lenticularized and/or aspherized to thin the lens periphery, have access to the 'tear pump' to reduce hypoxia under the lens periphery, and are generally not prescribed for extended wear. With high-minus hydrogel lenses, hypoxia of least magnitude is concentrated near the visual axis. Clinical signs and visual symptoms of central hypoxia, readily noted by the practitioner and patient, are minimal. Maximum hypoxia is concentrated in the corneal periphery and the greater hypoxic stress has more chance of drawing infiltration and vascularization across the limbus, especially at the superior cornea (De Donato, 1981; Gordon & Kracher, 1985). High-minus hydrogel lenses can be worn in daily wear, with special attention given to monitoring limbal and peripheral corneal abnormalities, but hydrogel lenses with refractive powers greater than −8 D are not recommended for extended wear. The power restriction for extended wear becomes −6 D in the vertical meridian of toric prism-ballasted hydrogel lenses (Westin *et al.*, 1989). Prism adds additional thickness to these lenses particularly at the inferior corneal position.

Finally, there is considerable variation in corneal response to hypoxia among the contact-lens-wearing population. Accounts of corneal requirements for oxygen usually do not include special requirements for the superior cornea. It was noted at the beginning of this chapter that the superior cornea was in a sort of 'double trouble', being far more hypoxic than the central or other peripheral corneal sites during day-time lens wear and slightly more hypoxic than the rest of the cornea during overnight wear. Thus, the minimum corneal requirement for oxygen is probably much higher than is currently realized, and particularly so for a significant minority of the population. It is imperative that the contact-lens-wearing patient's superior corneas be monitored for signs of hypoxic stress.

These aspects of oxygen transport through contact lenses make it necessary for critical clinical prescription and fastidious follow-through for each patient wearing contact lenses. Important though the practitioner's contact lens prescription may be, in terms of corneal oxygenation, it is made with an inadequate correspondance between oxygen transport characteristics of contact lenses and acceptability of wear for the individual patient. The practitioner can never predict with certainty how the individual cornea will react to the degree of hypoxia created by the contact lens. He or she does not really know how much oxygen the lens will supply, how much the lens will flex, how well it will wet on the eye, or how the eye will cope with its chronic presence.

This inability to focus considerable, yet inadequate, clinical and scientific knowledge for the benefit of the individual patient tends to drive practitioners to make selections about contact lens design and material based on hearsay, manufacturer claims, advertisements and pseudoscience articles published in trade journals. For these reasons the prescription of contact lenses is in some ways an art and not a science; this results in considerable inconsistency between decisions made by different prescribers, and confounds even the most practiced of contact lens practitioners.

ACKNOWLEDGMENT

I gratefully thank Dr Irving Fatt, as scientific reviewer, for his critical analysis of this chapter.

REFERENCES

Allaire, P.E., Allison, S.W. and Gooray, A.M. (1978) Tear film dynamics and oxygen tension under a circular contact lens. *American Journal of Optometry & Physiological Optics*, **54**, 617–26.

Ang, J.H.B. and Efron, N. (1989) Carbon dioxide permeability of contact lens materials. *International Contact Lens Clinic*, **16**, 48–57.

Barrer, R.M., Barrie, J.A. and Rogers, M.G. (1962) Permeation through a membrane with mixed boundary conditions. *Transactions of the Faraday Society*, **58**, 2473–83.

Benjamin W.J. (1982) *Corneal physiology under the closed eyelid of humans.* PhD dissertation, The Ohio State University, Columbus, Ohio.

Benjamin, W.J. (1986) The closed-lid tear pump during rigid extended wear. *International Eyecare*, **2** (4), 224–6.

Benjamin, W.J. and Hill, R.M. (1980) Ultrathins: The case for continuous care. *Journal of the American Optometric Association*, **51**(3), 277–9.

Benjamin, W.J. and Hill R.M. (1986a) Human corneal oxygen demand: the closed-eye interval. *Graefe's Archive for Clinical & Experimental Ophthalmology*, **224**, 291–4.

Benjamin, W.J. and Hill, R.M. (1986b) Closed-lid factors influencing human corneal oxygen demand. *Acta Ophthalmologica*, **64**, 644–8.

Benjamin, W.J. and Hill, R.M. (1988a) Human cornea: superior and central oxygen demands. *Graefe's Archive for Clinical & Experimental Ophthalmology*, **226**(1), 41–4.

Benjamin, W.J. and Hill, R.M. (1988b) Human cornea: individual responses to hypoxic environments. *Graefe's Archive for Clinical & Experimental Ophthalmology*, **226**(1), 45–8.

Benjamin W.J. and Rasmussen, M.A. (1985) The closed-lid tear pump: oxygenation? *International Eyecare*, **1**(3), 251–7.

Benjamin W.J. and Rasmussen, M.A. (1988) Oxygen consumption of the superior cornea following eyelid closure. *Acta Ophthalmologica*, **66**, 309–12.

Benjamin, W.J. and Simons, M.H. (1984) Extended wear of rigid lenses in aphakia: a preliminary report; and extended wear of oxygen-permeable rigid contact lenses in aphakia. *International Contact Lens Clinic*, **11** (1), 44–57; **11** (9), 547–61.

Benjamin, W.J., Mauger, T.F. and Hill, R.M. (1981) The devious deposit. *Contact Lens Forum*, **6**(8), 48–9.

Berger, R.E. (1974) Effect of contact lens motion on the oxygen tension distribution under the lens. *American Journal of Optometry & Physiological Optics*, **51**, 441–56.

Bourassa, S. and Benjamin, W.J. (1989) Compari-

Smelser, G.K. (1952) Relation of factors involved in maintenance of optical properties of the cornea to contact lens wear. *Archives of Ophthalmology*, **47**(3), 328–43.

Stefansson, E., Foulks, G.N. and Hamilton, R.C. (1987) The effect of corneal contact lenses on the oxygen tension in the anterior chamber of the rabbit eye. *Investigative Ophthalmology & Visual Science*, **28**, 1716–18.

Weissman, B.A. (1982) Designing uniform-thickness contact lens shells. *American Journal of Optometry & Physiological Optics*, **59** (11), 902–3.

Westin, E.J., McDaid, D. and Benjamin, W.J. (1989) Inferior corneal vascularization associated with extended wear of prism-ballasted toric hydrogel lenses. *International Contact Lens Clinic*, **16**, 20–2.

Winterton, L.C., White, J.C. and Su, K.C. (1987) Coulometric method for measuring oxygen flux and Dk of contact lenses and lens materials. *International Contact Lens Clinic*, **14**, 441–52.

Winterton, L.C., White, J.C. and Su, K.C. (1988) Coulometrically determined oxygen flux and resultant Dk of commercially available contact lenses. *International Contact Lens Clinic*, **15**, 117–23.

MECHANICAL PROPERTIES OF CONTACT LENSES

4

R.W.W. Stevenson

4.1 INTRODUCTION

The word polymer literally means 'many parts'. A polymeric solid material may be considered to be one that contains many chemically bonded parts or units, which themselves are bonded together to form a solid.

Plastics are a large and varied group of synthetic materials which are processed by forming or moulding into shape. Plastics can be divided into two classes, thermoplastic and thermosetting plastics, depending on how they are structurally chemically bonded. Thermoplastics, which include most of the polymers used for contact lenses, require heat to make them formable and after cooling, they retain the shape they were formed into. Most thermoplastics consist of very long main chains of carbon atoms covalently bonded together. The long molecular chains are bonded to each other by secondary bonds.

The gas permeability and the surface properties, including wettability, of contact lens materials have been discussed in Chapters 2 and 3. Other properties of contact lens materials are often ignored or regarded as being less important. However, with the ever-increasing number of hard gas permeable materials available for lens manufacture, and the more recent soft lenses having sophisti-cated production methods and thinner designs, it is now recognized that the mechanical properties of all lenses are important.

Factors such as the basic comfort of a lens, the optical performance of a lens in cases of corneal astigmatism, and the lens base-curve to cornea-fitting relationship, have all been shown to relate to the mechanical properties of lens materials. These properties include the modulus, toughness, form stability and ease of manufacture.

The fabrication of an article from a polymeric material in the bulk state involves deformation of the material by applied forces. Afterwards, the finished product is subjected to stresses and hence it is important to be aware of the mechanical properties of each material and understand the basic principles underlying their response to such forces.

The mechanical properties of elastic solids can be described by Hooke's Law, which states that applied stress is proportional to the resultant strain but is independent of the rate of strain. For liquids the corresponding statement is known as Newton's Law, with the stress now independent of the strain but proportional to the rate of strain. Both laws are valid only for small strains and whilst it is essential that conditions involving large stresses leading to eventual mechanical failure

Contact Lens Practice. Edited by Montague Ruben and Michel Guillon.
Published in 1994 by Chapman & Hall, London. ISBN 0 412 35120 X

be studied, it is also important to examine the response to small mechanical stresses.

In many cases a material may exhibit the characteristics of both a liquid and a solid, and is then said to be in a visco-elastic state. The response of polymers to mechanical stresses can vary widely and depends on the particular state the polymer is in at any given temperature. As a result of their chain like structures, polymers are not perfect elastic bodies and deformation is accompanied by a complex series of molecular re-arrangements.

Consequently, the mechanical behaviour of polymers is dominated by visco-elastic phenomenon in contrast to materials such as metal and glass where atomic adjustments under stress are more localized and limited.

4.2   LINEAR VISCO-ELASTIC BEHAVIOUR OF AMORPHOUS POLYMERS

A polymer can possess a wide range of material properties, and of these the hardness, deformability, toughness and ultimate strength are amongst the most significant when considering contact lenses. Certain features such as a high rigidity modulus and impact strength combined with low creep characteristics are desirable in a polymer, if eventually it is to be subjected to loading.

Unfortunately these are conflicting properties, as a polymer with a high modulus and low creep response does not absorb energy by deforming easily, and hence has poor impact strength. This means a compromise must be sought depending upon the use to which the polymer will be put, and this requires a knowledge of the mechanical response in detail.

With contact lens polymers, a low modulus will give a flexible lens assisting comfort, but may give poor lens parameter stability and possible material creep, as a result of external forces on the eye or in handling.

Clearly the comfort of a lens is of major importance to successful contact lens wear, which may be one main reason why the soft lens share of the total world-wide contact lens market has increased significantly in the 1990s. This includes countries like the UK which has traditionally favoured the hard lens since its introduction and development in the 1950s.

The mechanical properties of hard gas permeable and soft hydrogel lenses are inherently different and therefore need to be considered separately.

4.3   HARD GAS PERMEABLE OR RIGID GAS PERMEABLE (RGP)

The definition 'rigid gas permeable' (RGP) is now used routinely but can be misleading. The use of the term 'rigid' suggests or infers that such lenses will be resistant to bending or flexing which, as most contact lens practitioners will verify, is clearly not the case. These materials have changed significantly over the last 20 years since their introduction and have developed into complex polymers designed specifically for the production of contact lenses.

Two of the main mechanical properties of gas permeable lens materials are the modulus of elasticity and the hardness of the plastic. Some of the consequences of these two properties, which may be evident clinically, are flexing of lenses on toric corneas, the comfort or discomfort of a lens on insertion and the scratch resistance of a lens. The mechanical properties of a material, along with its permeability and surface characteristics, are therefore crucial to the clinical performance of an RGP contact lens.

The mechanical properties also determine the dimensional stability of the lens, a point which has significance to both manufacturers and clinicians. It was taken into consideration recently by the International Organization for Standardization (ISO) in developing new standards for rigid contact lenses, covering classification and tolerances for manufacture. (ISO 8321–1, 1991 and BS 7208, 1992).

The revised standards recognize that most of the newer custom-designed lens polymers are in fact more difficult for manufacturers to work with than PMMA. This is particularly so in the fact that the tolerance for the lens back optic zone radius has been doubled (now ± 0.05 mm), indicating that the dimensional stability of the group of RGPs is less than with PMMA. This point has undoubted clinical importance, in particular, to the verification, tolerances and fitting of rigid lenses.

The determination of some of the fundamental mechanical properties of contact lens materials is important when considering their relative properties and merits of various materials. In the engineering industry, test methods are well developed using prepared samples of the materials to be tested. This also applies to the plastics industry; however, in the contact lens industry, it may be more appropriate to test lenses rather than material samples, which can be difficult to obtain in the necessary forms.

One of the difficulties associated with the measurement of the mechanical properties of lens materials is that no single property measurement reflects accurately, the 'in eye' situation. Tensile strength indicates the resistance of the material to deformation under tension; tear strength the resistance of the material to tear propagation from a notch or imperfection (more relevant to soft lens materials), and rigidity modulus the resistance to deformation under compression.

The first two parameters relate to the behaviour of a lens material in handling and the third (modulus) indicates the extent to which various forces will deform it, most likely when in lens form. A hard or rigid material will have a high rigidity modulus, whereas a soft material will have a low modulus. Following on from this, and as suggested previously, a low rigidity modulus is likely to be associated with greater lens comfort. However, poorer visual results may be obtained when fitting astigmatic eyes, due to residual astigmatism resulting from

lens flexing. Again this has been traditionally a soft lens problem, but as indicated later, can also occur with RGPs, and in particular some of the recent high oxygen permeable (Dk) polymers, which have been described as flexible fluoropolymers (Isaacson 1988, 1989).

Mechanical property testing of materials in the engineering industry typically involves the application of a force or load to a sample and a measurement of the way in which the sample responds. Results are expressed as strength or modulus.

The strength of a material is defined as the force per unit area required to cause failure when the material is subjected to a test procedure, e.g. tensility, shear, impact, tear. The modulus is defined as the true stress (force per unit area) required to produce a true unit strain, i.e. deformation in the direction of the force, e.g. tensile modulus, rigidity modulus (Smith, 1990).

4.3.1 UNITS

One of the difficulties when comparing lenses is that units used in the measurement of 'stress' often differ. The SI unit of stress is now newtons per square metre (N/m^2) although MN/m^2 is more useful to contact lens materials (mega newtons per square metre $= 10^6$ N/m^2). However other units such as kg/mm^2 and dyn/cm^2 are also used and conversions may be necessary if comparison of materials is to be made:

$$1\ dyn/cm^2 = 0.1\ N/m^2 = 10^{-7}\ MN/m^2 = 1.02 \times 10^{-8}\ kg/mm^2$$

Values used may depend on the method used to test materials.

Materials can be tested under tension or compression and the results of these tests can give detailed information on the strength, deformation characteristics, stiffness and toughness of a material.

Tension

The tensile test provides a stress/strain curve as the load is applied and the associated measures are: (a) tensile strength (load at break/cross-sectional area); (b) tensile modulus (stress/strain); and (c) percentage elongation at break (extension at break/original length × 100%).

Compression

As previously indicated, unlike true elastic materials, most polymers are visco-elastic, that is they deform time-dependently when a load is applied and recover time-dependently when the load is removed, and this may result in a progressive deformation of the materials. In this way, stress/relaxation curves can be generated and these may be applicable to the contact lens industry.

Various instruments allow the indentation of any test sample by a small sphere under a small load. The recovery of the specimen can also be measured as a function of time. The value of the rigidity modulus indicates the force necessary to compress the material by a given amount.

Although it gives a good understanding of the flexibility of the material it bears no relationship to properties that are measured in tension. It is important to remember that on the eye, RGP lenses are acted upon by relatively small forces associated with lid blinking, lid tension, eye movements and the surface tension of tears. Some of the effects of these forces have been measured directly on the eye and they show interesting interactions between lid tension and corneal astigmatism (Wilson *et al.*, 1982).

The data derived from stress/strain measurements on thermoplastics are important from a practical viewpoint, providing as they do, information on the modulus, the brittleness and the ultimate and yield strengths of the polymer. By subjecting the specimen to a tensile force applied at a uniform rate and measuring the resulting deformation, a curve of the type shown in Figure 4.1, can be constructed.

The initial portion of the curve is linear and the tensile modulus E is obtained from its slope. The point L represents the stress beyond which a brittle material will fracture and the area under the curve to this point is proportional to the energy required for brittle fracture.

If the material is tough, no fracture occurs, and the curve then passes through a maximum or inflection point Y, known as the yield point. Beyond this, the ultimate elongation is eventually reached and the polymer breaks at B.

Rigidity modulus and related measurements have been made on a number of contact lens materials using a micro-indentation apparatus (Tighe, 1989a), a loading applied to prepared material samples (Fatt, 1988; Stevenson, 1988, 1991a), and to finished lenses by Fatt (1986, 1988). These measurements are discussed later (see page 75).

The widespread use of PMMA in industry made manufacturers of this material, carry out comprehensive engineering studies on its elastic behaviour. However, there have been very few published reports of RGP elastic moduli, mainly as a result of the

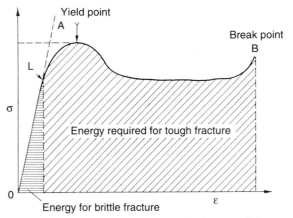

Figure 4.1 The response obtained when applying a load to a thermoplastic.

materials being custom designed for the contact lens industry.

4.3.2 FRACTURE CHARACTERISTICS OF POLYMERS

If mechanical testing of polymers goes beyond their elastic limit (i.e. beyond point L in Fig. 4.1) then their fracture characteristics can be evaluated. This can be useful for manufacturing purposes and may be relevant to patient handling of RGP lenses. That is, depending upon the shape of the curve in Figure 4.1 between L and B, materials can be classified as soft and weak, soft and tough, hard and brittle, hard and strong or hard and tough. The fracture characteristics of Boston Equalens were observed when loading samples of the material with weights up to 300 g (Stevenson, 1988).

Resistance to breakage is important for RGP materials to ensure durability in RGP lens usage. However, if this means increased flexibility and associated difficulty in masking corneal astigmatism and greater difficulty in lens manufacture then the balance of properties may be inappropriate. In designing new polymers for RGP lens use then this balance needs to be carefully considered.

4.3.3 HARDNESS TESTS

Hardness is a measure of the resistance of a material to permanent deformation. This property can be measured by forcing an indentor into the surface of a material. The indentor material is normally made of a material much harder than the material being tested. An empirical hardness number is calculated based on the cross sectional area or depth of the impression.

The four common hardness tests used in engineering and materials testing are Brinell, Vickers, Knoop and Rockwell. In these tests it is easier to measure a parallel-sided contact lens blank than a curved finished lens but the data is difficult to interpret. The tests

generally measure either the resistance of a material to indentation, the resistance of a material to scratching or the recovery from indentation.

Some hardness values for contact lens materials exist but they are difficult to relate to actual lens performance, for example, the scratch resistance of a lens. Mechanical failure with PMMA and RGP contact lenses usually relates to their breakage, chipping, scratching, crazing or distortion. The surface energy required to fracture an amorphous brittle glassy polymeric material such as PMMA is about 1000 times greater than that which would be required if the fracture involved just the simple breaking of carbon–carbon bonds on a fracture plane.

Thus, glassy polymeric materials such as PMMA are much tougher than inorganic glasses. The extra energy required to fracture thermoplastics is much higher because distorted localized regions called crazes form before cracking occurs. A craze in a glassy thermoplastic is formed in a highly stressed region of the material and consists of an alignment of molecular chains combined with a high density of interdispersed voids (Cowie, 1991). Contact lens practitioners will be familiar with the clinical presentation of this phenomenon, which is sudden discomfort, blurring of vision and an opaque stress pattern visible on examination of the PMMA or RGP lens. Checking the base curve of a lens in the radiuscope will confirm the distortion of a lens.

True crazing, usually as a result of patient mishandling (unintended bending or flexing of a lens) needs to be differentiated from the surface crazing referred to with some gas permeable lenses where surface breakdown or failure of the polymer occurs due to combination of lens manufacturing methods and deposits from the tear film. This has been explained by excessive heat during lens manufacture of certain materials. The interaction between the tears (and their constituents) and the polymer is crucial to the long-term mechanical performance of a lens.

The lathing techniques for gas permeable materials required to produce finished lenses take into account the differences in hardness found between materials. These differences can be assessed by looking at the swarf characteristics of materials such as the continuous strands found with PMMA or the powder effect produced with most of the RGP materials when cutting with a diamond tool. The assessment of swarf characteristics is a well established practice in the engineering industry when dealing with metals and the same phenomenon of continuous or particle swarf exists.

In fact, the powder effect of the swarf when producing lenses from polymer buttons is greatest with the highest *Dk* materials commonly used, and lathe speeds and depth of cut of the diamond tool can be adjusted to make allowance for such factors. This means that careful polishing techniques are also required to eliminate possible 'chipping' effects on the surfaces and edges of a lens. From a manufacturing point of view it would be ideal to have a gas permeable material with the machinability of PMMA. However, with the current range of silicone and fluorosilicone acrylate this remains a contradiction in terms.

4.3.4 MEASUREMENTS OF MECHANICAL PROPERTIES OF RGP LENS MATERIALS OR FINISHED LENSES

Experiments (Fatt, 1988; Stevenson, 1991b) have been conducted on both RGP lens materials and lenses, attempting to compare materials and to give useful information on mechanical properties helpful to both industry and the practitioner. These have concentrated mainly on the flexing characteristics of either materials or lenses. The term 'flexibility' should be used to define material characteristics and 'flexure' to define lens behaviour on the eye.

Flexure of PMMA lenses has been observed during the fitting of these lenses but rarely reported as a clinical problem. PMMA is a relatively stiff material (high Young's Modulus) and as PMMA lenses were relatively thick, flexure of a lens on the eye was small.

With the introduction of RGP lenses, flexure has become a more commonly observed problem. This results from the fact that RGP materials have a lower modulus than PMMA lenses and that they tend to be made thinner to maximize their oxygen transmissibility.

Methods of quantifying material flexibility should be developed so that manufacturers could then quote such details in the technical specification of their product. The most common measure used in the engineering field to describe the elasticity of a material is the Young's Modulus relating stress to strain as a result of loading a sample of a given material under specific experimental conditions. Stress/strain testing could be relatively easily standardized for contact lens materials and stress relaxation testing could also be useful to assess the likely plastic memory of lenses in different materials.

The Young's Modulus of Elasticity of a range of commercially available gas permeable contact lens materials has been measured in laboratory studies by Fatt (1988) and by Stevenson (1991a) using specially prepared samples of a range of gas permeable materials. Both studies found differences between materials such that groupings could be made on the basis of oxygen permeability. The total range in modulus across all materials measured was, however, relatively small (approximately 2×10^4 to 4×10^4 kg/cm^2).

The highest value of Young's Modulus in either of the studies was found with the lowest *Dk* (PMMA) and the lowest measured value with the highest *Dk* (Fluoroperm 90). The value for the 3M Fluorofocon A material correlated with its high *Dk* (100) although this material was not available in button form for laboratory testing and data was provided by the manufacturer.

These experimental results confirm that in the range of materials tested, the greater the oxygen permeability of a material the greater will be the flexibility. (See Stevenson and Ansell (1991) for details of the measurement of oxygen permeability.) This has significance when fitting and designing lenses for a toric cornea. Practitioners must balance the increase in centre thickness to offset flexing with the corresponding decrease in oxygen transmissibility. Conversely, it may be that lenses can be designed to flex where this would be an optical advantage. Material producers and lens manufacturers should provide Young's Modulus data to help practitioners more fully understand the materials they prescribe. However, as the Young's Modulus of materials does not vary widely, lens design features can be utilized to either enhance or minimize the likelihood of lens flexing.

An earlier study (Stevenson, 1988) determined the total bending of a sample of material to a relatively high load which meant that: (a) some samples broke under load; and (b) bending of the sample beyond the elastic limit of the material was produced. No attempt was made to quantify the modulus of elasticity. This type of mechanical testing, as suggested earlier, is designed to assess fracture resistance of polymers where the property of brittleness can be considered.

Questions have been raised in the literature regarding the difficulty of relating material measurements to subsequent lens performance where design factors may be as significant as material differences. This is undoubtedly the case, as when working with lenses of similar back vertex power, different designs can give different mechanical handling properties.

Fatt (1988) measured lens flexing *in vitro* by mechanically compressing the chord diameter of lenses and determining the force needed to produce the change in diameter.

His methodology involved the use of a keratometer to measure the front surface curvature of lenses under 'load' and is similar in concept to that used by lens manufacturers in the 'crimping' of material buttons to produce toric lenses.

Two main differences from the earlier reported experiments on fracture resistance were incorporated into this series of experiments.

First, if an assumption is made that the polymers to be tested and measured are perfect elastic bodies any assessment of the stress/strain relationship should be kept within their elastic limit. Hence the range of loads applied in stress/strain testing are much less than when testing fracture resistance. The actual range used in measuring Young's Modulus was 10–60 g, in 10 g intervals.

Preparation of samples is also very important to the measurement of the modulus of elasticity. Results of material flexibility can be obtained from 0.2 mm thick circular discs of material prepared from lens blanks. However, as has been pointed out by Fatt (1988), a significant increase in the sensitivity of the measuring technique can be obtained by using small rectangular plates such that more bending for a given load is obtained. Therefore, although they are more difficult to produce, rectangular flats of different thicknesses all 4 mm wide were prepared from standard contact lens buttons.

The loading device is applied as a knife edge across the width of a sample (Figure 4.2). Ideally, as in the engineering industry, rods of material would be the preferred form to test but rarely is it possible to obtain gas permeable materials in this form. A value for Young's Modulus (E) was calculated using the standard formula $E = L3/4ab3 \ (Y/W)$, where L is the separation of the supports, a is the width of the bar, b is the thickness of the bar and Y/W is the slope of the line relating bending to weight added. (Roark & Young, 1975).

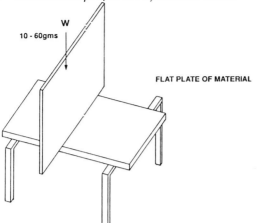

Figure 4.2 Schematic diagram of the measurement system for Young's Modulus.

Figure 4.3 shows two typical slopes obtained with comparable thickness samples of PMMA and Boston Equalens the difference reflecting the relative flexibility of those two materials. The value of each slope is the Y/W term substituted in the equation given above to calculate Young's Modulus (E). Figure 4.4 shows a bar chart of all the materials measured, the error bars being one standard deviation from the mean. The 3M Fluorofocon A material has no standard deviation shown since this was not an experimentally determined value.

The drop in the value for Young's Modulus

becomes significant at the Fluoroperm 30 material, suggesting that three main groupings of materials can be considered as far as flexibility is concerned. These would correspond to low-*Dk* materials (PMMA, Optacryl 18, SGP), medium-*Dk* materials (Paraperm EW, Boston Equalens, Fluorex700, Fluoroperm 30, 90), and high-*Dk* materials (3M Fluorofocon A). The high-*Dk* material information is only based on one type and therefore needs to be investigated with a larger range of materials in this group.

Clinically this would mean that standard thickness lenses in the first group would not flex but have low oxygen transmissibility, those in the middle group would flex in thin negative power design, but have moderate oxygen transmissibility, and those in the third group would flex in all powers but have high oxygen transmissibility. In terms of material classification it would appear from the results obtained in this experiment that most silicone acrylates would be in the first group, most fluorosilicone acrylates would in the middle group and the fluoropolymers in the last group.

Therefore polymer chemists in the devel-

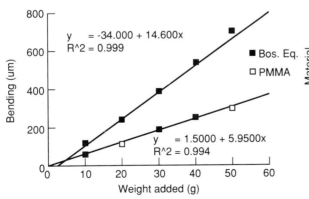

Figure 4.3 A comparison between PMMA and Boston Equalens to show the difference in slope for stress/strain testing.

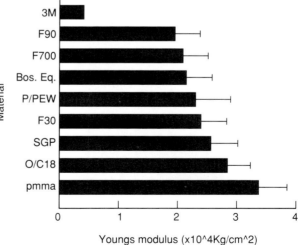

Figure 4.4 Young's Modulus measurements for the range of RGP materials tested.

opment of new gas permeable materials should consider the property of flexibility and to what extent practitioners view it as an advantage or disadvantage. The need to combine mechanical, physiological and optical properties is now well recognized.

The results of the experiments on modulus measurement confirm clinical observations with lenses. That is, the higher the oxygen permeability of the material the more flexible are lenses made from that material. One notable exception to this rule is CAB, which is a low-*Dk* material producing flexible lenses in standard thicknesses. This indicates that material chemistry is a major contributing factor to flexibility in addition to oxygen permeability. This has again been highlighted in recent literature (Swarbrick, 1993; Sobara *et al.*, 1992).

The cross-linking of a polymer controls the modulus, toughness and form stability. However, typically the undesirable results of increasing the cross-link density and increased brittleness, likely crazing and reduced oxygen permeability. The future requirement is therefore cross-linkers that are oxygen permeable to reverse the trend described.

Individual lens design has an important influence on flexing, centre thickness or average thickness being the most crucial lens parameter to balance oxygen transmissibility (*Dk/L*) and flexure. A personal clinical observation is that a thin toric base curve lens does not flex as much as a spherical design on an astigmatic cornea.

Previous publications (Harris & Chu, 1972; Harris *et al.*, 1987) have related the centre thickness of PMMA and low-*Dk* materials to flexing and residual astigmatism. Harris and Chu (1972) found that 0.13 mm was the crucial centre thickness of PMMA below which significant flexure occurred. Harris *et al.* (1987), using two different low-*Dk* silicone acrylates found 0.15 mm to be the critical centre thickness. It has also been shown that fitting lenses

steeper than the flattest '*K*' will cause more flexure (Herman, 1983; Stevenson & Cornish, 1990).

The main point of studies to determine modulus measurements should be to evaluate material characteristics using prepared samples rather than lenses, where lens design would be a difficult variable to control. When looking at flexing of lenses *in situ*, then of course fitting relationships are also crucial. At the present time it is recommended that manufacturers should quote values for the Young's Modulus of all materials allowing practitioners to predict those likely to flex when lenses are manufactured in a thin lens design to maximize oxygen transmissibility. This would be of particular importance when looking at new high *Dk* polymers being developed.

It may be that flexing is desirable in some clinical situations where induced astigmatism can be utilized. The question of induced astigmatism due to lens flexing is not a simple relationship and needs further examination. Preliminary results (Stevenson 1989; Stevenson, 1990; Sobara *et al.*, 1992) of flexing and induced astigmatism with high *Dk/L* (3M Fluorofocon A, 100 *Dk*) lenses show these lenses to have flexing characteristics somewhere between those of other gas permeable lenses and soft lenses. That is, they are likely to transmit some astigmatism but results can be variable and are subject dependent. Practitioners need to consider mechanical, optical and physiological factors when choosing and fitting hard gas permeable lenses, particularly with new generations of high oxygen permeable plastics.

4.4 HYDROGEL MATERIALS

Hydrogels are inherently different in their mechanical properties to rigid gas permeables. In their dehydrated state they are hard and brittle. Low water content hydrogels, such as PHEMA, are harder and more brittle than their higher water content counterparts in the dehydrated state.

When hydrated in water all hydrogels become soft and rubber-like, with a low tensile and tear strength. The lack of mechanical strength is the main limitation to the life of a soft lens. The low modulus also explains the comfort of such lenses but does mean that any corneal astigmatism is transferred through the lens as a result of the 'wrap' factor.

The mechanical strength of a soft hydrogel lens is controlled largely by its water content and overall thickness, although by manipulating the chemistry of the polymer it is claimed that newer higher water content materials can be produced with greater stability and tensile strength (e.g. Excelens, Ciba Vision; Omniflex, Allergan Hydron). The present trend to produce thinner soft lenses tends to over-ride the water content factor when considering mechanical strength.

This is demonstrated by the current range of disposable soft lenses all of which are easily damaged by repeated daily handling regardless of whether they are low water content (B & L Sequence) or medium to high water content (Acuvue, Johnson and Johnson; Focus, Ciba Vision). These disposable soft lenses have average thicknesses of 0.05 to 0.06 mm (at −3.00 D).

Questions have arisen regarding the quality of the edges of some of these lenses (Efron & Vays, 1992). As the manufacture of these lenses is based on a sophisticated moulding method it means that the possibility of damaged or wrinkled edges on removing the lens from the mould exists. Occasionally lenses are damaged on removal from their sealed pack, but as the individual lens cost is low and the relationship between edge defects and specific clinical problems is controversial and may have only moderate significance.

As discussed earlier, some independent studies have been done on the mechanical properties of gas permeable contact lens polymers, but little published work is available on the measurement of hydrogels used for contact lens production. Test methods for hydrogels are poorly defined mainly because the materials need to be in their hydrated state for results to be meaningful.

Manufacturers' literature has to be searched to obtain any information on materials, and even then it tends to have unspecified methodology and lacks a standardized format. To give some indication of differences between contact lens materials the two main properties of tensile strength and rigidity modulus are given in Table 4.1.

The effect of water content on the mechanical properties of hydrogels can be clearly seen from Table 4.2, which shows the typical values of tensile strength and elongation to break. The material elasticity increases and strength decreases with increasing water content. The data has been compiled from a range of manufacturers' technical publications.

Production methods for soft lenses include lathe cut, spin cast, static cast and melt pressed. As with gas permeable materials, lathe cutting involves the need to consider the mechanical properties of materials. Low water content materials tend to be harder and therefore more difficult to cut and polish whereas higher water content materials are softer and are easier to cut and polish.

Table 4.1 Tensile strength and rigidity modulus of different materials (units are dyn/cm^2)

	PMMA	Silicone elastomer	PHEMA
Tensile strength	5×10^7	10×10^7	0.5×10^7
Rigidity modulus	100×10^7	8×10^7	5×10^7

Table 4.2 The effect of the water content of hydrogels on their mechanical properties

	38%	60%	73%
Tensile strength (kg/cm^2)	6.5	4.6	3.6
Elongation to break (%)	110	155	206

Practitioners therefore need to consider the tensile modulus and elongation to break of all hydrogels, and it is recommended that manufacturers determine these values experimentally to allow data to be quoted in technical specifications for materials. The test method should also be known and units of measurement relevant to contact lens materials. Following a period of about 10 years when little change has been seen in new hydrogel development, there is good reason to hope that the next decade will see new innovation.

As pointed out by Tighe and Mishi (1988) and Tighe (1989b), the general understanding of biomaterials has been advancing whilst no new techniques for testing polymers have been developed. Most of the present methods are inappropriate to current requirements and it is important to ensure that the situation is remedied. The mechanical properties of contact lens materials are important to the industry, the practitioner and to the successful wearing of contact lenses.

REFERENCES

Cowie, J.M.G. (1991) *Chemistry and Physics of Modern Materials*, Chapman and Hall, New York.

Efron, N. and Veys, J. (1992) Defects in disposable lenses can compromise ocular integrity. *ICLC.*, **19**, 8–17.

Fatt, I. (1986) *Performance of Gas Permeable Hard Lenses on the Eye.* Transactions BCLA Conference, 32–7.

Fatt, I. (1988) Elasticity of rigid GP materials. *Optician*, **196**, 42–5.

Harris, M.G. and Chu, C.S. (1972) The effect of contact lens thickness and corneal toricity on flexure and residual astigmatism. *Am. J. Optom. Physiol. Opt.* **49**(4), 304–8.

Harris, M.G., Gale, B., Gansel K. and Slette, C. (1987) Flexure and residual astigmatism with Paraperm O2 and Boston 2 lenses on toric corneas. *Am. J. Optom. Physiol. Opt.* **64** 269–73.

Herman, J.P. (1983) Flexure of rigid contact lenses on toric corneas as a function of base curve fitting relationship. *J. Am. Optom. Assoc.*, **54**(3), 209–13.

Isaacson, W.B. (1988) New gas permeable materials for extended wear. *Optician*, **May 5**, 31–40.

Isaacson, W.B. (1989) Flexible fluoropolymers: a new category of contact lens. *Contact Lens Spectrum*, **Jan.**, 60–2.

ISO 8321-1 and BS 7208. *Contact Lenses.* **Part 1** (1992) Specification for rigid corneal and scleral contact lenses. **Part 2** (1991) Methods of assessing contact lens materials. **Part 3** (1992) Mehtods of testing for contact lenses. International Organization for Standardization and British Standards Institution.

Roark, R.J. and Young, W.C. (1975) *Formulas for stress and strain*, 5th edn, McGraw Hill, New York.

Smith, W.F. (1990) *Principles of Materials Science*, McGraw Hill Publishing Co, New York.

Sobara, L., Fonn, D. and MacNeill, ?? (1992) Effect of rigid gas permeable lens flexure on vision. *Optom. Vis. Sci.*, **69**(12), 953–8.

Stevenson, R.W.W. (1988) Flexibility of gas permeable lenses. *Am. J. Optom. Physiol. Opt.* **65**(11), 874–9.

Stevenson, R.W.W. (1989) *A Correlation of Contact Lens Material Elasticity with 'in-eye' Flexing of Lenses.* Paper presented at American Academy of Optometry meeting New Orleans, USA, December 1989.

Stevenson, R.W.W. (1990) Flexing of high *Dk* lenses. Paper presented at the American Academy of Optometry Annual Meeting, Nashville, USA.

Stevenson, R.W.W. (1991a) Young's Modulus measurements of gas permeable contact lens materials. *Optom. Vis. Sci.*, **68**(2), 142–5

Stevenson, R.W.W. (1991b) Elasticity of gas permeable lenses. *Optom. Vis. Sci.*, **68**(2), 142–5.

Stevenson, R.W.W. and Ansell, R.A. (1991) Polarographic oxygen measurements across gas permeable contact lenses *CLAO J.*, **17**(1), 36–40.

Stevenson, R.W.W. and Cornish, R. (1990) Fluorescein fitting patterns of RGP lenses. *Optician*, **February 2nd**, 31.

Swarbrick, H. (1993) Rigidity and stability are different [editorial]. *Clin. Exp. Optom.*, **76**(1), 1–2.

Tighe, B.J. (1989a) Contact lens materials. In *Contact Lenses* (eds. A. Stones and A.J. Phillips), Butterworths, London.

Tighe, B.J. (1989b) Hydrogel materials: the patents and the products. *Optician*, **June 2nd**.

Tighe, B.J. and Mishi, M. (1988) GP patents–patents, products and properties. *Optician*, **August 5th**.

Wilson, G.S. Bell, C. and Chotai, S. (1982) The effects of lifting the lids on astigmatism *Am. J Optom.*, **59**(8), 670–4.

PART THREE

Contact Lens Design Technology

INTRODUCTION

The design of contact lenses necessitates bringing together a multitude of disciplines. The contact lens designer first needs to understand the various aspects of material technology in order to fully appreciate the properties and limitations of the raw material he/she is given to work with. Such understanding involves a varied field of expertise, such as polymer chemistry, biochemistry, rheology, mechanical physics and microbiology (see Part II). The designer also needs to understand ocular anatomy, physiology and physical optics in order to set the goal for optimal contact lens design and judge how well these can be fulfilled by the material proposed.

The design of contact lenses falls into two broad categories: the design of prescription lenses by the contact lens practitioner for an individual patient, and the design of mass produced lenses by groups of scientists and technologists for a large population of patients. However, in both cases, the aims of those involved are the same; achieving good, stable vision during long-term comfortable wear, free of any adverse effect on the ocular tissues. The underlying principles to fulfil those requirements are therefore the same and directly applicable to both approaches to lens designing. In the initial chapter on lens design (Chapter 5), the authors consider lens designing from first principles, based upon the various disciplines mentioned earlier. Whereas the designs of rigid and soft lenses are treated separately, in each case an all encompassing method will enable the reader to understand any design proposed and

choose alternative suitable designs, if required. Following this initial general chapter, the kinetics of soft contact lens fitting is discussed in detail to help the contact lens practitioner understand how to manipulate soft lens design parameters in order to alter the lens mechanical performance (Chapter 6). The contact lens practitioner will also find useful a basic description of the effect of various contact lens parameters on both rigid and soft lens performance in the chapter on basic contact lens fitting (Chapter 27). A key aspect for most contact lenses is to produce an adequate optical correction; a specific chapter is therefore dedicated to contact lens optics (Chapter 7). This chapter considers the special aspects of contact lens optics whereby, due to the highly curved surfaces present and despite their extreme thinness, their optical effects are those of a thick lens.

However, it is the actual contact lens, and not its theoretical design, that performs on the eye. Hence, an accurate realization of the proposed design is essential. Several chapters have been dedicated to the verification of contact lenses. The verification also falls into two categories, quality assurance and quality control, that take place at the time of manufacturing and the verification of contact lenses carried out by the contact lens practitioner prior to contact lens dispensing to patients.

The verification of contact lenses has always been an important and integral part of contact lens manufacturing. However, it is with the advent of mass-produced lenses that the process has taken a new proactive role, whereby it is part of a feedback system that aims at controlling production at all times, in order to achieve the highest yield possible. The chapters on quality assurance and quality control (Chapters 8 and 9) deal with mass-produced contact lenses and differentiate between those measurements that are carried out on 100% of lenses produced (quality control), and those more specialized and necessary to release products in large batches that test small samples of representative lenses (quality assurance).

The verification of contact lenses in practice, while still remaining a very important aspect of contact lens dispensing, and universal for rigid contact lenses, is no longer carried out in 100% of soft contact lenses delivered. The reasons are multiple and include a better control of the manufacturing process, which makes measurement of all lenses unnecessary. There is extreme difficulty in achieving accurate measurements for some parameters, due to the very high lens flexibility and new dispensing methods, whereby patients are given multiple lenses at one time for regular replacement.

M. Guillon and W.A. Sammons

5.1 INTRODUCTION

There are three objectives in any lens design process. We can summarize these detailed considerations concisely by listing our three principal design criteria as comfort, safety and vision. These are not independent criteria – a very important fact, which is illustrated schematically in Figure 5.1. First, there is the need to maintain the integrity of ocular tissues. This involves the consideration, primarily, of minimizing mechanical trauma, maximizing gas transfer and eliminating corneal metabolic byproducts.

Mechanical trauma to the cornea and conjunctiva is caused by the transfer of pressure from the contact lens to the cornea where the back surface of the contact lens makes close contact with the cornea. During daytime wear, the movement of the lens during a blink leads to dynamic pressures in which contact forces exceed those pre-existing in the static mode (Hayashi, 1977). In this dynamic phase, contact-lens-induced pressure is distributed over most of the ocular surface as the pressure points move from place to place in response to lens excursions.

During overnight wear, when the eye is closed for long periods of time with very infrequent eye movements, as in sleep, the lens is in a static phase and the pressure is concentrated over the same ocular region under the continuous pressure of the lids (Fig. 5.2).

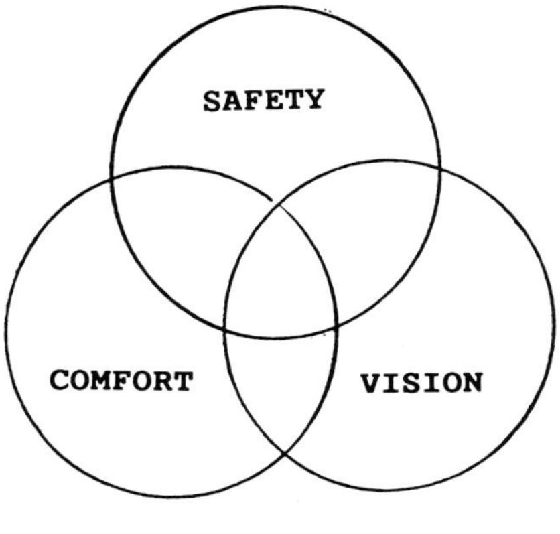

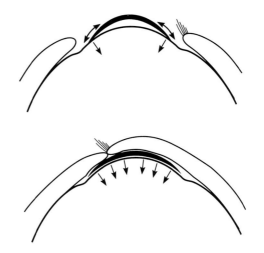

Figure 5.1 Schematic representation of contact lens design objectives.

Figure 5.2 Schematic representation of lid-induced pressure on contact lens.

Contact Lens Practice. Edited by Montague Ruben and Michel Guillon.
Published in 1994 by Chapman & Hall, London. ISBN 0 412 35120 X

Mechanical trauma to the lids is caused by the resistance of the lens to lid induced movement at blink. The front surface of the lens, and its edge, are contacted by both lids but predominantly the upper one during blink. Indeed, some front surface designs are such that the lid and lens co-operate in a predetermined manner to enhance movement of the lens during blink (Korb and Korb, 1970).

The contact forces themselves depend on the nature of the surfaces at the positions of contact, and are influenced by the relative shapes and curvatures of these surfaces, the rigidity of the lens material and the cornea, and the wettability of the system, which involves the tears as an essential lubricating agent. In order to minimize contact pressure, a lens design should be such that the curvatures of the principal contacting areas of the lens and the ocular surfaces are compatible with a low concentration of stress, in the static case, and allow smooth lens movement during the dynamic phase.

Corneal metabolism is critically dependent upon the supply, to the cornea, of an adequate amount of oxygen, and upon the outflow from the cornea of carbon dioxide. A contact lens is a barrier to these natural flows, and while the resistance to gas flow is intimately related to the solubility and diffusion constants of the lens material, for a given material, lens design ultimately controls gas flow. Gas flow is controlled in two ways, principally by minimizing thickness as gas flow is inversely proportional to thickness, but also by promoting tear exchange (see Chapter 47).

In a similar way to body implants, contact lenses, when first inserted become coated by a biofilm constituted mainly of mucopolysaccharides. This biofilm is essential to lens biocompatibility, giving to contact lenses their good lens-on-eye wettability. However, it is the denaturation of this biofilm under the effects of the wearing environment and of the care products

that leads to an undesirable coating of discrete or film-like deposits; both are potential causes of adverse effects by promoting additional mechanical trauma and producing toxic effects. Visual performance is also usually reduced by such deposits. Accordingly, one approach has been to develop materials with properties designed to prevent or delay the onset of the build-up of debris; another to replace contact lenses regularly, with the aim of disposal before there is any significant alteration in performance. A fact often ignored, however, is the significant contribution of the back surface which, by enhancing tear flow, promotes the early exit of contaminating materials from the system before they can become a problem. Similarly, specific front surface designs, minimizing zones of irregularity and discontinuity, help to prevent debris build-up.

The contact lens designer's next task is to consider the visual performance of the lens. Here we are concerned not only with achieving the required visual correction, but maintaining good, stable vision over the whole wearing period. Thus it is necessary to achieve a full sphero-cylindrical refractive correction and a retinal image whose quality is unimpaired by changes in aperture size, for example when the pupil is dilated under low ambient luminance. Historically, rigid lenses in particular have consisted largely of systems of co-axial spheres, with a central optical zone and a multiplicity of peripheral zones that have been necessary in order to match the lens to the shape of the corneal surface. This approach has often led to obtaining relatively small optic zones, which reduce performance under low luminance. An alternative approach, made possible by innovations in manufacturing technology, has been the use of aspheric surfaces, usually to help to reduce mechanical trauma. These surfaces, depending upon their characteristics, can lead either to image enhancement by the reduction of abberations, or to image degradation if induced aberrations are not controlled.

Finally we need to consider patient acceptance, which is concerned with subjective comfort, the ability to handle the lens and the level of care and maintenance required to be carried out by the patient, consistent with an adequate level of hygiene.

As previously mentioned, the three design criteria are not independent. For example, the strategy of introducing features to reduce mechanical trauma and promote smooth movement will be reflected not only in the maintenance of corneal integrity, but additionally in improved comfort to the patient. Likewise, the curves which help to match lens and corneal contour can also be of benefit to visual performance, and features that retard debris build-up on the lens surface help both to maintain good comfort and give good vision.

Good lens design, therefore, is based upon these three criteria, in an environment defined by the material's properties, the manufacturing technologies and the system geometries that we have at our disposal.

Contact lenses are often classified broadly into two major categories – 'rigid' and 'soft'. Other descriptions such as hard, flexible, hydrogel, elastomer, gas permeable, etc. may be more appropriate in specific contexts.

In this chapter, the two lens types whose design principles will be considered in detail are rigid gas permeable (RGP) and soft hydrogel lenses.

5.2 THE DESIGN OF RIGID GAS PERMEABLE LENSES

5.2.1 INTRODUCTORY REMARKS

In formalizing the design of rigid gas permeable (RGP) lenses it is both convenient and structurally sound to consider the two surfaces (front and back) of the lens separately.

Considering the back surface first, it is useful to divide this into four distinct zones: the central zone, the mid-periphery, the extreme periphery and the edge. The front surface design is usually considered in two zones, the central zone and peripheral portion. In this context the lens thickness is also discussed as part of the front surface design.

The lens design principles developed for RGP lenses in many instances do not usually specifically involve the lens material. The reason is that with the exception of oxygen permeability, many of the current daily and extended wear materials used have similar physical properties, or differences in physical properties that are not pertinent to lens design. A more influential factor is the lens wear modality. Over the years the design of RGP lenses has evolved, leading to optimization of lens performance for daily wear. The advent of highly gas permeable RGP materials has lead to their successful use in an extended wear modality (Guillon *et al.*, 1993only after specific modifications in lens design to address those specific requirements demanded by extended wear. Modifications are also treated in Chapter 43 on extended wear.

5.2.2 BACK SURFACE DESIGN

Central zone design

Traditionally, the role of the radius of curvature of the back surface optic zone (BOR) has been a major one, principally because lenses were usually spherical and fitting principles evolved around choosing a BOR, which bore a specific relationship to the central curvature of the cornea, the 'keratometric' or 'K' value. From the early days of PMMA, 'Rigid' lenses were fitted so that the lens BOR differed from 'K' by a specific amount. This led to the specification of the 'fitting increment', sometimes referred to as the 'bearing factor' and defined as the value (BOR–K) in millimetres (mm).

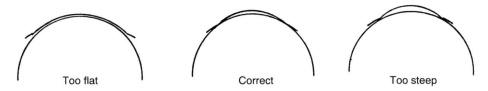

Too flat　　　　　　Correct　　　　　　Too steep

Figure 5.3 Schematic representation of a flat, correct and steep contact bearing relationship.

The criteria of acceptability which developed were based first upon achieving a stable positioning between blinks, and an adequate amplitude of lens movement following blinking and eye movements, and, second, on the absence of visible corneal disturbance following a period of wear. The lens designs developed to attain these acceptable performance criteria are therefore premised on dynamic behaviour and mechanical contact.

Both of these concepts have a common root cause, namely the pressure exerted by the contact lens on the eye. This pressure provides both the resistance to the desired movement and is the initiator of the corneal disturbance.

Rigid lenses are generally fitted such that the lens BOR is slightly steeper than the corneal 'K' value. Lenses fitted very much flatter than 'K' are uncomfortable, centre poorly and move excessively. Lenses which are fitted very much steeper than 'K' can be comfortable, and centre well, but they have too little movement and exert too great a pressure on the corneal tissues to be acceptable.

When the correct fitting increment is achieved, a small tear reservoir is created at the corneal apex. This reservoir is quantified by the thickness of the tear layer measured along the normal to the corneal surface at its apex; this measurement is known as the tear layer thickness (TLT) and is usually given in microns. An optimal fit is achieved when the TLT lies in the range 15 to 25 microns. This requirement is considered to be the first design criterion (Fig. 5.3).

With a co-axial spherical system, the fitting increment, and hence the BOR, (R_0), can be calculated from TLT, the diameter of the back optic zone (D_0) and the corneal 'K' value, using the sagittal depth relationship of two surfaces. The sag function, $S(A,B)$ (Fig. 5.4), is defined as the sagittal depth subtended by a circle of radius 'A' over a base chord 'B'. From the right-angled triangle $X^2 = A^2 - (B/2)^2$, and

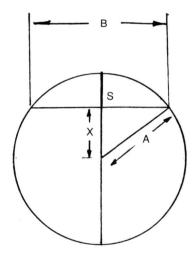

Figure 5.4 Spherical surface sagittal value representation.

$S = A-X$, therefore $S(A,B) = A - \sqrt{\{A^2 - (B/2)^2\}}$

Thus the TLT in the schematic diagram of a spherical lens of BOR(R_0) touching a spherical cornea of central radius 'K' is the difference between two sag functions, one for the lens optic zone and one for the cornea on the same chord (Fig. 5.5).

We therefore write: TLT = $S(R_0, D_0)$ – $S(K, D_0)$, where the sag functions are evaluated by substituting appropriately for 'A' and 'B'. If we now consider the fitting increment $(R_0 - K)$ mm, then a rough ratio between TLT mm and $(R_0 - K)$ mm can be calculated using the sag functions and the approximation $D = RK$. This ratio is of the order 1/8.

Thus we can say to a first approximation:

$$\text{TLT mm} = \frac{(R_0 - K)}{8} \text{ mm or}$$

$$\text{TLT } \mu m = \frac{(R_0 - K)}{8} \text{ mm} \times 1000 \qquad \text{(eqn 5.1)}$$

The contact lens does not touch the cornea at the corneal apex. There is the clearance of the TLT so the contact is further out in the periphery, usually at the edge of the optic zone. At that point a lid force normally applied to the cornea creates a pressure, when the patient blinks, that tends to compress the enclosed tear layer. When this force is removed, a negative pressure develops in the fluid that keeps the lens pressed against the cornea.

The corneal surface is not part of a sphere (see Chapter 17). For mathematical convenience, a number of functional representations of the cornea have been developed (Mandell and St Helen, 1971), their validity depending on the overall region of the cornea under consideration. For RGP lenses it is generally accepted that, because of their smaller diameter, a conic section, usually a prolate ellipse, is a good approximation for the corneal contour (Bennett, 1968). At any point along its surface a conic section is characterized by two instantaneous radii of curvature, referred to as the sagittal and tangential local radii. The former is related to the power of the surface at that point. The usual elliptical form of the cornea is such that the instantaneous sagittal curvature decreases as we move outwards from the apex, that is the cornea flattens, as the sagittal radius increases towards the periphery (Fig. 5.6), although in a few cases, the cornea steepens peripherally.

Clearly, therefore, a spherical curve with the same radius as the apical radius of the cornea must create a small apical clearance. A lens with a radius slightly steeper approaches the corneal surface even more quickly, producing a 'sharp' contact zone with its accompanying region of pressure concentration.

There are several ways to achieve the cor-

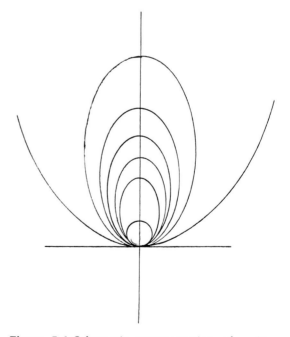

Figure 5.6 Schematic representation of various conic sections.

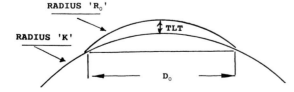

Figure 5.5 Tear layer thickness (TLT) representation.

rect contact lens back surface/corneal front surface interaction. This has led to the development of population-based lens designs aiming to fit a majority of patients and also to individualized designs to fit specific cases.

If we take the minimizing of local pressure at the zone of contact between the contact lens and the cornea as the key design criterion while the other lens fitting properties are respected, a central aspheric zone is a good possibility. A central aspheric zone designed to minimize pressure is generally a conic section which flattens at such a rate (the instantaneous curvature decreases away from the apex), that the contact between the lens and the cornea is spread over a band rather than concentrated at the edge of the optic zone.

We can demonstrate this approach by aiming for an optimum central TLT, and calculating the effect of lens geometry changes for four specific geometric combinations of the lens and corneal surface. These design combinations are:

1. A cornea assumed spherical and a lens with a spherical back optic zone.
2. A cornea assumed spherical and a lens with an aspheric back optic zone.
3. A cornea assumed aspheric and a lens with a spherical back optic zone.
4. A cornea assumed aspheric and a lens with an aspheric back optic zone.

The design parameters which remain constant within these shape choices are the central corneal radius, 'K' and the central TLT. The contact lens back optic radius (R_0), back optic diameter (D_0) and the eccentricity (E_0) of the contact lens become variable parameters which we can manipulate to obtain the optimum TLT for a cornea of any eccentricity.

In order to carry out calculations involving elliptical surfaces, we use the Sag function for a conic section. For convenience a Cartesian co-ordinate representation with the origin at the corneal apex is chosen (Fig. 5.7).

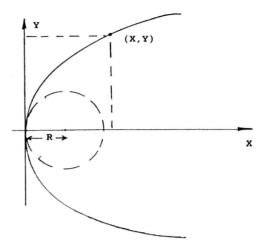

Figure 5.7 Cartesian co-ordinate representation of conic section with origin at surface apex.

Then: $Y^2 = 2RX - pX^2$, where 'R' is the radius of curvature at the apex (the apical radius) and 'p' is a shape constant indicative of the rate of change in curvature from the apex to the periphery. It is related to the conic eccentricity 'e' by the equation $p = 1 - e^2$.

From the above it is a straightforward matter to show that the sag function (S) for this conic representation is:

$$S(D,R,p) = R/p - \sqrt{\{R/p\}^2 - (1/p)(D/2)^2}\}$$
(eqn 5.2)

This confirms that for $p = 1$, ($e = 0$), the formula reduces to that previously derived for a circle $S(R,D)$.

For a prolate (flattening) ellipse, p lies between 0 and 1, whereas an oblate (steepening) ellipse with $p > 1$ is not often encountered as the corneal surface. Parabolic surfaces ($p = 0$), and hyperbolic surfaces ($p < 0$), are not usually encountered as representations of a normal cornea, or contact lens back optic zone (BOZ) surface – hence the limitation of the calculations to the four cases

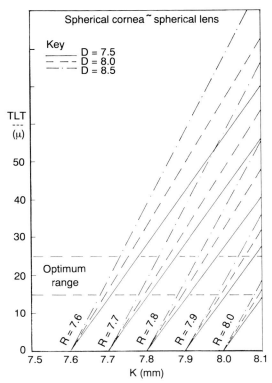

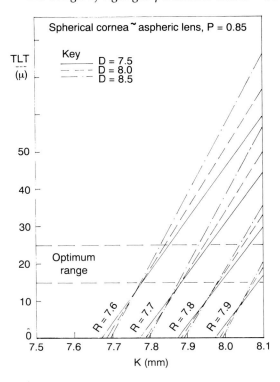

Figure 5.8 (a) Diagrammatic TLT representation for combinations of a spherical cornea and a spherical contact lens for back optic diameters of 7.5, 8.0, 8.5 mm.

Figure 5.8 (b) Diagrammatic TLT representation for combination of spherical cornea and aspheric contact lens ($P = 0.85$) for back optic diameters of 7.5, 8.0 and 8.5 mm.

previously listed. The values of TLT for the four combinations of lens and cornea shapes are thus given by the following set of equations:

1. $\text{TLT} = S(R_0 D_0) - S(K_F D_0)$
2. $\text{TLT} = S(R_0 D_0 p_0) - S(K_F D_0)$
3. $\text{TLT} = S(R_0 D_0) - S(K_F D_0 p_F)$
4. $\text{TLT} = S(R_0 D_0 p_0) - S(K_F D_0 p_F)$

where R_0, contact lens back optic radius; D_0, contact lens back optic diameter; P_0, contact lens back optic zone shape factor; K_F, apical corneal radius in flattest meridian; P_F, corneal shape factor in flattest meridian.

A set of graphs illustrates the effect of the various surface shapes on the choice of parameters required to achieve the optimum

TLT. The effect of 'aspherizing' (towards a prolate ellipse) the cornea with respect to the lens is to flatten the BOR towards 'K', whereas 'aspherizing' (towards a prolate ellipse) the lens with respect to the cornea steepens the BOR away from 'K' (Fig. 5.8).

Mid-peripheral zone design

For any specified central optic zone shape, it is necessary to generate a mid-peripheral zone that conforms to the cornea in that region in order to optimize the zone of contact by minimizing any local induced pressure. Several mid-peripheral zone designs are possible. Generally, but not necessarily, they should be tangential to the

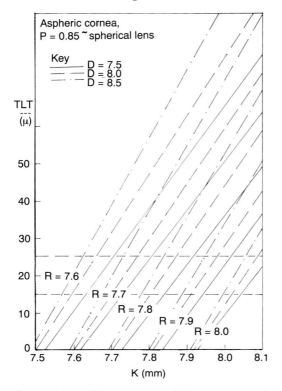

Figure 5.8 (c) Diagrammatic TLT representation for combination of aspheric cornea ($P = 0.85$) and spherical contact lens for back optic diameters of 7.5, 8.0 and 8.5 mm

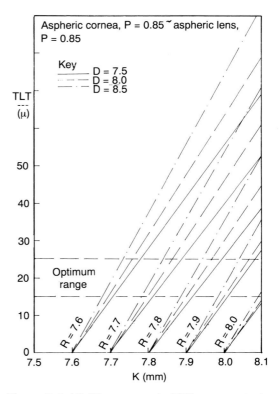

Figure 5.8 (d) Diagrammatic TLT representation for combination of aspheric cornea ($P = 0.85$) and aspheric contact lens ($P = 0.85$) for back optic diameters of 7.5, 8.0 and 8.5 mm.

central zone where these are contiguous. This zone is a region of flatter curvature than the central zone, and may be either spherical or aspheric, the latter a conic section in most cases. An extreme example of a specific conic surface would be a slice parallel to the cone surface, giving a mid-peripheral band which is geometrically flat in cross-section (Thomas, 1968). This mid-peripheral region of the lens surface serves to spread the contact over a larger area and thus reduces the contact pressure.

In order to understand how this construction works, we need to model the lens/cornea contact in terms of mechanics (Sammons, 1984b). There are two principal types of contact between two curved surfaces, 'counter-

formal' and 'conformal' (Fig. 5.9).

The first type of contact, called 'counterformal', refers to a contact where the curvatures of the two surfaces are orientated in *opposite* directions with respect to their common tangent at the point of contact. When this type of contact is encountered there is a dramatic increase in the local pressure in the region of contact. The second type of contact between surfaces is called 'conformal', and occurs when the curvatures are *similarly* orientated with respect to their common tangent. In the second arrangement there is still a pressure concentration (this cannot be avoided with differently curved surfaces), but the intensity of the pressure is very much less.

The designs of the mid-peripheral zone are

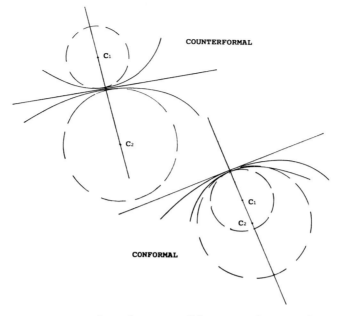

COUNTERFORMAL

CONFORMAL

Figure 5.9 Diagrammatic representation of two possible types of contact between curved surfaces: counterformal with surfaces orientated in opposite directions and conformal with surfaces orientated in same direction.

thus attempts to change a counterformal contact into a conformal one.

The simplest example of a construction of this kind is a central conic curve contiguous with another conic, to which it is tangential at the junction (Guillon *et al.*, 1981).

If we consider this junction to locate the notional BOZ diameter, the central region is defined by its apical radius R_0, diameter D_0 and shape factor 'p_0'. The intermediate zone is then defined by its apical radius R_1, diameter D_1 and shape factor p_1. For example, suppose that this zone is a parabola, with a shape factor $p_1 = 0$ (Fig. 5.10).

Taking the centre of the BOZ as the origin of co-ordinates, the ordinates of points on each of these two profile curves are given by the following equations:

$$Y_0 = \sqrt{\{(R_0/p_0)^2 - (X_0)^2/p_0\}} \qquad \text{(eqn 5.3)}$$

$$Y_1 = (R_p/p) + (1/(2R_p)) \times (D/2)^2 - (X_1)^2) \qquad \text{(eqn 5.4)}$$

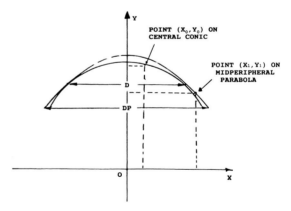

POINT (X_0, Y_0) ON CENTRAL CONIC

POINT (X_1, Y_1) ON MIDPERIPHERAL PARABOLA

Figure 5.10 Diagrammatic representation of tangential contact between elliptical corneal surface and parabolic mid-peripheral contact lens surface.

These equations confirm that when $X_0 = X_1 = D_0/2$, the ordinates Y_0 and Y_1, are equal. This is the point where the elliptical centre meets the flatter parabolic mid-region *tangentially*. A counterformal contact with the cornea has thus been changed into a conformal contact with a much reduced stress concentration (Fig. 5.11).

This construction needs to be used in co-operation with the principles discussed in the earlier section to adjust for optimum tear layer thickness and peripheral edge clearance.

Extreme peripheral zone design

The extreme periphery is defined as the region between the mid-periphery and the edge region and is composed of one or more annular zones near the outer edge of the lens. The width, radius and number of these zones are chosen to cause the back surface of the lens to clear the front surface of the cornea instead of digging into it. A clearance at the edge of the lens is therefore created in which a small reservoir of tears resides. This clearance is defined as the edge clearance (EC) and is given in microns. It is usually measured parallel to the axis of the lens, the axial edge clearance (AEC), or sometimes normal to the contact lens back surface, radial edge clearance (REC). These two values are related in the ratio REC = AEC × cos θ, θ being the half angle subtended by the lens diameter at the centre of the back optic. For conventional RGP lenses the ratio is of the order of 0.8. Excessive clearance, with an AEC greater than 150 μm, generally gives discomfort, and produces corneal desiccation, leading to 3 o'clock and 9 o'clock staining. Insufficient clearance with an AEC of less than 50 μm, usually leads to discomfort and corneal

trauma. The optimum AEC is in the range of 60–100 μm giving good comfort and fewest corneal problems. The calculation of this clearance again involves a collection of sag functions. We use the previous notation for the central zone (R_0, D_0, p_1) and intermediate zone (R_1, D_1, p_1) and extend this to a third zone (R_2, D_2, p_2).

For a bicurve with peripheral curve radius R_1, and overall diameter D_1, as illustrated, the peripheral edge clearance is (Fig. 5.12):

$$AEC = [S(K_F,D_1) - S(K_F,D_0) - S(R_1,D_1) - S(R_1,D_0)] \qquad \text{(eqn 5.5)}$$

For a tricurve, with peripheral curves R_1 and R_2, subtending diameters D_1 and D_2, the peripheral edge clearance is (Fig. 5.13):

$$AEC = [S(K_F,D_2) - S(K_F,D_0)] - [S(R_1,D_1) - S(R_1,D_0)] - [S(R_2,D_2) - S(R_2,D_1)] \qquad \text{(eqn 5.6)}$$

There is a recognizable pattern in this formulation and we can generalize to any number of peripheral curves up to 'n' and obtain the formula:

$$AEC = [S(K_F,D_n) - S(K_F,D_0)] - [S(R_n,D_n) - S(R_n,D_{(n-1)})] \qquad \text{(eqn 5.6)}$$

For elliptical curves, each Sag function is specified with an appropriate shape factor as before. Thus if p_F is the shape factor for the flattest meridian of the cornea and p_n the shape factor for the nth peripheral curve, we have:

$$AEC = [S(K_F,D_n,p_F) - S(K_F,D_0,p_F)] - [S(R_n,D_n,p_n) - S(R_n,D_{(n-1)}p_n)] \qquad \text{(eqn 5.7)}$$

A set of graphs is given for a simple bicurve fitted to a spherical cornea.

As the radius of the peripheral curve is increased (flattened), the edge clearance increases. Increasing the overall diameter, i.e. increasing the annular width of the peripheral curve, also produces an increase in edge clearance. If we now take the cornea to be aspheric, with a shape factor of 0.85, the effect of increasing the radius of the peripheral curve is the same as before, but the effect

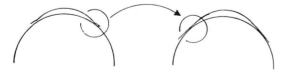

Figure 5.11 Diagrammatic representation of decrease in localized contact stress concentration produced by changing from a counterformal to a conformal mid peripheral curve.

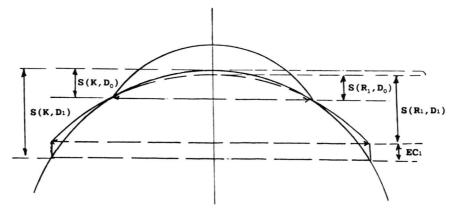

Figure 5.12 Diagrammatic AEC representation for a conic corneal surface and a spherical bicurve contact lens back surface.

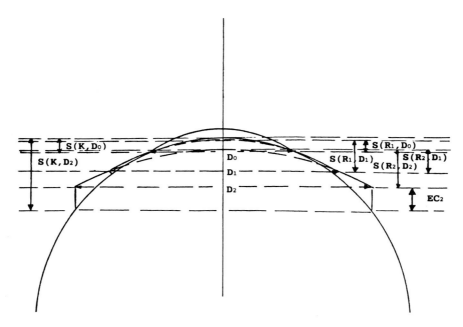

Figure 5.13 Diagrammatic AEC representation for a conic corneal surface and a spherical tricurve contact lens back surface.

of increasing the diameter is not so strong. For a given overall diameter, the edge clearance is smaller for the aspheric cornea ($p = 0.85$), than the spherical cornea, and as the diameter is increased, the increase in edge clearance is less rapid for the former (Fig. 5.14).

For a fixed back optic diameter (BOD), changes in the BOR will have no effect on the edge clearance as long as there is a positive TLT, and the zone of contact between the contact lens and cornea is situated at the edge of the BOZ. Likewise changes in the peripheral geometry will not usually influ-

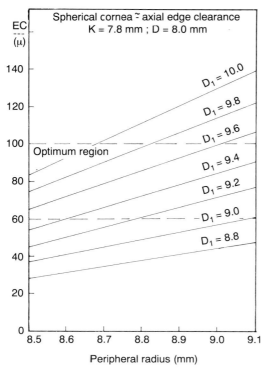

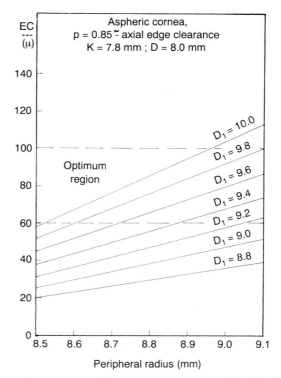

Figure 5.14 (a) Diagrammatic peripheral edge clearance representation for combination of spherical cornea and spherical contact lens for a fixed (8 mm) BOD.

Figure 5.14 (b) Diagrammatic peripheral edge clearance representation for combination of aspheric ($P = 0.85$) cornea and spherical contact lens for a fixed (8 mm) BOD.

ence the tear layer thickness. Thus, having selected a suitable BOD according to set criteria, the TLT and AEC may be 'fine tuned' independently.

Most commonly, contact lenses are produced with a central curve and multiple peripheral curves. In those cases a general contact with the cornea is created within the junction of the centre curve and along the innermost peripheral curve. This generates a zone of pressure, and a concentration of stress, which is influenced by the geometry and quality of the locus of contact. This arrangement is an example of counterformal contact. During manufacturing, an attempt is made to minimize this contact by creating a smooth radius instead of a 'sharp' edge.

Thus the back surface may be a single

curve or a combination of curves, but the objectives remain the same, to produce acceptable lens mobility, minimal corneal trauma due to mechanical pressure and to create optimal tear thicknesses between the contact lens and the cornea at the apex and the edge of the contact lens.

Additional design desiderata apply in the far periphery of the lens. Two important concepts which are influenced by the extreme periphery of the lens are tear exchange and the consequent elimination of debris, and the effect on the lens thickness profile. Increasing the AEC, in particular in association with increased peripheral width, helps to promote tear exchange at blink. This feature was particularly important with PMMA lenses where tear exchange was the main source of oxygenation of the central cornea. Changing the width or the radius of a peripheral curve causes the point at which the lens is thickest to move spontaneously from a point near the edge of the front optic zone to a point closer to the edge of the lens (Sammons, 1981b). This differs from the effect of changing other parameters, for example the front optic diameter, or the lenticular radius. In these cases the point of maximum thickness moves smoothly about the edge of the front optic zone. These parameters can vary by small amounts in the manufacturing process, so if we assert that the lid, during blinking, exerts most of its influence in the region of maximum thickness, changes in the peripheral values will affect the movement characteristics from lens to lens.

5.2.3 FRONT SURFACE DESIGN

Centre thickness

The principal role of the front surface is to establish the power of the lens, given the back optic radius, the lens thickness and the material refractive index.

The first step in designing the contact lens front surface is therefore to set the lens thickness. For negative contact lenses the centre thickness is set, whereas for positive lenses it is the thickness at the edge of the BOZ that is set.

Lens thickness affects a number of lens properties, principally the gas flow through the lens, a permeability property, and its flexibility or stiffness, a mechanical property. The proliferation of new rigid materials in the 1970s and 1980s was based largely upon the need for greater oxygen permeability to fulfil the normal physiological requirements. For these materials, an increased gas flow property was often associated with decreased lens rigidity. The lens designer was then faced with the task of assigning a minimal thickness to the lens so as to maxi-mize gas flow, which was sufficiently high to minimize flexure. If a lens is made too thin, its increased flexibility leads to the lens deforming under the lid induced pressure at blink creating poor vision and poor mechanical performance.

To set a thickness based upon gas flow properties one must understand the mechanism of gas transfer through a contact lens.

If the oxygen diffusion coefficient of the contact lens material is 'D', and its solubility co-efficient is 'k', then the parameter specifying the ability of the material to transmit oxygen is its permeability and is equal to their product 'Dk'. For a material of thickness 'L', the ability of that piece of material to transmit oxygen is the transmissibility and is the ratio Dk/L. Hence, the thinner the material the more oxygen is transmitted. For a contact lens whose thickness is not constant across its diameter, the 'effective' thickness or thickness that best relates to the lens' physiological performance is the 'average' thickness of the lens over a chosen diameter. Because the property of concern is gas flow, the correct average is obtained by calculating the harmonic mean lens thickness over the lens diameter (Sammons, 1980).

Because there is a need to transmit as much oxygen through the lens as possible in order to fulfil such corneal physiological requirements as those established by Holden and Mertz (1984) for both daily and extended wear, hydrogel lenses need to be made thin. These requirements, based on physiological needs, indicate that the minimal oxygen transmissibility criteria are $24.1 \pm 2.7 \times 10^{-9}$ (cm $\times$ ml O_2 $\times$ s^{-1} $\times$ $mmHg^{-1}$) to avoid contact lens induced daily wear oedema and $87.0 \pm 3.3 \times 10^{-9}$ (cm $\times$ ml O_2 $\times$ s^{-1} $\times$ $mmHg^{-1}$) to avoid contact lens induced extended wear oedema. Alternatively, a more attainable criteria for current soft contact lenses for extended wear is $34.3 \pm 5.2 \times 10^{-9}$ (cm $\times$ ml O_2 $\times$ s^{-1} $\times$ $mmHg^{-1}$) to achieve the 8% overnight oedema that is resorbed during open eye wear, and results in no contact lens induced oedema during open eye wear following closed eye wear. From those criteria we have established the minimal acceptable thickness for various RGP materials (Table 5.1). When considering mechanical properties one must understand that mechanical stiffness of a 'plate' of material in flexure, which is the most appropriate mode of deformation for a lens 'bent' over the cornea, is proportional to the cube of the thickness. Hence, if the lens is made very thin, the flexibility increases very rapidly indeed. For example, a 10% decrease in thickness, say from 0.11 mm to 0.10 mm, gives a 30% increase in flexibility. It has been demonstrated that there is a minimum thickness for obtaining the best performance with a rigid lens; for low-power, low-*Dk* silicone acrylate materials (Lydon & Guillon, 1984) that critical thickness is 0.12 mm. Of greater influence on the material rigidity is the decrease in rigidity for materials of higher *Dk* (Fatt, 1986; Stephenson, 1988). Even for material of the same family of polymers, there is a need to increase lens thickness for higher *Dk* lenses, the habitual increase being from 0.12 mm for *Dk* 40 to approximately 0.15 mm for *Dk* 70 or more. Lens thickness is also usually increased for larger diameter lenses by approximately 0.02 mm.

There are, however, exceptions to these rules between *Dk* and flexibility, as illustrated, for example, in the Boston range of material whereby Boston RX with a *Dk* of 45 can be made as thin as lenses in PMMA.

Centre thickness also influences lens volume, and therefore the total mass of the lens. Given the material density, then the centre thickness should be made sufficiently small, compatible with the requirements given above, to make the lens mass as small as possible so that it plays an insignificant role in lens centration. Lens mass consideration

Table 5.1 Minimal acceptable thickness for RGP materials

CONTACT LENS MATERIAL	*Dk*	0% Daily wear		4% Extended wear		8% (0% Resid) Extended wear	
		Mean	95% Range	Mean	95% Range	Mean	95% Range
Airlens	15.7b	65	84–53				
Albertor N	14.7a	61	79–50				
Boston II	11.6b	48	62–39				
Boston IV	19.6b	81	105–66				
Equalens	49.0a	203	262–166	56	61–52	143	205–110
Fluro O_2	36.5b	151	195–124	42	45–39	106	153–82
Fluroperm	63.0a	261	337–213	72	78–67	184	264–141
Menicon Ex	35.8b	148	191–121	41	45–38	104	150–80
Optacryl Ext	39.0a	162	209–132	45	49–42	114	163–87
Optacryl Z	55.0a	228	294–186	63	68–59	160	230–123
Paraperm EW	39.0a	162	209–132	45	49–42	114	163–87
Paraperm O_2	12.0a	50	64–41				
Quantum	45.0a	187	241–153	52	56–48	131	188–101
Toray A	131.0a	544	700–444	151	163–140	382	548–293

RGP material – maximum acceptable thickness in micron to fulfil Holden and Mertz criteria (Holden asnd Mertz, 1984) for: (1) 0% swelling during daily wear; (2) 4% swelling at waking during extended wear; (3) 8% swelling at waking during extended wear (equivalent to 0% residual swelling during open eye wear following extended wear). *Dk* values are given in $cm^2 \times s \times ml\ O_2 \times ml \times mmHg$. The values chosen were: (1) the mean values from Holden *et al.* (1990) whenever available; and (2) the mean values for the wet measurements from Winterton *et al.* (1988) when (1) not available.

is usually of secondary importance when setting the lens thickness, because for a given power requirement the possibility of manipulating these parameters is limited. This limitation is due to the similarity in specific weight and flexibility properties between the different materials available. There are two exceptions to this however, the butyrene and fluorocarbon materials. The former has a very low specific weight (0.97) compared to silicone acrylate materials, and a lens strength similar to PMMA, higher than the rigidity of silicone acrylate materials. This material is particularly useful when a lens is bulky and riding low. Both the high rigidity and low specific weight will contribute to reducing the weight and volume. Fluorocarbon, on the contrary, is highly flexible and has a high specific weight (1.58) and should generally be limited to low power lenses, and patients with low astigmatism ($<$ 1.50 D).

Central zone

The front optic zone (FOZ) is the central zone whose function is to provide the lens with an accurate, stable, refractive power which does not fluctuate during large lens excursions. This implies that the FOZ must be sufficiently large in relation to the pupil size so that visual performance is constant, even at low luminance, and glare is eliminated. The front surface is usually spherical, the least demanding shape to make and measure, but the use of non-spherical shapes can be considered in order to modify both the profile and optical characteristics of the lens. If the surface is considered to be spherical and the power of the lens is 'F' dioptres, the required front surface of curvature R_{a1} can be calculative from the formula:

$$R_{a1} = \frac{1 + ((N-1)/N{\cdot}T/R)}{(1/R_0) + (F/(1000{\cdot}(N-1)))} \qquad \text{(eqn 5.8)}$$

where N, refractive index; T, centre thickness.

Peripheral zone

Normally it is not possible to achieve a front surface which is a continuous single curve across the whole lens diameter. With most negative lenses this would give an unacceptably thick edge, and with most positive lenses excessive thickness at the geometric centre of the lens. Hence, whereas the optic zone should be as large as possible for a good visual performance, there are other issues, chiefly comfort and mechanical performance, which limit the size to which the FOZ can be made. A suitable peripheral zone of different curvature, known as lenticulation, is therefore introduced. Generally spherical, co-axial with the front and back surfaces, (no prism assumed), the geometry of the lenticular zone is usually determined by assigning a suitable value to the extreme edge of the lens.

A simple lenticulated front surface construction for a negative lens is given in Fig. 5.15.

If we fix the axial edge thickness (AET) as defined in Figure 5.15 the lenticular radius (R_{a2}) can be calculated from the following set of equations:

$$R_{a2} = \sqrt{((A - B)^2 + (D_{a1}/2)^2)}$$
$$A = R_0 + \text{AET} + S(R_1,D_0) - S(R_1 D_{a1}) - S(R_0,D_0)$$
$$B = [(A^2 - C^2) - (1/4)(Da_0^2 - (Da_1)^2)]/2{\cdot}(A - C)$$
$$C = R_0 + Ct - S(R_{a1}, D_{a0}) \qquad \text{(eqn 5.9–5.12)}$$

From these data it is possible to calculate the ordinate of any point on the front (Y_F), or back (Y_B), surface for a given radial distance 'X'. Their difference ($Y_F - Y_B$) gives the 'axial thickness' for any value of 'X' (Fig. 5.16).

By multiplying the axial thickness by the cosine of the angle between the axis and the normal to the front surface, that is $\cos(\arcsin (X/R_{a1}))$, we obtain a good approximation to the 'radial thickness' at 'X'. Radial thickness is the most appropriate thickness to use in gas transmission calculations because gases propagate normally to the surface and not along the

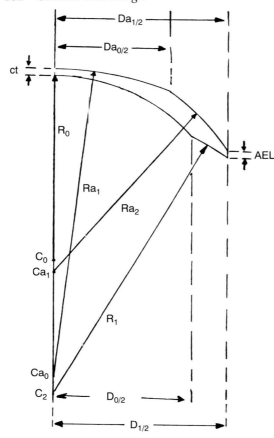

Figure 5.15 Lenticular front surface construction for a negative contact lens.

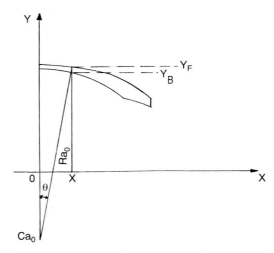

Figure 5.16 Contact lens section diagrammatic representation demonstration: the calculation of the axial edge thickness at any point of the lens.

geometric axis of the lens. There is, unfortunately, no handy algorithm with which to calculate the harmonic mean thickness of a contact lens. Unlike the arithmetic mean, which is found by integration, and is simply equal to lens volume divided by the back surface area, the harmonic mean has to be worked out numerically, point by point.

Variations can be made in the form of the lenticular zone which give the contact lens additional features; principally by the incorporation of an aspheric optic and/or peripheral zone. The aspheric front optic zone may be such that it produces its own peripheral flattening or steepening and in that way constitutes the lenticular construction. A steepening ellipse (oblate) will assist lenticulation for a negative lens, while a flattening conic (a prolate ellipse, parabola or hyperbola) will assist lenticulation for a positive lens. This latter construction has been used to make 'thin' aphakic lenses by designing a hyperbolic front surface, ($'p_1' = -1.25$) (Sammons, 1983; Bleshoy and Guillon, 1984). With such aspheric constructions, the lenticular 'junction' is made much smoother than the abrupt change in curvature and slope obtained with standard lenticulation.

The shape factor required to achieve the correct geometry with a single aspheric curve involving the optic zone and the lens periphery leads, in some cases, to a power gradient across the optic zone that adversely affects the patient's visual performance. In those cases an alternative strategy is to incorporate a separate lenticular curve with a common tangent to the optic curve where they meet at the edge of the optic zone. The lenticular curve may either be spherical or aspheric. The essential feature of this construction is that the centre of the lenticular curve is no longer on the axis but is offset. The lens profile can be modified by this means, so that the average thickness can be used to control gas flow, and the position of maximum thickness to influence lens movement.

Lens edge

The extreme edge of the lens is a combination of both front and back surface geometry and is designed principally to create comfort and provide minimal interference with the tear film. Traditionally the production of the lens edge has involved hand finishing or semi-automated finishing using various abrasive and polishing tools as part of a mechanical polishing process. The net result of that process is that the precise edge design is lost and its accurate description in terms of curves is impossible. The problem of precisely describing the lens edge was in the main solved by Mandell (1977) who removed the subjectivity of defining optimal lens edge by introducing a totally new reference system to quantify contact lens edges. The Mandell system, known as the boxing system (Fig. 5.17) identifies the extreme lens edge profile by four parameters: the edge height, 'H', and the edge thicknesses at 0.05, 0.20 and 0.50 mm, respectively, from the tip of the lens. The edge height is the distance of the extreme edge of the lens, that is the 'tip of the lens' measured normally to a template 0.50 mm long which is tangential to the lens back surface. The three lens thicknesses used to characterize the edge profile are also measured normally, with reference to the same template (Fig. 5.17).

Using the boxing system to characterize the lens edge of PMMA lenses, Mandell carried out an extensive clinical investigation of the comfort achieved with 20 different lens edge profiles. The optimal lens edge, that is the edge achieving the greatest comfort, was an edge with a height of 0.03 mm and thicknesses of 0.08, 0.14 and 0.16 mm at 0.05, 0.20

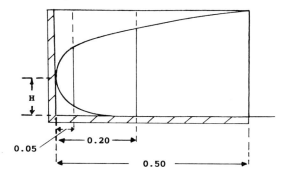

Figure 5.17 Mandell Box classification system for RGP lens edge profile.

and 0.50 mm, respectively, from the extreme edge (e) (Fig. 5.18) The key characteristics for a good edge were a thin profile with a rounded tip and an apex positioned closer to the back surface of the lens than to the front surface. Thick lens edge profiles (n) (Fig. 5.18), and in particular edge profiles with apex displaced towards the lens front surface (t) (Fig. 5.18), were particularly uncomfortable.

Recently Guillon and co-workers (Guillon *et al.*, 1987) developed a non-destructive method based on optical pachometry to characterize lens edges in a manner similar to

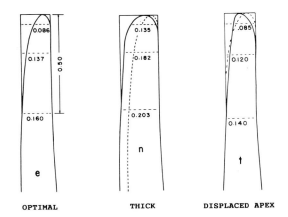

Figure 5.18 Diagrammatic edge profile representation of an optimal edge (e), a thick edge (n) and an edge with displaced apex (t) as regarded by Mandell (by courtesy of Mandell, 1974).

Mandell's Box System, using three RGP trial sets, made by different manufacturers from different materials, (two have a tricurve design and a third an aspheric design). The investigation showed that (Table 5.2): (a) the lens edges produced were fairly repeatable; (b) the average lens edge profiles for the three trial sets were very similar despite the markedly different nominal thicknesses supplied by the manufacturer (Fig. 5.19); and (c) the average edge profile was slightly thicker, but close to the Mandell ideal edge for PMMA lenses (0.095 versus 0.08 mm; 0.18 versus 0.14 mm and 0.20 versus 0.16 mm at 0.05, 0.20 and 0.50 mm, respectively, from the extreme edge) confirming that the Mandell profile is suitable for RGP lenses and should be a targeted design.

Confirmation of Mandell's ideal design that the position of the apex should be close to the lens posterior surface was given by La Hood (1988) who compared, in a masked fashion, the comfort achieved with four different PMMA edge profiles and found that a well rounded anterior edge was essential for good comfort for lenses of similar thickness.

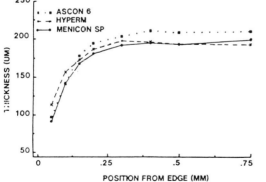

DIAGNOSTIC SETS AVERAGE EDGE SHAPE

Figure 5.19 Average edge thickness distribution from apex to 0.75 mm in from apex for three RGP diagnostic sets.

5.3 THE DESIGN OF HYDROGEL LENSES

5.3.1 INTRODUCTORY REMARKS

The discussion on the design of rigid lenses has laid down the basic ideas of how lens shape controls lens function. Much of the geometrical material is the same when hydrogel lenses are considered. However, the mechanics of a hydrogel lens when placed on the cornea impose quite a different set of criteria for creating a hydrogel lens design.

Contrary to RGP lenses, lens material plays a significant role in hydrogel lens design.

The variation in water content from 38 to 80% for current hydrogel materials imparts to those materials wide ranging physical properties that directly dictate lens design characteristics, two of which are of key influence. These are oxygen permeability and water pervaporation. Both properties increase with the level of hydrophilicity and decrease with increased lens thickness. These properties force the lens designer to make lens designs 'material specific', or at least specific to a narrow range of hydrophilicity, and lens design usually begins by consideration of the lens thickness. Because the lens thickness affects the lens mechanical performance the choice of the lens thickness profile must precede the choice of the exact back surface characteristics. Therefore the discussion of hydrophilic lens design will start with the lens thickness profile.

5.3.2 LENS THICKNESS

As with RGP lenses the contact lens oxygen transmissibility, for any given hydrogel material, is inversely proportional to the lens thickness. Like RGP lenses, the criteria to follow are those of Holden and Mertz (1984). The key aspect to remember when deciding upon a hydrogel contact lens thickness according to these criteria is that

Table 5.2 Material and lens design information in edge thickness study by courtesy of Guillon *et al.*, 1987)

Lens name	Manufacturer	*n*	Lens design	Nominal edge thickness
Ascon 6	Hecht Contact Linsen (Germany)	1.471	Aspheric	0.05 mm at 0.075 mm from edge
Hyperm	Hydron Europe (England)	1.470	Tricurve	0.14 mm
Menicon SP	Tokyo (Japan)	1.481	Tricurve	0.08 mm at 0.4 mm from edge

they do not apply just to the centre of the lens but also to the central 6 mm of the cornea. Thus such a criterion is debatable, and stricter criteria could be required to fulfil the corneal physiological requirements at all points over the cornea. At least one study (Guillon, 1982) using lenses of equal transmissibility over the cornea, but with different profiles, showed that: (a) the corneal swelling at any point was directly dependent upon the contact lens transmissibility at that point; and (b) the overall corneal physiological stress produced by lenses of equal transmissibility over the whole cornea was similar. Hence, one can take an extreme position and argue that the criteria suggested should apply to the thickest point of the lens over the cornea, the transmissibility over the central 6 mm diameter representing the criteria for the central corneal response for negative lenses. As the oxygen needs of the cornea appear to be similar over the whole corneal surface we suggest that to assess the overall contact lens induced corneal stress, the criteria chosen for oxygen transmissibility should be assessed over a diameter similar to the corneal diameter, 10 to 12 mm. Table 5.3 gives the thicknesses required to achieve the criteria indicated by Holden and Mertz (1984) for a low water (38%), a mid-water (55%) and a high water (70%)

content contact lens. These values are given for the average patient, and also for the 95% range of patients (± 2 standard deviation points) from the least to the most demanding patient in terms of oxygen consumption.

As can be seen from Table 5.3, the thickness required in some cases, whereas achievable with modern manufacturing techniques, are not acceptable because of the dehydration and flexure characteristics that such a thickness would give to the lens.

Several studies (Holden *et al.*, 1986; Zantos *et al.*, 1986; McNally *et al.*, 1987) have shown that below a critical thickness the lens performance is altered in such a way that it creates, in certain patients, unacceptable corneal staining. Several factors are included in this process, in particular localized lens dehydration (Guillon and Guillon, 1990), and unstable water flow at the lens surface (Fatt, 1990). The staining response is highly patient-dependent, some requiring fairly thick contact lenses to avoid epithelial staining. The staining response is also material- and environment-dependent; the higher water content material requires a greater thickness to avoid staining. Low hygrometry and high temperature environments produce the most staining when all other conditions are unchanged (Orsborn and Zantos, 1988).

Table 5.3 The thickness necessary to achieve the Holden and Mertz (1984) criteria

Contact lens type	Dk	0% Daily wear		8% (0% Residual) Extended wear	
		Mean	95% Range	Mean	95% Range
Acuvue	13.6	56	73–46	40	57–30
B&L 04	4.5	19	24–15	13	19–10
B&L U4	21.9	90	117–74	64	92–49
B&L 70	3.8	16	20–13	11	16–9
Cibasoft	4.5	19	24–15	13	19–10
CSI	8.2	34	44–28	24	34–18
Permaflex	21.1	88	113–72	62	88–47
Permalens	20.6	85	110–70	60	86–46

Hydrogel lens type acceptable thickness in micron to fulfil Holden and Mertz (1984) criteria: (1) 0% swelling during daily wear; (2) 8% swelling at waking during extended wear (equivalent to 0% residual swelling during open eye wear following extended wear). *Dk* values are given in $cm^2 \times ml\,O_2 \times ml \times mmHg$. All *Dk* values from Winterton *et al.* (1988).

Designs with current materials generally have minimal thickness 0.035 mm for low water content lenses (38%), 0.055 mm for mid-water content (55%) and 0.10 mm for high water content (70%).

Another feature of very thin lenses is their tendency to mould closely to the cornea and generate a high resistance to movement. Thus, while undoubtedly the gas transmission is higher, the lack of movement gives less opportunity for the dispersal of metabolic waste, and the overall lens performance suffers. There is clearly a need to balance the conflicting requirements of thickness and movement, just as in the case of the RGP lens, although the mechanisms for these two lens types are different.

The cause of this dehydration is still debatable, but certainly temperature (Fatt and Chaston, 1980a,b) and possibly pH, osmolarity and partial evaporation play a part.

5.3.3 BACK SURFACE DESIGN

With hydrogel lenses, the role of the back optic radius is of much less significance than is the case with rigid lenses. Hydrogel lenses, depending on their thickness, tend to 'mould' to the surface of the cornea, so that

the initial relationship between the BOR and the corneal curvature is lost. Originally, hydrogel lenses were considerably thicker than they are now, and were largely of lower water content, thus giving them much greater rigidity. The structural rigidity of a thin shell of material, already described for RGP lenses, is proportional to the cube of the thickness for bending stress. This bending stress is also proportional to the elastic modulus, which increases as the water content is made lower. For these thicker low

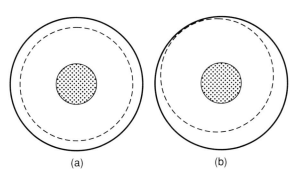

Figure 5.20 Diagrammatic representation of: (a) Optimally centring soft contact lens. (b) Decentred soft contact lens, still achieving full corneal coverage.

water contact lenses there was sometimes a meaningful 'fitting increment' relationship. In most cases, however, this parameter was often little more than a guide.

With soft lenses, the first requirement is adequate corneal coverage. This means that, in the static condition, the edge of the lens should overlap the cornea by at least 0.5 mm (Fig. 5.20). As lenses do not all settle perfectly in a central position, the soft lens diameter on the eye should be at least 13.6 mm, and preferably 14.0 mm, to satisfy a normal population of which the central diameter is 12.5 mm (Martin and Holden, 1985).

However, lenses tend to dehydrate when taken from the container and placed on the eye, and the amount of dehydration that takes place varies with the water content and the type of material in general (Fig. 5.21) (Brennan and Efron, 1987). High water content materials lose more water than those with low water content (Fatt and Chaston, 1980b). The net effect of this is a shrinkage in lens dimensions, so both the BOR (Chaston and Fatt, 1981) and lens diameter decrease. The implication when designing the contact lens is to consider the material factor when deciding upon the nominal contact lens diameter, which is usually measured, fully hydrated, in standard saline at 20 °C. Modern hydrophilic lenses of 38% water content are usually available with a 14.0 mm diameter, whereas high water content lenses most commonly have a diameter of 14.4 mm or more.

With a soft lens, when the lids close in blinking, the tears behind the lens are squeezed out by the force of the blink, and the lens is stretched by tangential membrane forces as the lens is moulded to align to the cornea. After the blink, the contraction of the lens back to its equilibrium form lags behind due to the visco-elastic nature of the material, so that the suction or squeeze pressure generated behind the lens remains and gives a resistance to motion which decreases with time (Fig. 5.22).

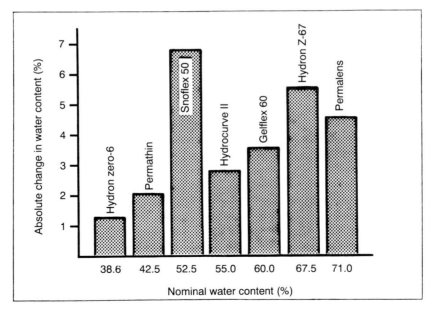

Figure 5.21 Dehydration characteristics (H_2O content diminution) for contact lenses made from materials of different water contents when going from vial to the eye (by courtesy of Brennan & Efron, 1987).

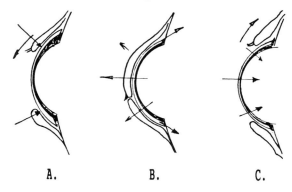

Figure 5.22 Force exerted by the lids during blink and material reaction creates a variable negative squeeze pressure: (a) before blink; (b) during blink; (c) on eye opening, behind the contact lens.

A lens is mobile only when the lid can generate enough force to overcome this suction effect and this is aided by a large fitting increment and by lens rigidity, but bearing in mind the limited usefulness of a 'fitting increment' approach, it has been found best to fit hydrogel lenses with a small positive fitting increment leading most commonly to a nominal BOR of 8.4 to 9.0 mm.

The squeeze pressure is highly dependent upon the lens rigidity. Below a certain threshold, for which Martin *et al.* (1989) give a value of 1370 dyn/cm^2, there is virtually no movement regardless of changes in lens BOR. The thinner the lens, the wider is this range of ineffective BOR flattening. For values above 1370 dyn/cm^2, increasing thickness is the most effective way of achieving lens movement.

Other factors, such as tear osmolarity, also affect hydrogel lens dimensions in a way that is not found with rigid lenses, so that lenses tend to tighten and shrink on the eye; if they are thin, and such tightening takes them below the threshold, then mobility is lost.

Contact pressure is less concentrated with hydrogel lenses due to their much lower mechanical stiffness and elastic modulus; a mechanical model which is an adaptation of the classic treatment of Hertz (1895) helps to

understand the phenomenon. According to this model, the maximum pressure generated over a small contact area between two curved surfaces of radii R_1 and R_2, whose elastic moduli are E_1 and E_2 respectively, is proportional to the quantity:

$$\sqrt{[E_1 E_2/(E_1 + E_2)\,(R_1 + R_2)/R_1 R_2]} \quad \text{(eqn 5.13)}$$

Thus if E_1 and R_1 refer to the lens, and E_2 and R_2 to the cornea, for a rigid lens $E_1 >> E_2$, so the overall modulus term is approximately equal to E_2. For a hydrogel, E_1 and E_2 are roughly equal and the overall modulus is $E_2/2$. Thus, for comparable curvatures, the maximum pressure for a rigid lens is about 1½ times that for a hydrogel.

Peripheral curves play a different role in the design of a hydrogel lens compared with a rigid lens. First, the hydrogel lens periphery is much simpler than RGP lens periphery. There is rarely more than one peripheral curve on the back surface of a hydrogel lens. This single zone can however, be manipulated to influence lens movement to a much greater extent than the RGP periphery, and can be very effectively controlled by varying its width and radius. The role of the peripheral curve is not to create a reservoir of tears at the lens periphery but to avoid undue pressure on the bulbar conjunctiva and so prevent movement. Overall sagittal depth can be varied with this parameter, but more important, we can control the effective overall diameter and through this the intensity of the suction force (Fig. 5.23).

The overall sagittal depth for a bicurve, with BOR parameters R_o and D_o, and peripheral curve parameters R_1 and D_1, is:

$$\text{Sag} = S(R_o,D_o) + S(R_1,D_1) - S(R_1,D_o)$$
$$\text{(eqn 5.14)}$$

The effective overall diameter is 'D_o', which is controlled by varying the width, W, of the peripheral curve. Hence effective diameter = $D_1 - 2W$.

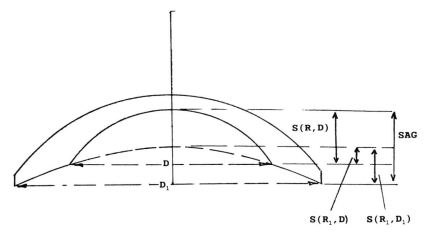

Figure 5.23 Diagram showing the relative sagitta of the contact lens back surface and cornea responsible for producing the negative squeeze pressure behind the contact lens.

5.3.4 FRONT SURFACE DESIGN

The factors which have to be considered in designing the front surface of a hydrogel lens are, in principle, the same as for the RGP lens. In the case of the hydrogel lens, the upper lid, in the open condition, covers more of the lens and this will have an effect on the means adopted to provide the lens with features which assist the top lid to develop movement. Such features include off-centre spherical and aspheric lenticular regions which distribute the mass differently near the periphery, and place the maximum lens thickness in a favourable position.

The soft lens edge shows more variation between lens designs than does its RGP counterpart. Many early soft lenses, which were usually fairly thick – 0.15 to 0.25 mm, compared to modern lenses which are generally less than 0.10 mm – were fabricated by lathing a dry precursor and hydrating this into the final soft lens. At the dry lens stage, the edge was prepared in much the same way as the then hard PMMA lens and the edge has followed very much the Mandell precepts. Soft lens fabrication techniques, however, were not limited to lathing, and edge forms which are characteristic of the

method of manufacture have been developed. The method which was used in parallel with the early lathed lenses was 'spin casting', and this method produced the familiar 'wafer-like' edge form. More recently, developments in cast moulding have yielded their own special forms. In one type of moulding process the lens is first produced in dry form, when it is possible to reshape the edge by polishing techniques before hydration. In another process, wet moulding, the lens is produced directly in its final hydrophilic form, so the edge is dependent on the mould design and the moulding process.

5.3.5 INFLUENCE OF MATERIAL ON DESIGN

The design of hydrophilic lenses is influenced by the hydration mechanism which swells the lens from the dry state to the soft wet lens. The dimensions increase by a specific amount which, ideally, is given by the 'swell factor' (SF):

$$SF = \frac{\text{wet dimension}}{\text{dry dimension}} \qquad \text{(eqn 5.15)}$$

and the power decreases by a specific amount, the 'power factor' (PF):

$$PF = \frac{\text{dry power}}{\text{wet power}} \qquad \text{(eqn 5.16)}$$

However, hydrophilic lenses do not swell from the dry form by the same amount in all directions. They have an anisotropic swelling behaviour (Sammons, 1981a), and this means that the diameter, thickness and associated radii of curvature require different swell factors. If we define fundamental swell factor components as shown in Fig. 5.24, then we can calculate the derived factor, which is appropriate to the radius.

If we assume that the swell factor is different in all the three axis directions, then the single swell factor defined above is replaced by a complicated nine-component hydration matrix operator. However, if we make some reasonable simplifying assumptions, i.e. the hydration is the same in all directions lying in the plane of the lens diameter, then the hydration operator is a simple 2×2 diagonal matrix (Fig 5.25).

The appropriate swell factors for the diameter, thickness and radius are then

$SF(\text{diameter}) = S_1$
$SF(\text{thickness}) = S_2$
$SF(\text{radius}) = (S_1)^2/S_2$

The power swell factor is given approximately by the formula:

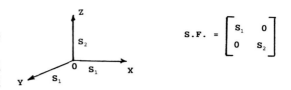

Figure 5.25 Figure showing the shape factor transformation from a xerogel to hydrated contact lens using a 2 × 2 matrix.

$$PF = SF(\text{radius})\,(N(\text{dry}) - 1)/(N(\text{wet}) - 1) \qquad \text{(eqn 5.17)}$$

The implications for design are related both to lens fit and visual performance. The hydration of a material with these anisotropic properties changes a spherical dry shape into a hydrated ellipse. This asphericity is sufficient to predict differences in base curve shape and visual aberrations from a lens designed purely on the assumption of isotropy.

A further structural feature of hydrophilic materials fabricated in the form of a thin lens which has design implications, is inhomogeneity (Sammons, 1984a; Sammons, 1989). This feature has been modelled in the form of a two-phase system, in which the outer region of the material, (the 'skin'), differs in swell behaviour from the central region, (the 'core') (Fig. 5.26).

Such a structure can result from a fabrication process such as moulding, in which the skin polymer is ordered differently from the

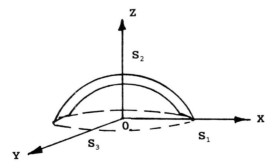

Figure 5.24 Diagram showing swell factors associated with the hydration of soft contact lenses initially produced as a xerogel.

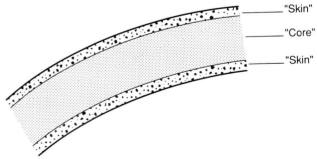

Figure 5.26 Diagrammatic representation of structural features of hydrogel materials.

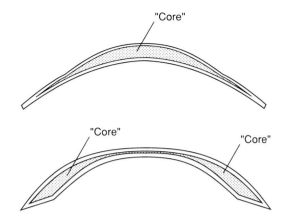

"Core"

"Core"   "Core"

Figure 5.27 Diagram showing the association of 'core' and 'skin' parts of a contact lens with different powers.

core material due to the effect of the nearby surfaces on polymerization. On the basis of this model the hydrated lens form would depend on the lens thickness, as the skin to core proportions would vary with the total thickness (Fig. 5.27).

The lens design will have to take this into account, otherwise a simple consequence of this is the different swell behaviour of plus and minus lenses which start out with, say, similar dry BOR.

REFERENCES

Bennett, A.G. (1968) Aspherical contact lens surfaces, part two. *Ophthal. Optician*, **30** (11), 1297–311.

Bleshoy, H. and Guillon, M. (1984) Aspheric aphakic soft lens design – clinical results. *J. Br. Contact Lens Assoc.* 7(1), 41–7.

Brennan, N.A. and Efron, N. (1987) Hydrogel lens dehydration: a material dependent phenomenon. *Contact Lens Spectrum*, **2**(4), 28–9.

Chaston, J. and Fatt, I. (1981) The influence of temperature on the base curve of hard plus soft contact lenses. *Int Contact Lens Clin.* 8(1), 42–50.

Fatt, I. (1986). Performance of gas permeable hard lenses on the eye. *Br. Contact Lens Assoc. Trans. Am. Clin. Conf.*, **9**, 32–7.

Fatt, I. (1989) A productive model for dehydration of a hydrogel contact lens in the eye. *J. Br. Contact Lens Assoc.*, **12**(2), 15–31.

Fatt, I. and Chaston, J. (1980a) The temperature of a contact lens in the eye. *Int. Contact Lens Clin.* 7(5), 195–8.

Fatt, I. and Chaston, J. (1980b) The effect of temperature or refractive index, water content and central thickness of hydrogel contact lenses. *Int. Contact Lens Clin.* 7(6), 250–5.

Guillon, M. (1982) Topographical study of corneal swelling for lenses of identical oxygen transmissibility. *J. Br. Contact Lens Assoc.*, **5**(4), 130–40.

Guillon, M., Lydon, D.P.M. and Sammons, W.A. (1983) Designing rigid gas permeable contact lenses using the edge clearance technique. *J. Br. Contact Lens Assoc.*, **6**(19), 22–6.

Guillon, M., Crosbie-Walsh, J. and Brynes, D. (1987) Application of pachometry to the measurement of rigid contact lens edge profile. *J. Br. Contact Lens Assoc.* **10**(2), 16–22.

Guillon, J.P., Guillon, M. and Malgouyres, S. (1990) Corneal desiccation staining with hydrogel lenses: tear film and contact lens factors. *Ophthal. Physiol. Opt.*, 10, 343–50.

Hayashi, T.T. (1977) *Mechanics of Contact Lens Motion.* PhD dissertation, University of California, Berkeley.

Hertz, H. (1895) *Gesammelte Werke*, **1**.

Holden, B.A. and Mertz, G.W. (1984) Critical oxygen levels to avoid corneal oedema for daily and extended wear contact lenses. *Invest. Ophthalmol. Vis. Sci.*, **1161–7**.

Holden, B.A., Sweeney, D.F. and Seger, R.G. (1986) Epithelial erosions caused by thin high water contact lenses. *Clin. Exp. Optom.*, **69**, 103–7.

Holden, B.A., Newton-Howes, J., Winterton, L., Fatt, I., Hamano, H., La Hood, D., Brennan, N.A. and Efron, N., (1990) The Dk project: an interlaboratory comparison of Dk measurements. *Optom. Vis. Sci.*, **67**, 476–81.

Korb, D.R. and Korb, J.E. (1970) A new concept in contact lens design parts 1 and 2. *J. Am. Optom. Assoc.* **41**, 1023–34.

La Hood, D. (1988) Edge shape and comfort of rigid lenses. *Am. J. Optom. Physiol. Opt.* **65**, 613–18.

Lydon, D.P.M. and Guillon, M. (1984) Effect of centre thickness variations on the performance of rigid gas permeable contact lenses. *Am. J. Optom. Physiol. Opt.*, **61**, 23–7.

Mandell, R.B. (1979) *Contact Lens Practice – hard and Flexible Lenses*, 2nd ed, CC Thomas, Springfield, LL.

Mandell, R.B. and St Helen, R. (1971) Mattre matical model of the corneal contour. *Br. J. Physiol. Opt.*, **26**, 183–97.

Martin, D.K., Boulos, J., Gan, J., Gauriel, K. and Harvey, R. (1989) A unifying parameter to describe the clinical mechanics of hydrogel contact lenses. *Optom. Vis. Sci.*, **66**, 87–91.

McNally, J.J., Chalmers, R. and Payor, R. (1987) Corneal epithelial disruption with extremely thin hydrogel lenses. *Clin. Exp. Optom.*, **70**, 106–111.

Orsborn, G.N. and Zantos, S.G. (1990) Corneal desiccation staining with thin high water content contact lenses. *Contact Lens Assoc. Ophthalmol. J.*, **14**, 81–4.

Sammons, W.A. (1980) Contact lens thickness and all that. *The Optician*, **December 5**.

Sammons, W.A. (1981a) A mathematical description of soft lens hydration, Part 1. *Am. J. Optom. Physiol. Opt.*, **58**, 718–24.

Sammons, W.A. (1981b) Thin lens design and average thickness. *J. Br. Contact Lens Assoc.*, **4**, 90–7.

Sammons, W.A. (1983) Thin aphakic soft lenses. *Am. J. Optom. Physiol. Opt.*, **60**, 100.

Sammons, W.A. (1984a) The naive cornea. *J. Br. Contact Lens. Assoc.*, **7**(4), 182–90.

Sammons, W.A. (1984b). Lens – eye geometry. *Proc. Europ. Contact Lens Soc. Ophthalmol. Helsinki,*

Sammons, W.A. (1989) The Nissel memorial lecture. Manufacturing – materials, methods and measurements. *J. Br. Contact Lens Assoc.*, **12**, 12–19.

Stevenson, R.V.W. (1988) Design considerations of gas permeable lenses. *J. Br. Contact Lens Assoc. Trans. Int. Conf.*, **11**, 29–33.

Thomas, P.F. (1968) The prescribing of 'Conoid' contact lens. *Contacto*, **12**(1), 66–9

Winterton, L.C., White, J.C. and Su, K.C. (1988) Contrometrically determined oxygen flux and resultant Dk of commercially available contact lenses. *Int. Contact Lens Clin.*, **15**, 117–23.

Zantos, S.G., Orsborn, G.N. and Walter, M. (1986) Studies on corneal staining with thin hydrogel contact lenses. *J. Br. Contact Lens Assoc.*, **9**, 61–4.

Y. Kikkawa

6.1 INTRODUCTION

The soft lens, after manufacture and obtaining its equilibrium in saline, achieves a form that is dependent upon several factors, such as material rigidity, elasticity, thickness distribution and resultant surface curvatures.

When the lens is introduced onto the eye one of the most important factors that governs its subsequent behaviour regarding fit on the eye is the elasticity of the lens. In most instances the lens takes on a different shape as it conforms to the eye surface. The primary mechanism is, however, the degree of mismatch between the eye surface shape and the lens form. The most important forces to be considered are those acting upon the peripheral portion of the lens.

6.2 METHODS OF LENS FIT

To understand the kinetics of lens fit the three variants of lens fit will be considered in a model. The three fits: steep, on keratometry (parallel) and flat are shown in Figure 6.1.

The shape of the hydrated lens in air or suspended in a saline solution is its natural form, free from all external forces which can deform the lens shape. In general such a lens, when placed on the eye, will deform to the eye shape. The spherical base curve of the lens does not conform to the aspherical eye surface.

A three-point fit exists by definition

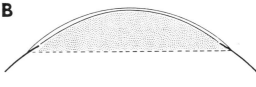

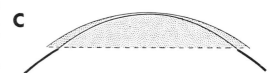

Figure 6.1 Three modes of fitting. (a) In an A-type fitting, the periphery of the lens is bent slightly outward, and the edge is stretched in circumferential direction. (b) In a B-type fitting, the inner surface of the soft lens coincides with the corneal contour. (c) In a C-type fitting, the lens periphery relaxes to adapt to the corneal contour. The dotted area shows the natural shape of the lens.

Contact Lens Practice. Edited by Montague Ruben and Michel Guillon.
Published in 1994 by Chapman & Hall, London. ISBN 0 412 35120 X

(Holden & Zantos, 1981) when touch occurs at the corneal apex and two points at the lens periphery. For the purpose of this argument, such a fit can occur with the soft lens without any stretching or relaxing of the lens. This condition can be expressed in mathematical terms using the *S* ratio (Campbell, 1984). The *S* factor is a parameter that expresses the soft lens deformation when on the eye. It is defined as follows:

S = the corneal circumference as measured at vault height of the lens/lens circumference at its edge off the eye.

Figure 6.1 illustrates the three types of fit. In an A-type fitting the lens periphery must stretch, as the lens diameter of the eye is less than the corneal diameter at the vault height of the lens. This produces a tight fit. In extreme cases the elastic forces will cause the lens to separate from the corneal apex. In these instances $S > 1$.

In the B-type fitting a three-point fit exists and $S = 1$. In the C-type fitting the edge of the lens is open and a flat fit exists; therefore $S < 1$. A portion of the lens periphery has an edge lift over the corneal surface. If the fit is excessively loose, the lens buckles and lifts away from the eye at the periphery.

6.3 RUBBER BAND MODEL

Let us consider an A-type fitting ($S > 1$). In this case, a concave lens is pressed down and stretched over a tear fluid covered surface of the cornea. Soft lenses are so thin that their resistance to flexure is insignificant compared to their resistance to stretching.

Let us envisage that the lens consists of many rubber bands which are stretched slightly at the periphery while the rest of the bands are still relaxed. An elastic force (*E*) develops in the stretched rubber band. The elastic force can be divided into tangential (*Et*) and normal (*En*) components (Fig. 6.2) (Kikkawa, 1979). An ideal elastic material will return immediately to its natural con-

figuration when external forces are removed. The stretched rubber band would therefore contract immediately and recover its natural shape, if there was no external resistance.

In proper fitting, the viscosity of the tear fluid behind the lens exerts a resistance to the tangential force (shearing force) (*Et*) of the rubber band. As long as *Et* is smaller than the viscous resistance (*VR*) of the tear fluid behind the lens, the rubber band stays on the corneal surface in a slightly stretched state, but if *Et* exceeds *VR*, the stretched rubber band slides over the corneal surface and contracts. Thus, the soft contact lens cannot be fitted steeper (tighter) beyond the critical condition where *Et* is in equilibrium with *VR* (*Et* = *VR*).

6.4 THE ROLE OF ELASTICITY ON CENTRATION

The criteria for the optimum fit are usually based on visual and physiological considerations. A lens is selected which will be the most stable and give the best vision and corneal tolerance.

On the open eye, the properly fitted lens is stable at the centred position. The lens is not fixed in this position but can be moved slightly with a small force. The force of the lid motion may move the lens from the centred position. However, it is desirable that the lens returns automatically to the same place on the cornea after a small displacement from the centred position.

The movement of the soft contact lens following a blink or after a displacement, and the eventual location of the lens, are determined by a complex interplay between the elastic (internal) forces of the lens, generated by deformation, and viscous resistance applied to the lens by the tear fluid behind the lens.

Let us first consider the elastic force of the lens itself. The role of tear viscosity will be discussed in the section on tear viscosity. The corneal contour has been described as consisting of two zones, a spherical corneal cap and the surrounding annular peripheral zone. The radius of curvature at the inner border of the peripheral corneal zone is 0.05 mm longer than the radius of the cap, and it gradually lengthens towards the sclera (Mandell, 1980). On blinking, the lens is dislocated slightly toward the peripheral cornea by lid movement, where the lens periphery is stretched because of the corneal topography. Thus, the elastic force of the rubber band in the lens periphery increases far beyond the critical value of normal fitting.

Elasticity of the soft contact lens is entropic in nature, like other polymers. On blinking, as the lens is stretched in a circumferential direction, the polymer molecules of the lens take a more ordered arrangement, i.e. entropy of the lens decreases. When a blink is over, the lens is released from the lid force, and entropy of the lens begins to increase; the lens tends to resume a state of less ordered molecular arrangement by thermal agitation. The ensuing elastic force (recentring force) pushes the lens toward the most stable position, the lens centred position, where stretching of the lens circumference is minimal.

Let us consider an A-type fitting, where $S > 1$. First, at the critical situation of fitting ($Et = VR$), an elastic recentring force works as soon as the lens leaves the centred position and draws back the lens to the centred position. Therefore the lens is very stable on the cornea. Second, at the fitting situation of $0 < Et < VR$, the lens can move easily within a certain range without any intervention of the recentring force. As the lens dislocates beyond this range, a recentring force begins to develop. In this case, the lens will centre well on the cornea but with a small lag in the downward direction due to gravity.

In a B-type fitting, where $S = 1$, the rubber bands remain unstretched ($Et = 0$), when the lens is put on the centre of the cornea. The lens can move easily without any resistance of recentring mechanism until the lens so

dislocates that Et surpasses VR. The recentring mechanism works only when the lens dislocates beyond this range.

When the lens is fitted as a C-type ($S < 1$), there will be no stretching in the lens periphery ($Et = 0$) until a significant decentration occurs, therefore recentring is very poor. Loose fitting lenses will lag downward significantly on the cornea in the straight ahead position and move easily to new positions.

For stable vision, good centration is essential. To accomplish this, the recentring mechanisms must work as soon as the lens is displaced from the centred position. Fitting in the critical situation will provide an automatic recentring feature to the lens.

Elastic forces generated by stretching in the lens periphery are the primary mechanism for centration and pump action (Kikkawa, 1979). S gives a measure of these forces in that they only exist for the lens if $S > 1$. Good fits seem to occur when S is about unity, or a little more (Campbell, 1984).

6.5 THEORETICAL AND CLINICAL BEST FIT

Considerations of the elastic forces generated by stretching in the lens periphery leads to the hypothesis that the best fit for stable vision is in a tight situation (Kikkawa, 1979), which calls for $S > 1$. Studies by many investigators and manufacturers have led to recommendations for fitting that indicate $S < 1$ is required for a good fit.

In general, the lens dimensions are measured when the lens is in equilibrium with saline in a container (100% humidity, 20 °C). When fitted on the eye, a soft lens undergoes dehydration and shrinkage by 4 – 10% due to elevated temperature and evaporation in low humidity conditions (Fatt & Chaston, 1982). Taking into account the dimensional changes, a mathematical calculation of change in S due to dehydration was done by Campbell (1984). Once the assumed lens comes to equilibrium with the atmospheric conditions, it does indeed fulfil Kikkawa's criterion that $S > 1$ for a good fit. In the case of the corneal fit, even though the lens fit is loose initially, e.g. $S = 0.98$, once the lens is in equilibrium with the atmosphere in low humidity conditions, S increases as a result of shrinkage due to dehydration, e.g. for a 4% shrinkage, S? (the new value of S) becomes 1.003. Thus a theoretical good fit criterion, $S > 1$ is reached in practice. On the other hand, the semi-scleral lenses, 14.5 mm in diameter, do not meet the theoretical best fit criteria when the lens comes to equilibrium, e.g. for $S = 0.98$, S? becomes 0.996.

6.6 FACTORS GOVERNING RECENTRATION

Different polymers have different elastic characteristics. The greater the modulus of elasticity of the lens material, the greater will be the recentring force for a given peripheral stretch. The peripheral thickness is also important as, for a unit stretch, more force will be supplied by the thicker lens.

The effective elastic modulus of the lens is proportional to the product of the Young's modulus of the lens and the local thickness of the lens. For a given lens, the elastic forces increase with the deformation. Therefore S is another factor to be considered. Within a certain range, as S increases, a great proportion of the lens is stretched when decentra-

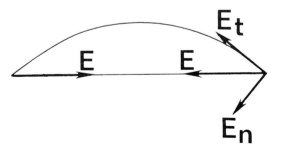

Figure 6.2 Elastic force of a stretched rubber band. The elastic force (E) can be divided into tangential (E_t) and normal (E_n) components.

tion occurs, thereby creating more recentring force.

6.7 TEAR VISCOSITY

The role of viscosity of the tear fluid behind the lens during lens motion will be considered. If there were no external forces exerted on the lens, the lens deformed by decentration would immediately recover its natural shape. In this process, parts of the lens would have to move along and away from the corneal surface. When a fluid is present behind the lens, viscous forces resist this motion. In the critical situation of fitting, the elastic force of a stretched rubber band (Et) is in equilibrium with the viscous resistance (VR) of the tears behind the lens.

Although the tear fluid is a complex chemical solution, its mechanical properties are usually supposed to be identical to those of water. For water, or any other Newtonian fluid, the shear stress is proportional to the rate at which the fluid is being sheared. The constant of proportionality is called the viscosity and is about 10^{-2} dyn/s/cm^2 for water.

Experiments on rabbit tears (Hamano & Mitsunaga, 1973) indicate that the magnitude of apparent viscosity is high at a slow shear rate, but it decreases abruptly on increasing the shear rate. At the velocity of the lid movement, the tear viscosity becomes close to that of water.

The mucous layer was recognized formerly as approximately 0.02–0.05 μm thick (Holly & Lemp, 1977). However, recent EM studies of the mucous layer of the tear film, employing a new technique, have revealed that the mucous layer may be far thicker than the formerly recognized value (Nichols *et al.*, 1985). Thus these investigators reported that the mucous film is 0.4–1 μm thick over the cornea and from 2 to 7 μm in the lower conjunctival fornix. Mucus constitutes a considerable part of the precorneal tear film, and plays a very important mechanical role; it cleans and lubricates the ocular surface while facilitating the sliding action of the eyelids; it is essential for contact lens fitting.

Let us consider a soft contact lens which is fitted at $S > 1$ (type A). The lens receives repeated pounding of the upper lid through blinking. The normal force exerted on the lens presses it in close conformity with the corneal and scleral surfaces. Tear viscosity resists the reduction in thickness of the tear fluid behind the lens. Furthermore, because the lens is always slightly stretched, even when the lens is in the centred position, the normal component of the lens elasticity, En, exerts continuous pressure on the tear film. Thus the peripheral portion of the lens may ride on the bottom of the tear film. The presence of a high concentration of mucin in the deep layer may give rise to large values of apparent viscosity. It is to be noticed that the reported tear viscosity was usually measured on collected tears, ie on the aqueous phase of tear film.

In the central area of the lens, in attempting to recover its natural shape by its elasticity, the lens may ride on the superficial layer of the tear film. When the lens is fitted as in a B type or C type, the normal force is not created at the lens periphery. The lens may ride lightly on the superficial layer of the tear film. It is likely that the tear fluid behind the lens behaves like water.

A meniscus exists at the edge of a soft lens, and may help to determine the thickness of the tear fluid behind the lens by creating a negative pressure. The stability of the lens increases with an increase in the total surface area of the lens. This is due in part to larger viscous resistance to the lens movement.

6.8 MOVEMENT OF THE LENS

In practice, the fitting characteristics of the soft contact lenses are evaluated primarily by its positioning and movement on the cornea. A well fitted lathe-cut or spin-cast lens will centre well on the cornea, with possibly a small lag in the downward direction. With a normal blink, the lens should move on the cornea, first upward as it is drawn with the upper lid and then downward from gravitation until the lens stabilizes on the cornea (Mandell, 1980). Analysis of the lens movement, especially of the lower edge by means of a video camera provides important and useful information.

Immediately after the blink, the lens is found to be located in the centre of the cornea. When the upper lid comes down to close the eye, a slight downward shift of the lens edge is elicited. The lens is forced to move towards the peripheral area of the cornea by lid motion. With the effects of the tangential and normal force, the lens circumference is so stretched that the elastic force increases beyond the critical value of normal fitting, because the cornea flattens more and more toward the periphery. When the eye opens again, the lens shifts upwards with the motion of the upper lid. Elastic contraction of the stretched lens periphery also assists the upward movement of the lens. However, the process is so quick that when blinking is over the lens is usually found to be located in the centred position as if there were no movement of the lens. Features of the lens movement in this example would suggest that the fitting be done in the critical situation ($Et = VR$).

The fact that the lens is displaced so little, even though there may be large relative motions between the lid and lens, is an indirect indication that, at least during the blink, the pre-lens tear film is substantially thicker than the post-lens tear film. In relation to this, it is known that tears are accumulated between the upper and lower lids when the eye is closed (Holly & Lemp, 1977).

In some cases, the lens remains centred but may ride a little low on the cornea. Just after the eye opens, the lens may be found slightly deviated upward from the corneal centre. Then the lens slides over the corneal surface by gravity until the lens stops moving as shown in Figure 6.3. With the next blink the lens is pushed further downward with the motion of the upper lid. Immediately following the blink, the lens is found to be located in a slightly deviated position again. The lens movement in this example would suggest the fitting in $0 < Et < VR$.

Sometimes the fit of the lens may be too tight or too loose. A tight lens does not appear to move on the cornea following a blink or after eye movement in any direction. A loose lens will lag downwards on the eye in the straight ahead position. In the case of extremely loose fitting, the lens will slide off the cornea entirely.

6.9   PUMP ACTION

During soft contact lens wear, oxygen can reach the cornea either by diffusion through the lens material or by freshly oxygenated tears being pumped under the lens during lens motion.

Pumping of oxygenated tears under the lens is supported by some experiments which demonstrate the circulation of instilled Fluorexon or the movement of blood cells in the tears (Carter, 1972). However, it has been shown that, regardless of fit, the magnitude of tear flow is small and contributes very little to the oxygen tension under the lens (Fatt & Lin, 1976; Decker *et al.*, 1978). The tear replenishment rate was determined with a slit lamp modified to serve as a fluorophotometer (Polse, 1979). Fractional tear volume replenishment rates under three different hydrogel lenses averaged 0.011 per blink. This data suggests that the amount of oxygen delivered to the cornea by tear pumping for gel lenses is relatively small.

On the other hand, it is known that if the fit of the lens is too tight, vision is slightly blurred. A tight soft lens tends to form an aspherical curve in the central area and is now steeper than the central corneal area and shows apical clearance that can be demonstrated by retinoscopy. Immediately after the blink there will be a temporary clearing of

vision; this lasts only a fraction of a second. The vision then returns to its original state. When the blink occurs, the upper lid smooths the lens across the cornea. During the brief period in which the lens is conforming to the cornea, the subjective vision acuity improves.

Immediately after the blink the lens remains in this state momentarily but soon reverts to its normal aspherical curve (Mandell, 1980). During this process, tears may collect beneath the apical clearance, and are then squeezed out from beneath the lens. This behaviour of the tight fitted lens suggests a possible mechanism of the tear pump. Although the example is concerned with too tight a situation, it is likely that a similar pump action may take place in a proper fitting, which is in fact a minimal steep situation.

On blinking, the upper lid presses the lens towards the cornea and pushes it downward, resulting in a slight displacement toward the peripheral cornea. The lens may conform so closely to the corneal contour that tears are squeezed out from beneath the lens; the rubber bands of the lens periphery are stretched beyond the critical condition of fitting ($Et > VR$), because the peripheral zone of the cornea flattens progressively towards the sclera. When the eye opens, the stretched lens resumes its original shape by virtue of its intrinsic elasticity. During this process, tears would be sucked behind the lens. In this manner, the lid and the lens work together as a pump and exchange some tear fluid behind the lens.

The soft lens has to meet some requirements in order to perform a pump action. The lens has to be fitted as in an A-type. The effective elastic modulus of the peripheral portion of the lens must be large enough to provide a necessary elastic force for a pump. The central portion of the lens must be sufficiently rigid to recover the original shape. In addition, the magnitude of the elastic forces that are determining

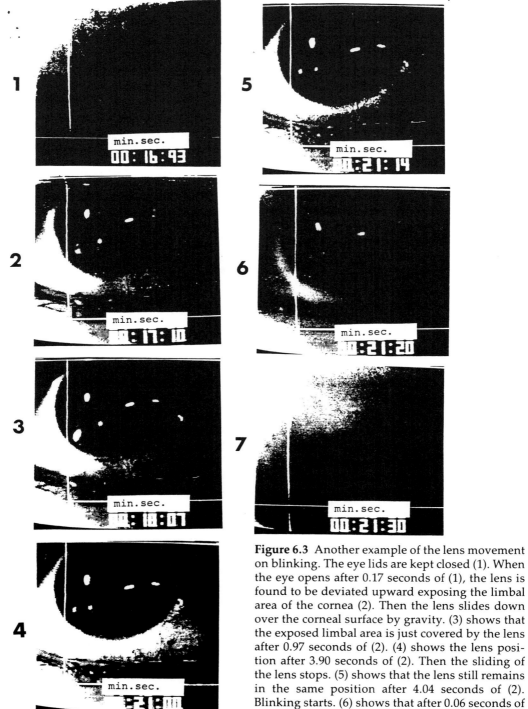

Figure 6.3 Another example of the lens movement on blinking. The eye lids are kept closed (1). When the eye opens after 0.17 seconds of (1), the lens is found to be deviated upward exposing the limbal area of the cornea (2). Then the lens slides down over the corneal surface by gravity. (3) shows that the exposed limbal area is just covered by the lens after 0.97 seconds of (2). (4) shows the lens position after 3.90 seconds of (2). Then the sliding of the lens stops. (5) shows that the lens still remains in the same position after 4.04 seconds of (2). Blinking starts. (6) shows that after 0.06 seconds of (5), the lens is pushed downward by the closing lid. After 0.1 second of (6), the eyelids are completely closed (7).

the recovery of the natural shape is related to the degree of deformation of the lens on fitting.

If the lens fitting meets the requirements mentioned above, tears would be drawn back through a very thin channel of tear fluid around the lens periphery. However, the flow rates of tears would be very low. Experimental studies suggest that the amount of oxygen delivered to the cornea by tear pumping for gel lenses is relatively small and that oxygen received by the cornea covered by a gel lens comes primarily by diffusion through the material.

Even the most gas permeable lens cannot ensure entirely trouble-free results. If for some reason the soft lens stops moving, a major accumulation of epithelial debris underneath the lens may occur. Debris accumulation is considered to be an important contributor to complications with extended wear. The material is mucus, polymorphonuclear leucocytes and exfoliated epithelial cells and must be evacuated by pump action.

The mucus plays an essential role not only in the maintenance of the hydration of the cornea and conjunctiva, and in the stability of the tear film, but also in the defensive process of the oculopalpebral environment (Liotet *et al.*, 1985). Mucins are synthesized in the goblet cells of the conjunctiva and become the gel-forming component in the mucous layer of the tear film. Other constituents that have been identified in the mucous layer are immunoglobulins, salts, urea, glucose, leucocytes, tissue debris and enzymes such as betalysin, peroxidase and lysozyme (Nichols *et al.*, 1985).

Blinking produces mild mechanical agitation of the mucous layer and body temperature favours thermal dissociation of mucous gels. Both of these factors could cause the dispersal of some mucin molecules in the tear film where the aqueous and mucous layers meet (Nichols *et al.* 1985). The dispersed mucous gels contain-

ing mucins and other important components can be supplied behind the lens by virtue of pump action.

Chloride transport may promote corneal deturgescence and play a role in epithelial wound healing (Fogle & Neufeld, 1979). These important functions of the cornea may possibly be initiated by catecholamines in the tears (Trope & Runfrey, 1984) via the β-receptor adenyl cyclase mechanism. Catecholamines could be supplied to the corneal epithelium by pump action of the lens.

Even with high oxygen permeable lenses, the other functions of the tear pump should be kept in mind to obtain physiological functional fitting of the soft contact lenses.

REFERENCES

Campbell, C. (1984) The fit of soft contact lenses. *Int. Contact Lens Clin.*, **11**(4), 219–40.

Carter, D.B. (1972) Use of red blood cells to observe tear flow under contact lenses. *Am. J. Optom.*, **49**, 617–18.

Decker, M., Polse, K.A. and Fatt, I. (1978) Oxygen flux into the human cornea covered by a soft contact lens. *Am. J. Optom. Physiol. Opt.*, **55**, 285–93.

Fatt, I. and Chaston, J. (1982) Swelling factors of hydrogels and the effects of deswelling (drying) in the eye on power of a soft contact lens. *Int. Contact Lens Clin.*, **9**(3), 146–153.

Fatt, I. and Lin, D. (1976) Oxygen tension under a soft or hard gas permeable contact lens in the presence of tear pumping. *Am. J. Optom. Physiol. Opt.*, **53**, 104–11.

Fogle, F.A. and Neufled, A.H. (1979) The adrenergic and cholinergic corneal epithelium. *Invest. Ophthalmol. Vis. Sci.*, **18**, 1212–15.

Hamano, H. and Mitsunaga, S. (1973) Viscosity of rabbit tears. *Jap. J. Ophthalmol.*, **17**, 290–9.

Holden, B.A. and Zantos, S.G. (1981) The conformity of soft lenses to the shape of the cornea. *Am. J. Optom. Physiol. Opt.*, **58**(2), 139–43.

Holly, F.J. and Lemp, M.A. (1977) Tear physiology and dry eyes. *Surv. Opthalmol.*, **22**, 69–87.

Kikkawa, Y. (1979) Kinetics of soft contact lens fitting. *Contacto*, **23**(4), 10–17.

Liotet, S., Triclot, M.P., Perderiset, M., Warnet,

V.N. and Laroche, L. (1985) The role of conjunctival mucous in contact lens fitting. *CLAO Journal*, **11**, 149–54.

Mandell, R.B. (1980) *Contact Lens Practice*. Charles C Thomas, Springfield, IL.

Nichols, B.A., Chiappino, M.L. and Dawson, C.R. (1985) Demonstration of the mucous layer of the tear film by electron microscopy. *Invest. Ophthalmol. Vis. Sci.*, **26**, 464–73.

Polse, K.A. (1979) Tear flow under hydrogel contact lenses. *Invest. Ophthalmol. Vis. Sci.*, **18**, 409–13.

Trope, G.E. and Runfey, A. (1984) Catecholamine concentration in tears. *Exp. Eye Res.*, **39**, 247–50.

CONTACT LENS OPTICS 7

C. Fowler

7.1 INTRODUCTION

A knowledge of the optics of contact lenses is essential for anyone involved in their fitting. This chapter attempts to give a straightforward review of the basics of this subject, but for more comprehensive information, the references should be consulted.

The sign convention for optical calculations and diagrams is as follows:

1. In diagrams, incident light is considered to travel from left to right.
2. Distances measured in the same direction as incident light are considered to be positive, in the opposite direction to incident light negative.
3. Distances are measured from the surface under consideration.

Unless otherwise specified, the 'power' of a contact lens is assumed to be the back vertex power (BVP) measured in air. Terminology is as specified in BS 3521: *Terms relating to ophthalmic optics and spectacle frames. Part 3 1988: Glossary of terms and symbols relating to contact lenses.*

The author's interest in the optics of contact lenses was inspired by A.G. Bennett, to whom much gratitude must go for his assistance in the preparation of this chapter.

7.2 EFFECTIVITY OF CORRECTING LENS

The effective power of a correcting lens will depend on its distance from the eye. As there is often a 10–15 mm difference between the position of the spectacle plane and the cornea, there will naturally be a difference between the power of a contact lens *in situ* and that of a spectacle lens required to cor-

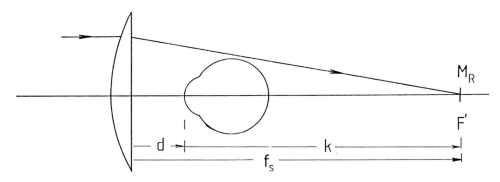

Figure 7.1 Variables used in the calculation of effectivity of the correcting lens at the eye.

Contact Lens Practice. Edited by Montague Ruben and Michel Guillon.
Published in 1994 by Chapman & Hall, London. ISBN 0 412 35120 X

rect the same eye. In Figure 7.1, a correcting spectacle lens is shown positioned at a distance 'd' from the corneal apex of a reduced eye. A focal length of f_s will be required to image distant objects at the far point (M_R) of the eye. In other words, the focus F' of the lens should coincide with M_R.

The distance of the eye from M_R is given by k, and the reciprocal of this value, K, is the ocular refraction. The relationship between the ocular and spectacle refraction is given by:

$$K = \frac{F_s}{1-dF_s} \qquad \text{(eqn 7.1)}$$

For example, if the spectacle refraction is −5.00 D at 13 mm from the cornea, then the ocular refraction will be −4.70 D. Alternatively, a spectacle refraction of +5.00 D at 13 mm from the cornea indicates an ocular refraction of +5.35 D.

Thus it is general good practice to record the distance from the eye at which a trial lens is used, and this is essential for lens powers over 5.00 D if significant errors are to be avoided.

Note that the BVP of the contact lens in air is not necessarily the same as the ocular refraction. Any liquid lens formed by the tears beneath the contact lens also has to be taken in consideration.

7.3   CONTACT LENS POWER CALCULATION

Because of their steep curves, and hence very short radii of curvature in relation to axial thickness, it is necessary to treat contact lenses as 'thick' lenses. This means that in determining the required surface powers for the lens, the thickness is taken into consideration, and not ignored, as in 'thin' lenses.

The calculation to be performed by the manufacturer is this: the back optic zone radius (BOZR) of a contact lens is fixed by the fitting relationship required, and the BVP. The lens refractive index (n) is fixed by the lens material, and the axial thickness (t_c) by the lens design. The problem then is to calculate the front optic zone radius (FOZR) required for the lens to give the correct BVP.

This problem can be considered as the reverse of the effectivity problem described earlier. It is possible to solve this type of problem by reversing the light path through the contact lens, so that the change of vergence at each surface is calculated with light incident at the rear surface. Allowance must be made

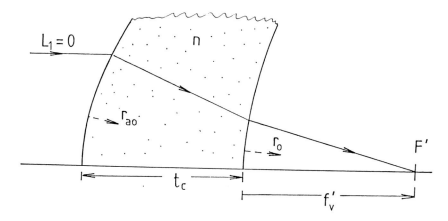

Figure 7.2 Calculation of FOZR (r_{ao}) required to give a desired back vertex focal length (f_v) for parallel incident light ($L_1 = 0$) at the front surface.

for the 'reduced thickness' (t_c/n) between the lens surfaces. The front surface power is calculated so that light emerges parallel (zero vergence) under these conditions (Fig. 7.2).

However, a simpler approach is to use the formula:

$$F_{ao} = \frac{F'v - F_o}{1 + (t_c/n)(F'_v - F_o)} \qquad \text{(eqn 7.2)}$$

Note that t is in metres.

For example:
$F'v$ (BVP) $= -8.00$ D;
r_o (BOZR) $= 8.00$ mm;
$t_c = 0.30$ mm;
$n = 1.49$;
r_{ao} (FOZR) $= ?$
where r_o is in millimetres, since:

$$F_o = \frac{1000(1-n)}{r_o}$$

thus $F_o = -61.25$ D.

Substituting in the above expression:

$$F_{ao} = \frac{(-8.00 + 61.25)}{1 + \dfrac{(0.0003)(-8.00 + 61.25)}{1.49}}$$

$$F_{ao} = 52.69$$

Therefore:

$$\text{FOZR } (r_{ao}) = \frac{1000(n-1)}{F_{ao}}$$
$$= 9.30\text{mm}$$

The power of the front surface calculated here ($+52.69$ D) is seen to be weaker than the value of $+53.25$ D indicated by simply applying thin lens theory.

7.4   LIQUID LENS POWERS

In the case of hard contact lenses, it will be apparent that the total power effect of the contact lens on the eye is a combination of the refractive power of the lens plus any lens effect from the layer of tear fluid between the contact lens and the cornea, shown diagrammatically in Figure 7.3. In the case of a lens with BOZR shorter than the corneal radius this will result in a positive liquid lens and, as shown in Figure 7.3, a lens with BOZR longer than the corneal radius will result in a negative power liquid lens.

The effective power of this liquid lens can be calculated by assuming that the contact lens and the liquid lens are both surrounded

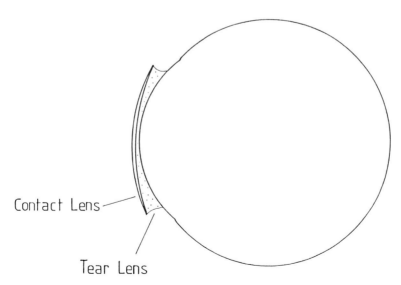

Figure 7.3 Schematic illustration of the formation of a liquid tear lens between contact lens and cornea.

by a very thin film of air. Thus the total power of the system is then simply the sum of each of the individual components, measured in air.

Example

A hard contact lens with BOZR 8.0 mm, is fitted on an eye with a central keratometry reading of 7.8 mm. What is the power of the liquid lens?

We first have to assume a value for the mean refractive index of tears. This is generally taken as 1.336. Hence in air:

Front surface power $= 1000(n-1)/ r_{ao} = 336/8.0 = +42.00$ D
Rear surface power $= 1000(1-n)/r_o = 336/7.8 = -43.08$ D

Total thin lens power $= -1.08$ D

This gave rise to the approximate relationship that was used extensively in fitting of hard (PMMA) contact lenses: *A difference of 0.05 mm between BOZR of a hard contact lens and keratometry reading is equivalent to 0.25 D of liquid lens power.*

This rule should be used carefully, particularly with very steep or very flat corneas. For example, a lens with BOZR of 6.8 mm fitted on a cornea of radius 7.0 mm will have a liquid lens power in air of +1.41 D, and not + 1.00 D as the approximate rule would suggest. Another example, using much flatter curves would be of a lens with BOZR of 9.0 mm fitted on a cornea with radius 9.2 mm. This would give a liquid lens power of +0.81 D, as opposed to +1.00 D if the approximate rule is used.

7.5 CORRECTION OF ASTIGMATISM AND TORIC LENSES

The use of a spherical hard contact lens on an astigmatic cornea gives very effective correction of corneal astigmatism. This might seem surprising, as the corneal refractive index is 1.376, compared with 1.336 for tears. From this relationship, it might be assumed that a spherical lens would only neutralise 336/376 × 100 or 90% of the corneal astigmatism. However, it is generally assumed that the rear surface of a typical cornea neutralizes some 10% of the astigmatism introduced by the front surface of the cornea.

Example

A spherical rear surface hard contact lens has a BOZR of 8.00 mm, and is used on an eye with keratometry readings of 7.50 and 8.00 mm.

The rear surface of the contact lens and the front surface of the tear lens are both spherical, and hence can be ignored in the calculation of astigmatism:

	Index	Astigmatism
Cornea	1.376	(50.13– 47.00) = 3.13 D
Rear surface tear lens	1.336	–(44.80–42.00) = –2.80 D

It is assumed that 10% of the corneal astigmatism (– 0.31 D) will be corrected by the rear surface of the cornea.

Any astigmatism not corrected by the contact lens in this case would be known as residual astigmatism.

However, it is extremely unlikely that a spherical lens would give an adequate fit in this case, therefore a rear toroidal surface might be used instead. If this is fitted in alignment, the powers of the liquid lens can be ignored, as this simply becomes an afocal layer sandwiched between the contact lens and the cornea:

	Index	Astigmatism
Cornea	1.376	(50.13 – 47.00) = 3.13 D
Rear surface contact lens	1.490	– (65.33 – 61.25) = – 4.08 D

an increase of –1.28 D

Thus in this case, the higher refractive index

of the hard contact lens over-corrects the corneal astigmatism, giving rise to induced astigmatism. This may well require the use of a toroidal front surface in order to correct the unwanted astigmatism.

Occasionally, scleral lenses are used with rear toroidal surfaces for the correction of astigmatism. In air, the back surface power of an acrylic contact lens is $-490/r_o$ dioptres (r_o in millimetres), but in contact with tears fluid it is:

$$-\frac{(490-336)}{r_o} \text{ or } \frac{-154}{r_o}$$

The power of the rear surface is hence reduced by a factor of 490/154 or 3.18. Thus to produce a desired cylinder power of C dioptres when *in situ*, the back surface should be made 3.18 C dioptres when measured in air. A general expression for this ratio, for any contact lens material of refractive index *n* is:

$$\frac{1000\,(n-1)}{1000\,(n-1)-336}$$

In the case of soft contact lenses, a spherical lens will mould itself to a toric cornea, transmitting the corneal astigmatism. Designs are produced commercially with either a front surface toric or a rear surface toric, the other surface being spherical. However with these designs it is likely that the lens will end up as bi-toric on an astigmatic eye as it moulds to the shape of the cornea. One advantage of a front surface toric is that lens designs of this type can also be used to correct for lenticular astigmatism, as well as corneal astigmatism. Front and back surface torics are stabilized by using techniques such as truncation and prism ballasting.

The theoretical ideal for a soft lens with a rear surface toric would be one with a high water content, as here the refractive indices of the contact lens and cornea would be the closest.

7.6 BIFOCAL CONTACT LENSES

Contact lens bifocals of conventional (refractive) designs are manufactured in both fused and solid varieties. Because of the neutralizing effects of tears, a front and rear surface solid hard bifocal contact lenses require different treatment.

For example, if a front surface addition of +2.00 D is required on a 1.490 refractive index lens with a FOZR of 7.90, then this will require a radius of 7.65 mm for the segment, as these radii are equivalent to +62.03 D and +64.06 D, respectively.

However, if a rear surface bifocal with an addition of +2.00 D is made from the same refractive index material and a BOZR of 7.45 mm, then account must be taken of the refractive index of tears. Thus addition required in air is 2.00 × 3.18 = 6.36 D. A BOZR of 7.45 mm gives a power in air of $-490/7.45 = 65.77$ D. Hence near vision area must have a power in air of = −59.41 D.

$$\text{Required radius} = \frac{-490}{-59.41} = 8.25 \text{ mm}$$

7.7 MAGNIFICATION EFFECTS OF CONTACT LENSES

The differences in retinal image magnification with spectacle and contact lenses have important clinical considerations. Two types of magnification related to a correcting lens on an eye are conventionally described – spectacle magnification and relative spectacle magnification.

7.7.1 SPECTACLE MAGNIFICATION

This is the ratio of the image size in the corrected eye to the image size in the uncorrected eye. The retinal image in the uncorrected eye may be blurred, as in myopia, or sharp, as in hypermetropia neutralized by accommodation. To cover both possibilities, the size is defined by rays from the object's extenities, passing through the centre of the eye's entrance pupil. These measure the distance between the centres of the limiting blur circles, whatever their size. In Figure 7.4, a spectacle lens is shown correcting a hypermetropic eye. The angular subtense of a distant object at the entrance pupil centre is given by <H'EF', and the angular subtense of the image in the far point plane by <H'SF'.

Hence spectacle magnification is given by:

$$<\text{H'SF'} = \frac{f_s}{f_s - a_s} = \frac{1}{1 - aF_s} \qquad \text{(eqn 7.3)}$$
$$<\text{H'EF'}$$

Note that the value of a is in metres in this expression. This applies to a thin lens and is known as the power factor (P). For a spectacle lens, the magnification due to lens form known as the shape factor (S) can be readily calculated from the expression:

$$S = \frac{1}{1 - (t_c/n)F_{ao}} \qquad \text{(eqn 7.4)}$$

The shape factor can become quite large in spectacle lenses. In contact lenses, a more complex expression is required for the calculation of S, but the values are always small,

around 1.01 for corneal lenses, although scleral lenses can have values nearly up to 1.05.

From the expression for the power factor it will be appreciated that any correcting lens will have some spectacle magnification, unless implanted within the eye, in which case the value of a will be very close to zero. Positive power lenses will have magnification of greater than 1, negative power lenses magnification of less than 1. However, in the case of a contact lens, a will be reduced to about 3 mm, whereas the spectacle lens value is usually 10–15 mm more than this.

Figure 7.5 shows the values of spectacle magnification, calculated for a range of lens powers, in both contact lenses and spectacle lenses. Lens form and thickness have both been taken into account, typical values having been assumed throughout.

7.7.2 RELATIVE SPECTACLE MAGNIFICATION

This is the ratio of the image size in the corrected eye to image size in the 'standard' emmetropic eye. Expressions for relative

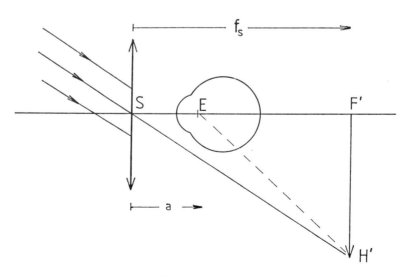

Figure 7.4 Calculation of spectacle magnification.

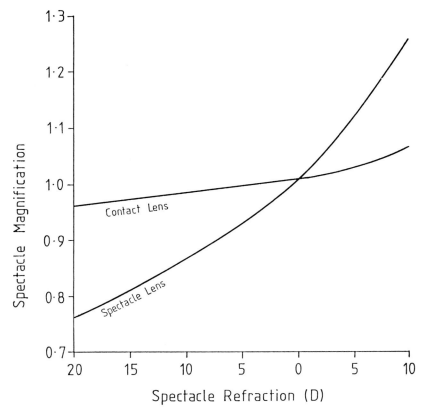

Figure 7.5 Variation of spectacle magnification with spectacle refraction, for typical contact lenses and spectacle lenses (from Ruben, 1975).

spectacle magnification (RSM) can be derived from the following variables:

F: Equivalent power of eye/correcting lens system.
F_o: Power of the emmetropic schematic eye.
F_e: Power of ametropic eye.
F_s: Spectacle refraction.
d: Distance from spectacle plane to first principal point of the eye.

The following derivation assumes a thin correcting lens, ignoring the shape factor, which however, is almost negligible in the case of contact lenses.

For a distant object, the size of an image is directly proportional to the equivalent focal length of the lens, and hence inversely proportional to the equivalent power. From this:

$$RSM = F_o = \frac{F_o}{F_s + F_e - dF_sF_e} \qquad \text{(eqn 7.5)}$$

This expression can be further simplified depending on whether the ametropia is axial or refractive.

In the case of refractive ametropia:

$$F_o = F_e + K \qquad \text{(eqn 7.6)}$$

thus:

$$RSM = \frac{F_e + K}{F_s + F_e - dF_sF_e} \qquad \text{(eqn 7.7)}$$

substituting K:

$$K = \frac{F_s M}{1 + dF_s} \qquad \text{(eqn 7.8)}$$

$$RSM = \frac{1}{1 - dF_s} \qquad \text{(eqn 7.9)}$$

As the values of d and a would differ by only about 1.5 mm, this means that the relative spectacle magnification is similar to the spectacle magnification in refractive emmetropia

In the case of purely axial ametropia, then F_e is the same as F_o and the expression for RSM can be simplified to:

$$RSM = \frac{1}{1 - (f_o + d)F_s} \qquad \text{(eqn 7.10)}$$

where f_o is the anterior focal length of the eye. If the spectacle lens is fitted in the anterior focal plane of the eye so that $d = f_o$ (approximately 15 mm from the corneal vertex), then the above expression will evoluate as unity, indicating that the image size in the same as in an emmetropic eye.

Applying these expressions to contact lenses:

1. The power of the lens *in situ* is K, which here replaces F_s.
2. The distance d from the back vertex of the fluid lens to the eye's first principal point is only about 1.55 mm. Hence, if the term $d\,F_s F_e$ is ignored.

$$RSM \approx \frac{F_o}{K + F_e} \qquad \text{(eqn 7.11)}$$

Axial error

$F_e = F_o$, and if F_o is taken as $+60$ D:

$$RSM \approx \frac{60}{K + 60} \approx \frac{1}{1 + 0.017K} \approx 1 - 0.017K$$

Refractive error

$$F_e = F_o - K \text{ or } F_o = F_e + K \qquad \text{(eqn 7.12)}$$

Substituted in the above, this gives RSM = 1. This result could have been predicted because the eye with purely refractive error has the same axial length as the standard emmetropic eye, and when its cornea is reshaped to give the correct power, the eye is virtually made into the standard emmetropic model.

In practical terms, the magnification effects of most interest are:

Myopia

Figure 7.5 shows that, as myopia increases, contact lenses give a progressively larger image size than the equivalent spectacle correction. This could be useful in improving visual acuity.

Aphakia

As shown in Figure 7.6, the percentage increase in retinal image after cataract removal, which renders an eye aphakic, can give rise to a considerable change in retinal image size. These graphs show the percentage increase in retinal image size in eyes corrected by spectacle or contact lenses.

It should be pointed out that the graph lines are the means of the possible spread of values, which vary with the optical dimensions of the given eye. For spectacle lenses, possible spread is of the order of ±15%. For example, the percentage increase for the previously emmetropic eye would range from about 20 to 50%. For contact lenses, the possible spread is only about ±2%.

For the majority of individuals, who had a spectacle refraction of less than ±5 dioptres, a contact lens correction will clearly give a corrected image size closest to that of the previous spectacle refraction. This is of particular benefit to the bilateral aphakic, where the use of a contact lens correction on the

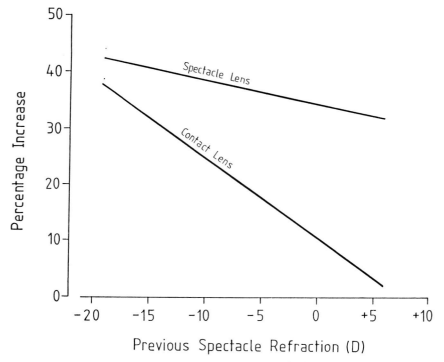

Figure 7.6 Percentage increase in retinal image size of aphakics for both contact lens and spectacle lens corrections (from Ruben, 1975).

aphakic eye will often permit binocular vision. If a spectacle correction were used, this would render binocular vision impossible due to a disparity in image size.

Anisometropia

In order to equalize retinal image sizes, spectacles would be the best form of correction if the emmetropia was mainly axial, and contact lenses if the emmetropia was mainly refractive. However, an alternative view is that of Halass (1959), who proposed that the main object in the correction of anisometropia should be to disturb as little as possible the retinal image sizes in uncorrected eyes. On this basis, contact lenses with their relatively insignificant spectacle magnification are advantageous in all cases of anisometropia. This view has been supported by Winn *et al.* (1986).

Marked astigmatism

In marked astigmatism, the spectacle magnifications in the two principal meridians are unequal, causing distortion of the retinal image, especially if these meridians are oblique. This defect is greatly lessened by contact lenses; though the wearer may take time to accustom himself to the new imagery.

7.8 SOFT LENS OPTICS

Soft contact lenses are affected by temperature, water content and bending.

7.8.1 TEMPERATURE

Optical plastics have a variation of refractive index due to lens temperature, the index decreasing as the temperature increases. However, at the temperatures likely to be encountered by a soft contact lens, the effect on power is small.

7.8.2 WATER CONTENT

A soft contact lens containing saline will have a lower refractive index as the water (saline) content increases. However, this is not necessarily a constant value. On the eye, soft lenses tend to lose water content, and Ford (1976) has shown that due to the change of refractive index and loss of thickness that this entails, the power of the lens will increase. Brennan *et al.* (1987) found that thick and thin lenses of the same material dehydrated to an equal extent, and also that the decrease in water content was not predictable on the basis of a knowledge of the initial water content.

7.8.3 LENS BENDING

If a soft contact lens moulded itself perfectly to the front surface curvature of the cornea, then it can be shown that a loss of positive power, or an increase in negative power should result. However, in practice it appears that the situation is more complex then this.

One explanation for the power changes that are found is the presence of a tear lens in many cases (Weissman & Zisman, 1981). However, Chaston and Fatt (1980) do not accept this hypothesis, and experimental evidence for a lack of tear lens was given by Holden and Zantos (1981).

Bennett (1976) gave a model for the change in power ($\triangle F'_v$) when a contact lens with a back radius of r_2 is deformed to a new radius r_2':

$$\triangle F'_v = -300 \, t_c \, (1/r_2'^2 - 1/r_2^2) \qquad \text{(eqn 7.13)}$$

A number of other mathematical models have been given for the change in curvature and power when a soft lens is flexed (see Chaston & Fatt, 1980, for review), however these all assume that the lens surfaces are spherical.

7.9 ACCOMMODATION AND CONVERGENCE WITH CONTACT LENSES

7.9.1 ACCOMMODATION

The accommodative effect required to view a near object can be measured either relative to the eye (ocular accommodation) or relative to the spectacle plane (spectacle accommodation). In clinical examination, it is this latter value that is measured, but for comparisons between contact lenses and spectacle lenses, the ocular accommodation is more useful.

Consider a myope, – 6.00 DS spectacle refraction at 12 mm from the cornea, viewing an object 250 mm from the spectacle plane.

Spectacles

The spectacle lens will form an image of the near object with vergence $L' = L + F = -4.00 + (-6.00) = -10.00$. Thus the image is formed at $1000 - 10 = -100$ mm from the spectacle plane or -112 mm from the cornea. The ocular refraction (K) is -5.60, and the vergence of the image at the eye is $1000/-112 = -8.93$. Thus:

$$\text{Accommodation} = -5.60 - (-8.93)$$
$$= 3.33 \, \text{D}$$

Contact lenses

With little error we can assume that the contact lens wearer is very similar to the emmetrope. Thus the eye looks directly at the object, which has a vergence at the eye of $1000/-262 = -3.82$. Thus:

$$\text{Accommodation} = 3.82 \, \text{D}$$

Thus in this case the contact lens wearer will

have to exert 0.49 D more accommodation when wearing contact lenses than with spectacles. Note that this example ignores form and thickness of correcting lenses.

Figure 7.7 shows the ocular accommodation that is required by spectacle wearers for two different fixation distances. Lens form and thickness are taken in account. This figure shows the advantage in terms of low accommodation that is enjoyed by myopes when wearing spectacles; this advantage will be lost on switching to contact lenses.

7.9.2 CONVERGENCE

There will naturally be a difference in the convergence requirements of spectacle and contact lens correction. With spectacles, the eyes are rotating behind fixed lenses, but with variable induced prismatic effects; with contact lenses the lenses move with the eyes, giving effectively zero induced prism.

In Figure 7.8, a spectacle-wearing myope is shown converging through an angle θ to view the image (b') of an object (h) formed by the spectacle lens.

Consider, as in the example given for accommodation that the spectacle refraction is -6.00 D at 12 mm from the eye. Assume that the eye is viewing a near object 250 mm from the spectacle plane, and that the centre of rotation of the eye is 15 mm behind the cornea. If the interpupillary distance is 70 mm, then the convergence can be calculated as follows:

Spectacles

In Figure 7.8 the spectacle lens is fitted at a distance z from the centre of rotation of the eye, which in this case is 27 mm. Assuming that myope is converging to the mid-line, the object size (h) will be half the interpupillary distance or 35 mm:

$$\text{The image size } h' = l' \times \frac{h}{l} = \frac{-100 \times 35}{-250}$$
$$= 14.0 \text{ mm}$$

$$\text{Angle of convergence, } \tan \theta = h'/(z-l')$$
$$= 14/(27=100)$$
$$= 0.1102$$

Thus $\theta = 11.0\triangle$

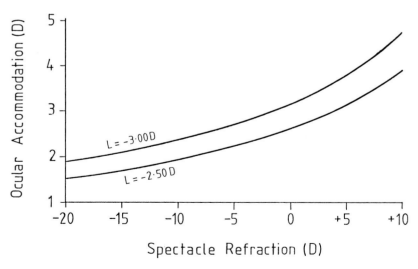

Figure 7.7 Graph showing the relationship between ocular accommodation and spectacle refraction for near objects at 333.33 mm ($L = -3.00$) and 400 mm ($L = -2.50$) (from Ruben, 1975).

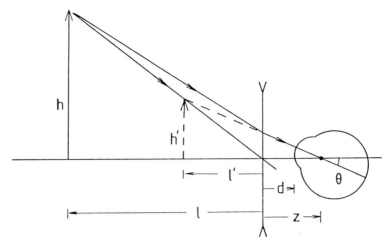

Figure 7.8 Calculation of convergence required to view a near object.

Contact Lenses

As with accommodation, assume that the eye is emmetropic and looking directly at the object. Thus for each eye:

Angle of convergence, $\tan \theta = h/(z-l)$
$$= 35/(27{=}250)$$
$$= 0.1264$$

Thus $\theta = 12.6\triangle$

Thus, with contact lenses, this myope will have to converge by nearly $1.6\triangle$ more than the spectacle lens wearer, as well as needing more accommodation. This could be predicted qualitatively as the contact lens wearer does not have the prismatic effect of spectacle lenses to aid convergence. In the case of a hypermetrope, the situation is reversed, so that a contact lens wearer will require less accommodation and less convergence than a spectacle lens wearer.

It was pointed out by Stone (1967) that the ratio of convergence to accommodation remains substantially the same for both myopes and hypermetropes on changing from spectacles to contact lenses.

7.10   ASPHERIC CONTACT LENSES

Aspheric rear surface hard contact lenses are increasingly being used in order to provide a better fit on the aspheric cornea. For many years, manufacturers of hard contact lenses used multiple concentric spherical curves in order to give a pseudo-aspheric rear surface, as these designs were much easier to produce than a true aspheric curve. However with modern lathe technology, this is no longer the case.

The simplest type of aspheric curve is the conic section, which can be described (Baker, 1943) in x, y co-ordinates, with the origin at the vertex to the surface by:

$$y^2 = 2r_ox - px^2 \qquad \text{(eqn 7.14)}$$

In this expression, r_0 is the vertex radius of the curve, and p is the parameter describing the type of conic curve:

$P>1$ Oblate ellipsoid.
$P=1$ Spherical.
$1<p<0$ Ellipsoid.
$p=0$ Paraboloid
$p<0$ Hyberboloid

The cornea is an ellipsoid with a *p* in the region of 0.75, although there is considerable individual variation. Thus by changing the *p* value of the rear surface of a lens, a design can be produced with any desired axial edge lift, for a given BOZR r_0.

More control on the shape of the aspheric curve is given by the use of a polynomial equation for a surface:

$$x = Ay^2 + By^4 + C_y{}^6 + D_{y8} \ldots$$

In this case A, B, C, D are aspheric co-efficients. The series can be extended as far is required. A conic surface can be considered as a special case of a polynomial with only one aspheric co-efficient. An example of a lens using a polynomial rear surface is the Bausch and Lomb 'Quantum' design (Atkinson, 1989).

7.11 DIFFRACTIVE OPTICS AND CONTACT LENSES

Although bifocal contact lenses have been available for many years with solid or fused segments, analagous to spectacle types, there have been developed recently contact lenses that work by diffraction of light, rather than refraction. Freeman (1984) has shown a design method for such a lens. The basic principles of diffractive lenses (also known as zone plates) have been known for many years. Wood (1898) drew a series of concentric rings on a white sheet of paper such that the radii were proportional to the square root of the integer numbers 1, 2, 3, 4, etc. Spaces between the alternate rings were blackened, and then the diagram photographically reduced, such that the radius of the first black/white zone equals:

$$\pm \sqrt{(2f\lambda)}$$

where *f* is the focal length, and λ is the design wavelength in the visible spectrum. The light is bent by the narrow gaps between successive rings acting as a series of variable width diffraction gratings

Because of this, these devices are very wavelength-dependent. Negative diffraction also takes place, so that equal energy goes into forming the +f and −f images. Additionally, there are positive and negative second-, third-, fourth-, etc. order diffraction images, all decreasing the clarity of the optical system. An additional, major problem is that about one-third of the light is directly transmitted by zero order diffraction. This latter problem can be overcome by the use of alternate zones of difference thickness, rather than black/white (Figure 7.9), but this still leaves equal energy going into negative and positive first-order diffraction. The solution of Freeman to this problem was to make a stepped zone plate, so that the majority of light at the design wavelength (400 nm) is transmitted by positive first-order diffraction, and the unwanted diffractive effects are reduced. Also, at 600+ nm, the diffractive image will be much reduced in intensity, but zero-order transmission will be enhanced. Thus a lens with two completely different focal powers is possible.

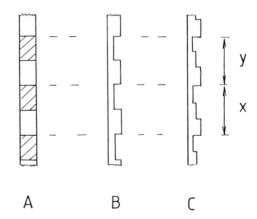

Figure 7.9 Sections through parts of various types of diffractive lens, where *x* and *y* are successive zones. A, alternate black/white zone plate; B, lens with thickness variation; C, lens with 'stepped' thickness variation.

7.12   CALCULATION OF AXIAL EDGE LIFT – COMPUTER PROGRAM

It is useful to know when fitting a multi-curve contact lens what the axial edge lift will be when fitted to an alignment on the central curve. The following short computer program (see Fowler, 1985 for method of calculation) will calculate axial edge lift for any number of curves up to ten. The program is written in BASIC and should run on most personal computers:

```
10 DIM r(10): DIM y(10): DIM d(10)
15 k=0
20 INPUT "No of curves"; n
30 FOR i = 1 TO n STEP 1
35 PRINT "curve no."; i
40 INPUT "Radius (mm)" ; r(i)
50 INPUT "Diameter (mm)"; d(i)
55 y(i)=d(i)/2
60 NEXT i
65 L=y(n)
70 FOR i=1 TO n STEP 1
80 IF i=1 THEN a(1)=0
100 IF i<>1 THEN a(i)=r(i–1)–SQR(r(i–1)^2–
y(i–1)^2)–(r(i)–SQR(r(i)^2–y(i–1)^2))
105 PRINT a(i)
110 r=r(i)
120 k=k + a(i)
220 IF L<=y(i) THEN 300
250 NEXT i
300 s=r–SQR(r^2–L^2)+k
301 IF L>r(1) THEN 305
302 t=r(1)–SQR(r(1)^2–L^2)
303 q=t–s
304 PRINT "Edge Lift ="; q
305 PRINT "y="; L
306 PRINT "Sag ="; s
310 END
```

REFERENCES

Atkinson, T.C.O. (1989) Towards a new gas permeable lens geometry. *The Optician*, **197** (5158), 13–15, 17.

Baker, T.Y. (1943) Ray tracing through non-spherical surfaces. *Proc. Phys. Soc.*, **LV**, 361–4.

Bennett, A.G. (1976) Power changes in soft contact lenses due to bending. *Ophthalmic Optician*, **16** (22), 939–47.

Brennan, N.A., Lowe, R., Efron, N., Ungerer, J.L. and Carney, L.G. (1987) Dehydration of hydrogel lenses during overnight wear. *Am. J. Optom. Physiol. Opti.*, **64** (7), 534–9.

Chaston, J. and Fatt, I. (1980) The change in power of soft lenses. *The Optician*, **180** (4663), 12–21.

Ford, M.W. (1976) *Changes in Hydrophlic Lenses when Placed in the Eye*. Paper at a joint International Congress of the Contact Lens Society and the National Eye Research Foundation, Montreux, Switzerland.

Fowler, C.W. (1985) Some notes on the construction of 'zonal aspheric' aphakic spectacle lenses. *Ophthal. Physiol. Opt.*, **5** (3), 343–6.

Freeman, M.H. (1984) Bifocal contact lens having diffractive power. *UK Patent Application 2 129 157 A*, The Patent Office, London.

Halass, S. (1959) Aniseikonic lenses of improved design and their application. *Aust. J. Optom.*, **43**, 417–20; 469–71.

Holden, B.A. and Zantos, S.G. (1981) On the conformity of soft lenses to the shape of the cornea. *Am. J. Optom. Physiol. Opti.*, **58** (2), 139–43.

Ruben, M. (1975) *Contact Lens Practice*, Baillière Tindall, London.

Stone, J.S. (1967) Near vision difficulties in non-presbyopic corneal lens wearers. *Contact Lens*, **1**(2), 14–16; 24–5.

Weissman, B.A. and Zisman, F. (1981) Effective powers of flexible contact lenses. *Am. J. Optom.*, **58** (1), 2–5.

Winn, B., Ackerley, R.G., Brown, C.A., Murray, F.K., Paris, J. and St John, M.F. (1986) The superiority of contact lenses in the correction of axial anisometropia. *Transactions of the British Contact Lens Association Annual Clinical Conference 1986*.

Wood, R.W. (1898) Phase reversal zone-plates and diffraction-telescopes. *Philos. Mag. J. Sci.*, **45** (5th series), 511–22.

QUALITY ASSURANCE AND QUALITY CONTROL FOR VOLUME LENS MANUFACTURING

8

W.S. Gibson

8.1 DEFINITIONS

8.1.1 QUALITY

The *Oxford English Dictionary* defines quality as 'degree of excellence' or general excellence.

8.1.2 QUALITY CONTROL

Quality control (QC) is the aggregate of activities and operational techniques concerned with producing a specified article within design parameters. In continuous production it includes:

1. Inspection.
2. Adjustment to process settings.
3. Removal of defectives.
4. Rectification of defective items.

Quality control may be performed by people or by machines; in either case, feedback of information from inspection is fundamental to determine process adjustments. Inspection is most effective when performed automatically or by the process operator to shorten the feedback time. An independent inspection team is less effective at achieving control.

8.1.3 QUALITY ASSURANCE

Quality assurance (QA) is the aggregate of the activities performed in providing evidence and confidence that the quality intended has been achieved. It includes:

1. Raw material acceptance and vendor appraisal.
2. In-process release of components.
3. Finished product appraisal and release/rejection.
4. Failure investigations.
5. Authorization of product specifications and quality standards (quality manual).
6. Verification of equipment calibration.
7. Verification of all quality activities.

8.1.4 QUALITY OF DESIGN AND QUALITY OF CONFORMANCE

Product users understand quality mainly in terms of quality of design; producers understand quality in terms of conformance to design.

Design quality is set by the technical resource of a company, for example whether the product is designed to be a lounge chair or a kitchen chair, or alternatively a luxury motor car or a delivery van.

Contact Lens Practice. Edited by Montague Ruben and Michel Guillon. Published in 1994 by Chapman & Hall, London. ISBN 0 412 35120 X

Quality of conformance is the degree to which the product is free from defects and thereby fulfils its design concept. This chapter is solely concerned with the latter – quality of conformance – as viewed by the producer. Measurement of this quality and application to the benefit of the user and the producer falls to the quality assurance team; clearly, objectivity and impartiality are ideal requirements, although the necessary proximity to design, production and financial teams can challenge attainment of these ideals. A properly balanced relationship with marketing and customer service, to emphasize the user's viewpoint of quality, is also necessary to effective quality assurance

8.2 ESTABLISHING A QUALITY POLICY FOR CONTACT LENS PRODUCTION

8.2.1 GENERAL CONSTRAINTS

There are no major differences between producing contact lenses and producing most other consumer goods, such as bars of soap, razor blades or ball-point pens. They have commonalities of production, e.g.:

1. Basic starting materials.
2. Process equipment to convert materials.
3. Instruments to measure the results.
4. Packaging processes.
5. Human operatives.

Faulty materials, processes and instruments can lead to the production of defective products as, also, can adventitious damage and human error.

8.2.2 STATUTORY REQUIREMENTS

United States of America – Food and Drug Administration

Specific requirements arise for contact lenses as these are regulated in the USA. Premarketing approval is required and hydrophilic soft lenses must be sterile. Furthermore, medical device Good Manufacturing Practices must be followed in production (CFR 21 Pt 820, 1978):

1. All starting materials must be properly qualified and approved before manufacture.
2. All finished products must be evaluated and approved for release and distribution by an independent quality assurance unit.
3. Equipment must be suited to its purpose and maintained and calibrated at regular intervals.

Rest of the world

Only minor regulations currently apply to contact lenses, for example in Germany lenses must comply with labelling regulations for 'fictitious drugs' under the German drug law. The Council of the European Communities has adopted Council Directive 93/42/EEC of 14 June 1993 concerning medical devices. When passed into the national laws of the member states (January 1995), this directive will govern the production and supply of contact lenses in the community.

Despite the current absence of significant regulations, the supply of contact lenses to the end user is normally restricted to optometric practices having professionally qualified staff who are accountable to a government department, and thus 'regulated' indirectly, and also to the requirements of their professional body.

8.2.3 INTERNATIONAL AND NATIONAL STANDARDS

The American National Standards Institute has published standards for hard and for soft contact lenses (ANSI Z80.2, 1989; ANSI Z80.6, 1983; ANSI Z80.8, 1986). The British Standards Institution has published a contact lens standard (BS7208) establishing a method of classifying contact lens material, a specification – including tolerances – for rigid contact lenses and providing test methods for contact lenses.

The European Community's Standards Body CEN (*Comité Européen de Normalisation*) will be adopting the ISO standards now being developed for contact lens specifying requirements and test methods. The EN standards will be those regarded for the purpose of assessing contact lenses by member states.

ISO 9000: 1987 series (EN 29000: 1987 series) provides guidance on quality systems. When the Council Directive 93/42/EEC is fully implemented, producers of contact lenses will have to ensure that their quality systems conform to the requirements of the relevant part of EN 29000 or its equivalent.

8.2.4 COMPANY CONSTRAINTS

Consumerism, product liability laws, marketing goals (image, growth and pricing) and feedback from customers all contribute to forming a quality policy for a company.

8.2.5 QUALITY POLICY AND QUALITY MANUALS

Quality policy

A written policy forming part of a quality manual crystallizes the general and statutory requirements and constraints shown above into broad quality objectives for manufacturing. The first part of the quality manual may follow these headings:

1. Introduction – company description.
2. Scope – products involved.
3. General requirements – quality policy.
4. Quality system – who is responsible and for what.
5. Organization – human resources and training.
6. Quality plans – work instructions.
7. Documentation – drawings, batch records, calibration.
8. Change control procedures – relating to policy.
9. Rework procedures and disposal of non-conforming items.
10. Warranties, return goods procedures and product recalls.
11. Quality system audits – periodic reviews to check operating effectiveness.

CORRECTIVE ACTION PROCEDURES
Operating quality manuals

In the subsequent parts of the quality manual the specific goals of the quality system will be stated. Several separate sub-manuals usually prove necessary, for example:

1. Purchasing quality agreements, raw material acceptance procedures and vendor quality system auditing.
2. Calibration procedures and periodic instrument servicing.

Table 8.1 Final GP lens verification

Characteristics	Nominal values	Tolerances	Test methods	Sampling levels
BOZR (mm)	8.00; 8.10; 8.20	±0.05	Radiuscope	GII
DIA (mm)	7.8; 8.2	±0.1	Travelling microscope	S4
Power (dioptres)	Plano to −10.00 in 0.25 steps	±0.125	Focimeter with 5 mm aperture	GII
Centre thickness (mm)	0.15	±0.02	Dial gauge	S4

3. In-process quality control procedures, e.g. statistical process control, 100% inspection, etc.
4. Finished product verification and release.
5. Process validations (e.g. sterilizers).
6. Subcontractor quality assurance.
7. Environmental controls.
8. Process and product change control procedures.

In these manuals, there should be stated the specific goals which must be met and the methods of assuring them. For example, a company may require its finished gas permeable lens to be labelled with back optic zone radius (BOZR), total diameter (dia) and spherical refractive power in the discrete values:

BOZR 8.00, 8.10, 8.20. . .
dia 7.8, 8.2
power in 0.25 steps

Tolerances need to be provided because the measuring equipment will have finer precision (able to measure BOZR in 0.02 steps or diameter in 0.05 steps) and the lens may be expected to have actual parameter values off the discrete values. Typical tolerances might be:

BOZR ± 0.05 mm
dia ± 0.10 mm
power ± 0.125 D

Part of the finished product verification manual would then look like Table 8.1. The sampling level column states the intensity with which inspection is to be performed. These important sampling terms are explained in ISO 2859–1: 1989. Test methods will require clear descriptions and may be elaborated in a special test method manual or included in those manuals which refer to them.

8.3 CONTACT LENS MANUFACTURING PROCESSES

The earliest procedure was for rigid lenses

1. Polymerization of liquid monomer.
2. Machining (turning) the base curve, the peripheral curves and the edge.
3. Polishing base curves and the edge.
4. Mounting the base curve component.
5. Machining the front surface and lenticulation.
6. Polishing the front surface.
7. Demounting, cleaning.
8. Inspection.
9. Packaging.

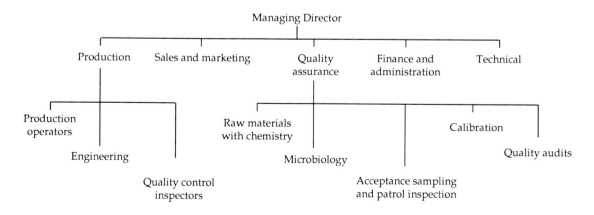

Figure 8.1 Organization chart for volume contact lens manufacturing.

A similar set of procedures is followed for lathe-cut hydrophilic lenses, to which is added, in place of packaging:

1. Hydration/extraction
2. Inspection (100% refractive power measurement).
3. Washing, packaging and labelling.
4. Sterilization.

Although it is beyond the scope of this chapter to explain the reasons, it is a fact that despite the controls exercised during polymer blank manufacturing and during the dry soft lens manufacturing steps, it is not feasible to anticipate the hydrated lens power that will result for any one lens to the required accuracy. A low water content polymer lens may have a dry (zerogel) power of 4.2 D, which on hydration becomes 3.0 D. Greater changes than this example take place for higher water content polymer lenses. In consequence, 100% measurement of finished lens wet power is essential to labelling each lens accurately. Assurance of the correctness

of the final label parameters is more critical than with rigid lenses or with most consumer products.

Spin casting of hydrophilic lenses follows a similar sequence amounting to several steps:

1. Production of spin casting moulds by injection moulding into metal mould tools.
2. Preparation of liquid polymer batch.
3. Injection, spinning and curing of polymer into moulds.
4. Inspection after spin casting (e.g. centre thickness).
5. Hydration/extraction.
6. 100% inspection (power).
7. Washing, packaging and labelling.
8. Sterilization.

Cast moulding of hydrophilic lenses is also similar except that two plastic components are produced and the liquid polymer is placed between the matching pairs and cured without spinning. Edge polishing the moulded lenses

Table 8.2 Accountabilities of quality control and quality assurance

Quality control	Quality assurance
	Approves sources of raw materials (vendor approval)
	Identifies and approves batches of raw materials
Works with standards supplied	Supplies and maintains quality standards, product specifications, and tolerances (operating quality manual)
100% inspection of lenses	Checks QC records and tests samples, patrol inspection and acceptance sampling
Accepts good lenses individually	Accepts batches of good lenses collectively and authorizes release
Rejects bad lenses individually	Rejects batches of lenses which have defectives exceeding permitted limits
Calibrates own equipment	Checks that properly calibrated equipment is in use (patrol inspection)
	Evaluates sterility of soft lens batches and authorizes release
	Audits the quality function and keeps watch on compliance to good manufacturing practices
	Investigates failures

may be done before hydration.

In planning QC and QA procedures for contact lenses, the particular process steps above will be the basis for what is done. To this must be added several procedures which indirectly control in-process and finished product quality, for example:

1. Raw material qualification/acceptance.
2. Environmental control/monitoring.
3. Evaluation of wash water quality.
4. Sterilizer validation.
5. Final product sterility evaluation.

In the next section, the allocation of these responsibilities and tasks between QC and QA is shown.

8.4 ORGANIZATION, ACCOUNTABILITIES AND DUTIES OF QC AND QA TEAMS

8.4.1 ORGANIZATION AND QUALIFICATIONS OF QC AND QA

A suitable organization chart for volume lens manufacturing is shown in Figure 8.1. The independence and authority of quality assurance is emphasized by its direct line into the chief executive.

Whereas Quality Control lens inspectors need normally only have training on the job, some quality assurance personnel will certainly need qualifications gained in technical college or university. A national qualification such as the Certificate in Quality Control (Institute of Quality Assurance) is desirable for laboratory technicians who are concerned with fine metrology and calibration; alternatively, a microbiological or chemical qualification is desirable for technicians assessing contamination or purity.

8.4.2 ACCOUNTABILITIES OF QC AND QA

Table 8.2 compares the accountabilities of QC and QA. The responsibility for fulfilling the company's quality policy does not rest only with QC and QA through their account-abilities satisfying the customers' needs and desires requires the continual input of Technical, Engineering, Production, Purchasing, Inventory and Sales teams as well.

Figure 8.2 shows how some of the accountabilities of QC and QA work along with production activities for lathe-cut soft lenses.

8.4.3 DUTIES OF QUALITY CONTROL TEAM

The work of the quality control team is closely associated with production, and they report to the Production Director under a Chief Inspector. This association means that QC will measure and inspect all lenses to segregate good ones from bad ones and feedback their findings to the process operator. This may seem outdated practice but it is not always possible to inspect lenses after each process step and the process must be allowed to run on for quite some time before feedback is possible. For example, errors in mounting base curve components (voids in mounting wax, particles trapped in mounting wax or non-coaxiallity) cannot be detected by inspection until both diameter and front surface machining processes have been completed. Indeed, imperfections in the mounting wax will not be inspectable until front surface polishing, edging and demounting steps are complete. In this example, the feedback loop will not take seconds, but probably hours.

The application of statistical quality control techniques (Grant & Leavenworth, 1988) is not wide in volume lens production, although some processes do lend themselves well to it, for instance:

1. Control of base curve machining.
2. Final diameter machining.
3. Centre thickness control of spin casting.

8.4.4 DUTIES OF THE QUALITY ASSURANCE TEAM

Figure 8.3 shows a typical allocation of QA resources to their major duties.

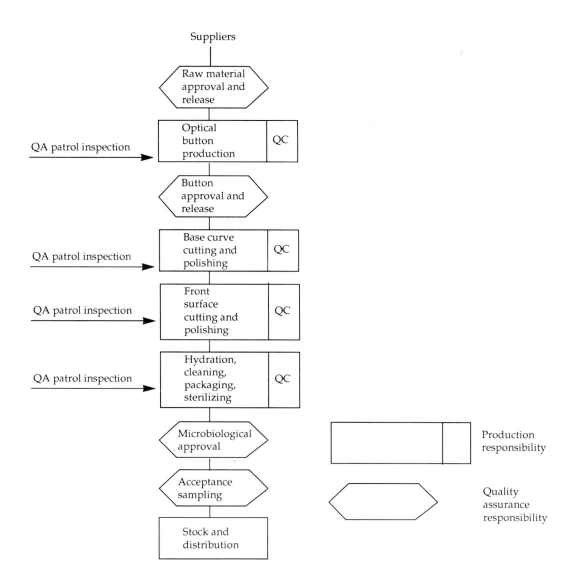

Figure 8.2 Lens manufacturing sequence showing quality assurance's role.

Specifications

Continual review and refinement of the specifications of starting materials, packaging materials and intermediate and finished product need the attention of the quality engineering function. Input from Regulatory, Marketing, Technical, Materials and Production departments create the need for change.

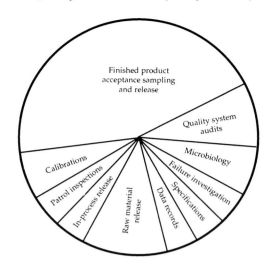

Figure 8.3 Allocation of quality assurance resources.

Thus new indirect materials such as solvents will need evaluation for safety and suitability and may affect acceptance procedures. QA will work with the sponsoring department to ensure that company objectives are met and that appropriate documentation is in place before authorization of changes.

Raw material acceptance and vendor appraisal

QA determines the acceptability of the ingredients of both the product and its packaging. Each batch of materials received will be tested and will not be released for production until it is approved. This duty means that standards of quality for the material must be agreed with the supplier. These standards are fully documented to eliminate arbitrary decision making, and there must be regular liasion with vendors to ensure that the requirements are understood.

In-process release

The polymerized monomer in the form of the optical button is the basic substance which contacts the eye. The correctness of the for-

mulation and its physicochemical properties must be independently verified by QA before lenses are made from the polymer. Individual groups of buttons are given release status by QA.

Patrol inspection and calibration

Adherence to good manufacturing practices (GMPs) requires a certain state of mind in the production worker and supervisor. When problems demand the special attention of the employees, it is inevitable that some relaxation of the GMPs will ensue. QA maintains a regular patrol to continually remind people of the quality objectives. Particular surveillance is made of:

1.   Raw material labelling and button batch identification.
2.   Production specifications and record keeping, process settings (e.g. autoclave pressure and timer controls).
3.   Environmental conditions, including temperature and humidity, control of waste and employee attire and cleanliness.
4.   Production and quality control instruments – these are checked regularly to ensure that valid results are being obtained.

Finished product release

QA has the sole authority to release or to reject finished lenses. Following 100% inspection by quality control, batches of lenses are passed to QA, who measure conformance to design by taking statistically valid samples. The technique is more fully described later. Either the batch is released for distribution or, if the criteria are not met, it is returned to production quality control, who may decide that removal of defectives by inspection is possible or that reprocessing is feasible and appropriate. Reworked batches must again be submitted to QA for further acceptance sampling before release can be decided upon. In the case of a defective batch which cannot be improved, the whole batch will be quarantined pending destruction under supervision by QA.

Final approval and release of lenses for distribution forms the greater proportion of the QA department's work and reflects the importance which attaches to making and supplying these sterile medical devices which are fitted to millions of people. Inadequate or improper control of this step could be hazardous to lens users and to the company's fortunes in the marketplace.

Microbiology

The main duty is to evaluate the sterility of each sterilization batch of soft lenses. Three options exist:

1. Sterility testing of finished product following a pharmacopoeial monograph (USP XX1, 1985).
2. By including product units inoculated with biological indicators (*B. stearothermophilus*) in the batch and testing these for viability.
3. By reviewing records of the time and temperature cycle to which the load was exposed.

One or more of these can be followed to reach a level of confidence in batch sterility. It is considered good manufacturing practice to have a knowledge of the nature and extent of biological contamination in the lens package before sterilization and the QA microbiologist should monitor this regularly once or twice a week.

Similarly, potential sources of contamination should be monitored microbiologically, i.e. lens washing water and the air in the washing/packaging area. This knowledge will help to minimize contamination once the major causes are identified.

Failure investigation and data records

Internal and external failures must be reviewed by QA and properly documented and investigated. Corrective action to future production should ensue. These actions may take the form of changes to a product specification, a test method, a raw material specification or a processing method.

Batch records are kept by QA (including certain production department records) and these enable the details of each batch to be retrieved if, as may happen, a lens is the subject of a complaint. Quantities of similar lenses can be established and the dates of manufacturing, together with the lot numbers of direct and indirect material. If necessary part or all of the batch could be recalled or withheld from further distribution with help from these data records.

8.5   ACCEPTANCE SAMPLING

The appraisal technique used to determine suitability of lenses for final distribution is called acceptance sampling. In repetitive high volume production, human errors and machine failures result in a few defective units randomly scattered throughout the product. Soft contact lens production is not exempt from these problems. The quality control team at each process step certainly remove the vast majority of defectives, but a few inevitably get through. Other kinds of defect not visible or not inspectable by non-destructive methods creep into some units, a particularly notorious example of the latter being the 'wrong lens in the bottle', meaning that the lens parameters are not the same as those on the vial label. This example of a defective unit actually costs opticians valuable chair-time, and they may even have to ask a patient to return another day if they have not got the lens they thought they had. Acceptance sampling can regulate the amount of error and defects in lenses and the cost of having such a system is usually amply rewarded by savings for both the practitioner and the manufacturer.

8.5.1 ACCEPTANCE SAMPLING TECHNIQUES

Well defined techniques emerged in the USA, Canada and UK during the Second World War and were published as various defence and military standards. There are two subdivisions:

1. Acceptance sampling by attributes.
2. Acceptance sampling by variables.

Modern standards are ISO 2859–1: 1989 for 'attributes' and ISO 3951 for 'variables'.

An attribute is a product characteristic which can be judged 'right' or 'wrong', that is, acceptable or defective. An example would be a finished contact lens which was either torn (defective) or not torn (acceptable). A variable is a measurable product characteristic (diameter, power, BOZR); it can provide information about product quality conformance (to a given tolerance) and the combined data of several items teaches us about the process or measuring equipment or the inspector as well. Variables are often treated like attributes and reduced to simple good/bad classifications.

These standards are soundly based in statistical probability theory (Caplen, 1988, Juran & Gryna, 1988). They give guidance on:

1. Classification of defects by seriousness.
2. Assigning Acceptable Quality Levels – AQLs.
3. Sampling plans.
4. Decision making on acceptance.

8.5.2 DISADVANTAGES OF BATCH ACCEPTANCE SAMPLING

Although the use of batch acceptance sampling procedures for releasing large numbers of contact lenses to distribution has been practiced by many producers, this chapter's author prefers to use continuous sampling wherever possible, both to expedite delivery and to minimize the number of lenses held in batch acceptance after processing is completed. Alternatively, ways may be available of eliminating the testing of product totally. Thus, for example, the periodic validation (i.e. qualification) of the process, combined with continuously accurate process control and monitoring of process conditions for each batch treated in the wet stream sterilization process (autoclaving) can provide all the assurance required to declare lenses 'sterile' on the same day the batch is sterilized; whereas product testing or the use of biological indicators requires incubation for 14 days or longer before 'sterility' can be decided. The latter can result in long delivery times for non-stock lenses and custom made lenses.

8.5.3 QUALITY IMPROVEMENT TECHNIQUES

The use of acceptance sampling procedures has received the serious criticism that it gives the supplier a right to make and supply a proportion of bad lenses. This criticism is much reduced if the supplier is continually reviewing the process defect levels and, more importantly, progressively reducing the alloted AQLs. Even so, this does not directly address corrective action on the causes.

A better way to meet the customers' needs and desires is to implement a continuous quality improvement programme involving all those persons/departments (e.g. design, engineering, purchasing, production and quality assurance) whose work bears on the process where defective lenses arise. Small interdisciplinary teams would correlate defects with their sources and look for ways of controlling these to eliminate further defects.

The concept of 'zero defects', as the performance standard, should be nurtured in everyone's mind; mistakes are caused by lack of knowledge and lack of attention, and can be avoided. Perfection may never be achieved but neither should it be assumed impossible.

Continuous quality improvement programmes form part of the overall business strategy known as Total Quality Management which has proved to be a powerful way of delivering quality product (Crosby, 1979; Deming, 1986; Juran and Gryna, 1988; Oakland, 1990).

REFERENCES

ANSI-Z80.2 (1989) *Rigid Contact Lenses – Prescription Requirements for Ophthalmic Lenses*. American National Standards Institute Inc., New York.

ANSI-Z80.6 (1983) *Conventional Hard Plastic Contact Lenses – Physicochemical Properties*. American National Standards Institute Inc., New York.

ANSI-Z80.8 (1986) *Ophthalmic Soft Contact Lenses – Prescription Requirements*. American National Standards Institute Inc., New York.

BS 7208 Part 1 (1992) (same as ISO 8321-1:1991) *Contact Lenses-Specification for Rigid Lenses*. British Standards Institution, London.

BS 7208 Part 2 (1991) *Contact lenses. Method of classifying contact lens materials*.

BS 7208 Part 3 (1992) *Contact lenses. Methods of test for contact lenses*.

Caplen, R.H. (1988) *A Practical Approach to Quality Control* (4th ed), Business Books Ltd, London.

CFR 21 820 (1978) *Code of Federal Regulations – Title 21 – Food and Drugs – Part 820, Manufacturing, Packing, Storage and Installation of Medical Devices. Regulations Establishing Good Manufacturing Practices*. US Department of Health, Education and Welfare, *The Federal Register*, **43** (141).

Council of the European Communities (1993) *Council Directive 93/42/EEC of 14 June 1993 concerning medical devices*. OJ No. L 169, 12 July.

Crosby, P.B. (1979) *Quality is free*. McGraw-Hill Book Company, New York.

Deming, W.E. (1986) *Quality, Productivity and Competitive Position*. MIT Center for Advanced Engineering Study, Cambridge, Massachusetts.

Grant, E.L and Leavenworth, R.S. (1988) *Statistical Quality Control* (6th ed), McGraw-Hill Book Company, New York.

ISO 2859-1 (1989) (same as BS 6001 Part 1:1991) *Sampling procedures for inspection by attributes. Specification for sampling plans indexed by acceptable quality level (AQL) for lot-by-lot inspection*. British Standards Institution, London.

ISO 3951 (equivalent to BS 6002:1979 *Specification for sampling procedures and charts for inspection by variables for percent defective*). British Standards Institution, London.

ISO 9000 (1987) *Quality Systems – Guidelines for Selection and Use* (same as BS 5750: Part 0: Section 0.1: 1987 and EN 29000–1987).

ISO 9001 (1987) *Quality Systems–Model for Quality Assurance in Design/Development, Production, Installation and Servicing* (same as BS 5750: Part 1: 1987 and EN 29001–1987).

ISO 9002 (1987) *Quality Systems–Model for Quality Assurance in Production and Installation* (same as BS 5750: Part 2: 1987 and EN 29002–1987).

ISO 9003 (1987) *Quality Systems–Model for Quality Assurance in Final Inspection and Test* (same as BS 5750: Part 3: 1987 and EN 29003–1987).

ISO 9004 (1987) *Quality Systems – Guide to quality management and quality systems elements* (same as BS 5750: Part 0: Section 0.2: 1987 and EN 29004).

Juran, J.M and Gryna, F.M (1988) *Juran's Quality Control Handbook* (4th Edn), McGraw-Hill Book Company, New York.

Oakland, J.S. (1990) *Total Qality Management*. Nichols Publishing Co., New York, NY.

USP XXII (1990) *United States Pharmacopeia*. United States Pharmacopeial Convention Inc., Rockville, MD.

R.M. Pearson

9.1 THE IMPORTANCE OF IN-PRACTICE QUALITY CONTROL

Responsibility for the quality and subsequent clinical performance of contact lenses rests with the practitioner who supplies them. It is, therefore, essential that every contact lens is measured and inspected carefully to determine both its quantitative and qualitative adequacy prior to being issued to the patient. Lenses may be obtained from a company using high volume mass production methods and such firms generally undertake rigorous quality assurance checks upon a statistically valid sample of each production run. Nevertheless, the possibility remains that an inaccurate or poorly made lens, which was not included in this sample, will be sent to the practitioner. On the other hand, small laboratories may use less sophisticated manufacturing equipment and procedures and these might lead to inconsistent standards, again presenting the possibility of an unsatisfactory lens being supplied to the practitioner.

It is, of course, imperative that the practitioner undertakes fitting with trial lenses of exactly known specification. Unfortunately, studies by Fletcher and Nisted (1961) and Shanks (1966) demonstrated that such lenses were frequently supplied with incorrect dimensions. Despite the advent of computer-controlled lathes and other automated manufacturing procedures, it is clear that the difficulty of poorly made lenses remains (McMonnies, 1989). A brief time invested in checking both trial and prescription lenses may save a greater amount of time being wasted at after-care visits in resolving unnecessary problems.

The back optic zone radius (BOZR) and back optic zone diameter (BOZD) are arguably the most important dimensions in determining the fit of a corneal lens and the former is vulnerable to change and distortion over a period of time. Verification of BOZR should accordingly be an essential feature of the routine after-care examination of the patient. Measurement of BOZR can resolve the problem of lenses misplaced in a fitting set by the practitioner or a pair of lenses, perhaps of similar power, transposed by the patient.

It is not uncommon to be asked by a patient to provide after-care for lenses fitted elsewhere of unknown specification. Competent clinical care can only be provided in such cases if an attempt is made to ascertain the dimensional and optical properties of the present lenses. Although the major part of the specification can usually be determined without too much difficulty, identification of the material may not be possible. Attempts have been made to develop simple methods

Contact Lens Practice. Edited by Montague Ruben and Michel Guillon.
Published in 1994 by Chapman & Hall, London. ISBN 0 412 35120 X

for practice use to establish the identity of the material on the basis of specific gravity (Refojo & Leong, 1984) but such tests are imprecise (Morton *et al.*, 1987). A further complication in this approach is the advent of materials such as the fluoropolymer Boston Equalens (Polymer Technology Inc.), which has the same specific gravity of 1.18 as polymethyl methacrylate (PMMA).

An alternative approach to the identification of material from which a lens has been manufactured is measurement of refractive index. A hand refractometer (Atago N3000) was used by Hodur *et al.* (1992) who found that fluoropolymer materials had a value of less than 1.460 and silicone–acrylate polymers had a value of 1.460, or more. A refractive index of 1.490 indicated that the material was PMMA.

9.2 CALIBRATION OF MEASUREMENT INSTRUMENTS

Of the various rôles of contact lens measurement, that of greatest value is the confirmation that a newly made pair conform accurately to the specification ordered. Certain tolerance limits on dimensional and optical properties must be accepted by both manufacturers and practitioners and they should realistically reflect accuracy of lens measurement and limits of accuracy in fitting. Both the International Standards Organization and several national standards bodies have addressed the problem of formulating valid tolerance limits. The implementation of such limits is dependent upon the use of specified measurement procedures and the use of properly calibrated instruments. Regrettably, the importance of calibration has been neglected in the past and this probably explains at least some of the disputes between between practitioner and laboratory over a lens specification. Calibration is the process of identifying errors inherent in the use of an instrument by a particular operator. The general procedure

for calibration can be summarized as follows:

1. A minimum of three test pieces of known accuracy are required for each type of instrument. Suitable test objects are mentioned in the description of equipment which follows.
2. Ten independent readings of each test piece are made and the mean value for each is calculated. The expression 'independent' signifies that the test piece is removed from the instrument then repositioned between each reading.
3. The accurately known values for each test piece are plotted against the mean measured values in order to obtain a calibration curve. Subsequently measured lens values are corrected by reference to this curve.

Alternatively, the same data can be used to perform a least-squares linear regression and the slope and intercept values can be used to

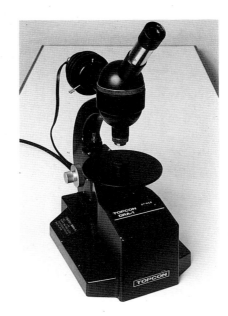

Figure 9.1 An optical spherometer. The instrument illustrated is a Topcon Digital Radiusmeter (model DRA-1) which has a digital display of radius.

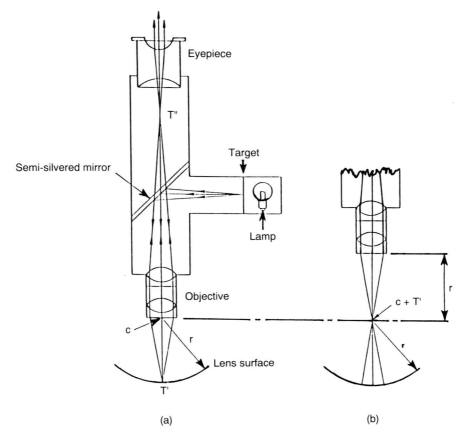

Figure 9.2 The optical system of the optical spherometer showing the formation of the surface (a) and aerial (b) images of the target (T).

calculate correct values from measured readings. This calibration process should be repeated at intervals or if there is a new individual using the instrument.

In this account of in-practice quality control, emphasis will be placed on recommended methods which, when calibrated for a particular user, allow implementation of the corresponding tolerance limits which are stated.

9.3   MEASUREMENT OF RADII

The exploitation of Drysdale's principle to the measurement of contact lens radii was first described by Bier (1958). The optical spherometer (Figs. 9.1 and 9.2) is essentially a microscope of which either the body or the stage supporting the lens can move vertically. Light from an illuminated spoke pattern target (T) is reflected down the microscope body by means of a semi-silvered mirror to be imaged by the microscope objective. When the focus is coincident with the lens surface, light is reflected along the diametrically opposite path forming images at both at T and T". The latter image coincides with the first principal focus of the eyepiece so that the observer sees a sharp image of the target (Figs. 9.2(a) and 9.3). The distance between the microscope and the lens surface is increased, either by raising the microscope or by lowering the stage, until the image formed by the objective (T') is coincident with the centre (C) of the surface (Fig. 9.2(b)). Light from the target becomes incident upon the surface normally and is reflected back along its own path to again form images at T and T″ (Figs. 9.2(b) and 9.4(a,b,c)). The distance through which the microscope or stage has been moved corresponds to the radius (r) of curvature of the contact lens.

The microscope objective normally has a magnification of × 10, or more, and a numerical aperture of 0.25, or greater. From both theoretical and experimental evidence, it was concluded by Charman (1972) that, due to diffraction effects, the use of an objective with a numerical aperture of less than 0.15 would result in a spread of measurements of more than 0.02 mm. The total magnification of the microscope is usually at least ×100 and the real image of the target object should be less than 1.2 mm in diameter. The radius is displayed either upon an analogue dial gauge or an electronic digital display.

The optical spherometer is commonly referred to as a 'Radiuscope', the trade name

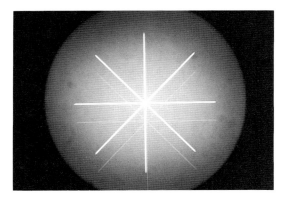

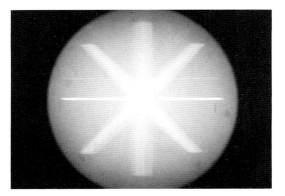

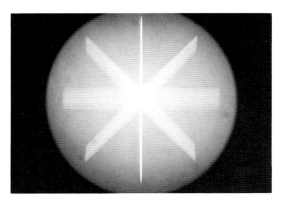

Figure 9.4 (a) The aerial image formed by a lens with a spherical back optic zone radius. (b) and (c) show the aerial images of the steep and flat meridians of a toric lens.

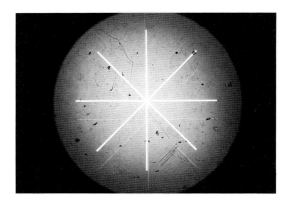

Figure 9.3 View through the eyepiece of the surface image. Note the particles of surface debris and minor scratches.

of an instrument introduced by the American Optical Co.

9.3.1   CALIBRATION

Three high quality crown glass concave test plates are required with radii of approximately 6.5, 8.0 and 9.5 mm, the accuracy and sphericity of each being certified by a recognized test laboratory such as the National Physical Laboratory of the UK (Fig. 9.5).

9.3.2   BACK OPTIC ZONE RADIUS (BOZR)

The measurement procedure is as follows:

1. A few drops of water are placed in the concave recess of the lens support (Fig. 9.6) to reduce reflection from the front surface of the lens. Too much water on the support will allow the lens to move around while it is being measured.
2. The lens, which must be clean and dry, is placed with its front surface in contact with the water upon the support. The lens must be handled with care to avoid flexing, which might result in spurious readings of toricity.
3. The support is placed upon the stage of the spherometer and centred approximately.
4. The microscope is focused upon the aerial image at the centre of the back surface of the lens and the stage is

adjusted until the image of the spoke-patterned target appears exactly centred within the field of observation. A well-made spherical lens will permit sharp focus to be obtained simultaneously of all the radial lines of the target.

5. The radius display is set to zero.
6. The microscope is next focused using the fine adjustment control upon the surface of the lens. Particles of debris and scratches facilitate identification of this image. The radius value displayed is noted.

Three readings of BOZR are taken. Each of these must be obtained by focusing first upon the aerial image and then upon the surface image or vice versa. Repetition of measurements in the same sequence should minimize errors due to backlash in the focusing system. A note should be made of the quality of the aerial image, which will be degraded in the case of a poorly made lens.

The target imaged on the surface of either a

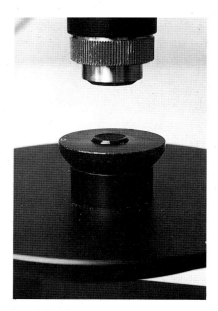

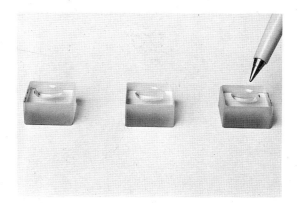

Figure 9.5 Three crown glass concave test plates used for calibration of the optical spherometer.

Figure 9.6 The lens support used for measurement of back optic zone radius.

toric or warped lens can be uniformly focused. There will, however, be two different positions in which the aerial image can be brought into focus so that first one spoke of the target is focused and then the perpendicular one.

Tolerance limits for BOZR are ±0.05 mm for gas permeable hard lenses and ±0.025 mm for PMMA lenses.

9.3.3 BACK PERIPHERAL RADIUS (BPR)

The instrument is focused upon the surface image and the lens support is repositioned beneath the microscope objective and tilted so that the target is imaged upon the periphery of the lens. The peripheral surface to be measured must be perpendicular to the axis of the instrument. The first aerial image brought into focus may be that due to the back optic zone radius. Further movement of the instrument allows the corresponding image of the back peripheral radius to be focused.

In practice, both the narrow width of peripheral curves and the presence of blending usually renders their measurement impossible. Tolerance limits of ±0.20 mm for BPR are accordingly only applicable to peripheral zones 1 mm, or more, wide.

9.3.4 FRONT OPTIC ZONE RADIUS (FOZR)

It is unnecessary to measure the front optic zone radius of a lens if the back optic zone radius, geometrical centre thickness and back vertex power are within tolerance limits and of acceptable image quality. It is, however, useful to measure the FOZR in the case of lenses giving a poor visual performance, especially in the case of front surface toric designs.

The lens is placed with a little water beneath its back surface upon a convex-shaped lens support (Fig. 9.7). The measurement procedure is essentially similar to that for BOZR but the relative positions of

the aerial and surface images are transposed.

9.3.5 ALTERNATIVE METHODS

Several companies have produced a device which can be clamped to the head-rest of an ophthalmometer in order to measure the BOZR of a corneal lens. Commonly these devices incorporate a mirror at 45 degrees to the optical axis of the instrument, which reflects light from the instrument to the lens which floats on a drop of water upon a vertical support (Fig. 9.8). For most, but not all, keratometers it will be necessary to modify the radius scale reading, as these instruments are primarily intended for the measurement of convex surfaces. In clinical practice, it is inconvenient repeatedly to attach and remove such a device to the head-rest. This problem does not arise in industry, and some firms measure BOZR with a keratometer dedicated to this purpose.

If necessary, the range of the instrument

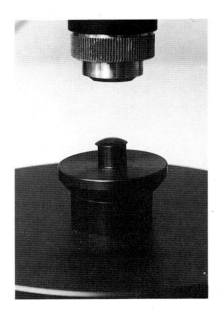

Figure 9.7 The lens support used for measurement of front optic zone radius.

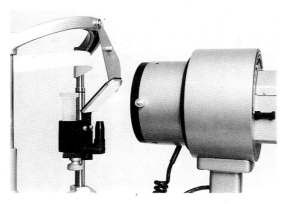

Figure 9.8 Contact lens support with mirror attached to the head-rest of a keratometer in order to measure back optic zone radius (Tama Inc. Con-ta-chek).

can be extended by mounting an auxiliary lens, such as one from a trial case, in front of the objective. A positive lens allows steeper radii to be measured and a negative lens extends the range of flatter radii which can be measured. Calibration with test spheres is required to validate the use of such auxiliary lenses.

The keratometer measures radius utilizing two points on either side of the lens axis which are separated by a distance of approximately 3 mm – hence, narrow curves such as peripheral radii cannot be measured by this means.

A now obsolete instrument, the Toposcope, described by Blackstone (1966) used interference patterns to produce moiré fringes. As the instrument measured only one meridian at a time, verification of toric lenses or detection of induced toricity was difficult. Janoff (1977) concluded from a small pilot study that the Toposcope had comparable accuracy to that of the optical spherometer.

The Radius Checking Device introduced by Sarver and Kerr (1964) is essentially a lens of known power and curvature upon which the lens to be measured is placed. Between the device and the lens is liquid with the same refractive index as the contact lens. BOZR is deduced from differences in the power measured on the focimeter of the device, the contact lens and the lens mounted upon the device (Dickins, 1966a). BOZR values obtained by this method do not correlate strongly with those obtained with the optical spherometer (Dickins, 1966b).

9.3.6 THE INFLUENCE OF THE STATE OF HYDRATION UPON BOZR

The fact that the BOZR of corneal lenses flattens as a result of hydration appears first to have been reported by Bailey (1960). Lenses made from PMMA have been observed to flatten on hydration from 0.02 to more than 0.10 mm. depending upon their centre thickness (Jessen, 1961; Salvatori, 1961; Black; 1962). Lenses made from cellulose acetate butyrate (CAB) undergo even greater curvature change as a consequence of hydration (Pearson, 1978; Sarver *et al.*, 1978; Stone, 1978; Smith, 1979, 1981). High minus power lenses (–15.00 D) made from siloxane methacrylate flatten by up to 0.15 mm and fluoropolymer lenses of similar power flatten by up to 0.34 mm (Kerr & Dilly, 1988). The occurrence of 'radical flattening' in medium and high powered minus lenses made from a range of siloxane methacrylate and fluoropolymer lenses has similarly been reported by Walker (1988). Particularly dramatic changes in BOZR may occur if the lens is stored in an inappropriate solution such as an alcohol based cleaner (Lowther, 1987).

In view of the influence of hydration upon curvature, radii should either be measured dry (i.e. at an ambient level of hydration) or following 24 hours immersion in a suitable liquid. After this period, radii are assumed to have attained equilibrated, hydrated values.

9.3.7 ASPHERIC BACK SURFACES

Aspheric back surface corneal lenses such as the Con-o-coid design (Nissel, 1967) made their appearance in the late 1960s. At that period, due to the exclusive use of PMMA as a contact lens material, lenses of small total diameter were favoured in an endeavour to minimize corneal hypoxia (Sarver, 1966; Kirsch, 1967). Use of small lenses tended to negate the potential advantages of aspheric constructions so they achieved relatively little popularity. The advent of materials having significant oxygen permeability has permitted the fitting of lenses with larger diameters leading to a reawakened interest in aspheric designs.

Two alternative methods of measurement of aspheric back surfaces were devised and evaluated by Defazio and Lowther (1979). One of these consisted of an optical spherometer with a stage which could be inclined to permit measurement of sagittal radius at five known distances from the back vertex of the lens. As the support was tilted, the stage was moved laterally so that the target was still incident perpendicularly to the lens surface. The eccentricity, or *e* value, of the back surface of some aspheric corneal lenses was calculated from the back vertex radius and saggital radius values. Their second method was based upon a comparison of measurements of back surface radius made with an optical spherometer used in the conventional manner with those from an ophthalmometer which was assumed to have measured radius at an approximate distance of 1.5 mm from the back vertex of the lens. This approach proved to be of doubtful value, whereas the modified optical spherometer was considered to be accurate and capable of detecting variations in asphericity across the back surface of a lens. This is an important consideration because several contemporary lens designs described as 'aspheric' cannot be represented as simple conic sections.

A simple interferometric technique was used by Garner (1981) to determine the eccentricity of aspheric back surface lenses. The contact lens was placed upon precision convex test plates of successively flatter curvature and a low power stereomicroscope

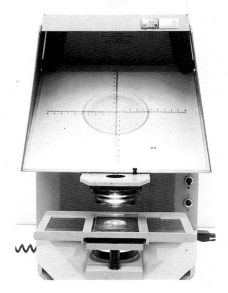

Figure 9.9 An optical projector (Carl Zeiss, Jena) for measurement of diameters.

equipped with a graticule eyepiece was used to measure the diameter of the interference fringes or the diameter of the band of optical contact between the lens and each test plate. A low pressure sodium lamp provided the necessary monochromatic illumination.

A swivelling contact lens support which is attached to an ophthalmometer in order to measure sagittal radii at up to 25 to 30 degrees from the back vertex of the lens has been described by Wilms (1981). From this data, the eccentricity of an aspheric back surface can be calculated.

9.4 MEASUREMENT OF DIAMETERS

9.4.1 TOTAL DIAMETER

Total diameter is best measured using an optical projection system having a magnification of 15 ×, or more. The lens is positioned so that its image can be focused sharply upon a screen equipped with a linear scale (Fig. 9.9). The precision of each measurement should be ± 50 μm. Tolerance limits for total diameter are ± 0.10 mm.

9.4.2 ALTERNATIVE METHODS

Total diameter is commonly measured using a gauge which is made of plastic or metal into which a V-shaped channel has been cut (Fig. 9.10). The lens is placed back surface downwards at the widest end of the channel and the gauge is inclined at an angle of about 45 degrees so that the lens slides towards the narrow end until it stops. Total diameter is read from the scale along the side of the channel. In order that the lens can move freely under the influence of gravity, both it and the gauge must be clean and dry.

A popular alternative to the V-gauge is a hand-held measuring magnifier with an eyepiece which can be focused upon a linear scale, usually 20 mm in length, having intervals of 0.10 mm. The lens is placed with its back surface towards the scale and kept in place by one finger (Fig. 9.11). The scale is most easily seen against a bright background or a light source such as a tubular fluorescent lamp.

With each method, the lens should be measured at four locations, rotating it 45

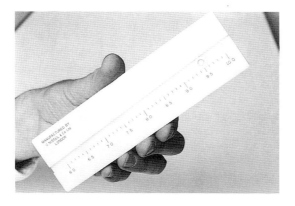

Figure 9.10 A V-channel gauge used for measurement of total diameter. The metal ring is a test piece for calibration.

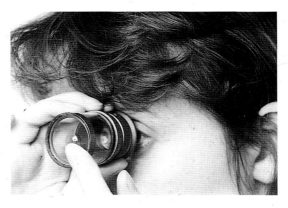

Figure 9.11 A hand-held measuring magnifier used for determination of diameters.

degrees before each measurement, in order to confirm that its shape is symmetrical.

9.4.3 CALIBRATION

Suitable test pieces are circular with a minimum range of three different diameters corresponding to the range likely to be measured.

The three methods described above have been compared by Port (1987a) who concluded that a high quality V-gauge was the most effective and the hand magnifier was the least effective due to problems of parallax, lens movement during measurement and low (4×) magnification. Despite the evidence of this study, standards bodies maintain a preference for diameter measurements using a projection instrument.

9.4.4 OTHER DIAMETERS

Back optic zone diameter and back peripheral zone diameters can be measured using either the measuring loupe or a projection system in a similar manner to measurement of total diameter. In practice, location of these diameters may be difficult due to blending of the transitions. Measurements should be repeated in different meridians in order to verify that the back optic zone is circular. If the lens has a spherical back optic zone radius and a toric periphery, the back optic zone will, naturally, be oval in shape.

The same problem may be encountered in the measurement of the front optic zone diameter of lenticular lenses and care and skill are required so that the front and back diameters are distinguished correctly. When using a hand magnifier, these diameters may be more easily discerned if the lens is moved slightly against an illuminated background.

In the case of lenses with sharp transitions, the following tolerance limits are applicable:

Back optic zone diameter ± 0.20 mm
Back peripheral zone diameter ± 0.10 mm
Front optic zone diameter ± 0.20 mm

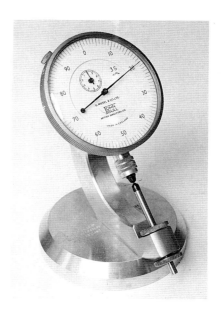

Figure 9.12 A dial gauge for measurement of geometrical centre thickness. Between the anvil and plunger is a precision engineering shim being used for calibration.

9.5   MEASUREMENT OF THICKNESS

Thickness is measured using either an analogue dial gauge or a digital gauge, having an anvil and plunger with smooth surfaces in order to avoid damage to the lens (Fig. 9.12).

9.5.1   CALIBRATION

Appropriate test pieces for calibration are a minimum of three engineering shims, the nominal thicknesses of which should represent the range of contact lens thicknesses to be measured.

9.5.2   GEOMETRICAL CENTRE THICKNESS

The contact lens is placed centrally upon the anvil of a thickness gauge and the previously raised spring-loaded plunger is lowered gently into contact with its surface. Three independent readings are taken and the mean value is corrected using the calibration data. The precision of such measurements is ± 5 μm. Tolerance limits for geometrical centre thickness are ± 0.02 mm.

9.5.3   ALTERNATIVE METHODS

The optical spherometer can be used to measure apparent or actual geometrical centre thickness. In the former approach, the lens is placed upon the support used for back optic zone radius measurement but without water between them. Having centred the lens, the instrument is focused in turn upon its front and back surfaces. The instrument reading, which is the apparent thickness, is multiplied by the refractive index of the contact lens material to obtain true thickness.

To measure geometrical centre thickness directly, a flat, polished support is required and the optical spherometer is focused upon it. The lens is placed front surface downwards on this support and the spherometer is focused on the back surface. The instrument reading is the actual geometrical centre thickness of the lens.

Centre thickness can also be determined by means of a lens measure which is normally used to establish the surface curvature of spectacle lenses. One dioptre on the scale corresponds approximately to 0.10 mm when measuring thickness. Great care must be exercised with this method to ensure that the pins do not scratch the lens surface.

9.5.4   EDGE THICKNESS

Two problems have frustrated the acceptance of valid tolerance limits for edge thickness. The first of these has been a failure to distinguish between axial edge thickness, which is measured parallel to the lens axis, and radial edge thickness, which is measured at a normal to the front surface of the lens. The former dimension is commonly used in computations by the manufacturing industry, while the latter is the dimension actually measured. The second difficulty has been that of specifying precisely the distance from the edge of the lens to which the measured value applies. In an attempt to overcome this problem, a positional micrometer has been developed (Port, 1987b), which permits measurement along an axis which closely approximates to radial thickness at an accurately determined distance from the lens edge (Fig. 9.13).

A modified digital pachometer has been used by Guillon *et al.* (1986) to measure axial edge thickness but the sophistication of this system precludes its application in clinical practice.

9.6   MEASUREMENT OF DIOPTRIC AND PRISMATIC POWER

Dioptric and prismatic power are measured using a focimeter (lensometer) equipped with a contact lens support having a central aperture with a diameter between 4.00 and 5.00 mm. The height of the support should be about 0.55 mm less than that used with spectacle lenses (Fig. 9.14). Measurement is facilitated by the use of a vertically orien-

(a)

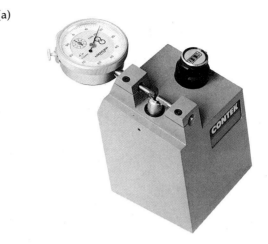

(b)

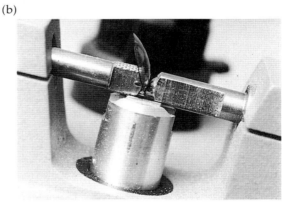

Figure 9.13 (a) A dial gauge and positional micrometer for measurement of radial edge thickness (Contek). (b) shows the positioning of the lens.

tated instrument, a standard feature of projection type instruments.

9.6.1   CALIBRATION

The test lenses should span a wide range of nominal back vertex powers such as –20 D, –10 D, +10 D, +20 D and each should be certified by a recognized institution such as

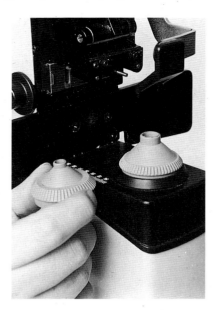

Figure 9.14 The spectacle and contact lens supports of a focimeter equipped with both (Topcon LM-6).

the National Physical Laboratory of the UK.

9.6.2   BACK VERTEX POWER

The contact lens is placed with its back surface upon the support and three independent readings are taken. The arithmetic mean of these values is calculated and corrected using the calibration curve. The lens must be positioned with care since clumsy handling might distort it and induce a false cylindrical reading.

In the case of steep corneal lenses and most scleral lenses, their back vertex will not be in the plane of the focimeter stop. While this is of little consequence with low powered lenses, a greater positive or smaller negative reading will be obtained in the case of high powers. An attempt has been made to overcome this problem in the contact lens support, manufactured by Rodenstock (Fig. 9.15). This device ensures that irrespective of their back optic zone radii, lenses are positioned at a constant distance from the standard lens of the focimeter. As the back optic zone radius of a lens is selected on the rotating scale, the lens support rises in the case of flat values, or moves downwards for steeper ones. An alternative method of dealing with this problem is to place the contact lens with its front surface downwards to measure its front vertex power (Fv). Back vertex power (F'v) is then calculated from the following equation:

$$Fv = \frac{F1}{1 - t_c/n\ F1} + F2 \qquad \text{(eqn 9.1)}$$

where F1 is the front surface power:

$$F1 = Fv - \frac{F2N}{1 - t_c/n\ F2} \qquad \text{(eqn 9.2)}$$

and F2, back surface power (D); t_c, geometrical centre thickness (m); n, refractive index.

Four illustrations of the application of this equation are given in Table 9.1, taking in each case a back optic zone radius (r_0) of 7.80 mm and a refractive index of 1.47.

These examples show that the difference between measured front and calculated back vertex power increases with geometrical centre thickness and is likely to be of greatest

Table 9.1 Applications of eqn 9.2

r_o	t_c	Measured Fv (D)	Calculated F'v (D)
7.80	0.60	+20.00	+21.17
7.80	0.49	+10.00	+10.44
7.80	0.12	−10.00	−10.09
7.80	0.10	−20.00	−20.14

significance in the case of high plus power corneal lenses and all scleral lenses.

Any cylinder measured should be compared with the original order since it is sometimes a manifestation of poor manufacture or of clumsy handling during measurement.

When measuring power, the sharpness of the target image should be noted as an indication of the quality of lens manufacture.

Tolerance limits for back vertex power are shown in Table 9.2.

9.6.3 MEASUREMENT OF PRISMATIC POWER

The lens must be centred carefully upon the focimeter support to measure prismatic power. Positioning may be facilitated by marking the geometrical centre thickness with a dot.

Tolerance limits for prescribed prismatic power are shown in Table 9.3.

9.6.4 BIFOCAL LENSES

In the case of fused and front surface addition solid bifocals, the addition power can be measured directly using the focimeter. For a solid bifocal of the back surface addition type, addition power measured in air will be 3.51 times greater than its effective power on

Table 9.2 Tolerance limits

	Tolerance limits (D)
Back vertex power	
Plano up to 7 D	±0.12
above 7 D up to 14 D	±0.25
above 14 D	±0.50
Cylinder power	
Plano up to 2 D	±0.25
above 2 D up to 4 D	±0.37
above 4 D	±0.50
Cylinder axis	±5°

Table 9.3 Tolerance limits for prescribed prismatic power

Prismatic power	Tolerance limits
Up to 1△	±0.25△
above 1△	±0.50△
base/apex direction	±5°

the eye, assuming that it was made from a material having a refractive index of 1.47.

9.7 EDGE LIFT

Two methods of measurement of axial edge lift utilizing the optical spherometer have been described by Stone (1975).

In the first method, the contact lens is positioned on the support used for measurement of BOZR and a microscope cover glass is placed over the lens. The instrument is focused upon the lower surface of the cover glass and then upon the back surface of the lens. The distance travelled by the microscope corresponds to the overall sagitta (OS) of the lens at a diameter approximating to its total diameter (TD).

The axial edge lift (AEL) at the approximate total diameter is calculated as follows:

AEL = calculated sagitta of BOZR at TD − measured OS   (eqn 9.3)

This method has been employed (Pearson, 1990) to obtain data on the axial edge lift at the total diameter of several proprietary designs of gas permeable corneal lenses. The procedure used was found to be both simple and reliable.

In an alternative method, the lens is placed back surface downwards upon a flat anvil and the optical spherometer is focused upon the surface of the anvil and then upon the apex of the front of the lens. The distance travelled by the microscope is equal to the overall sagitta plus the geometrical centre thickness. Deduction of the latter value from the instrument reading allows use of the above equation. Axial edge lift could be measured at other diameters using anvils with diameters smaller than the total diameter of the lens. The same method can be used to determine radial edge lift (REL) which is calculated as follows:

$$REL = \frac{\sqrt{(BOZR - OS)^2 + \dfrac{(anvil\ diameter)^2}{2}} - BOZR}{}$$

9.8 INSPECTION OF EDGE PROFILE

The shape of any contact lens edge can have a significant influence upon its comfort in wear.

It has been suggested that edge quality may be assessed by rubbing the lens edge on the wrist or fingers, or by a trial period of wear in the practitioner's eye. Such tests are capable of disclosing grossly unacceptable edge forms but the actual profile is not determined.

An impression of the lens edge in dental stone (model plaster) can provide a permanent record. Transient impressions can be obtained more quickly by the use of modelling clay (Plasticine®) or a silicone elastomer material. The impression can be inspected or photographed at high magnification. The process is time-consuming since it should be repeated several times around the circumference of the lens to ensure consistency of shape.

A simpler and quicker method is to inspect the lens using the magnification of a hand loupe, projection magnifier, slit-lamp microscope or stereomicroscope. At higher magnifications, it is helpful to support the lens on a holder, which tilts to permit observation from the front around to the back surface of the lens and which rotates to allow inspection around its circumference (Fig. 9.16).

In the 'light intersection method' of Forst (1972), the lens is placed in a wet cell filled with liquid having the same refractive index

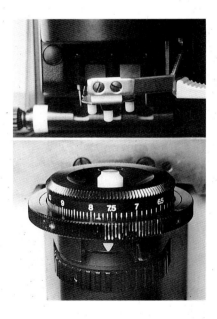

Figure 9.15 The Rodenstock device which ensures that contact lenses are supported at a constant distance from the standard lens of the focimeter.

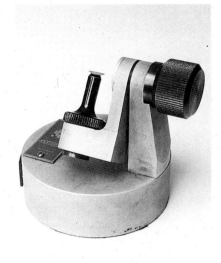

Figure 9.16 A lens support which rotates and swivels to facilitate inspection of the edge of a corneal lens.

as that of the contact lens (e.g. *p*-Xylol in the case of PMMA lenses). Lens profile is observed with a slit-lamp microscope at 40 × or projected onto a screen at 100 ×. The lens can be rotated on its support within the cell (Fig. 9.17).

The various methods of edge inspection have been the subject of an extensive review by Smart (1984).

9.9 SURFACE QUALITY AND POLISH

Inspection of new lenses using the stereomicroscope or slit-lamp microscope is important (Fig. 9.18). A magnification of 20 × or more is essential to detect surface defects which have been caused by poor manufacture such as:

1. Pitting.
2. Burning and mottling.
3. Scratches.
4. Lathe marks.
5. Incomplete polishing.

Such problems will be missed if the lens is examined at the low magnification provided by a hand loupe. Surface burning or mottling results from excessive heat during manufac-

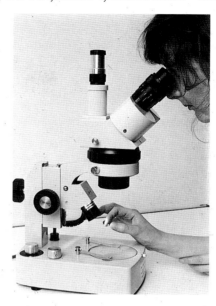

Figure 9.18 The surface of a corneal lens being inspected with the aid of a zoom stereomicroscope.

ture and is likely to cause poor *in vivo* wetting.

At after-care examinations, inspection using darkfield conditions helps in the detection and examination of surface deposits. It is important to look for surface degradation described as cracking or crazing. According to Lembach *et al.* (1988), this problem is related to lens wear rather than being a primary defect in the material. In contrast, Phillips and Gascoigne (1988) suspected that some fault in the polymer is implicated.

9.10 THE VERIFICATION OF SCLERAL LENSES

In view of the very limited use of scleral lenses in conventional optometric practice, their verification is described only briefly. The following dimensions may be measured in exactly the same manner as corneal lenses:

1. Back optic zone radius using the optical spherometer.

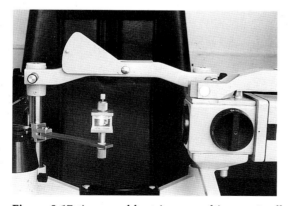

Figure 9.17 A corneal lens immersed in a wet cell filled with liquid having the same refractive index as the lens. The illumination system of the slit-lamp is positioned on one side of the cell and the microscope on the opposite side.

Table 9.4 Dimensional tolerance limits for corneal lenses

Dimension	Tolerance limits	Recommended method	Comments
Radii			
Back optic zone radius	± 0.05 mm ⎫	Optical spherometer	For PMMA lenses, tolerance limits are ± 0.025 mm
Back peripheral radius	± 0.10 mm ⎬		Applies to lenses with sharp transitions with peripheral zones wider than 1 mm
Diameters			
Back optic zone diameter	± 0.20 mm ⎫		
Back peripheral zone diameter	± 0.10 mm	Optical projector	Applies to lenses with sharp transitions
Front optic zone diameter	± 0.20 mm		
Total diameter	± 0.10 mm ⎭		
Thickness			
Geometrical centre thickness	± 0.02 mm	Dial or digital gauge	

2. Back scleral size and total diameter using an optical projection system.
3. Geometrical centre thickness using a dial gauge.
4. Optical properties determined on the focimeter.

Since a typical value for the back scleral radius of a preformed lens is 13.50 mm, a specially made lens support is likely to be required to enable the optical spherometer to focus in turn upon both the surface and aerial images (Stone, 1964).

The basic optic diameter is formed by the junction of the back optic and scleral surfaces and, due to the presence of a transition which may be about 2.00 mm wide, it is impossible to measure this dimension directly. Stone (1964) has described a suitable method of measurement involving the use of a series of test spheres corresponding to a range of back scleral radii and a micrometer. It should be emphasized that together with back optic zone radius, the basic optic diameter is of great importance in determining the nature of the fit of the optic zone.

Table 9.5 Optical tolerance limits for corneal and scleral lenses

Optical property	Tolerance limits
Back vertex power	
Plano up to 7 D	±0.12 △
above 7 D up to 14 D	±0.25 △
above 14 D	±0.50 △
Cylinder power	
Plano up to 2 D	±0.25 △
above 2 D up to 4 D	±0.37 △
above 4 D	±0.50 △
Cylinder axis	±5°
Prescribed prism	
up to 1 δ	±0.25 △
above 1 δ	±0.50 △
Base/apex direction	±5°
Prismatic error	
back vertex power up to 6 D	±0.25 △
back vertex power above 6 D	±0.50 △

In the case of impression lenses, it is the vertex clearance which, together with back optic zone radius, governs the optic zone fit.

Table 9.6 Dimensional tolerance limits for scleral lenses

Dimension	Tolerance limits (mm)	Recommended method
Radii		
Back optic zone radius	±0.10 ⎫	
Back scleral radius	±0.10 ⎭	Optical spherometer
Diameters		
Basic optic diameter	±0.20	Micrometer
Back scleral size	±0.25 ⎫	
Total diameter	±0.25 ⎭	Optical projector
Thickness		
Geometrical centre thickness (of optic zone)	±0.02	Dial or digital gauge
Clearance		
Vertex clearance from cast	±0.20	Dial or digital gauge

Vertex clearance is the distance from the front surface of the cast to the back surface of the scleral lens, measured at the geometric centre of the back optic zone. It can be determined after Bennett (1966) as follows:

1. Measure the geometrical centre thickness (1) of the lens.
2. Measure the height of the cast from base to vertex (2) using a dial gauge or micrometer.
3. Measure the height from the base of the cast to the front vertex of the lens (3) which is mounted upon it, using the same instrument.

Then, vertex clearance = 3 – 1 – 2

For ease of reference, dimensional tolerance limits for corneal lenses are summarized in Table 9.4. Optical tolerance limits for corneal and scleral lenses are shown in Table 9.5 and Table 9.6 lists tolerance limits for scleral lenses.

ACKNOWLEDGEMENTS

The author is indebted to the British Standards Institution for permission to cite tolerance limits from British Standard, BS 7208: Part 1: 1989. Mr Michael Sheridan, formerly Senior Lecturer, Department of Optometry, University of Bradford, kindly supplied the diagram upon which Figure 9.2 is based. Photography of equipment was undertaken by Mr C.N. Miller of City University, London.

REFERENCES

Bailey, N.J. (1960) Contact lenses must be kept wet. *J. Am. Optom. Ass.*, **31**, 985.

Bennett, A.G. (1966) *Optics of Contact Lenses*. Association of Dispensing Opticians, London.

Bier, N. (1958) Two new contact lens instruments for measuring the corneal radius of contact lenses. *Optician*, **136** (3512), 31–2.

Black, C.J. (1962) Clinical procedure. *Trans. Am. Acad. Ophthal. Otol.*, **66**, 290–4.

Blackstone, M. (1966) The toposcope examined. *Optician*, **152** (3928), 38–39.

Charman, W.N. (1972) Diffraction and the precision of measurement of corneal and other small radii. *Am. J. Optom.*, **49**, 672–80.

Defazio, A.J. and Lowther, G.E. (1979) Inspection of back surface aspheric contact lenses. *Am. J. Optom. Physiol. Optics*, **56**, 471–9.

Dickins, R. (1966a) An investigation into the accuracy of the radius checking device. *Optician*, **151** (3911), 265–9.

Dickins, R. (1966b) Further results using the radius checking device. *Optician*, **152** (3932), 135–7.

Fletcher, R.J. and Nisted, M. (1961) The accuracy of corneal lenses. *Ophthal. Optician*, **1**, 217–19.

Forst, G. (1972), Randprofil-Betrachtung einer Contactlinse – eine einfache Anordnung für den Praktiker. *Die Contactlinse*, 6(1), 6–9.

Garner, L.F. (1981) A simple interferometer for hard contact lenses. *Am. J. Optom. Physiol. Optics*, 58, 944–50.

Guillon, M., Crosbie-Walsh, J. and Byrnes, D. (1986) Application of pachometry to the measurement of hard contact lens edge profile. *Transactions of the British Contact Lens Association Annual Clinical Conference*, British Contact Lens Association, London, 56–9.

Hodur, N.R., Jurkus, J. and Gunderson, G. (1992) Rigid gas permeable lens identification using refractometry. *Int. Contact Lens Clinic*, 19, 71–4.

Janoff, L.E. (1977) A pilot study of the comparison of validity and reliability between the Radiuscope and Toposcope. *Int. Contact Lens Clinic*, 4, 68–73.

Jessen, G.N. (1961) New bifocal lens technique results in more comfortable single vision lenses. *Contacto*, 5(7), 237–43.

Kerr, C. and Dilly, P.N. (1988) Problems of dimensional stability in RGPs. *Optician*, 195 (5134), 21–3.

Kirsch, M.S. (1967) Small lenses may convert large numbers. Contact lens 'failures' may yet succeed. *J. Am. Optom. Ass.*, 38, 219–20.

Lembach, R.G., McLaughlin, R. and Barr, J.T. (1988) Crazing in a rigid gas permeable contact lens. *CLAO J.*, 14, 38–41.

Lowther, G.E. (1987) Effect of some solutions on HGP contact lens parameters. *J. Am. Optom. Ass.*, 58, 188–92.

McMonnies, C.W. (1989) Quality control for gas permeable hard lens manufacture. *Clin. Exptl. Optom.*, 72, 15–18.

Morton, J.M., McMahon, T.T. and Farber, M.D. (1987), Effectiveness of the Opti-mis system in differentiating PMMA from rigid gas permeable contact lenses. *CLAO J.*, 13, 197–202.

Nissel, G. (1967), Aspheric contact lenses. *Ophthal. Optician*, 7, 1007–10.

Pearson, R.M. (1978) Dimensional stability of lathe cut C.A.B. lenses. *J. Am. Optom. Ass.*, 49, 927–9.

Pearson, R.M. (1990) Measurement of axial edge lift of rigid corneal lenses. *Clin. Exptl. Optom.*, 172–7.

Phillips, A.J. and Gascoigne, K. (1988) Surface cracking of RGP materials. *Clin. Exptl. Optom.*, 71, 198–203.

Port, M.J.A. (1987a) The measurement of rigid contact lens diameters. *J. Br. Contact Lens Ass.*, 10, 23–6.

Port, M.J.A. (1987b) A new method of edge thickness measurement for rigid lenses. *J. Br. Contact Lens Ass.*, 10, 16–20.

Refojo, M.F. and Leong, F-L. (1984) Identification of hard contact lenses by their specific gravity. *Int. Contact Lens Clinic*, 11, 79–82.

Salvatori, P.L. (1961) The effect of hydration upon corneal radius. *J. Am. Optom. Ass.*, 32, 644.

Sarver, M.D. (1966), Comparison of small and large corneal contact lenses. *Am. J. Optom.*, 43, 633–652.

Sarver, M.D. and Kerr, K. (1964) A radius of curvature measuring device for contact lenses. *Am. J. Optom.*, 41, 481–9.

Sarver, M.D. et al. (1978), Stability of CAB contact lenses with hydration. *J. Am. Optom. Ass.*, 49, 1377–80.

Shanks, K.R. (1966) A comparison of corneal lenses supplied to identical specification. *Br. J. Physiol. Optics*, 23, 50–4.

Smart, C.F.G. (1984) The edge form of contact lenses. *Contact Lens J.*, 12(10), 10–17.

Smith, H.C. (1979) A study of the stability of lenses fabricated from cellulose acetate butyrate. *Int. Contact Lens Clinic*, 6(4), 60–3.

Smith, H.C. (1981) A study of the effect of time on the flattening due to hydration of CAB material, *Int. Contact Lens Clinic*, 8(2), 55–8.

Stone J. (1964) Checking preformed contact lenses. *Br. J. Physiol. Optics*, 21, 264–86.

Stone, J. (1975) Corneal lenses with constant axial edge lift. *Ophth. Optician*, 15, 818–24.

Stone, J. (1978) Changes in curvature of cellulose acetate butyrate lenses during hydration and dehydration. *J. Br. Contact Lens Ass.*, 1(1), 22–35.

Walker, J. (1988) Radical flattening – a laboratory enigma. *Optician*, 195 (5142), 21–23.

Wilms, K.H. (1981) Topometry of the cornea and contact lenses with new equipment. *Ophthal. Optician*, 49, 672–80.

CLINICAL PRACTICE

M.J.A. Port

10.1 INTRODUCTION

There is a body of opinion that implies it is not worthwhile verifying the dimensions of a soft lens, prior to putting the lens on the eye of the wearer for an *in vivo* assessment. Indeed, most contact lens practitioners probably follow this approach on the grounds of expediency. In an ideal world, we should not need to check lens parameters if we have faith in the manufacturer's ability to reproduce lenses to a given specification. For a contact lens manufacturer whose production involves batch runs (one material, one design, one power) the reproducibility is related to the acceptable quality level (AQL) that a company has adopted.

In some types of manufacture, e.g. intraocular lenses, there is complete reliance on production quality control. The surgeon does not check the lens power on a focimeter before inserting the sterile lens permanently into the eye. The surgeon has faith that the specifications are within acceptable tolerances.

The advent of disposable lenses (e.g. AcuVue (Vistakon), NewVues (Ciba Vision), SeeQuence (Bausch & Lomb), Calendar (Pilkington)) means that the wearer usually has a supply of identical lenses to use when a worn lens has been in use for a prescribed period of time. The conventional method of storing the lenses is in 'blister packs'. The sterile lenses are sealed in saline 'blisters' at the factory. Verification and resealing is not possible. Thus, the wearer has a supply of lenses which have only been subjected to the factory's quality assurance (QA) procedures and the fit of one lens has been seen on the eye by the practitioner. Inevitably a small percentage of lenses will be outside the specification either in terms of dimensions, power or finish. However, in a competitive world, the manufacturer can ill afford to have an AQL below that of his rivals and may even have an incentive to raise it! Practitioners soon see if a product's reproducibility is poor and can switch to alternatives if the resulting problems render the design impractical and inconvenient.

In the contact lens field, automated lens production has been well established for two decades, notably the spin casting technique. Lenses such as Bausch & Lomb's 'U' series have established a reputation for being reliable in terms of quality and fit. Several factors affect the AQL. A company wishes to have a competitive product. It therefore needs a QA scheme which does not throw out too many lenses (the unit production cost is higher) or throws out too few (poorer quality product). If batches are not sampled frequently enough or rigorously enough, then production time and materials can be

Contact Lens Practice. Edited by Montague Ruben and Michel Guillon.
Published in 1994 by Chapman & Hall, London. ISBN 0 412 35120 X

wasted if a fault occurs. Chapter 8 deals with QA in more detail.

Let us return to some basic notions. The contact lens practitioner has a trial set or inventory of lenses. These are normally kept at room temperature (15 ° to 25 °C). During the fitting of lenses, a lens is placed on the eye and allowed to equilibrate with the ocular environment. The most important change occurring is the temperature rise of the lens. This will be approximately 15 °C and with most conventional hydrogel materials this implies that the water content will become smaller, the sequelae being that the lens' dimensions reduce and the lens may well become tighter on the eye. This effect is usually greater with higher water content materials than with low water content materials. After a given time the practitioner assesses the lens fit and decides if it is acceptable. The specifications of the lens at room temperature are given on a lens order. The realistic assumption is then made that a lens made to an identical specification will eventually fit the wearer equally well. Hence one needs to know the correct specification of the trial lenses. Let us take an example of a manufacturer who makes lenses with back optic zone radii (BOZR) in 0.3 mm steps, e.g. 8.4, 8.7, 9.0 and 9.3 mm. If the radius of the 8.7 mm trial lens was 0.15 mm flatter (8.85 mm) than the labelled value, then a perfectly accurate prescription lens, supplied on the basis of the trial lens value, may fit too tightly on the eye. How would the practitioner deal with this 'mysteriously tight' lens? If he relied solely on the *in vivo* information he might order a replacement lens, only to find the same situation again. If he then ordered a 9.00 mm radius lens, the problem might be solved but it could be a looser fit than his 8.85 mm trial lens.

Another example (using the same fitting set) might be as follows. The lenses labelled 8.7 mm (but actually 8.85 mm) and 9.0 mm radius appear to fit an eye equally well; the 9.3 mm radius lens is too loose, the 8.4 mm

lens is too tight. If the practitioner orders the 8.7 mm, the fit of the lens supplied may be too tight.

Similar problems can arise with replacement lenses. If an original lens (fitting correctly) was labelled 8.7 mm radius but actually was 8.55 mm and a replacement lens was 8.85 mm instead of 8.7 mm, then again the practitioner may be perplexed as to why the fitting characteristics are different. Without verification of all the lenses involved, the difference in radius of 0.3 mm between original and replacement would not be appreciated. The practitioner can be frustrated as to why he cannot get a replacement to fit like an original. In fact, it is my view that with most of today's relatively thin and flexible lenses we do not need fitting steps of 0.3 mm and 0.2 mm. First, if we have a fitting interval of 0.3 mm (as in the above example) then a lens with a BOZR of 8.85 mm, having a radius tolerance of ± 0.15 mm could fit into either the 8.7 mm or 9.0 mm batches. To avoid this, the tolerance on radius would need to be ± 0.10 mm. Evidence collected by me from the same lenses being measured at various laboratories, using similar equipment under standard conditions, suggests that it is extremely difficult to get this level of agreement on the measurement of radius. A tolerance should take account of measurement methods and production variations. It seems sensible to widen the fitting intervals to 0.4 mm or 0.5 mm so that practical and achievable tolerances of ± 0.15 mm and ±0.20 mm can be applied.

To have data to support claims of lenses being supplied outside of tolerance limits is extremely convincing. Many practitioners simply inform the manufacturer that 'the lens does not fit well'. Most companies, wishing to minimize aggravation and preserve good customer relations, will simply supply a replacement.

The same arguments used above in terms of curvature can be applied to power. The BVP of trial lenses should be checked. In the case of high power lenses in particular, the correct size focimeter stop should be used. If a trial lens was labelled –6.00 D but was actually –6.25 and the over-refraction was –2.00 D, then the lens ordered would be –8.00 D. If the lens supplied was –7.75 D then the supplied lens, on the eye, will give the patient a 0.50 D blur.

Not knowing the lens parameters before the patient comes to the practice wastes patient time if there is a lens error and the practitioner loses credibility. Time can also be saved if a practitioner does not have to resort to frequent use of exchange schemes for ordered lenses which are not fitting well or give blurred vision:

Rule 1: 'Verify your trial sets' – particularly for curvature, diameter and power (using a known solution, tonicity, pH and temperature).
Rule 2: 'Verify your supplied lenses' – again in a known environment.

10.2 WHICH PARAMETERS ARE WORTH CHECKING?

Besides the nature of the material itself, the dimensions/parameters which affect the fit of the lens are:

1. Shape of back surface.
2. Total diameter.
3. Thickness profile.

A correct lens power is necessary to correct the wearer's refractive error. The lens *thickness* will affect its gas transmissibility (Dk/t), movement and comfort. The lens must be *free from defects* which would cause discomfort, poor vision, or damage ocular tissues. The *colour* of the lens and the size of coloured zones may be important.

It is very common for manufacturers to quote typical Dk values for the centre thickness of a –3.00 D lens. There may be no problem with hypoxia in the centre of the corneal – particularly with minus powered

lenses, but lack of knowledge regarding the peripheral lens thickness may give rise to peripheral hypoxia with some designs on some patients' eyes.

It is important, at this stage, to appreciate the relationship between thickness and radius. A very thin lens will wrap itself around the cornea very effectively. A thicker lens will not have this ability and the back surface shape becomes more critical. It is not necessary to have such a tight tolerance on back surface shape if the thickness is very small and the material is very flexible. Additionally, the radius itself is a factor. A lens with a BOZR of 7.3 mm powered at +28.00 will be relatively stiff. A 9.3 mm radius lens, 0.05 mm thick, powered at – 1.00 D will be relatively flexible. Lenses which are very thin (0.03 to 0.05 mm) are generally more difficult to verify. Fortunately, when considered clinically, the absolute dimensional values are less critical than those for a thick lens.

10.3 CALIBRATION OF EQUIPMENT

At the outset, it must be stated that this is a neglected area of contact lens metrology. Instruments, such as focimeters, require very little calibration – particularly for the commonly encountered powers (between – 10.00 and + 10.00 D) and users tend to forget the calibration process. If this is not done there can be large discrepancies between operators (even if the same type of equipment is used). Where there is an operator involved to assess a subjective end point, calibration must involve the operator *and* the instrument. The test pieces used for calibration should have confirmed traceability so that their accuracy can be known. When plotting a calibration curve, it is important to look at the general shape of the curve. Where the shape is essentially linear, a least squares, best fit line can be used (Fig. 10.1). Where the data is not linear and linear regression cannot be used, the points should be simply joined and intrapolation used (Fig. 10.2). Alternatively a

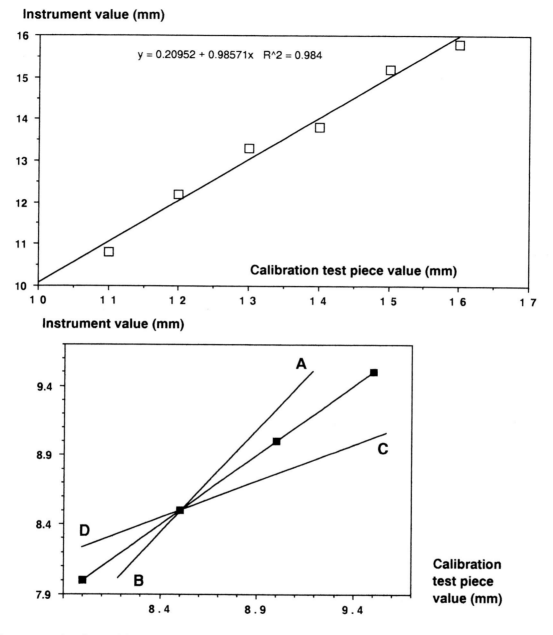

Figure 10.1 (Top) A calibration curve for total diameter. Six test pieces have been used to cover the range of the instrument and a best fit line has been constructed. Each data point would represent a mean of 10 independent measurements, for example. (Bottom) The solid squares show the mean instrument values for four radius test pieces. The best fit line enables the operator to convert instrument values to calibrated values. If only one test piece is used then any number of lines could be drawn through this one data point (8.5 mm in the diagram). The lines AB and CD are just two examples. Establishing that the instrument is accurate at one point does not imply that it is accurate throughout its range.

polynomial expression can be found to fit the data. This is done very simply if a computerized curve-fitting program is used. The author uses Cricketgraph™ very successfully for this purpose.

10.4 MEASUREMENT TECHNIQUES FOR CURVATURE DETERMINATION

10.4.1   THE BACK SURFACE SHAPE

Variation in back surface shape is necessary to fit different shaped eyes. Most eyes tend to flatten from the centre of the cornea towards the limbus and sclera. Soft lenses may have aspheric back surfaces or they may have a series of concentric spherical curves which flatten in radius from centre to edge. In the case of a multicurve back surface the back optic zone radius (BOZR) is specified and a given lens series may have anything from one to six different BOZR values; the BOZD

is usually 10 or 11 mm. The verification of the BOZR is carried out using one of two broad principles – one mechanical and one optical.

There are two traditional arguments regarding radius determination. First, measurement in air or in saline, and second, sagitta determination versus ophthalmometry.

The reason for in-air measurement is speed. The disadvantage is that soft lenses in air dehydrate quickly (Port, 1980a) and lose their shape. The use of optical methods means that toroidal surfaces can be measured and this is impossible with sagitta methods. However, the reflection from the hydrogel lens/saline interface is very small and this coupled with reflections from the front surface of the lens, can make the method difficult at times. There are two other techniques which have been reported, but are not in widespread use. One is the Drysdale principle (Chamarro, 1974; Steel & Noack, 1977; Drysdale, 1900) and the other is a template

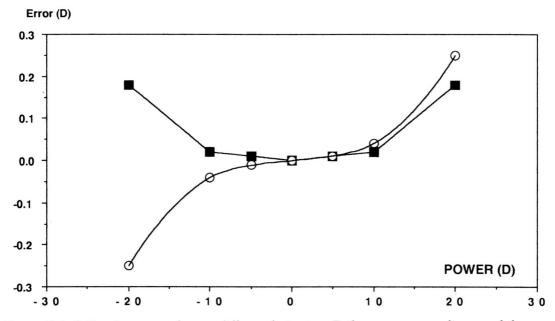

Figure 10.2 Calibration curves for two different focimeters. Both curves are non-linear and the use of linear regression to establish a best fit line is inappropriate. One can either join the points (solid squares) and intrapolate where necessary, or, fit a mathematical curve which has a polynomial equation (open circles).

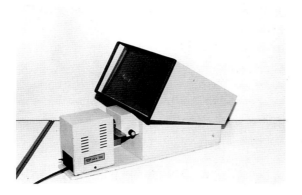

Figure 10.3 The Hydro-Vue™ soft lens analyser. This is an in-saline device where the image of the lens on a spherical dome is projected on to a translucent screen.

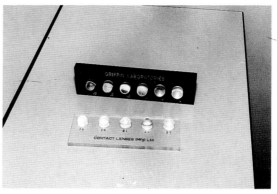

Figure 10.4 Hemispherical domes with different radii of curvature were the first development in the checking of back optic zone radius. The lens was transferred from dome to dome until the best match was found. This in-air method is not reliable with thin lenses and is not in current use.

matching technique (as used in the Söhnges projection system (Söhnges, 1973; Loran, 1974; Koetting, 1981a) and the American Hydro-Vue™ device (Fig. 10.3). In the latter case (Elmstrom, 1979; Lester & Lester, 1979; McDonald, 1981; Davis & Anderson, 1982), lenses are placed over hemispherical domes of different curvatures. The dome providing the best match gives the curvature of the lens surface. Although the dome and lens are in saline, there is no temperature control of the saline. The system uses a projection system and light from the projector lamp must warm up the saline unless a heat filter is incorporated. With lenses being generally thinner now than in the past, the lenses tend to wrap around the dome with the implication that some lenses fit a range of domes quite well. Template matching in air (Wodack, 1972) was the first simple method of verifying the posterior curvature (Fig. 10.4) but with the advent of thinner lenses and lenses of higher water content, its usefulness declined in favour of more applicable methods.

10.4.2   SAGITTA METHODS

The principle is to measure the sagitta above a known chord. In practice, this means supporting the soft lens on the circular face of a

vertical cylinder (usually 8.0 to 10.0 mm) and gauging the distance from the centre of that face to the apex of the posterior lens surface. This distance (sagitta) can be converted to a radius value (r) using the expression:

$$r = s/2 + d^2/8s \qquad \text{(eqn 10.1)}$$

where s is the measured sagitta and d is the diameter of the chord (lens support).

In-air sagitta methods

All these systems use the electrical conductivity of hydrogel lenses to complete an electrical circuit. With the lens supported on a metallic cylinder, a central probe is moved upwards towards the apex of the posterior surface. When it just touches the lens, a circuit is completed and a meter or LED indicates the completed circuit. The apparatus designed by Wöhlk in Germany and Kelvin in the UK was similar and used this concept. The notion was taken further by the French company Medicornea, with their BC-Tronic (Duprat & Joinet, 1979; Koetting, 1981b). In this case the probe was adjusted manually but a transducer was used to measure the sag and a digital display indicated the result. Probably the most sophisticated design was the SM 100 by Neitz of Japan. The central probe movement was automated. When electrical contact with the lens was made, the probe reversed to its starting position. A digital display of sag or radius was given (Port, 1980b).

It has been found (Port, 1980b) that the main problem with in-air systems was the sagging of the lens on the support resulting in flat readings. Saline, being a denser medium supports the lens shape much better and also prevents dehydration.

In-saline sagitta methods

The mechanical determination of sagitta in saline was pioneered by two people. One was Peter Höfer (1977) in Germany and the other was John Coy in the UK. Coy, whilst working for Contact Lenses (Manufacturing) Ltd. designed a device (Fig. 10.5) which had a mechanically operated central probe and a telescope arrangement with which to view the lens apex and assess the point when the probe touches the lens. The lens support was too small and there was no simple way to centre the lens on it. When he left the company he evolved the design. The probe adjustment remained essentially the same, the lens support became larger (8.5 mm) and the the end-point was determined from a projection system where the image was viewed on a screen. Perhaps the major step forward was his excellent, patented, centration device. This enables the soft lens to be centred accurately on the lens support prior to measurement. The only exception to this is when soft lenses with prism are measured. The current model of his 'Optimec' (Fig. 10.6) uses a 10 mm lens support. Ancillary attachments have further improved the equipment. There is now the option for the saline wet cell to be temperature controlled and a filter system can be attached to keep the measurement saline clear. Besides BOZR, other con-

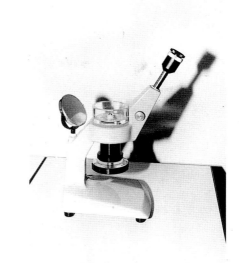

Figure 10.5 One of the original radius measurement devices designed by John Coy for Contact Lenses (Manufacturing) Ltd. The central lens support was too small and it was extremely difficult to centre the lenses. The operator used the integral telescope to assess when the central probe just touched the back vertex of the lens.

tact lens dimensions and properties can also be measured or assessed. The Optimec™ equipment is highly recommended as it is simple to use and performs its function well (Port, 1981a, 1982). The instrument must be calibrated carefully to reduce systematic error. The apparatus is now in widespread use by laboratories and practitioners.

With the Optimec system, the major operator variable which could affect random errors is the assessment of endpoint when the probe touches or lifts the lens. Some operators will try and see the probe just touch the apex of the back surface (Fig. 10.7) and some will look for one edge of the lens lifting slightly. With very thin lenses, the latter method is not reliable as the probe can distort the centre of the lens before an edge lifts. Conversely, with some lens powers and lenticular designs it is quite difficult to see

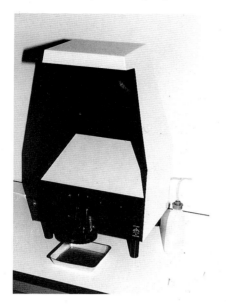

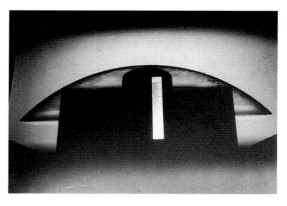

Figure 10.7 The back optic zone radius of a soft lens being measured on an Optimec device. The soft lens is resting on the 10 mm cylinder and the central probe can be seen near the back vertex of the lens. It is also possible to assess the edge profile of the lens.

Figure 10.6 A current Optimec soft lens analayser. This model has two wet cells – one to measure the back optic zone radius and centre thickness, the other to measure total diameter and to carry out inspection of the surfaces.

the probe and the lens apex clearly to make a good assessment of touch.

To overcome the mechanical limitations of the sagitta method Port (1976, 1979) described a method of determining sagitta using ultrasound. As the velocity of sound in saline varies with temperature it is essential to have a saline wet cell which is temperature controlled to ± 0.5 °C for this method. The quality and design of the transducer used are of paramount importance. The ultrasound beam must reflect from the lens apex and a beam which is too strongly focused gives reflections from paraxial regions of the lens. The Panametrics device (Patella *et al.*, 1982) is used quite widely but the Optison (Port, 1981b) has now been discontinued.

The Kelvin company designed an instrument which also did not rely on mechanical applanation of the lens surface. The principle utilized was that of proximity gauging but

the effect of different water content materials meant that calibration with anything other than the same hydrogel material was impossible (Port, 1983).

10.4.3   OPTICAL METHODS

Athough the Drysdale method has been mentioned, there are other optical methods which have been used viz interferometry (El-Nashar & Larke, 1980) and Moiré fringes (Rotlex Optics Ltd, 1991). These have been used primarily in research applications.

The ophthalmometer (keratometer) is conventionally used to measure the central curvature of the cornea (convex) but can be used to measure the corresponding area of the back surfaces of a soft lens. The soft lens has to be immersed in saline (at room temperature) so that the shape of the lens is normal. The use of the instrument to determine the BOZR was reported in 1973 (Chaston, 1973; Forst, 1973) and subsequent modifications to the keratometer method have been described (Vögel, 1977). With some keratometers, the light source has to be modified (Chaston & Fatt, 1979) as the original source gives rise to very low intensity images. The Zeiss Jena ophthalmometer (Fig. 10.8) employs a high intensity light source which has a neutral density filter *in situ* for conventional corneal keratometry. For measuring the curvature of soft lenses in saline, the filter is removed.

The usual instrument scale cannot be used directly as it is relates to surfaces in air:

1. **Advantages of the keratometer method**: suitable instrument may be available; toroidal surfaces can be measured.
2. **Disadvantages**:
   light source may be inadequate;
   only central 3 mm of surface is sampled;
   reflections from anterior surface of lens may lead to confusion (Forst, 1974);
   saline wet cells are not temperature controlled;
   centration of lenses is time consuming.

Although it is theoretically possible to convert the normal keratometer scale to take account of curved surfaces in saline, it is worthwhile calibrating the instrument with a series of rigid surfaces in saline (Holden, 1975). These

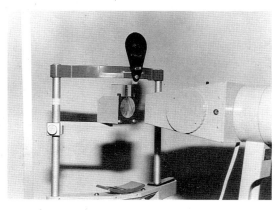

Figure 10.8 A wet cell (filled with saline and holding the soft lens) is clamped to the headrest of a Zeiss Jena ophthalmometer to enable the Back Optic Zone Radius to be measured. The instrument value for the soft lens in saline would not be accurate as the instrument conventionally determines radius values (of the cornea) in air.

reference surfaces are preferably precision surfaces made from glass. Probably the most convenient optical method is to use the Rodenstock CES ophthalmometer. This has an alternative objective lens so that recalibration for surfaces in saline is unnecessary.

10.4.4   DISPUTING BOZR VALUES

Before disputing radius values the following questions should be answered and recorded:

1. Has the machine been calibrated correctly and recently by its operator? Are the reference pieces of known accuracy?
2. Is the radius being assessed indirectly by sagitta determination or keratometry? If the former, which diameter lens support was used and which apparatus?
3. What temperature was used for measurement?
4. If standard ISO saline was not used, what formulation was used?
5. Was the lens 'conditioned' by storing it in measurement saline for 2–3 hours before measurement at the measurement temperature?
6. Is the lens inside out?
7. Were three independent measurements taken? ('Independent' implying that the lens was removed from the appararatus and replaced, between measurements).
8. Was the arithmetic mean or median value found?

Example

The three independent readings were 8.60, 8.75 and 9.20 mm. The arithmetic mean is 8.85 mm and the median value is 8.75 mm. If the radius specification was 8.60 mm and the tolerance ± 0.15 mm, then a result based on the mean value would fail the lens whilst one based on the median would pass the lens. In order to reduce the effect of 'outliers', the median value is recommended. To minimize the variations that can occur, it is recommended that national or international guidelines on the appropriate measuring methods are followed.

10.4.5 ASPHERIC SURFACES

The verification of aspheric concave surfaces is more difficult. The radius of curvature is flattening gradually from the centre to the edge of the lens. Two aspects are important – the apical radius and the degree of flattening (eccentricity, for conoid sections). Optical methods using the ophthalmometer or radiuscope will give information about the central (apical) curvature but little information regarding the change in shape. If sagitta is determined, information regarding shape may be missed. However, Ciba Vision have two elliptical series – a 'flat' and a 'steep' and Bausch & Lomb have favoured a 'sag 0', 'sag 1' and 'sag 2' description. In the latter case, 'sag 0' has a smallest sagitta value and 'sag 2' the largest. It is interesting to note that most large volume manufacturers utilize the sagitta measurement when checking samples from batches. If the total diameter of the lens and back surface geometry are known, the total back surface sagitta can be computed and this is verified during quality control procedures. As far as I know, there are no instruments commercially available to specifically measure the total sag of the lens' back surface. Precision instrument manufacturers, e.g. Mitutoyo, produce high quality projection systems which can be used for this purpose.

For the practitioner, it is quite simple to measure the sag above a 10 mm chord (a cylinder whose diameter is 10 mm) and this is recommended. The main reason for doing this is only to distinguish between different series and to check ordered lenses against trial lenses. In the case of aspheric surfaces, the absolute curvatures are not so important but the sags measured should be comparable.

With an aspheric back surface the term 'equivalent spherical radius' (ESR) is useful. If one measured the sag (s) of an aspheric lens above a given chord (d) the use of the normal expression for spherical surfaces is:

$$ESR = s/2 + d^2/8s \qquad \text{(eqn 10.2)}$$

Thus, for aspheric surfaces it is recommended to measure the sag above a known chord and /or convert this to an ESR. It would be extremely useful for manufacturers of such lenses to provide the kind of table shown in Table 10.1. It may be necessary to establish from manufacturers' information if the sag of the back surface varies with power (Port, 1992) for a given total diameter and lens series. All reputable manufacturers should have this data available.

10.5 DETERMINATION OF LENS DIAMETERS

In terms of lens dimensions, the total diameter has the largest numerical value. This implies that any changes affecting the lens dimensions will be more easily apparent by diameter changes as opposed to radius and thickness changes. Coupled to this, the measurement of diameter is considerably simpler than the measurement of thickness or radius. It is strongly advised that total diameter is the dimension to monitor if one is looking at dimensional changes in hydrogel lenses.

There are two approaches to total diameter measurement. First, to look at the lens from the side, and second, to take a plan view of

Table 10.1 Sample table for details of aspheric surfaces

Chord diameter (mm)	Flat series		Steep series	
	Sag	ESR	Sag	ESR
8.0				
8.5				
9.0				
9.5				
10.0				

the lens. The advantage of the first method is to enable the edge profile of the lens to be assessed at the same time. The advantages of the second method are that measurements in more than one meridian are possible to enable a check for lens ovality to be made, and the lens surfaces can be inspected for quality.

Calibration test pieces for diameter should be thin metal discs. Three diameters should suffice: 13.00 mm, 14.00 mm and 15.00 mm, accurate to ± 0.01 mm.

Total diameter and radius are connected when the fit of the lens on the eye is considered. Although it is possible to reject a lens because it is outside the tolerance limits for a particular dimension it is occasionally useful to think of the combined effects of radius and diameter. If a lens is smaller than specified, it will tend to be looser on an eye. If the radius is steeper than specified, the lens will tend to be tighter. Thus if dimensions are a little wrong in this combination, the effect of lens fit may be hardly any different from the specified lens. If a lens is both smaller in size and flatter in radius, or larger in size and steeper in radius, then these combinations are unlikely to produce well fitting lenses.

Soft lenses are immersed in saline and an image of the lens is projected onto a screen. A magnification of 10× to 20× is recommended. The Zeiss Dokumator (Fig 10.9) has been used in this way. This is an instrument designed as a microfiche reader. It only needs a wet cell to hold the lens and saline. A largest scale interval should be 0.10 mm. The scale can either be incorporated into the floor of the wet cell or printed on the screen.

If one is measuring dimensions such as front optic zone diameter, tinted zone (inside and outside) diameters the lens should be imaged from its back or front. The Optimec™ system is best suited to total diameter measurement (Fig. 10.10).

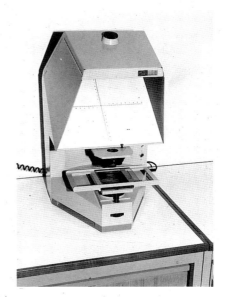

Figure 10.9 The Zeiss Dokumator. A wet cell containing the lens and saline is placed on the microfiche platen. In this example, the measurement scale is printed on the screen. The instrument has been used for many years in the industry and profession for measuring total diameter and lens inspection.

10.6 DETERMINATION OF LENS THICKNESS

It is possible to measure the lens thickness while the lens is in saline. The Optimec™ projection system does this but the resolution of thickness is poor for lenses < 0.1 mm substance. Although in-saline methods using microscopes have been tried, it is difficult for the operator to focus on a lens/saline interface.

Most methods measure the lens in air. A simple and cheap method is to use a radiuscope as a travelling microscope (the magnification of which is usually 75× to 100×). The microscope is first focused on a flat, polished, horizontal piece of black PMMA and the instrument zeroed. The soft lens should have the surface saline removed with a tissue. It is then placed convex side down on

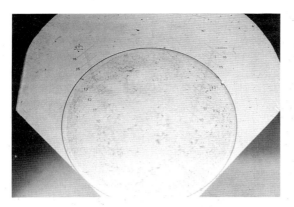

Figure 10.10 A soft lens in an Optimec instrument. This wet cell gives a plan view of the lens. The diameter can be measured in two perpendicular meridians to check for ovality. The focus can be adjusted to view the lens matrix and the surfaces. In this example, the soft lens is very dirty and there is a small piece of the edge missing. Besides being useful to the practitioner for measurement purposes, such projection systems can be useful to demonstrate aspects of the lens which would otherwise be difficult for a wearer to see macroscopically.

the PMMA with the apex along the optical axis of the radiuscope. The instrument is then focused on the concave side of the lens. The vertical movement of the radiuscope gives the thickness. This should be repeated at least three times and the median value obtained. The method will overestimate the thickness if there is a small lake of saline left in the concave side of the lens. Conversely, the thickness will be underestimated if it has dehydrated. A similar method was described by Port (1990).

Most other methods use a micrometer of some description. The soft lens is usually mounted on a spherical dome which has a radius close to that of the lens. Prior to mounting the lens, the micrometer is zeroed on the apex of the dome. When the lens is *in situ*, the sensor of the micrometer is carefully lowered towards the anterior apex of the lens. The thickness is recorded when the sensor just touches the surface of the lens.

The end-point can be visual (with the aid of some magnifier or telescope), an electrical circuit can be completed (Fatt, 1977) or a low force gauge can be employed, e.g. the Rehder gauge. All methods that rely on a sensor applanating a surface are likely to have an error which reduces the measurement value. It is easy for the sensor to indent the material and register a thickness less than the true value. Gauging can be employed to measure the geometric centre thickness or the radial thickness of the periphery. In the latter case the lens and its support is rotated the appropriate amount. Data concerning the peripheral thickness is not always obtainable from the manufacturer and it is often this dimension which gives corneal hypoxia problems with minus powered contact lenses. To be in a position to calculate the peripheral oxygen transmissibility can be useful with problem cases.

10.7   MEASUREMENT OF LENS POWER

The measurement of lens power is apparently a simple measurement. However, in the case of soft lenses, it is often quite difficult and inconsistent (Shepherd, 1992). Although one can measure power of soft lenses in saline (Pearson, 1980), the conversion factor to give a power in air is between 4× and 8× for most materials. Thus any errors are magnified and much more precise methods are needed for this approach. In reality, the vast majority of power measurements are made in air. A normal focimeter, fitted with a contact lens stop is used. Practically, the problems are related to a heterogeneous surface quality. The image is degraded by surface saline, incomplete and variable drying. Any poor polishing of the lens surface whilst it is in the zerogel state will be magnified when the lens is hydrated. High water content lenses, having greater swell factors, tend to have slightly poorer images. High plus lenses tend to have slightly poorer images than high minus lenses. This is presumably due to the fact that the plus lenses have smaller radii of curvature on the front surface and these are more difficult to polish than the relatively flat anterior surfaces of minus lenses. Fuzzy images and double images may indicate poor optical quality. If the image is poor try soaking the lens again and re-drying the surfaces with a clean paper tissue before taking another power measurement. A lens could be rejected for poor image quality and/or incorrect power. There is probably more variation in images of toric lenses then in spherical lenses. It is important to locate any reference marks on a toric lens as the cylinder axis is designated in relation to the reference marks. The reference marks are located at 90 ° or 180 ° on the focimeter. The Tori-Check™ is a useful device (Fig. 10.11) to aid the axis location and ensures that the lens itself is not distorted during measurement. It can be used for both toric and spherical lenses.

10.8 MEASUREMENT OF WATER CONTENT

There are several reasons why it may be necessary to assess the water content of a hydrogel lens. For most practitioners and laboratories a hand held refractometer (Fig. 10.1) is quite suitable (Efron & Brennan, 1985). It will give results which are within 2% of a gravimetric method. Until the present time there has been a relationship between *Dk* and water content so that knowing one, the other can be predicted with reasonable certainty. However, new soft lens materials being developed may invalidate this assumption.

10.9 LENS DEFECTS

Defects are uncommon in new lenses. In used lenses one may see cracks, splits, chips, discoloration and deposits. It is best to view these from a plan view and to be able to focus through the lens. In some cases it is better to view against a dark field and in others against a light field. In the former case, the lens is illuminated from the side.

Some practitioners will examine the lens on the eye for material defects. The slit lamp has variable magnification and illumination and can be very useful for this purpose. A device known as the View-All™ (Fig. 10.13) is also used in conjunction with a slit lamp. There is enough time to examine the lens thoroughly without it drying out and examination is better than with the lens on the eye.

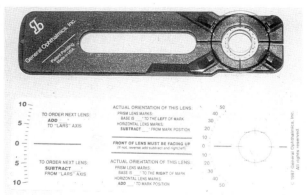

Figure 10.11 The Tori-Check lens holder. Soft lenses can be positioned on a focimeter accurately to measure power, cylinder axis and prism.

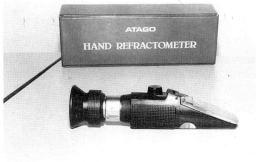

Figure 10.12 An example of a hand refractometer. It is an inexpensive device which can be used to measure the water content of soft lenses.

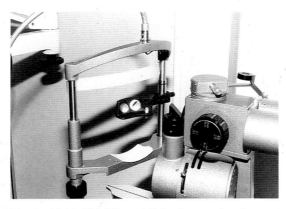

Figure 10.13 The View-All device used to inspect lens surfaces. The lens holder is clamped to the headrest of the slit lamp. Direct, retro-, and dark field illumination of the lens is possible.

Edges of a soft lens can sometimes be the cause of discomfort. In order to examine the edge of a soft lens, viewing has to occur from the side. A projection device is therefore suitable and the lens should be in saline. Using this method it is only possible to view two points on the lens at any one time. The operator should therefore make a point of turning the lens around on its support as there is no reason to belive that the edge profile is always the same at all points on the lens edge.

10.10 CONTACT LENS STANDARDS

There are a number of soft lens standards being revised or initiated at the present time. A list of relevant Draft International Standards (DIS) is given by Port (1991). Requirements for soft lenses will be given together with test methods for various dimensions, parameters and properties.

REFERENCES

Chamarro, T.C.J. (1974) Las lentes de contact flexibles merced a un sencillo sistema optico pueden ser meridas y controladas. *J. Gaceta. Optica*, **36**, 31–5.

Chaston, J. (1973) A method of measuring the radius of curvature of a soft contact lens. *The Optician*, **165** (4271), 8–12.

Chaston, J. and Fatt, I. (1979) Optical measurement of front and back radius of soft contact lenses in saline. *Int. Contact Lens Clin.*, **6**, 136–42.

Davis, H.E. and Anderson, D. (1982) The soft lens analyser. *Int. Contact Lens Clin.*, **9**(1), 11–18.

Drysdale, C.V. (1900) On a simple direct method of measuring the curvature of small lenses. *Trans. Opt. Soc.*, **2**, 1–12.

Duprat, A. and Joinet, B. (1979) Determination of soft lens parameters. *Contacto*, **23**(3), 39–40.

Efron, N. and Brennan, N.A. (1985) Simple measurement of oxygen transmissibility., *Aust. J. Optom.*, **68**, 27–35.

El-Nashar, N.F. and Larke, J.R. (1980) Interference measurement of soft lenses. *J. Br. Contact Lens Assoc.*, **3**, 64–70.

Elmstrom, G. (1979) Hydrophilic lens analyser. *J. Am. Optom. Assoc.*, **50**, 757.

Fatt, I. (1977) A simple electrical device for measuring thickness and sagittal height of gel contact lenses. *The Optician*, **173**(4474), 23–4.

Forst, G. (1973) Kritischer Vergleich der verschieden Messfahren zur ermitlung der Krummungs radien von weichen Contactlinsen. *Die Contactlinse*, **4**, 4–11.

Forst, G. (1974) New methods of controlling soft lens quality. *Contacto*, **18**(6), 6–9.

Höfer, P. (1977) Toleranzen und Messmoglichkeiten von harten und weichen Contaclinsen. *Die Contactlinse*, **2**(3), 24–7.

Holden, B.A. (1975) An accurate and reliable method of measuring soft lens curvatures. *Aust. J. Optom.*, **58**, 443–9.

Koetting, R.A. (1981a) Clinical use of the Söhnges Kontramess system for measuring contact lenses. *Am. J. Optom. Physiol. Opt.*, **58**, 633–4.

Koetting, R.A. (1981b) Clinical use of the Medicornea BC Tronic unit for measuring soft lenses. *Am. J. Optom. Physiol. Opt.*, **58**, 631–2.

Lester, R. and Lester, S. (1979) The soft lens analyser. *Contact Lens Forum*, **4**(2), 85.

Loran, D.F.C. (1974) The determination of hydrogel contact lens radii by projection. *Ophthal. Optician*, **14**, 980–5.

McDonald, R. (1981) Clinical applications of the soft lens analyser. *Am. J. Optom. Physiol. Opt.*, **58**, 626–30.

Patella, V.M., Harris, M.G., Wong, V.A. and Yuen, D.C. (1982) Ultrasonic measurement of soft lens base curves. *Int. Contact Lens Clin.*, **9**, 41–53.

Pearson, R.M. (1980) Wet cell measurement of soft lens powers. *J. Br. Contact Lens Assoc.*, **3**, 15–16.

Port, M.J.A. (1976) New methods of measuring hydrophilic contact lenses. *Ophthal. Optician*, **16**, 1078–82.

Port, M.J.A. (1979) The measurement of soft lens surfaces using ultrasound. *Contacto*, **23**, 5–9.

Port, M.J.A. (1980a) Curvature changes in dehydrating soft lenses. *J. Br. Contact Lens Assoc.*, **3**, 168–76.

Port, M.J.A. (1980b) The radius measurement of soft lenses in air. *J. Br. Contact Lens Assoc.*, **3**, 168–76.

Port, M.J.A. (1981a) The Optimec contact lens analyser. *The Optician*, **181**(4683), 11–14.

Port, M.J.A. (1981b) Assessing a new soft lens radiuscope; the AMS Optison. *The Optician*, **181** (4726) 11–14.

Port, M.J.A. (1982) A comparison of two soft lens radiuscopes. *J. Br. Contact Lens Assoc.*, **5**, 107–16.

Port, M.J.A. (1983) Soft lens radius measurement using proximity gauging. *Ophth. Physiol. Opt.*, **3**, 167–74.

Port, M.J.A. (1990) Measurement of centre thickness in soft lenses. *Contact Lens J.*, **18**(3), 69–74.

Port, M.J.A. (1991) Contact lens verification. *The Optician*, **202**(5318), 15–20.

Port, M.J.A. (1992) New Vues disposable lens: BOZR variations. *Contact Lens J.*, **20**(3), 6–9.

Rotlex Optics Ltd (1991) *The OMS 100 system.* Company literature.

Shepherd, D. (1992) Precision of power measurement of hydrogel contact lenses. *The Optician*, **204** (5358), 37–8.

Söhnges, C.P. (1973) The Söhnges control and measuring unit for hard and soft lenses. *Die Contactlinse*, **2**, 30–3.

Steel, W.H. and Noack, D.B. (1977) Measuring the radius of curvature of soft lenses. *App. Opt.*, **16**, 778.

Vögel, A. (1977) Mesung von weichen Contactlinsen mit dem ophthalmometer nach Littmann. *Suddeutsche Optikerzeitung*, **1**(15 Jan.), 78–82.

Wodak, G.M. (1972) Instrumentation for flexible lenses. In *Soft Contact Lenses* (ed. A.R. Gassette and H.E. Kaufman), C.V. Mosby Co., St Louis.

M. Sheridan

11.1 GENERAL COMMENTS AND PRINCIPLES

Before discussing the detailed provisions of national and international standards it may be appropriate to consider why standards are necessary.

No manufactured object will conform exactly to the specification to which it is made. It is therefore necessary to decide what is the maximum permissible deviation from the specification beyond which the product becomes unacceptable. The following factors, often overlooked in discussions on standards, must be taken into consideration:

1. *The effect on performance.* A deviation from specification which has an adverse effect on the performance of the contact lens is unacceptable. Conversely there is no point in setting extremely tight tolerances if these cannot be justified in terms of their effect on performance.

2. *The effect on cost.* Accuracy costs money both directly, since high precision in manufacture requires high technology equipment and/or highly skilled staff, and indirectly, since the higher the precision required the more lenses will be rejected at final inspection.

3. *The accuracy of available methods of measurement.* For manufacturing purposes, there must be readily available methods of checking compliance with the stan-

dard at appropriate stages of manufacture. Ideally, these methods should also be available to practitioners wishing to check lenses on delivery. The tolerance specified for any dimension must be greater than the experimental error of the method of measurement; in general it should be at least double that value. It is meaningless to specify a tolerance without specifying the method by which the dimension or property can be objectively measured. For example, BS 7208, Part 1 (1992a) *Specifications for rigid corneal and scleral lenses*, which is identical to ISO 8321–1 (1991), is completed by BS 7208, Part 3 (1992b) which describes the test methods to be used in checking compliance. If no objective method of measurement exists then no tolerance can be specified. If the available methods of measurement are of low accuracy a large tolerance must be specified however desirable a small tolerance might be on other grounds.

4. *The smallest step used in prescribing.* The tolerance should not be such that two identical lenses could be supplied in response to a prescription calling for a difference between the right and left eyes. For example, if a prescription calls for back vertex powers of R + 1.00 D, L + 1.25 D a tolerance on back vertex power ± 0.12 D allows a pair of lenses of + 1.12 D to be supplied, the

Contact Lens Practice. Edited by Montague Ruben and Michel Guillon.
Published in 1994 by Chapman & Hall, London. ISBN 0 412 35120 X

right lens complying with the positive tolerance and the left lens with the negative. It may not be possible to apply this principle if the result of doing so conflicts with the tolerance dictated by the accuracy of available methods of measurement. BS 7208, Part 1 (1992a) for example, specifies a power tolerance of ± 0.12 for rigid lenses with powers between $+$ and $- 5.00$ D, a power range within which a prescribing interval of 0.25 D is common. This is a recognition of the fact that few commercially available focimeters will measure power to the order of accuracy (± 0.03 D), which would permit a tolerance of ± 0.06 D. Similar considerations apply to the tolerances for the back optic zone radius of corneal lenses of ± 0.025 mm for those made of PMMA and ± 0.05 mm for those of gas permeable material, in spite of the fact that this dimension is generally prescribed in steps of ± 0.05 mm. Before arriving at these decisions, members of the responsible BSI subcommittee HCC 78/1 carried out extensive and time-consuming experiments on the accuracy of measurement obtainable with readily available instruments. The problem described above, where a pair of identical lenses could be supplied although the prescription for the right and left eyes is not identical could be avoided by requiring that, where a pair of lenses is supplied, any deviation from the specification must be in the same direction for each lens. This has not proved acceptable to manufacturers, especially at international level, and of course could not apply to replacement lenses, which are usually ordered singly. A detailed discussion of the problems touched on above appears in subclause 8.6 of BSO, Part 3 (1981) *Methods of verifying compliance with requirements.*

11.2 DEVELOPMENT OF CONTACT LENS STANDARDS

11.2.1 BRITISH STANDARDS

Until 1980 ophthalmic standards were national standards; they were developed by each country independently to meet its own requirements and generally without reference to standards developed in other countries. In the United Kingdom, a group of British Standards relating to spectacles and contact lenses was published in the early 1960s. Contact lens nomenclature and methods of specification were dealt with in section 14 and Appendix B of BS 3521 (1962). The rapid technological developments in contact lenses made it necessary by 1979 to issue an updated version as a separate Part 3 of a revised BS 3521. Dimensional and optical tolerances for contact lenses were published as BS 5562 (1978).

11.2.2 INTERNATIONAL STANDARDS

General organization

In 1980 the International Standards Organization created two new subcommittees of its Technical Committee 172: Optics and Optical Instruments Subcommittees 7 and 8. Subcommittee 8 (SC8), 'Ophthalmic optics', has three working groups. Working group 1 (WG1) is responsible for developing International Standards for contact lenses. Subcommittee 7 (SC7), originally entitled 'Other optical instruments', but subsequently re-named 'Ophthalmic, endoscopic and metrological instruments and test methods', deals with contact lens testing through two working groups. Working group 4 (WG4), 'Test instruments and test methods for contact lenses', is responsible for developing standards for methods of measurement and inspection of contact lenses while working group 5 (WG5), 'Chemical and biological test methods for contact lenses', is concerned with the biocompatibility and possible toxicity of contact lens materials.

This division of labour has not proved entirely successful. WG1 of SC8 began work in 1980 and by 1982 had produced two draft standards, one for nomenclature and one for dimensional and optical tolerances, based on of BS 3521, Part 3 and BS 5562, respectively, but modified to accommodate differences between United States and European practice. These drafts failed to achieve enough support to become International Standards and when WG4 of SC7 was set up in 1983 its attempts to produce standards for methods of measuring contact lens parameters soon made it apparent that earlier standards for dimensional and optical tolerances were often based upon assumptions about the accuracy and reliability of methods of measurement which were not easy to justify. This realization led to the withdrawal of BS 5562 in 1985. With hindsight, WG4 should have preceded WG1.

Contact lens testing methods standards

The heavy workload which has fallen upon WG4 of SC7 can be appreciated from the list of projects which have reached an advanced stage of development. These include the following Draft International Standards which are presently at the voting stage by the different national bodies.

Determination of vertex power	ISO DIS 9337
Determination of curvature	ISO DIS 10338
Determination of diameters	ISO DIS 9338
Determination of thickness of rigid contact lenses	ISO DIS 9339–1
Determination of strains	ISO DIS 9340
Determination of inclusions and surface inspections of rigid contact lenses	ISO DIS 9341
Determination of spectral and luminous transmittance	ISO DIS 8599
Determination of oxygen permeability and transmissibility with the Fatt method	ISO DIS 9913–1
Determination of refractive index of contact lens materials	ISO DIS 9914
Determination of water content of soft lenses	ISO DIS 10339
Saline solution for contact lenses	ISO DIS 10344

Working group 5, set up in 1985, deals with both contact lens materials and contact lens care products. This working group is concerned with all test methods covering microbiological efficacy, leachable of impurities and shelf life. Also over the last two years, this working group has been involved also with the clinical evaluation of both contact lenses and contact lens products. In general, progress is slow in this working group because of: (a) the very divergent national standards in the area of microbiology; (b) the lack of recognized test methods for efficacy testing such as *in vitro* cleaning efficacy of contact lens cleaners and; (c) the enormous work needed to prepare an all encompassing standards for clinical testing of the various products available. However, working group 5 has already produced a number of Draft International Standards test methods:

Determination of biological compatibility	ISO DIS 9394
Determination of cytotoxicity of contact lens materials, Part 1: Agar overlay test and growth inhibition test	ISO DIS 9363–1
Determination of biological compatibility of contact lens material – testing of the contact lens system by ocular study with rabbit eyes	ISO DIS 9394
Solvent extraction	ISO DIS 10340

Contact specification and manufacturing standards

Progress in WG1 of SC8 has been slowed by the need to await the completion by WG4 of SC7 of time-consuming programmes of experiments necessary to establish the true accuracy and reliability of the methods of measurement. Since 1984, meetings of these two working groups have been arranged to take place consecutively and this arrangement, together with a considerable overlap of membership, has all but eliminated the potential inefficiency of the splitting of responsibility for lenses and test methods.

The constraint of test method has not applied to nomenclature and International Standard 8320, *Contact lenses – vocabulary and symbols* was published in 1986. However, because of the many developments that have taken place since 1986, this standard needed very rapid major additions and revisions. This standard is therefore presently being reviewed by WG1 SC8 under the five-year rule, which allows for revision of any standard five years after publication.

Terminology concerning the classification of materials has now been worked upon for several years. Unfortunately two fundamentally different nomenclatures have been proposed, one of European origin, which has the broad support of Euromcontact, the Association representing the European contact lens industry, and the other based upon the American Food and Drug Administration system. It will therefore be some time before a standard becomes available. A major difficulty for these classification systems is the need to accommodate the new families of materials that are constantly being developed.

As the main obstacle to progress in issuing a contact lens specification standard is the difficulty of measuring soft lenses, WG1 of SC8 decided to develop a two-part standard; Part 1 dealing with rigid and Part 2 with soft lenses. The *Rigid Contact Lenses – Specifica-*tion, after some delay in reaching agreement, not on the tolerances to be applied, but on the recommended methods of specification, has been finally published as International Standard ISO 8321–1 (1991). In the meantime, the United Kingdom, France and the United States have produced national standards for rigid contact lenses which, although not identical in content, have set national standards tolerances in close conformity with those of the International Standard.

Progress in developing an International Standard specification for soft lenses has been much slower, principally because of the difficulty in establishing reliable and available test methods for measuring their dimensions and powers, but a Committee Draft (the earliest stage in the preparation of an International Standard) was approved for circulation in October 1989 and is currently under review to be released as a DIS in 1993.

11.2.3 EUROPEAN STANDARDS

Until 1989 the European Committee for Standardization (Comité Européen de Normalisation (CEN)), had not attempted to produce European standards for contact lenses. However, as long ago as 1985, the European Commission had decided that in implementing the single European act, to be in place by 1993, CEN should (with CENELEC, which is responsible for electrical standards) be responsible for publishing harmonized European standards. These standards will then be referred to in EEC Directives on matters such as health and safety and products conforming to those standards will be presumed to meet the legal requirements of the Directives. An important difference between a European standard (EN) and an International Standard is that once approved by a weighted majority vote an EN must be adopted without deviation as the national standard of all member countries of the EEC, replacing any pre-existing national standard even if the country concerned voted against its adoption. In contrast, adoption of an International Standard is entirely voluntary, although is has been the policy of the British Standards Institution in recent years to adopt and dual number any International Standards for which the United Kingdom cast an affirmative vote, for example ISO 8320–1986, which became BS 3521, Part 3 (1988).

The potential conflict between CEN and ISO standards was minimized by the declared intention of CEN to adopt ISO standards wherever practicable but the implementation of the European single market in 1993 imposes a timetable on CEN working groups concerned with standards in areas which are the subject of• EEC Directives to which their ISO counterparts are not subject. CEN TC/170, 'Ophthalmic optics', held its first meeting in June 1989, shortly after the issue of a Draft Directive on non-active medical devices. It set up two working groups dealing with contact lens standards. WG4 combined the functions of the ISO groups SC7/WG4 and SC8/WG1 under the title 'Physical requirements, test instruments and test methods for contact lenses'. WG5 has the title 'Chemical and biological requirements and test methods for contact lenses and care products', a field of activity very similar to that of ISO/SC7/WG5. By September 1990, these groups had made substantial progress on a large number of EN relating to contact lenses, largely based on the ISO work referred to above and there was every prospect at that stage that a large battery of European contact lens standards would be completed in 1991. As Draft International Standards, although at the penultimate stage of development, were still subject to revision, it was by no means certain that the final European and International standards would be identical. The creation of a European consensus and the level of activity in Europe has had a powerful influence in the ISO decision to approach CEN and enquire on the possibility of having joint meetings and working groups. The first joint meeting took place in March 1992 in San Francisco. Current DIS and CEN preliminary standards are therefore harmonized and the information given for ISO is now directly applicable to CEN standards.

REFERENCES

BS 3521 (1962) *Glossary of terms relating to ophthalmic and spectacle frames*. British Standards Institution, London.

BS 5562 (1978) *Specification for contact lenses*. British Standards Institution, London.

BS 3521 (1979) Part 3. *Glossary of terms relating to ophthalmic and spectacle frames Part 3. Contact lens nomenclature and methods of specification*. British Standards Institution, London.

BSO (1981) Part3. *Drafting and presentation of British Standards*. British Standards Institution, London.

BS 7208 (1992a) Part 1. *Contact Lenses. Part 1. Specifications for rigid corneal and scleral contact lenses*. British Standards Institution, London.

BS 7208 (1992b) Part 3. *Contact Lenses. Part 3. Methods of test for contact lenses*. British Standards Institution London.

International Standard Organization (1986) ISO 8320. *Contact lenses vocabulary and symbols*. International Standard Organization for Standardization.

International Standardization (1991) ISO 8321–1. *Optics and Optical Instruments – Contact Lenses – Part 1: Specification for rigid corneal and scleral contact lenses*. International Organization for Standardization Organization.

oxygen uptake dominates the philosophy of contact lens research and will be found again and again in this text.

It is possible for those not possessing a basic knowledge of biochemistry to understand the mechanisms involved. Thus the simple approach is to appreciate that the vital cells of the cornea, i.e. epithelial, keratocytic and endothelial, have different functions and metabolic demands upon nutrition and oxygen. The epithelial cell is chiefly concerned with protection and therefore rapid reproduction of the basal cell, whereas the keratocyte is a dormant inflammatory cell better described as a fibrocyte and able to secrete collagen when required. The endothelial cell is not able to reproduce itself and thus is specialized. It is concerned with water metabolism, which is a most important role maintaining a transparent cornea. The enzymatic cycles required to utilize oxygen and break down glucose and/or glycogen so that the cells remain viable and functional are most complicated and finely tuned to limited ranges of oxygen tension. In brief, the highest oxygen intake is required by the epithelial cells, then by the keratocytes and finally by the endothelium, which can subsist at the lowest intake level, but this is a simplistic explanation and details which can even involve the organelles (mitochondria) are to be found in Chapters 15 and 42. The state of anoxia or more commonly, hypoxia gives different corneal signals of distress (Chapter 45), depending upon which layer of the cornea is affected. The term physiological stress indicates a reversible condition. Beyond this begins irreversible tissue and cell changes best described as pathology or disease.

Another basic anatomical consideration is the shape or form of the front of the eye. This given information not only in descriptive terms but in detailed measurements.

Chapters 16 and 17 give several methods of determining the topography of the eye.

There are also obvious measurements such as the palpebral fissure and limbal diameters. Because of racial and age characteristics there exist big variations in the eye size. Then there are the characteristics of corneal abnormalities, such as high myopia and keratoconus, that will markedly alter the corneal shape. Injury and surgical procedures can also produce abnormal shapes. The topography and the recording of such measurements has a role in clinical practice quite apart from contact lens practice.

The fitting of a contact lens (especially a rigid lens) and the initial and follow-up examinations all depend upon accurate topography, whether in its simple form as keratometry, for research or for more complicated procedures. Such techniques have been utilized as a basis for automated fitting (Chapter 27). If the uninitiated practitioner considers the cornea to be a tilted ellipsoid, then it will be appreciated that topography is an essential role in understanding the corneal shape.

The anatomy of the body, and in particular of the eye, gives information on the gross and minute structure but often omits details concerning the lubrication fluids essential for function. It is perhaps obvious that a joint of a limb must have such fluids. It is perhaps not so obvious that the eye is a moving organ and the lids also move, often several times a minute. The lubricant is the tears. The contact lens is an additional moving part and its ultimate success depends very much upon the quality and quantity of tears (Chapter 21). The analysis of the tears and their glands of formations in both normal and abnormal states is possibly the most important factor. The physiology and examination of tears establishes how the integrity of the corneal surface and the contact lens surface depends on the tears. Indeed the use of so many substitute tear preparations (Chapter 25 and 26) supports the notion that lubrication is of tantamount importance to the contact lens wearer.

From the early days of contact lens usage it was realized that the lens could not function in isolation. There are many preparations that are now essential to the correct use of the device. These are best dealt with later in the text under the heading of cleaning and disinfection (Chapter 25). More information also will be found in Chapter 47.

MICROSCOPIC ANATOMY AND ULTRASTRUCTURE OF THE CORNEA, CONJUNCTIVA AND LIDS

Brenda J. Tripathi, R.C. Tripathi and N.S.C. Borisuth

12.1 THE CORNEA

The cornea is a transparent, a vascular, visco-elastic tissue with a smooth, convex external surface and a concave internal surface. The primary function of the cornea is optical; with a refractive index of 1.376, the cornea accounts for some 70% (45 dioptres) of the total refractive power of the dioptric system of the eye.

When the lids are open, the cornea is separated anteriorly from the air only by the pre-corneal tear film (6–20 μm in thickness), which provides an even surface for the passage of light at the air–cornea interface. The precorneal tear film is also the main vehicle for the supply of nourishment to the corneal epithelium, and for the removal of surface detritus, as well as for maintaining the non-keratinized state of the kerato-conjunctival epithelium.

12.1.1 SURFACE MICRO-ANATOMY

The cornea occupies one-sixth (1.3 cm^2) of the total surface area of the fibrous coat of the globe. Viewed anteriorly *in vivo*, the vertical diameter of the cornea is smaller than the horizontal diameter (average 10.6 mm and 11.7 mm, respectively, in men; in women, each is 0.1 mm smaller). The radius of curva-ture of the anterior surface in the central area of the adult male cornea is 7.8 mm; the sclera has a curvature of 11.5 mm. However, the flattening of the anterior sclera and periph-eral cornea and the sinking effect of the external sulcus prevent the cornea from pro-truding much beyond the scleral surface.

In the central or optical zone (about 4 mm in diameter), the thickness of the cornea is 0.52 mm, with little difference between men and women. In the periphery, the cornea thickens to 0.97 mm as it merges with the conjunctiva, episclera and sclera. The growth of the cornea is most rapid during the first 6 months after birth and reaches its final size at about 6 years of age, a fact to be borne in mind in the fitting of contact lenses to children.

12.1.2 MICROSCOPIC ANATOMY

Structurally, the cornea is composed of four layers (Fig. 12.1): (a) an epithelial layer with a basement membrane; (b) the stroma with its anterior Bowman's zone; (c) Descemet's mem-brane, which is the basement membrane of the corneal endothelium; and (d) endothelium.

Epithelium

The multilayered corneal epithelium is

Contact Lens Practice. Edited by Montague Ruben and Michel Guillon.
Published in 1994 by Chapman & Hall, London. ISBN 0 412 35120 X

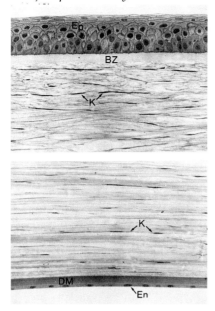

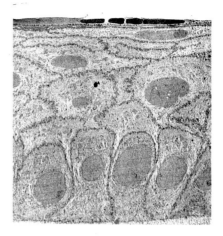

Figure 12.2 Transmission electron micrograph of corneal epithelium. The superficial zone has two to three layers of squamous cells. Prior to exfoliation, the surface cells become pyknotic. The mid-zone is composed of two or three layers of polygonal 'wing' cells. The tall, cuboidal basal cells constitute the germinative layer (original magnification ×3000).

Figure 12.1 Sectional view of the cornea. The anterior surface is covered by a multilayered epithelium (Ep) that rests on a tenuous basement membrane which, in turn, is attached to the acellular collagenous Bowman's zone (BZ). The collagenous lamellae in the anterior stroma are arranged irregularly and contain keratocytes (K). The posterior surface of the cornea is covered by a single layered endothelium (En) that rests on a thickened basement membrane, Descemet's membrane (DM) (original magnification × 500).

derived from surface ectoderm and is probably the most regularly organized stratified squamous epithelium in the body. It is uniformly thick (50–60 μm) and consists of five to six nucleated layers (Fig. 12.2) that are continuous with the epithelium of the bulbar conjunctiva at the limbus. The epithelium occupies about 10 per cent of the total corneal thickness. Based on its morphological organization, the epithelium can be divided into three zones.

Superficial Zone

The superficial zone has two to three layers of thin, polygonal squamous cells formed by the progressive flattening of daughter epi-

thelial cells which originate from the deepest layer (Fig. 12.1). When studied by scanning and transmission electron microscopy, the superficial cells have straight lateral borders and slightly curved anterior surfaces. The cells measure 45–50 μm in length and 4–5 μm in thickness; their flattened nuclei are about 25 μm long and both nuclei and cytoplasm stain well with Giemsa and with haematoxylin and eosin. Although clinical and light-microscopic examination of the cornea shows its anterior surface to be completely smooth, electron microscopy of well-preserved specimens reveals that the outermost cells possess a dense arrangement of small surface projections or microvilli (0.5–1 μm high and 0.5 μm thick) and microplicae (0.5 μm high, 0.5 μm thick and 1–3 μm long), the latter being abundant at the cell junctions (Figs 12.3 and 12.4). The morphogenesis of these configurations is not clearly understood; one view is that they result from the preservation of the digitated or corrugated pattern of the cell border exposed by the exfoliating squamous cells. The role of these projections is to increase the absorptive surface area and the diffusion of the tear fluid, as well as the retention of the mucoid layer of the tear film.

Electron microscopy demonstrates an additional structural specialization of the surface epithelial cells, which is probably related to the deep layer of the precorneal tear film. Ultrastructurally, it is observed that the osmiophilic outer leaflet of the anterior cell membrane of the most superficial squamous cell layer is of increased thickness (6–7 nm instead of the usual thickness of 3–4 nm), so that the unit membrane of this region is 10 nm rather than the usual 7.5 nm thick. The thickened outer layer of the squamous cell membrane supporting the precorneal tear film may form a structural basis for the osmiophilic and PAS-positive layer of phospholipids. Scanning electron microscopy of the surface layer shows cells of 'light', 'intermediate' and 'dark' shades, which are

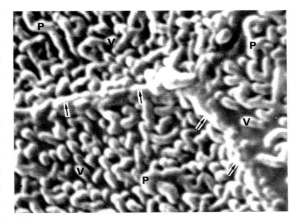

Figure 12.4 Higher magnification of the surface of corneal epithelium showing microvilli (V) and microplicae (P). At the cell junctions, microplicae predominate and cause a ridge-like appearance of the border (arrows) (original magnification ×120 000).

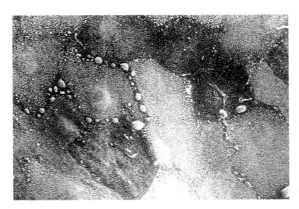

Figure 12.3 Scanning electron micrograph of surface layer of corneal epithelium showing 'light', 'intermediate', and 'dark' shades of cells. This differential appearance of the cells is attributed to the degree of electron scatter caused by microvilli and microplicae on the cell surface. The blebs seen at the cell borders probably represent early or oedematous changes (original magnification × 2000).

attributable to differences in the degree of secondary electron scatter caused by the cell surface irregularities. Thus, the greater the number of surface projections, the more the electrons are scattered and the 'lighter' the appearance of the cells (Fig. 12.3). When the surface epithelial cells are viewed with the optical beam of a specular microscope, this phenomenon is reversed.

The distinguishing features of the surface epithelial cells are the aggregations of glycogen granules and numerous cytoplasmic vesicles that are adjacent to Golgi complexes. The vesicles measure between 0.18 and 0.36 μm in diameter; they may be observed to open into the lateral and posterior intercellular spaces more often than onto the external surface. A granular material can frequently be seen in the lumina of these vesicles. Although the prominent Golgi complexes and vesicles are implicated in the secretion of glycoproteins, their contribution to the precorneal tear film remains to be determined. The epithelial cells also synthesize mitogenic factors.

Each day, the cornea sheds approximately

in the merging of the basal lamina to the underlying Bowman's zone. Because the attachment of the basal lamina to the basal cells and to Bowman's zone is extremely firm, mechanical scraping of the epithelium usually leaves behind the basement membrane together with the hemidesmosomal component of the basal cells. Lipid solvents loosen the cohesion between the epithelium and its basement membrane. With age, the basement membrane becomes irregular and multilaminar; its thickness increases, and patches of oxytalan fibres and calcific spherules may appear in the peripheral zone of the cornea. In the presence of oedematous and inflammatory processes, the basal lamina tends to separate from the underlying Bowman's zone, but remains attached to the corneal epithelium.

Following injury, the newly formed base-

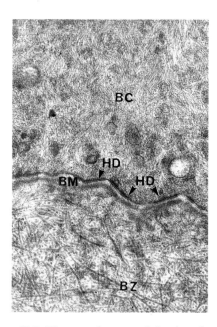

Figure 12.7 The attachment of the basal corneal epithelial cells (BC) to their basement membrane (BM) is mediated by hemidesmosomes (HD). BZ, Bowman's zone of anterior stroma. Transmission electron micrograph (original magnification × 45 000).

ment membrane may take four to six weeks to re-establish its firm connection with the basal cells and Bowman's zone. After epithelial erosion over a large area, therefore, the contact lens wearer should respect this time interval before recommencing wear. The application of growth-promoting and cell-adhesion factors that enhance cell–basement membrane attachment may minimize this time interval.

The structural integrity and the normal functioning of the corneal epithelium are especially important in determining the patient's tolerance for contact lenses. The use of daily-wear hard or extended wear soft contact lenses may exacerbate problems of dry eyes. The mechanical effect of these lenses can result in suppression of surface cell desquamation and reduction in the number of microplicae and microvilli, thus causing the cell surface to become smooth. Rupture of the anterior corneal epithelium by poorly fitted contact lenses can be diagnosed by staining with dyes (such as fluorescein and Rose-Bengal) and causes epithelial oedema (Sattler's veil). The latter condition is best visualized by the slit-lamp technique of sclerotic scatter. In the early stages, intracellular oedema is reversible, but if it is allowed to progress, hydropic degeneration and disruption of the cell membrane may occur, giving rise to liquefaction, degeneration and cystic changes in the epithelium. Disruption of the epithelium is followed by a rapid regenerative response, which can lead to the restoration of the normal thickness of the cornea in a few days if the wound is small (2–3 mm diameter), but may take several weeks if the denudation is massive. In the early stages of regeneration, the epithelium can be dislodged easily, a point of clinical significance for recommencement of contact lens wear. The form (hard versus soft) and size (corneal versus scleral) of the contact lenses worn also determine their interference with normal epithelial biochemistry and physiology (see Chapters 14 and 15). If there is a defect in the epithelium resulting from contact lens wear, it may give rise to localized stromal oedema, which resolves as the epithelial defect is repaired. This further underscores the anterior barrier function of the corneal epithelium.

Stroma

The corneal stroma or substantia propria, which constitutes approximately 90% of the thickness of the cornea, is composed largely of 200 to 250 collagenous lamellae and their resident, corneal corpuscles or keratocytes. The most anterior part of the stroma, 8–14 μm in diameter and known to light microscopists as Bowman's membrane, was originally considered to be a special hyaline and homogeneous corneal membrane (see Fig. 12.1). Electron microscopists, however, prefer the term Bowman's zone or layer because it is composed of a homogeneous, acellular feltwork of randomly orientated, uniform collagen fibrils of 14–19 nm diameter, that exhibit an embryonic microperiodicity (Fig. 12.8). The interstices between the fibrils are filled with a glycosaminoglycan ground substance which is similar histochemically to that of the remainder of the stroma. However, the staining of Bowman's layer is less metachromatic than that of the corneal stroma. By slit lamp biomicroscopy, Bowman's zone is more translucent than is the deeper corneal stroma.

Posteriorly, the collagenous feltwork of Bowman's zone becomes increasingly regular and merges imperceptibly with the underlying anterior stroma (Fig. 12.8), making it difficult to detach. At the periphery of the cornea, Bowman's zone becomes thinner and less dense; the collagen fibrils have a loose arrangement and they gradually merge with those of the conjunctiva. The tapering of the peripheral Bowman's zone is produced by a gradual loss of some of the posterior collagen. Even though Bowman's zone is perforated by numerous branches of fine

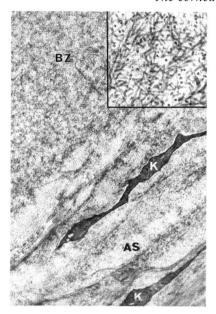

Figure 12.8 Bowman's zone (BZ) of anterior stroma (AS) is composed of an acellular feltwork of collagen fibrils that are orientated randomly (inset, original magnification × 45 000). K, keratocytes. Transmission electron micrograph (original magnification × 14 000).

non-medullated nerves that are in transit to the epithelium, it offers considerable resistance to mechanical trauma and to passage of bacterial and other foreign particles. Once destroyed, however, its typical architecture is not renewed, and the defect is filled either by the downgrowth of the epithelium or by the formation of scar tissue.

The substantia propria deep to Bowman's zone is composed of collagen bundles which are arranged in intertwining layers or lamellae (see Fig. 12.1) with a thickness of about 2 μm and a width of 9–260 μm; they extend across the entire diameter of the cornea. The lamellae in the anterior stroma are arranged in a less orderly manner than are those in the posterior stroma. The collagen bundles of the anterior lamellae are of irregular width and spacing; they branch and anastomose with other layers or insert into Bowman's zone

(Fig. 12.9). In the deep corneal stroma, the lamellae are of almost uniform thickness and become arranged in a more orderly fashion parallel to the corneal surface. Surgically, this organization is confirmed by a greater ease of dissection of the corneal lamellae of the posterior than of the anterior stroma. In paraffin sections, artefactual clefts in the stromal lamellae usually occur from separation in the plane of the keratocytes as a result of processing. The lamellae themselves do not readily come apart, because of the interlacing pattern of the bundles, and probably limit artefactual clefts over any great distance.

At a normal or raised intraocular pressure, Bowman's zone is under tension and appears smooth when viewed from its anterior surface. In the presence of hypotony and corneal indentation, however, the prominent oblique lamellae of the anterior stroma are relaxed, and a polygonal ridged mosaic pattern manifests itself on the corneal surface (Fig. 12.10). This phenomenon may be observed transiently during applanation tonometry, and on gentle massaging of the cornea through the lids, as well as in some cases of contact lens wear, probably indicating compression of the epithelium against the mosaic pattern.

Within each lamella, broad bands of parallel collagen fibrils crisscross at nearly right angles to the fibres in the adjacent lamellae. Most fibrils have a uniform diameter that ranges from 19 nm anteriorly to 34 nm posteriorly, but a few fibrils may measure 60–70 nm. In the posterior cornea

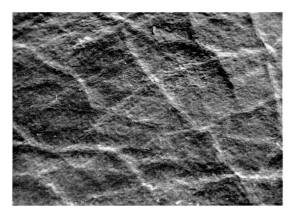

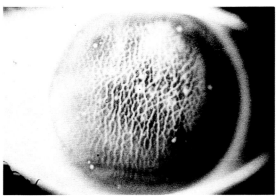

Figure 12.9 Transverse section of human cornea viewed by polarized light. In the anterior stroma, the collagenous lamellae criss-cross and are orientated obliquely, eventually terminating in Bowman's zone. In the deeper stroma, the lamellae are organized regularly and parallel to the corneal surface (original magnification × 300).

Figure 12.10 (a) The anterior corneal mosaic as revealed by scanning electron microscopy (original magnification × 65). (b) Clinical appearance of the mosaic demonstrated with fluorescein in the conjunctival sac after rubbing the upper lid over the cornea (from Bron, 1970.)

overlying Descemet's membrane, electron microscopy demonstrates a thin transition zone containing fibrils with a diameter of 10 nm. The size of human corneal collagen fibrils falls within the same range as that of other vertebrate species, and they share embryonic characteristics such as microperiodicity (ranging from 62–64 nm), a small diameter, and an extremely slow turnover rate. The corneal stroma is composed primarily of interstitial collagen type I, along with smaller amounts of collagens type III, IV, V, VI and VIII. The fibrils within the bundles of collagen are coated with and separated from one another by a cementing ground substance that consists predominantly of glycosaminoglycans (GAGs) and glycoproteins (amounting to 4 to 5% of the dry weight of the cornea). The constituents of the GAGs are keratan sulphate (50–60%), chondroitin-4-sulphate (25%), small amounts of low sulphated dermatan sulphate and non-sulphated chondroitin, and heparan sulphate. The regularity of the arrangement and thickness of collagen fibrils and lamellae is affected by various physiological (sleep, pregnancy) and disease processes (such as mechanical or chemical trauma, infections and dystrophies) and may lead to blurring and loss of transparency of the cornea. The thickening of the cornea during sleep may be due to lid closure, which prevents the evaporation of water from the cornea. A similar phenomenon may occur with contact lens wear, because large lenses prevent rapid evaporation of water from the cornea.

The orderly array of corneal lamellae with the ground substance interposed between individual collagen fibrils creates a three-dimensional diffraction grating. With the fibrils separated by a distance of about 200 nm (less than half the wavelength of light), this arrangement provides the structural basis for corneal transparency (see Chapter 1).

The cellular component of the substantia propria consists largely of fixed, modified fibrocytic cells known as keratocytes or corneal corpuscles, which constitute about 3 to 5% of the total stromal volume. By slit-lamp biomicroscopy and in histological sections, the keratocytes are characterized by their flattened, thin, irregular profiles that are orientated parallel to the corneal surface (see Fig. 12.1); however, the intralamellar location of the cell bodies is revealed by electron microscopy (Fig. 12.11). Flat sections of the cornea show that the keratocytes at the same level communicate with the adjacent cells via long cytoplasmic processes that are occasionally joined by zonulae occludentes; however, the individual borders are distinct and the cells do not form a syncytium. A space of 20 nm usually separates the keratocytes where they meet one another. Gap junctions between adjacent cells provide cell-to-cell communication.

Keratocytes contain a flattened, centrally located nucleus with one to three nucleoli. Each cell is widened in the nuclear region, where it measures between 1 and 2 μm in diameter. However, the cytoplasm is scanty around the nucleus and may be as thin as 0.1 μm; elsewhere, the cytoplasm contains an

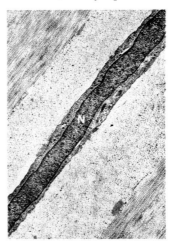

Figure 12.11 Transmission electron micrograph showing the intralamellar location of keratocytes. These modified fibrocytic cells have a thin, flattened profile with a central nucleus (N) (original magnification × 18 000).

extensive array of intracellular organelles, especially RER, Golgi complexes, glycogen granules and ribosomes. Although the metabolic rate of keratocytes is low, they are responsible for the continuous synthesis and secretion of ground substance. Normally, the cells do not undergo mitosis but following injury to the cornea, they may proliferate rapidly. Extracellular material of microfibrillar structures juxtaposed to the keratocytes probably represents tropocollagen fibrils and an early precursor form of ground substance. Other cellular components of the stroma include occasional wandering cells (leucocytes and macrophages), and unmyelinated nerves.

Descemet's membrane

Descemet's membrane is a specialized basement membrane of the corneal endothelium that lines the posterior boundary of the corneal stroma (see Fig. 12.1). Its abrupt peripheral termination marks the peripheral boundary of the cornea. Under the light microscope, Descemet's membrane appears as a thick, glassy membrane that demonstrates no apparent substructure. It is quite unusual because of its thickness and structure and its positive staining with PAS. Ultramicroscopy with dark ground illumination and with polarization microscopy has shown Descemet's membrane to be composed of stratified layers. Electron microscopy confirms this observation, thereby providing a histological and embryological basis for differentiating it into two zones. The anterior one-third of Descemet's membrane is a banded zone that consists of atypical collagen fibrils which are arranged in a hexagonal pattern and are interconnected with nodes and internodes of electron-dense material. This creates a lamellar pattern of equilateral triangles with sides of 100–110 nm, as seen in transverse sections of the membrane. The posterior two-thirds of Descemet's membrane, known to electron microscopists as the posterior non-banded

zone, is homogeneous and fibrillogranular; it is mainly responsible for the age-dependent increase in thickness, as well as for abnormal formation of Descemet's membrane, in the presence of endothelial dysfunction. In general, Descemet's membrane is composed of about 73% collagen (primarily type IV and type VIII) and 27% glycosaminoglycans. The residues galactose, glucose, mannose, glucosamine and galactosamine account for 14% of the dry weight of the membrane, thus explaining its intense PAS positivity.

The synthesis of the anterior banded zone begins during embryonic (second month of gestation) and fetal life. The banding pattern is apparent by the eighth month of gestation. The posterior non-banded zone is formed postnatally as a secretory product of the corneal endothelium. Descemet's membrane increases in thickness from about 3 μm at birth to 5 μm in childhood, and to 8–12 μm in adulthood.

Although Descemet's membrane appears dense morphologically, it is readily permeable to solutes and particles of the dimensions of colloids. The membrane is extremely resistant to inflammatory processes and is indigestible by proteases or chemical agents, a characteristic that is useful in its isolation from the rest of the cornea. Unlike Bowman's zone, it readily regenerates after pathological destruction; this supports the concept that it is a secretory product of the corneal endothelium. Descemet's membrane can be easily separated from the underlying endothelium and also from the overlying stroma. When cut, the edges of the membrane tend to curl toward the stroma (and may form a scroll) even though it contains no true elastic tissue. In patients with disorders of the corneal endothelium, Descemet's membrane shows certain characteristic alterations in its constituents.

Corneal endothelium

The corneal endothelium lines the posterior surface of the cornea and forms the anterior boundary of the aqueous cavity of the anterior chamber (see Fig. 12.1). Based on its morphological appearance, the corneal endothelium is more like a mesothelium than like an endothelium. However, we determined recently that the corneal endothelium develops from neural-crest-derived mesenchymal cells that migrate from the margins of the rim of the optic cup into the developing eye at the 12 mm (5 week) stage of embryogenesis. Indeed, the neural-crest origin of the corneal endothelium raises the question as to its 'endothelial' designation.

The corneal endothelium comprises a single layer of approximately 500 000 closely fitted flattened, polygonal cells, each 18–20 μm wide, that constitute the 11 mm diameter of the continuous cellular membrane. Specular microscopy and phase contrast micrography show that the corneal endothelium forms a regular mosaic (Fig. 12.12). The hexagonal pattern of the peripheral endothelial cells is less regular than that in the central endothelium. At birth, the cells are as thick as Descemet's membrane (about 3 μm) but increase to 5–6 μm in adulthood, and eventually flattening with advancing age.

Electron-microscopic studies reveal extremely tortuous, but parallel cell borders.

The interdigitations continue along the lateral cell membranes almost to the anterior chamber, where a marginal fold is frequently seen (Fig. 12.13). The endothelial cells are connected by junctional complexes that include zonulae occludentes, maculae occludentes, and rare desmosomes that bridge the normal gap of approximately 25–40 nm between the interdigitating membranes of adjacent cells. Toward the apical surface, the intercellular space narrows to 3 nm, and the borders of the cells are joined by maculae occludentes and gap junctions similar to terminal bars (zonulae occludentes) elsewhere in the body. Terminal bars constitute the endothelial barrier during the fourth and fifth months of gestation, which coincides with the commencement of aqueous humor circulation. Functionally, the zonulae occludentes form a barrier to molecules of colloidal dimension, such as Thorotrast (10 nm diameter).

The cell membrane in the corneal endothelium is a typical unit membrane, having numerous pinocytotic vesicles on its apical,

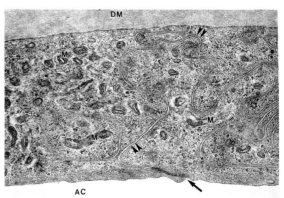

Figure 12.13 Section of corneal endothelium as seen by transmission electron microscopy. Adjacent cell borders are parallel but tortuous (arrowhead) and, at the border of the anterior chamber (AC), are joined by a zonula occludentes (arrow). The cell cytoplasm contains abundant mitochondria (M). DM, Descemet's membrane (original magnification × 40 300).

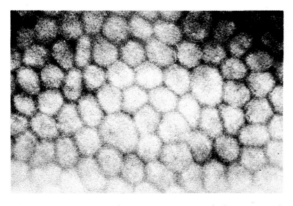

Figure 12.12 Specular microscopy of the corneal endothelium *in vivo* reveals the regular mosaic of polygonal cells.

lateral, and basal sides. The apical surface shows 20 to 30 microvillous projections per cell that measure 0.1–0.2 μm in width and 0.5–0.6 μm in height. Internally, the cells contain a centrally located, oval nucleus of 7 μm diameter and abundant intracellular organelles that signify their active involvement in transport and protein synthesis for secretion. The number of mitochondria in corneal endothelial cells is striking; they are more numerous than in any other ocular cells, with the exception of the ellipsoids of the retinal photoreceptor cells. The elongated mitochondria possess a matrix of increased intracristal density, accompanied by slight dilatation of their intercristal spaces, and therefore, they differ from mitochondria in cells of other ocular tissues (except in keratocytes) in their response to fixation. There is an extremely well-developed Golgi apparatus in the usual perinuclear position, and multivesicular bodies are present as well. Some cells have a pair of centrioles situated posteriorly in the cytoplasm, with a cilium projecting into the anterior chamber. Occasionally, phagocytosed pigment granules of uveal origin may be located in the cytoplasm of corneal endothelial cells. The condensation of cell cytoplasm along the apical border lies in juxtaposition to the zonulae occludentes and resembles the arrangement of the terminal web of intestinal cells. The basal aspect of the cells is somewhat undulating and is applied closely to the posterior surface of Descemet's membrane; the two are joined by modified hemidesmosomes or focal condensations of the plasma membrane.

In children below six years of age, the cell size and density in the corneal endothelium are fairly constant. In infants less than a year old, the mean cell population density (CPD) is close to 4500 cells/mm² (range 3000 cells/mm² to 5500 cells/mm²). In the next five years, the CPD reduces to about 3500 cells/mm² in the central region of the cornea. Between 5 and 50 years of age, however, there is much heterogeneity (1000 to 3500 cells/mm²) in the cell population density. By early adulthood, the mean CPD is close to 3000 cells/mm², in the fourth decade, it is further reduced to 2500 cells/mm², and it may decrease to below 2000 cells/mm² in old age.

Mitoses occur in young endothelial cells but are extremely rare in adult cells. Thus, a cell loss is generally compensated by remodelling of the adjacent cells, which spread and thin out. This physiological response does not alter the hexagonal shape of the cell population albeit at larger cell volumes and areas than were originally present. In older eyes, the cells may enlarge unevenly and form an irregular mosaic pattern. The resulting heterogeneity in cell size and the emergence of large cells is regarded as an indicator of inadequacy of the normal endothelial response to insult. The endothelium maintains a balance between its leakiness and its pump function; this plays a major role in the regulation of corneal hydration. If the normal metabolism of the cornea is interfered with, the structural and functional integrity of the corneal endothelium may be disrupted; this invariably leads to stromal oedema and swelling thereby compromising the functional capacity of the corneal endothelium to maintain transparency of the cornea.

On applanation, a peculiar feature of the posterior corneal surface in individuals past the age of 25 years is the presence of concentric undulations, termed posterior corneal rings (PCRs). Each ring appears as a pair of featureless dark bands separated by a ribbon of visible endothelial cells. Under identical applanating pressures, the PCRs appear at similar positions in the same cornea, but are considered distortion artefacts in normal eyes. In certain pathological states, the PCRs may be a characteristic feature that can be present even in children and therefore, may have some diagnostic value.

In many wearers of contact lenses (the type, form, and fitting of the lens worn obviously being important), the appearance of transitory spots called blebs in different locations of the endothelium may be observed. The nature of these blebs remains to be determined; they are believed to be localized enlargements of the intercellular endothelial spaces caused by hypoxia or accumulation of lactate. Of more pressing concern is the observation of polymegethism or loss of the regular mosaic pattern in long-term wearers of polymethylmethacrylate (PMMA), rigid gas permeable and hydrophilic contact lenses. The mean endothelial cell density is unchanged from that of non-wearers; but a heterogeneity of cell shapes and irregularity of the posterior corneal surface become apparent. While these alterations may be harmless, they can overtax the endothelial function and exacerbate the changes that occur with ageing.

Peripheral cornea

The human cornea is approximately 50% thicker towards the periphery as compared to the central region. The epithelium in the periphery consists of ten or more layers due largely to an increased number of wing cells (Fig. 12.14). The basal lamina assumes a multilaminar configuration and thickens more conspicuously with age than does the central cornea. Bowman's layer becomes less dense and thinner in the periphery, and cells and even capillaries may appear in its meshes. The stromal thickness gradually increases to almost 1 mm near the limbal periphery. The corneal lamellae and their constituent fibrils are not as regularly orientated as they are in the stroma, and their structure gradually approaches the form seen in the sclera. Larger fibrils, 60–70 nm in diameter appear, and the regular spacing between the fibrils is lost. The tips of the limbal vascular arcade are seen at the edge of the peripheral stroma and, at this region, the incoming myelinated nerve fibers lose their myelin sheath. At the edge of the cornea,

Descemet's membrane shows thickening and accumulation of wide-spaced collagen as it frays out into the trabecular sheets.

Just inside the peripheral cornea, in individuals more than age 20, the corneal endothelial cells become slightly attenuated and can recreate their prenatal activities by producing foci of excessive basement membrane material, similar to that seen in the anterior banded zone. By light microscopy, these nodular thickenings can be identified as Hassel–Henle warts. The warts are dome-shaped thickenings of Descemet's membrane, which protrude into the anterior chamber and are covered by a distinctly altered corneal endothelium. Whereas such bodies in the periphery of Descemet's membrane are considered a normal or physiological change with ageing, their presence in the central or axial cornea gives rise to a clinical entity known as cornea guttata. The dome-shaped excrescences of Hassel–Henle bodies

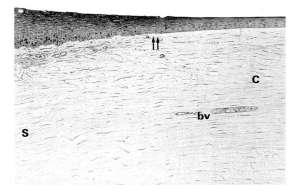

Figure 12.14 Sectional view of anterior corneoscleral limbus showing transition of corneal epithelium (right) into conjunctival epithelium (left), termination of Bowman's zone (arrow), and beginning of conjunctival stroma. The conjunctival stroma, fascia bulbi, and episclera fuse at the epithelial ridge to form dense tissue. The collagen lamellae of the peripheral corneal stroma (C) merge imperceptibly with those of the scleral stroma (S). Note also terminal blood vessels (bv) of the peripheral corneal arcade (original magnification × 260).

have multiple crevices and fissures, into which myriad endothelial cell processes project. The fissures may contain endothelial cell debris, which is interpreted as degenerated fragments of pinched-off cytoplasmic projections.

12.2 THE CONJUNCTIVA

12.2.1 SURFACE MICRO-ANATOMY

The conjunctiva is a thin, transparent mucous membrane that lines the posterior surface of the eyelids (palpebral conjunctiva), is reflected on itself to form the fornices, and covers the anterior surface of the sclera (bulbar conjunctiva). The conjunctiva forms an uninterrupted membrane that lines the large space of the conjunctival sac; at the lid margin, its epithelium joins the epidermis (mucocutaneous junction), whereas, at the corneal margin, the conjunctiva is continuous with the corneal epithelium (Fig. 12.14). At the lacrimal punctum, the mucous membrane is continuous with the membrane lining the lacrimal canaliculi. On the nasal side of the globe and at the edge of the caruncle,

the conjunctiva forms a crescent (plica semi-lunaris), which is a vestige of the nictitating membrane of lower animal species.

The palpebral conjunctiva, which lines the inner surface of the lids, can be subdivided into three anatomical zones (Fig. 12.15). The marginal conjunctiva commences at the intermarginal zone of the lids, where the stratified epithelium of the skin continues as that of the conjunctiva. It runs along the under-surface of the lids until it merges with the tarsal conjunctiva, the transition being marked by the sub-tarsal sulcus. This groove runs parallel to the lid margin. The richly vascularized tarsal conjunctiva firmly adheres to the tarsal plates and continues as the orbital conjunctiva, which extends from the upper border of the tarsal plate to the fornix. The orbital conjunctiva loosely covers the smooth muscles of Müller and is thrown into horizontal wrinkles during opening of the lid.

The forniceal conjunctiva appears as a loosely disposed fold that is maintained independently of the movement of the globe or lid. This tethering action is provided by the fascial insertion of the levator and supe-

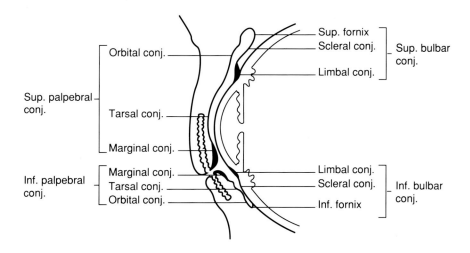

Figure 12.15 Diagrammatic representation of the conjunctival sac and its regional topography as seen in a vertical section of a closed eye.

rior rectus muscles into the superior fornix, and by the attachment of the suspensory ligament of Lockwood to the inferior fornix. The lateral fornix is a recess lying between the lateral canthus and the globe. The medial fornix, which does not form a recess, contains the caruncle (see page 213) and plica semilunaris (Fig. 12.16).

The bulbar or scleral conjunctiva is the thinnest region of the mucous membrane, such that underlying vessels and white sclera are easily visualized. Except toward the limbal region, where the conjunctiva and Tenon's capsule merge for a distance of about 3 mm, the bulbar conjunctiva is connected loosely to the underlying fascia bulbi which, in turn, forms a lax attachment to the underlying episclera and sclera.

12.2.2 MICROSCOPIC ANATOMY

The conjunctiva, like other mucous membranes in the body, consists of epithelium and a substantia propria. The thickness of the epithelium varies from region to region, being thinnest in the bulbar region (two cell layers) and thickest at the limbal

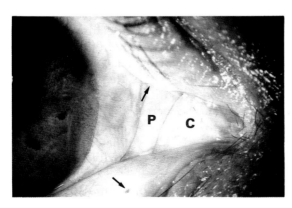

Figure 12.16 Gross appearance of medial canthus showing plica semilunaris (P) and caruncle (C). The punctum of the upper lid is seen as a slight indentation (arrowhead), whereas the lower lid has been pulled slightly inferiorly to reveal this structure (arrow).

conjunctiva (up to 15 layers). The tarsal conjunctiva of the upper lid consists of two layers of cells, but in the lower lid it is three to four cell layers thick, with an intervening central polygonal layer. The ultrastructure of the epithelium is similar to that of the cornea. The superficial cells contain some glycogen, but their surfaces are not as smooth as those of the corneal cells. In the basal layer of the conjuntiva, the cells are smaller and more closely packed than are the germinal cells of the cornea (see page 198). Their basement membrane, however, has a similar thickness and structure as that of the cornea.

The ultrastructure of the limbal epithelial cells differs from their corneal counterparts in that the conjunctival cells have larger mitochondria and their cytoplasmic filaments are in dense bundles, some of which are associated with desmosomes. The interdigitating cell membranes and their associated junctional complexes are like those of the cornea. The surfaces of the superficial cells show a similar arrangement and density of microplicae and microvilli as are seen in the corneal epithelium. However, the rate of turnover of conjunctival cells is slower than that of the cells of the corneal epithelium. The continuous bathing by the tears prevents conjunctival keratinization similar to that of the cornea.

Melanin granules are present in the cuboidal basal cells, and occasionally in the middle (wing-cell) layer of the conjunctival epithelium. Lymphocytes and melanocytes are also seen in the basal and suprabasal layers of the limbal conjunctiva but these cells lack abundant tonofilaments and do not form a specialized attachment with the adjacent epithelial cells. Melanocytes contain few filaments, and their cytoplasm appears less dense than that of the basal epithelial cells. Langerhans' cells, which are frequently encountered within the epithelium, display dilated Golgi zones, numerous striated cytoplasmic rodlets referred to as Langerhans'

12.3 THE EYELIDS

12.3.1 EXTERNAL SURFACE

The eyelids are two modified folds of skin that serve to protect the eye, distribute tears over its anterior surface and limit the entry of the light into the eye. The upper lid is connected to the eyebrow, which separates it from the forehead, whereas the lower lid merges with the skin of the cheek. The naso-jugal and malar folds mark the inferior extent of the lower lid (Fig. 12.20).

The horizontal orbito-palpebral sulcus divides each eyelid into a palpebral (tarsal) portion and an orbital portion. The palpebral part, which lies in contact with the globe, is involved in reflex blinking. The orbital portion extends between the orbital margin and the globe. The superior palpebral sulcus is well defined and lies 2–3 mm above the cutaneous insertion of the levator palpebrae muscles. The poorly defined inferior palpebral sulcus is formed by the cutaneous insertion of the orbicularis oculi muscle.

Palpebral fissure

When open, the two lids expose an elliptical or almond-shaped area of the keratoconjunctiva known as the palpebral fissure. The size of this aperture varies with age ranging from 10 mm × 19 mm in the newborn to 15 mm × 30 mm in the adult. The shape of the palpebral fissure varies according to the racial characteristics of the individual; in Caucasians it follows mainly superior and inferior sinusoidal lines, the greatest opening being slightly lateral to the midpoint of the horizontal width of the fissure.

Laterally and medially, the fissure terminates at the meeting points of the two lids, called the canthi or angles. The medial canthus is elliptical and surrounds the 'tear lake' or lacus lacrimale. Two structures can be identified in the lacus lacrimale: (a) The plica semilunaris is a vestige of the nictitating

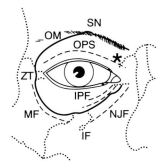

Figure 12.20 Diagrammatic representation of the surface anatomy of the eyelids and their relationships with the orbital margins and sutures of the bones. OM, orbital margin; SN, supraorbital notch; OPS, orbitopalpebral sulcus; NJF, nasojugular folds; MF, malar folds; IPF, intrapalpebral folds; IF, infraorbital foramen; ZT, zygomatic tubercle. Asterisk denotes area of orbital fat herniation.

membrane of lower animal species and represents a fold of mucous membrane (see also page 208); (b) The lacrimal caruncle is a small, pink elevation of modified lid tissue that extends medially from the plica semilunaris to the medial canthus (see Fig. 12.16). It is covered by stratified epithelium which, like that of the lid margin, does not undergo keratinization, probably because it is constantly bathed by the tear fluid in the lacus lacrimale. The surface epithelium of the caruncle contains abundant goblet cells, and there are many adenoidal invaginations of the epithelium into the substantia propria. The caruncle contains approximately 15 to 20 hair follicles with associated large, modified sebaceous and sweat glands, as well as occasional tubulo-racemose, serous glands resembling accessory lacrimal glands (Fig. 12.21). The substantia propria of the caruncle is composed of connective and fatty tissue and a few smooth-muscle fibres. Rarely, foci of cartilage may be discovered

The lateral canthus lies about 5 mm from the lateral orbital rim and forms an acute angle, ranging from 30 to 60 degrees, depending on how wide the eye is open. In

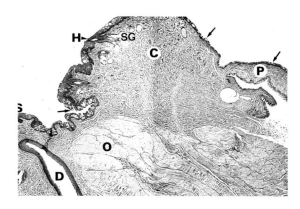

Figure 12.21 Horizontal section passing through the plica semilunaris (P) and caruncle (C) containing hair follicles, sebaceous and sweat glands. O, orbicularis muscle; D, duct of common canaliculis; H, hair follicle; SG, sebaceous glands; S, skin at medial canthus. Arrows denote goblet cells (original magnification × 140).

Caucasian and black individuals, with the eyes open, the lateral canthi are somewhat higher than the medial canthi. This relationship is reversed when the eyes are closed. In oriental individuals, the lateral canthus is 4–5 mm higher than the medial canthus, imparting the characteristic slant to the palpebral fissure. Furthermore, the curve of the medial angle of the palpebral fissure may be partly obscured by a vertical skin fold (epicanthus) that is normally present in fetal life and in orientals, but it disappears in Caucasians and blacks, with the development of the nose bridge.

The shape of the human eye as it appears through the palpebral fissure is very expressive and shows the various moods of the individual; if contact lenses produce abnormalities of the fissure, such as rigidity, the normal look of the eye will be affected. It is worth noting that the degree of tightness of the lids may be a guide to the choice of diameter of corneal lenses. Because the lower lid margin almost rests on the limbus it is very unlikely that any scleral lens would

have a haptic chord inferiorly that exceeds 9 mm; the superior haptic chord rarely exceeds 11 mm. The haptic area according to the outline of the conjunctival sac will not exceed 14 mm laterally and 7 mm nasally. Given a limbal diameter and average chords of the above dimensions, the overall sizes for scleral lenses can be determined from the anatomical outline of the conjunctival sac.

Lid margin

The palpebral margin of the eyelid is approximately 2 mm wide and 25–30 mm long. The superior and inferior puncta lacrimalia, which are the openings of the lacrimal canaliculi, are located in a small eminence, the papilla lacrimalis, some 5 mm from the medial canthus. The puncta drain the tears from the lacus lacrimalis through the corresponding canaliculi into the lacrimal sac, and they divide the lid margins into ciliary and lacrimal portions. The ciliary part of the eyelid margin is the lateral five-sixths of the free margin of the lid and contains two to three layers of eyelashes (cilia) as well as the openings of the tarsal glands. The medial one-sixth of the eyelid, or the lacrimal portion, has no cilia or gland openings.

The upper cilia, which are directed upward, are longer than the lower lashes, which curve downward. There are as many as 150 cilia in the upper lid and 75 in the lower lid. The cilia pass into the lid margin obliquely in front of the palpebral muscle of Riolan and attach to the follicle (which has no erector muscle) anterior to the tarsus. The intermarginal sulcus, or grey line, is a landmark of the lid margin and is located between the opening of the tarsal glands and the cilia. An incision along this line divides the eyelids into an anterior leaf containing skin, muscle and cilia, and a posterior leaf containing fibrous tissue, the tarsal plate (glands and openings) and the conjunctiva. The orifices of the tarsal glands mark the mucocutaneous junction of the skin epithelium with the conjunctival mucous membrane.

12.3.2 MICROSCOPIC ANATOMY

On the outside, the eyelids are lined by keratinizing surface epidermis with associated adnexal structures, and on the inside, by a non-keratinizing conjunctival epithelium. From their superficial (anterior) to deep (posterior) surfaces, the lids consist of tissues in four principal planes (Figs 12.22 and 12.23): cutaneous, muscular, fibrous, and conjunctival. The lids contain a variety of glands which open at the lid margin.

Cutaneous tissue

The eyelids are covered by a loose, elastic skin (the thinnest in the body) that permits extreme swelling under pathological conditions and a subsequent return to normal shape and size. The cutaneous tissue is semi-transparent and consists of epidermis, dermis, and fat-free subcutaneous areolar tissue (Fig. 12.24). The blood vessels appear as dark blue channels.

Epidermis

The epidermis (0.9 mm thick) consists mainly of six to seven layers of a stratified squamous epithelium with a keratinized surface. The cells are organized as follows: (a)

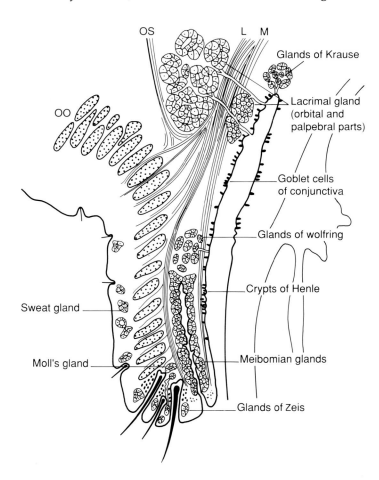

Figure 12.22 Diagrammatic representation of upper eyelid in vertical section. L, levator muscle; M, Müller muscle; OO, orbicularis oculi; R, muscle of Riolan; OS, orbital septum.

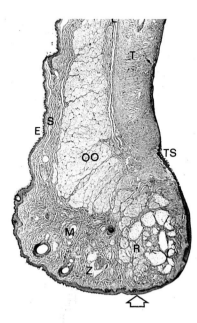

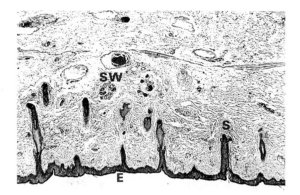

Figure 12.24 Section of lid skin showing its thin subcutaneous areolar tissue and absence of subcutaneous fat. It contains the usual pilosebaceous units and vessels, but the hairs are small. S, sebaceous gland associated with hair follicle; SW, sweat gland in the dermis; E, epidermis (original magnification X 64).

Figure 12.23 Vertical section of lower half of upper lid showing its anatomical constitution. E, epidermis; S, subcutis; R, muscle of Riolan; L, levator muscle; OO, orbicularis oculi; T, tarsal plate containing meibomian gland which opens at the lid margin; Z, gland of Zeis; M, gland of Moll; TS, subtarsal sulcus. Arrow denotes the junction of conjunctival (right) and epidermal (left) epithelia (original magnification X 62).

the stratum basale (germinativum) constitutes the basal layer of columnar cells, which are thrown into papillary projections and attach to a thin, wavy basement membrane via hemidesmosomes. Myriad desmosomes along the lateral and upper surfaces of the basal cells bind adjacent cells of the layer; (b) the stratum spinosum (spongiosum) consists of three to four layers of polygonal cells, which are bound firmly together by a system of filament-filled cytoplasmic spines and desmosomes that punctuate the cell surface and present a prickly appearance by light microscopy; (c) the stratum granulosum is a poorly-defined layer of flattened, polygonal cells that contain centrally located nuclei and cytoplasm filled with coarse basophilic keratohyalin granules; (d) the stratum lucidum is

less apparent in the epidermis of the eyelids than it is in thick skin elsewhere in the body. It consists primarily of densely packed filaments embedded in an electron-dense matrix; (e) the stratum corneum (surface layer) consists of an anuclear cornified flattened layer of cells or 15 to 30 keratin lamellae.

At the mucocutaneous junction on the lid margin, the granular and keratin layers disappear. The hairs on the lid skin are small, and their roots are connected to small sebaceous glands. Sweat glands are abundant, but small. The nasal eyelid is smoother and contains more hairs and sebaceous glands than does the skin on the temporal side.

Dermis

The dermis is composed of connective tissue and contains blood vessels, lymphatics, nerves, and large melanocytes. In the lids, the outer papillary dermis is not well developed because of the absence of prominent epidermal rete ridges, so that there is an imperceptible merging of the papillary dermis with the deep reticular dermis.

Hypodermis

The underlying subcutaneous areolar layer (hypodermis) consists of loose connective tissue without fat, thus permitting the thin layer of skin to be separated easily from the underlying muscle by oedematous fluid. This layer wrinkles in old age and is responsible for the appearance of 'crow's feet'. The dermis contains hair follicles, under-developed sweat and sebaceous glands, pigment cells and mast and plasma cells. The palpebral fissure, ciliary margins of the lids and medial and lateral angles lack this areolar layer, thus causing the thin cutaneous portion to be directly adherent to the underlying muscle layer.

Muscular tissue

The muscles of the eyelid comprise the striated orbicularis oculi and the levator palpebrae superiosis, as well as the small palpebral smooth muscle of Müller. Together, they are involved in maintaining eyelid tone, full opening and closure of the lids, and reflex blinking and flickering.

The orbicularis oculi (Fig. 12.25) is a thin, sphincter-like striated muscle that covers the lids and extends over the orbital rim. It is innervated by the facial nerve (CN VII) and can be divided into palpebral, orbital and lacrimal portions. The palpebral part of the orbicularis oculi muscle is arranged approximately parallel to the palpebral fissure, forming two half-ellipses. A small, isolated bundle of muscle fibres of the palpebral portion is called the ciliary bundle (muscle of Riolan). The orbital portion of the orbicularis oculi surrounds the orbital margin, and covers the cheek, eyebrows and forehead. In contrast to other regions of this muscle, the orbital division is separated from the overlying cutaneous tissue by a layer of fat. The lacrimal part of the orbicularis oculi (the muscle of Horner) arises from the posterior lacrimal crest of the lacrimal bone and inserts into the connective tissue surrounding the upper and lower canaliculi and the medial border of the tarsal plates.

The levator palpebrae superiosis lies anterior to the superior rectus muscle and is innervated by the superior division of the oculomotor nerve (CN III). At the level of the superior fornix, approximately 1 cm behind the orbital septum, the levator palpebrae superiosis expands into a broad aponeurosis. Superiorly, the upper border of the levator aponeurosis fuses with the orbital septum, whereas its central fibres enter the upper eyelid above the tarsal plate to terminate mainly in cutaneous (skin of the pretarsal region of the lids) and osseous (orbital tubercle of the zygomatic bone) insertions. Secondary insertions of the levator muscle are often directed to the lower one-third of the anterior surface of the tarsal plate and to the conjunctiva in the region of the fornix (see Fig. 12.22). The levator is probably responsible for the almost involuntary retraction of the lids during blinking, and for the varying width of the palpebral fissure in emotional states, such as fear and excitement.

The palpebral muscles of Müller, one each in the upper and lower lids, are thin, flat sheets of smooth (unstriated) muscle that lie deep to the orbital septum (see Fig. 12.22). They are innervated by the sympathetic fibres that enter along with branches of the ophthalmic artery. The fascicles of smooth muscle of the superior palpebral muscle lie posterior to the levator aponeurosis and deep to the substantia propria of the forniceal conjunctiva (Fig. 12.26). The smooth muscle fibres arise directly from the striated fibres of the levator palpebrae, a unique example in human anatomy of such an arrangement between these disparate muscle types. The palpebral muscle is inserted into the upper margin of the tarsal plate. The inferior palpebral muscle of Müller is less well defined than the superior one. Because of the absence of the levator muscle in the lower lid, the

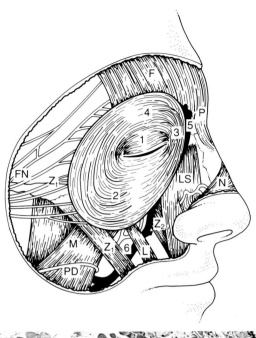

inferior palpebral muscle arises from the fascial sheath of the inferior rectus muscle and from its expansion into the inferior oblique. Directed toward the lower fornix, the fibres split into two lamellae, one attaching to the bulbar conjunctiva and the other inserting into the lower tarsal plate in the lid.

The cytological features of the striated- and smooth-muscle tissues of the lid are somewhat similar to their counterparts elsewhere in the body. The orbicularis oculi and levator palpebrae muscles are composed of characteristic long, cylindrical, multi-nucleated cells that show cross-striations when stained with haematoxylin and eosin. By electron microscopy, the sarcoplasm of each fibre is found to contain myofibrils 1–2 µm in diameter, which are

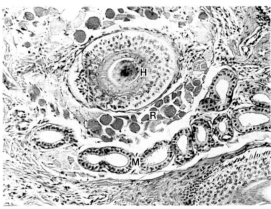

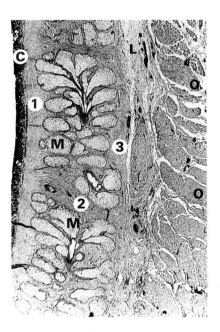

Figure 12.25 (a) Front view of dissected orbital and related facial structures depicted semi-schematically. 1, orbicularis (palpebral part); 2, orbicularis (orbital part); 3, medial palpebral ligament; 4, corrugator supercilii; 5, angular vein; 6, facial vein; F, frontalis; P, procerus; N, compressor naris; LS, levator labii superioris; Z, zygomaticus major; M, masseter; PD, parotid duct; Z, zygoma; FN, rami of facial nerve. (b) Section of lid margin showing muscle bundles of Riolan (R) traversed by hair follicle (H). Note the associated coiled gland of Moll (original magnification × 205).

Figure 12.26 Vertical section of lid showing the tarsal plate containing meibomian glands (M). Note the vertical orientation of compact connective tissue on the inner (1) and outer (3) surfaces of the plate, and sagittal orientation of central zone (2). C, conjunctiva; L, levator aponeurosis; O, orbicularis oculi muscle bundles (original magnification × 51).

composed of sarcomeres in an end-to-end, chain-like arrangement. The cells of the smooth muscles of Müller contain the characteristic thin and thick myofilaments (5 to 7 nm and 12 to 16 nm, respectively), fusiform densities, pinocytotic vesicles, plasmalemmal hemidesmosomes, a centrally located ellipsoidal or cigar-shaped nucleus and an enveloping basement membrane.

The various actions of the muscles of the eyelids provide for a range of protective movements. Blinking, flickering and full closure of the lids are associated with some rotation of the eyeball upward and inward (Bell's phenomenon). In flicker, there is a rapid synchronous movement of the upper lids, whereas full closure of the lids involves the orbital portion of the orbicularis and palpebral muscles, and often the frontalis and corrugator muscles. These movements may be voluntary or reflex; the latter occurs as part of normal periodic blinking or as a protective reflex, varying from a blink to full closure of the lids, depending on the exciting stimulus. It is not uncommon for contact lens practitioners to encounter a problem of prolonged blepharospasm in patients prior to the initial insertion of the lenses. During the adaptation period, a close watch should be kept on blinking frequency, which may increase if the lens is too mobile, or diminish if there is a decrease in the critical sensation of the cornea, conjunctiva, and lids.

Fibrous tissue

The fibrous layer of the eyelid consists of four main structures: (a) the orbital septum, which lines the orbital rim; (b) the tarsal plates; (c) the medial palpebral ligament; and (d) the lateral palpebral ligament.

Orbital septum

The orbital septum (see Fig. 12.22) is a thin, fibro-elastic membrane that is attached to the periorbita, which lines the entire margin of the orbit (Fig. 12.27). In the upper lid, the superior orbital septum blends with the tendon of the levator palpebrae superiosis and superior tarsus; in the lower lid, the inferior orbital septum fuses with the inferior tarsus. Laterally, the orbital septum combines with some fibres of the palpebral portion of the orbicularis oculi to form the lateral palpebral raphe. The orbital septum is perforated by many vessels and nerves entering the lid from the orbit, including the lacrimal and supra-orbital vessels and nerves, the supratrochlear artery and nerve, the trochlear nerve, and the anastomosis between the angular and ophthalmic veins. The orbital septum separates structures in the orbit from those in the eyelid and serves as an effective barrier to the extension of inflammation and extravasations in either direction.

Tarsal plates

The tarsal plates consist of non-cartilagenous, compact, fibrous tissue, which, together with some elastic tissue, forms the main supporting structure of the lid (see Fig. 12.26). The plates are curved on their inner aspects to conform to the shape of the globe. The tarsal plate in the upper lid is larger (1 mm thick) than that in the lower lid. The inferior tarsal plate presents a flattened, band-shaped profile, with a width of 5 mm in the central region. The outer surface of the superior tarsus is covered by the levator aponeurosis, which inserts into the lower third of the plate. In the lower lid, because of the absence of the levator muscle, the orbicularis oculi covers the inferior tarsus. The orbital septum, together with the palpebral portion of the inferior orbicularis oculi and the fascial expansion from the inferior rectus, inserts into the lower border of the inferior tarsus. The medial and lateral extensions of the tarsal plates attach to the orbital margin via the medial and lateral palpebral ligaments,

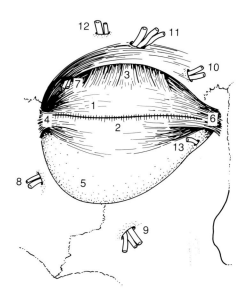

Figure 12.27 View of orbital septum from front with orbicularis oculi removed. 1, upper tarsal plate and lid margin; 2, lower tarsal plate and margin; 3, levator aponeurosis; 4, lateral canthal ligament; 5, orbital septum; 6, medial canthal ligament; 7, lacrimal artery and nerve; 8, zygomatic-facial artery and nerve; 9, infra-orbital artery and nerve; 10, supratrochlear atery and nerve; 11, supraorbital artery and nerve; 12, frontal artery and nerve; 13, palpebral artery (courtesy of Paul Henkind 1982).

respectively. Each plate is pierced by nerves, vessels and lymphatics.

The fibro-elastic connective tissue of the tarsus is arranged approximately in three planes. On both the outer and inner surfaces of the tarsal plates, highly regimented collagen fibrils of uniform diameter (60–70 nm) are oriented vertically, whereas in the central part they are directed sagittally. The tarsal glands that occupy a great portion of the central region of the tarsal plate are surrounded by a dense feltwork of elastic tissue.

Medial palpebral ligament

The medial palpebral ligament connects the tarsal plates to the frontal process of the maxilla, at the medial canthus anterior to the lacrimal sac. At its origin, the medial palpebral ligament divides into anterior and posterior lamellae. The ribbon-like anterior portion passes to the anterior lacrimal crest, then splits into the upper and lower lids, and attaches to the medial tarsal plates. The anterior lamella provides a part of the origin of the palpebral (or lacrimal) portion of the orbicularis oculi muscle. The posterior lamella runs between the anterior and posterior lacrimal crests, thereby spanning the lacrimal fossa.

Lateral palpebral ligament

The lateral palpebral ligament is a single band, 7 mm long and 2.5 mm wide, to which the pretarsal fibres of the orbicularis oculi muscle as well as the lateral extremities of the tarsal plate are attached. The upper border of the ligament blends with the more fully developed lateral horn of the levator aponeurosis, and together they attach to the orbital tubercle of the zygomatic bone. The inferior border of the lateral palpebral ligament merges with the suspensory ligament of Lockwood, which is the fused fascial sheath of the inferior rectus and inferior oblique muscles.

Conjunctival tissue of the lid.

See page 209.

Glands of the eyelid

The glands of the eyelid secrete numerous products that provide lubrication and antibacterial properties to the anterior surface of the eye. The glands of Zeis (sebaceous) and the glands of Moll (sweat) are associated with the eyelashes; the meibomian glands are associated with the tarsal plates; and the accessory lacrimal glands of Krause and Wolfring are associated with the conjunctival fornices (see Fig. 12.22).

Meibomian glands

The meibomian (tarsal) glands are modified sebaceous glands that appear as yellow vertical streaks deep to the conjunctiva. Corresponding to the size of the tarsal plate, the glands of the upper lid are longer and more numerous than are the glands of the lower lid (from 25 to 30 and from 20 to 25, respectively). The meibomian glands consist of a single row of straight canals that are oriented vertically to the lid margin and terminate as minute orifices on the lid margin along its entire length (Fig. 12.28). Each gland consists of a central duct into which numerous acini or saccules (up to 30 in the larger glands) of varying shapes and sizes open. Each saccule is composed of glandular epithelial cells; those at the periphery are cuboidal in shape and non-lipidized, but those located centrally are polygonal and contain fat. Under the electron microscope, the single outside layer of germinal cells contains scattered tonofilaments, and is supported by a multilaminar basement membrane without a myoepithelial layer. The intralobular sebaceous cells contain numerous lipid vacuoles and abundant smooth endoplasmic reticulum. The lining of the ducts is formed by four layers of cuboidal cells which increase to six near the orifices of the glands, where the cells are keratinized (Fig. 12.28b). Surrounded by lymph spaces, the glands are supplied with nerves and blood vessels. The secretory product, sebum, which is released by a holocrine process, is composed of a complex mixture of lipids that contains cholesterol, fatty acids, triglycerides, waxes, and squalene. Besides providing lubrication to the lid margin, sebum forms an essential component of the precorneal tear film, that retards the evaporation of the aqueous compartments of tears.

Glands of Zeis

The glands of Zeis are unilobular, rudimentary sebaceous glands that open into the

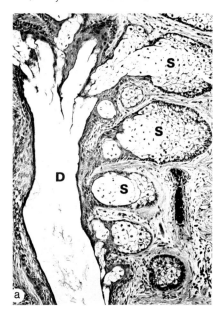

Figure 12.28 (a) Section of meibomian gland showing a number of saccules (S) with disintegrating secretory cells. The meibomian secretion, sebum, that results from disintegration of cells is poured into the ducts (D) which are lined by stratified squamous epithelium (original magnification × 205).

follicles or cilia by means of short ducts (Fig. 12.29). Each gland consists of an outer, marginal layer of cuboidal cells that divide, differentiate, degenerate and eventually secrete sebum as they migrate toward the secretory duct. The cells in the centre of the lobules contain myriad lipid droplets and abundant rough and smooth endoplasmic reticulum. The secretion provides lubrication to the eyelashes.

Ciliary glands of Moll

The ciliary or tarsal glands of Moll are large, modified sweat (apocrine) glands. They consist of unbranched, sinuous tubules, 1.5–2 mm long, and may be considered as sweat glands of the glomerular type that have become arrested in their develop-

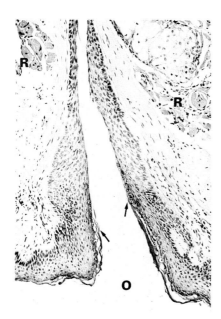

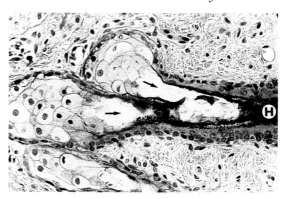

Figure 12.29 Section of ciliary gland of Zeis. The glands are associated with the hair follicles (H) through short ducts. The cytoplasm of the mature secretory cells of the gland disintegrate and their nuclei become pyknotic as they move (arrow) toward the duct to produce the sebaceous secretion (original magnification × 512).

Figure 12.28 (b) Section of lid passing through opening of tarsal gland. Toward the external orifice (O), the duct of the epithelium thickens and the surface cells become keratinized (arrows). R, muscle of Riolan (original magnification × 205).

ment. Each gland has a fundus, a body, an ampullary region and a neck. The secretory portions of the glands of Moll are lined by a single layer of cylindrical epithelial cells that is supported by a layer of myoepithelial cells and basement membrane (Fig. 12.30). The cytoplasm of the glandular cells is deeply eosinophilic. The secretory cells manifest various stages of metabolic activity, some being flat to cuboidal, others being more columnar, with apical granules. Electron microscopy shows tonofilaments dispersed singly, well-developed Golgi complexes, and light and dark secretory granules. The tubules of the glands of Moll open into the ducts of the glands of Zeis, into the hair follicles near the lid margin, or even onto the surface of the lid between two cilia (see Figs 12.22 and 12.23). Secretion occurs by a merocrine process.

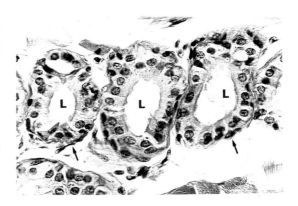

Figure 12.30 Section of ciliary gland of Moll showing lumen (L) lined by cylindrical epithelial cells supported by a layer of flattened myoepithelial cells and basement membrane (arrows) (magnification × 900).

Accessory lacrimal glands

The accessory lacrimal glands of Krause and Wolfring are intimately connected to the conjunctival fornices. They are associated with the lacrimal secretions and provide the baseline secretion of tears under sympathetic control.

12.3.3 BLOOD SUPPLY AND LYMPHATICS OF THE EYELID

The blood supply to the eyelids derives mainly from the ophthalmic and lacrimal arteries. The anastomoses between the lateral and medial palpebral branches of these arteries are formed from the submuscular areolar tissue, which contains the tarsal arcades. The venous drainage of the lids is via the ophthalmic vein and into other veins (angular and frontal) that drain the temple and forehead. The veins are arranged into pre- and post-tarsal plexuses. The lymphatics of the lateral segment of the lids drain into the preauricular and parotid nodes. The medial segment drains into the submaxillary lymph nodes.

ACKNOWLEDGEMENT

Many of the figures included in this chapter are adapted from Tripathi, R.C. and Tripathi, B.J. (1984) Anatomy of the human eye, orbit, and adnexa. In *The Eye, vol. IA.* (ed. H. Davson), Academic Press, New York.

BIBLIOGRAPHY

Alexander, R.A. and Garner, A. (1983) Elastic and precursor fibres in the normal human eye. *Exp. Eye Res.*, **36**, 305–15.

Beems, E.M. and Van Best, J.A. (1990) Light transmission of the cornea in whole human eyes. *Exp. Eye Res.*, **50**, 393–5.

Bergmanson, J.P.G. (1991) Histopathological analysis of corneal endothelial polymegathism. *Cornea*, May, 1991.

Buck, R.C. (1986) Ultrastructure of conjunctival epithelium replacing corneal epithelium. *Curr. Eye Res.*, **5**, 149–59.

Cavanagh, H.D., Jester, J.V., Esspian, J., Shields, W. and Lemp, M.A. (1990) Confocal microscopy of the living eye. *CLAO J.*, **16**, 65–73.

Diereck, H.G. and Missotten, L. (1992) Is the corneal contour influenced by a tension in the superficial epithelial cells? A new hypothesis. *Refract. Corneal Surg.*, **8**, 54–9.

Doughty, M.J. (1992) Concerning the symmetry of the hexagonal cells of the corneal endothelium. *Exp. Eye Res.*, **55**, 145–54.

Duke-Elder, S. and Wybar, K.C. (1961) The anatomy of the visual system. In *System of Ophthalmology, vol. II.* CV Mosby Co., St Louis.

Fine, B.S. and Yanoff, M. (1979) *Ocular Histology. A Text and Atlas*, (2nd ed.), Harper & Row, Publishers, Inc., Maryland.

Fonn, D. and Gauthier, C. (1991) Prevalence of superficial fibrillary lines of the cornea in contact lens wearers and non-wearers. *Cornea*, **10**, 507–10.

Giasson, C. and Forthomme, D. (1992) Comparison of central corneal thickness measurements between optical and ultrasound pachometer. *Optom. Vis. Sci.*, **69**, 236–41.

Guillon, M. Lydon, D.P. and Wilson C. (1986) Corneal topography: a clinical model. *Opthalmic Physiol. Opt.*, **6**, 47–56.

Hitzenberger, C.K., Drexler, W. and Fercher, A.F. (1992) Measurement of corneal thickness by laser Doppler interferometry. *Invest. Opthalmol. Vis. Sci.*, **33**, 98–103.

Hodson, S.A. and Sherrard, E.S. (1988) The specular microscope: its impact on laboratory and clinical studies of the cornea. *Eye*, **2(Suppl)**, S81–97.

Hogan, M.J., Alvarado, J.A. and Weddell, J.E. (1971), *Histology of the Eye. An Atlas and Textbook*. W.B. Saunders Company, Philadelphia.

Holly, F.J. (1987) Tear film physiology. *Int. Opthalmol. Clin.*, 27, 2–6.

Jacobiec, F.A. (1982) *Ocular Anatomy, Embryology, and Teratology*. Harper & Row Publishers, Inc., Philadelphia.

Jue, B. and Maurice, D.M. (1986) The mechanical properties of the rabbit and human cornea. *J. Biochem.*, **19**, 847–53.

Kwok, L.S. (1990) Measurement of corneal diameter [letter]. *Br. J. Opthalmol.*, **74**, 63–4.

Lemp, M.A. and Mathers, W.D. (1991) Conrad Berens Lecture. Renewal of the corneal epithelium. *CLAO J.*, **17**, 258–66.

Madigan, M.C., Holden, B.A. and Kwok, L.S. (1987) Extended wear of contact lenses can compromise corneal epithelial adhesion. *Curr. Eye Res.*, **6**, 1257–60.

Malik, N.S., Moss, S.J., Ahmed, N., Furth, A.J., Wall, R.S. and Meek, K.M. (1992) Ageing of the human corneal stroma: structural and biochemical changes. *Biochim. Biophys. Acta.*, **1138**, 222–28.

Maurice, D.M. and Monroe, F. (1990) Cohesion strength of corneal lamellae. *Exp. Eye Res.*, **50**, 59–63.

McCartney, M.D., Wood, T.O. and McLaughlin, B.J. (1987) Freeze-fracture label of functional and dysfunctional human corneal endothelium. *Curr. Eye Res.*, **6**, 589–97.

McCulley, J.P. (1989) The circulation of fluid at the limbus (flow and diffusion at the limbus). *Eye*, **3**, 114–20.

Murphy, C., Alvarado, J., Juster, R. and Maglio, M. (1984) Prenatal and postnatal cellularity of the human corneal endothelium. *Invest. Ophthalmol. Vis. Sci.*, **25**, 312–22.

Scott, J.E. and Bosworth, T.R. (1990) The comparative chemical morphology of the mammalian cornea. *Basic Appl. Histochem.*, **34**, 35–42.

Steuhl, K.P. (1989) Ultrastructure of the conjunctival epithelium. *Dev. Ophthalmol.*, **19**, 1–104.

Tripathi, B.J. and Tripathi, R.C. (1990) Embryology of the anterior segment of the human eye. In *The Glaucomas*, vol. 2 (eds R. Ritch, M.B. Shields and T. Krupin), Mosby, St Louis.

Tripathi, R.C. (1973) Applied physiology and anatomy. Tears, cornea, conjunctiva, and ocular adnexa. In *Contact Lens Practice* (ed. M. Ruben), Bailliere Tindall, London, pp. 24–55.

Tripathi, R.C. and Tripathi, B.J. (1984) Anatomy of the human eye, orbit, and adnexa. In *The Eye*, *vol. Ia* (ed. H. Davson), Academic Press, New York

Tseng, S.C. (1989) Concept and application of limbal stem cells *Eye*, **3** 141–57.

Tuft, S.J. and Coster D.J. (1990) The corneal endothelium. *Eye*, **4** 389–424.

Van Buskirk, E.M. (1989) The anatomy of the limbus. *Eye*, **3** 101–8.

Wigham, C.G. and Hodson, S.A. (1987) Physiological changes in the cornea of the ageing eye. *Eye*, **1** 190–6.

Wilson, S.E. and Klyce, S.D. (1991) Advances in the analysis of corneal topography. *Surv. Ophthalmol.*, **35**, 269–77..

G. Ruskell and J.G. Lawrenson

13.1 INNERVATION OF THE CORNEA

The cornea is innervated by the ophthalmic division of the trigeminal nerve. The nasociliary branch of the ophthalmic nerve is the source of all somatic sensory nerves of the eye. Branches from the nasociliary nerve either pass directly to the eye as long ciliary nerves or pass through the ciliary ganglion and enter the eye together with postganglionic parasympathetic fibres in several short ciliary nerves. Long and short ciliary nerves commonly join before penetrating the sclera in a ring around and close to the optic nerve. They advance in the suprachoroid and enter the ciliary body where sensory fibres, destined for the cornea, separate from the much larger parasympathetic content of the ciliary nerves. Shortly after their separation the sensory fibres enter the sclera as numerous fine nerves, often using the same conduits as the anterior ciliary arteries and venules, and advance radially to the corneal stroma (Fig. 13.1). Most cross from sclera to cornea in the outer half, the more superficial of them often having first reached the episclera. A few small fibre bundles enter conjunctival epithelium within 1 mm of the cornea and continue into corneal epithelium rather than the stroma (Zander & Weddell, 1951; Lim & Ruskell, 1978) (Fig. 13.2). A suggestion that access for all corneal nerve fibres is via this route (Lim & Ruskell, 1978) is now know to be false.

A circumcorneal arrangement of nerves is demonstrable in gross preparations, using such stains as methylene blue or acetylcholinesterase. This arrangement is composed of an episcleral pericorneal plexus and a subconjunctival plexus or bundles (Attius, 1912; Zander & Weddell, 1951); the two are interconnected. A few scleral branches may pass superficially and contribute to the pericorneal arrays and subsequently turn forward into the cornea at a superficial level – those

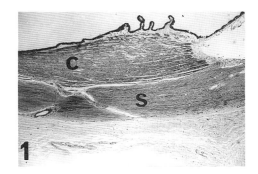

Figure 13.1 Meridional section through the anterior segment of the coat of the eye. The 'vermiform' structure leaving the ciliary muscle (c) and penetrating the sclera (s) is a ciliary nerve branch destined for the cornea via the episclera. An anterior ciliary vein occupies the same conduit (magnification × 25).

Contact Lens Practice. Edited by Montague Ruben and Michel Guillon.
Published in 1994 by Chapman & Hall, London. ISBN 0 412 35120 X

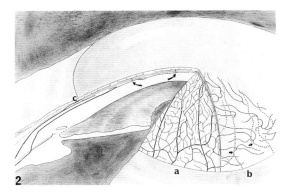

Figure 13.2 Anterior view of the eye showing the distribution of corneal nerves. A segment is removed to reveal the cornea in section. In an adjacent segment opposite the limbus at (a) the epithelium is removed to show the distribution of stromal nerves. In the segment opposite (b) epithelial nerves are added with the broken lines representing the principle stromal nerves; examples of penetration of Bowman's layer are arrowed. Penetration is again shown in the corneal section (larger arrows), and direct access of a nerve fibre bundle from the conjunctiva to the corneal epithelium is indicated at (c). The drawing is based on the nerve pattern seen in rabbit and human cornea (modified from Ruskell, 1989).

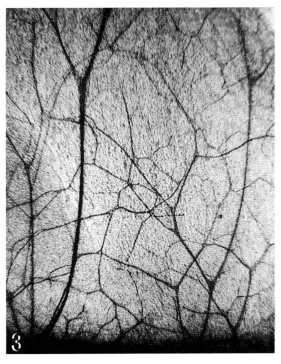

Figure 13.3 Nerves of the corneal stroma of a rabbit stained with acetylcholinesterase. They radiate from the darkened limbal tissue below (magnification × 34).

passing directly into the corneal epithelium are an example of this. However, most of the pericorneal nerves tend to follow the course of limbal blood vessels and are predominantly autonomic and vasomotor. The claim that a fraction of the nerves entering the cornea come from sources other than the ciliary nerves (Attius, 1912) has not been confirmed (Zander & Weddell, 1951). The superficial circumferential pattern terminates at the corneal margin and nerve distribution in the cornea itself is predominantly radial. But, as can be seen in Figure 13.3, branches of the principal nerves disperse in a variety of directions.

The 50–80 precorneal nerve trunks contain a mixture of myelinated and, more numerous, unmyelinated fibres, enclosed by a perineurium and packed with endoneurial collagen (Fig. 13.4). Only the nerve fibres progress into the cornea and any myelin quickly terminates. The initial path of nerve fibre bundles in the cornea may be seen with the biomicroscope as dull white spikes for a fraction of a millimetre and sometimes substantially longer. Their visibility is presumably due to light reflection from the Schwann cell sheaths of larger fibre bundles, rather than to the persistence of myelin.

Unmyelinated nerve fibre bundles contain between one and eight axons and as many as 20 bundles are initially grouped together in the larger corneal nerves. Much overlapping occurs and junctions between nerves are quite common. Some penetrate to the centre of the cornea and beyond. This arrangement explains why sensitivity, although reduced,

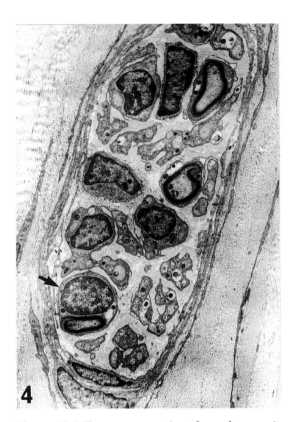

Figure 13.4 Transverse section through an episcleral nerve shortly before entering the cornea. It contains three myelinated fibres (one with a Schwann cell nucleus is arrowed) and numerous unmyelinated nerve fibre bundles. A thick perineurium encloses the nerve (magnificataion × 5300).

persists in all areas of the cornea subsequent to large, full-penetration, perilimbal incisions (Schirmer & Mellor, 1961). All nerves move to a more superficial position to become confined to the anterior third of the stroma, and a subepithelial plexus of nerves is formed. Single nerve fibres issue from the large radial nerves or the plexus, often at right angles, and divide a number of times. These are assumed to terminate in the stroma. In our preparations the single axons are beaded (Fig. 13.5) and not in the form of simple fine threads as described by Zander

and Weddell (1951). Beading also occurs along axons of the plexus nerves. The axoplasm is composed largely of neurofilaments, and mitochondria occur at infrequent intervals; this pattern is interrupted at the beads which are packed with mitochondria and often contain a few vesicles (Fig. 13.6). Matsuda (1968) claimed that beads or varicosities fall into two groups – one with and the other without vesicles – and he attributed different functions to them. However, it remains unclear whether or not the difference in form is attributable to sampling from single rather than serial sections; the latter might reveal similar organelles in all beads. As nerves penetrate deeper into the cornea they tend to flatten between or within stromal lamellae (Fig. 13.7).

Nerves from the subepithelial plexus pass superficially and penetrate Bowman's layer to enter the epithelium (Fig. 13.8). Schwann cells are shed before or during their passage through this layer. Generally they consist of small groups or leashes of naked axons that turn into the plane of the epithelium at basal cell level close to or on

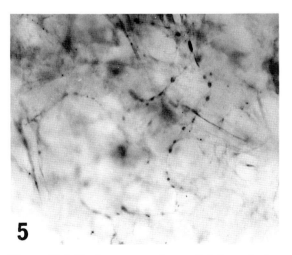

Figure 13.5 Varicose axons immediately underlying Bowman's layer. They appear to run singly and presumably terminate in this position. Whole mount, gold chloride (magnification × 720).

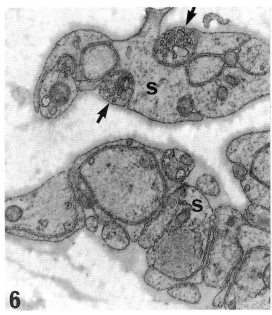

Figure 13.6 Nerve fibre bundles of the corneal stroma close to the limbus. Note the prominence of Schwann cell sheaths (s), a substantial variation in axon diameters and the presence of small agranular vesicles in some axons (arrows) (magnification × 22 700).

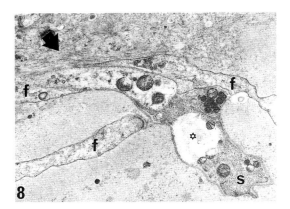

Figure 13.8 A nerve fibre bundle entering Bowman's layer (top left) from the stroma. Each of the five axons in the bundle contains mitochondria; one is practically filled with them, another (asterisk) appears to have swollen and contains few organelles, and the uppermost axon, which is turning into Bowman's layer, also contains vesicles. The lowermost axons are ensheathed by a Schwann cell (s) and the bundle is accompanied by fibroblast processes (f) that continue into Bowman's layer. The random orientation of collagen fibrils of Bowman's layer is discernible (arrow) (magnification × 17 000).

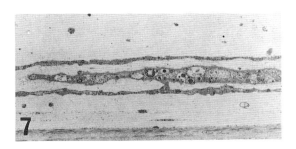

Figure 13.7 A nerve fibre bundle, remote from the limbus, is flattened in the plane of the cornea (magnification × 6300).

the basement membrane (Fig. 13.9). They usually divide into smaller groups upon entry and run a lengthy and surprisingly straight course, maintaining their position close to the basement membrane. Single axons separate from the bundle and terminate locally.

The relationship between axons and the basal epithelial cells varies. Single or multiple axons may lie between the cell and its basement membrane or between cells. Others deeply invaginate the cells, lying within a fold of the plasma membrane; the axon or axons are tightly enclosed as are the apposed cell membranes forming the channel connecting the axon chamber to the surface of the cell (Fig. 13.10). The channel commonly displays a series of sharp convolutions and it is bridged by gap junctions and desmosomes (Fig. 13.11). Some axons turn superficially towards the corneal surface (Fig. 13.12). Schimmelpfennig (1982) found evidence that axons passing towards the surface are numerous, but in our experience they have a relatively low frequency and the bulk of epithelial axons remain close to the basement membrane.

An agreed morphological or biochemical

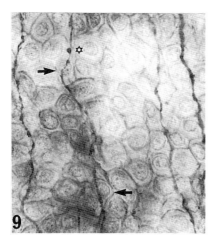

Figure 13.9 Varicose axons with a common direction at basal cell level. Each of the four strands may represent more than a single axon. Note that they mainly pass between basal cells but sometimes appear to traverse cells (arrows). The dense dark spot (asterisk) indicates an axon orientated perpendicular to the plane of the cornea. Whole mount, gold chloride (magnification × 680).

et al., 1982; Stone & Kuwayama, 1985) and calcitonin gene-related peptide (Stone & McGlinn 1988; Uusitalo *et al.*, 1989) immunoreactive nerves of trigeminal origin are described in the human cornea. They are present in the stroma and in the epithelium. However, it is unlikely that the two reactions indicate separate groups of sensory fibres, because it is known that both neuropeptides occur in the same neuron in experimental animals (Lee *et al.*, 1985; Gulbenkian *et al.*, 1986). The specific local functional roles of the neuropeptides is not known. The proportion of nerves showing these reactions is a small fraction of the total corneal innervation, and presumably sensory nerves of a different character may be present.

Whether or not the human cornea has sympathetic innervation remains uncertain. A histochemical technique providing evidence for a sympathetic innervation in subprimate mammalian species fails to do so when applied to monkey and human

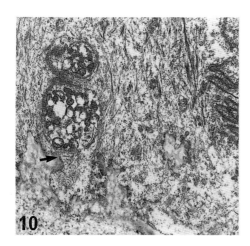

Figure 13.10 Two epithelial axons sectioned at varicosities and packed with mitochondria. They invaginate a basal cell, and the periaxonal spaces are exposed to the cell surface through a short narrow channel (arrow) (magnification × 12 800).

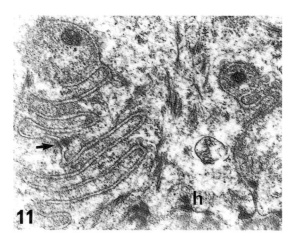

Figure 13.11 Two more examples of axons invaginating a basal cell. The axons are sectioned at intervaricose level and contain mainly neurofilaments and microtubules. The circuitous channel on the left, linking the periaxonal space to the cell base is bridged by a desmosome (arrow). h, basal hemidesmosome (magnification × 41 700).

subdivision of corneal nerve terminals in man has not been found. Substance P (Tervo

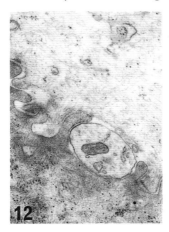

Figure 13.12 Axon with several agranular vesicles near the surface of the cornea; the lighter cell above was adjacent to a squamous surface cell (magnification × 37 500).

corneas (Ehinger, 1964, 1971; Laties & Jacobowitz, 1966), yet application of a modified version of the technique is claimed to give a positive result in man (Toivanen *et al.*, 1987). On the other hand, neuropeptide-Y-like immunoreactive nerves closely parallel sympathetic nerve distribution in the eye, and none could be found in human corneas (Stone, 1986).

Cataract surgery and other procedures requiring incision of the limbus incur the severance of a large fraction of the nerves serving the cornea, and in penetrating keratoplasty the nerves of the donor cornea are totally severed and destroyed. The capacity of nerves to regenerate in these circumstances is limited. Progress of reinnervation may be inferred from sensitivity monitoring following the lesion. Corneal touch sensitivity close to a limbal lesion is reduced to half the normal level and subsequent testing shows little improvement (Draeger, 1984). Recovery of sensitivity following corneal grafts is practically nil in some cases and slow and fractional in others (Ruben & Colebrook, 1979; Lyne, 1982). These observations parallel the very few

nerves seen in corneal grafts obtained less than three years after operation (Tervo *et al.*, 1985), yet in a single clear cornea with a 29-year-old graft, epithelial innervation was almost normal, whereas few stromal nerves had regenerated.

The possibility that the maxillary nerve is the source of some corneal nerves cannot be discounted. Fibres from a maxillary root to the ciliary ganglion found in monkeys, continue in the short ciliary nerves (Ruskell, 1974). Their terminations within the eye remain unknown but the cornea is a likely target.

13.2   INNERVATION OF THE TRABECULAR MESHWORK

Because the ciliary muscle inserts into the uveal part of the trabecular meshwork, any nerve fibres present may represent looping or misdirected fibres properly belonging to the ciliary muscle. But fibres of terminal form have been located well forward of the muscle, and the possibility of a function specific to the trabeculae cannot be ignored. They are present in the uveal and scleral trabeculae and immediately beneath the inner wall of the canal of Schlemm in monkeys (Ruskell, 1976), but their frequency is low (Fig. 13.13). Of the sympathetic, parasympathetic (of pterygopalatine ganglion origin) and sensory terminals found, only the latter were found regularly. In man, sympathetic adrenergic nerves are usually absent (Ehinger, 1971) or few (Stone, 1986) (assuming that fibres immunoreactive to neuropeptide Y are sympathetic). Moderate numbers of substance P-like immunoreactive fibres, and therefore probably sensory, are present (Stone & Kuwayama, 1985). The frequency and apparent variability of trabecular terminals hinders consideration of their possible roles and does not permit disciplined speculation. This must await more detailed and comprehensive study.

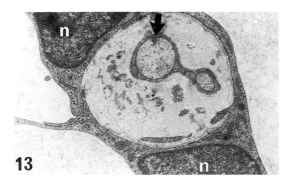

Figure 13.13 Two axons, ringed and separated by a Schwann cell process, within a trabecula. A few vesicles are present in the larger axon (arrow). The nuclei of two trabecular endothelial cells are shown (n) (magnification × 9900).

13.3 INNERVATION OF THE CONJUNCTIVA

It has now been established that the conjunctiva receives a tripartite nerve supply; conjuctival nerve fibres are classified as sensory, sympathetic or parasympathetic. The sensory nerves are trigeminal in origin and reach the conjunctiva principally via branches of the ophthalmic nerve. The traditional view is that the inferior conjunctiva is served, additionally, by the infra-orbital branch of the maxillary nerve (Duke-Elder & Wybar, 1961). However, Oduntan (1987), tracing Wallerian degeneration following maxillary neurectomy in monkeys, questioned the constancy of the maxillary contribution, which when present was found to be minor.

There is some evidence that the bulbar and limbal conjunctiva receive their sensory supply via ciliary nerve branches that penetrate the sclera from an intra-ocular position anteriorly in monkeys (Ruskell & Simons, 1990). Presumably, nervous activity arising from stimulation of the bulbar conjunctiva would therefore, in part, be transmitted through the eye.

Evidence for a sympathetic innervation of the conjunctiva was presented by Ehinger (1971) who demonstrated catecholaminergic

and, by implication, sympathetic fibres in relation to conjunctival blood vessels. Further evidence for a sympathetic supply issuing from the superior cervical ganglion has been obtained from degeneration studies in monkeys (Macintosh, 1974), from tracer experiments in rabbits (Ten Tusscher et al., 1988), and combined immunohistochemical and denervation studies in rats (Luhtala et al., 1991).

Parasympathetic nerve fibres of facial nerve origin are known to innervate the eye and orbital structures (Ruskell, 1965, 1970). Such fibres, relaying in the pterygopalatine ganglion (PPG), are known to project to conjunctival blood vessels (Macintosh 1974; Ruskell, 1985; Ten Tusscher et al., 1988). Vasoactive intestinal polypeptide (VIP) has been identified as a neurohumour localized in ocular parasympathetic nerve endings of PPG origin (Uddman et al., 1980) and it is known to be a potent vasodilator in the eye (Nilsson & Bill, 1984). The concentration of VIP in the rabbit conjunctiva was reduced following PPG lesions (Butler et al., 1984) but, surprisingly, conjunctival nerves displaying VIP immunoreactivity have not been identified so far in man (Miller et al., 1983).

The general form and distribution of conjunctival nerve fibres and their terminals in man is similar to that described in monkeys (Macintosh, 1974; Ruskell, 1985; Oduntan, 1987). Nerves of various calibres, containing both myelinated and unmyelinated fibres and invested with a perineural sheath (Fig. 13.14), are present within the deep fibrous layer of the conjunctiva, where they frequently lie adjacent to conjunctival blood vessels. In addition, single and small groups of nerve fibres (with or without a perineurium) and nerve terminals are widely distributed throughout the substantia propria, with greatest concentration close to the basal epithelial layer (Fig. 13.15) and within the adventitia of blood vessels (Fig. 13.16). Although nerves fibres terminate at all levels of the substantia propria but few enter the epithelium – those that do are confined to the basal layer (Fig. 13.17). Nerve endings are located in the walls of arterioles and capillaries where sympathetic parasympathetic and sensory terminals have been identified (Macintosh, 1974). The presence of a sensory supply to conjunctival blood vessels is supported by studies on the distribution of the neuropeptides substance P and calcitonin gene related peptide (Stone & Kuwayama, 1985; Stone & McGlinn, 1988; Luhtala *et al.*, 1991). These biologically active peptides are known to localize in ocular sensory nerves (Stone *et al.*, 1987).

Accounts of conjunctival innervation describe two forms of nerve termination – free nerve endings and corpuscular (compact) nerve endings. The term 'free nerve ending' describes terminals showing the minimal degree of structural specialization, where an axon ends blindly with sparse cellular wrappings. Free nerve endings arise from both unmyelinated and myelinated

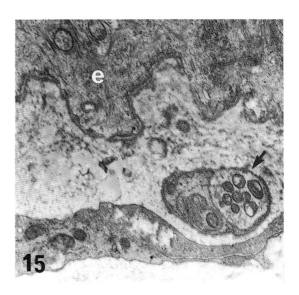

Figure 13.15 A subepithelial unmyelinated nerve fibre bundle including a large axon terminal varicosity (arrowed) underlying limbal conjunctival epithelium (e). The varicostiy contains several mitochondria (magnification × 16 257).

axons, and account for the mode of termination of all autonomic fibres and the majority of sensory fibres. A feature of the axon terminal is the presence of beads or varicosities (Figs 13.15 and 13.17). Varicosity content cannot generally be used to distinguish sensory from autonomic terminals, but those containing small granular vesicles are, in our experience, highly suggestive of sympathetic terminals (Ruskell, 1981).

Nerve endings of corpuscular form represent the terminal morphology of a proportion of human conjunctival sensory nerves, although surprisingly they are not found in the conjunctiva of other primates. They were first described in the mid-nineteenth century (Krause, 1859), and subsequent accounts express various opinions as to the precise morphology and relative incidence of these complex nerve endings (see Duke-Elder & Wybar, 1961 for a summary). Corpuscular nerve endings are distributed throughout the bulbar conjunctiva (Fig. 13.18), where

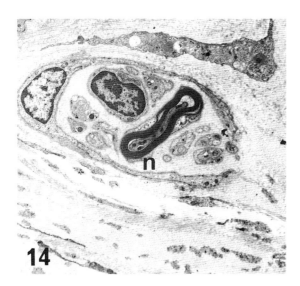

Figure 13.14 Electron micrograph of a mixed nerve from deep in conjunctival stroma. An incomplete perineural sheath encloses a single myelinated nerve fibre (n) and several unmyelinated fibres (magnification × 9661).

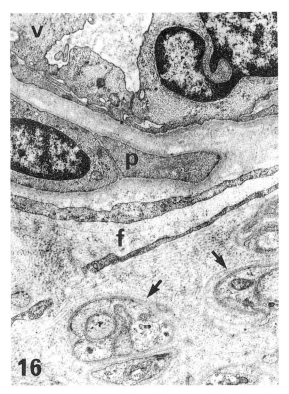

Figure 13.16 Unmyelinated nerve fibre bundles (arrowed) adjacent to a conjunctival capillary. v, vascular endothelium; p, pericyte; f, fibrocyte processes (magnification × 11 216).

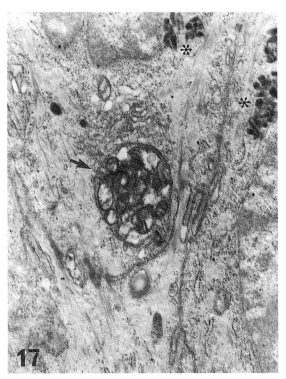

Figure 13.17 Intra-epithelial axon terminal varicosity (arrowed) enclosed by a basal epithelial cell. Note compound melanosomes (asterisks) within epithelial cells (magnification × 19 501).

they are most numerous in the upper temporal quadrant (Ciaccio, 1874; Oppenheimer *et al.*, 1958). In addition, they are commonly found at the eyelid margin (Munger & Hulata, 1984) and at the limbus (Lawrenson & Ruskell, 1991) where they show a close association with the conjunctival palisades of Vogt. Corpuscles are often found within the connective tissue ridges which make up the palisades (Fig. 13.19). Each corpuscle is usually served by a single nerve fibre (Fig. 13.20), which loses its myelin sheath upon entering the corpuscle. This afferent fibre subsequently branches to give rise to a variable number of axon terminal varicosities containing an accumulation of mitochondria. Both terminal and preterminal axons are surrounded by Schwann-like supporting cells, and the whole corpuscle is enclosed by a thin fibrocyte capsule (Figs. 13.21 and 13.22).

The sensory innervation of the conjunctiva provides the mucous membrane with the ability to detect changes in its environment. The sensory receptors are capable of responding to the sensory modalities of touch, pain, warmth and cold. Although subordinate to the cornea in its sensitivity to touch and pain, the conjunctiva appears to be superior in differentiating temperature (Kenshalo, 1960). Terminal form within the conjunctiva cannot as yet be related to function, although free nerve endings in the skin have been implicated in the mediation of a full range of modalities. The function of

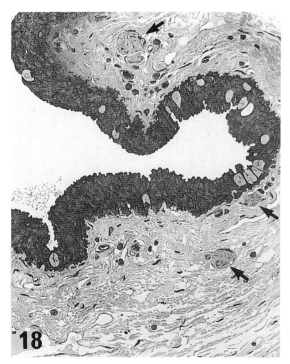

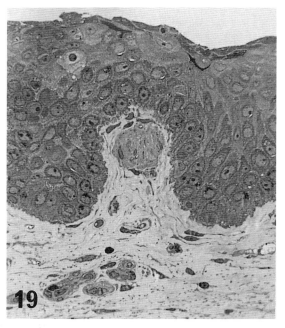

Figure 13.18 Three corpuscular nerve endings (arrowed), assumed to be sensory receptors, in the bulbar conjunctiva at varying distances from the goblet cell-containing epithelium (magnification × 182).

Figure 13.19 Corpuscular receptor in the limbal conjunctiva. The corpuscle is located within a stromal elevation which forms a palisade of Vogt (magnification × 469).

corpuscular nerve endings found within the conjunctiva has been considered by various investigators and suggestions include mechanoreception (Krause, 1859) and cold reception (Strughold & Karbe, 1925). In contrast, Oppenheimer and co-workers (1958) claimed that rather than representing specific receptors, such nerve endings are the product of cyclic degenerative and regenerative changes taking place within sensory nerve terminals. However, our own observations of a normal appearance of axoplasm in all or most of these putative receptors discourages acceptance of this dismissal of their functional relevance. Furthermore, a recent study of the limbal touch sensitivity (Lawrenson & Ruskell, 1993) has provided some indirect evidence of a role for corpuscular nerve endings in mechanoreception. The palisade zone was found to have a higher touch sensitivity than the adjacent conjunctiva, which may be related to the concentration of sensory corpuscles in this zone.

Sensory nerves of the conjunctiva mediate a local inflammatory response to a variety of noxious stimuli (Lewis, 1937). This phenomenon, known as neurogenic inflammation, is characterized by vasodilation and increased permeability, which are thought to be mediated specifically by sensory nerves containing the neuropeptide substance P and calcitonin gene-related peptide (Unger & Butler, 1988). These neuropeptides can act on blood vessels, or indirectly by stimulating the release of vasoactive substances from mast cells. The vascular sympathetic and parasympathetic terminals are responsible for vessel constriction and dilation respectively.

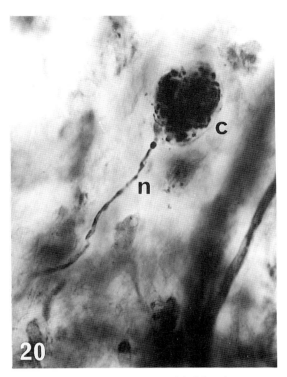

Figure 13.20 Whole-mount gold chloride preparation of a corpuscular receptor showing the afferent nerve fibre (n) and connective tissue capsule (c). Detail within the corpuscle is obliterated by the dense staining pattern (magnification × 540).

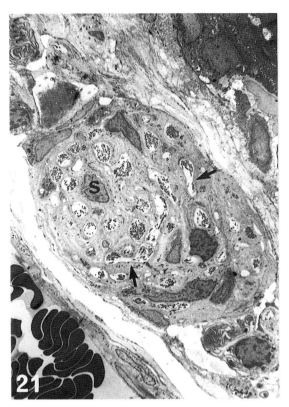

Figure 13.21 Electron micrograph of a corpuscular receptor. The interior of the corpuscle displays axon terminal varicosities (arrowed) and Schwann-like accessory cell nuclei (s) (magnification × 1637).

REFERENCES

Attius, G. (1912) Die Nerven der hornhaut des Menschen. *Graefes Arch. Ophthalmol.*, **83**, 207–316.

Butler, J.M., Ruskell, G.L., Cole, D.F., Unger, W.G., Zhang, S.Q., Blank, M.A., McGregor, G.P. and Bloom, S.R. (1984) Effects of VII (facial) nerve degeneration on vasoactive intestinal polypeptide and substance P levels in ocular and orbital tissues for the rat. *Exp. Eye Res.*, **39**, 523–32.

Ciaccio, G.V. (1874) Osservazioni intorno alla struttora della congiuntiva umana. *Mem. Accad. Bologna. Sci. Fis. 5th Ser.*, **10**, 409–524.

Draeger, J. (1984) *Corneal Sensitivity: Measurement and Clinical Importance*. Vienna, Springer Verlag.

Duke-Elder, S. and Wybar, K.C., (1961) *System of Ophthalmology. Vol II. The anatomy of the visual system*. London, Henry Kimpton.

Ehinger, B. (1964) Ocular and orbital vegetative nerves. *Acta Physiol. Scand.*, **Suppl. 67**, 1–35.

Ehinger, B. (1971) A comparative study of the adrenergic nerves to the anterior eye segment of some primates. *Z. Zellforsch. Mikroskop. Anat.*, **116**, 157–97.

Gulbenkian, S., Merighi, A., Wharton, J., Varndell, I.M. and Polak, J.M. (1986) Ultrastructural evidence for coexistence of calcitonin generelated peptide and substance-P in secretory vesicles of peripheral nerves in guinea pig. *J. Neurocytol.*, **15**, 535–42.

Kenshalo, D.R. (1960) Comparison of the thermal sensitivity of the forehead, lip, conjunctiva, and cornea. *J. Appl. Physiol.*, **15**, 987–91.

Krause, W. (1859) Über Nervenendigungen. *Z.*

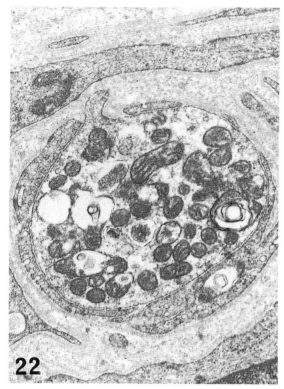

Figure 13.22 Detail of a terminal varicosity from a corpuscle. Accumulated small mitochondria, neurofilaments and neurotubules are present in the axoplasm. The varicosity is surrounded by cytoplasmic processes derived from the Schwann-like cells (magnification × 25 000).

Ration. Med. 3rd Ser., **5**, 28–43.

Laties, A.M. and Jacobowitz, D. (1966) A comparative study of the autonomic innervation of the eye in monkey, cat and rabbit. *Anat. Rec.*, **156**, 383–96.

Laties, A.M., Stone, R.A. and Brecha, N.C. (1981) Substance-P like immunoreactive nerves in the trabecular meshwork. *Invest. Ophthalmol. Vis. Sci.*, **21**, 484–6.

Lawrenson, J.G. and Ruskell G.L. (1991) The structure of corpuscular nerve endings in the limbal conjunctiva of the human eye. *J. Anat.*, **177**, 75–84.

Laerenson, J.G. and Ruskell, G.L. (1993) Investigation of limbal touch sensitivity using a Cochet–Bonnet aesthesiometer. *Br. J. Ophthalmol.*, **77**, 339–43.

Lee, Y., Takami, K., Kawai, Y., Girgis, S., Hillyard, C.J., MacIntyre, I., Emson, P.C. and Tohyama, M. (1985) Distribution of calcitonin-gene-related peptide in the rat peripheral nervous system with reference to the coexistence with substance-P. *Neuroscience*, **15**, 1227–37.

Lewis, T. (1937) The nocisensor system of nerves and its reactions. *Br. Med. J.*, **1**, 431–5.

Lim, C.H. and Ruskell, G.L. (1978) Corneal nerve access in monkeys. *Graefes Arch. Ophthalmol.*, **208**, 15–23.

Luhtala, J., Palkama, A. and Uusitalo, H. (1991) Distribution and origin of substance P, CGRP, neuropeptide Y immunoreactive nerves in the rat conjunctiva. *Invest. Ophthalmol. Vis. Sci.*, **32**, 1285.

Lyne, A. (1982) Corneal sensitivity after surgery. *Trans. Ophthalmol. Soc. U.K.*, **102**, 302–5.

Macintosh, S.R. (1974) The innervation of the conjunctiva in monkeys. *Graefes Arch. Ophthalmol.*, **192**, 105–16.

Matsuda, H. (1968) Electron microscopic study of the corneal nerve with special reference to its endings. *Jap. J. Ophthalmol.*, **12**, 163–73.

Miller, A.S., Coster, D.J., Costa, M. and Furness, J.B. (1983) Vasoactive intestinal polypeptide immunoreactive nerve fibres in the human eye. *Aust. J. Ophthalmol.*, **11**, 185–93.

Munger B.L. and Halata, Z. (1984) The sensorineural apparatus of the human eyelid. *Am. J. Anat.*, **170**, 181–204.

Nilsson, S.F.E. and Bill, A. (1984) Vasoactive intestinal polypeptide (VIP) effects in the eye and on regional blood flow. *Acta physiol. Scand.*, **121**, 385–92.

Oduntan, A.O. (1987) *Aspects of the structure and innervation of the primate conjunctiva and its response to denervation*. PhD Thesis, City University, London.

Oppenheimer, D.R., Palmer, E. and Weddell G. (1958) Nerve endings in the conjunctiva. *J. Anat.*, **92**, 321–52.

Ruben, M. and Colebrook, E. (1979) Keratoplasty sensitivity. *Br. J. Ophthalmol.*, **12**, 163–73.

Ruskell, G.L. (1965) The orbital distribution of the sphenopalatine ganglion in the rabbit. In *The Structure of the Eye, vol. II* (ed. J.W. Rohen) Schattauer Verlag, Stuttgart, pp. 355–68.

Ruskell, G.L. (1970) An ocular parasympathetic pathway of facial nerve origin and its influence on intra-ocular pressure. *Exp. Eye. Res.*, **10**, 319–30.

Ruskell, G.L. (1974) Ocular fibres of the maxillary nerve in monkeys. *J. Anat.*, **118**, 195–203.

Ruskell, G.L. (1976) The source of nerve fibres of the trabeculae and adjacent structures in monkey eyes. *Exp. Eye Res.*, **23**, 449–59.

Ruskell, G.L. (1981) Innervation of the anterior segment of the eye. In *Basic Aspects of Glaucoma Research* (ed. E. Lütjen-Drecoll), Schattauer Verlag, Stuttgart, pp. 49–66.

Ruskell, G.L. (1985) Innervation of the conjunctiva. *Trans. Ophthalmol. Soc. U.K.*, **104**, 390–5.

Ruskell, G.L. (1989) Anatomy and physiology of the cornea and related structures. In *Contact Lenses. A Textbook for Practitioner and Student* (3rd ed), (eds. A.J. Philips and J. Stone), Butterworth & Co., London.

Ruskell, G.L. and Simons, T. (1990) Distribution of scleral sensory nerves to the cornea and adjacent structures. *Ophthal. Physiol. Opt.*, **10**, 409.

Schimmelpfennig, B. (1982) Nerve structure in human central corneal epithelium. *Graefes Arch. Ophthalmol.*, **218**, 14–20.

Schirmer, K.E. and Mellor, L.D. (1961) Corneal sensitivity after cataract extraction. *Arch. Ophthalmol.*, **65**, 433–6.

Stone, R.A. (1986) Neuropeptide Y and the innervation of the human eye. *Exp. Eye Res.*, **42**, 349–55.

Stone, R.A. and Kuwayama, Y. (1985) Substance P-like immunoreactive nerves in the human eye. *Arch. Ophthalmol.*, **103**, 1207–11.

Stone, R.A. and McGlinn, A.M. (1988) Calcitonin gene-related peptide immunoreactive nerves in human and rhesus monkey eyes. *Invest. Ophthalmol. Vis. Sci.*, **29**, 305–10.

Stone, R.A. Laties, A.M. and Brecha, N.C. (1982) Substance-P like immunoreactive nerves in the anterior segment of the rabbit, cat, and monkey eye. *Neuroscience*, **7**, 2459–68.

Stone, R.A. Kuwayama, Y. and Laties, A.M. (1987) Regulatory peptides in the eye. *Experientia*, **43**, 791–800.

Strughold, H. and Karbe, M. (1925) Vitale Färbung des Auges und experientelle untersuchungen der gefärblen Nervenelemente. *Z. Biol.*, **83**, 297–308.

Ten Tusscher, M.P.M., Klooster, J. and Vrenson, G.F.J.M. (1988) The innervation of the rabbit's anterior eye segment. A retrograde tracing study. *Exp. Eye Res.*, **46**, 717–30.

Tervo, K., Tervo, T., Eranko, L., Vannas, A., Cuello, A.C. and Eranko, O. (1982) Substance P-like immunoreactive nerves in the human cornea and iris. *Invest. Ophthalmol. Vis. Sci.*, **23**, 671–4.

Tervo, T., Vannas, A., Tervo, K. and Holden, B. (1985) Histochemical evidence of limited reinnervation of human corneal grafts. *Acta Ophthalmol.*, **63**, 207–14.

Toivanen, M., Tervo, T., Partanen, M., Vannas, A., and Hervonen, A. (1987) Histochemical demonstration of adrenergic nerves in the stroma of the human cornea. *Invest. Ophthalmol. Vis. Sci.*, **28**, 398–400.

Uddman, R., Alumets, J., Ehinger, B., Hananson, R. *et al.*, (1980) Vasoactive intestinal polypeptide nerves in ocular and orbital structures of the cat. *Invest. Ophthalmol. Vis. Sci.*, **19**, 878–85.

Unger, W.G. and Butler, J.M. (1988) Neuropeptides in the uveal tract. *Eye*, **2 (suppl.)**, S202–S212.

Uusitalo, H., Krootila, K. and Palkama, A. (1989) Calcitonin gene-related peptide (CGRP) immunoreactive sensory nerves in the human and guinea pig uvea and cornea. *Exp. Eye. Res.*, **48**, 467–75.

Zander, E. and Weddell, G. (1951) Observations on the innervation of the cornea. *J. Anat.*, **85**, 68–98.

CORNEAL PHYSIOLOGY AND BIOPHYSICS

14

L.S. Kwok

14.1 INTRODUCTION

Our understanding of corneal physiology and biophysics has advanced considerably in the last few years. An accelerating factor in the emergence of these exciting developments has been the introduction of powerful techniques in molecular biology, cellular biophysics and high resolution electrophysiology. Recent developments are emphasized in this review, which is selective rather than comprehensive; the treatises by Maurice (1984), Worthington (1984) and O'Leary (1985a, b) are recommended to complement the present material.

14.2 CORNEAL CELLULAR PHYSIOLOGY

The mechanisms of interactions between corneal cells, basement membranes and extracellular matrices, are being elucidated with new techniques in molecular biology. These are of fundamental importance to understanding processes such as corneal development, cell migration and corneal wound healing (Mattey & Garrod, 1984; Akiyama *et al.*, 1990b). One example is the recent application of the polymerase chain reaction to amplify nucleic acid sequences such as the herpes viral genome to detect herpes virus in the corneal epithelium (Crouse *et al.*, 1990).

New specular microscopic techniques allow the visualization and morphometry of superficial corneal epithelial cells in the living eye (see Lemp *et al.*, 1990). In older patients in the fifth to sixth decade, Tsubota *et al.* (1991) reported that the average area of superficial corneal epithelial cells (821 ± 203) μm^2 in diabetic aphakic patients was greater than normal (648 ± 152 μm^2 average size). Paradoxically, the corneal epithelium in the presence of either aphakia or diabetes alone has normal-sized cells (643 ± 125 μm^2 and 658 ± 146 μm^2 average area, respectively). Why corneal epithelial cells are larger in combined diabetes and aphakia is unclear. However, larger corneal epithelial cells (818 ± 187) μm^2 are also reported in aphakic extended soft contact lens wear (Lemp *et al.*, 1990). In younger phakic patients, extended soft contact lens wear also increases the area of superficial corneal epithelial cells (Lemp *et al.*, 1990). Diabetes or extended contact lens wear probably affects the cellular physiology of the corneal epithelium in aphakia, but the biological significance of areally larger epithelial cells remains to be established. Soft contact lens wear in rabbits produce alterations to corneal enzyme activities and epithelial thinning (Cejková *et al.*, 1988).

The cytochemistry of the surface of the corneal epithelium is important to understanding how the cornea resists invasion by

Contact Lens Practice. Edited by Montague Ruben and Michel Guillon.
Published in 1994 by Chapman & Hall, London. ISBN 0 412 35120 X

tear-borne bacteria and other harmful exogenous entities. The sialic acid membrane receptor has been implicated in the mediation of *Pseudomonas aeruginosa* adherence in pre-adult mouse corneas (see Hazlett *et al.*, 1987), and the higher density of sialic acid receptors in the adult cornea apparently protects against *Pseudomonas* invasion (Hazlett & Mathieu, 1989). *Pseudomonas* appears to bind preferentially to basal and wing cells of cultured rabbit corneal epithelium but not to adult superficial cells (Spurr-Michaud *et al.*, 1988; Klotz *et al.*, 1989) especially at sites on the cell periphery, whereas *Staphylococcus aureus* binds randomly over the cell surface (Panjwani *et al.*, 1990). Apparently, *Pseudomonas* has an affinity for membrane receptors involved in cell–cell or cell–substratum interactions; corneal adherence is enhanced when epithelial integrity is breached to expose deeper epithelial cells (Klotz *et al.*, 1989). The devastating ocular parasite *Acanthamoeba* can bind to the anterior corneal surface and eventually penetrate into the corneal epithelium, even in the absence of preceding tissue trauma (Stopak *et al.*, 1991). The invading *Acanthamoeba* parasite consumes living corneal epithelial cells. This profoundly disturbs the cellular cytoskeleton, which is surrounded by tremendous intracellular trafficking of water and metabolites necessary for normal cell function (Goodsell, 1991). Such disruption of intracellular organization in the superficial corneal epithelium is particularly perilous, because destabilization of intracellular filaments such as actin will affect the integrity of the epithelial tight junctions (Rojanasakul & Robinson, 1991) and hence compromise the superficial epithelial cell barrier, the major site of corneal resistance to ionic molecules (Ehlers, 1970; Fee & Edelhauser, 1970; Klyce, 1972). Stromal penetration with poor clinical prognosis will eventuate if the infection is not controlled (Hirst *et al.*, 1984; Stopak *et al.*, 1991). Recent evidence suggests that the *Acanthamoeba* parasite might directly contribute to stromal lesions by releasing collagenase, thus attracting neutrophil infiltrates which release collagenolytic enzymes resulting in collagenolysis and stromal thinning (He *et al.*, 1990). Degradation and loss of corneal stroma in inflammatory corneal disease is thought to be due mainly to the liberation of proteolytic enzymes by invading polymorphonuclear leucocytes (PMNs) (Trinkhaus-Randall *et al.*, 1991).

An interesting finding is a 70 kDa collagen binding glycoprotein in chick corneal epithelial cell membranes (Sugrue, 1987). If this acts as a collagen receptor, it could link the intracellular milieu with extracellular collagen matrices, and play a role in corneal morphogenesis, or wound healing (Sugrue & Hay, 1986).

The mammalian corneas system includes the presence of the degradative enzyme acetylcholinesterase. High levels of acetylcholine in rabbit and bovine corneal epithelium may modulate cyclic GMP (Walkenbach & Ye, 1991), but clear-cut physiological role has yet to be established. In the developing chick cornea, levels of acetylcholine peak in the middle of corneal maturation and coincide with events such as increased epithelial innervation and corneal transparency (Sturges & Conrad, 1987).

The basement membrane of the human corneal epithelium is thinner and more uniform centrally, becoming thicker and interdigitated peripherally (McTigue & Fine, 1966). Glycoprotein microfibres are also seen peripherally, and only appear centrally in acute keratoconus, when the central basement membrane becomes thickened (Brewitt & Reale, 1981). The basement membrane is characterized by numerous hemidemsosomes, which are areas of focal attachment of anchoring fibrils between the corneal epithelium and the underlying stroma (Gipson *et al.*, 1987; Tisdale *et al.*, 1988). Extended soft contact lens wear in cat corneas causes a decrease in the number of hemidesmosomes per unit length of basement membrane

(Madigan, 1989), which explains why the contact lens wearing corneal epithelium is less adherent than normal (Madigan *et al.*, 1987). Adhesion structures in the healed corneal epithelium can take 12 months to recover (Gipson *et al.*, 1989). Contact lens wear initiates a sequence of unknown biochemical events in the cat cornea which reduce the epithelial hemidesmosome density. Changes in extracellular matrix components could be translated into intracellular events in corneal epithelial cells by modulated basement membrane proteins such as integrin which are linked to the epithelial cytoskeleton (Trinkhaus-Randall *et al.*, 1990). Extracellular fibronectin is involved in cell shape and movement, as well as the formation and development of extracellular matrices (Mattey & Garrod, 1984).

In the normal cornea, type I collagen fibrils are an important contributor to stromal structure. In the rabbit and avian cornea, type VI collagen is located between the type I fibrils (Linsenmayer *et al.*, 1986; Cintron & Hong, 1988; Hirano *et al.*, 1989) and may play a structural role. In connective tissues, the collagen fibrils eventually degrade to be replaced by new fibrils. This turnover is achieved by the presence of type I collagen-degrading enzymes. In cultured rabbit corneal cells, Fini and Girard (1990) reported enzymes able to degrade type IV, V and VII collagen. The first two collagenases were thought to be synthesized by corneal epithelial cells, and the latter by stromal fibroblasts (Fini & Girard, 1990).

The corneal stroma in keratoconus contains several abnormal proteins together with reduced levels of normal proteins (Panjwani *et al.*, 1989). A major proteoglycan of the cornea, keratan sulphate proteoglycan (KSPG) has an altered keratan sulphate arrangement in keratoconus (Funderburgh *et al.*, 1989; Sawaguchi *et al.* 1991). The subnormal biostructural properties of the cornea in keratoconus are presumably linked to an abnormal KSPG function.

The developing mammalian eye shows an age-associated decrease in corneal endothelial cell density (ECD), which attains an adult value of around 250 000 cells/cm^2 (Bahn *et al.*, 1986.) The posterior surface of the cat, rabbit, and human cornea increases in area by 210%, 130% and 17% from the infant to adult (areas of 2.8 cm^2, 2.3 cm^2 and 1.2 cm^2, respectively: see Kwok, 1984; Bahn *et al.*, 1986). In the non-human cornea, the areal increase can account for about 80% of the adult ECD, and since the total number of endothelial cells per cornea is calculated to increase, mitosis is calculated to contribute 20% of the ECD (Bahn *et al.*, 1986). The human cornea shows a net loss of almost half its original endothelial cells, which could account for most of the lowered adult ECD. Bahn *et al.* (1986) concluded that if mitosis exists in the developing human corneal endothelium it must be have a minor effect, which is more than compensated for by the cell loss. The analysis of Bahn *et al.* (1986) can only be approximate, because it does not allow for the possibility that neighbouring cells may join to form larger endothelial cells: if mitosis is present, its contribution would be under-estimated.

The morphology of the corneal endothelium is altered by contact lens wear (Schoessler & Woloschak, 1981). Intermediate filaments which form a stable part of the cytoskeleton in corneal endothelium (Risen *et al.*, 1987) must depolymerize to effect a long-term shape change in corneal endothelial cells. The migration and shape change of rat corneal endothelial cells after a cryo-injury is known to involve reorganization of intracellular microtubules rather than microfilaments (Gordon & Staley, 1990) but could represent a different condition. Polymegethous corneal endothelial changes were reported by Carlson *et al.* (1988a) in patients who had worn contact lenses for 2 to 23 years; endothelial fluorescein permeability was unchanged, and no other significant physiological changes were found. While a multitude of morphological changes are reported, the biological basis and physiological significance of these observations remains poorly understood. Polse *et al.* (1990) have identified hypoxia as the primary causative factor, but the underlying aetiology is scarcely understood. Major enzymes involved in glucose breakdown were significantly affected by closed-eye soft contact lens wear (Kilp *et al.*, 1985). Stromal oedema in rabbit corneas during soft contact lens wear was preceded by changes in corneal enzymes, including impairment of corneal endothelial Na^+K^+-ATPase (Cejková *et al.*, 1988). Corneal pH is often mentioned as an important facet, but stromal pH only changes from a normal pH 7.5 (open eyes) to pH 7.4 during eyelid closure (Bonanno & Polse, 1987). The rabbit corneal endothelium is able to maintain normal permeability for external pH in the range 6.5 to 8.5 (Gonnering *et al.*, 1979) sustaining a maximal corneal endothelial potential difference (Fischbarg & Lim, 1974; Lyslo *et al.*, 1985). When endothelial pumping was briefly impaired by 10^{-6} M ouabain, the pH of the rabbit corneal endothelium remained unchanged, as did the endothelial intracellular potential (Bowman *et al.*, 1984). Transient dark guttate-like spots in the corneal endothelium of novice soft contact lens wearers were first reported by Zantos and Holden (1977). The physiological significance of this transient phenomenon is unclear since it does not appear in adapted lens wearers. Madigan (1989) recently reported the same phenomenon in monkey eyes, opening the possibility of a useful animal model for investigation.

Sodium hyaluronate (NaHA) is injected into the anterior chamber to protect the corneal endothelium during anterior eye surgery. A coating of viscous NaHA of 2 150 000 molecular mass acts as a shock absorber of blunt trauma and also preserves the water permeability of rabbit corneal endothelium (Miyauchi & Iwata, 1984). Interestingly, the mammalian corneal endothelium has surface sites that bind hyaluronate, raising the possibility that native hyaluronate coats the posterior corneal surface and that the corneal endothelium catabolizes hyaluronate (Madsen *et al.*, 1989). Integrin receptors are reported in human corneal endothelium (Lauweryns *et al.*, 1991) but their role in endothelial adhesion and wound healing remains to be studied further. Endocytosis in the corneal endothelium (Kaye & Donn, 1965) was re-examined in rabbit eyes by Raphael and McLaughlin (1990), but questions regarding possible mediation by membrane receptors and the physiological relevance to endothelial transport remain unresolved.

Corneal oxygen is usually regarded as an important imperative in contact lens considerations but paradoxically the physiological breakdown of molecular oxygen generates free radical species capable of great oxidative cell damage (Srivastava *et al.*, 1989; Farber *et al.*, 1990). Oxidative free radical damage, especially the response of the corneal endothelium to H_2O_2 has been studied intensely because of the implications for lens cataract formation (see Hull, 1990). Tear lactoferrin (Boonstra & Kijlstra, 1987) may help protect the cornea against oxidative damage by scavenging oxygen radicals (Kuizenga *et al.*, 1987). The enzyme superoxide dismutase (SOD) is present in the non-human cornea but its activity decreases with age (Crouch *et al.*, 1984). SOD scavenges the harmful superoxide radical, but forms intracellular hydrogen peroxide (H_2O_2), which is toxic in greater than micromolar amounts. Fortunately, H_2O_2 can be vanquished rapidly by other intracellular scavenging pathways mediated by catalase and glutathione peroxidase. Catalase is present in the mammalian cornea (Atalla *et al.*, 1987) and protects against superoxide damage in the corneal endothelium (Hull *et al.*, 1984). Both catalase and SOD are found in the human cornea but their activities are very low (Mayer, 1980; Hayden *et al.*, 1990). Although catalase, SOD and the enzyme glutathione peroxidase can protect the cornea by scavenging harmful free radicals, their interactions and specific roles are poorly understood especially in the human eye (see Kwok & Klyce, 1992). High intracellular levels of oxidants such as H_2O_2 can damage cell membranes through lipid peroxidation. Aldehyde dehydrogenase in the cornea (Holmes & VandeBerg, 1986; Holmes *et al.*, 1989) mitigates the effects of membrane lipid peroxidation by detoxifying the aldehyde by-products (Abedinia *et al.*, 1990).

14.3 CORNEAL WOUND HEALING

14.3.1 CORNEAL CYTOTOXICITY

Alkaline chemical injuries of the cornea disrupt the basement membrane of the corneal epithelium (Hirst *et al.*, 1981; Gartaganis *et al.*, 1987). Alkali degradation of corneal collagen is thought to liberate an attractant for PMNs which are lysed, releasing hydrolytic enzymes leading to collagen loss and possible stromal ulceration (Pfister *et al.*, 1988). It is possible that in the cornea injured with sodium hydroxide, hydroxide ions can be stored in the cornea (for later release) bonded to corneal collagen and glycosaminoglycans (Whikehart *et al.*, 1991). The rabbit cornea takes 6 months to recover normal epithelial thickness following an alkali wound; this appears to coincide with renormalization of anterior stromal hydration (Chung *et al.*, 1988). Chemical cautery was used by Culton *et al.* (1990) in the rat cornea to re-examine the effect of oxygen on corneal neovascularization. No difference was found in the degree of neovascularization in the rat cornea under anoxia when compared with normal oxygen. The corneal cytoxicity of various chemicals is sometimes ascertained by scanning electron microscopy of the corneal epithelium. Unfortunately, it may be difficult to establish unambiguous damage thresholds because of artefacts (Maclean & Haining, 1971). One preferred alternative is to examine the effect on corneal electrical resistance and ion transport (Burstein & Klyce, 1977). This method offers greater sensitivity to changes induced in the intact corneal epithelium by tears-side addition of an agent. Perturbations to the corneal epithelial membranes induced by *t*-butyl hydroperoxide (an organic hydrogen peroxide) are reversed within an hour providing the dose does not exceed 1–2 mM (Kwok & Klyce, 1992). Corneal epithelial toxicity studies are often undertaken with superficial circular wounds used to ascertain the effect on wound closure rate. To improve current methods in use, Kwok (1991b) has recently proposed a more accurate analysis of the areal closure rate which is typically nonlinear. The healing cornea re-epithelializes at a time-varying cell migration rate (Kwok & Madigan, 1986) with a shifting rate of protein synthesis (Zieske *et al.*, 1987). A time-varying cellular migration rate is reported in healing corneal endothelium (Miyata *et al.*, 1990).

14.3.2 CONTACT LENS-INDUCED CELL DEATH

There is little doubt that contact lens wear can lead to death of corneal cells, especially in cells of the corneal epithelium. Soft contact lens wear can significantly affect corneal epithelial cell integrity and physiology (see Kwok, 1983; Holden *et al.*, 1985; Friedlander & Zimny, 1989). In rabbits according to Cejková *et al.* (1988) soft contact lens wear leads to corneal damage which is 'very similar to that evoked by other traumas such as mechanical or chemical damage'. Mechanical destruction of rabbit corneal epithelium took longer than normal to heal in contact lens wear (Kilp *et al.*, 1985). Chemicals could cause cell damage by overwhelming the cellular defence mechanisms to cause cell death. Another lethal cell mechanism is apoptosis, where cell death is triggered by some stimulus e.g. hypoxia, leading to cell 'suicide' (Kerr *et al.*, 1972; Boobis *et al.*, 1989). Madigan

(1989) using electron microscopy found intra-epithelial vacuoles within the wing and superficial cells following soft contact lens wear on the monkey cornea. Condensed or involuted epithelial cells (a possible feature of apoptosis) were also found in contact lens-wearing cat corneas. Madigan's (1989) suggestion that apoptosis may be the basis of contact lens-induced epithelial microcysts deserves confirmation in the human cornea.

14.3.3   SUPERFICIAL INJURIES

The cornea shows remarkable rapidity in repairing superficial injuries. A light scratch to the cat corneal epithelium *in vitro* immediately caused a fall in corneal resistance, which was reversed within 1 h (Kwok, 1986). The rabbit corneal endothelium shows a similar response (Fukami *et al.*, 1988). The rabbit corneal epithelium is apparently able swiftly to re-establish its barrier properties even after superficial chemical injury (Wolosin, 1988; Sokol *et al.*, 1990). Presumably the process includes regeneration of the tight junction complexes between superficial cells. The cornea *in vivo* is exposed to various nutrients and agents such as epidermal growth factor (EGF) in the tears (Ohashi *et al.*, 1989), which would favour rapid corneal repair. EGF promotes epithelial wound healing and its release by the lacrimal gland is increased during reflex tearing, but its concentration still falls (van Setten, 1990). A rapid corneal repair response would greatly assist contact lens wear to successfully surmount the many possible modes of epithelial cell injury (see Kwok, 1985b, c).

Painful stimuli which cause excitement or annoyance were found to diminish the mitotic rate in the rat corneal epithelium, which is apparently an adrenergic response since it can be simulated by adrenaline (Friedenwald & Buschke, 1944). Significantly, contact lens wear also affects the mitotic rate of corneal epithelium (Hamano & Hori, 1983; Hayashi *et al.*, 1985). This may impair the corneal response of contact lens-associated epithelial cell injury, since mitosis is the primary mechanism for re-establishing normal corneal epithelial thickness (Thompson *et al.*, 1991). Labelling of mitosing rat corneal epithelial cells with ^{3}H-thymidine indicates that about 50% of basal cells are replaced every 3 days, with more mitosis seen peripherally (Cenedella & Fleschner, 1990). A disturbance of corneal epithelial cell turnover by contact lens-induced hypoxia (Kwarecki & Krawcyzk, 1989) may present a form of cellular stress insofar as the extended lifetime could age the epithelium and adversely affect epithelial cell defences.

Epithelial cells migrate to re-establish corneal confluency in the healing cornea after epithelial scraping. In the rabbit cornea, cell regeneration and differentiation is derived ultimately from the limbal stem cells (Chen & Tseng, 1990). Epithelial cells at the leading edge of movement have different membrane–protein receptors than normal superficial epithelial cells (Gipson *et al.*, 1983; McLaughlin *et al.*, 1986), but it is uncertain whether these are normally deeper in the epithelium, or represent a cell surface change. The complex cellular events in the healing corneal epithelium are partially known, and involve extracellular components such as fibronectin (Fujikawa *et al.*, 1981), cell surface receptors such as integrin (Gipson & Spurr-Michaud, 1988; Trinkhaus-Randall *et al.*, 1990; Päällysaho & Williams, 1991) and vinculin (Soong, 1987; Zieske *et al.*, 1988) and intracellular enzymes such as calcium-activated calpain (Shearer *et al.*, 1990). Watanabe *et al.* (1988) suggested that fibronectin (FN) may be applied clinically where adhesion of the corneal epithelium is abnormal or retarded. In vitamin A deficiency, application of FN accelerated corneal epithelial healing in the rat (Watanabe *et al.*, 1991). Delayed re-epithelialization was found in retinol deficiency (El-Ghorab *et al.*, 1988), and topical therapy with vitamin A is a possibility because it is a cofactor for corneal epithelial growth and function and is normally present as retinol in the tears (Ubels & MacRae, 1984).

Membrane-bound receptors for low-density lipoprotein were found in cultured corneal endothelial cells (Elner *et al.*, 1991). In human corneal endothelium, cells adjacent to a scratch injury site significantly increased their low-density lipoprotein uptake. Most likely the migrating or compromised cells had increased receptor densities which elevated the intracellular supplies of amino acids, fatty acids and free cholesterol from lipoprotein hydrolysis (Elner *et al.*, 1991). Corneal endothelial wound healing can be pharmacologically modified by EGF (Jumblatt *et al.*, 1988; Joyce *et al.*, 1989) raising the future possibility of clinical treatment with growth factors like EGF. A prostaglandin membrane receptor was found in rabbit corneal endothelium (Jumblatt & Paterson, 1991). The prostaglandin receptor is coupled to cyclic AMP synthesis, and is believed to be involved in maintaining the characteristic polygonal endothelial cell shape (Jumblatt *et al.*, 1988).

14.4 PHOTOTHERAPEUTIC CORNEAL SURGERY

The controlled application of 193 nm ultraviolet laser energy to the living cornea is capable of precise sculpturing of the corneal tissue for refractive correction (Krueger *et al.*, 1985). The word 'precise' here is used to denote repeatability. In regard to *accuracy*, the actual correction is highly dependent on several procedural variables (Gaster *et al.*, 1989). However, it is worth mentioning that corneal incisions can be measured to within 5–10 μm with femtosecond optical ranging (Stern *et al.*, 1989). Ocular optics considerations in postoperative vision (for example, Hemenger *et al.*, 1990) need greater research attention, especially to what long-term results are actually achieved in refractive surgery.

Corneal scars have been recently treated with phototherapeutic keratectomy using 193 nm excimer laser surgery (Sher *et al.*, 1991). The corneal epithelium was removed prior to photoablation, and although the cornea was re-epithelialized within 4 to 5 days without induced scarring, Sher *et al.* (1991) recommended in retrospect that the epithelium should be kept intact for best results. In a previous study of corneal photoablation, Tuft *et al.* (1989) noted that collagen remodelling in the rabbit corneal stroma was only initiated after complete re-epithelialization. A persistent subepithelial haze of unknown origin was noted, which was partly ameliorated by postoperative steroid treatment. The anterior proliferation of stromal keratocytes with large vacuoules found in photoablated rabbit cornea (Gaster *et al.*, 1989) could account for the subepithelial haze.

The results reported by Sher *et al.* (1991) were encouraging, but several problems appeared. The majority of patients had eye pain, some severe, and generally at a level greater than that experienced in radial keratotomy. Some patients even required narcotic analgesia during the initial 24 to 48 hours after the operation. A hyperopic shift was found in about half the patients and a secondary hyperopic steepening procedure was recommended after the primary myopic ablation. Corneal scars in adult rabbit cornea contain unusual proteoglycan structures (Funderburgh *et al.*, 1988). Healing takes 2 years to restore normal patterns of proteoglycan stromal composition, and involves movement of existing corneal proteoglycans, *de novo* macromolecular synthesis, and a partial reactivation of biosynthetic mechanisms usually present in the younger, developing cornea (Cintron *et al.*, 1990). Thus, the age of the scar and its varying biochemical composition at the time of surgical intervention may affect the clinical success of treatment of corneal scars.

The biological effects of laser energy directed at the cornea are largely unknown, and more animal experiments are required (see for example, Mecke *et al.*, 1991). A thorough understanding of the likely long-term effects of phototherapeutic procedures on the cornea is essential if tissue side effects are to be minimized, and clinical objectives met. The short wavelength radiations involved can damage cellular DNA and even jeopardize long-term corneal transparency (Applegate & Ley, 1991). The effect on DNA is particularly important, as little data are available on the mutagenic effects of laser corneal surgery.

14.5   CORNEAL BIOPHYSICS

14.5.1   CORNEAL EPITHELIAL BIOMECHANICS

The resistance of rabbit corneal epithelium to stretching was recently determined in isolated corneas (Kwok, 1991a). The modulus of elasticity was estimated to be of the order of 10^4 Pa in the tangential direction (running limbus to limbus). This modulus is one order of magnitude less than that reported for the rabbit corneal stroma (Jue & Maurice, 1986), and indicates that for the same tangential stress the epithelium will undergo greater elongation.

Despite this difference in moduli, the presence of an intact corneal epithelium could have an effect on the overall biomechanical behaviour of the cornea. The corneal epithelium would be expected to modify the expansion of the underlying stroma by restraining its physical excursions.

14.5.2   CORNEAL STROMAL BIOMECHANICS

The modulus of elasticity of corneal stroma is of the order of 10^5 Pa, but the value determined experimentally depends on the tangential stress applied to the tissue. Corneal stress–strain relationships were examined by Jue and Maurice (1986) in intact human and rabbit eyes. Corneal distensions and initial

tensions of Descemet's membrane were found to differ: the rabbit corneal stroma began to accept additional tension only after a calculated strain of 9% in Descemet's membrane; the human corneal stroma accepted tension immediately. The authors cautioned against extrapolation of rabbit corneal biomechanics to the human situation.

The tangential tension exerted by the intraocular pressure on the stroma is relatively uniform throughout the stromal depth (McPhee *et al.*, 1985) and is essentially borne by the collagen fibrils. An important implication of this distribution is that the epithelial basement membrane, and hence the epithelium, must also be under tangential tension in the limbus-to-limbus direction (Kwok, 1991a).

14.5.3   STROMAL BIOPHYSICS

The quasi-regular spacing of the collagen fibrils of the corneal stroma is the basis of stromal transparency (Maurice, 1957). McCally and Farrell (1988) have elaborated on various aspects of the biophysics of minimal light scattering as the basis of stromal transparency.

The corneal stroma contains proteoglycans (PGs) in the interfibrillary matrix, the two major types being the keratan sulphate proteoglycan (KSPG) and the chondroitin sulphate proteoglycan (CSPG). These are large macromolecules approaching 50 000 units of molecular mass, and are largely responsible for the stromal swelling pressure (see below). One end of the protein core of the proteoglycan is covalently attached to the collagen fibril (Scott & Haigh, 1985), while the other end containing the glycosaminoglycan (GAG) side-chains is projected radially. At physiological pH, carboxylic and sulphonic acid groups in the GAGs dissociate and adopt a net negative charge. The bulk charge for most corneas at pH 7.4 is around 0.05 mole e^-/kg stromal fluid (see Maurice, 1984). Since the PGs are attached at regular intervals along the collagen fibril (Scott &

Haigh, 1985; Hirsch *et al.*, 1989) each collagen fibril roughly resembles a bottle brush in three dimensions. If the PGs have sufficient rigidity, it is possible that the PG structures could generate long-distance influence on neighbouring collagen fibrils. In particular, a structural influence of the corneal PGs (Hart & Farrell, 1971) could explain the curious spatial uniformity of interfibrillary spacing during corneal swelling. Prolonged immersion of pieces of corneal stroma produces a biphasic time course of swelling (Kwok, 1986). The biphasicity could be explained by an uncoupling of the stromal PG complex due to salt degradation and subsequent loss of long-distance interaction between collagen fibrils (Kwok, 1990).

In the intact cornea, the compressive effect of the intraocular pressure on the stroma is greatest at the endothelial side falling to zero at the epithelium (Berkley, 1971). A gradient in fluid pressure (or imbition pressure IP) was found in the rabbit corneal stroma with a central pressure of -5.7 kPa (-42.7 mmHg) falling to -2.4 kPa (-17.8 mmHg) peripherally (Wiig, 1989). Since IP = IOP–SP (see Maurice, 1984), where IOP is the intraocular pressure and SP is the swelling pressure, an IP of greater magnitude in the central cornea would imply a greater SP centrally than peripherally if the same IOP operated at both locations. This could not be accounted for by differences in local stromal hydration, which is similar anteriorly (central versus peripheral) and in the wrong direction posteriorly (Kikkawa & Hirayama, 1970). Otherwise, a greater IOP effect must be postulated peripherally.

Microfibres of type VI collagen in the interfibrillary space (Linsenmayer *et al.*, 1986; Cintron & Hong, 1988; Hirano *et al.*, 1989) may also play a structural role. An orthogonal network of microfibrils is reported in the chick corneal stroma (Bruns *et al.*, 1987) but the chick cornea is a poor biostructural model for the human corneal stroma, which is less organized. Clusters of proteinaceous microfibrils of unknown function are reported between stromal lamellae and near keratocytes in the rabbit cornea (Carlson & Waring, 1988). The abnormal collagen arrangement in macular corneal dystrophy (Quantock *et al.*, 1990) could be due to the breakdown of PG structures mediating interfibrillary collagen spacing.

Recent developments in confocal microscopy have enabled high resolution imaging of the cornea *in vitro* (Masters & Paddock, 1990; Xiao *et al.*, 1990). Fine filaments were observed throughout the corneal stroma (but were highest near Descemet's membrane), as well as extensive interconnecting processes between stromal keratocytes; even nerve plexuses were resolved.

The corneal stromal fluid is comprised of two fractions: the 'free' water is the major portion and behaves similarly to bulk water, and 'bound' water wherein dissolved molecules move around less freely. These fractions can be discriminated with a variety of techniques including proton NMR spectroscopy (Masters *et al.*, 1983), differential scanning calorimetry (DSC) Castoro *et al.*, 1988) and isothermal thermogravimetry. Unfortunately, the estimated fractions will depend on the method of measurement: the DSC method measures non-freezable water. The 'bound' water is associated with structural elements such as collagen fibrils, perhaps arranged like a cylinder concentric with the long axis of the fibril. Each measurement technique can be imagined to intersect different cylinders around the fibril leading to different estimates of 'bound' water. The exchange between the free fluid fraction and external fluid will be more rapid than the exchange between the two stromal fractions. However, of paramount importance is the physiological relevance and plausibility of the fraction estimated as 'bound' water. As far as mobile small ions are concerned, around 8–10% of total stromal fluid can be considered 'bound' at normal hydration (3.4 kg H_2O/kg dry mass). The free fraction of stromal fluid is the solvent volume for osmotic effects and is important to stromal swelling pressure (see below).

14.6 CORNEAL PERMEABILITY

14.6.1 NORMAL CORNEA

The cornea is significantly more permeable to nonelectrolytes than the conjunctiva, by at least one order of magnitude (Huang *et al.*, 1989; see Maurice (1991) for a discussion of this article). Damage to the anterior or posterior epithelial layers of the cornea leads to tissue swelling (Maurice & Giardini, 1951). The corneal epithelium contains the site of greatest electrical resistance in the cornea (Fee & Edelhauser, 1970; Klyce, 1972). The superficial cells, interconnected by tight junctions form the primary site (Klyce, 1972). The superficial cells in the rabbit cornea are relatively more dehydrated than the basal and wing cells, with the dry mass content of the superficial cells being 50% greater than that of basal cells (Chung *et al.*, 1988). The hydration of superficial epithelial cells is normally comparable with the hydration of the anterior stroma (Chung *et al.*, 1988).

Desquamation of superficial epithelial cells is a normal event in the turnover of corneal epithelium, but the mandatory desmosomal detachment of the departing cell (Hazlett *et al.*, 1980) is exquisitely timed with the re-establishment of epithelial integrity (Wolosin, 1988; Sokol *et al.*, 1990). The desquamating epithelial cell undergoes changes to its plasma membrane, as evidenced by increased binding of the lectin probe concanavalin A (Bonvicini *et al.*, 1983). Calcium in the tears is associated with normal surface cell exfoliation in the corneal epithelium (O'Leary *et al.*, 1985). Perfusion of the excised rabbit cornea with a calcium-free 165.8 mM saline solution (0.97% solution by weight) for 150 min was found to induce abnormal sloughing of surface epithelial cells (Bergmanson & Wilson, 1989), but the physi-

ological implications for the living human cornea are not known.

The corneal endothelium is the principal entry site for corneal glucose (see Maurice, 1984; DiMattio, 1984) and is reported to have a transmembrane–protein glucose transporter which allows the passage of water molecules (Fischbarg *et al.*, 1987). Although water permeation was only demonstrated for osmotically-induced flows, the glucose transporter may mediate most of the water flow through the corneal endothelium. The corneal endothelium forms a functional syncytium presumably via intercellular gap junctions (Rae *et al.*, 1989b) but the physiological ramifications of such good cell-to-cell coupling are yet to be fully explored.

Sodium fluorescein is a widely used ophthalmic probe of membrane permeability. For doses expected in clinical and research practice, fluorescein is confirmed to have no deleterious ocular effects as evidenced from corneal endothelial electrical potential measurements (Akiyama *et al.*, 1990a).

14.6.2 PATHOLOGICAL CHANGES

The corneal epithelial barrier is altered in diseases such as diabetes (Göbbels *et al.*, 1989) and Graves' ophthalmopathy (Khalil *et al.*, 1990) as evidenced by a subnormal resistance to fluorescein. However, Stolwijk *et al.* (1990) found a normal fluorescein permeability in the corneal epithelium of diabetic patients, but epithelial permeability to one drop of 0.4% oxybuprocaine HCl was twice the normal value. The corneal epithelium in diabetes shows abnormal fragility (O'Leary & Millodot, 1981), and has abnormal wound repair (Fukushi *et al.*, 1980). Pathophysiological changes such as increased glucose storage (Friend *et al.*, 1981), and subnormal oxygen uptake (Graham *et al.*, 1981) indicate that abnormal cell functions are associated with the permeability changes.

The permeability to non-electrolytes of the rabbit corneal endothelium is claimed to increase during intraocular inflammation (Macdonald *et al.*, 1987). Exposure of rabbit eyes to 300 nm UV-B radiation in doses of 0.1 to 0.5 J/cm² induced temporary corneal swelling, which was attributed to increased endothelial permeability due to cell membrane damage (Riley *et al.*, 1987).

14.6.3 CHANGES IN WOUND HEALING

The permeability of healed rabbit corneal epithelium to non-electrolytes after an epithelial scraping is initially elevated after re-epithelialization (Huang *et al.*, 1990) but recovers to normal within a week (Thoft & Friend, 1975; Huang *et al.*, 1990). The regenerating rabbit corneal epithelium after scraping loses its adrenaline sensitivity for at least 1–2 months (Kikkawa & Morimoto, 1980). This implies that chloride transport is directly affected, since it is exogenous adrenaline which normally decreases epithelial chloride resistance (Klyce & Wong, 1977). Although the regenerating corneal epithelium after wounding is initially thin, electrophysiological functions such as the transepithelial potential remain operational but only subnormally (Okuhara & Kikkawa, 1968). Epithelial ion transport after myopic keratomileusis surgery in rabbit corneas began to recover epithelial adrenaline sensitivity at 25 days (Marcus *et al.*, 1983).

The rabbit corneal epithelium has a gradient of hydration with the lowest hydration found anteriorly in the superficial cells (Chung *et al.*, 1988). After re-epithelialization of an alkali wound, the rabbit corneal epithelial cells become more hydrated taking up to 6 months to recover (Chung *et al.*, 1988). Presumably, the epithelial barrier is also affected after regeneration.

The healed cat cornea is able to tolerate a postoperative decrease in endothelial cell density of 60%, following mechanical scraping (Landshman *et al.*, 1988). A greater decrease, where endothelial cell densities fell below 105 000 cells/cm², resulted in increased postoperative corneal thickness. The decompensation was attributed to greater numbers of giant endothelial cells, which apparently compromised the endothelial barrier.

14.6.4 CHEMICALLY-INDUCED CHANGES

Proper regulation of epithelial cell volume is essential in maintaining the epithelial barrier function. Epithelial oedema will result if the normal homeostatic mechanisms (see below) are overwhelmed, as in the case of a severe alkali wound (Chung *et al.*, 1988). The application of tears-side *t*-butyl hydroperoxide (*t*BHP) induced a permeability increase in the rabbit corneal epithelium, as well as abnormal oscillations of corneal thickness (Kwok & Klyce, 1992). The rabbit corneal epithelium responded to *t*BHP with immediate and reversible falls in electrical potential difference (PD) and short circuit current, providing that the dose did not exceed 1 mM *t*BHP (Kwok and Klyce, 1992). Epithelial Na⁺K⁺-ATPase generates the epithelial PD and irreversible alterations occurred at doses exceeding 1 mM *t*BHP indicating H_2O_2 modification of Na⁺K⁺-ATPase (Garner *et al.*, 1986). An increased epithelial conductance was due to unnamed effects in the anterior corneal epithelial membranes. An extremely high dose of 8.8 mM H_2O_2 was reported to penetrate the cornea and impede the function of the corneal endothelium (Yuan & Pitts, 1991). Such a clinical occurrence would be exceptional and unlikely since this dose equals 300 ppm, and was applied for 10 min/day for 5 days (Yuan & Pitts, 1991). Acute reactions by patients to H_2O_2 associated with contact lens wear are occasionally reported in the clinical literature (Knopf, 1984) but the long-term consequences of corneal exposure to small amounts of H_2O_2 are unknown.

Addition of 50 µM H_2O_2 to the aqueous humour halves the resistance of the rabbit corneal endothelium to the penetration of nonelectrolytes like inulin and mannitol (Riley & Giblin, 1983). The endothelial Na^+K^+-ATPase is apparently unaffected by small amounts of H_2O_2, so the altered permeability is due to membrane changes (Welsh *et al.*, 1985), or perhaps modulation of the bicarbonate pump. Glucose in the aqueous humour can protect the rabbit corneal endothelium from the deleterious effects of H_2O_2.

14.7   CORNEAL ION TRANSPORT

14.7.1   EPITHELIAL ION TRANSPORT

In the rabbit corneal epithelium, chloride is transported into the tears (van der Heyden *et al.*, 1975) at levels modulated by exogenous adrenaline (Klyce & Wong, 1977). The suspected location of a chloride ion channel in the tears-side membrane of corneal epithelium (Festen & Slegers, 1979) was confirmed by Marshall and Hanrahan (1991) using voltage-clamped gigaohm sealed patches of cultured corneal epithelium. Possible sources of exogenous adrenaline are the tears (Trope & Rumley, 1984), and adrenergic nerves in the human corneal stroma (Toivanen *et al.*, 1987). Adrenaline can enhance intracellular cyclic AMP by stimulating β-adrenergic receptors in the corneal epithelium (Fogle & Neufeld, 1979), which are predominantly of the $β_2$ subtype (Walkenbach *et al.*, 1984). Increased intracellular cyclic AMP will increase the tear-side chloride permeability of the corneal epithelium, favouring greater efflux of chloride into the tears (for reviews, see Reinach, 1985; Klyce & Bonanno, 1988). The activation of the β-adrenoreceptor system has the ability to thin a swollen rabbit cornea (Klyce, 1977), but would play a secondary role since its rate is equivalent to less than 5% of the rate known for the endothelial HCO_3^- transport mechanism. Additionally, the human corneal epithelium appears to transport chloride into the stroma and sodium into the tears (Fischer *et al.*, 1978), so the applicability of the rabbit corneal findings to human corneal function is unclear.

The basal cells of the rabbit and bullfrog corneal epithelium contain a potassium conducting channel (Klyce, 1972; Festen & Slegers, 1979; Carrasquer *et al.*, 1987). The potassium channel was thought to face the stroma and Rae *et al.* (1990a) recently confirmed this location using voltage-clamped patches of basal cell membrane. Such a conductance would be expected to recycle potassium ions from the corneal stroma for subsequent extrusion by the stromally-facing Na^+K^+-dependent ATPase electrogenic pump located in the basal cells. The Na^+K^+-ATPase pump generates the bulk of the transcorneal potential difference (TCP) of 20–40 mV in rabbits (aqueous side positive). The cornea seems different in carnivorous mammals: the human cornea has a far lower TCP of around 0–1 mV (Fischer *et al.*, 1974, 1978) and similar TCPs were reported in cat corneas (Ehlers, 1970; Kwok, 1986). The TCP is sensitive to oxygen (Ehlers & Ehlers, 1966) and is reduced in contact lens wear (see Kwok, 1983).

The pH of rabbit corneal epithelium in cultured cells was found to be 6.87 ± 0.02 using a dual wavelength photometer technique (Korbmacher *et al.*, 1988). This agrees with a pH of 6.5 reported by Krejci (1972), but is somewhat lower than a pH of 7.34 ± 0.03 reported by Bonanno and Machen (1989), who used an identical photometric procedure. The pH of rabbit corneal epithelium appears to be normally more acidic than the tears, which have a pH in the range of 7–7.5 (Krejci, 1972). The normal human tears have a pH of around 7.5 (Carney *et al.*, 1989). Intracellular pH in rabbit corneal epithelium is regulated by a basal cell Na^+/H^+ exchanger, which extrudes intracellular protons (H^+ ions) while bringing in extracellular sodium ions (Korbmacher *et al.*, 1988; Bonanno & Machen, 1989). Intracellular pH may affect the epithelial transport of ions like chloride, and hence modify functions such as hydration control (Klyce, 1977). Intracellular pH in the rabbit corneal epithelial basal cell is regulated by co-operative Na^+–K^+ and K^+–H^+ exchangers; inhibition of these mechanisms will acidify the basal cell interior (Bonanno & Machen, 1989; Bonanno, 1991). Enhancement of anaerobic glycolysis by anoxia, or application of cyanide elevates epithelial production of lactate which is transported into the stroma by a lactate–H^+ cotransporter (Bonanno, 1990; Chen & Chen, 1990).

14.7.2 STROMAL ION TRANSPORT

The osmotic effect of stromal accumulation of epithelially-generated lactate during anterior hypoxia is widely believed to be the basis of contact lens-induced corneal oedema (Refojo, 1975; Klyce, 1981). In the rabbit cornea, around 95% of total lactate is normally found in the corneal stroma (Chen & Chen, 1990). Of the total rabbit corneal lactate formation, 47% was formed in the corneal epithelium, 32% in the stroma and 21% in the endothelium. Epithelial lactate was shown to be transported into the stroma by a proton–lactate pump. That 79% of corneal lactate production is normally associated with the corneal epithelium and stroma is not surprising since the total stromal cell volume (Kaye, 1966) is comparable to total epithelial cell volume (Huff, 1990b). Lactate itself was confirmed to have no directly detrimental effects on corneal function (Huff, 1990a). Of the total exogenous glucose provided to the isolated cornea, the epithelium consumed about half.

The presence of a fixed negative charge enables the stromal movement of ions and water to be calculated by modelling the corneal stroma as an ion-exchange matrix (Maroudas, 1968, 1975). In this model, the fixed negative charge in the corneal stroma attracts counterions such as Na^+ to preserve bulk electroneutrality in the stromal fluid. Additionally, Cl^- would be attracted to any fixed positive charges in the corneal stroma. In the cornea *in vivo*, the aqueous humour will host many of the mobile ions. At steady state, the mobile ions will be distributed according to the Gibbs–Donnan distribution, the simplest form of which is:

$$[Na^+]_i \times [Cl^-]_i = [Na^+]_o \times [Cl^-]_o \quad \text{(eqn 14.1)}$$

where the concentrations are in moles/litre, subscript *i* refers to the stroma, and *o* refers to the external solution. Experimental determinations indicate an excess of Na^+ in the corneal stroma exceeding the concentration calculated from eqn 14.1. This extra fraction is required to neutralize the fixed stromal charge, and the (mainly sodium) ions immobilized in the stromal matrix represent an hyperosmotic force which generates an osmotic pressure. The fluid entering from the external solution creates a swelling pressure. The expansive force found in isolated corneal stroma from the osmotic pressure is around 8 kPa (60 mmHg) but figures can vary according to measurement methods.

Equation 14.1 can be used to derive an expression to calculate the fixed stromal charge and the osmotic pressure generated (Hodson, 1971). The result indicated good agreement with experimental swelling pressures, and calculated a charge of 0.048 mole e^-/l (Hodson, 1971). A recent determination in bovine corneal stroma reported a charge of 0.0395 mole e^-/l (Hodson *et al.*, 1991), somewhat lower than expected but which could be due to the osmometric method used. On theoretical grounds, it appears that the stromal charge may have an anomalous dependency on temperature (Kwok & Klyce, 1990). A corneal stromal charge that increased with falling temperature can account for apparently conflicting results in the past. The molecular biophysics of this temperature effect remains to be found, but it probably originates in conformational changes in stromal proteoglycans.

The Gibbs–Donnan result (eqn 14.1) can be used to accurately model corneal stromal swelling, but a previous attempt (Elliott *et al.*, 1980) neglected factors such as the 'bound' fluid fraction in the stroma and calculated low stromal charges. The situation for the cornea *in vivo* is different because gradients of water pressure and hydration are present, and has yet to be rigorously described.

14.7.3 ENDOTHELIAL ION TRANSPORT

The physiological functions of the so-called corneal endothelium suggest that 'posterior corneal epithelium' (Stocker, 1954) is a better description. As outlined below, the barrier and ion transport properties of the corneal endothelium are primarily directed towards controlling stromal hydration and preserving stromal transparency. In that sense, it differs little in principle to the purpose and mission of the corneal epithelium. The term corneal endothelium is now so well entrenched that it has become routine jargon, and will be used here.

In 1873, Theodore Leber demonstrated that the corneal endothelium contains the primary mechanism for corneal hydration control (see Stocker & Reichle, 1974). Leber's crude experiments were later refined by several workers who confirmed the endothelial site of the fluid pump (for example Itoi *et al.*, 1964; Mishima & Kudo, 1967; Hoshino, 1968; Maurice, 1972). Many of the basic principles governing the corneal endothelial transport of ions and fluid evolved from the rabbit corneal model (see Fischbarg *et al.*, 1985). The rabbit corneal endothelium actively mediates an efflux of fluid from the corneal stroma equal to about 7 $\mu l/cm^2/h^1$ (Baum *et al.*, 1984; Kuang *et al.*, 1990). Mathematically this is equivalent to a thickness change of 70 $\mu m/h$. Opposing this outwards pump is an inwards fluid 'leak' from the aqueous humor into the corneal stroma. At steady-state stromal thickness, the fluid loss due to the pump is offset by the fluid gain of the 'leak'.

Bicarbonate dependency

A bicarbonate transporter is the primary corneal endothelial mechanism responsible for moving fluid out of the stroma (Fischbarg & Lim, 1974; Hodson, 1974). The corneal endothelium shows a net transport of bicarbonate into the aqueous humour (Hodson & Miller, 1976) and inhibition of bicarbonate translocation retards water efflux (Harris *et al.*, 1956; Fischbarg & Lim, 1974) and instigates stromal swelling (Hull *et al.*, 1977). The net amount of bicarbonate solute translocated into the aqueous humour can be calculated to satisfactorily account for experimentally determined 'pump' rates (Liebovitch & Weinbaum, 1981).

A bicarbonate-dependent K^+ pump which transports K^+ into cultured bovine corneal endothelial cells was reported by Savion *et al.* (1989). This K^+ pump is ouabain-insensitive but must be electroneutral because ouabain can completely abolish the corneal endothelial potential difference (PD) (Fischbarg & Lim, 1974).

Transendothelial potential difference

A small electrical PD of around −0.5 mV is measured across the corneal endothelium of the rabbit, bovine, human and cat eye (Fischbarg, 1972; Hodson, 1974; Wigham & Hodson, 1981a,b; Kwok, 1986). The endothelial PD is negative on the aqueous side – of opposite direction to the transepithelial PD, whose magnitude is 40–80 times larger in the rabbit eye but of comparable magnitude in the human and cat eye (see Fischer *et al.*, 1978; Kwok, 1986). The endothelial PD is temperature sensitive and falls with decreased temperature (Hodson, 1975). The PD was decreased in cultured bovine corneal endothelial cells exposed to hypotonic media, and bicarbonate sensitivity was diminished (Coroneo *et al.*, 1989), an effect possibly mediated by a membrane ion channel.

The removal of stromal fluid through the corneal endothelium is coupled to bicarbonate translocation and is also associated with the small endothelial PD (Fischbarg & Lim, 1974; Hodson, 1974). However, the PD is not generated by the bicarbonate transporter which is electroneutral. This explains why inhibition of endothelial bicarbonate supply by the carbonic anhydrase inhibitor 10^{-7} M ethoxyzolamide represses the endothelial pump (Barfort & Maurice, 1974), but has little effect on the transendothelial potential difference (Fischbarg & Lim, 1974). The corneal endothelial PD principally arises from activity of endothelial Na^+K^+-ATPase (see Fischbarg *et al.*, 1985). Immunohistochemical probes confirm the presence of carbonic anhydrase, a bicarbonate–chloride exchanger and Na^+K^+-ATPase in human corneal endothelium, which are located primarily on the aqueous-side of the endothelium (Holthöfer *et al.*, 1991).

Transendothelial electrical resistance

The corneal endothelial electrical resistance or conductance are good indicators of corneal endothelial permeability, owing to the correspondence between endothelial permeability and ionic fluxes (Hodson & Wigham, 1983). The corneal endothelium resistance is reported in the range 20 to 70 ohm cm^{-2} in the presence of adenosine (see Fischbarg & Lim, 1984). Comparable but slightly higher resistances were reported in the cat corneal endothelium (Kwok, 1986). Lower resistances are found when adenosine is omitted from the Ringer solution bathing the isolated corneal endothelium (Fischbarg & Lim, 1984). The endothelial resistance is temperature sensitive and rises with decreased temperature (Hodson, 1975).

Using the patch clamp technique,* Liebovitch *et al.*, (1987) modelled the molecular kinetics of ion channels as they gated between open and shut states. An unconventional fractal scaling model was introduced. Ion channel kinetics of a potassium channel and non-selective cation channel have been characterized in the endothelial membrane facing the aqueous in rabbit cornea (Rae *et al.*, 1989a, 1990b).

Corneal endothelial pH

The rabbit corneal endothelium has an intracellular pH of around 7.1 for an ambient pH of 7.5 (Bowman *et al.*, 1984). Endothelial PD is greatest when the external pH is in the range 7.3 to 8 (Fischbarg & Lim, 1974; Lyslo *et al.*, 1985). The corneal endothelial pH is responsive to external levels of H^+, falling to pH 6.6 when the external pH is 7.0 (Bowman *et al.*, 1984). To account for this effect, a Na^+/H^+ exchanger is hypothesized (Fischbarg *et al.*, 1985), which transports H^+ out of the endothelium. The endothelial PD also falls with pH (Fischbarg & Lim, 1974; Lyslo *et al.*, 1985) suggesting that the electrogenic endothelial Na^+K^+-ATPase is indirectly coupled to the Na^+/H^+ exchanger.

The short-circuited corneal endothelium

Details of the exact mechanism of transendothelial ion flow remain unresolved. Wigham and Hodson (1985) used the classic Ussing technique of electrically short-circuiting the corneal endothelium to calculate the net ionic flow. In an electrically 'tight' cell layer such as the corneal epithelium, the short-circuit current (SCC) equals the net flow of ions through the layer. However, the endothelium is of very low resistance and the meaning of the SCC, and its relationship to the physiological (open circuit) condition is disputed (Fischbarg & Lim, 1984). In the young rabbit cornea, Wigham and Hodson (1985) measured an SCC that was equivalent to a net ionic current of 5×10^{-14} mol/m^2. The net HCO_3^- flux was measured at 3.4×10^{-14} mol/m^2, which could not entirely account for the

---

* The patch clamp technique, developed in Germany, captures a small piece (a 'patch') of cell membrane in a micropipette to measure an electrical current of a few picoamps as one or more ion channels open. The membrane is held at an electrically constant voltage, or voltage 'clamp' (see Rae *et al.*, 1988; Liebovitch & Tóth, 1990).

endothelial SCC. The short-fall could be made up by a net flow of another anion such as Cl^- in the same direction as HCO_3^-, or by a net cation flow of Na^+ in the opposite direction. No net Cl^- flux was detected, and the net Na^+ flux was only 0.08×10^{-14} mol/m^2 into the stroma, the correct direction, but too small to account for the difference. It should be emphasized that such simple balance sheet calculations ignore several subtle mechanisms which are operating under conditions where a voltage is imposed across the endothelium. One possible factor for example is the different mobilities of the ions, which may affect the overall calculation. The short-circuit technique yields different net fluxes than reported under open-circuit conditions (see Fischbarg & Lim, 1984). Other criticisms can be advanced:

In Hodson's technique the electrical resistance of the corneal endothelium R_e is in series with the corneal stroma R_{str} and resistance of the solutions R_{sol}, but the electrical current required to short the endothelium is given by $SCC = V_e/R_e$ where V_e is the open-circuit potential difference. But in each cornea, R_e is only known at the end of the experiment, so it must be *estimated* at the start; this is done by assuming that $R_{str} + R_{sol}$ is constant across all corneas so $R_e = R_{tot} - (R_{str} + R_{sol}) = R_{tot} - $ constant, where R_{tot} is the total resistance for a particular cornea. Unfortunately, stromal resistance R_{str} can vary by up to 12% (Maurice, 1961; Green, 1967), and in the absence of solution stirring, the unstirred fluid layer resistance R_{sol} could also vary. If high stromal resistance corneas had high V_e values and hence high SCC levels, then if stromal resistance is assumed constant, the SCC estimated from $V_e/(R_{tot} - $ constant) will be lower than the actual value $V_e/(R_{tot} - R_{str} - R_{sol})$. Thus, in the studies of Hodson and Wigham (1985) and Wigham and Hodson (1985), if high resistance corneas had high resistance stromas, it is possible that the SCC in these specimens was under-estimated. Overall, this would bring the SCC and net bicarbonate fluxes closer to agreement.

The endothelial 'pump-leak' controversy

The 'pump-leak' concept has been disputed lately. Doughty and Maurice (1988) claimed that the fluid pump in the rabbit corneal endothelium was not bicarbonate dependent; Doughty (1989) alleged that in rabbit corneas previously stored at 4 °C some were able to deturgesce in the absence of measurable endothelial pump activity. The criticism of both studies is the possibility of confounding artefacts in the apparatus used to quantify endothelial pump rate. In that system, corneal endothelial pump rate is inferred from the movement of a meniscus of a liquid column continuous with the aqueous side of the perfused cornea (see Fig. 1 of Baum *et al.*, 1984). The problem is that the epithelium is typically removed, so the corneal stroma will swell; the stroma is constrained anteriorly, so will expand posteriorly registering as a 'pump rate'. Continuous stromal swelling would explain why Doughty and Maurice (1988) measured a gradually increasing 'pump rate' at zero bicarbonate levels. Another possible problem with the technique is the uncertainty of the stromal fluid compartment adjacent to Descemet's membrane, which must be at steady state to justify the analysis adopted. The corneal stroma has a gradient of hydration across its thickness (Castoro *et al.*, 1988) and does not swell uniformly throughout its thickness, but shows a spatial variation (Kikkawa & Hirayama, 1970; Wilson *et al.*, 1984). It is assumed in the Doughty and Maurice (1988) system that stromal gradients in hydration and swelling are dissipated, and stromal fluid flow stabilized. However, the absence of an epithelium would affect the biomechanics of the corneal tissue (Kwok, 1991a) and influence stromal fluid flows. The methods and conclusions of Doughty (1989) can be similarly criticized. The corneal endothelial pump rate was recently reported to be abolished when carbonic anhydrase inhibitors (which decrease bicarbonate levels) were applied to rabbit corneas (Kuang *et al.*, 1990). This finding confirms the bicarbonate-dependency of the corneal endothelial pump, and casts a further doubt on the contrary Doughty and Maurice (1988) claim. To date, the 'pump-leak' hypothesis remains the best framework for exploring details of stromal deturgescence by the corneal endothelium.

Endothelial hypoxia

The corneal endothelium runs the risk of a dysfunctional fluid pump under hypoxic conditions (Mishima & Kudo, 1967; Dikstein & Maurice, 1972) associated with contact lens wear. Contact lenses applied to rabbit corneas caused a 30% drop in endothelial oxygen partial pressure (Stefánsson *et al.*, 1987), and the corneal endothelium could theoretically approach anoxia during anterior hypoxia (Kwok, 1985a). Under normoxic conditions the corneal endothelial production of lactate is depressed (the Pasteur effect), but the generation of cellular energy in the form of ATP through the tricarboxylic acid cycle (TCA) is so efficient (36–38 mole of ATP per mole of glucose) that oxidative phosphorylation usually accounts for less than half of corneal glucose breakdown (Riley, 1982). The diminution of corneal respiration will favour greater anaerobic glycolysis and more lactate production, but generation of ATP is less efficient (two moles of ATP per mole of glucose). If the corneal glucose supply can accommodate an increased rate of consumption to maintain ATP generation, the corneal endothelial pump should be minimally affected. The rabbit aqueous humour apparently contains sufficient glucose to minimize the effect of short-term hypoxia on corneal ATP. The activity of rabbit corneal endothelial Na^+K^+-ATPase as reflected in the intrac-

ellular potential was apparently little affected by the absence of external oxygen for an hour (Bowman *et al.*, 1984). When corneal respiration was suspended by a 1 h exposure to sodium cyanide, the ratio of ATP/ADP only fell by 20% (Masters *et al.*, 1989). (Cyanide disrupts the electron transport chain impairing ATP generation via oxidative phosphorylation; see Stryer, 1988.) Similarly, the de-epithelialized isolated rabbit cornea shows minimal swelling when exposed to potassium cyanide (Riley & Winkler, 1990). However, in that study the aqueous-side perfusate was continuously replaced at a rate equivalent to five times normal anterior chamber volume per hour, essentially ensuring a constant glucose supply. Taking the result of Masters *et al.* (1989), a fall in corneal ATP of around 20% in the living eye during contact lens wear may impede endothelial pumping and affect corneal hydration. Green *et al.* (1990) halved the level of oxygen exposed to the rabbit cornea and found that the net bicarbonate efflux increased by about two-thirds, while net sodium efflux fell by about one-fifth. It is uncertain what effects were involved, but an increased bicarbonate flux would be expected to create an efflux of fluid from the corneal stroma. For obscure reasons, the human corneal endothelial fluid pumping shows long-term endurance in anterior hypoxia with contact lens wear while endothelial morphology shows a considerable transient sensitivity (Zantos & Holden, 1977) and then an acquired polymegethism (Schoessler & Woloschak, 1981). The diabetic corneal endothelium shows long-term changes in morphology in the human (Schultz *et al.*, 1984), and has a subnormal deswelling capacity in the diabetic rabbit (Herse, 1990). This was attributed to altered Na^+K^+-dependent ATPase. However, endothelial pumping could also be impaired by lowered cellular ATP due to diminished glucose uptake by the diabetic corneal endothelium.

Corneal endothelium in disease

Ouabain binds to membrane Na^+K^+-ATPase and is capable of inhibiting activity, but has little effect on the permeability of the corneal endothelium (Mishima & Trenberth, 1968). The radio-active marker ^3H-ouabain has been used to label the location and spread of Na^+K^+-ATPase. The areal density of labelling is referred to as the 'pump site density', a potentially confusing term since the endothelial bicarbonate transport is the endothelial pump directly associated with water movement. The endothelial pump site density was claimed to be subnormal in dysfunctional corneas such as those with Fuch's endothelial dystrophy, and bullous keratopathy (McCartney *et al.*, 1987) where corneal detumescence is demonstrably subnormal (Mandell *et al.*, 1989; Polse *et al.*, 1989). Reduced pump site density is also reported in the corneal endothelium in intraocular inflammation in the rabbit eye (Macdonald *et al.*, 1987). However, these analyses assume that ouabain binds 1:1 to Na^+K^+-ATPase, but there could be a fraction of endothelial Na^+K^+-dependent ATPase that is ouabain insensitive. Even if the 1:1 binding assumption is correct, there is no guarantee that the same ratio applies in the diseased cornea. Exogenous factors such as diet can affect corneal endothelial cell density (Nadakavukaren *et al.*, 1987). The Na^+K^+-dependent ATPase activity in the cornea of diabetic rabbits is less than normal (Herse, 1990). This was claimed to explain the increased stromal hydration, but increased endothelial permeability can not be ruled out since the diabetic corneal endothelium has increased polymegethism and pleomorphism (Meyer *et al.*, 1988). The rate of the HCO_3^- transport, which determines transendothelial fluid transport, was also not considered.

Chondroitin sulphate (CS), a GAG found in the corneal stroma and sometimes included into commercial corneal preservation media (Stein *et al.*, 1988), was reported to stimulate (in an unknown way) the rabbit corneal endothelial potential (Koniarek *et al.*, 1988). If the oedematous cornea loses stromal GAGs into the aqueous humour (Kangas *et al.*, 1990), an intriguing possibility arises. CS leaching out of an oedematous corneal stroma will encounter the corneal endothelium and stimulate the endothelial potential difference. This will increase endothelial fluid pumping (which is correlated positively with potential difference; Barfort & Maurice, 1974; Fischbarg & Lim, 1974) and thus act to oppose further corneal swelling. Could such a negative feedback loop exist in the intact cornea as an emergency resort to keep stromal swelling in check?

Muscarinic cholinergic receptors which regulate intracellular cyclic GMP have been reported in bovine corneal endothelium (Walkenbach & Ye, 1991).

14.7.4 MACROSCOPIC ION TRANSPORT

Over 35 years ago, Kronfeld (1956) proposed that corneal thickness be used as an indicator of corneal physiology during contact lens wear. The measurement of corneal thickness, or pachometry, has become a useful research and clinical tool. Unfortunately, pachometry-based clinical assessment requires careful interpretation to avoid false negatives. In corneas with abnormally low endothelial permeability (measured with fluorescein) following penetrating keratoplasty, no correlation is found with corneal thickness (Bourne & Brubaker, 1983). In patients aged 5 to 79 years, the corneal endothelial permeability to fluorescein was found to increase by 23% with age, but corneal thickness was not found to change with age (Carlson *et al.*, 1988b). Thus, a cornea may have an apparently normal thickness when the endothelial permeability is abnormal.

The older human cornea is reported to show a slower recovery from induced oedema than the deswelling rate found in younger corneas (Polse *et al.*, 1989). Detumescence of swelled corneas with Fuch's dystrophy is also subnormal (Mandell *et al.*, 1989).

It is unclear whether hyperosmotic drops applied to the corneal surface can sustain a useful change in corneal thickness. Chan and Mandell (1975) instilled a total of 1000 drops of a 2% solution of saline onto the corneas of three subjects over 20 mins, and induced a 1–3% change in corneal thickness. However, after an hour the thickness reversed to baseline levels. In rabbit eyes cryo-injured to induce corneal swelling, Insler *et al.* (1987) suggested that 2% and 5% saline drops were equally effective in deswelling oedematous corneas. Unfortunately, they were unable to statistically substantiate an improvement over balanced saline control drops due to the variability of results.

14.8 CONCLUSIONS

14.8.1 CLOSING THE CREDIBILITY GAP: THE FUTURE

The goal of laboratory-based corneal research is to help further our understanding of ocular biological processes. The hope is that this will lead to effective clinical strategies in treatment of corneal disease. Unfortunately, the clinician is often alienated by the esoteric nature of much of laboratory research in corneal physiology and biophysics. The uncertain extrapolation of necessary animal studies to the clinical situation is exacerbatory but improved research techniques will hopefully propitiate the clinician.

The reader will correctly gather from this selective overview that present research findings are far from definitive. Our current understanding of corneal physiology and biophysics and the effects of contact lenses remains incomplete and answers demand analyses at the molecular level. Fortunately, we now have the research technology available.

ACKNOWLEDGMENTS

I thank various colleagues for kindly providing reprints and preprints of their research. This work was supported in part by a University of Houston Research Initiation Grant, and my thanks to Dr Stephen D. Klyce for postdoctoral sponsorship at the LSU Eye Center where experiments and ideas for this work began with support in part from USPHS grants EY03311 and EY02377 from the National Eye Institute.

REFERENCES

Abedinia, M., Pain, T., Algar, E.M. and Holmes, R.S. (1990) Bovine corneal aldehyde dehydrogenase: the major soluble corneal protein with a possible dual protective role for the eye. *Exp. Eye Res.*, **51**, 419–26.

Akiyama, R., Koniarek, J.P. and Fischbarg, J. (1990a) Effect of fluorescein on the electrical potential difference across isolated rabbit corneal endothelium. *Invest. Ophthalmol. Vis. Sci.*, **31**, 2593–5.

Akiyama, S.K., Nagata, K. and Yamada, K.M. (1990b) Cell surface receptors for extracellular matrix components. *Biochim. Biophys. Acta*, **1031**, 91–110.

Applegate, L.A. and Ley, R.D. (1991) DNA damage is involved in the induction of opacification and neovascularization of the cornea by ultraviolet radiation. *Exp. Eye Res.*, **52**, 493–7.

Atalla, L., Fernandez, M.A. and Rao, N.A. (1987) Immunohistochemical localization of catalase in ocular tissue. *Curr. Eye Res.*, **6**, 1181–7.

Bahn, C.F., Glassman, R.M., MacCallum, D.K., Lillie, J.H., Meyer, R.F., Robinson, B.J. and Rich, N.M. (1986) Postnatal development of corneal endothelium. *Invest. Ophthalmol. Vis. Sci.*, **27**, 44–51.

Barfort, P. and Maurice, D. (1974) Electrical potential and fluid transport across the corneal endothelium. *Exp. Eye Res.*, **19**, 11–19.

Baum, J.P., Maurice, D.M. and McCarey, B.E. (1984) The active and passive transport of water across the corneal endothelium. *Exp. Eye Res.*, **39**, 335–42.

Bergmanson, J.P.G. and Wilson, G.S. (1989) Ultrastructural effects of sodium chloride on the corneal epithelium. *Invest. Ophthalmol. Vis. Sci.*, **30**, 116–21.

Berkley, D.A. (1971) Influence of intraocular pressure on corneal fluid pressure, tissue stress and thickness. *Exp. Eye Res.*, **11**, 132–9.

Bonanno, J.A. (1990) Lactate-proton cotransport in rabbit corneal epithelium. *Curr. Eye Res.*, **9**, 707–12.

Bonanno, J.A. (1991) K^+ – H^+ exchange, a fundamental cell acidifier in corneal epithelium. *Am. J. Physiol.*, **260** (Cell Physiol., **29**), C618–C625.

Bonanno, J.A. and Machen, T.E. (1989) Intracellular pH regulation in basal corneal epithelial cells measured in corneal explants: characterization of Na/H exchange. *Exp. Eye Res.*, **49**, 129–42.

Bonanno, J.A. and Polse, K.A. (1987) Measurement of in vivo corneal stromal pH: open and closed eyes. *Invest. Ophthalmol. Vis. Sci.*, **28**, 522–30.

Bonvicini, F., Versura, P., Caruso, F., Maltarello, M.C., Caramazza, R. and Laschi, R. (1983) Lectin receptors on human corneal epithelium: visualization by fluorescence microscopy and electron microscopy. *Cornea*, **2**, 237–41.

Boobis, A.R., Fawthrop, D.J. and Davies, D.S. (1989) Mechanisms of cell death. *Trends Pharmacol. Sci.*, **10**, 275–80.

Boonstra, A. and Kijlstra, A. (1987) Guinea pig tears contain lactoferrin and transferrin. *Curr. Eye Res.*, **6**, 1115–23.

Bourne, W.M. and Brubaker, R.F. (1983) Decreased endothelial permeability in transplanted corneas. *Am. J. Ophthalmol.*, **96**, 362–7.

Bowman, K.A. Elijah, R.D., Cheeks, K.E. and Green, K. (1984) Intracellular potential and pH of rabbit corneal endothelial cells. *Curr. Eye Res.*, **3**, 991–1000.

Brewitt, H. and Reale, E. (1981) The basement membrane complex of the human corneal epithelium. *Graefes Arch. Klin. Exp. Ophthalmol.*, **215**, 223–31.

Bruns, R.R., Press, W. and Gross, J. (1987) A large-scale, orthogonal network of microfibril bundles in the corneal stroma. *Invest. Ophthalmol. Vis. Sci.*, **28**, 1939–46.

Burstein, N.L. and Klyce, S.D. (1977) Electrophysiologic and morphologic effects of ophthalmic preparations on rabbit corneal epithelium. *Invest. Ophthalmol. Vis. Sci.*, **16**, 899–911.

Carlson, E.C. and Waring, G.O., III. (1988) Ultrastructural analyses of enzyme-treated microfibrils in rabbit corneal stroma. *Invest. Ophthalmol. Vis. Sci.*, **29**, 578–85.

Carlson, K.H., Bourne, W.M. and Brubaker, R.F. (1988a) Effect of long-term contact lens wear on corneal endothelial morphology and function. *Invest. Ophthalmol. Vis. Sci.*, **29**, 185–93.

Carlson, K.H., Bourne, W.M., McLaren, J.W. and Brubaker, R.F. (1988b) Variations in human corneal endothelial cell morphology and permeability to fluorescein with age. *Exp. Eye Res.*, **47**, 27–41.

Carney, L.G., Mauger, T.F. and Hill, R.M. (1989) Buffering in human tears: pH responses to acid and base challenge. *Invest. Ophthalmol. Vis. Sci.*, **30**, 747–54.

Carrasquer, G., Nagel, W., Rehm, W.S. and Schwartz, M. (1987) Microelectrode studies of potential difference responses to changes in stromal K^+ in bullfrog cornea. *Biochim. Biophys. Acta*, **900**, 258–66.

Castoro, J.A., Bettelheim, A.A. and Bettelheim, F.A. (1988) Water gradients across bovine cornea. *Invest. Ophthalmol. Vis. Sci.*, **29**, 963–8.

Cejková, J., Lojda, Z., Brunová, B., Vacík, J. and Michálek, J. (1988) Disturbances in the rabbit cornea after short-term and long-term wear of hydrogel contact lenses. *Histochemistry*, **89**, 91–7.

Cenedella, R.J. and Fleschner, C.R. (1990) Kinetics of corneal epithelium turnover in vivo: studies of lovastatin. *Invest. Ophthalmol. Vis. Sci.*, **31**, 1957–62.

Chan, R.S. and Mandell, R.B. (1975) Corneal thickness changes from bathing solutions. *Am. J. Optom. Physiol. Opt.*, **52**, 465–9.

Chen, C.-H. and Chen, S.C. (1990) Lactate transport and glycolytic activity in the freshly isolated rabbit cornea. *Arch. Biochem. Biophys.*, **276**, 70–6.

Chen, J.J.Y. and Tseng. S.C.G. (1990) Corneal epithelial wound healing in partial limbal deficiency. *Invest. Ophthalmol. Vis. Sci.*, **31**, 1301–14.

Chung, J.-H., Fagerholm, P. and Lindström, B. (1988) Dry mass and water content in the corneal epithelium and superficial stroma during healing of corneal alkali wounds. *Exp. Eye Res.*, **46**, 705–15.

Cintron, C. and Hong, B.-S. (1988) Heterogeneity of collagens in rabbit cornea: type VI collagen. *Invest. Ophthalmol. Vis. Sci.*, **29**, 760–6.

Cintron, C., Gregory, J.D., Damle, S.P. and Kublin, C.L. (1990) Biochemical analyses of proteoglycans in rabbit corneal scars. *Invest. Ophthalmol. Vis. Sci.*, **31**, 1975–81.

Coroneo, M.T., Helbig, H., Korbmacher, C. and Wiederholt, M. (1989) Effect of hypotonic media on the membrane voltage of cultured bovine corneal endothelial cells. *Curr. Eye Res.*, **8**, 891–9.

Crouch, R.K., Patrick, J., Goosey, J. and Coles, W.H. (1984) The effect of age on corneal and lens superoxide dismutase. *Curr. Eye Res.*, **3**, 1119–23.

Crouse, C.A., Pflugfelder, S.C., Pereira, I., Cleary, T., Rabinowitz, S. and Atherton, S.S. (1990) Detection of herpes viral genomes in normal and diseased corneal epithelium. *Curr. Eye Res.*, **9**, 569–81.

Culton, M., Chandler, D.B., Proia, A.D., Hickingbotham, D. and Klintworth, G.K. (1990) The effect of oxygen on corneal neovascularization. *Invest. Ophthalmol. Vis. Sci.*, **31**, 1277–81.

Dikstein, S. and Maurice, D.M. (1972) The metabolic basis to the fluid pump in the cornea. *J. Physiol.*, **221**, 29–41.

DiMattio, J. (1984) In vivo entry of glucose analogs into lens and cornea of the rat. *Invest. Ophthalmol. Vis. Sci.*, **25**, 160–5.

Doughty, M.J. (1989) Physiological state of the rabbit cornea following 4 °C moist chamber storage. *Exp. Eye Res.*, **49**, 807–27.

Doughty, M.J. and Maurice, D. (1988) Bicarbonate sensitivity of rabbit corneal endothelium fluid pump in vitro. *Invest. Ophthalmol. Vis. Sci.*, **29**, 216–23.

Ehlers, N. (1970) Intracellular potentials of the corneal epithelium. *Acta Physiol. Scand.*, **78**, 471–7.

Ehlers, N. and Ehlers, D. (1966) An apparatus for studies on explanted corneae. *Acta Ophthalmol.*, **44**, 539–48.

El-Ghorab, M., Capone, A., Jr., Underwood, B.A., Hatchell, D.L., Friend, J. and Thoft, R.A. (1988) Response of ocular surface epithelium to corneal wounding in retinol-deficient rabbits. *Invest. Ophthalmol. Vis. Sci.*, **29**, 1671–6.

Elliott, G.F., Goodfellow, J.M. and Woolgar, A.E. (1980) Swelling studies of bovine corneal stroma without bounding membranes. *J. Physiol.*, **298**, 453–70.

Elner, S.G., Elner, V.M., Pavilack, M.A., Davis, H.R., Cornicelli, J.A. and Yue, B.Y.J.T. (1991) Human and monkey corneal endothelium expression of low-density lipoprotein receptors. *Am. J. Ophthalmol.*, **111**, 84–91.

Farber, J.L., Kyle, M.E. and Coleman, J.B. (1990) Biology of disease: mechanisms of cell injury by activated oxygen species. *Lab. Invest.*, **62**, 670–9.

Fee, J.P. and Edelhauser, H.F. (1970) Intracellular electrical potentials in the rabbit corneal epithelium. *Exp. Eye Res.*, **9**, 233–40.

Festen, C.M.A.W. and Slegers, J.F.G. (1979) The influence of ions, ouabain, propranolol and amiloride on the transepithelial potential and resistance of rabbit cornea. *Exp. Eye Res.*, **28**, 413–26.

Fini, M.E. and Girard, M.T. (1990) Expression of collagenolytic/gelatinolytic metalloproteinases by normal cornea. *Invest. Ophthalmol. Vis. Sci.*, **31**, 1779–88.

Fischbarg, J. (1972) Potential difference and fluid transport across rabbit corneal endothelium. *Biochim. Biophys. Acta*, **288**, 362–6.

Fischbarg, J. and Lim, J.J. (1974) Role of cations, anions and carbonic anhydrase in fluid transport across rabbit corneal endothelium. *J. Physiol.*, **241**, 647–75.

Fischbarg, J. and Lim, J.J. (1984) Fluid and electrolyte transports across corneal endothelium. *Curr. Top. Eye Res.*, **4**, 201–23.

Fischbarg, J., Hernandez, J., Liebovitch, L.S. and Koniarek, J.P. (1985) The mechanism of fluid and electrolyte transport across corneal endothelium: critical revision and update of a model. *Curr. Eye Res.*, **4**, 351–60.

Fischbarg, J., Liebovitch, L.S. and Koniarek, J.P. (1987) Inhibition of transepithelial osmotic water flow by blockers of the glucose transporter. *Biochim. Biophys. Acta*, **898**, 266–74.

Fischer, F., Voigt, G., Liegl, O. and Wiederholt, M. (1974) Effect of pH on potential difference and short circuit current in the isolated human cornea. *Pflügers Arch. Eur. J. Physiol.*, **349**, 119–31.

Fischer, F., Schmitz, L., Hoff, W., Schartl, S., Liegl, O. and Wiederholt, M. (1978) Sodium and chloride transport in the isolated human cornea. *Pflügers Arch. Eur. J. Physiol.*, **373**, 179–88.

Fogle, J.A. and Neufeld, A.H. (1979) The adrenergic and cholinergic corneal epithelium (Editorial). *Invest. Ophthalmol. Vis. Sci.*, **18**, 1212–14.

Friedenwald, J.S. and Buschke, W. (1944) The effects of excitement, of epinephrine and of sympathectomy on the mitotic activity of the corneal epithelium in rats. *Am. J. Physiol.*, **141**, 689–94.

Friedlander, P. and Zimny, M.L. (1989) Effects of soft contacts of differing thickness on corneal wound healing in rabbits. *Invest. Ophthalmol. Vis. Sci.*, **30**, 2138–47.

Friend, J., Kiorpes, T.C. and Thoft, R.A. (1981) Diabetes mellitus and the rabbit corneal epithelium. *Invest. Ophthalmol. Vis. Sci.*, **21**, 317–21.

Fujikawa, L.S., Foster, C.S., Harrist, T.J., Lanigan, J.M. and Colvi, R.B. (1981) Fibronection in healing rabbit corneal wounds. *Lab. Invest.*, **45**, 120–9.

Fukami, H., Laing, R.A., Tsubota, K., Chiba, K. and Oak, S.S. (1988) Corneal endothelial changes following minor trauma. *Invest. Ophthalmol. Vis. Sci.*, **29**, 1677–82.

Fukushi, S., Merola, L.O., Tanaka, M., Datiles, M. and Kinoshita, J.H. (1980) Reepithelization of denuded corneas in diabetic rats. *Exp. Eye Res.*, **31**, 611–21.

Funderburgh, J.L., Cintron, C., Covington, H.I. and Conrad, G.W. (1988) Immunoanalysis of keratan sulfate proteoglycan from corneal scars. *Invest. Ophthalmol. Vis. Sci.*, **29**, 1116–24.

Funderburgh, J.L., Panjwani, N., Conrad, G.W. and Baum, J. (1989) Altered keratan sulfate epitopes in keratoconus. *Invest. Ophthalmol. Vis. Sci.*, **30**, 2278–81.

Garner, M.H., Garner, W.H. and Spector, A. (1986) H_2O_2-modification of Na, K-ATPase: alterations in external Na^+ and K^+ stimulation of K^+ influx. *Invest. Ophthalmol. Vis. Sci.*, **27**, 103–7.

Gartaganis, S.P., Margaritis, L.H. and Koliopoulos, J.X. (1987) The corneal epithelium basement membrane complexes after alkali burn: an ultrastructural study. *Ann. Ophthalmol.*, **19**, 263–8.

Gaster, R.N., Binder, P.S., Coalwell, K., Berns, M., McCord, R.C. and Burstein, N.L. (1989) Corneal surface ablation by 193 nm excimer laser and wound healing in rabbits. *Invest. Ophthalmol. Vis. Sci.*, **30**, 90–8.

Gipson, I.K. and Spurr-Michaud, S.J. (1988) Localization of the β_1 subunit of integrin in stationary and migratory corneal epithelium of the rat [abstract]. *J. Cell Biol.*, **107**, 151a.

Gipson, I.K., Riddle, C.V., Kiorpes, T.C. and Spurr, S.J. (1983) Lectin binding to cell surfaces: comparisons between normal and migrating corneal epithelium. *Dev. Biol.*, **96**, 337–45.

Gipson, I.K., Spurr-Michaud, S.J. and Tisdale, A.S. (1987) Anchoring fibrils form a complex network in human and rabbit cornea. *Invest. Ophthalmol. Vis. Sci.*, **28**, 212–20.

Gipson, I.K., Spurr-Michaud, S.J., Tisdale, A.S. and Keough, M. (1989) Reassembly of the anchoring structures of the corneal epithelium during wound repair in the rabbit. *Invest. Ophthalmol. Vis. Sci.*, **30**, 425–34.

Göbbels, M., Spitznas, M. and Oldendoerp, J. (1989) Impairment of corneal epithelial barrier function in diabetics. *Graefe's Arch. Clin. Exp. Ophthalmol.*, **227**, 142–4.

Gonnering, R., Edelhauser, H.F., Van Horn, D.L. and Durant, W. (1979) The pH tolerance of rabbit and human corneal endothelium. *Invest. Ophthalmol. Vis. Sci.*, **18**, 373–90.

Goodsell, D.S. (1991) Inside a living cell. *Trends Biochem. Sci.*, **16**, 203–6.

Gordon, S.R. and Staley, C.A. (1990) Role of the cytoskeleton during injury-induced cell migration in corneal endothelium. *Cell Motil. Cytoskel.*, **16**, 47–57.

Graham, C.R., Richards, R.D. and Varma, S.D. (1981) Oxygen consumption by normal and diabetic rat and human corneas. *Ophthal. Res.*, **13**, 65–71.

Green, K. (1967) Solute movement across the constituent membranes of the cornea. *Exp. Eye Res.*, **6**, 79–92.

Green, K., Cheeks, L., Armstrong, E., Berdecia, R., Kramer, K. and Hull, D.S. (1990) Effect of pO_2 and metabolic inhibitors on ionic fluxes across the isolated rabbit corneal endothelium. *Lens Eye Toxicol. Res.*, **7.**, 103–19.

Hamano, H. and Hori, M. (1983) Effect of contact lens wear on the mitosis of epithelial cells: preliminary report. *CLAO J.*, **9**, 133–6.

Harris, J.E., Gehrsitz, L. and Gruber, L. (1956) The hydration of the cornea. II. The effect of the intraocular pressure. *Am. J. Ophthalmol.*, **42** (Part II), 325–9.

Hart, R.W. and Farrell, R.A. (1971) Structural theory of the swelling pressure of corneal stroma in saline. *Bull. Math. Biophys.*, **33**, 165–86.

Hayashi, T., Tada, T. and Kishimoto, H. (1985) H^3-thymidine incorporation into corneal epithelia of rabbits under continuous wear of oxygen-permeable hard contact lenses. *J. Jpn. Contact Lens Soc.*, **27**, 153–8.

Hayden, B.J., Zhu, L., Sens, D., *et al.* (1990) Cytolysis of corneal epithelial cells by hydrogen peroxide. *Exp. Eye Res.*, **50**, 11–16.

Hazlett, L.D. and Mathieu, P. (1989) Glycoconjugates on corneal epithelial surface: effect of neuraminidase treatment. *J. Histochem. Cytochem.*, **37**, 1215–24.

Hazlett, L.D., Spann, B., Wells, P. and Berk, R.S. (1980) Desquamation of the corneal epithelium in the immature mouse: a scanning and transmission microscopy study. *Exp. Eye Res.*, **31**, 21–30.

Hazlett, L.D., Moon, M.M., Strejc, M. and Berk, R.S. (1987) Evidence for N-acetylmannosamine as an ocular receptor for *P. aeruginosa* adherence to scarified cornea. *Invest. Ophthalmol. Vis. Sci.*, **28**, 1978–85.

He, Y.-G., Niederkorn, J.Y., McCulley, J.P., Stewart, G.L., Meyer, D.R., Silvany, R. and Dougherty, J. (1990) In vivo and in vitro collagenolytic activity of *Acanthamoeba castellanii. Invest. Ophthalmol. Vis. Sci.*, **31**, 2235–40.

Hemenger, R.P., Tomlinson, A. and McDonnell, P.J. (1990) Explanation for good visual acuity in uncorrected residual hyperopia and presbyopia after radial keratotomy. *Invest. Ophthalmol. Vis. Sci.*, **31**, 1644–6.

Herse, P.R. (1990) Corneal hydration control in normal and alloxan-induced diabetic rabbits. *Invest. Ophthalmol. Vis. Sci.*, **31**, 2205–13.

Hirano, K., Kobayashi, M., Kobayashi, K., Hoshino, T. and Awaya, S. (1989) Experimental formation of 100 nm periodic fibrils in the mouse corneal stroma and trabecular meshwork. *Invest. Ophthalmol. Vis. Sci.*, **30**, 869–74.

Hirsch, M., Nicolas, G. and Pouliquen, Y. (1989) Interfibrillary structures in fast-frozen, deep-etched and rotary-shadowed extracellular matrix of the rabbit corneal stroma. *Exp. Eye Res.*, **49**, 311–15.

Hirst, L.W., Kenyon, K.R., Fogle, J.A., Hanninen, L. and Stark, W.J. (1981) Comparative studies of corneal surface injury in the monkey and rabbit. *Arch. Ophthalmol.*, **99**, 1066–73.

Hirst, L.W., Green, W.R., Merz, W., Kaufmann, C., Visvesvara, G.S., Jensen, A. and Howard, M. (1984) Management of Acanthamoeba keratitis: a case report and review of the literature. *Ophthalmology*, **91**, 1105–11.

Hodson, S. (1971) Why the cornea swells. *J. Theor. Biol.*, **33**, 419–27.

Hodson, S. (1974) The regulation of corneal hydration by a salt pump requiring the presence of sodium and bicarbonate ions. *J. Physiol.*, **236**, 271–302.

Hodson, S. (1975) The regulation of corneal hydration to maintain high transparency in fluctuating ambient temperatures. *Exp. Eye Res.*, **20**, 375–81.

Hodson, S. and Miller, F. (1976) The bicarbonate ion pump in the endothelium which regulates the hydration of rabbit cornea. *J. Physiol.*, **263**, 563–77.

Hodson, S. and Wigham, C. (1983) The permeability of rabbit and human corneal endothelium. *J. Physiol.*, **342**, 409–19.

Hodson, S.A. and Wigham, C.G. (1985) A difference between net bicarbonate flux and short-circuit current across rabbit corneal endothelium. *J. Physiol.*, **369**, 111P. (Abstr.)

Hodson, S., O'Leary, D. and Watkins, S. (1991) The measurement of ox corneal swelling pressure by osmometry. *J. Physiol.*, **434**, 399–408.

Holden, B.A., Vannas, A., Nilsson, K., Efron, N., Sweeney, D., Kotow, M., La Hood, D. and Guillon, M. (1985) Epithelial and endothelial effects from the extended wear of contact lenses. *Curr. Eye Res.*, **4**, 739–42.

Holmes, R.S. and VandeBerg, J.L. (1986) Ocular NAD-dependent alcohol dehydrogenase and aldehyde dehydrogenase in the baboon. *Exp. Eye Res.*, **43**, 383–96.

Holmes, R.S., Cheung, B. and VandeBerg, J.L. (1989) Isoelectric focusing studies of aldehyde dehydrogenases, alcohol dehydrogenases and oxidases from mammalian anterior eye tissues. *Comp. Biochem. Physiol.*, **93B**, 271–7.

Holthöfer, H., Siegel, G.J., Tarkkanen, A. and Tervo, T. (1991) Immunocytochemical localization of carbonic anhydrase NaK-ATPase and the bicarbonate chloride exchanger in the anterior segment of the human eye. *Acta Ophthalmol.*, **69**, 149–54.

Hoshino, T. (1968) Role of the limiting membranes of the cornea in regulation of corneal hydration. *Folia Ophthalmol. Jpn.*, **19**, 276–82.

Huang, A.J.W., Tseng, S.C.G. and Kenyon, K.R. (1989) Paracellular permeability of corneal and conjunctival epithelia. *Invest. Ophthalmol. Vis. Sci.*, **30**, 684–9.

Huang, A.J.W., Tseng, S.C.G. and Kenyon, K.R. (1990) Alteration of epithelial paracellular permeability during corneal epithelial wound healing. *Invest. Ophthalmol. Vis. Sci.*, **31**, 429–35.

Huff, J.W. (1990a) Effects of sodium lactate on isolated rabbit corneas. *Invest. Ophthalmol. Vis. Sci.*, **31**, 942–7.

Huff, J.W. (1990b) Contact lens-induced edema *in vitro*: Ion transport and metabolic considerations. *Invest. Ophthalmol. Vis. Sci.*, **31**, 1288–93.

Hull, D.S. (1990) Oxygen free radicals and corneal endothelium. *Trans. Am. Ophthalmol. Soc.*, **88**, 462–511.

Hull, D.S., Green, K., Boyd, M. and Wynn, H.R. (1977) Corneal endothelium bicarbonate transport and the effect of carbonic anhydrase inhibitors on endothelial permeability and fluxes and corneal thickness. *Invest. Ophthalmol. Vis. Sci.*, **16**, 883–92.

Hull, D.S., Green, K. and Hampstead, D. (1984)

Potassium superoxide induction of rabbit corneal endothelial cell damage. *Curr. Eye Res.*, **3**, 1321–8.

Insler, M.S., Benefield, D.W. and Ross, E.V. (1987) Topical hyperosmolar solutions in the reduction of corneal edema. *CLAO J.*, **13**, 149–51.

Itoi, M., Komatsu, S. and Tanda, I. (1964) Water pump in the cornea: preliminary report. *Jpn. J. Ophthalmol.*, **8**, 212–18.

Joyce, N.C., Matkin, E.D. and Neufeld, A.H. (1989) Corneal endothelial wound closure in vitro: effects of EGF and/or indomethacin. *Invest. Ophthalmol Vis. Sci.*, **30**, 1548–59.

Jue, B. and Maurice, D.M. (1986) The mechanical properties of the rabbit and human cornea. *J. Biomech.*, **19**, 847–53.

Jumblatt, M.M. and Paterson, C.A. (1991) Prostaglandin E_2 effects on corneal endothelial cyclic adenosine monophosphate synthesis and cell shape are mediated by a receptor of the EP_2 subtype. *Invest. Ophthalmol. Vis. Sci.*, **32**, 360–5.

Jumblatt, M.M., Matkin, E.D. and Neufeld, A.H. (1988) Pharmacological regulation of morphology and mitosis in cultured rabbit corneal endothelium. *Invest. Ophthalmol. Vis. Sci.*, **29**, 586–93.

Kangas, T., Edelhauser, H.F., Twining, S.S. and O'Brien, W.J. (1990) Loss of stromal glycosaminoglycans during corneal edema. *Invest. Ophthalmol. Vis. Sci.*, **31**, 1994–2002.

Kaye, G.I. (1969) Stereological measurement of cell volume fraction of rabbit corneal stroma. *Arch. Ophthalmol.*, **82**, 792–4.

Kaye, G.I. and Donn, A. (1965) Studies on the cornea. IV. Some effects of ouabain on pinocytosis and stromal thickness in the rabbit cornea. *Invest. Ophthalmol.*, **4**, 844–52.

Kerr, J.F.R., Wyllie, A.H. and Currie, A.R. (1972) Apoptosis: a basic biological phenomenon with wide-ranging implications in tissue kinetics. *Br. J. Cancer*, **26**, 239–57.

Khalil, H.A., van Best, J.A. and de Keizer, R.J.W. (1990) The permeability of the corneal epithelium of Graves' ophthalmopathy as determined by fluorophotometry. *Doc. Ophthalmol.*, **73**, 249–54.

Kikkawa, Y. and Hirayama, K. (1970) Uneven swelling of the corneal stroma. *Invest. Ophthalmol.*, **10**, 735–41.

Kikkawa, Y. and Morimoto, K. (1980) Potential difference and short-circuit current of the regenerating corneal epithelium. *Proceedings of the IVth International Congress for Eye Research*, p. 39. (Abstract.)

Kilp, H., Helsig-Salentin, B. and Framing, D. (1985) Metabolites and enzymes in the corneal epithelium after extended contact lens wear. *Curr. Eye Res.*, **4**, 738–9.

Klotz, S.A., Au, Y.-K. and Misra, R.P. (1989) A partial-thickness epithelial defect increases the adherence of *Pseudomonas aeruginosa* to the cornea. *Invest. Ophthalmol. Vis. Sci.*, **30**, 1069–74.

Klyce, S.D. (1972) Electrical potentials in the corneal epithelium. *J. Physiol.*, **226**, 407–29.

Klyce, S.D. (1977) Enhancing fluid secretion by the corneal epithelium. *Invest. Ophthalmol. Vis. Sci.* **16**, 968–73.

Klyce, S.D. (1981) Stromal lactate accumulation can account for corneal oedema osmotically following epithelial hypoxia in the rabbit. *J. Physiol.* **321**, 49–64.

Klyce, S.D. and Bonanno, J.A. (1988) Role of the epithelium in corneal hydration. In *The Cornea: Transactions of the World Congress on the Cornea III* (ed. H.D. Cavanagh), Raven Press, New York, pp. 159–64.

Klyce, S.D. and Wong, R.K.S. (1977) Site and adrenaline action on chloride transport across the rabbit corneal epithelium. *J. Physiol.*, **266**, 777–99.

Knopf, H.L.S. (1984) Reaction to hydrogen peroxide in a contact-lens wearer. *Am. J. Ophthalmol.*, **97**, 796.

Koniarek, J.P., Lee, H.-B., Rosskothen, H.D., Liebovitch, L.S. and Fischbarg, J. (1988) Use of transendothelial electrical potential difference to assess the chondroitin sulfate effect in corneal preservation media. *Invest. Ophthalmol. Vis. Sci.*, **29**, 657–60.

Korbmacher, C., Helbig, H., Förster, C. and Wiederholt, M. (1988) Characterization of Na^+/H^+ exchange in a rabbit corneal epithelial cell line (SIRC). *Biochim. Biophys. Acta*, **943**, 405–10.

Krejci, L. (1972) Changes of pH associated with experimental trauma and acute elevation of intraocular pressure. *Ophthal. Res.*, **3**, 193–7.

Kronfeld, P. (1956) Discussion to: Von Bahr, G. Corneal thickness: its measurement and changes. *Am. J. Ophthalmol.*, **42**, 251–66.

Krueger, R.R., Trokel, S.L. and Schubert, H.D. (1985) Interaction of ultraviolet laser light with the cornea. *Invest. Ophthalmol. Vis. Sci.*, **26**, 1455–64.

Kuang, K., Xu M., Koniarek, J.P. and Fischbarg, J. (1990) Effects of ambient bicarbonate, phosphate and carbonic anhydrase inhibitors on fluid transport across rabbit corneal endothelium. *Exp. Eye Res.*, **50**, 487–93.

Kuizenga, A., van Haeringen, N.J. and Kijlstra, A. (1987) Inhibition of hydroxyl radical formation by human tears. *Invest. Ophthalmol. Vis. Sci.*, **28**, 305–13.

Kwarecki, K. and Krawcyzk, J. (1989) Comparison of the circadian rhythm in cell proliferation in corneal epithelium of male rats studied under normal and hypobaric (hypoxic) conditions. *Chronobiol. Intern.*, **6**, 217–22.

Kwok, L.S. (1983) Review: the effect of contact lens wear on the electrophysiology of the corneal epithelium. *Aust. J. Optom.*, **66**, 138–41.

Kwok, L.S. (1984) Calculation and application of the anterior surface area of a model human cornea. *J. Theor. Biol.*, **108**, 295–313.

Kwok, L.S. (1985a) Endothelial oxygen levels during anterior corneal hypoxia. *Aust. J. Optom.*, **68**, 58–62.

Kwok, L.S. (1985b) Modeling the electrophysiology of the corneal epithelium and its response to cellular injury. *Am. J. Optom. Physiol. Opt.*, **62**, 538–44.

Kwok, L.S. (1985c) Effect of epithelial cell injury on anterior corneal oxygen flux. *Am. J. Optom. Physiol. Opt.*, **62**, 642–7.

Kwok, L.S. (1986) *Physiological Properties of the Normal and Healed Cat Cornea.* PhD Thesis, University of New South Wales, Sydney, Australia.

Kwok, L.S. (1990) Application of catastrophe theory to corneal swelling. *Proc. Royal Soc. Lond.* B, **242**, 141–7.

Kwok, L.S. (1991a) Hydro-elastic deformation of rabbit corneal epithelium by intraocular pressure. ARVO Abstracts. *Invest. Ophthalmol. Vis. Sci.*, **32**, 888.

Kwok, L.S. (1991b) Kinematics of epithelial wound closure in the rabbit cornea. *Doc. Ophthalmol.*, **77**, 1–38.

Kwok, L.S. and Klyce, S.D. (1990) Theoretical basis for an anomalous temperature coefficient in swelling pressure of rabbit corneal stroma. *Biophys. J.*, **57**, 657–62.

Kwok, L.S. and Klyce, S.D. (1992) Physiological effects of tert-butyl hydroperoxide on the rabbit corneal epithelium. *CLAO J.*, **18**, 97–100.

Kwok, L.S. and Madigan, M. (1986) A new analysis of wound closure kinematics in the cat and rabbit corneal epithelium. *Clin. Exp. Optom.*, **69**, 4–12.

Landshman, N., Ben-Hanan, I., Assia, E., Ben-Chaim, O. and Belkin, M. (1988) Relationship between morphology and functional ability of regenerated corneal endothelium. *Invest. Ophthalmol. Vis. Sci.*, **29**, 1100–9.

Lauweryns, B., van den Oord, J.J., Volpes, R., Foets, F. and Missotten, L. (1991) Distribution of very late activation integrins in the human cornea: an immunohistochemical study using monoclonal antibodies. *Invest. Ophthalmol. Vis. Sci.*, **32**, 2079–85.

Lemp, M.A., Mathers, W.D. and Sachdev, M.S. (1990) The effects of contact lens wear on the morphology of corneal surface cells in the human. *Trans. Am. Ophthalmol. Soc.*, **88**, 313–25.

Liebovitch, L.S. and Tóth, T.I. (1990) Using fractals to understand the opening and closing of ion channels. *Ann. Biomed. Eng.*, **18**, 177–94.

Liebovitch, L.S. and Weinbaum, S. (1981) A model of epithelial water transport: the corneal endothelium. *Biophys. J.*, **35**, 315–38.

Liebovitch, L.S., Fischbarg, J. and Koniarek, J.P. (1987) Ion channel kinetics: a model based on fractal scaling rather than multistate Markov processes. *math. Biosc.*, **84**, 37–68.

Linsenmayer, T.F., Bruns, R.R., Mentzer, A. and Mayne, R. (1986) Type VI collagen: immunohistochemical identification as a filamentous component of the extracellular matrix of the developing avian corneal stroma. *Dev. Biol.*, **118**, 425–31.

Lyslo, A., Kvernes, S., Garlid, K. and Ratkje S.K. (1985) Ionic transport across corneal endothelium. *Acta Ophthalmol.*, **63**, 116–25.

Macdonald, J.M., Geroski, D.H. and Edelhauser, H.F. (1987) Effect of inflammation on the corneal endothelial pump and barrier. *Curr. Eye Res.*, **6**, 1125–32.

Maclean, H. and Haining, W.M. (1971) Scanning electron microscopy of cornea. *Trans. Ophthalmol. Soc. U.K.*, **91**, 31–40.

Madigan, M.C. (1989) *Cat and Monkey Cornea as Models for Extended Wear Hydrogel Contact Lens Wear in Humans.* PhD Thesis, University of New South Wales, Sydney, Australia.

Madigan, M.C., Holden, B.A. and Kwok, L.S. (1987) Extended wear of contact lenses can compromise corneal epithelial adhesion. *Curr. Eye Res.*, **6**, 1257–60.

Madsen, K., Schenholm, M., Jahnke, G. and Tengblad, A. (1989) Hyaluronate binding to intact corneas and cultured endothelial cells. *Invest. Ophthalmol. Vis. Sci.*, **30**, 2132–7.

Mandell, R.B., Polse, K.A., Brand, R.J., Vastine, D., Demartini, D. and Flom, R. (1989) Corneal hydration control in Fuch's dystrophy. *Invest. Ophthalmol. Vis. Sci.*, **30**, 845–52.

Marcus, S., Candia, O., Swinger, C. and Barker, B. (1983) Epithelial ion transport in rabbit corneas after myopic keratomileusis. ARVO Abstracts. *Invest. Ophthalmol. Vis. Sci.*, **24**, 67.

Maroudas, A. (1968) Physicochemical properties of cartilage in the light of ion exchange theory. *Biophys. J.*, **8**, 575–95.

Maroudas, A. (1975) Biophysical chemistry of cartilaginous tissues with special reference to solute and fluid transport. *Biorheology*, **12**, 233–48.

Marshall, W.S. and Hanrahan, J.W. (1991) Anion channels in the apical membrane of mammalian corneal epithelium primary cultures. *Invest. Ophthalmol. Vis. Sci.*, **32**, 1562–8.

Masters, B.R. and Paddock, S. (1990) *In vitro* confocal imaging of the rabbit cornea. *J. Microsc.*, **158**, 267–74.

Masters, B.R., Subramanian, V.H. and Chance, B. (1983) Rabbit cornea stromal hydration measured with proton NMR spectroscopy. *Curr. Eye Res.*, **2**, 317–21.

Masters, B.R., Ghosh, A.K., Wilson, J. and Matschinsky, F.M. (1989) Pyridine nucleotides and phosphorylation potential of rabbit corneal epithelium and endothelium. *Invest. Ophthalmol. Vis. Sci.*, **30**, 861–8.

Mattey, D.L. and Garrod, D.R. (1984) Role of glycosaminoglycans and collagen in the development of a fibronectin-rich extracellular matrix in cultured embryonic corneal epithelial cells. *J. Cell Sci.*, **67**, 189–202.

Maurice, D.M. (1957) The structure and transparency of the cornea. *J. Physiol.*, **136**, 263–86.

Maurice, D.M. (1961) The use of permeability studies in the investigation of submicroscopic structure. In *The Structure of the Eye* (ed. G.K. Smelser), Academic Press, London and New York, pp. 381–91.

Maurice, D.M. (1972) The location of the fluid pump in the cornea. *J. Physiol.*, **221**, 43–54.

Maurice, D.M. (1984) The cornea and sclera. In *The Eye, Vol. 1b* (ed. H. Davson), Academic Press, Orlando, pp. 1–158.

Maurice, D. (1991) Letter to the editor; reply. *Invest. Ophthalmol. Vis. Sci.*, **32**, 2163; 2166.

Maurice, D.M. and Giardini, A.A. (1951) Swelling of the cornea *in vivo* after the destruction of its limiting layers. *Br. J. Ophthalmol.*, **35**, 791–7.

Mayer, U. (1980) Comparative investigations of catalase activity in different ocular tissues of cattle and man. *Graefes Arch. Klin. Exp. Ophthalmol.*, **213**, 261–5.

McCally, R.L. and Farrell, R.A. (1988) Interaction of light and the cornea: light scattering versus transparency. In *The Cornea: Transactions of the World Congress on the Cornea III* (ed. H.D. Cavanagh), Raven Press, New York, pp. 165–71.

McCartney, M.D., Robertson, D.P., Wood, T.O. and McLaughlin, B.J. (1987) ATPase pump site density in human dysfunctional corneal endothelium. *Invest. Ophthalmol. Vis. Sci.*, **28**, 1955–62.

McLaughlin, B.J., Barlar, E.K. and Donaldson, D.J. (1986) Wheat germ agglutinin and concanavalin A binding during epithelial wound healing in the cornea. *Curr. Eye Res.*, **5**, 601–9.

McPhee, T.J., Bourne, W.M. and Brubaker, R.F. (1985) Location of the stress-bearing layers of the cornea. *Invest. Ophthalmol. Vis. Sci.*, **26**, 869–72.

McTigue, J.W. and Fine, B.S. (1966) The basement membrane of the corneal epithelium. *Sixth International Congress for Electron Microscopy*, Kyoto, pp. 775–6.

Mecke, H., Schünke, M., Schnaidt, S., Freys, I. and Semm, K. (1991) Width of thermal damage after using the YAG contact laser for cutting biological tissue: animal experimental investigation. *Res. Exp. Med.*, **191**, 37–45.

Meyer, L.A., Ubels, J.L. and Edelhauser, H.F. (1988) Corneal endothelial morphology in the rat. Effects of aging, diabetes, and topical aldose reductase inhibitor treatment. *Invest. Ophthalmol. Vis. Sci.*, **29**, 940–8.

Mishima, S. and Kudo, T. (1967) In vitro incubation of the rabbit cornea. *Invest. Ophthalmol.*, **6**, 329–39.

Mishima, S. and Trenberth, S.M. (1968) Permeability of the corneal endothelium to nonelectrolytes. *Invest. Ophthalmol.*, **7**, 34–43.

Miyata, K., Murao, M., Sawa, M. and Tanishima, T. (1990) New wound-healing model using cultured corneal endothelial cells. 1. Quantitative study of healing process. *Jpn. J. Ophthalmol.*, **34**, 257–66.

Miyauchi, S. and Iwata, S. (1984) Biochemical studies on the use of sodium hyaluronate in the anterior eye segment: IV. The protective efficacy of the corneal endothelium. *Curr. Eye Res.*, **3**, 1063–7.

Nadakavukaren, M.J., Fitch, K.L. and Richardson, A. (1987) Dietary restriction retards age-related decrease in cell population of rat corneal endothelium. *Proc. Soc. Exp. Biol. Med.*, **184**, 98–101.

Ohashi, Y., Motokura, M., Kinoshita, Y., Mano, T.,

Watanabe, H., Kinoshita, S., Manabe, R., Oshiden, K. and Yanaihara, C. (1989) Presence of epidermal growth factor in human tears. *Invest. Ophthalmol. Vis. Sci.*, **30**, 1879–82.

Okuhara, S. and Kikkawa, Y. (1968) Studies on the potential difference of the regenerating epithelium of the cornea. *Acta Ophthalmol. Soc. Jpn.*, **72**, 990–3.

O'Leary, D.J. (1985a) Anatomy and physiology of the epithelium. In *The Eye in Contact Lens Wear* (ed. J.R. Larke), Butterworths, London, pp. 59–88.

O'Leary, D.J. (1985b) Stroma and Bowman's layer. In *The Eye in Contact Lens Wear* (ed. J. R. Larke), Butterworths, London, pp. 123–46.

O'Leary, D.J. and Millodot, M. (1981) Abnormal epithelial fragility in diabetes and contact lens wear. *Acta Ophthalmol.*, **59**, 827–33.

O'Leary, D.J., Wilson, G. and Bergmanson, J. (1985) The influence of calcium in the tear-side perfusate on desquamation from the rabbit corneal epithelium. *Curr. Eye Res.*, **4**, 721–31.

Päällysaho, T. and Williams, D.S. (1991) Epithelial cell-substrate adhesion in the cornea: Localization of actin, talin, integrin, and fibronectin. *Exp. Eye Res.*, **52**, 261–7.

Panjwani, N., Drysdale, J., Clark, B., Alberta, J. and Baum, J. (1989) Protein-related abnormalities in keratoconus. *Invest. Ophthalmol. Vis. Sci.*, **30**, 2481–7.

Panjwani, N., Clark, B., Cohen, M., Barza, M. and Baum, J. (1990) Differential binding of *P. aeruginosa* and *S. aureus* to corneal epithelium in culture. *Invest. Ophthalmol. Vis. Sci.*, **31**, 696–701.

Pfister, R.R., Haddox, J.L., Lam, K.-W. and Lank, K.M. (1988) Preliminary characterization of a polymorphonuclear leukocyte stimulant isolated from alkali-treated collagen. *Invest. Ophthalmol. Vis. Sci.*, **29**, 955–62.

Polse, K.A., Brand, R.J., Mandell, R.B., Vastine, D., Demartini, D. and Flom, R. (1989) Age differences in corneal hydration control. *Invest. Ophthalmol. Vis. Sci.*, **30**, 392–9.

Polse, K.A., Brand, R.J., Cohen, S.R. and Guillon, M. (1990) Hypoxic effects on corneal morphology and function. *Invest. Ophthalmol. Vis. Sci.*, **31**, 1542–54.

Quantock, A.J., Meek, K.M., Ridgway, A.E.A., Bron, A.J. and Thonar, E.J.- M.A. (1990) Macular corneal dystrophy: reduction in both corneal thickness and collagen interfibrillar spacing. *Curr. Eye Res.*, **9**, 393–8.

Rae, J.L., Levis, R.A. and Eisenberg, R.S. (1988) Ionic channels in ocular epithelia. In *Ion Channels*, Vol. 1 (ed. T. Narahashi), Plenum Press, New York, pp. 283–327.

Rae, J.L., Dewey, J. and Cooper, K. (1989a) Properties of single potassium selective ionic channels from the apical membrane of rabbit corneal endothelium. *Exp. Eye Res.*, **49**, 591–609.

Rae, J.L., Lewno, A.W., Cooper, K. and Gates, P. (1989b) Dye and electrical coupling between cells of the rabbit corneal endothelium. *Curr. Eye Res.*, **8**, 859–69.

Rae, J.L., Dewey, J., Rae, J.S., Nesler, M. and Cooper, K. (1990a) Single potassium channels in corneal epithelium. *Invest. Ophthalmol. Vis. Sci.*, **31**, 1799–809.

Rae, J.L., Dewey, J., Cooper, K. and Gates, P. (1990b) A non-selective cation channel in rabbit corneal endothelium activated by internal calcium and inhibited by internal ATP. *Exp. Eye Res.*, **50**, 373–84.

Raphael, B. and McLaughlin, B.J. (1990) Adsorptive and fluid phase endocytosis by cultured rabbit corneal endothelium. *Curr. Eye Res.*, **9**, 249–58.

Refojo M.F. (1975) Metabolic-dependent osmotic mechanism for the maintenance of corneal deturgescence *in vivo*. Unpublished paper, given at the Cornea Conference, Boston.

Reinach, P.S. (1985) Roles of cyclic AMP and Ca in epithelial ion transport across corneal epithelium: a review. *Curr. Eye Res.*, **4**, 385–97.

Riley, M.V. (1982) Transport of ions and metabolites across the corneal endothelium. In *Cell Biology of the Eye* (ed. D. McDevitt), Academic Press, New York and London, pp. 53–95.

Riley, M.V. and Giblin, F.J. (1983) Toxic effects of hydrogen peroxide on corneal endothelium. *Curr. Eye Res.*, **2**, 451–8.

Riley, M.V. and Winkler, B.S. (1990) Strong Pasteur effect in rabbit corneal endothelium preserves fluid transport under anaerobic conditions. *J. Physiol.*, **426**, 81–93.

Riley, M.V., Susan, S., Peters, M.I. and Schwartz, C.A. (1987) The effects of UV-B irradiation on the corneal endothelium. *Curr. Eye Res.*, **6**, 1021–33.

Risen, L.A, Binder, P.S. and Nayak, S.K. (1987) Intermediate filaments and their organization in human corneal endothelium. *Invest. Ophthalmol. Vis. Sci.*, **28**, 1933–8.

Rojanasakul, Y. and Robinson, J.R. (1991) The cytoskeleton of the cornea and its role in tight junction permeability. *Int. J. Pharm.*, **68**, 135–49.

Savion, N., Farzame, N. and Berlin, H.B. (1989) Characterization of bicarbonate-dependent potassium uptake in cultured corneal endothelial cells. *Invest. Ophthalmol. Vis. Sci.*, **30**, 690–7.

Sawaguchi, S., Yue, B.Y.J.T., Chang, I., Sugar, J. and Robin, J. (1991) Proteoglycan molecules in keratoconus corneas. *Invest. Ophthalmol. Vis. Sci.*, **32**, 1846–53.

Schoessler, J.P. and Woloschak, M.J. (1981) Corneal endothelium in veteran PMMA contact lens wearers. *Int. Contact Lens Clin.*, **8** (6), 19–25.

Schultz, R.O., Matsuda, M., Yee, R.W., Edelhauser, H.F. and Schultz, K.J. (1984) Corneal endothelial changes in type I and type II diabetes mellitus. *Am. J. Ophthalmol.*, **98**, 401–10.

Scott, J.E. and Haigh, M. (1985) 'Small' proteoglycan:collagen interactions: keratan sulphate proteoglycan associates with rabbit corneal collagen fibrils at the 'a' and 'c' bands. *Biosc. Rep.*, **5**, 765–74.

Shearer, T.R., Azuma, M., David, L.L., Yamagata, Y. and Murachi, T. (1990) Calpain and calpastatin in rabbit corneal epithelium. *Curr. Eye Res.*, **9**, 39–44.

Sher, N.A., Bowers, R.A., Zabel, R.W., Frantz, J.M., Eiferman, R.A., Brown, D.C., Rowsey, J.J., Parker, P., Chen, V. and Lindstrom, R.L. (1991) Clinical use of the 193-nm excimer laser in the treatment of corneal scars. *Arch. Ophthalmol.*, **109**, 491–8.

Sokol, J.L., Masur, S.K., Asbell, P.A. and Wolosin, J.M. (1990) Layer-by-layer desquamation of corneal epithelium and maturation of tear-facing membranes. *Invest. Ophthalmol. Vis. Sci.*, **31**, 294–304.

Soong, H.K. (1987) Vinculin in focal cell-to-substrate attachments of spreading corneal epithelial cells. *Arch. Ophthalmol.*, **105**, 1129–32.

Spurr-Michaud, S.J., Barza, M. and Gipson, I.K. (1988) An organ culture system for study of adherence of *Pseudomonas aeruginosa* to normal and wounded corneas. *Invest. Ophthalmol. Vis. Sci.*, **29**, 379–86.

Srivastava, S.K., Ansari, N.H., Liu, S., Izban, A., Das, B. and Szabo, G. (1989) The effect of oxidants on biomembranes and cellular metabolism. *Molec. Cell. Biochem.*, **91**, 149–57.

Stefánsson, E., Foulks, G.N. and Hamilton, R.C. (1987) The effect of corneal contact lenses on the oxygen tension in the anterior chamber of the rabbit eye. *Invest. Ophthalmol. Vis. Sci.*, **28**, 1716–19.

Stein, R.M., Bourne, W.M. and Campbell, R.J. (1986) Chondroitin sulfate for corneal preservation at 4 °C: evaluation by electron microscopy. *Arch. Ophthalmol.*, **104**, 1358–61.

Stern, D., Lin, W.-Z., Puliafito, C.A and Fujimoto, J.G. (1989) Femtosecond optical ranging of corneal incision depth. *Invest. Ophthalmol. Vis. Sci.*, **30**, 99–104.

Stocker, F.W. (1954) The endothelium of the cornea and its clinical implications. *Trans. Am. Ophthalmol. Soc.*, **51**, 669–786.

Stocker, F.W. and Reichle, K. (1974) Theodor Leber and the endothelium of the cornea. *Am. J. Ophthalmol.*, **78**, 893–6.

Stolwijk, T.R., van Best, J.A., Boot, J.P., Lemkes, H.H.P.J. and Oosterhuis, J.A. (1990) Corneal epithelial barrier function after oxybuprocaine provocation in diabetics. *Invest. Ophthalmol. Vis. Sci*, **31**, 436–9.

Stopak, S.S., Roat, M.I., Nauheim, R.C., Turgeon, P.W., Sossi, G., Kowalski, R.P. and Thoft, R.A. (1991) Growth of Acanthamoeba on human corneal epithelial cells and keratocytes in vitro. *Invest. Ophthalmol. Vis. Sci.*, **32**, 354–9.

Stryer, L. (1988) *Biochemistry*. W.H. Freeman, New York.

Sturges, S.A and Conrad, G.W. (1987) Acetylcholinesterase activity in the cornea of the developing chick embryo. *Invest. Ophthalmol. Vis. Sci.*, **28**, 850–8.

Sugrue, S.P. (1987) Isolation of collagen binding proteins from embryonic chicken corneal epithelial cells. *J. Biol. Chem.*, **262**, 3338–43.

Sugrue, S.P. and Hay, E.D. (1986) The identification of extracellular matrix (ECM) binding sites on the basal surface of embryonic corneal epithelium and the effect of ECM binding on epithelial collagen production. *J. Cell Biol.*, **102**, 1907–16.

Thoft, R.A and Friend, J. (1975) Permeability of regenerated corneal epithelium. *Exp. Eye Res.*, **21**, 409–16.

Thompson, H.W., Malter, J.S., Steinemann, T.L. and Beuerman, R.W. (1991) Flow cytometry measurements of the DNA content of corneal epithelial cells during wound healing. *Invest. Ophthalmol. Vis. Sci.*, **32**, 433–6.

Tisdale, A.S., Spurr-Michaud, S.J., Rodrigues, M., Hackett, J., Krachmer, J. and Gipson, I.K. (1988) Development of the anchoring structures of the epithelium in rabbit and human fetal corneas. *Invest. Ophthalmol. Vis. Sci.*, **29**, 727–36.

Toivanen, M., Tervo, T., Partanen, M., Vannas, A.

and Hervonen, A. (1987) Histochemical demonstration of adrenergic nerves in the stroma of human cornea. *Invest. Ophthalmol. Vis. Sci.*, **28**, 398–400.

Trinkhaus-Randall, V., Newton, A.W. and Franzblau, C. (1990) The synthesis and role of integrin in corneal epithelial cells in culture. *Invest. Ophthalmol. Vis. Sci.*, **31**, 440–7.

Trinkhaus-Randall, V., Liebowitz, H.M., Ryan, W.J. and Kupferman, A. (1991) Quantification of stromal destruction in the inflamed cornea. *Invest. Ophthalmol. Vis. Sci.*, **32**, 603–9.

Trope, G.E. and Rumley, A.G. (1984) Catecholamine concentrations in tears. *Exp. Eye Res.*, **39**, 247–50.

Tsubota, K., Chiba, K. and Shimazakai, J. (1991) Corneal epithelium in diabetic patients. *Cornea*, **10**, 156–60.

Tuft, S., Zabel, R.W. and Marshall, J. (1989) Corneal repair following keratectomy: a comparison between conventional surgery and laser photoablation. *Invest. Ophthalmol. Vis. Sci.*, **30**, 1769–77.

Ubels, J.L. and MacRae, S.M. (1984) Vitamin A is present as retinol in the tears of humans and rabbits. *Curr. Eye Res.*, **3**, 815–22.

van der Heyden, C., Weekers, J.F. and Schoffeniels, E. (1975) Sodium and chloride transport across the isolated rabbit cornea. *Exp. Eye Res.*, **20**, 89–96.

van Setten, G.-B. (1990) Epidermal growth factor in human tear fluid: increased release but decreased concentrations during reflex tearing. *Curr. Eye Res.*, **9**, 79–83.

Walkenbach, R.J. and Ye, G.-S. (1990) Muscarinic receptors and their regulation of cyclic GMP in corneal endothelial cells. *Invest. Ophthalmol. Vis. Sci.*, **31**, 702–7.

Walkenbach, R.J. and Ye, G.-S. (1991) Muscarinic cholinoceptor regulation of cyclic guanosine monophosphate in human corneal epithelium. *Invest. Ophthalmol. Vis. Sci.*, **32**, 610–15.

Walkenbach, R.J., Gibbs, S.R., Bylund, D.B. and Chao, W.-T.H. (1984) Characteristics of β-adrenergic receptors in bovine corneal epithelium: comparison of fresh tissue and cultured cells. *Biochem. Biophys. Res. Comm.*, **121**, 664–72.

Watanabe, K., Nakagawa, S. and Nishida, T. (1988) Chemotactic and haptotactic activities of fibronectin for cultured rabbit corneal epithelial cells. *Invest. Ophthalmol. Vis. Sci.*, **29**, 572–7.

Watanabe, K., Frangieh, G., Reddy, C.V. and Kenyon, K.R. (1991) Effect of fibronectin on corneal epithelial wound healing in the vitamin A-deficient rat. *Invest. Ophthalmol. Vis. Sci.*, **32**, 2159–62.

Welsh M.J., Shasby, D.M. and Husted, R.M. (1985) Oxidants increase paracellular permeability in a cultured epithelial cell line. *J. Clin. Invest.*, **76**, 1155–68.

Whikehart, D.R., Edwards, W.C. and Pfister, R.R. (1991) Sorption of sodium hydroxide by type I collagen and bovine corneas. *Cornea*, **10**, 54–8.

Wigham, C. and Hodson, S. (1981a) The effect of bicarbonate ion concentration on trans-endothelial short circuit current in ox corneas. *Curr. Eye Res.*, **1**, 37–41.

Wigham, C. and Hodson, S. (1981b) Bicarbonate and the trans-endothelial short circuit current of human cornea. *Curr. Eye Res.*, **1**, 285–90.

Wigham, C. and Hodson, S. (1985) The movement of sodium across short-circuited rabbit corneal endothelium. *Curr. Eye Res.*, **4**, 1241–5.

Wiig, H. (1989) Cornea fluid dynamics. I. Measurement of hydrostatic and colloid osmotic pressure in rabbits. *Exp. Eye Res.*, **49**, 1015–30.

Wilson, G., O'Leary, D.J. and Vaughan, W. (1984) Differential swelling in compartments of the corneal stroma. *Invest. Ophthalmol. Vis. Sci.*, **25**, 1105–8.

Wolosin, J.M. (1988) Regeneration of resistance and ion transport in rabbit corneal epithelium after induced surface cell exfoliation. *J. Membr. Biol.*, **104**, 45–55.

Worthington, C.R. (1984) The structure of cornea. *Quart. Rev. Biophys.*, **17**, 423–51.

Xiao, G.Q., King, G.S. and Masters, B.R. (1990) Observation of the rabbit cornea and lens with a new real-time confocal scanning optical microscope. *Scanning*, **12**, 161–6.

Yuan, N. and Pitts, D.G. (1991) Residual H_2O_2 compromises deswelling function of in vivo rabbit cornea. *Acta Ophthalmol.*, **69**, 241–6.

Zantos, S.G. and Holden, B.A. (1977) Transient endothelial changes soon after wearing contact lenses. *Am. J. Optom. Physiol. Opt.*, **54**, 856–8.

Zieske, J.D., Higashijima, S.C., Spurr-Michaud, S.J. and Gipson, I.K. (1987) Biosynthetic responses of the rabbit cornea to a keratectomy wound. *Invest. Ophthalmol. Vis. Sci.*, **28**, 1668–77.

Zieske, J.D., Bukusoglu, G. and Gipson, I.K. (1988) Synthesis of vinculin is enhanced during corneal epithelial migration. ARVO Abstracts. *Invest. Ophthalmol. Vis. Sci.*, **29** (Suppl.), 53.

BIOCHEMICAL ASPECTS OF THE CORNEA

B.R. Masters

15.1 INTRODUCTION.

This chapter is intended to serve as a guide to the literature on the biochemistry of the cornea. Due to the size limitations of the chapter, the author has chosen to emphasize the role of oxygen and respiratory metabolism. Contact lens wear has a multitude of biochemical effects on the cornea (O'Leary, 1985; and Hamano & Kaufman, 1987; Holden *et al.*, 1987). Some of the effects are transitory and others are long term; adaptive mechanisms also occur. Therefore, the time course of biochemical assays is important. Finally, the scientist and the clinician must determine if the biochemical changes are important to the function and structure of the cornea. Small changes in enzyme activity may be critical for corneal function; alternatively, relatively large changes in metabolite concentration or enzyme activity may have little consequence for corneal function and transparency.

15.2 BIOCHEMISTRY OF THE CORNEA

This chapter will serve a guide to the literature on biochemistry and the regulation of metabolism. It will cover the biochemical pathways (Reinach & Pasnikowski, 1963; Reich & Sel'kov, 1981; Riley, 1982; Stanifer *et al.*, 1983; Sies, 1985; Edelhauser *et al.*, 1986;

Klyce & Beuerman, 1988; Scholte, 1988; Reim, 1989) and describe the regulation and control of metabolic function. (Atkinson, 1977; Sies, 1982, 1985). Many articles on the biochemistry of the cornea discuss only the former aspects; it is the regulation of cellular biochemistry that is important for the contact lens scientist.

15.3 OXYGEN AND RESPIRATORY METABOLISM

We need oxygen for life; but why? How is oxygen used by the cells in the body? What are mitochondria, and how do they function? These questions are discussed in this section (Perkins, 1964; Keilin, 1966; Gilbert, 1981a,b,c; Kanfer & Turo, 1981).

Lavoisier proposed that there is a combustion of food in the body, but incorrectly placed the site in the blood. It was Spallanzani who correctly placed respiration in the tissues. Almost a decade later, in 1884, MacMunn discovered the heme pigments, which we now call cytochromes. In 1925, Warburg concluded that aerobic cells contain Atmungsferment, which is cytochrome oxidase. At about the same time, Keilin (1966) was able to characterize the absorption spectrum of the oxidized and reduced cytochromes. These investigations formed the basis for the optical measurement of cellular respiration

Contact Lens Practice. Edited by Montague Ruben and Michel Guillon.
Published in 1994 by Chapman & Hall, London. ISBN 0 412 35120 X

that developed into the modern non-invasive optical methods to measure cellular oxidation. Lehninger and Kennedy demonstrated that mitochondria were the sites of ATP synthesis, as well as the sites for the citric acid and fatty oxidation biochemical pathways. In the 1960s Chance, using new dual wavelength spectrophotometric methods, demonstrated the sequence of the electron transport chain in mitochondria as follows:

Substrates → pyridine nucleotides → flavoproteins → cyt b → cyt c → cyt a → cyt a3 → oxygen

The carrier of chemical free energy is ATP which is formed continuously and converted into adenosine diphosphate (ADP) and free energy, which is used for active transport, mechanical work and biosynthesis. Cells derive useful free energy from the oxidation of substances such as glucose and fatty acids. Electrons are ultimately transferred from the substrates to oxygen with the concomitant formation of ATP and the reduction of oxygen to water. This process is called oxidative phosphorylation (Reinach & Pasnikowski, 1963). However, the electron transfer is not direct from the substrates to oxygen; the electrons are transferred in a step wise fashion through a series of electron carriers. The pyridine nucleotides (NADH) and the flavins ($FADH_2$) are the main electron carriers for the oxidation of substrates.

The major electron acceptor in the oxidation of substrates is nicotinamide adenine dinucleotide (NAD^+). The nicotinamide ring of the NAD^+ accepts two electrons and a hydrogen ion in the oxidation of substrate. The resulting species is the reduced form of the electron carrier, and is called NADH. An important property for our optical studies is that the molecule NADH exhibits a strong fluorescence centred at 450 nm when excited with light of about 366 nm (Chance, 1976; Laing et al., 1980; Masters, 1984a). The NAD^+ shows almost no fluorescence under the same conditions. This property forms the biochemical basis of a fluorescence method to measure the respiratory activity of cells by measuring their intrinsic fluorescence. This method is called redox fluorometry.

Flavin adenine dinucleotide (FAD) is the other major electron carrier in the oxidation of substrates. FAD is a component in a variety of flavoproteins and forms the prosthetic group of succinate-Q reductase. FAD is the oxidized form and the reduced form is $FADH_2$. The isoalloxazine ring of FAD can accept two electrons to form the reduced form. There is a series of flavoproteins which undergo electron transfer reactions. The optical property of interest is that the oxidized form (FAD) has a strong fluorescence in the region of 550 nm when excited with light of 450 nm. The reduced form of the molecule ($FADH_2$) shows very weak fluorescence. Electrons from NADH are transferred to the respiratory chain at NADH-Q reductase, which is also named NADH dehydrogenase. Two electrons from NADH are accepted by the flavin mononucleotide (FMN), which forms the prosthetic group of NADH-Q reductase to yield the reduced form, $FMNH_2$.

Reductive biosynthesis requires NADPH in addition to ATP. The reduced form of nicotinamide adenine dinucleotide phosphate is $NADP^+$. While NADPH carries electrons in a similar manner to NADH, there is an important difference. NADH is used primarily for the production of ATP, while NADPH is used almost exclusively for reductive biosynthesis.

There are some additional biochemical aspects of metabolism that require mention: oxidative phosphorylation, glycolysis and finally the pentose phosphate pathway. Oxidative phosphorylation is the biochemical process in which ATP is synthesized as electrons are transferred from NADH or $FADH_2$ to oxygen by a series of electron carriers. This process occurs in respiratory assemblies located in the inner membrane of the mitochondria. The reactions of the citric acid cycle and fatty acid oxidation occur in the mitochondrial matrix. In the process of oxidative phosphorylation, the electron-transfer potential of the electron carriers NADH and $FADH_2$ is converted to the phosphate-transfer potential of ATP.

Electrons are transferred from NADH to oxygen by a respiratory chain. The respiratory chain in the mitochondria is made up of three enzyme complexes that are linked by two mobile electron carriers. The protein complexes are NADH-Q reductase, cytochrome reductase and cytochrome oxidase. The two mobile carriers are ubiquinone and cytochrome c. Ubiquinone also transfers electrons from $FADH_2$ to cytochrome reductase.

The generation of ATP, which accompanies the flow of electrons along the respiratory chain from NADH to oxygen, occurs at three sites along the chain. These sites can be specifically blocked by inhibitors which are specific for each site. Electron transfer between NADH-Q reductase and ubiquinone (QH_2) can be inhibited by rotenone or amytal. Electron transfer between QH_2 and cytochrome c can be inhibited by antimycin A. And electron transfer between cytochrome oxidase and oxygen can be inhibited with cyanide, azide or carbon monoxide. In fact, this is the chemical basis of carbon monoxide poisoning.

ATP can also be synthesized by glycolysis. Glycolysis is a set of chemical reactions in which glucose is converted to pyruvate with the production of ATP. One of the by-products from this sequence of reactions is the conversion of NAD^+ into NADH. This is the source of the cytoplasmic NADH. Glycolysis is the prelude to the citric acid cycle and the electron transport chain. There are two main functions of glycolysis: to generate ATP and to produce NADH which is used in cellular synthesis (actually NADPH).

Finally, the role of the pentose phosphate pathway in the synthesis of NADPH should be reviewed. NADPH has similar fluorescence spectral properties as NADH in solution. However, there are differences in their biochemical utilization: NADH is oxidized by the mitochondrial respiratory chain to generate ATP, and NADPH is used in reductive biosynthesis as a hydride ion donor. The main functions of the pentose phosphate pathway are the generation of NADPH and the synthesis of five-carbon sugars. The pentose phosphate pathway is reversibly linked to the glycolytic pathway. It should be noted that the rate of the pentose phosphate pathway is regulated by the concentration of $NADP^+$ in the cytosol.

15.4 NON-INVASIVE METHODS TO STUDY RESPIRATORY METABOLISM

The basic principle of redox fluorometry may be described as follows: the intensity of the fluorescence signal from the reduced pyridine nucleotides is an indicator of the degree of respiratory function occurring within the cell (Chance, 1976; Masters 1981a,b,c, 1982a,b, 1984a,b,c, 1986, 1988a,b,c, 1990b,c, Masters *et al.*, 1980, 1983a,b, 1987, 1989). The intensity of fluorescence is given by the product of the incident light intensity, the quantum yield of the fluorescence and the concentration of the fluorescing molecule. Several molecular species contribute to the measured 'pyridine nucleotide fluorescence'. The list of contributing molecular species includes bound and free species of both NADH and NADPH and other chromophores, which are usually labelled non-specific fluorescence.

The cellular concentration of NADH is determined by the difference between the rates at which reducing equivalents are supplied by the dehydrogenases and the rate of transfer of these reducing equivalents to the mitochondrial respiratory chain. If the rate of supply exceeds the rate of transfer, the cell redox state becomes more reduced; if the transfer rate exceeds the supply rate, the cell redox state becomes more oxidized. The cell redox state responds to alterations in the mitochondrial workload and to the availability of oxygen and metabolic substrates. Increased intracellular work loads result in more oxidation of the pyridine nucleotides; decreased workloads result in more reduction of the pyridine nucleotides. The cell redox level is very sensitive to the concentration of oxygen, and therefore the fluorescence of the reduced pyridine nucleotides can serve as an optical probe of oxygen concentration.

What can be measured in the tissue is the following: the fluorescence intensity from the reduced pyridine nucleotides NAD(P)H. This intensity may have components from both the cytoplasmic and the mitochondrial spaces. What is not directly measured is the ratio of $NAD^+/NADH$. In order to measure this quantity it is necessary to measure the tissue under conditions in which the pyridine nucleotides are fully reduced and fully oxidized. While the fully reduced state is easily obtained (anoxia or cyanide inhibition of cytochrome oxidase) the fully oxidized state is more difficult to obtain even with the use of uncoupling agents. Chemical analysis of the cells can aid in the interpretation of the optical results, although they measure different components and cannot be directly compared to the fluorometric measurements. The main advantage of optical studies, in spite of the previously mentioned limitations, is that they provide a real-time, non-invasive signal, which under careful experimental analysis, can be used to measure cellular respiratory function and, in ocular tissue, provide a functional measure of cell function in the normal and pathological living eye.

15.5 APPLICATIONS TO THE CORNEA

The first study on the intrinsic fluorescence emission from the cornea was performed at liquid nitrogen temperatures in order to enhance the intensity of the mitochondrial signals (Nissen *et al.*, 1980). A comparison of the emission spectra from both the epithelial and the endothelial sides of the cornea and frozen suspensions of mitochondria indicated that the signals were from the mitochondria. The authors also concluded from the flavoprotein/pyridine nucleotide redox ratio that the endothelial cells were more oxidized than the epithelial cells. While the redox fluorescence from the epithelial side was mainly from the epithelial cells, the signal from the endothelial side also included signals from the stroma. The redox signals were further characterized in a study of redox signals from freeze trapped rabbit and rat corneas that were subjected to hypoxia or histotoxic anoxia prior to freezing. This study found that inhibiting electron transport in the mitochondria resulted in a 26 per cent increase of fluorescence intensity from the pyridine nucleotides in the epithelium and only a 16 per cent increase in the fluorescence intensity from the endothelium. Both anoxia from nitrogen and cytochrome oxidase inhibition with sulphide gave similar results.

The next set of investigations addressed the relationship between alterations of the mitochondrial redox state of the rabbit corneal endothelium and physiological function, specifically transendothelial potential difference, and rates of endothelial fluid transport (Masters *et al.*, 1982b). These studies showed that amobarbital (an inhibitor of mitochondrial electron transport at site I) results in a decrease of the rate of transendothelial fluid transport, and a dose-dependent increase in the fluorescence intensity from the reduced pyridine nucleotides. A second study using perfused rabbit cornea related the changes in both the redox fluorescence intensity from reduced pyridine nucleotides and oxidized flavoproteins to measured values of transendothelial potential difference (Masters *et al.*, 1983b). The mitochondrial respiratory chain inhibitors of electron transport, azide, cyanide, amytal and sulphide, were incubated with perfused corneas and the fluorescence was measured from the reduced pyridine nucleotides and the oxidized flavoproteins as a function of inhibitor concentration. The Law of Mass Action was used to determine the inhibition constant and the number of moles of inhibitor bound per mole of inhibited enzyme for each inhibitor. The latter quantity was approximately 1. It was found that the change in transendothelial potential difference was proportional to the log of the inhibitor concentration. This study supports the correlation between corneal redox state measured from intensity measurements and corneal endothelial transport function.

Several subsequent reports involved calibration studies of the redox fluorescence intensity of corneal epithelial cells as a function of the oxygen tension at the anterior corneal surface (Masters, 1986, 1988b). In studies using a perfused rabbit corneal preparation it was demonstrated that both nitrogen and cyanide result in identical increases in the fluorescence intensity. Upon removal from the epithelial surface it was found that both nitrogen and cyanide (an inhibitor of cytochrome oxidase in the mitochondria) result in a reversible return to the baseline fluorescence intensity. It was suggested that the oxygen titration curve can be used to calibrate a nitrogen hypoxic stress test to determine epithelial oxygen concentrations, i.e. under a contact lens (Masters, 1988b).

The first *in vivo* application of redox fluorometry to evaluate the redox state of the corneal epithelium of a living rabbit involved intensity measurements from the oxidized flavoproteins. The passage of hydrated nitrogen over the corneal epithelial surface of a live rabbit resulted in a 20 per cent decrease of fluorescence intensity. The was completely reversed when hydrated air was substituted for the nitrogen. This study demonstrated the feasibility of *in vivo* noninvasive redox fluorometry measurements of corneal epithelium.

The next set of investigations addressed the question of whether we investigate the possibility of heterogeneity of respiratory function among a population of corneal endothelial cells (Masters, 1988c). There was evidence that mitochondrial function might vary between normal and pathological endothelial cells in Fuchs' dystrophy. It was reasonable to assume that endothelial cells may show variations in respiratory function, depending on their degree of 'stress'. A second question concerned the ability to perform the redox fluorescence measurements on the individual layers (and eventually the single cells) of the corneal epithelium. While the early applications of redox fluorometry to the cornea resolved the epithelium from the stroma and from the endothelium it was always known that the different cell layers in the epithelium have different rates of oxygen consumption and enzyme activity. For example, the basal cells are the sites of mitotic activity and show a high degree of biosynthesis; the superficial epithelial cells show less metabolic activity.

There was a continuous improvement of the ability to optically section the living cornea to perform the redox fluorometric measurements on thinner optical sections of the cornea. The details of an optically sectioning fluorescence microscope have been reported previously. The main improvements included the following: high numerical aperture objectives, improved antireflection coatings on optical surfaces, improved reflection coatings on mirrors, a smaller slit height and improved photodetector instrumentation. The rapid development of confocal microscopes has permitted submicron optical sectioning of the cornea (Masters, 1990a). The use of a confocal microscope coupled to a redox fluorometer would allow measurements to be made of the individual cells in the endothelium and the cells of the component layers of the corneal epithelium. A clinical redox fluorometer based on a confocal microscope is under development (Masters, 1990b).

A study of the effects of contact lenses on the oxygen concentration and epithelial mitochondrial redox state of rabbit cornea was performed (Masters, 1988b). The purpose of this study was to demonstrate that the oxygen concentration at the corneal epithelial surface under various contact lenses could be monitored non-invasively *in vivo*, and that the resulting degree of epithelial hypoxia could be determined and correlated with the oxygen transmission properties of the contact lens. A relationship was found between the degree of epithelial hypoxia and the *Dk* of the contact lens material.

There were two other significant observations from this *in vivo* study. The first was that the fluorescence from the stromal region did not significantly change during the time course of the epithelial hypoxia. This is similar to the results found using perfused corneas in which the mitochondrial cytochrome oxidase was inhibited with cyanide. Second, it was noted that the fluorescence intensity from the endothelial cell layer did not change significantly during the period in which the contact lens resulted in a significant change in the fluorescence intensity from the corneal epithelium. Within the resolution of these measurements, which were repeated several times on different rabbits, it may be concluded that the redox state of the corneal endothelium in the rabbit is not dependent on the source of oxygen from the tear-side of the cornea. This observation should be taken as preliminary.

The correlation between the redox state as determined by non-invasive redox fluorometry and its physiological correlates such as effects on the rate of transendothelial fluid transport, and the magnitude of the transendothelial potential difference were investigated by Masters *et al.* (1983a). It was found that azide-induced histotoxic anoxia decreased the rates of transendothelial fluid transport and transendothelial potential difference in a dose-dependent manner. A similar dose-dependent effect was found between the azide concentration and the inhibition of endothelial transport function.

To validate *in situ* corneal redox fluorometry, the redox state and the phosphorylation potential of freeze trapped rabbit corneal epithelium, stromal and endothelium were studied using quantitative histochemical methods (Masters *et al.*, 1989). The results indicated that the corneal endothelium is in a more oxidized state than the corneal epithelium, the rabbit epithelium is less sensitive to hypoxia than the endothelium, and this difference is reflected in alterations of phosphorylation potential induced by hypoxia. The similarly high efficiencies of both layers in maintaining relatively high ATP levels during histotoxic hypoxia is most likely a result of compensatory ATP generation by enhanced glycolysis. The samples from the stroma that were analysed for pyridine nucleotides gave results similar to the blanks. This is consistent with the fluorometric results, which show no significant changes in the fluorescence intensity of the stromal region with shifts in the mitochondrial redox state. Possible explanations for this result have been discussed. Furthermore, aerobic–anoxic transitions altered the concentrations of NADH and NAD$^+$ but did not alter the concentration of NADPH and NADP$^+$. This is consistent with the known biochemical roles of these nucleotides.

Can we compare microchemical analysis of the pyridine nucleotides and redox fluorometry measurements? No, there is not a direct comparison between results on the pyridine nucleotides obtained from these two methods. The apparent discrepancy is due in part to the fact that the biochemical method measures the free NADH and NAD$^+$ present in both the cytoplasmic and the mitochondrial space. The great advantage of the biochemical method is that it can measure the content of the individual pyridine and adenine nucleotides, since the analytical methods are based on highly specific enzyme cycling reactions. However, the redox fluorometric measurements mainly involve the bound pool of mitochondrial NADH. The intensity of the fluorescence from the reduced pyridine nucleotides is greatly affected by protein binding. Therefore, the change in intensity of the reduced pyridine nucleotide is subject to multiple interpretation: a change in the redox state of the bound nucleotide or a change in the binding. The experimental resolution of this ambiguity in physical interpretation of the intensity measurements could possibly be elucidated with the use of fluorescence life-time measurements, which are sensitive to the physical state of the fluorescing molecule. Within the above-mentioned limitation of physical interpretation of the fluorescence intensity it should be stated that the real advantage of the technique of redox fluorometry is its non-invasive character.

This summary of the role of oxidative metabolism in the function of the cornea stressed oxygen; other metabolites and regulatory pathways are also important in our further investigations of the effects of contact lenses on the cornea (Edelhauser *et al.*, 1986; Tuberville *et al.*, 1986; Abraham *et al.*, 1987; Hayashi & Kenyon, 1988; Akahoshi *et al.*, 1989).

REFERENCES

Abraham, N.G., Lin, J.H.-C, Dunn, M.W. and Schwartzman, M.L. (1987) Presence of heme oxygenase and NADPH cytochrome P-450(c) reductase in human corneal epithelium. *Invest. Ophthalmol. Vis. Sci.*, **28**, 1464–72.

Akahoshi, T., Ohara, K. and Masuda, K. (1989) Enzyme cytochemical observation of the corneal cytochrome c oxidase under contact lens wear. *Invest. Ophthalmol. Vis. Sci.*, **30** (Suppl.), 258.

Atkinson, D.E. (1977) *Cellular Energy Metabolism and its Regulation.* Academic Press, New York.

Chance, B. (1976) Pyridine nucleotide as an indicator of the oxygen requirements for energy-linked functions in mitochondria, *Circ. Res.*, **38** (5 Suppl.1), I31–8.

Edelhauser, H.F., Geroski, D.H., Glasser, D.B. and Matsuda, M. (1986) Physiologic techniques for evaluation. In *Corneal Surgery: Theory, Technique, and Tissue* (ed. F.S. Brightbill), The C.V. Mosby Company, St Louis, pp. 627–36.

Fischbarg, J., Hernandez, J., Liebovitch, L.S. and Koniarek, J.P. (1985) The mechanism of fluid and electrolyte transport across corneal endothelium: critical revision and update of a model. *Curr. Eye Res.*, **4**, 351–60.

Gilbert, D.L. (1981a) Oxygen: an overall biological view. In *Oxygen and Living Processes. An Interdisciplinary Approach* (ed. D.L. Gilbert), Springer-Verlag, New York, pp. 376–92.

Gilbert, D.L. (1981b) Perspectives on the history of oxygen and life. In *Oxygen and Living Processes. An Interdisciplinary Approach* (ed. D.L. Gilbert). Springer-Verlag, New York, pp. 1–43.

Gilbert, D.L. (1981c) Significance of oxygen on earth. In *Oxygen and Living Processes. An Interdisciplinary Approach* (ed. D.L. Gilbert). Springer-Verlag, New York, 73–101.

Hamano, H. and Kaufman, H.E. (1987) *The Physiology of the Cornea and Contact Lens Applications.* Churchill Livingstone, New York.

Hayashi, K. and Kenyon, K.R. (1988) Increased cytochrome oxidase activity in alkalai-burned corneas. *Curr. Eye Res.*, **7**, 131–8.

Holden, B.A., Brennan, N.A., Efron, N. and Swarbrick, H.A. (1987) The contact lens: physiological considerations. In *Contact Lenses* (eds. J.V. Aquavella and G.N. Rao), J.B. Lippincott Company, Philadelphia, pp. 1–38.

Kanfer, S. and Turo, N.J. (1981) Reactive forms of oxygen. In *Oxygen and Living Processes. An Interdisciplinary Approach* (ed. D.L. Gilbert). Springer-Verlag, New York, pp. 47–64.

Keilin, D. (1966) *The History of Cell Respiration and Cytochrome.* Cambridge University Press, London.

Klyce, S.D. and Beuerman, R.W. (1988) Structure and function of the cornea. In *The Cornea* (eds. H.E. Kaufman, B.A. Barron, M.B. McDonald and S.R. Waltman), Churchill Livingstone, pp. 3–54.

Laing, R.A., Fischbarg, J. and Chance, B. (1980) Noninvasive measurements of pyridine nucleotide fluorescence from the cornea. *Invest. Ophthalmol. Vis. Sci.*, **19**, 96–102.

Masters, B.R. (1984a) Noninvasive corneal redox fluorometry. *Curr. Top. Eye Res.*, **4**, 139–200.

Masters, B.R. (1984b) Oxygen tensions of rabbit corneal epithelium measured by non-invasive

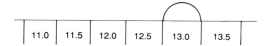

Figure 16.1 Measurement of the horizontal visible iris diameter (HVID).

nate measurement errors caused by the distance between scale and cornea: the millimetre scale is mounted in the anterior focal plane of a positive lens of power about 6.50 D, while a small aperture is placed in the posterior focal plane. Corneal reflection PD gauges, which employ the same telecentric principle, may be similarly used, while their internal light source may be helpful. Both instruments may also aid in measuring the vertex distance between spectacle trial lenses and the cornea. Some slit lamps have eyepiece graticules (reticles) to enable measurements to be undertaken, at a magnification of about 10x.

Mandell (1965a) showed that the HVID was approximately 0.7 mm smaller than that measured from profile photographs of the cornea. Impression casts of the eye were used by Obrig (1942), who showed that the average horizontal corneal diameter from limbus to limbus was 13.5 mm, while the vertical diameter was 11.9 mm.

16.1.2   MEASUREMENT OF PUPIL DIAMETER

Comparison of the patient's pupil with a series of graded circles gives sufficient precision for contact lens fitting. Measurement in average consulting room illumination and in reduced illumination should be made: in the latter case, illumination of the

eye by the UV lamp gives enough light for the practitioner to estimate the pupil diameter, either by illuminating the iris or by making the crystalline lens fluoresce. A large pupil will need a lens with a larger optic zone and good centration in order to avoid flare.

16.1.3   PALPEBRAL APERTURE AND LID POSITION

While, in principle, a measurement of the vertical palpebral aperture may be easily made, the patient may either tend to stare wide or to close the lids when a ruler is placed close to the eye. It is of greater clinical use to mark the average open eye lid position on a circle indicating the cornea, as in Figure 16.3. This both indicates whether or not either lid may support the contact lens centrally on the cornea and gives a ready comparison for the aperture when a lens has been placed on the eye.

16.2   HISTORY AND DEVELOPMENT OF KERATOMETRY AND KERATOSCOPY

The first record of the determination of the central corneal radius by utilizing its relationship with the size of the image formed by reflection at its anterior surface, was made by Scheiner in 1619. His work was overlooked until recognized by Levene in 1965 and by Wittenberg and Ludlam in 1966. In order to try to detect changes in corneal curvature on accommodating, Ramsden, in 1796, attempted to quantify

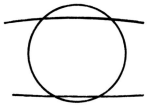

Figure 16.3 Typical record of lid positions with respect to the limbus.

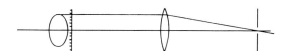

Figure 16.2 The Wessely keratometer.

the image size by means of a microscope with a measuring graticule in the eyepiece (Mandell, 1960; Levene, 1977). Apart from this, measurement of the radius of curvature of the cornea in excised eyes was attempted as early as 1832 by Krause, who described the anterior corneal surface as spheroidal and the posterior surface as paraboloidal. Kohlrausch (1840) appears to have been the next person to determine the corneal radius in the living eye by direct measurement of the reflected image of a given sized object, viewed through a telescope at a known distance from the eye. This basic method is still employed today over a century later. Senff in 1846 recognized the peripheral flattening of the cornea and produced measurements of its ellipticity, as well as establishing that the apex of the cornea does not always coincide with its intersection with the visual axis.

Although credit for the first keratoscope is usually given to Plácido (1880a, b). Levene (1965) has shown that Henry Goode invented the first hand keratoscope in 1847 when he diagnosed astigmatism by utilizing a luminous square reflected from the cornea. However, Plácido in 1882 was the first to use photographic keratoscopy, although Javal independently developed a photokeratoscope a little later in the same year. At first square targets and the familiar circular targets were used. De Wecker and Masselon in 1882 employed a square target in their astigmometer. Gullstrand (1896), formerly credited with the invention of the photokeratoscope, also used a square target.

Shortly after the first keratoscope was used, measurements of corneal curvature were made easier by the development of the ophthalmometer by Helmholtz in 1854. This incorporated a doubling device using glass plates to facilitate measurement of the mobile image reflected from the human cornea. Javal and Schiötz converted the idea into a practical clinical instrument in 1881. This instrument is essentially the same as several available today. Modern refinements include internally illuminated mires instead of external illumination by candle or gas flame.

From this time onwards many studies of corneal curvature were made. Mathematical formulae to describe its curvature were produced and its departure from an ellipsoidal shape was noted. It was generally agreed that the cornea had a more spherical central zone, surrounded by an annulus where more rapid flattening took place, and that the flattening was not symmetrical. This has been described in Chapter 00.

By the end of the nineteenth century a considerable number of investigations had been made and figures were amassed giving variations of central corneal curvature in several populations. The work of Donders (1864), Sulzer (1891, 1892) and Steiger (1895) established a mean value of approximately 7.8 mm for the central radius of the anterior corneal surface, slightly flatter in men than women, and ranging from 7.1 mm to 8.4 mm. Physiological with-the-rule corneal astigmatism (greater power in the vertical meridian than in the horizontal) of an average value of 0.75 D had been established by Nordensen (1883) and Steiger (1895). The reduction of this astigmatism with age, and the trend towards against-the-rule astigmatism, had also been demonstrated by Steiger and others.

The keratometer was beginning to be used for contact lens work in the 1920s when afocal scleral lenses were fitted, the power being provided entirely by the liquid lens. Heine (1929) produced a scale (Fig. 16.4) which enabled the back optic radius of the necessary afocal contact lens to be selected using the corneal radius and the ocular refraction. Keratometry is still used for power calculation purposes today. Some modern keratometers or ophthalmometers (the terms are now synonymous) are shown in Figures 16.5, 16.6 and 16.7.

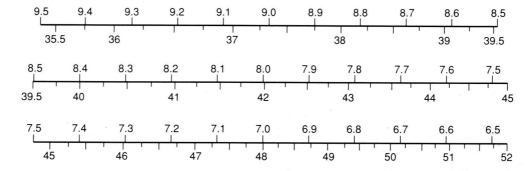

Figure 16.4 Heine's double scale. The upper figures are the radii of corneal curvature in millimeters, the lower the corresponding dioptric power in air. $n = 1.336$.

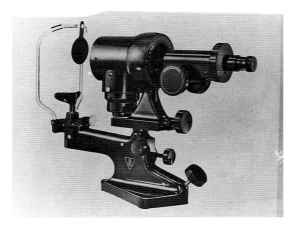

Figure 16.5 The Bausch and Lomb keratometer (reproduced by courtesy of Reichert Jung).

16.3 OPTICAL PRINCIPLES OF KERATOMETRY

16.3.1 THE KERATOMETER FORMULA

Because the front surface of the cornea acts as a convex mirror its radius of curvature may be measured by a relatively simple optical method. This is illustrated in Figure 16.8.

BQ is an object of size h. Rays from B and Q directed towards C, the centre of curvature of the corneal surface, strike the surface normally and are reflected back along their original paths. Rays from B and Q directed towards F', the principal focus of the corneal

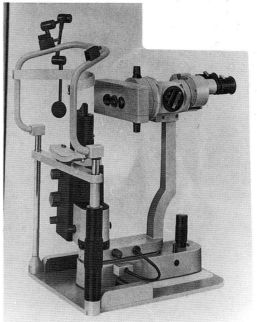

Figure 16.6 The Zeiss keratometer (reproduced by courtesy of Zeiss (Oberkochen) Ltd).

surface, are reflected parallel to the optical axis (which passes through F' and C). Thus the virtual image formed by reflection at the corneal surface is B'Q' of size h'.

It can be seen that the points of reflection, Y and Z, or the rays directed towards F' have the same separation as the image height h'.

be seen from the similar triangles YF′Z and BF′Q that:

$$\frac{h'}{h} = \frac{f'}{x} \text{ and thus } \frac{h'}{h} = \frac{r'}{2x}$$

Now, if the object BQ is sufficiently distant from the surface, the image B′Q′ is formed in a plane very close to the focal plane F′. The distance d between object and image may, therefore, be assumed to equal x, with an error of only 0.16 mm if $d = 100$ mm and 0.2 mm if $d = 80$ mm. Making this substitution, it can be seen that:

$$r = \frac{2dh'}{h} \tag{eqn 16.1}$$

This is known as the keratometer formula. It assumes first-order or paraxial theory: that is, it does not take into account aberrations which occur and which alter the size of the image. These will be dealt with later (see page 297).

In practice, the separation BQ is the distance between the two test objects, termed mires (from the French for targets) of a keratometer. The image B′Q′ is both small and virtual and therefore has to be observed and magnified by a long focus microscope (or short focus telescope). The distance d is a constant of the instrument, and is measured from the plane of the mires to the focusing plane of the instrument.

16.3.2 OBSERVATION AND DOUBLING

Besides allowing observation of the reflected mire images, B′ and Q′, the optical system of a keratometer must allow measurement of their separation, h'. Because the reflected images from the cornea are never quite stationary this measurement is most easily carried out by using a doubling system. Even though the doubled images move, because they move together it is possible to judge whether they are separated, overlapped or adjacent to one another. Again the optical

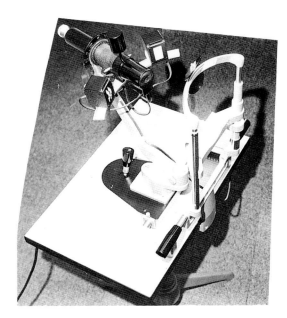

Figure 16.7 The Haag–Streit Javal–Schiötz keratometer.

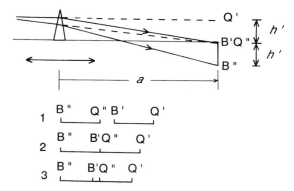

Figure 16.8 The basic principles of keratometry: $AC = r = \dfrac{2dh'}{h}$

The distance from A, the vertex of the cornea, to F′ is the focal length f' which is half the radius of curvature, r. If the distance between object plane BQ and focal plane F′ is x, it may

principle is simple and is illustrated in Figure 16.9 in which it is assumed that a prism is used for doubling, although other methods of doubling the image are sometimes used.

Here a prism of power P prism dioptres occupies half the aperture through which image B'Q' is observed at a distance a. Through the prism the image B'Q' is seen displaced by its own height h' to B''Q'' and the doubled image is seen correctly displaced, as shown in the lower part of Figure 16.9. Since this displacement depends entirely on the power of the prism P and the distance a at which it is used, then provided h' and a are in cm:

$$\frac{P}{100} = \frac{h'}{aa} \text{ and } h' = \frac{aP}{100}$$

Thus h' may be measured in terms of a and P. When using prisms to achieve doubling, P is obviously a fixed value and a is varied by moving the prism along the optical axis of the instrument to obtain the correct amount of doubling, thereby enabling indirect measurement of h'.

16.3.3 TYPES OF DOUBLING.

Reference to the keratometer formula, eqn 16.1, shows that r, the radius of curvature of the corneal surface, is dependent on three parameters d, h and h'. Since d is a fixed value for any one instrument, it is only necessary to fix either h or h' and measure the other to obtain r. If the mire separation, h, is fixed then to determine r from h' some variable system of doubling must be employed. But if the image size, h', is fixed the doubling must also be fixed, and variable mire separation used to determine r.

16.3.4 VARIABLE DOUBLING

When the mires have a constant separation as in the Bausch and Lomb keratometer and its many derivatives, the Rodenstock and the two Zeiss instruments, the doubling is varied in order to determine h'. The control knob is linked mechanically to the doubling system, and either carries the curvature graduations itself or drives a separate indicator scale. The keratometer formula shows that the radius is directly proportional to h', so in these instruments the radius scale is linear.

In the Bausch and Lomb keratometer the doubling is achieved by the use of four apertures placed between the two objectives of the viewing telescope (Fig. 16.10). Apertures C and D contain base-in and base-down prisms, respectively. The mire image is viewed through all four apertures. Aperture C causes a doubled image in the horizontal plane and aperture D in the vertical plane. Apertures A and B do not contain prisms and do not therefore displace the image, but give rise to two closely over-

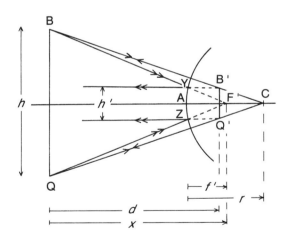

Figure 16.9 The prism doubling principle of the image h'. (1) separated images; (2) aligned images; (3) overlapped images.

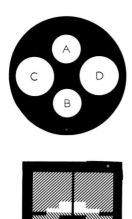

Figure 16.10 The objective apertures of the Bausch & Lomb keratometer.

lapped direct images unless the telescope is in sharp focus. (This is the Scheiner principle used in range finders and other optical instruments). Figure 16.11 shows the appearances seen. The doubling is varied by movement along the axis of the prisms behind apertures C and D. To equate the image path length, two parallel plane glass blocks are placed behind apertures A and B.

The Rodenstock C-BES keratometer uses tilting glass plates to provide the doubling, a technique first used for this purpose by Helmholtz in 1854. Their obliquity (Fig. 16.12) may be adjusted to provide variable

doubling in the form of a linear rather than angular displacement of the mire image. The inner plate rotates in one direction, while the outer rotates in the opposite direction. The two parts of the outer plate act like a Scheiner disc aperture to enable precise setting of the instrument's focus. Mires similar to those of either the Haag–Streit or Zeiss instruments described below are available.

The Zeiss ophthalmometers G and H utilize a reflecting prism system to double the mire images, two lenses which move perpendicular to the axis to vary the amount of doubling, and then a further reflecting prism system to reunite the doubled images. The optical system is shown in Figure 16.13. The instrument differs from the Bausch and Lomb keratometer in that the final setting is made by superimposing one mire image on the other – a single cross within a hollow cross – rather than by juxtaposition of the images. A similar system was used in the Gambs ophthalmometer and in the Guilbert–Routit topographical ophthalmometer.

A second Zeiss instrument (Fig. 16.14), manufactured both as a complete instrument and as an attachment to their slit lamp 30 SL/M, also employs Helmholtz tilted plates. The mires are of the cross-within-a-cross type, and their images are viewed through one eyepiece, while the scales are viewed through the other. Zeiss have named this instrument a keratometer to differentiate it from their ophthalmometer.

16.3.5 FIXED DOUBLING

In the Javal–Schiötz keratometer, such as the instruments made by Haag–Streit and Sbisa, the doubling is fixed and provided by a Wollaston double image prism (Fig. 16.15). Descriptions of this prism, which depends on the birefringence of quartz, may be found in textbooks on optics. Fixed

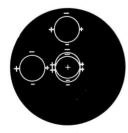

Figure 16.11 Non-focused mires (Bausch & Lomb).

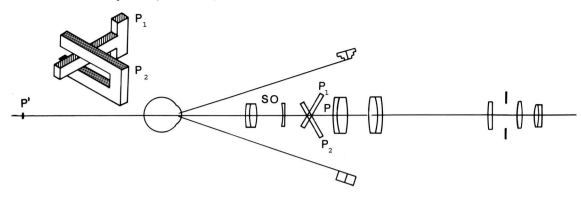

Figure 16.12 The optical principles of the Rodenstock C – BES ophthalmometer. The inset shows the Helmholtz doubling plates, redrawn from information kindly supplied by Rodenstock (UK) Ltd.

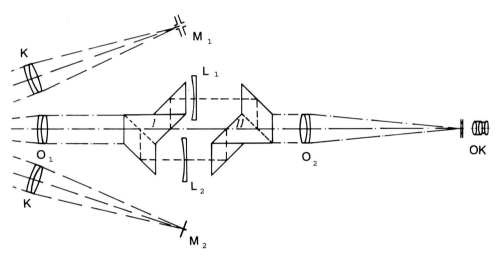

Figure 16.13 The optical system of the Zeiss (Oberkochen) ophthalmometers, G and H, reproduced by courtesy of Carl Zeiss (Oberkochen) Ltd.

doubling provides a simpler optical system than variable doubling. The image height h' is adjusted by varying the separation h of the mires. These are linked mechanically to the radius cursor indicating the radius. The keratometer formula shows that the mire separation is inversely proportional to the radius of curvature of the cornea. Hence, the scales on these instruments show a relatively linear corneal power calibration and a non-linear radius one.

16.3.6 TOROIDAL CORNEAS: SETTING THE DOUBLED IMAGE

Figures 16.16, 16.17 and 16.18 show the types of mire used in various keratometers, the object size h, being indicated in each case. When reflected from a toroidal cornea these mires appear distorted (Fig. 16.19) unless the meridian in which they lie corresponds with one of the principal meridians of the surface being measured. It is not possible to obtain a

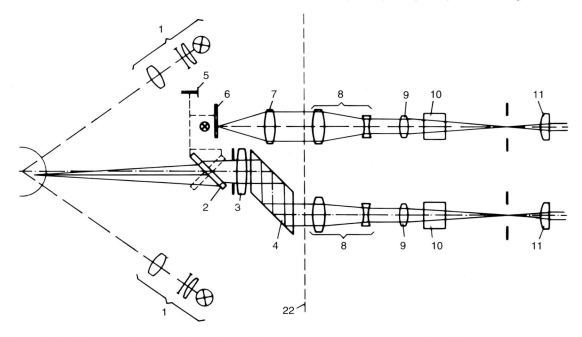

Figure 16.14 The optical system of the Zeiss (Oberkochen) keratometer, reproduced by courtesy of Carl Zeiss (Oberkochen) Ltd.

correct alignment of the doubled images unless the mires are situated along a principal meridian. The mires and doubling system are therefore rotated about the optical axis of the instrument until their images no longer appear distorted, and until appearances are similar to those shown in Figure 16.20 are achieved. Alignment of the doubled images may then be made (Fig. 16.21).

After locating and measuring the radius of curvature along one principal meridian the instrument is then rotated through 90° (or approximately so) to locate and measure the other principal meridian. However, the Bausch and Lomb instrument has an annular mire with two reference marks, a + sign and a − sign, projecting from it in the horizontal and vertical meridians. It also has vertical and horizontal doubling systems. It is therefore only necessary to rotate the instrument about its axis to locate one principal meridian and the other is automatically lined up

and visible at the same time. It is consequently know as a 'one-position' instrument, whereas most keratometers are 'two-position' instruments.

In the Javal–Schiötz instrument, the inner edges of the mires are brought into apposition. If the flattest meridian is measured first, then the mire images will initially overlap when the instrument is rotated to the steeper meridian. Traditionally, one mire is stepped, each step approximating to one dioptre of corneal astigmatism.

The meridian indicator in some instruments is poorly designed, pointing at 90° on the scale when the mires are in the horizontal plane. Addition or subtraction of 90° is necessary to give the true meridian.

Where the corneal surface is neither spherical nor toroidal, as for example in keratocunus or other conditions giving rise to surface irregularity, it is usually impossible to align the mires so as to arrive at a

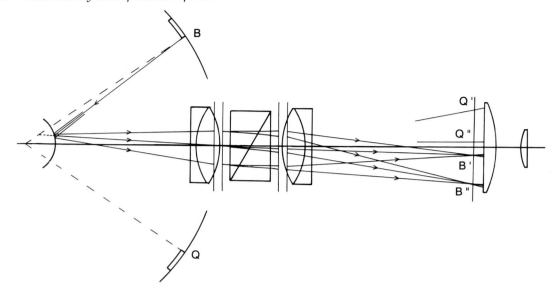

Figure 16.15 The optical system of the Javal–Schiötz keratometer.

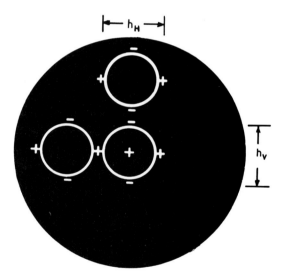

Figure 16.16 The mire of the Bausch & Lomb keratometer. The central cross in the middle of the lower right circle indicates the eyepiece graticule. Ideally, the mires should be positioned as indicated in the field of view when taking readings.

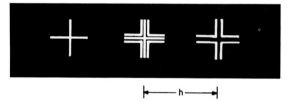

Figure 16.17 The mire of the Zeiss instruments.

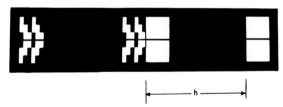

Figure 16.18 The mire of the Haag–Streit keratometer.

16.4 MEASUREMENT OF CORNEAL POWER

Most keratometers are so constructed that the mires are reflected from two small zones of cornea falling within the central area in front of the pupil. The exact size and location of

satisfactory doubled and aligned image, and accurate measurements are therefore impossible.

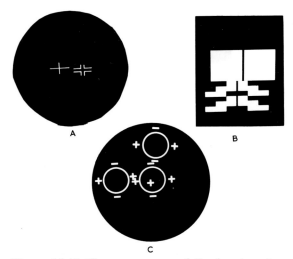

Figure 16.19 The appearance of the keratometer mires when reflected from an astigmatic cornea. (A) Zeiss mires. (B) Javal–Schiötz mires. (C) Bausch & Lomb mires. All are incorrectly aligned.

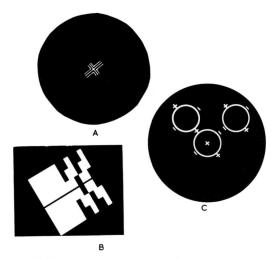

Figure 16.21 The appearance of the keratometer mires when both are correctly orientated and aligned along the corneal meridian.

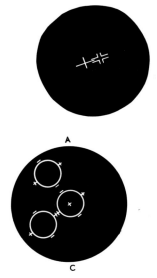

Figure 16.20 The appearance of the keratometer mires when correctly orientated along the corneal meridian.

these reflecting areas will be discussed later (see pages 298–90). It is this central area of the cornea which contributes to the total refracting power of the eye and is combined, with the crystalline lens, in the formation of the retinal image at the macula. The power and the astigmatism of the cornea in this area are therefore of interest.

The keratometer measures the radius of curvature of the anterior corneal surface, but most keratometers are also calibrated to read total corneal power. To do this an assumption must be made that the back surface of the cornea has a negative power of approximately one tenth that of the positive power of the front surface. Therefore instead of calibrating the instruments for the true refractive index of the cornea (1.376), which would give a reading of the front surface power, a lower notional refractive index is assumed. Most instruments use 1.3375, although Zeiss assume 1.332 and the American Optical Company use the refractive index of the tear fluid, 1.336.

Since the last value is also the index of the aqueous humour, it has been adopted as the notional index of the cornea in calculations for the power of intra-ocular implants and would appear to be the most sensible to employ for keratometer calibration.

The usual relationship between power F,

radius r and refractive index n, is used in calibration:

$$F = \frac{n-1}{r}$$

(eqn 16.2)

where F is in dioptres and r in metres. Since F is inversely proportional to r, it will be noted that the power and radius scales of keratometers have their maximum and minimum values at opposite ends (Fig. 16.22), a fact which can be overlooked and so lead to incorrect readings of either radius or power.

As an approximate rule, a difference of 0.2 mm between the radii of the meridians of a cornea corresponds to 1 D of astigmatism, irrespective of which value of index is used (compare Figs. 16.4 and 16.22). This easily remembered approximation is also valid for the tears lens power given by a difference in front and back radii, and the required change in rigid lens BVP with changes in BOZR. During the preliminary assessment of a prospective contact lens patient, the corneal astigmatism should be compared with the ocular refraction (i.e. the spectacle refraction effective in the plane of the cornea after allowing for vertex distance; see Chapter 00).

16.4.1   DIFFERENCES IN POWER READINGS

When power readings are used instead of radius readings another possible source of error arises. It is common in the United States for keratometer power to be given rather than radius. (The keratometer power is also used to describe the surface curvature of contact lenses which have a completely different refractive index, leading to more confusion.) Thus in addition to different instruments using different areas of cornea and therefore obtaining different radius and power readings on a given cornea, some instruments use different indices of calibration: 42 D on one keratometer does not necessarily imply the same radius of curvature as 42 D on another keratometer. The

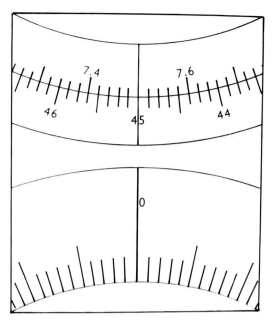

Figure 16.22 The instrument geared to give visual results in radii, dioptres and meridians. The lower scale gives the meridian reading and the upper gives corneal radius (mm) and power (D).

error in radius due to using the wrong index is of the order of 0.13 mm (Stone, 1962). This means that a contact lens specified assuming an index of 1.3375 but measured with an instrument calibrated for 1.332 would be over 0.1 mm too flat.

It is essential, therefore, to know the index of calibration of the instrument being used and if possible to convert all powers to radii. In any case, the total power of corneas given by keratometers is an assumed power. Two corneas having the same front surface radius might well have different back surface radii and thicknesses and so have completely different total corneal powers, but in each case the keratometer would read the same value.

16.5   SOURCES OF ERROR IN KERATOMETRY

Most of the errors are of an optical nature, but mechanical errors in using an instrument may also be made. The movable parts of a keratometer which determine the accuracy of the reading obtained are the focusing control and either the doubling device or the mire separation control, depending on whether the instrument has variable or fixed doubling. Even in the best engineered instruments these controls are liable to backlash or 'play' which can introduce error if they are not used correctly. To minimize error in those instruments where the scale and cursor are attached to or driven by the control knob rather than being integral with the mires, all settings should be made by rotating the controls from one direction. When a setting is over-run and a control knob must be reversed in order to come back to the setting, then backlash error is introduced. If this occurs the setting must be over-run again in the reverse direction and the setting made by turning the control knob in the original direction. The magnitude of the error caused by backlash depends entirely on the amount of freedom of movement of the control knob before it operates the movable mechanism of the instrument.

16.5.1 ERRORS DUE TO OPTICAL CAUSES

Optical sources of error are greater on some instruments than others. The basic optical system used in most keratometers is shown in Figure 16.23. From this it can be seen that the image h'', formed by the objectives O of the telescope must be viewed by means of the eyepiece E. There is only one position of h'' which allows the instrument to be operated at its correct working distance d. However, there are a number of positions of h'' nearer to the eyepiece than the correct position, in which h'' may be seen clearly by an observer who uses his accommodation. When h'' is formed too close to the eyepiece the instrument is used at too short a working distance. Because the mires are also now closer to the cornea and therefore subtend a larger angle, and second, the keratometer objective gives a greater magnification, an enlarged image is formed at the eyepiece. A longer radius of curvature and lower corneal power than the correct value is indicated.*

To overcome this most instruments have an eyepiece containing a cross-wire or graticule in the plane of which h'' should be formed. Before using the instrument the eyepiece should first be adjusted by the observer so that this cross-wire is seen clearly with the accommodation relaxed. This is best done by first rotating the eye lens of the eyepiece anticlockwise which brings it nearer to the observer and renders the vergence of the light reaching the observer too positive. This discourages accommodation

---

* Rabbetts (1977) showed that a 5 D eyepiece focusing error could, with some instruments, lead to an error of more than 0.05 mm in measured radius. The induced error is a function of the eyepiece power because the lower the power, the longer the travel per dioptre of adjustment. A high power eyepiece, however, gives a dimmer image and a smaller field of view.

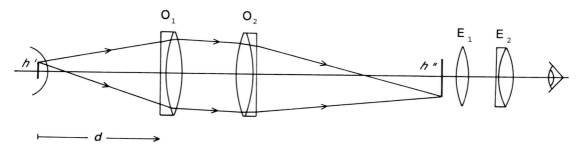

Figure 16.23 The basic viewing system. O_1O_2 objective system; E_1E_2 eye piece system; h' corneal image.

and puts the cross-wire out of focus. Then if the observer keeps both eyes open and relaxes accommodation by apparently staring into the distance, and slowly turns the eye lens inwards or clockwise until the cross-wire is first seen sharply focused, the eyepiece will be correctly adjusted for that observer. Even so, the observer must continue to make sure that, during the use of the instrument, to observe the mire images the cross-wire is kept sharply in focus by keeping the accommodation relaxed. To ensure that the final mire images h'' are formed in the plane of the cross-wire, a slight lateral movement of the observer's head while looking through the instrument will demonstrate whether or not there is any parallax between the two. If there is, the instrument and not the eyepiece must be refocused until there is no parallax. Even when used as carefully as this small errors can occur due to the depth of focus of the observer's eye. A diffusely lit background for focusing the graticule is conveniently provided by switching the instrument on and viewing the patient's closed lids.

At this juncture it may be as well to point out that a great deal of time and trouble may be saved in locating the subject's cornea if a light from a pen torch or ophthalmoscope is shone through the eyepiece. The image of this light formed by the keratometer's optical system can be brought onto the cornea by the height and direction adjustments of the instrument. Manufacturer's instructions regarding the setting up of instruments in order to locate the cornea to be measured do not always allow sufficiently precise positioning, and a lot of time can be wasted by the beginner in simply finding the patient's eye. The patient then views a small light or mirror placed centrally in front of the keratometer's objective.

It is also evident that focusing the instrument is critical if h'' is to be formed in the correct plane without inducing the observer's accommodation. Having adjusted the eyepiece to suit his own refractive error and with accommodation relaxed, the observer should therefore start with the instrument at a greater distance from the cornea than is required. Then the instrument should be slowly moved towards the cornea until the mire images are first seen sharply. Further forward movement of the instrument will only induce the observer's accommodation and again result in too large a radius reading and too low a power reading being obtained.

The Zeiss G and H ophthalmometers have a system in which the doubling device is situated between the two objective lenses of the telescope and in the focal plane of the first objective lens. This ensures that the amount of doubling will give correct alignment, even if the mires are out of focus and even if the observer's accommodation is active. The mires are collimated, and thus subtend a constant angle at the cornea irrespective of the working distance. It is therefore unnecessary to have an adjustable eyepiece with a graticule and so the eyepiece is then fixed.

An alternative technique for maintaining valid readings in the presence of instrument focusing errors is provided by Rodenstock in their C-BES instrument. As shown in Figure 16.12, a supplementary objective SO is placed in front of the Helmholtz tilting plates so that these are imaged at P' behind the patient's eye. If the instrument is moved too close to the eye, the mires subtend too large an angle at the cornea, but their image is now further from P', the instrument's effective entrance pupil, and hence subtends a smaller angle. These two factors are designed to be self-compensating.

The Bausch and Lomb, and Rodenstock keratometers employ the Scheiner principle to assist accurate focusing so that the mire image viewed directly is only seen single when sharply focused. This to some extent offsets the disadvantage of a one-position instrument, which is that the focus setting made for one meridian tends to be used quite incorrectly for the other meridian. A toroidal cornea forms reflected images of the mires in different planes in the two principal meridians and to obtain accurate readings the instrument must be separately focused for each meridian. If, as is usually done, the horizontal setting is made first and the cornea has with-the-rule astigmatism, then the steeper vertical meridian forms an image which can be brought into focus by use of the observer's accommodation, but this will make the radius reading for the steeper meridian inaccurate. Too long a radius is recorded for the steeper meridian unless careful refocusing is carried out.

Depending on the quality of the optical system of a keratometer, error can also be introduced if the mire images are not kept in the centre of the field of view, as the aberrations of the optical system and the slightly oblique viewing can lead to distortion of the images and alterations in their size. It is therefore wise to adjust all instruments carefully to ensure that the images occupy a central position. To assist this the subject should be requested to keep as still as possible and to gaze steadily at the fixation target with the other eye occluded. If this is not done the eye being measured may wander, especially if it is the non-dominant eye, and a measurement of a paracentral area of the cornea may inadvertently be made by the observer. It is also well worth taking time to instruct the patient to keep his head firmly in the rest.

Other small errors can occur in setting the doubled images of the mires. Those instruments which employ a vernier setting, such as the now obsolete Guilbert–Routit model of the Javal–Schiötz type instrument, permit the most accurate setting to be made. The Zeiss and Gambs instruments require a single cross to be placed centrally within a double cross and small inaccuracies can occur. The Bausch and Lomb keratometer requires superimposition of crosses and lines, but this can be improved by masking off part of the mires so as to allow vernier settings (Shick, 1982). The Javal–Schiötz mires which should be placed just adjacent to one another have been coloured red and green by Haag–Streit and Sbisa, so that if they are overlapped a yellow band is seen. However some observers find the colouring of the mires causes them to appear in different planes due to the chromatic aberration of the observer's eye, and this then creates difficulty in focusing.

Charman (1972) applied diffraction theory to the keratometer, and showed that in the absence of all other errors, the resulting tolerance on focusing could give an error for a single reading with the Bausch and Lomb instrument of $\pm$ 0.04 mm. Clark (1973) reviewed many articles on the experimental determination of the instrument's repeatability; many of the workers cited had found an average figure of 0.015 mm for the standard deviation of a series of readings. Since 95% of a normal deviation lies within two standard deviations from the mean value, Charman's and Clark's results are in good agreement, and suggest that, provided a number of readings are taken, keratometry provides a good estimate of corneal curvature.

It was pointed out on page 287 that the keratometer formula assumes that the reflection from the corneal surface is within the paraxial zone. Because of the short radius of curvature of the cornea, about 8 mm, and height of incidence on the surface, paraxial formulae are inappropriate. Bennett (1966) has shown how trigonometrical ray-tracing procedures may be used to derive more accurate calibration formulae, and how errors of the order of 4–5% may be introduced if these are ignored. He has pointed out that a radius of 8 mm may be recorded as less than 7.7 mm if paraxial formulae are used. In practice, prototype instruments are almost certainly calibrated on test spheres.

Additional slight errors, which are impossible to avoid, occur because the cornea is not truly spherical or toroidal. For purposes of contact lens fitting, however, the central area of the cornea may be assumed to be spherical or toroidal as long as the possible errors introduced by this assumption are known and, if necessary, allowed for.

Using a two-position keratometer, it is often found that the principal meridians of the cornea are not perpendicular. Thus maximum and minimum radius readings may be different with a one-position keratometer because the latter assumes perpendicular principal meridians.

16.5.2   ZONES USED FOR REFLECTION

Studies of corneal topography from Gullstrand's time onwards have shown that the cornea flattens gradually from apex to limbus. This flattening is not constant or symmetrical in all meridians, nor does the apex of the cornea coincide with the position at which the visual axis intersects it. Mandell and St Helen (1969) found no significant pattern in the position of the corneal apex with respect to the fixational axis. Sheridan and Douthwaite's (1989) analysis of 56 eyes showed, however, that in the horizontal meridian, the corneal pole was displaced approximately 5° temporal to the fixation axis (see also Chapter 00). Keratometers used in the conventional way are centred about the subject's visual axis and directed towards the corneal surface at its point of intersection. However, the mires are reflected from small areas about 1.5 mm on either side of this point, so that the keratometer does not actually record the radius of the portion of cornea towards which it is directed. Also since the areas used for reflection are asymmetrical with respect to the corneal apex they are likely to have slightly different radii of curvature. Figure 16.24 shows a typical cornea, flattening gradually from the apex outwards. The area AA has a centre of curvature at C*a* and area BB a centre of curvature at C*b*. The keratometer interprets the radius of the central portion as having its centre of curvature at C*o*,

the position of intersection of the perpendicular bisectors of areas AA and BB. In other words it is the angle which areas AA and BB make with the optical axis of the instrument which determines the radius of curvature recorded. The central area of the cornea, between the areas used for forming the reflected images of the mires, could have a very small steep apex as shown by the broken line in Figure 16.24 but as this is not used in forming the mire images its radius is not recorded.

Figure 16.25 shows how light from the mires, M, of a keratometer, is reflected at the cornea and passes back to the objective of the instrument. It is apparent that the extent *w* and separation *m* of the zones of the corneal surface used for reflecting the mires depend on the curvature of the cornea, the size and separation of the mires and the size of the objective and its distance from the cornea. Different instruments therefore use different zones of reflection in determining the corneal radius, and since the cornea is aspheric it is not surprising that different instruments record different radii of curvature for the same cornea.

Mandell (1964), Lehman (1967) and Ehrlich and Tromans (1988) have studied the differ-

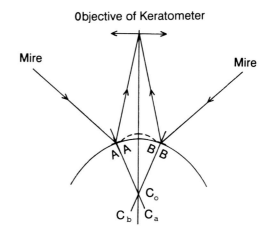

Figure 16.24 The zones of the cornea used in keratometry.

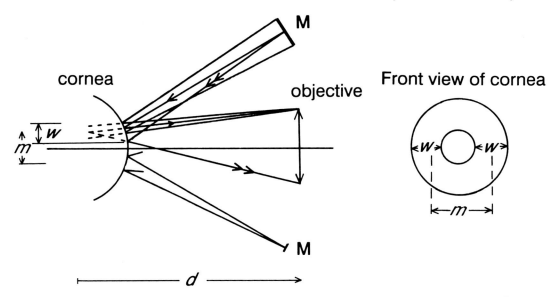

Figure 16.25 Details of the annulus of the cornea reflecting rays. w, corneal zones; m, distance between zones.

ences between various keratometers. Figure 16.26 combines their findings to show the separation (m) of the centres of these zones of reflection. Of the instruments used it can be seen, as Lehman concluded, that the Haag–Streit instrument has the most constant separation of the two zones. This is because it is a fixed doubling instrument, all the others having variable doubling. The Gambs keratometer (no longer in production) uses zones of reflection closer to the corneal apex than other instruments.

Using eqn 16.4 (see page 302), for a relatively aspheric cornea with a p-value of 0.6, a cornea with an apical radius of 8.0 would have a sagittal* radius at a chord diameter of 2.0 mm of 8.025 mm and at 3.0 mm of 8.056 mm. This would suggest that the differences indicated by instruments in correct

calibration on the same test sphere should be no more than about 0.03 mm, though on deformed corneas, as in oedema and keratoconus, larger discrepancies may well occur. Conversely, two corneas giving the same reading but at these two different chord diameters may have apical radii differing by 0.05 mm.

Lehman also measured the width (w) of the reflection zones and showed that over the entire range of curvatures the Bausch and Lomb keratometer used zones of 0.1 mm width, the Zeiss and Gambs models 0.2 to 0.3 mm and the Haag–Streit 0.3 to 0.4 mm. While the whole of this zone may be used to observe distortion of the Javal–Schiötz mire, the width that is used when setting the instrument will be less because it is only the inner edges that are apposed.

16.5.3 GRADUATION OF POWER, RADIUS AND AXIS SCALES

Some instruments have scales which are much easier to read than others, and some

---

* Because of the oblique incidence of the light reflected at the cornea, the mires form tangential and sagittal astigmatic images. Although the instrument is set using the tangential image, Bennett and Rabbetts (1991) have shown that the instrument effectively measures the sagittal radius when used in the normal way.

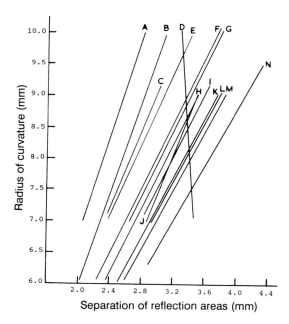

Figure 16.26 Comparison of separation distance (*m*) for 12 different keratometers. A, Gambs; B, Zeiss keratometer; C, American Optical Company; D, Haag–Streit; E, Zeiss ophthalmometers G and H; F, Humphrey Auto-Keratometer; G, Guilbert–Routit topographical, used conventionally; H, Nidek KM 800; I,J,L, Bausch & Lomb; K, Nidek ARK-2000; M, Topcon CK 1000; N, Canon RK1. (A, D, E, G, I, L after Lehmann, 1967; C,J after Mandell, 1964; B and F from manufacturers' data and the remainder from Ehrlich & Tromans, 1988.)

are more finely graduated than others. Poorly constructed scales are another possible source of error in keratometry. For contact lens work, radii of curvature should, ideally, be recorded to 0.01 mm.

16.6   CALIBRATION OF KERATOMETERS

Where possible practitioners should check the calibration of their own instruments using accurately machined steel balls as test surfaces. Manufacturers of ball bearings guarantee their top-grade balls for both sphericity and diameter to within ± 0.001 mm. Sets can be obtained with

diameters in 1 mm steps covering the range of radii measured by keratometers, and beyond. Thus individual users may measure and allow for both instrument and user error.

To test calibration the instrument should be carefully adjusted by the user; the radius of each steel ball is measured five times and a mean value recorded. A graph may then be plotted of mean recorded radius against actual radius as shown in Figure 16.27. If there is a constant error over the entire range of radii (see slope A) it may be possible on certain instruments to alter the position of the recording scale to allow for this. If, however, the error is variable (as for example in slope B) it is best to use the plotted graph to obtain actual radius readings on each occasion.

The alignment of the mires and doubling system should also be checked while viewing the steel ball: the meridian indicator lines should be in a straight line, as in Figure 16.20, and not suggest an astigmatic surface, as in Figure 16.19.

When several people use the same instrument, the eyepiece (if adjustable)

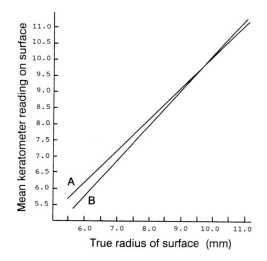

Figure 16.27 Recording keratometer error. A, constant error; B, variable error.

must be preset for each individual before taking a reading. A steel ball of known radius is used and the instrument scale preset to record this value. The instrument is then set up correctly and focused by the observer to view the mire images. If these are not aligned correctly but are too far apart, the eyepiece should be screwed outwards (anticlockwise) and the instrument simultaneously refocused until alignment is achieved. Screwing the eyepiece inwards and simultaneous refocusing may give a correct setting if the mire images overlap. Having set up the instrument in this way it may then be used in the normal manner, provided that the eyepiece is left in this calibrated position.

The obvious disadvantage of this method is that the eyepiece graticule can no longer be seen sharply focused and therefore the observer has no check that his accommodation is fully relaxed. Also, if the instrument is a one-position model having two perpendicular doubling systems, it may be necessary to re-adjust and refocus the eyepiece for each doubling system.

To record radii steeper than the range of the instrument allows, a low power positive lens of about + 1.25 D is placed just in front of the keratometer objective and a series of steep steel balls of known radii are observed. Their radii, as recorded by the instrument viewing through the + 1.25 D lens are flatter than their true values and therefore fall within the instrument range. Thus a graph may be plotted of recorded values against actual values as shown in Figure 16.28. Provided the same + 1.25 D lens is always used the instrument and graph may be used subsequently to measure steep radii quite readily. A − 1 D lens may be used to extend the range in the opposite direction, when flat radii will be recorded as steeper than they really are. The Bausch and Lomb instrument can be fitted with such lenses to extend its range to measure very steep or flat corneas.

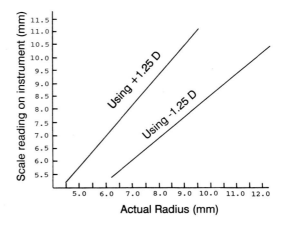

Figure 16.28 A typical graph to give the radius with + 1.25 or − 1.00 D added to the objective. Extended range is 4.5–12 mm of radius of curvature.

16.7 KERATOMETRY ADAPTED FOR PERIPHERAL CORNEAL MEASUREMENT

There are several approaches to analysing the peripheral corneal contour. A conventional keratometer may be used with the subject's fixation displaced from the normal position, analysis of photo keratographs (Chapter 00), and modified or specialized keratometers.

16.7.1 PERIPHERAL FIXATION

It has already been explained that keratometers cannot be used accurately if the surface being measured does not have a constant radius of curvature. In spite of this some instruments provide peripheral fixation points in order to allow measurement of peripheral areas of the cornea. Despite their inaccuracy these readings do have a definite use in that any curvature changes which take place in a specific area of cornea can be recorded numerically: for example flattening or steepening due to contact lens wear and during the healing of corneal wounds. The value of such readings using ordinary keratometers must be to a certain extent qualitative. Discs incorporating peripheral fixation points can be attached to several keratometers, for example the Bausch and Lomb, and Rodenstock instruments.

If the cornea is assumed to be an ellipsoid of revolution, then peripheral keratometry can give an indication of the asphericity of the cornea. Baker (1943) derived a general equation for any conic section with its apex at the co-ordinate origin and vertex radius r_0:

$$y^2 = 2r_0x - px^2 \qquad \text{(eqn 16.3)}$$

The value given to the parameter p determines the type of conic section (Fig. 16.29). A value of one gives a circular cross-section, while a positive value less than one gives ellipses with curvature flattening away from the apex, typical of the human cornea. Other writers use the term Q for $(p-1)$, some the term 'eccentricity' either for e equalling $(1-p)$ or for e equalling $(1-p)^2$.

At any point P, away from the vertex of the surface, there are two radii of curvature, the sagittal and the tangential. In Figure 16.30, the line PN is normal to the surface at P. The sagittal arc SPS is formed by rotating P

around the axis AA', and thus has a radius of curvature $r_s = PC_s$. Mathematically, this is given by:

$$r_s = \{r_0^2 + (1-p)y^2\}^{1/2} \qquad \text{(eqn 16.4)}$$

The tangential radius r_t is that of the arc TPT in the plane of the diagram, with centre of curvature at C_t. The radius r_t can be calculated from that of r_s by the equation.

$$r_t = r_s^3/r_0^2 \qquad \text{(eqn 16.5)}$$

With a non-astigmatic or 'spherical' cornea, the tangential radius in the periphery may be measured by displacing fixation away from the centre along the plane of the mires. If fixation is made on a point approximately mid-way between the nasal mire and the centre of the telescope objective, then the light from the nasal mire will be reflected off the centre of the cornea, while the other mire image will be formed by reflection approximately 3 mm temporal to the corneal apex. Assuming the variation in corneal curvature over the central 3 mm diameter zone to be negligible, the resulting peripheral reading will be the mean of the central radius and that of the peripheral area reflecting the other

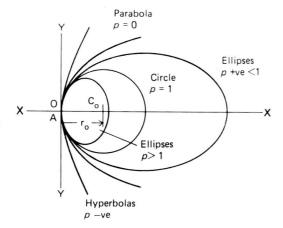

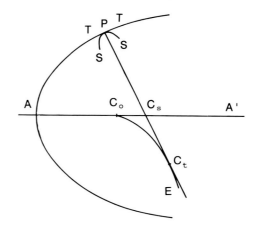

Figure 16.29 Conic sections all having the same radius of curvature r_0 at the pole. A schematical aspherical cornea showing peripheral flattening or steepening of curvature is formed by revolution of the curve about the x-axis (reproduced by kind permission of Mr A. G. Bennett).

Figure 16.30 The sagittal and tangential radii of curvature at a peripheral point on an aspheric surface. Centres of curvature C_s (sagittal) and C_t (tangential). Arcs SS and TT are in the mutually perpendicular sagittal and tangential planes.

mire. An example will serve to illustrate this:

Central keratometer reading (C)   8.00 mm
Peripheral keratometer reading (M) 8.20 mm
(the mean of 8.00 and 8.40 mm)

Thus the peripheral area used for mire reflection has a radius P of 8.4 mm. In other words, P = M + (M − C).

More peripheral readings may be obtained by fixation of the nasal mire, or beyond. The difference in size of the images reflected by the 'central' and peripheral zone of the cornea is readily apparent. Mandell (1962) discusses some of the approximations that are made in this simple calculation, while a scheme for calculating the departure of the corneal contour from that of a circle using the Rodenstock instrument is given by Wilms and Rabbetts (1977).

The sagittal radius in the periphery may be obtained by displacing fixation perpendicularly to the plane of the mires: Figure 16.31 illustrates the attachment to the Zeiss keratometer. A similar device may also be fitted to their ophthalmometer.

Sheridan and Douthwaite (1989), citing Bennett's (1987) previously unpublished analysis, showed that if an ellipsoid is viewed at an angle θ from its axis of revolution, the height y of the peripheral point P is $r_s \sin \theta$. Knowing the central and peripheral keratometry reading, r_0 and r_s respectively, Baker's equation may be re-arranged to give the parameter p:

$$p = 1 - \left\{ \frac{r_s^2 - r_o^2}{r_s^2 \sin^2 \theta} \right\}$$

As most corneas are toroidal, Wilms and Rabbetts (1977) showed that a correction factor of the numerical difference between the steep and flat central keratometry readings has to be added to or subtracted from the peripheral sagittal readings. Thus in Figure 16.32, illustrating with-the-rule astigmatism, H and V are the central keratometry radii. The keratometry reading, r_v, obtained with the mires in a vertical plane at P_N in the nasal periphery is governed both by the corneal toricity and the corneal flattening. The sagittal radius, r_s, is obtained by adding the difference (H–V) to r_v.

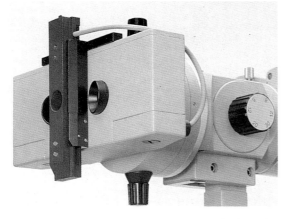

Figure 16.31 The fixation device attached to the Zeiss keratometer for sagittal radius measurement. Reproduced by courtesy of Zeiss (Oberkochen) Ltd.

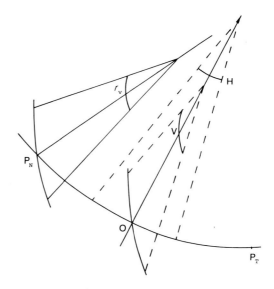

Figure 16.32 The sagittal keratometry measurement at a peripheral point P_N of the cornea, showing with-the-rule astigmatism. H and V are the central keratometry radii, and r_v is the keratometry reading taken with the mires in a vertical plane.

Conversely, the sagittal radius for a point above or below the visual axis is obtained by subtracting (H–V) from the instrumental reading.

Means of the two sets of readings taken on either side of the normal fixation axis should normally be used, though analysis of keratographs (see Chapter 17) shows that the flattening is rarely equal on opposite sides of the corneal pole.

16.7.2 SPECIALIZED INSTRUMENTS

Bonnet and Cochet (1962) developed the now obsolete topographical keratometer manufactured by Gilbert Routit. To isolate a small area of the cornea, only single mire was used for peripheral readings, a separate doubling system being incorporated to allow one end of the single mire's image to coincide with the other. A fuller description of this and some other instruments is given by Stone (1975).

The converse approach was made by Douthwaite and Sheridan (1989). A Bausch and Lomb instrument was modified by increasing the separation of the minus signs (see Fig. 16.16) to give reflection areas about 6 mm apart. The doubling prism in this meridian was also modified. The corneal curvature is first measured conventionally in the meridian with the plus signs of the mire. The instrument is then rotated through 90°, and the same meridian measured with the large mire, both readings being taken with central fixation. The corneal asphericity (*p*-value) in this meridian may then be calculated from these two readings. Good agreement was obtained with results from other techniques.

Ryland (1910) and Bennett (1964) have independently suggested a Drysdale-type keratometer; (this principle, applied to the microspherometer, is described in Chapter 00). Douthwaite (1987) modified this principle by incorporating a cylindrical or Stokes lens behind the microscope objective which

therefore forms two astigmatic focal line images. If the instrument as a whole is moved to place the image nearest the objective on the corneal surface, the cylindrical lens can then be adjusted to position the other image at the centre of curvature of the corneal surface. This simultaneous setting of the mire reflections is necessary to reduce errors caused by patient movement, for the same reason that the normal keratometer incorporates a doubling system. Because only a small reflection zone is employed, topographical keratometry should be possible with this type of instrument.

By arranging the orientation of the mires to be parallel and perpendicular to the displacement of fixation, peripheral small mire keratometry can automatically give the sagittal and tangential radii of curvature. Because the centre of curvature of the tangential arcs do not lie on the axis of the cornea, the corneal profile is an evolute (Fig. 16.33).

16.8 AUTOMATED INSTRUMENTS

Various electronic instruments have become available for the measurement of the corneal radius. Because of the speed of electronic recording, conventional doubling systems are unnecessary, but the instruments have to

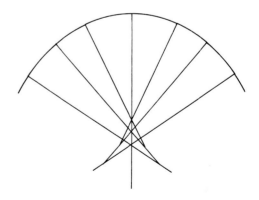

Figure 16.33 Simulation of the corneal curvature using an evolute of centres which become offset when the region measured is peripheral.

determine both the meridians and radii. The first automated instrument was the Humphrey Auto-Keratometer.

This instrument projects three beams of near infrared light onto the cornea in a triangular pattern about 3 mm in diameter. One beam is positioned on either side of the fixational axis, with the third below it. After reflection, they are received by directional photosensors, which effectively isolate rays making a predetermined angle with the instrument's optical axis. In principle, although the ray paths are reversed, this recalls a variable doubling keratometer in which the mires subtend a constant angle at the cornea.

Figure 16.34 shows a simplified scheme of ray paths in one of the three beams. The source S is a light-emitting diode (LED) focused by condenser L to form an image S′ on the instrument's axis. This image, in turn, acts as an object for projector lens P which forms a second image S″ behind the patient's eye. One ray RH of the reflected beam – not necessarily the central one through L – passes into the detector D at the predetermined angle. In general, skew reflection takes place unless the meridians of the corneal astigmatism are exactly horizontal and vertical.

The precise location of the reflection point R on the cornea is determined by the position of the rotating chopper C, which sweeps across all three beams and is imaged in the plane of the cornea by projector lens P. Since the image S″ lies on the axis at a known position, the angle at which the incident ray GR meets the cornea can also be determined. From the information provided by all three beams, the principal radii and meridians of the cornea on the visual axis can then be calculated by the internal computer.

Peripheral readings may then be taken with the subject's fixation directed in turn at 13.5° to either side of the central fixation mark. Their purpose is to provide the additional data needed to determine the quasi-ellipsoidal surface giving the best fit to the cornea. The parameter *e* defining the 'shape' of this hypothetical surface in its horizontal meridian is included in the print-out, together with the estimated position of its apex relative to the visual axis. The calculated principal radii and meridians at the apex of this surface are also recorded in addition to those measured on the visual axis of the true cornea. A more detailed account of this instrument is given by Rabbetts (1985).

The Canon Auto-Refractor/Keratometer RK-1 provides two concentric ring mires for reflection at the corneal surface. Annular lenses of cylindrical cross-section collimate the mires, thus partially compensating for the short working distance of 45 mm. The inner mire is transilluminated by a circular fluorescent tube, and focused by means of a closed circuit television system. When correctly positioned, an electronic flash behind the outer mire is triggered. The resulting mire image falls onto a photodetector subdivided into five sectors.

In general, this image will be elliptical – the co-ordinates of its centre and shape are calculated from the relative amounts of radiation falling on each sector of the photodetector. In turn, the corneal meridians and radii may be determined. Descriptions of the earlier Auto-Keratometer K-1 are given by Port (1985) and Stockwell (1986). Ehlrich and Tromans (1988) found the repeatability of measurements on

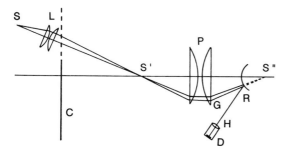

Figure 16.34 Principle of the Humphrey Auto-Keratometer (drawn from information kindly provided by Humphrey Instruments Inc).

both steel balls and normal, non-contact-lens-wearing corneas to be slightly better with this instrument than those made with a conventional one position keratometer.

At the date of publication, other auto-keratometers are manufactured by Nidek and Topcon.

16.9   USE OF THE KERATOMETER AFTER CONTACT LENS WEAR

16.9.1   REFRACTIVE CHANGES RELATIVE TO KERATOMETRY

After wearing contact lenses many patients experience blurred vision with the spectacles that previously afforded them good visual acuity. If this is due to light scatter in corneal oedema, then visual acuity cannot be restored to normal with correcting lenses. In rigid lens wear, oedema can usually be detected by using the scleral scatter illumination technique with the slit lamp biomicroscope. If, however, the blurring is due to change in corneal curvature, it should be detectable with a keratometer; for example, if a person has become 1 D more myopic then the corneal radius would be decreased by about 0.2 mm. Any blur caused by induced corneal irregularity should also show up with the keratometer, provided it is in the area used for reflection. From this point of view, retinoscopy can provide a superior quality control for the corneal contour because it allows inspection of the whole pupillary aperture. Irregularities of mire image formation are often due to oedema or moulding of the cornea to the contact lens. Keratometry and/or retinoscopy is therefore essential for the follow-up care of the patient.

The ring mire of the Bausch and Lomb type instrument is often recommended for its ability to demonstrate corneal distortion because the mire image loses its circular shape. The ring is reflected from a complete annular zone of the cornea, and therefore inspects a larger area of the cornea than a two position instrument which samples only four elemental zones within this annulus. Conversely, the Scheiner disc doubling of the ring mire with a distorted cornea can lead to uncertainty in setting the focus, it being impossible to obtain a single image of the whole circle. Distortion of the mires of other instruments is very nearly as obvious.

16.10   USE OF THE KERATOMETER IN SURGERY

As a simplification, the eye's refractive error is governed by four factors, the focusing ability of the cornea and crystalline lens, and the depth of the anterior chamber and overall length of the eye.

In cataract surgery in which the natural lens is replaced with an implant, sometimes called pseudophakia, the required dioptric power for the lens can be calculated if the corneal power and axial length are measured. Based on a statistical analysis of postoperative assessments, Retzlaff *et al.* (1981) have derived formulae for various types of implant. A typical one for posterior chamber lenses is:

$$F_i = 116.8 - 2.5 \ axial \ length - 0.9F_c$$

where F_i and F_c are the implant and corneal powers, respectively. A more rigorous optical treatment of this subject has been given by Bennett and Rabbetts (1989).

During the operation, care has to be taken when suturing the incision to avoid distorting the cornea. A ring type mire is provided in, for example, the Keeler Amoils Astigmometer, which is attached to the operating microscope. A comparison ring placed in the eyepiece can be tilted with respect to the optical axis to estimate the amount of corneal distortion.

16.11   MEASUREMENT OF CONTACT LENSES

In the same way that the keratometer is used to observe the cornea and measure its curvature, so it may be used for observing and measuring contact lenses. They are best mounted horizontally and viewed through a 45° inclined mirror, as shown in Figure 16.35. In measuring the back optic zone radius (BOZR) of a lens, it must be remembered that the area of surface used for reflection is outside the paraxial region. Since the spherical aberration introduced by a concave surface is different from that of a convex surface, a correction factor must be applied to the radius measurement obtained for concave surfaces. The optical theory underlying the difference in measurement between convex and concave surfaces has been fully dealt with by Emsley (1963), whose findings have been confirmed by Bennett (1966). They have shown that, on average, 0.03 mm must be added to the radius recorded by the Bausch and Lomb keratometer when measuring concave surfaces.

Calibration tables are provided by the

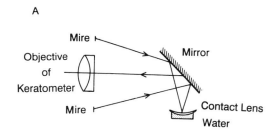

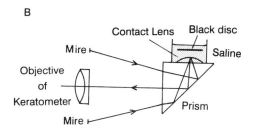

Figure 16.35 The keratometer used for contact lens measurement. (A) A front-surface silvered mirror for verifying the BOZR of rigid lenses. (B) A prism and saline cell for checking soft lenses. The position of the mires in both illustrations is diagrammatic – they will usually be placed in a horizontal plane.

manufacturer, and have been published by Mandell (1965b). A practitioner can easily produce a calibration graph for his own instrument by measuring a series of trial lenses on the keratometer, and having the same lenses measured on an optical microspherometer or radiuscope (see Chapter 00) by a laboratory. Because of their stability of radius, low power PMMA lenses may be better for this purpose than gas permeable lenses.

Disturbing reflections from the front surface can be minimized by mounting the lens in a drop of water or petroleum jelly. The front surface radius may be measured similarly, but no correction factor need be applied. Alternative methods of mounting the lens are to use surface tension to hold the lens in place in a depression on the vertical face of a bar attached to the headrest, or to hold the lens onto a flat bar with double-sided adhesive tape and add a drop of viscous wetting solution between the lens and tape to reduce the front surface reflection. Careful cleaning is subsequently needed.

Soft lenses may be similarly measured, but in this case a reflecting prism is used to direct the light upwards, while the lens is placed concave side down in saline in a wet cell on top of the prism. A black disc immersed in the saline above the lens is used to eliminate light reflected from the surface of the saline, while reflections from both surfaces of the lens are seen. With a negative power lens, it is the smaller image that is measured, since it is reflected by the steeper back surface. Conversely, it is the larger image in positive lenses. Because the lens is measured in saline, the resulting findings need to be multiplied by the reciprocal of the refractive index of saline, i.e. approximately 4/3. Also, as only the central few millimetres of the lens are being measured, the results may not be relevant to soft lens fitting where it is the average radius over a 10 to 12 mm chord which governs the sag or vault height of the lens. A keratometer with small, bright mires is essential. The Rodenstock BES instrument may be fitted with a supplementary lens system which both compensates the instrument for focusing errors (see page 297) and magnifies the mire image so that the radius scale reads correctly without conversion. An auxiliary system may also be fitted to the Zeiss Ophthalmometer so that it also indicates the correct radius.

16.12 THE ULTRAVIOLET LAMP

Rigid lens fitting has traditionally been verified by instilling a drop of a dilute solution of fluorescein sodium, and observing the brightness of the fluorescing tear layer trapped under the contact lens with a lamp emitting long wavelength ultraviolet (UV-A) and short wavelength blue light. Special fluorescent tubes are used, one mounted above and below a low powered magnifier used to aid observation. One of the earliest lamps of this type was the Burton lamp, and this name is often applied generically. Campbell and Patella (1986) showed that the minimum thickness of tears film under a lens that could be detected with this technique was 0.0022 mm, while the gradation of intensity could be seen up to a thickness of 0.02 mm.

Figure 16.36 shows that a dilute solution of fluorescien absorbs radiation maximally between 485 and 500 nm, and re-emits greenish light at a peak wavelength of between 525 and 530 nm (Pearson, 1984). The ultraviolet-emitting tubes provide peak radiation at 350 nm (Fig. 16.37), though there are small subsidiary emissions at 405 and 435 nm from the mercury vapour spectrum.

In order to provide greater contrast, the blue radiation can be absorbed by tinting the magnifying glass yellow or covering it with a yellow filter, thus leaving only the emitted green light to be seen. Possible filters are Kodak Wratten 15 (gelatin), Schott OG30

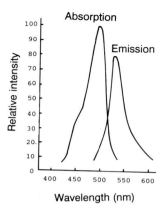

Figure 16.36 The absorption and emission spectrum of fluorescein sodium (redrawn from Pearson, 1984, by kind permission of the British Contact Lens Association).

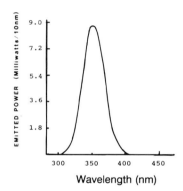

Figure 16.37 The emission spectrum of a 'Blacklight Blue' miniature tubular fluorescent lamp. This diagram omits representation of the residual mercury spectrum and is based on data provided by Thorn EMI Lighting LT and GTE Sylvania Ltd (redrawn from Pearson, 1984, by kind permission of the British Contact Lens Association).

(glass) or Lee Filter's 101* (coated polyester) (Fig. 16.38). The same filters may be used to advantage in visual and photographic observation with the slit lamp.

Many of the early gas permeable materials, with their pale and often blue tints, have a

* Obtainable from Lee Filters, Central Way, Walworth Industrial Estate, Andover, Hants, SP10 5AN, England.

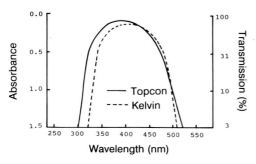

Figure 16.38 The absorption spectrum of yellow barrier filters (redrawn with addition from Pearson, 1984, by kind permission of the British Contact Lens Association).

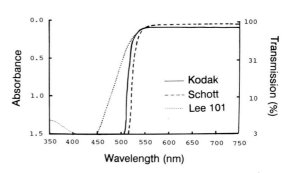

Figure 16.39 Absorbance/transmission characteristics of blue filters in slit lamp microscopes. (redrawn from Pearson, 1984, by kind permission of the British Contact Lens Association).

higher UV transmission than the grey-brown PMMA 912 material (Allen, 1986). This may explain why, for example, slight apical clearance of a PMMA lens appears as a greater clearance in a nominally identical gas permeable lens. Conversely, some modified PMMA and an increasing number of gas permeable materials incorporate UV absorbing filters. This prevents the UV radiation from reaching the fluorescein under the lens, apart from the capillary ring around the lens edge.

One alternative technique is to use the blue filter on the slit lamp. This should preferably not have a significant secondary red transmission as occurs with cobalt blue glass: the red light is reflected by the melanin pigment in the patient's iris. Figure 16.39 shows that the blue transmission from two manufacturers' filters covers the absorption spectrum of the fluorescein.

Another possibilty would be to replace the ultraviolet tubes with white ones covered with blue filter material, for example Lee Filter's 132 medium blue or 119 dark blue. Some ultraviolet lamps are fitted with four tubes, giving the practitioner the choice of keeping the UV and covering the white tubes, or replacing the UV tubes and retaining the white. The writer finds that the white tubes are too bright for many patients, and therefore has covered them with neutral filter.

REFERENCES

Allen, N.C. (1986) Ultraviolet transmission properties of some contact lens materials. *Optom. Today*, **26**, 571–2.

Baker, T.Y. (1943) Ray tracing through non-spherical surfaces. *Proc. Phys. Soc.*, **55**, 361–4.

Bennett, A.G. (1964) A new keratometer and its application to corneal topography. *Br. J. Physiol. Optics.*, **21**, 234–8.

Bennett, A.G. (1966) The calibration of keratometers. *Optician*, **151**, 317–22.

Bennett, A.G. (1987) Drysdale-type keratometer: determination of *p*-value. (Personal communication).

Bennett, A.G. and Rabbetts, R.B. (1989) *Clinical Visual Optics*, 2nd ed. Butterworths, London, pp.270–3.

Bennett, A.G. and Rabbetts, R.B. (1991) What radius does a conventional keratometer measure? *Ophthal. Phsiol. Opt.*, **11**, 239–47.

Bonnett, R. and Cochet, P. (1962) New method of topographical ophthalmometry: its theoretical and clinical applications. *Am. J. Optom.*, **39**, 227–51.

Campbell, C. and Patella, M. (1986) The minimum observable fluorescein film thickness. *Optician*, **192**, 5071, 32.

Charman, W.N. (1972) Diffraction and the precision of measurement of corneal and other small radii. *Am. J. Optom.*, **49**, 672–80.

Clark, B.A.J. (1973) Keratometry: a review. *Aust. J. Optom.*, **56**, 94–100.

de Wecker, L and Masselon, J (1882) Astigometre

de De Wecker et Masselon. *Ann. Oculist*, **88**, 44.

Donders, F.C. (1864) *On the Anomalies of Accommodation and Refraction*. New Sydenham Society, London.

Douthwaite, W.A. (1987) A new keratometer. *Am. J. Optom.*, **64**, 711–15.

Douthwaite, W.A. and Sheridan, M. (1989) The measurement of the corneal ellipse for the contact lens practitioner. *Opthal. Physiol. Opt.*, **9**, 239–42.

Emsley, H.H. (1963) The keratometer: measurement of concave surfaces. *Optician*, **146**, 161–8.

Ehrlich, D.L. and Tromans, C. (1988) The Canon RK-1: Keratometry mode evaluation. Poster: *The International Contact Lens Centenary Congress*, London.

Goode, H. (1847) On a peculiar defect of vision. *Trans. Camb. Phil. Soc.*, **8**, 493.

Gullstrand, A. (1896) Photographische-Ophthalmometrische und Klinische Untersuchungen uber die Hornhautrefraktion. *K. Svenska Vetensk Acad. Handl.*, **28**, 7.

Gullstrand, A. (1909) Appendix to Helmholtz (1909).

Heine, L. (1929) Die Korrectur samlicher Ametropien durch gesechliffene Kontaktschalen. *Bericht. Kong. Ophthal.*, **1**, 232.

Helmholtz, H. von. (1909/1962) *Handbuch der Physiologischen Optic*. Translated as *Treatise on Physiological Optics* (ed. J.P.C. Southall), Dover Publications, London.

Javal, A. and Schiotz, I. (1881) Un ophthalmometre practique. *Trans. Int. Med. Congr. London*. **3**, 30.

Kohlrausch (1840) cited in Helmholtz (1909/1962).

Krause, C. (1832) Bemerkungwyn uber den Bau und die Dimensionen des menschlichen Augen. *Meckels Arch. Anat. Physiol.*, **6**, 86.

Lehman, S.P. (1967) Corneal areas used in keratometry. *Optician*, **154**, 261–4.

Levene, J.R. (1965) The true inventors of the keratoscope. *Br. J. Hist. Sci.*, **2**, 324–42.

Levene, J.R. (1977) *Clinical Refraction and Visual Science*, Butterworths, London, pp. 128–31.

Mandell, R.B. (1960) Jessie Ramsden – inventor of the ophthalmometer. *Am. J. Optom.*, **37**, 633–8.

Mandell, R.B. (1962) Reflection point ophthalmometry. *Am. J. Optom.*, **39**, 513–37.

Mandell, R.B. (1964) Corneal areas used in keratometry. *Am. J. Optom.*, **41**, 150.

Mandell, R.B. (1965a) *Contact Lens Practice, Basic and Advanced*. Thomas, Springfield, IL, pp. 48–50.

Mandell, R.B. (1965b) *Contact Lens Practice, Basic and Advanced*. Thomas, Springfield, IL, pp. 453–5.

Mandell, R.B. and St Helen, R. (1969) Position and curvature of the corneal apex. *Am. J. Optom.*, **46**, 25–9.

Nordensen, E. (1883) Recherches ophthalmometriques sur l'astigmatism de la cornee humaine chez les ecoliers de 7 a 20 ans. *Ann. Oculist*, **89**, 341.

Obrig, T.E. (1942) *Contact Lenses*, 1st edn, Chilton, Philadelphia, p. 23.

Pearson, R.M. (1984) The mystery of the missing fluorescein. *J. Brit. Contact Lens Ass.*, **7**, 122–5.

Plácido, A. (1880a) Novo instrumento de esploracao de cornea. *Periodico Oftalmol. Pract.*, **5**, 27–30.

Plácido, A (1880b) Novo instrumento par analyse immediate das irregularidades de curvatura da cornea. *Periodico Oftalmol. Pract.*, **6**, 44–9.

Plácido, A. (1882) Correspondence. *Zentbl. Prakt. Augenheilk.*, **6**, 157.

Port, M (1985) The Canon Auto-keratometer K1. *J. Brit. Contact Lens Ass.*, **8**, 79–85.

Rabbetts, R.B. (1977) Comparative focusing errors of keratometers. *Optician*, **173** (4482), 28–9.

Rabbetts, R.B. (1985) The Humphrey Auto-keratometer. *Ophthal. Physiol. Opt.*, **5**, 451–8.

Retzlaff, J., Sanders, D. and Kraff, M. (1981) *A Manual of Implant Power Calculation: SRK formula*. Medford, Oregon. Published by the authors.

Ryland, H.S. (1910) On ophthalmic instruments. *Trans. Opt. Soc. Am.*, **12**, 105–12.

Scheiner, C. (1619) *Oculus Sive Fundamentum Opticum*. Innsbruck.

Senff, R. (1846) quoted by Helmholtz (1909/1962).

Shick, C. (1962) A simple mire modification to improve keratometer efficiency. *J. Am. Optom. Ass.*, **34**, 388.

Sheridan, M. and Douthwaite W.A. (1989) Corneal asphericity and refractive error. *Ophthal. Physiol. Opt.*, **9**, 235–8.

Steiger, A. (1895) *Beitrage zur Physiologie und Pathologie der Hauthorn-refraction*. Wiesbaden.

Stockwell, H. (1986) From old ophthalmometers to new keratometers. *Optician*, **191** (5041), 18–24.

Stone, J. (1962) The validity of some existing methods for measuring corneal contour compared with suggested new methods. *Br. J. Physiol. Optics.*, **19**, 205–30.

Stone, J. (1975) Keratometry. In *Contact Lens Prac-*

tice: Visual, Therapeutic and Prosthetic (ed. M. Ruben), Bailliere Tindall, London, pp. 104–29.

Sulzer, D. (1891/92) La forme de la cornee humaine et son influence sur la vision. *Arch. Ophthal., Paris*, **11** (419); 12, 32.

Wilms, K.H. and Rabbetts, R.B. (1977) Practical concepts of corneal topography. *Optician*, **174** (4502), 7, 8, 12, 13.

Wittenberg, S. and Ludlam, W.M. (1966) Derivation of a system for analysing the corneal surface from photokeratoscopic data. *J. Opt. Soc. Am.*, **56**, 1612–15.

M. Guillon and A. Ho

17.1 INTRODUCTION

17.1.1 AIMS AND APPLICATIONS

The aim of photokeratoscopy is to measure and describe accurately the shape of the corneal front surface in all meridians. Although a difficult task due to the complex shape of the cornea, photokeratoscopy has numerous useful applications. These can be classified as follows:

Monitoring of corneal changes

A number of eye surgeries (both corneal and intraocular) are accompanied post-surgically by changes in the shape of the cornea. These changes to the corneal topography may be unintentional; as in the case of cataract extractions (Smith, 1977), or intentional; in the form of refractive surgery (McDonnell & Garbus, 1988). Changes in corneal topography are also seen in certain corneal diseases such as keratoconus. The close monitoring of any changes is essential to patient management for three main reasons:

1. In baseline (pre-surgery) examinations as a reference for further/future measurements. This is also important as a safe-guard in any possible legal developments.
2. To monitor the progress of any pathology or in surgical cases of surgical operations, to ensure that any procedures used do not create any unacceptable/adverse effects.
3. To assess the duration of the post-surgical stabilization period in order to establish the optimum period before prescribing follow-up treatments (e.g. optical appliances).

Contact lens fitting

Corneal topography influences the choice of the posterior contact lense surface geometry, e.g. radii of curvature. This is particularly important in the fitting of rigid lenses (Moss, 1959; Von Fieandt 1965; Brungardt, 1965; Kemmetmuller, 1984; Kivayev *et al*, 1985). In routine practice, clinicians assess the fit of contact lenses by subjective assessment of the fluorescein pattern of the tear layer situated between the contact lens and the cornea (Phillips, 1980). An exact knowledge of the patient's corneal surface shape would render this choice less empirical (Amiard & Cochet, 1972). Similarly, lens designers can benefit from the knowledge of the corneal shape of large patient populations when designing lenses to provide optimal fitting characteristics (Bibby, 1976b).

Corneal optical modelling

The front surface of the cornea is the most powerful ocular refractive surface and a

Contact Lens Practice. Edited by Montague Ruben and Michel Guillon.
Published in 1994 by Chapman & Hall, London. ISBN 0 412 35120 X

major determinant of the optical performance of the eye. A knowledge of its exact geometric form is therefore essential to any modelling of the optical system of the eye (El Hage, 1971; Lotmar, 1971; Klyce, 1989).

17.1.2 MEASUREMENT PRINCIPLES

Photokeratoscopy and keratometry are based on a similar principle, making use of the reflective property of the corneal front surface (Duke-Elder, 1970; Borish, 1975). In both techniques, information regarding corneal shape is obtained by measuring the size of the image of the target formed by corneal reflection. In keratometry the central corneal radii are calculated from measurements made with a single target (Clark, 1973b). In keratoscopy a series of targets, usually circular, are used. This arrangement of targets allows both the central and peripheral corneal curvature, and consequently the corneal topography, to be assessed (Clark, 1973c).

Keratoscopy may be carried out qualitatively with the use of equipment which involves nothing more than a Placido disk (Klein, 1958; Levene, 1962). However, it is when a recording of the image created by the cornea of the target is made and subsequently used for quantitative measurements of corneal topography that the true potential of keratoscopy is realized.

Photokeratoscopy hence involves the measurement or estimation of the sizes of the optical images of a series of targets created by corneal reflection. Traditionally, a photographic record is made using a flash tube light source in order to eliminate eye movements. The measurements and calculations are then made from the photographs. Recently, the advances made in microprocessing have made it possible for the keratoscopic image to be captured electronically and analysed on line using high-speed, modern personal computers with dedicated programs. The new instruments are known as video keratoscopes.

The methods used to convert measurements of image size to local corneal radii, and subsequently corneal topography, involves the application of geometrical optics. However, when we consider the complexity of the contour of the anterior surface of the cornea and the limitations of the photokeratoscopic system it is possible to understand the many problems associated with photokeratoscopy.

The problems, and the instrument designs and special features employed to overcome or minimize these problems will be discussed in this chapter.

17.2 INSTRUMENTATION

17.2.1 GENERAL FEATURES

Introduction

Historical notes

The invention of photokeratoscopy cannot be attributed to any particular individual. A review of the literature points to a series of developments that have evolved into modern photokeratoscopy.

Scheiner, in the seventeenth century, and Senff (1846) in the nineteenth century, were apparently the first to analyse the shape of the cornea and compare it to an ellipsoid (Bonnet & Cochet, 1962).

The invention of the concentric ring target which is the basis of modern keratoscopes is variously attributed to Amsler (Bonnet & Cochet, 1962) and to Goode (1847) (Clark, 1973c).

Placido, 1880 is thought to be the first to have produced a photokeratoscope; this instrument was used for qualitative analysis of keratoconic corneas by Javal (Holden, 1970; Clark, 1973c).

Gullstrand in 1896 (translated by Ludlam, 1966; Ludlam & Wittenberg, 1966a) was the first to achieve quantitative photokeratoscopy. He analysed the data obtained using a flat target instrument consisting of four concentric rings that covered a diameter of approximately 4 mm. By the judicious choice of additional fixation points he was able to obtain information covering the whole cornea (Ludlam & Wittenberg, 1966b).

From these early instruments further improvements have been made resulting in the sophisticated instruments of today. These improvements will be discussed in the ensuing sections.

Photokeratoscope subsystems

Photokeratoscopes are basically composed of three sub systems (Fig. 17.1):

The photokeratoscopic target The photokeratoscopic target is the object which is imaged by the cornea. The measurement of the image of this target is the basis for the determination of corneal parameters.

The optical system The role of the optical system is to focus the image of the target produced by the cornea onto the recording plane. The optical system also enables the operator to focus the instrument correctly.

The recording system The recording system creates a permanent record (photographic, electronic/digital signal, etc.) of the image of the target produced by the cornea and the optical system. It is this permanent record

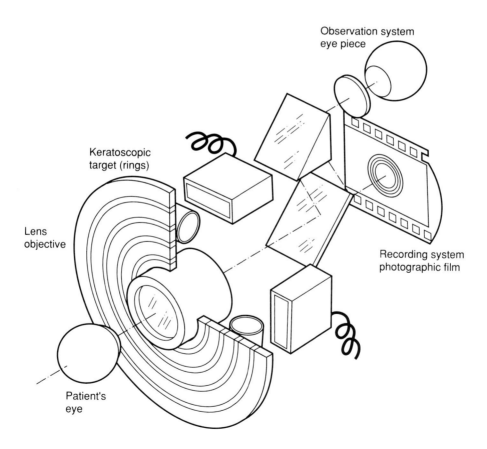

Figure 17.1 Photokeratoscope main component systems.

which is used for analysis.

We will describe and assess the general features of the photokeratoscope according to the above three subsystems.

Targets

Photokeratoscopic targets can be classified according to three major features: (1) target locus; (2) target type; and (3) target illumination.

Target locus describes the geometric surface on which the individual targets are positioned (e.g. hemispherical, cylindrical).

Target type refers to the geometrical shape of the individual targets (e.g. rings, bars).

Target illumination refers to whether the target's behaviour as a light source for the recording system can be equated to a diffusive or a directional source.

Target locus

The target locus is the target feature that has the greatest influence on the instrument's performance because it controls the extent of corneal coverage by the target and also affects the shape of the image field (e.g. plane, curved) formed by the optical system. Therefore, classification of photokeratoscopes may be based on the target locus, the geometric surface on which the target is built.

Target loci can be classified into five groups: (1) plane; (2) hemispherical; (3) cylindrical; (4) ellipsoidal; and (5) others.

Plane targets Plane targets are often referred to as flat targets (Table 17.1). A flat target is the simplest target locus to produce and the earliest used. Its invention has been attributed to Amsler (Bonnet & Cochet, 1962). A review of the literature showed an abundance of instruments built with such a target (Clark, 1973c). However, it has the greatest number of limitations. First, only limited corneal coverage is possible; practically never more than 60% of the cornea (Aan De Kerk *et al.*, 1973). Second, curvature of field of the image produced by the cornea for a plane object makes it impossible to attain correct focus for the entire target (Knoll *et al.* 1957).

Hemispherical targets In order to increase corneal coverage by the target, Berg (in 1929) proposed a hemispherical target (Bonnet & Cochet, 1962; Holden, 1970; Clark, 1973c) that provides up to 80% corneal coverage (Donaldson, 1972). Such a target also tends to decrease the curvature of field of the image.

Cylindrical target Dekking in 1930, proposed that the curvature of the image surface of a flat target produced by the cornea was in the same direction as the cornea and suggested the use of a cylindrical target to overcome this problem. This design improved results with regard to image focus and also enabled full corneal coverage (Ludlam & Wittenberg, 1966c; Aan De Kerk *et al*, 1973).

Ellipsoidal target Further investigation of the problem of a flat field image led Ludlam (Ludlam & Wittenberg, 1966c) to suggest the use of an ellipsoid of revolution for a target locus to obtain a plane image. Such a target locus, however, can only truly provide a flat image field for a cornea with a specific profile.

Other targets Two other targets have been described which give good results: a cardioid (Amiard, 1972, 1973) and projected targets (Westheimer, 1965; El Hage, 1971; Clark, 1972; Fujii *et al.*, 1972).

Target type

Two types of targets have been used: (1) rings; and (2) lines, bars and points.

Ring targets These offer the greatest advantages and are the most commonly used photokeratoscopic targets. In particular, each

Table 17.1 Classification of photokeratoscopes according to target locii

Target	Qualitative experimental instrument	Quantitative experimental instrument	Qualitative commercial instrument	Quantitative commercial instrument
P L A N E	Streiff J, 1900 Hartinger, 1930 Von der Heydt, 1932 Howard, 1936 Kokott, 1938 Streiff EB, 1938 Fincham, 1953 Phillips & Hansell, 1954 Hansell, 1956 Stein, 1958 Reynolds & Kratt, 1959 Perth Photokeratoscope, 1961 Norton & Sullivan, 1962 Zingara, 1963 Brown, 1969	Gullstrand, 1896 AIM Keratograph, 1956 Keeler Keratoscope, 1958 Photo-Electronic Keratoscope (PEK) of Reynolds, 1959	Zeiss Reflectograph, 1930 Photokeratoscope, 1980	Nidek Sun PKS-1000 Photokeratoscope
H E M I S P H E R E		Berg, 1929 Lenoble, 1952 Knoll, Stansson & Weeks, 1957 Stone, 1962 Donaldson, 1972		Corneascope photokeratoscope of International Diagnostic Instruments
C Y L I N D R I C A L	Dekking, 1930 Eye Hospital Rotterdam Photokeratoscope	Knoll Bausch & Lomb Photokeratoscope, 1961 Ludlam & Wittenberg, 1966 Mandell, 1968 El Hage Photokeratoscope (EHP), 1976 Photokeratoscope (EHP), 1976	Bausch & Lomb Photokeratoscope, 1963	
E L L I P S O I D		Holden Photokeratoscope, 1970		Wesley Jessen Photokeratoscope, 1967 Computed Anatomy TMS-1 corneal modelling system EyeSys ES100 corneal topography and analysis system Visioptic EH-270 computerized corneal topographer
O T H E R		Cardioid target keratoscope of Amiard, 1972. Projected target keratoscope of Westheimer, 1965		

The date indicates the first reference to the instrument in the literature. The instruments are divided into experimental and commercially available instruments and are further divided into instruments that only produce photokeratoscopic images for observation and those that produce a numerical representation of the cornea.

ring, being an infinite number of points, carries information in any meridional direction. This is particularly important when analysing distorted corneas (e.g. keratoconus) where the information required for the analysis cannot be limited to two perpendicular meridians (Cohen *et al.*, 1984).

Further, with ring targets there is no need to determine the direction of the principal meridians by keratometry prior to undertaking photokeratoscopy.

Following Gullstrand's suggestion (Ludlam & Wittenburg, 1966a) the target rings are sometimes constructed with a thin black line at the centre of the illuminated ring to improve the focusing accuracy. The Wesley–Jessen Photoelectric Keratoscope (PEK) was the first commercial instrument incorporating such a feature.

Line, bar and point targets

Small thin line (or bar) and point targets, usually situated on two perpendicular arms which can be rotated, are found in a few photokeratoscopes (Berg photokeratoscope, Ysoptic Keratometre, Holden photokeratoscope). However, due to their limitations of measuring only two meridians (usually at 90 degrees), they are not included in any modern instrument.

Two other parameters to consider when assessing photokeratoscopic targets are the diameter of the central ring and the distance between successive rings.

The central ring should be as small as possible in order to give accurate information on the central radii of curvature of non-spherical surfaces.

The distance between successive rings should be as small as practicable in order to maximize the number (density) of data points. This is important when fitting curves to any meridional section. In addition, some methods of analysis are based on determining the mean value between successive rings. In those cases, smaller separations of

the rings will provide a greater accuracy.

Nature of the target illumination

The nature of the light produced by the target rings can either be: (1) diffuse; or (2) directional. These two types of illumination can be achieved by either frontal illumination of the target surface (e.g. Brown photokeratoscope (Brown, 1969)) or by transmission through a transparent or translucent target medium (e.g. Nidek PKS-1000 photokeratoscope).

Diffusive illumination Diffuse target illumination is used in the majority of photokeratoscopes. Light rays emanating from such objects are multi-directional so that at least some rays will pass through the nodal point of the optical system (assuming a standard arrangement of optical components in the photokeratoscope). With this optical arrangement, the image size of the photographic record is generally proportional to the location and size of the photokeratoscopic target.

Directional illumination Three types of photokeratoscope fall into this category: externally illuminated, collimated and projected focal targets. Externally illuminated targets were proposed and assessed by El Hage (1971). However, no instrument of this design is known. Collimated targets are found in a few instruments: (Amiard, 1972; 1973; Fuji *et al.*, 1972). The only photokeratoscope to feature a projected focal (autocollimating) target is the Clark Photokeratoscope (Clark, 1972).

The general aim of the use of these types of target illumination is to reduce the effect of, or to eliminate certain parameters during analysis.

The design of the light source for illuminating the target will depend upon the nature of that target. Obviously, the source must illuminate the whole target and must ensure that at least some of the light rays produced by the target will pass through to the recording system after reflection at the cornea. For the diffusive targets such a condition is always met, but precautions must be taken when designing light sources for instruments with reflective targets.

Optical system

The optical system of the photokeratoscope has two functions:

1. To bring the image of the target produced by the cornea into focus in the recording plane (target imaging system).
2. To enable the operator to focus the instrument accurately on to the image produced by the cornea (viewing system).

Target imaging system

Three general types of target imaging systems are encountered in photokeratoscopy. It is essential to know the exact nature of any optical arrangement used as the choice of the method of data analysis depends in part upon the nature of the optical system itself.

The three optical systems encountered are:

1. The non-telecentric systems that are found in the majority of instruments built and in all those commercially available.
2. The telecentric system, which has the advantage of eliminating errors in results otherwise introduceable by errors in focusing (EI Hage (EHP) photokeratoscope, Ysoptic Photokeratometre and Westheimer photokeratoscope).
3. Other systems are mainly of the autocollimating type, of which the autocollimating system of Clark appears to have the best potential.

Regardless of the type of target imaging system used there are a number of common requirements:

Working distance and magnification The working distance is usually defined by the target location, the latter of which is generally designed to give as large a corneal coverage as possible, while taking into consideration the patient's facial anatomical features.

The magnification is usually chosen to give optimal coverage of the recording system by the target images. In general, the highest magnification fulfilling the requirement is chosen in order to maximize resolution.

Both above requirements are dependent upon the focal length of the optical system. Typically the optical system is a long focusing microscope with a working distance of 5 cm to 30 cm and a linear magnification of ×1 to ×5.

Depth of focus and depth of field For accurate focusing, the optical system must have a narrow depth of focus. However during recording, the depth of field in the image plane must be maximal to compensate for the non-aplanatic nature of the image. These conflicting requirements can be met by using a wide aperture optical system to which a small aperture is automatically incorporated during image recording.

Aberration control The off-axis monochromatic aberrations are the major aberrations affecting the quality of photokeratoscopic recordings (Amiard & Cochet, 1972).

Curvature of field is the most problematic of these aberrations. In practice, curvature of field can be minimized in two ways. First, the optical system can be designed to provide a flat image of the target. This requires consideration of both the target locus and the curvature of field of the image of the target created by the cornea and the optical system of the photokeratoscope. (Systems delivering flat image fields generally can only be achieved with some degradation in astigmatism.) Second, a small aperture size can be used in the recording system in order to improve the depth of field.

Coma is another prominent aberration in the optical system of the photokeratoscope. Although the effect of this aberration appears severe through the view finder (especially in instruments which do not use ring targets), experience of the authors suggests that the effect of coma on the accuracy of data collection is minimal. This is true provided that the estimation of ring sizes is made at the head of the coma flare; among most the accuracy of the resultant measurement is generally not affected. Because of the skewed comatic distribution of light, this can be accomplished readily. Further, the tail of the coma flare can be reduced with the cor-

rect choice of aperture size, and film exposure and development.

The major effect of the other off-axis aberrations (astigmatism, distortion) is to alter the linear magnification of the different target rings. Their effects can be minimized by appropriate calibration and measurement procedures (Amiard & Cochet, 1967).

Viewing system

The photokeratoscope viewing system has several features that are common to other ophthalmic instruments.

The light source is usually a fluorescent tube, and is often annular.

A fixation system is incorporated in order

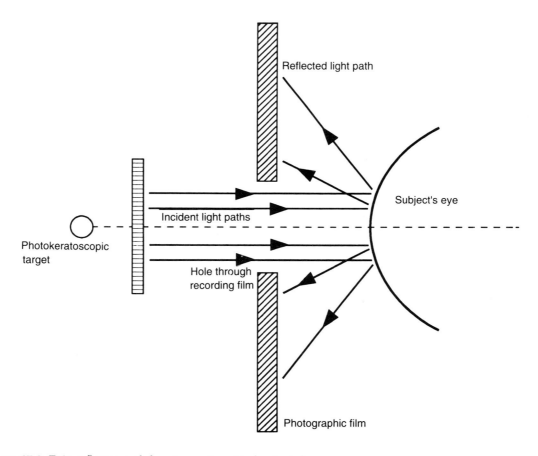

Figure 17.2 Zeis reflectograph keratoscopic optical principle.

to locate corneal features accurately and repeatably.

With some instruments, vignetting by the nose is a problem. A fixation point situated temporally to the main optical system of the photokeratoscope is habitually used to overcome that problem (Amiard, 1972, 1973). An alternative procedure to avoid vignetting is to keep the fixation coaxial with the photokeratoscope's main optical system and position the patient slightly side-on to the target.

A number of focusing aids such as ametropia correction, magnifying eye piece, split prism, ground glass focusing screen and alignment cross have been used. In all cases, the viewing system should operate at full aperture in order to allow critical focusing.

Recording system

As its name suggests, photokeratoscopy involves the photographic recording of the keratoscopic image. However, in at least three experimental instruments (Westheimer, 1965; El Hage, 1976; Gormley *et al.*, 1988) and in all the latest commercial instruments (Topographic Modeling System TMS-1, EyeSys video keratoscope, Visioptic EH-270 Computerised Corneal Topographer) an electronic recording system has been incorporated.

The advantages of electronic recording are obvious. Such systems offer immediate availability of results and enable direct data analysis. Only technological limitations, not permitting as high a resolution as the photographic system, have hindered its wider use in the past. But as demonstrated by the current instruments, advancements in technology (and particularly in the area of computing and electronics), has remedied this problem.*

A wide range of photographic systems has been used to record photokeratoscopy data.

---

* The accuracy of the recently developed Corneal Modeling System (Gormley *et al*, 1988; Hannush *et al*, 1989) is a clear indication that the photographic media will soon be rendered obsolete by fully electronic/digital instruments.

However, we will limit our discussion to a number of features that are known to optimize the performance of such a system.

Light source

All modern photokeratoscopes utilize an electronic flash as a light source. These flashes deliver as much light as necessary (keeping in mind other limits including the maximum safety level to light exposure of various ocular tissues) and, through their short duration (1/1000 s or less), they eliminate all problems associated with eye movements. The videokeratoscopes incorporate CCD video cameras; in two out of the three systems commercially available, these are sensitive enough to respond to the constant white light source also used for focusing (The Visioptic Corneal Topographer EH-270 utilizes an electronic flash). The eye movement problems are eliminated by instantaneous electronic image capture.

Optimally the peak emission wavelength of the illumination system should be chosen to match the peak sensitivity of the recording medium.

Filters

In some instruments filters are incorporated to improve the image quality by transforming the system to a near monochromatic system (Clark, 1972). However, filters must be chosen carefully, with a spectral bandwidth matching the emission peak of the light source. Further, if interference filters are used, the direction of all possible light paths must be considered.

Recording media

Photographic film

1. Film type. Black and white negatives and prints, and colour prints, have all

been used in photokeratoscopy. We personally favour the direct use of black and white negatives during measurement and analysis as they afford a high contrast and require no further steps which can introduce additional sources of errors (e.g. enlargement magnification errors and dimension instability of the medium). One-step prints such as Polaroid print films can also provide these advantages.

All current instruments use Polaroid-type instant processing films or plates. Clinically, this is essential as it gives the operator instant feed back on the suitability of the record. For this reason commercial photokeratoscopes utilize fine grain Polaroid films originally designed for landscape and aerial photography.

2. Film size. It is preferable to use large or medium format systems (such as 6 cm × 9 cm) rather than the conventional 35 cm format. With the larger formats, a greater overall magnification is possible. For example, the Wesley–Jessen negative image on a 6 cm × 9 cm format has a linear magnification of approximately × 5, while the Nidek photokeratoscope using an 8.5 cm × 10.8 cm format (two records per frame) has a magnification of approximately × 2.6. This improves resolution, thus reducing percentage error of measurement.

3. Film speed. The main concern regarding the high film speed required in some cases is the accompanying larger film grain that may limit resolution. However, film grain is not usually a limiting factor with modern films.

Video recording The recording media for the video system is the CCD camera. Because of the high resolution required to obtain sufficient accuracy when determining the corneal topography only high or very high resolution systems with at least 512 pixels per recording cell in the horizontal and vertical directions are suitable. In one instrument (Computer Anatomy TMS-1 keratoscope) 1500 pixels are used. The dynamic (brightness) range and resolution of each pixel is of consideration. Localization of image peaks and target edges is more accurate with a higher dynamic range. It is also possible to utilize amplitude interpolative algorithms to localize image peaks or target edges between pixels, provided a sufficiently high dynamic resolution is available. The CCD camera can either be colour or black and white, the latter however suffices as the information used only needs to be monochromatic. The image formed on the recording cells is then captured via a dedicated electronic digitizing board.

17.2.2 SPECIFIC INSTRUMENTS

Introduction

As we have seen, photokeratoscopes can be systematically divided into three subsystems, the main classification being concerned with variations in targets and the associated imaging system. This section gives a listing of all known instruments according to these two classifications.

Research and experimental instruments

A review of the literature (Morris, 1956; Knoll *et al*, 1957; Holden, 1970; El Hage, 1971; Amiard & Cochet, 1972; Clark, 1973c) revealed a plethora of photokeratoscopes. The majority of these instruments remained experimental prototypes and were never distributed commercially. Some, however, had unique features worthy of mention. For clarity, we have classified them according to their target design (Table 17.1) and have listed them in chronological order with regard to the first reference of the instrument appearing in the literature.

Of the instruments listed, some no longer available are worthy of special comment. The discussion of these instruments will be presented according to their target types:

Plane target instruments

1. The Zeiss reflectograph, 1930 (Morris, 1956; Clark, 1973c) was in fact a reverse flat target (Fig. 17.2). The target was situated where the plane of the film is normally positioned and vice versa. The light reaches the cornea via a central aperture through the film plate.
2. The photokeratoscope of Kokott 1938 (Clark, 1973c) used a pair of cameras which gave a stereoscopic pair of photographs of the corneal images.
3. The Fincham Photokeratoscope 1953 (Fincham, 1953) has been the bench mark for flat target photokeratoscopes since its introduction and has been the subject of several copies: the Hansell Photokeratoscope in 1956 (Brown, 1969); the Perth Photokeratoscope (Plummer & Lamb, 1961); the Brown Photokeratoscope (Brown, 1969); and one which became commercially available: AIM Keratograph (Morris, 1956).
4. The Norton-Sullivan Photokeratoscope (Norton & Sullivan, 1962) was the first to incorporate a Polaroid camera back.
5. A compact (and therefore portable) photokeratoscope based on a 35 mm camera with extension bellows and readily available components was designed and constructed by Sivak (1977).
6. A device for converting a Topcon photo-slit-lamp to a photokeratoscope was designed and constructed by Cotran and Miller (1987). A modification unit of this kind may be a cost and space efficient method of attaining corneal topographical examination in the clinical practice.

Hemispherical target instruments

The Donaldson photokeratoscope had two photographic systems (Donaldson, 1954) that enabled stereoscopic corneal shape reproduction.

Cylindrical target instruments

The Knoll, Bausch and Lomb Photokeratoscope (Knoll, 1961) was the basis of the Ludlam and Wittenberg, the Mandell's and El Hage (El Hage, 1972b) photokeratoscopes and gave full corneal coverage by the target with the exception of vignetting by the nose. Excellent results have been reported with this type of instrument.

Ellipsoidal target instruments

The Holden Photokeratoscope (Holden, 1970) was fairly large in construction in order to enable the precise location of individual target rings. It also incorporated a relocatable fixation light which enabled the operator to locate the position of the corneal apex.

Other instruments

The Clark Photokeratoscope (Clark, 1972) utilized a projected target system whereby an image of the actual target was projected onto the cornea. The 'photokeratometre' of Ysoptic (Amiard, 1972, 1973) used a cardioid target surface (closely approaching an ellipsoid) which purportedly provided an optimally flat corneal image.

Commercial instruments

Six instruments are presently available commercially:

1. The PEK photokeratoscope from Wesley–Jessen Incorporated of Chicago, Illinois (Bibby, 1976a).
2. The PKS-1000 Photokeratoscope from Nidek Incorporated of Palo Alto, California; previously distributed as the Sun Photokeratoscopy (Sun Contact Lens Company of Kyoto, Japan).

Table 17.2 Commercially available instruments

Features	Instruments		
	Corneascope	PEK	PKS

Commercial photokeratoscope instruments

Features	Corneascope	PEK	PKS
Target shape	Hemispherical	Ellipsoid	Elliptical
Target type	Reflective	Diffusive	Diffusive
Corneal coverage	Model 900 7 mm Model 1200 10.9 mm	9 mm	10 mm
Centre ring	3 mm	3 mm	2 mm
Number of rings	9 (model 900) 12 (model 1200)	9	10
Recording system	Polaroid Type 108 or 699 (possible computer storage)	Polaroid-High Contrast Land Projection Film 146	Polaroid Type 667 (possible computer storage)
Output of results	Local 'power or 'radii' for each ring in 8 major meridians	Apical radius and shape factor for each principal meridian	Local 'radii' of principal meridians and 3D graphics display
Claimed accuracy	Same as keratometer ±0.25–0.50D	Repeatability ± 0.18 D central K ± 0.05 shape factor at 95% confidence level	Precision ± 0.03 mm for central cornea 0.07/0.08 mm for peripheral cornea

	Corneal modeling system TMS	Eye Sys ES-100	Visioptis EH-270

Commercial videokeratoscopic instruments

Features			
Target shape	Conical	Conical	Conical
Target type	Diffusive	Projected	Diffusive
Corneal coverage	11 mm × 14 mm	9.6 mm	>10.0 mm
Centre ring		0.7 mm	0.31 mm
Number of rings	25 (standard model) 32 (contour model)	On the Eyesis, the analysis is based on the edges between rings. Hence corneal points are obtained for each half meridian	22
Recording system	Super resolving CCD video camera 1000 × 1500 pixels	High resolution CCD video camera	High resolution CCD video camera
Output of results	Digital information and colour coded topographic maps	Digital information and colour coded topographic maps	Digital information and colour coded top0graphic maps
Claimed accuracy	Accuracy ± 0.2 D	Resolution 0.01 D Reproductibility ± 0.25 D	Resolution ± 0.2 D

3. The Corneascope from International Diagnostic Instruments Ltd of Broken Arrow, previously distributed by the Kera Corporation of Santa Clara, California (Rowsey *et al*, 1981; Petricciani *et al*, 1985).
4. The Corneal Modeling System TMS 1 (Fig. 17.3) from Computed Anatomy Incorporated, New York, NY (Gormley *et al*, 1988).
5. The ES100 Corneal Topographic System (Fig. 17.4) from EyeSys Laboratories, Houston, Texas.
6. The EH-270 Computerised Corneal Topographer from Vision Optics Inc. (Fig. 17.5) Houston, Texas.

Each photographic instrument is also available as a part of a package for which the manufacturer undertakes the analysis of the photokeratographs and provides the practitioner with a mathematical representation of the patient's corneal shape. Analysis systems for on-site data analysis are also available. The analysis systems are the Kerascan from the International Diagnostic Company, the System 2000 from Wesley–Jessen and the Pal 250 from the Nidek Corporation. All the video systems incorporate an on-line PC based data analysis system that gives both graphic representation of the corneal topography and numerical values.

The features of these six instruments are summarized in Table 17.2.

17.3 METHODS OF ANALYSIS

The single most complex phase in photokeratoscopy is data analysis. The rapidity of development and the intensity with which improvement is sought in all facets of data analysis (including algorithm, hardware and software) bears witness to this (Townsley, 1970; Clark, 1973a; Klyce, 1984; Gormley *et al.* 1988; Busin *et al.*, 1989).

Analysis begins with the measurement of photographic or electronic records of target

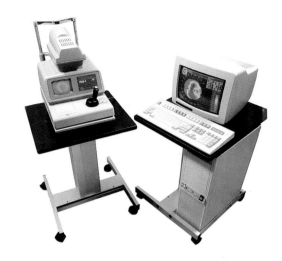

Figure 17.3 Computer Anatomy Incorporated Corneal Modeling System TMS-1 video keratoscope.

images formed by corneal reflection and is completed with a description of the corneal shape. The steps include: (1) data collection; (2) computation; and (3) presentation of results.

17.3.1 DATA COLLECTION

There are two steps in data collection; initially the obtention of a record (photographic or electronic) of the image given by the cornea of the instrument's target followed by the measurement of this record to obtain data values for the analytical parameters. There are two types of parameter: (1) fixed; and (2) variable. Those of relevance will be considered in Table 17.3.

Fixed parameters

The fixed parameters are the instrument specifications. The values of the fixed parameters (for the purpose of data analysis) are assumed to remain constant. For example, the locations of the target rings are considered to be fixed parameters as they are relatively fixed with

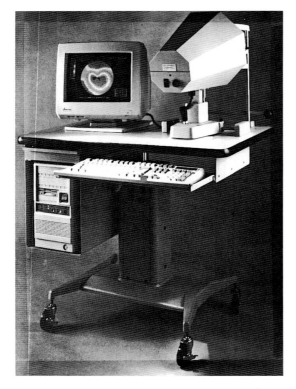

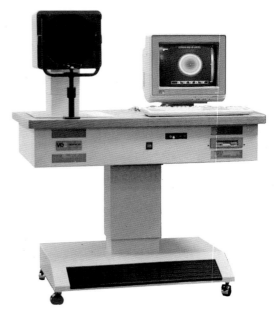

Figure 17.5 Visioptics Incorporated, Computerised Corneal Topographer EH-270 video keratoscope.

Figure 17.4 EyeSys Laboratories ES100 video keratoscope.

respect to the subject's eye and the optical system of the photokeratoscope. Typically, these fixed parameters are measured or are known accurately during the construction of the instrument (Ludlam *et al.*, 1967).

Some fixed parameters may vary during instrument use. However, because these variations are small or not estimable, the parameters are assumed to be constant. For example, the magnification of the photographic system, although theoretically fixed by the focal length of the photographic lens and the subject's eye to film plane distance, may change by a minute amount due to focusing errors.

Variable parameters

In a valid measurement system, the variable parameters are related to corneal topography. The purpose of data collection is to measure these variable parameters in order to calculate the corneal topography.

These measurements may involve either analysis of photographic records or electronic output. In the former case, the records may be measured using a travelling or projection microscope (Wesley–Jessen) or an image analyser (Nidek Corporation). In the latter case, the output from electronic photo-arrays is directly transmitted to a computer for analysis (Westheimer, 1965; El Hage, 1976).

Two examples of variable parameters are the recorded size of the corneal image of the target and the direction of light rays following reflection at the cornea.

17.3.2   COMPUTATION

During computation measured parameters are processed mathematically or graphically (Mandell & York, 1969; York, 1969) to derive a description of the topography of the measured

Table 17.3 Parameters included in keratoscopic data analysis

	Fixed parameters	Variable parameters
Instrument target	Location, diameter, reflected/diffused target	
Optical system	Lens focal length, aperture size, magnification, film/photocell/plane distance	Fixation direction/ angle, corneal apex centration, corneal curvature topography
Measurement system	Calibration constants, magnification	
Subject's eye		Object's focus plans

cornea. The choice of computational method is important as the accuracy and validity of the photokeratoscopic results depend upon it.

A large number of analytical techniques (Ludlam & Wittenberg, 1966b; Townsley, 1970; Clark, 1973a; Klyce, 1984; Gormley, 1988; Busin *et al.*, 1989) are available to determine the corneal surface topography. The choice of analytical techniques are, to some extent, limited by the type of instrument used (El Hage, 1971). For each instrument type, however, it is possible to account for any number of parameters in order to increase the accuracy (albeit at the expense of increasing the complexity) of the analysis. Conversely it is possible to omit or make assumptions for other parameters in order to simplify the analysis at the cost of reducing the accuracy.

Requirements

An appropriate computation system must: (1) minimize data distortion; and (2) employ minimal and only valid assumptions.

Data distortion

Data distortion refers to the loss of validity of the computed results as a true representation of the actual corneal shape. Data distortion mainly occurs as a result of the choice of an incorrect or inappropriate computational method or due to numerical computational errors. Other sources of data distortion include the use of inappropriate assumptions, and systematic errors which may occur during any part of the data acquisition phase.

Assumptions

The use of inappropriate assumptions will lead to data distortion (Ludlam & Wittenberg, 1966b; Mandell & York, 1969; York, 1969; Edmund, 1986). Generally, the greater the number of assumptions made, the more probable the computed description of corneal surface will deviate from the true corneal surface. The number of assumptions also determines the scope of a computational method. The greater the number of assumptions the more limited will be the applicability of the computation method.

For these reasons, the introduction of any assumption must be assessed critically before incorporation into an analysis method. Obviously, any assumption made must be consistent with the data acquisition system, the instrument type and the corneal model used (Ludlam & Wittenberg, 1966b).

General analysis methods

Computational methods found in the

literature fall into the following categories: (1) calibration with reference spheres; (2) slope of the surface method; (3) curve matching; and (4) others.

Calibration with reference spheres

Calibration with reference spheres is the earliest method used to analyse photokeratoscopic data; it is similar to the method used to derive keratometry results by Scheiner (Wittenberg & Ludlam, 1966). Basically, the recorded corneal image is compared to the reflected image of the same target produced by a reference sphere. The radius of curvature of the sphere with the same size reflected image as the corneal image is recorded as the radius of curvature of the cornea. For photokeratoscopy, where up to 32 rings have been used as targets, each ring may be used to obtain a separate 'local' radius of curvature.

This method is acceptable near the geometric axis but is inappropriate for the other regions of the corneal surface. From geometric principles the centres of the spheres representing each local radius of curvature must lie on the geometric axis. This assumption is inappropriate for the cornea for which the centres of curvature of the peripheral surface do not lie on the axis but form an evolute away from the axis (Bennett, 1968) (Fig. 17.6).

Further, the method assumes that the image forming property of the cornea at the point of reflection is similar to that of a sphere at the same point (Mandell & York,

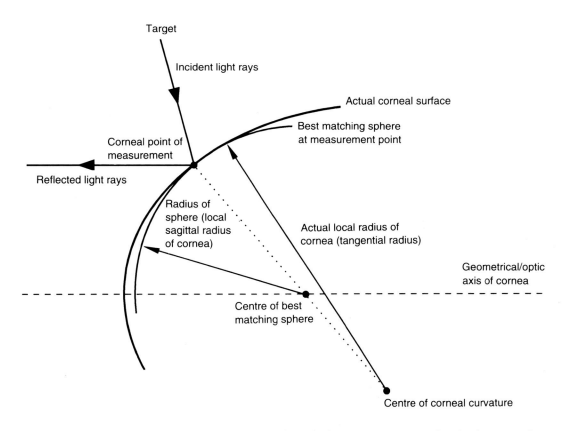

Figure 17.6 Geometric principle of peripheral corneal image formation assuming local reference sphere.

1969; Edmund, 1986). This assumption is also unacceptable as the true surface shape at the region near the point of reflection is different from the curve of the reference sphere (Wittenberg & Ludlam, 1966). In particular, the tangential* radius of curvature of the cornea at any point is different from the radius of the matching reference sphere (Bennett, 1968).

In fact, with this method, the only parameters which are identical between the corneal surface measured and the matching reference sphere are the ray height and the slope of the tangent to the surface at the point of reflection. These parameters can be used as the basis for a computational method.

Slope of surface method

This is the most frequently described and employed computational method (Westheimer, 1965; Wittenberg & Ludlam, 1966; El Hage, 1972a; Fujii *et al.*, 1972).

When a ray travels from a target to the cornea and after reflection passes through the optical system of the photokeratoscope, its path can be traced by applying optical and geometric principles (Fig. 17.7). If the position of the cornea, the angles of the incident and the reflected rays to the optical axis, and the location of the target are known, then the angles of incidence and reflection to the cornea can be calculated. From these parameters, the slope of the normal at the point of reflection, and therefore the slope of the tangent to the surface, may be calculated. By repeating this calculation for each point of reflection for the different target rings, a set of data containing the position of the point of reflection and the corresponding slope of the tangent may be generated.

If an assumption is made that the sectional

curve along a meridian of the corneal surface is representable by a (or a series of) differentiable mathematical function (the topographical function) then the first derivative of this function represents the slope of the tangent to the surface (Westheimer, 1965). Therefore, by numerical integration of a set of data containing the slope of the tangent at each point of reflection with respect to the position of the point of reflection, the topographical function describing the corneal shape can be obtained.

This procedure may be applied to different corneal sectional curves belonging to different meridians until a three-dimensional representation of the entire corneal surface is obtained.

With this method of computation, if a single topographical function is used, one major assumption made is that the corneal curve can be represented by a continuous function. Generally, this assumption is appropriate provided the measured cornea is relatively free from any severe distortions as may be present in some abnormal corneal conditions, such as keratoconus. In the cases where this assumption may be suspected not to be robust, it can either be made valid or be eliminated altogether in the following ways.

Being a physical structure with no sharp edges (except perhaps immediately following corneal surgery) the anterior cornea is a continuous surface in the mathematical sense. Any apparent discontinuities in any resultant topographical function is a result of the limited number of target rings used. Therefore, for even a severely distorted cornea, a continuous mathematical function to describe the topography can be achieved provided a sufficient number of target rings are used.

If, due to the instrument's limitation, a significantly large number of target rings cannot be incorporated, the assumption of continuity can be eliminated by using a series (many) of mathematical functions (e.g. polynomials) to fit the surface. In this variation, the topo-

---

* The geometrical descriptions 'tangential radius' and 'saggital radius' are used throughout this chapter. In some texts, the corresponding descriptions 'instantaneous/local radius' respectively are used.

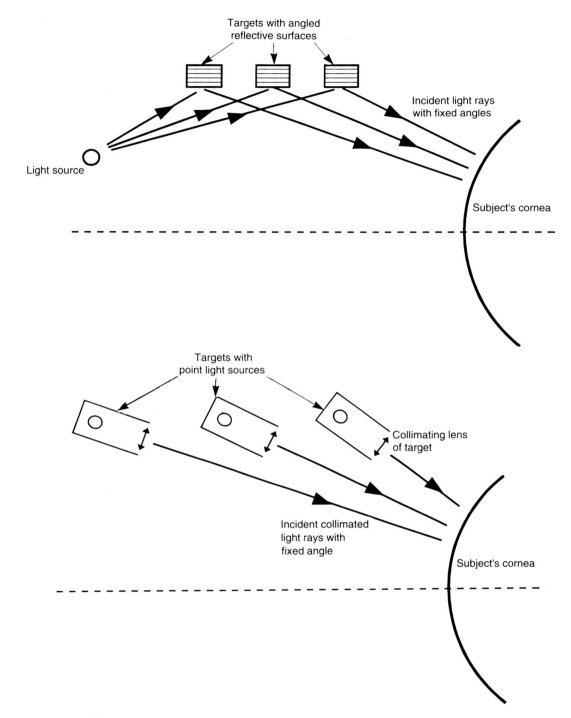

Figure 17.11a b Photokeratoscopic target image arrangement for (a) EI Hage system, (b) Fujii system.

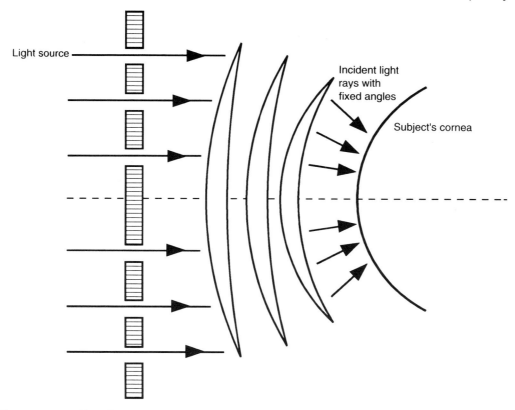

Figure 17.11c Photokeratoscopic target image arrangement for Clark System.

bration is also important in establishing the accuracy of both the instrument and the computational method used. Regular calibration also ensures minimum data distortion and checks on changes or drifts in the parameters of the instrument.

Although calibration is most commonly carried out on glass or steel spheres, for maximum validity, calibrators with the shape of a typical cornea should be used. Therefore calibration should be carried out on ellipsoid standards with central radii and eccentricity resembling those of the eye (Mandell & York, 1969; York, 1969). If the computational method adopts a general mathematical model for the eye (e.g. a catenary), then the surface of the calibration standard should match that general model.

The ideal standards should be made from dimensionally stable, scratch-proof, glossy materials such as pyrex or zerodur. Their dimensions should be measured regularly using methods such as interferometry to guard against dimensional variations. These reference surfaces should be kept and measured under constant environmental conditions.

17.3.3 PRESENTATION OF RESULTS

General comments

At the end of computation, a decision needs to be made concerning the method of presentation of results. This decision is not a trivial one as the method of results presentation must:

1. Provide a quick and easily recognizable description of the measured corneal topography.
2. Provide the maximum amount of information regarding the cornea measured.
3. Facilitate further analysis of corneal topography as required.

Regardless of the method of presentation chosen, consistency must be kept within any study to allow the comparison of results of different corneas. Given the conflicting requirements in (1) and (2) above, it is obvious that no single method of presentation of results can satisfy all requirements.

Description of methods

The methods of presentation of results can be categorized loosely as: (1) surface/curve fitting to data points; (2) distinct data points; and (3) parametric descriptions.

Surface/curve fitting to data points

This method initially provides the locations of the corneal surface points measured. By assuming that the cornea has a continuous surface the method attempts to interpolate between points, which renders the corneal topographical results easy to visualize. For this reason, this method lends itself well to representation by computer graphics (Dingeldein & Klyce, 1988).

However, by making this assumption, information presented may be misleading in that discontinuous surfaces, as for a post-surgical cornea, may be falsely displayed as being continuous. The validity of this method thus depends on the type of instrument used and the degree of sophistication of the curve/surface fitting algorithm.

Distinct data points

Validity of information is retained by keeping the measurement points unjoined rather than producing a visual, contour map-type of presentation (Clark, 1974a). At least this method cannot introduce any misleading information: falsely fitting continuous surfaces when the corneal surface may be a discontinuous one or ignoring fine topographical details. Certainly this method makes no assumption about the nature of the surface in between the measured points.

One such method is to record the departure of the corneal surface from a standard surface, for example, a reference sphere (Pulvermacher & Rott, 1972; Clark, 1974a; Doss *et al.*, 1981) or an ellipse (Bibby, 1976b).

However, with this method there is necessarily a larger amount of data to process to obtain useful comparisons between corneas, the number of data points to process depending upon the number of target rings and meridians used.

Variations of this method of data description include the presentation of a topographical map of either the local radius of curvature or the local refractive power (Fry, 1975a, b; Klyce, 1984; Maguire *et al.*, 1985).

Parametric description

In these methods of presentation, a mathematical model is adopted for the corneal shape. Individual corneas are then described by the set of parameters which approximates that cornea under the mathematical model.

The main difference between this approach and surface/curve fitting to data points are that in the curve fitting interpolative method, the values of the individual data (surface) points are retained (or at least are not altered) so that the accuracy of any subsequent analysis required does not suffer. Mathematical interpretation of surface details is limited to the intervals between points. In the parametric description method, the general mathematical model is fitted to the corneal surface. For this reason, the value of each surface point is replaced (implicitly) by the expected value of that point under the adopted/assumed model.

Certainly this method greatly simplifies data recording and any subsequent analysis since the follow-up analysis may be applied to the individual parameters (as compared to the much large number of surface points). This may be an important consideration in epidemiological applications. This method, however, in order to achieve a simplified analysis necessarily ignores a large amount of information regarding the corneal topography.

Many mathematical models have been described and used, ranging from the ellipse to more complex functions including a catenary and an Ignesi curve (Himi *et al.*, 1981).

This method of presentation may be extended by employing published abstract mathematical/geometrical concepts in order to facilitate subsequent data handling and analysis. One such method for describing the corneal topography has been proposed by Cohen *et al.*, (1984), which eliminates the need for recording large numbers of corneal surface co-ordinates and which also does not assume any general model for the corneal surface. A number of indices describing various features of the corneal surface measured are calculated. These indices can then be used for parametric or non parametric statistical analysis.

The main drawback of parametric methods of presentation is that the descriptive parameters/indices may not define a unique corneal surface in that a number of different corneal topographies may have the same descriptive parameters. Because of this, the original corneal shape cannot be reconstructed from the parameters.

Discussion

Applications of the photokeratoscopic results play a major role in the selection of the method of presentation. For instance, if the results are to be used in a numerically descriptive form (e.g. epidemiological survey) for which statistical analyses may need to be carried out, then the relative advantages of keeping all topographical data points must be weighed against the relative simplicity of employing a general corneal model. The parametric descriptive method may be the better choice in this case (Guillon *et al* 1986).

If the aim of photokeratoscopy is to analyse the corneal topography of individual corneas as, for example, in designing the optimum back surface shape of a contact lens, then it may be preferable to keep all measurements in the form of topographical co-ordinates. In this way, lens fitting parameters such as surface clearance, tear layer thickness and shape can be calculated directly from the data. If this method of data presentation is employed, a further decision will need to be made in selecting the co-ordinates system of measurement to use, e.g. longitudinal/axial or with respect to a reference surface. For instance, in examining the tear layer thickness, the deviation of a surface along the normals to a reference surface would have greater validity than the equivalent longitudinal measurement (Tomlinson & Bibby, 1977).

For optical analysis (e.g. in trigonometrical ray tracing of the eye), the important information includes the topographical co-ordinates of the surface points and the angle or slope of the tangent and normal to any point along the surface. Because in many cases a continuous refracting surface is assumed, there is no other choice but to fit a continuous surface to the measured points. However, even given this constraint, the type of surfaces fitted will still depend upon the level of sophistication required in the optical model.

17.4 ACCURACY AND REPEATABILITY

17.4.1 GENERAL PRINCIPLES

The usual method to assess the overall accuracy and repeatability of a keratoscopic sys-

Table 17.4 Summary of sources of errors

Type of error	Parameter	Class	Source of error	Method of error prevention/detection/ minimization
Instrument	Magnification	Systematic	Object and image	Careful accurate construction, assessment measurement, check of instrument, specifications
	Target rings	Systematic	Roundness, concentricity, alignment of rings, diameter position	
Data acquisition	Focus	Random	Interobserver differences	Train observers Implement rigid criteria
	Focus	Random	Depth of focus	Focus using the wide aperture exposure with small aperture
	Focus	Both	Curvature of field of corneal image	Improve optical system, optimize target locus, implement rigid criteria
	Focus	Random	Eye movement	Electronic flash exposure
	Alignment	Random	Interobserver	Train observers, implement rigid criteria
	Alignment	?	Corneal assymetry/ astigmatism	?
	Alignment	Random	Eye movement	Electronic flash exposure
	Corneal records photographic/ electronic	Random	Resolution of medium halation	Use slow fine grain film with thin film base of denser photocell arrays
	Corneal records photographic/ electronic	Random ?	Location of film plane photocells	Careful checks film, pressure plates/ transparent fil slide
		Random and systematic	Diffraction aberrations	Use optimum aperture, improve optical system
Data storage	Photographic record dimensions	Random and systematic	Dimension stability/ standardize temperature and humidity during measurement	Test film stability per film type and batch
Data retrieval	Measurement of records	Random	Interobserver	Train observers, standardize record measurement procedures
		Random and systematic	Accuracy of measurement device	Use accurate/calibrated equipment only, calibrate regularly
		Random	Determination of actual centre of lines	Obtain good quality photographs, use dark lines on rings as guide, improve optical system

Type of error	Parameter	Class	Source of error	Method of error prevention/detection/ minimization
	Random	Defining centre of cornea for semi-meridian	?	
Data computation and analysis	Computation	Systematic	Method of computation	Use appropriate method
		Random and systematic	Incorrect assumptions, approximations	Use appropriate assumptions and general models
		Random and systematic	Numerical operations, EG truncation	Double precision, check accuracies of mathematical functions
		Random and systematic	Integration/ differentiation e.g. quadrature vs spline fit	Check numerical analytic
		Systematic	Type of general model or reference surface	Select reference surface with similar parameters to cornea and model adopted

tem is to compare the results from a number of photographs of one or more reference surfaces and corneas.

Numerous claims have been made in the literature regarding mainly the accuracy, but also, the repeatability of photokeratoscopic systems. However, with perhaps a few exceptions (Ludlam *et al.*, 1967), the information given was either incomplete and/or was derived in a manner which departed from standard methods, making it difficult and sometimes impossible to calculate the instrument's true accuracy and/or repeatability. Some authors, often the instrument's designers, depart from accepted metrological techniques in the determination of accuracy and repeatability and, in so doing, tend to overestimate the performance of the instrument tested.

The accuracy (sometimes called validity) of an instrument indicates the closeness between the mean measured value and the true value of the parameter measured. The repeatability of a measurement (often called reliability or precision) indicates the ability of the instrument to duplicate its own results (ISO 3534, 1982). In other words 'the accuracy is a measure of an instrument's ability to tell the truth, whereas repeatability is a measure of its ability to stick to the same story' (Hayward, 1977). From the definitions it is obvious that in order to determine the accuracy of an instrument one must first know the 'true' value of the parameters measured. Hence, the accuracy of a photokeratoscope can only be determined for reference surfaces such as steel balls or glass spheres of known radii. Repeatability on the other hand can be measured for both reference surfaces and the *in vivo* corneas.

Most papers quote the standard deviation of a series of measurements as the repeatability of an instrument. It is, however, the usual convention in metrology to report accuracy and repeatability of an instrument at the 95% confidence level; this is obtained by multiplying the standard deviation by the corresponding Student *t* value.*

As this is not the place to detail the methodology to measure accuracy and repeatability, the interested reader should consult metrology texts (e.g. Campion, 1973; Dietrich, 1973). However, it is useful to be familiar with the two types of uncertainties which affect measurements; namely random and systematic uncertainties. Repeatability refers only to random uncertainties, while accuracy is concerned with both. Hence the accuracy of an instrument can never be better than its repeatability. It should be noted that some authors describe instrument performance in terms of resolution, which should not be confused with accuracy nor repeatability. Resolution describes the smallest difference that the instrument can detect. Accuracy can never be better than resolution but can be significantly worse.

The accuracy achievable with any instrument depends upon both the hardware available and the various steps taken from image acquisition to its analysis. The various types of errors encountered and their sources are summarized in Table 17.4.

17.4.2 INFORMATION CURRENTLY AVAILABLE

For comparison, the information reported in the literature on accuracy and repeatability is given in summarized form in Table 17.5. The references cited for each method in Table 17.5 are the earliest published works in which the basic method was first applied to corneal topography. A brief outline of the method is given in the second column. The accuracy quoted is the best and worst case claimed in the published works in which the method was first applied to corneal topography. Where no quantitative estimates of accuracy were found, the most reasonable subjective estimate was given.

A number of comments can be made about the information in Table 17.5. Some authors quoted instrumental errors. In these cases we assumed that the results obtained referred to the instrument accuracy. In many cases no data was given to support the claims made for the accuracy (Knoll, 1961; Clark, 1973c, 1974a; El Hage, 1976; Doss *et al.*, 1981) and also for repeatability (Clark, 1973c; Klyce, 1984).

In a number of cases where data are given and claims made, the two did not agree and we have subsequently recalculated the relevant parameters as follows:

1. Doss *et al.* (1981) reported for the measurement of a reference sphere of nominal radius 9.52 mm an average measured radius of 9.663 ± 0.2385 mm for the nine rings. The standard deviation alone gives an instrument repeatability of ± 0.477 mm on the radius. The data thus gave an accuracy of $((9.663 - 9.52)^2 + (0.477)^2)^{1/2} = 0.498$ mm.

2. Ludlam *et al.* (1967) did not analyse their data fully. By meaning in quadrature the standard deviations reported for the two reference steel balls measured we obtain a repeatability at 95% confidence level of ± 0.00896 mm (SD ± 0.00448 mm) for the image of the first ring and ± 0.04016 mm (SD ± 0.02008 mm) for that of the sixth ring. A similar computation for a cornea gives repeatability of ± 0.0122 mm (SD ± 0.0061 mm) for the first ring and ± 0.044 mm (SD ± 0.0472 mm) for the sixth ring.

3. Klyce (1984) reported for a reference sphere of 8.100 mm nominal radius, and measured radii of 8.137 ± 0.015 mm and 8.138 ± 0.020 mm. This data gives a mean systematic uncertainty of

---

* The 95% confidence level calculated gives a range approximately ×2 the range obtained by taking the standard deviation.

Table 17.5 Summary of published data on accuracy and repeatability of specific photokeratoscopes

Instrument	Reference	Accuracy	Repeatability
Gullstrand (E)	Gullstrand, 1896	Claim: Average ± 0.0025 mm for image of photokeratograph of steel balls	
Sun PKS – 1000 Photokeratoscope (C)	Sun Contact Lens	Claim: 1% error on radii 7.00–8.00 mm. No supporting evidence	
	Klyce, 1984		Measurement: $n = 2$ photographs, no difference between mean for reference sphere
Berg Photokeratoscope (E)	Clark, 1973	Measurement: ± 0.2 D error (equivalent to ± 0.04 mm radius) on glass lens	
Corneascope or Photokeratoscope (International Diagnostic Instrument) (C)	Doss *et al.*, 1981	Measurement: ± 2.7 to 4.7% on power. Claim: Overall accuracy ± 2 to 5% with possible improvement to an accuracy of ± 0.5% Measurement: reference steel balls nominal radius = 9.52 mm measured radius = 9.663 ± 0.2385 mm	
Knoll Bausch & Lomb	Knoll, 1961	Claim: approximately ± 0.2 mm	
Photokeratoscope (C)	Ludlam *et al.*, 1967		Measurement: ± 0.030 mm for central ring ± 0.036 mm for periphery for 95% confidence level for reference sphere
Mandell Photokeratoscope (E)	Mandell and St Helen, 1968 Mandell and St Helen, 1971	Measurement: + 1% on ring diameter of photokeratographs of reference steel balls Claim: ± 0.25% possible if careful focusing applied	Measurement: 1) ± 0.12% (on average change 0 to 0.53%) on ring diameter from 5 photokeratographs of a steel reference ball 2) ± 0.21% (range 0.21% (range 0.02 to 0.58%) as above for corneal surface

Instrument	Reference	Accuracy	Repeatability
El Hage Photokeratoscope (EHP) (E)	El Hage, 1976	Claim: Less than ± 0.01 mm at the extreme corneal periphery	
Wesley-Jessen Photokeratoscope	Bibby and Townsley, 1976	Measurement: 1) ± 0.0036 to ± 0.0122 mm on saggital values at the 95% confidence level 2) ± 0.18 D on central curvature and ± 0.08 on shape factor at the 95% confidence level	
Holden Photokeratoscope	Holden, 1970	Measurement: 1) ± 0.0009 mm SD on central ring and ± 0.0032 mm SD on peripheral ring of steel ball photokeratograph (equivalent to ± 0.022 mm ± 0.26%) 2) ± 0.0012 mm SD on diameters of central ring and ± 0.0052 mm SD on peripheral ring of corneal photokeratograph (equivalent ± 0.023 mm 0.25%)	
Photokeratometre Ysoptic (C)	Clark, 1973	Claim: ± 0.01 mm (SD) error	Claim: Precision ± 1%
Computer Anatomy TMS1	Computer Anatomy Inc.	Claim: ± 0.2 D	Claim: Resolution ± 0.20 D
EyeSys ES100	EyeSys Laboratories		Claim: Resolution ± 0.01 D Reproducibility ± 0.25 D
Visioptics EN270	Visioptics Inc.		Claim: Resolution ± 0.20 D

± 0.075 mm and a random uncertainty of ± 0.045 mm, hence an accuracy of $((0.045)^2 + (0.075)^2)^{1/2} = 0.0875$ mm.

4. Maguire *et al.* (1985) reported that their instrument achieved a video digitizer resolution of 2000 pixels per frame corresponding to a resolution of 7.5 μm in the photokeratograph. They claim this to be equivalent to an error of an accuracy of 0.3 D, for a 40 D surface, This 0.3 D is probably the instrument resolution in equivalent dioptric units. Their paper has no information from which accuracy could be calculated.

17.4.3 ACCURACY REQUIREMENTS

The usefulness of photokeratoscopic information in any application is limited by its accuracy. For example, one important application is the determination of the corneal shape in view of designing optimally fitting rigid lenses (Moss, 1959: Cochet & Amiard, 1969; Amiard, 1972; Wilms, 1974, 1981; Bibby, 1976a, b; Muckenhirn, 1981; Guillon *et al.*, 1983; Kemmetmuller, 1984; Kivayev *et al.*, 1985; Manabe *et al.*, 1986). For this application a useful system will need to have an accuracy commensurate with this task.

The most critical aspect in rigid lens fitting is the distance between the contact lens back surface and the corneal front surface at the apex, often called the central tear layer thickness (TLTc). Experienced practitioners by subjective assessment of fluorescein patterns can differentiate between the fit of two lenses differing by as little as 0.05 mm in back optic radius (BOR). Thus, arguably, any photokeratoscopic system intended for this purpose should have an accuracy in radius of curvature equivalent to (or finer than) 0.05 mm. In terms of linear dimensions, this corresponds, for a typical lens with an 8.00 mm back optic diameter, to a difference in TLTc variation of 10.0 μm to 6.8 μm over the normal range of BOR from 7.20 mm to 8.40 mm, respectively. Therefore, the required system will need an accuracy of approximately 0.025 mm radius determination.

Note that, in this application, the accuracy required depends greatly on the clinically significant difference for the control variables. For example, although practitioners can detect differences of 0.05 mm BOR, this difference in contact lenses may cause little difference in performance. The above calculations were greatly simplified and were intended solely for illustration.

In another example, the application may be for optical ray-tracing of an eye model.

In this case, the two controlling variables are location of surface points and surface slope at those points. For the second variable, the cornea has typically a 10° slope (normal with respect to the geometrical axis) at the mid-periphery. In order to resolve a 0.25 D change in refractive power at this point, the slope of the surface will need to be measured with an accuracy of 0.05° (3 minutes).

Based on the information in Table 17.4, one may argue that photokeratoscopy will need further improvement before either of the two applications described can be tackled with confidence.

17.5 NON-PHOTOKERATOSCOPIC METHODS

17.5.1 GENERAL COMMENTS

There are a number of noteworthy methods of corneal topographic analysis which do not involve photokeratoscopy (Table 17.6). Although this chapter deals only with photokeratoscopy, by examining the accuracy, validity and practicality of non-photokeratoscopic methods the relative merits of both photokeratoscopy and non-photokeratoscopy techniques can be assessed.

One point which must be borne in mind is that although many of the listed methods can purportedly record the cornea in three dimensions, problems still exist as to how quantitative data can be extracted from the resultant topographical records. For example, holographic recordings or cast impressions of several test eyes can be made. However, comparisons between these eyes cannot be made unless topographical data in some quantitative form (e.g. sag heights or local radii of curvature) can be obtained from the recordings. The discussion concerning methods of data presentation for photokeratoscopy should also

Table 17.6 Brief notes on non-photo and video keratoscopic methods

Methods	Advantages	Disadvantages	Accuracy
Peripheral keratometry	Relatively simple instrumentation	Equivalent radii at periphery not necessarily true, local radii of curvature, computation very involved	
Autocollimation	No calculation of results required–direct reading of 'local radius'	Symmetry about optical point assumed, only one radius measurement per aperture, eye movement a problem	Depends upon aperture size, lens aperture, define area of surface used. As good or better than keratometer?
Interferometry (common path)	Less affected by movement	Needs diffusing surface?	Potential wavelength accuracy
Interferometry (projected dual beam)		Needs diffusing surface, must be very stable	
Holography	Three dimensional recording and presentation	Subject must be very stable, needs further work before data usable	Potentially very accurate
Moire fringes (toposcope)	No integration in analysis, valid for very uneven surfaces	Needs diffuse surface, field of view depends on aperture, less accurate at corneal apex	$\pm$ 5 µm for 7.50 mm radius
Stereo photogrammetry	Good at recording severe departures from normality e.g. keratoconus	Needs diffuse surface	$\pm$ 30 µm for 8 mm radius
Profile method (direct)	Simple analysis	Horizontal meridians difficult to evaluate	Depends on recording medium, potentially accurate
Profile method (optic section)	Slit lamp or special camera		$\pm$ 5 µm on sag $\pm$ 12.5 µm on radius
Profile method (Schiempflug)	Specialized instrument	Need to reconstruct actual curvation from apparent curvature	
Casting/moulding		Only gross irregularity detectable, deformation of cornea shape by mould material, shrinkage, needs further work before data usable.	Poor repeatability

Methods	Advantages	Disadvantages	Accuracy
Fluorescein methods	Shows up small irregularities well	Lens must not distort, sensitivity depends on reference contact lens shape	Subjective judgement better than ± 0.05 mm radius

be considered for the non-photokerato-scopic methods.

A number of methods have been described. Most of these are optical (peripheral keratometry, autocollimation, corneal profile, moiré fringes, stereophotogrammetry, interferometry and holography, and fluorescence methods (Stone, 1962; Clark, 1973d; Borish, 1975; Smith, 1977)), while one is physical/mechanical (casts/moulding, although the use of fluorescein may also be classified as being a physical method as contact is made with the eye). As one important criteria of corneal topographical assessment is that test cornea must not be distorted, the physical methods may not be suitable.

17.5.2 PERIPHERAL KERATOMETRY

Peripheral keratometry involves the measurement of local radii of curvature (Douthwaite, 1987b; Grosvenor, 1961; Wilms, 1974, 1981; Wilms & Rabbetts, 1977; Campbell, 1982; Kemmetmuller, 1984). To facilitate this, a series of peripheral fixation points are added to the keratometer (Grosvenor, 1961; Mandell, 1961, 1962). The validity of the measurement can be improved with this method by using a small mire keratometer (Fry, 1975b; Douthwaite, 1987b). From the set of measured local radii of curvature and their angular positions relative to the primary visual axis, the approximate corneal topography can be reconstructed (Borish, 1975). However, there are a number of limitations that affect the validity of this method. In particular, two major limitations imposed are:

1. An assumption is made that the actual surface at the point of measurement is spherical (or is at least symmetrically disposed about the point of measurement). Because the cornea approximates an ellipse (Holden, 1970; Guillon *et al.*, 1986), this assumption can only be met at the corneal apex and therefore is inappropriate in general.

2. If the surface is described by a mathematical function, the local radius of curvature is a composite variable consisting of the first (slope) and second (acceleration) derivative of that function (Thomas, 1975). Because the two derivatives have been reduced to a single quantity, it is impossible mathematically to extract the exact parent function describing the corneal surface from the local radii of curvature. An approximation of the corneal surface, however, can be obtained (in polar co-ordinates) provided certain assumptions about the geometry of eye movement are accepted (Fry, 1975b). Analysis of data from peripheral keratometry can be simplified if a general model (e.g. ellipse) for the corneal shape is adopted (Douthwaite & Sheridan, 1989).

17.5.3 AUTOCOLLIMATION

Autocollimation uses the Drysdale method to measure the radius of curvature of a surface (Bennett, 1964; Douthwaite, 1987a) (Fig. 17.12). Basically, the local radius of curvature at a given point of reflection is measured as the distance between the focal plane of the optical system and the corneal apex when autocollimation is achieved.

For different aperture sizes used, different

Table 17.7 Central keratometric measurement for the normal Caucasian population

	Mean ± SD (mm)	95% Range (mm)	Absolute range (mm)
Kiely *et al.* (1984) (*n* = 196 eyes)	Horizontal meridian 7.79 ± 0.26	7.27–8.31	7.10–8.75
	Vertical meridian 7.69 ± 0.28	7.12–8.24	7.06–8.66
Guillon *et al.* (1986) (*n* = 220 eyes)	Flat meridian 7.87 ± 0.25	7.37–8.37	7.14–8.54
	Steep meridian 7.70 ± 0.27	7.16–8.24	7.03–8.46

(Guillon *et al.*, 1986) in the flattest meridian and at 7.69 mm and 7.70 mm respectively in the steepest meridian. The difference between those central meridional values, which represent the central corneal astigmatism, peaks at 0.1 mm but is highly patient-dependent, as illustrated by a standard deviation of ± 0.15 mm, which indicates a 95% range of 0.00 mm to 0.45 mm (Guillon *et al.*, 1986). The corneal periphery is most often best represented by a flattening (oblate) ellipse (Table 17.8) with mean shape factors $p = 0.80$ (Kiely *et al.*, 1984) or $p = 0.83$ (Guillon *et al.*, 1986). However, both studies report a wide range of p values with a significant number of corneas that show no peripheral change in radii of curvature and other corneas that are steeper at the periphery than at the centre. The distribution of the differ-

ence in shape factor between the flat and steep meridians (Table 17.8) shows that the flattening or steepening of the cornea is not always the same in the two meridians of the same cornea. Neither of the two studies report any systematic differences between males and females.

The two characteristics of the peripheral cornea have significant implications. The difference in peripheral flattening between corneas with identical central radii of curvature explains why, to achieve a given fluorescein pattern (hence a given central tear layer thickness) for corneas that have identical central radii of curvature, one may require in extreme cases rigid gas permeable lenses with back optic radii that differ by as much as 0.3 mm. The difference in peripheral flattening between two merid-

Table 17.8 Peripheral corneal asphericity (p value) for the normal Caucasian population

Authors	Mean ± SD (p)	95% Range (p)	Absolute range (p)
Kiely *et al.* (1984) (*n* = 196 eyes)	Horizontal meridian 0.80 ± 0.15	0.50–1.10	0.48–1.13
	Vertical meridian 0.80 ± 0.22	0.36–1.24	−0.11–1.52
Guillon *et al.* (1986) (*n* = 200 eyes)	Flat meridian 0.83 ± 0.13	0.57–1.09	0.21–1.20
	Steep meridian 0.81 ± 0.16	0.49–1.13	0.11–1.16

ians of the same cornea explains why two corneas with similar amounts of moderate corneal astigmatism (e.g. 0.4 mm difference in k readings) may need different lens designs to achieve a good peripheral fit. In such a case, a cornea with a similar rate of flattening in both principal meridians or a greater flattening in the steepest meridian can usually be adequately fitted with a spherical back surface contact lens. On the contrary, a cornea with a more rapid rate of flattening in the flattest meridian than in the steepest meridian will require a toric back surface or toric peripheral back surface contact lens to achieve an adequate fit.

The main demographic factor that has been relatively well investigated is the racial difference in corneal topography. A Japanese population study has shown that, on average, they have a much steeper central cornea than Caucasians, with a mean of 7.54 mm, but have a similar span of measurements to the Caucasian population (Hamano & Tanaka, 1968). Population studies with Chinese subjects also show a statistically significant difference in the central and peripheral cornea compared to Caucasians (Lam & Loran, 1991). On average, Chinese corneas are slightly steeper, by ≈ 0.10 mm, and show less peripheral corneal flattening. Changes with age have also been fairly well documented and indicate that the peripheral (Vihlen & Wilson, 1983) and central cornea (Hirsch, 1959) flatten with age.

The studies concerned with the systematic effects of different factors, other than race and age, have used relatively small samples and therefore are difficult to extrapolate for the overall population. Kiely (Kiely *et al.*, 1982b), has suggested a steepening of both the horizontal and vertical central meridians during the day. The variations in corneal shape were large and not systematic. On the contrary Clark (1973f) reported a decrease in corneal asphericity throughout the day and Reng-

storff (1972) a constant corneal asphericity throughout the day. Similarly, the studies dealing with menstrual cycle variations (Soni, 1982; Kiely *et al.*, 1983) do indicate some fluctuations but their samples are too small to be representative.

Finally, associations have been suggested between corneal thickness and curvature (Hovding, 1983) and between refractive error and corneal curvature (Sheridan & Douthwaite, 1989). Thick corneas are slightly flatter than thin corneas (Hovding, 1983); whereas the difference between emmetropes, hyperopes and myopes resides into differences in central radii of curvatures and indicates similar peripheral flattening (Sheridan & Douthwaite, 1989).

REFERENCES

Aan De Kerk, A.L. Verhallen, J. and Vijfvinkel, G. (1973) A new portable photokeratoscope. *Med. Biol. Illust.*, **23**, 206–9.

Amiard, H. (1962) *Aspects geometriques de l'adaptation*. Le Contact Paris, Laboratoires Ysoptic, No. 9, 1–12.

Amiard, H. (1972) *Pratique de la photokeratometrie*. Le Contact Paris, Laboratoires Ysoptic, No. 29, 1–15.

Amiard, H. (1973) Pratique de la photokeratometrie. *Opticien Lunetier*, **244**(5), 41–5.

Amiard, H. and Cochet, P. (1972) *Photokeratometrie*. Le Contact Paris, Laboratoires Ysoptic, No. 25, 1–16.

Bennett, A.G. (1964) A new keratometer and its application to corneal topography. *Br. J. Physiol. Opt.*, **21**, 234.

Bennett, A.G. (1968) Aspherical contact lens surfaces. Part two. *The Ophthalmic Optician*, **30** (11), 1297–311.

Bibby, M.M. (1976a) The Wesley–Jessen System 2000 Photokeratoscope. *Contact Lens Forum*, **1** (11), 37–45.

Bibby, M.M. (1976b) Analysis and description of corneal shape. *Contact Lens Forum*, **1** (12), 27–35.

Bibby, M.M. (1976c) Computer assisted photokeratoscopy and contact lens design. *The Optician* **171** (4423), 37–43; **171** (4424), 11–15; **171** (4425), 22–3; **171** (4426), 15–17.

Bille, J.F., Dreher, A.W., Sittig, W.F. and Brown, S.I. (1987) 3D corneal imaging using the laser tomographic scanner (LTS). *Invest. Ophthalmol. Vis. Sci..*, **Suppl. 28**, 223.

Bonnet, R. and Cochet, P. (1962) New method of topographical ophthalmometry – its theoretical and clinical applications. *Am. J. Optom. Arch. Am. Acad. Optom.*, **39** (5), 227–51.

Borish, I. (1975) Ophthalmometry. In *Clinical Refraction* (3rd edn), Professional Press, Chicago, pp. 617–67.

Brown, N. (1969) A simplified photokeratoscope. *Am. J. Ophthalmol.*, **68** (3), 517–19.

Brown, N. (1972) An advanced slit image camera. *Br. J. Ophthalmol.*, **56**, 624–31.

Brungardt, T.F. (1965) Sagittal height of the cornea. *Am. J. Optom. Arch. Am. Acad. Optom.*, **42** (9), 525–33.

Brungardt, T.F. (1981) A corneal topographical model and fitting conclusion. *Am. J. Optom. Physiol. Opt.*, **58** (2), 136–8.

Busin, M., Wilmanns, I. and Spitznas, M. (1989) Automated corneal topography: computerized analysis of photokeratoscope images. *Graefe's Arch Ophthalmol.*, **227**, 230–6.

Campbell, C.E. (1982) Measuring eccentricity. *Contacto*, **26** (5), 4–8.

Campion, P.J. (1973) *A Code of Practice for the Detailed Statement of Accuracy.* London, Her Majesty's Stationery Office.

Chander, M. Bindal, M.M., Kulshreshtha, A. and Agarwala, B.K. (1976) Photokeratography using moire techniques. *Applied Opt.*, **15** (12), 2964–5.

Charman, W.N. (1972) Diffraction and the precision of measurement of corneal and other small radii. *Am. J. Optom. Physiol. Opt.*, **49**, 672–9.

Clark, B.A.J. (1966) *The Determination of Corneal Topography.* Master's Thesis, University of Melbourne, Sydney, Australia.

Clark, B.A.J. (1972) Autocollimating photokeratoscope. *J. Opt. Soc. Am.*, **62** (2), 169–76.

Clark, B.A.J. (1973a) Systems for describing corneal topograpy. *Aust. J. Optom.*, **56**, 48–56.

Clark, B.A.J. (1973b) Keratometry – a review. *Aust. J. Optom.*, **56**, 94–100.

Clark, B.A.J. (1973c) Conventional keratoscopy – a critical review. *Aust. J. Optom.*, **56**, 140–55.

Clark, B.A.J. (1973d) Less common methods of measuring corneal topography. *Aust. J. Optom.*, **56**, 182–92.

Clark, B.A.J. (1973e) Some experiments in corneal interferometry. *Aust. J. Optom.*, **56**, 448–53.

Clark, B.A.J. (1973f) Time variations in observed corneal topography. *Aust. J. Optom.*, **56**, 443–7.

Clark, B.A.J. (1974a) Validation testing of the auto-collimating photokeratoscope. *Aust. J. Optom.*, **57** (1), 22–7.

Clark, B.A.J. (1974b) Controversy on keratoscopy. Reply to comments by Townsley. *Aust. J. Optom.*, **57** (4), 122–6.

Cochet, P. and Amiard, H. (1969) Photography and contact lens fitting. *Contacto*, **13** (7), 3–9.

Cohen, K.L., Tripoli, N.K., Pellom, A.C., Kupper, L.L. and Fryczkowski, A.W. (1984) A new photogrammetric method for quantifying corneal topography. *Invest. Ophthalmol. Vis. Sci.*, **25** (3), 323–30.

Cotran, P. and Miller, D. (1987) An adaptation of the Topcon slit lamp for photokeratoscopy. *CLAO J.*, **13** (5), 277–9.

Dietrich, C.F. (1973) *Uncertainty Calibration and Probability.* London, Adam Hilger.

Dingeldein, S.A. and Klyce, S.D. (1988) Imaging of the cornea. *Cornea*, **7** (3), 170–82.

Donaldson, D.D. (1972) A new camera for medical stereophotography with special reference to the eye. *Arch. Ophthalmol.*, **52**, 564–70.

Doss, J.D., Hutson, R.L., Rowsey, J.J. and Brown, D.R. (1981) Method for calculation of corneal profile and power distribution. *Arch. Ophthalmol.*, **99** (7), 1261–5.

Douthwaite, W.A. (1987a) A new keratometer. *Am. J. Optom. Physiol. Opt.*, **64** (9), 711–15.

Douthwaite, W.A. (1987b) Corneal topography. *Contact Lens J.*, **15** (6), 7–12.

Douthwaite, W.A. and Sheridan, M. (1989) The measurement of the corneal ellipse for the contact lens practitioner. *Ophthalmol. Physiol. Opt.*, **9**, 239–42.

Dragomirescu, V., Hockwin, O., Koch, H.R. and Sasaki, K. (1980) Development of a new equipment for rotating slit image photography according to Scheimpflug's principle. *Interdiscipl. Topics Geront. (Kerger Basel)*, **13**, 118–30.

Duke-Elder, S. (1970) The dioptric imagery of the eye. In *System of Ophthalmology, Vol. V Ophthalmic Optics and Refraction*, Henry Kimpton, London, pp. 93–150.

Edmund, C. (1986) The significance of using different methods for analysing photokeratoscopic data. *Acta Ophthalmologia*, **64** (9), 97–100.

Edmund, C. (1987) Location of the corneal apex and its influence on the stability of the central corneal curvature. A photokeratoscopy study. *Am. J. Optom. Physiol. Opt.*, **64** (11), 846–52.

Edmund, C. and Sjøntoft, E. (1985) The central-peripheral radius of the normal corneal curvature. A photokeratoscopic study. *Acta Ophthalmologia*, **63**, 670–7.

El Hage, S.G. (1971) Suggested new methods for photokeratoscopy. A comparison for their validities Part I. *Am. J. Optom. Arch. Am. Acad. Optom.*, **48** (11), 897–912.

El Hage, S.G. (1972a) Differential equation for the use of the diffused ring photokeratoscope. *Am. J. Optom. Arch. Am. Acad. Optom.*, **49** (5), 422–36.

El Hage, S.G. (1972b) A new conception of the corneal topology and its application. *Optica Acta*, **19** (5), 431–3.

El Hage, S.G. (1976) A new photokeratoscopic technique. *Optical Engineering*, **15** (4), 308–11.

Fincham, E.F. (1953) The photokeratoscope. *Med. Biol. III*, **3**, 87.

Fry, G.A. (1975a) Photokeratoscopy with a telecentric camera. *Optometric Weekly*, **66** (8), 201–3.

Fry, G.A. (1975b) Analysis of photometric data. *Am. J. Optom. Physiol. Opt.*, **52** (5), 305–12.

Fujii, T., Maruyama, S. and Ikeda, M. (1972) Determination of corneal configuration by the measurement of its derivatives. *Optica Acta*, **19**, 425–30.

Furakawa, R.E., Polse, K.A. and Emori, Y. (1976) Slit lamp fluorophotometry. *Optical Engineering*, **15** (4), 321–4.

Girard, J.L. and Soper, W.J. (1962) *Corneal Contact Lenses*. CV Mosby Co, St Louis.

Gormley, D.J., Gersten, M., Koplin, R.S. and Lubkin, V. (1988) Corneal modeling. *Cornea*, **7** (1), 30–5.

Grosvenor, T. (1961) Clinical use of the keratometer in evaluating the corneal contour. *Am. J. Optom. Arch. Am. Acad. Optom.*, **38** (5), 237–46.

Guillon, M., Lydon, D.P.M. and Sammons, W.A. (1983) Designing rigid gas permeable contact lenses using the edge clearance technique. *J.Br. Contact Lens Assoc.*, **6**(1), 19–26.

Guillon, M., Lydon, D.P.M. and Wilson, C. (1986) Corneal topography: A clinical model. *Ophthalmic Physiol. Optics*, **6**, 47–56.

Gullstraud, A. (1896) Photographic–ophthalmometric and clinical investigation of corneal refraction. Part 1. (Translated by Ludlam, W.M. 1966) *Am. J. Optom. Arch. Am. Acad. Optom.*, **43**, 143–214.

Hamano, J. and Tanaka, K. (1968) Examination of patients after extended wear of contact lenses. *Contacto*, **12**, 3–8.

Hannush, S.B., Crawford, S.L., Waring, G.O. III, Germmill, M.C., Lynn, M.F. and Nizam, A. (1989) Accuracy and precision of keratometry, photokeratoscopy and corneal modeling on calibrated steel balls. *Arch. Opthalmol.*, **107**, 1235–9.

Hannush, S.B., Crawford, S.L., Waring, G.O. III, Germmill, M.C. Lynn, M.F. and Nizam, A. (1990) Reproductibility of normal corneal power measurements with a keratometer, photokeratoscope and video imaging system. *Arch. Opthalmol.*, **108**, 539–44.

Hayward, A.T.J. (1977) *Repeatability and Accuracy*. Mechanic Engineering Publications, London.

Himi, T. Mizutani, Y. and Fujiwara, Y. (1981) Corneal curvature: its calculated model formula. *Contacto*, **25**, 15–18.

Hirsch, M.J. (1959) Changes in astigmatism after the age of forty. *Am. J. Optom. Arch. Am. Acad. Optom.*, **36**, 395–405.

Holden, B.A. (1970) *A Study of the Development and Control of Myopia and the Effects of Contact Lenses on Corneal Topography*. PhD Thesis, The City University, London.

Hovding, G. (1983) A clinical study of the association between thickness and curvature of the central cornea. *Acta Ophthalmologica*, **61**, 461–6.

ISO 3534 (1982) *International Standard Organization Statistics Vocabulary and Symbols*. International Organization for Standardization.

Kawara, T. (1984) Corneal topography using moire contour fringes. *Appl. Opt.*, **18**(21), 3675–8.

Kemmetmuller, H. (1984) Accurate fitting of new gas permeable contact lenses by means of inproved keratometry. *Contact Lens J.*, **12**(7), 5–17.

Kiely, P.M., Smith, G. and Carney, L.G. (1982a) The mean shape of the human cornea. *Optica Acta*, **29**, 1027–40.

Kiely, P.M., Carney, L.G. and Smith, G. (1982b) Diurnal variations of corneal topography and thickness. *Am. J. Optom. Physiol. Opt.*, **59**, 976–82.

Kiely, P.M., Smith, G. and Carney, L.G. (1984) Mechanical variations of corneal shape. *Am. J. Optom. Physiol. Opt.*, **61**, 619–26.

Kiely, P.M., Carney, L.G. and Smith, G. (1983) Menstrual cycle variations of corneal topography and thickness. *Am. J. Optom. Physiol. Opt.*, **60**, 822–9.

Kivayev, A.A., Ososkov, G.A. and Shapiro, E.L. (1985) Corneal topography investigation and principles of contact lenses design on the basis of photokeratometry. *Contact Lens J.*, **13**(8), 1–14.

Klein, M. (1958) A new keratoscope with self luminous Placido disc. *Br. J. Ophthalmol.*, **42**, 380–1.

Klyce, S.D. (1984) Computer-assisted corneal topography. High resolution graphic presentation and analysis of keratoscopy. *Invest. Ophthalmol. Vis. Sci.*, **25**(12), 1426–35.

Klyce, S.D. (1989) The topography of normal corneas. *Arch. Opthalmol.*, **107**(4), 512–18.

Knoll, H.A. (1961) Corneal contours in the general population as revealed by the photokeratoscope. *Am. J. Optom. Arch. Am. Acad. Optom.*, **38**(7), 389–97.

Knoll, H.A., Stimson, R. and Weeks, C.L. (1957) New photokeratoscope utilising a hemispherical object surface. *J. Opt. Soc. Am.*, **47**(3), 221–2.

Lam, C.S.Y. and Loran, D.F.C. (1991) Designing contact lenses for oriental eyes. *J. Br. Contact Lens Assoc.*, **14**(3), 109–14.

Levene, J.R. (1962) An evaluation of the hand keratoscope as a diagnostic instrument for corneal astigmatism. *Br. J. Physiol. Opt.*, **19**, 237–49.

Lotmar, W. (1971) Theoretical eye model with aspherics. *J. Opt. Soc. Am.*, **61**(11), 1522–9.

Ludlam, W.M. and Kaye, M. (1966) Optometry and the new metrology. *Am. J. Optom. Arch. Am. Acad. Optom.*, **43**(8), 525–8.

Ludlam, W.M. and Wittenberg, S. (1966a) Photokeratoscopy – one of Gullstrand's contributions to the measurement of ocular components. *Canadian J. Optom.*, **28**(2), 47–50.

Ludlam, W.M. and Wittenberg, S. (1966b) The effects of measuring corneal toroidicity with reference to the line of sight. *Br. J. Physiol. Opt.*, **23**(2), 178–85.

Ludlam, W.M. and Wittenberg, S. (1966c) Measurements of the ocular dioptric elements utilising photographic methods. Part II, Corneal – theoretical considerations. *Am. J. Optom. Arch. Am. Acad. Optom.*, **43** (4), 249–67.

Ludlam, W.M., Wittenberg, S., Rosenthal, J. and Harris, G. (1967) Photographic analysis of the ocular dioptric components. Part III. The acquisition, storage, retrieval and utilization of primary data in photokeratoscopy. *Am. J. Optom. Arch. Am. Acad. Optom.*, **44** (4), 276–96.

McDonnell, P.J. and Garbus, J. (1989) Corneal topographic changes after radial keratotomy. *Ophthalmology*, **96** (1), 45–9.

McMonnies, C.W. (1971) Corneal curvature from profile measurements. *Aust. J. Optom.*, **54**, 153–223.

Maguire, L.G., Singer, D.E. and Klyce, S.D. (1985) Graphic presentation of computer analyzed keratoscope photographs. *Arch. Opthalmol.*, **105**, 223–30.

Manabe, R., Matsuda, M. and Suda, T. (1986) Photokeratoscopy in fitting contact lens after penetrating kerataoplasty. *Br. J. Ophthalmol.*, **70**, 55–9.

Mandell, R.B. (1961) Methods to measure the peripheral corneal curvature. *J. Am. Optom. Assoc.*, **33**, 137; **33**, 585; **33**, 889.

Mandell, R.B. (1962) Reflection point ophthalmometry. A method to measure corneal contour. **39** (10), 513–37.

Mandell, R.B. (1966) Corneal curvature measurements by the aid of Moire fringes. *J. Am. Optom. Assoc.*, **37** (3), 219–20.

Mandell, R.B. and St Helen, R. (1968) Stability of the corneal contour. *Am. J. Optom. Arch. Am. Acad. Optom.*, **45** (12), 797–805.

Mandell, R.B. and St Helen, R. (1971) Mathematical model of the corneal contour. *Br. J. Physiol. Opt.*, **26**, 183–97.

Mandell, R.B. and York, M.A. (1969) A new calibration system for photokeratoscopy. *Am. J. Optom. Arch. Am. Acad. Optom.*, **46** (6), 410–17.

Morris, J.W. (1956) Observing, measuring and recording the curvature of the cornea. A description of the AIM Keratograph. *The Optician*, **131**, 341–3.

Moss, H.I. (1959) A clinical experimental study of corneal contours in the fitting of contact lenses. *Am. J. Optom. Arch. Am. Acad. Optom.*, **36** (6), 313–17.

Muckenhirn, D. (1981) Fitting individual contact lenses with the use of computer tonometry. *Contacto*, **25** (6), 28–34.

Norton, H.J. and Sullivan, C.T. (1962) A modern photographing keratoscope. *Am. J. Ophthalmol.*, **53**, 371–3.

Petricciani, J.C., Ditto, J.R. and Collins, W.B. (1985) Elucidating the cornea. *Contact Lens Forum*, **10** (6), 41–7.

Phillips, A.J. (1980) Corneal lens fitting. In *Contact Lenses: A textbook for practitioner and student. Vol 1, Background Pre-fitting Care and Basic Hard Lens Techniques* (2nd edn) Butterworth, London.

Plummer, R. and Lamb, A. (1961) Method for keratographic recording. *Br. J. Ophthalmol.*, **45**, 312–15.

Pulvermacker, H. and Rott, P. (1972) A new method for adjusting the eye in photokeratoscopy. *Optica Acta*, **19** (5), 435–7.

Rengstorff, R.H. (1972) Diurnal constancy of corneal curvature. *Am. J. Optom. Physiol. Opt.*, **49**, 1002–5.

Richards, D.W., Russell, S.R. and Anderson, D.R. (1988) A method for improved biometry of the anterior chamber with a Scheimpflug technique. *Invest. Ophthalmol. Vis. Sci.*, **29**, 1826–35.

Ritz, N.W. (1963) Keratoscopic photographs of the cornea. *The Optician*, **144** (3744), 657–9.

Rowsey, J.J., Reynolds, A.E. and Brown, R. (1981) Corneal topography. Corneascope. *Arch. Ophthalmol.*, **99** (6), 1093–100.

Rowsey, J.J., Monlux, R., Balyeat, H.D., Stevens, S.X., Gelender, H., Holladay, J., Krachmer, J.H., Laibson, P., Lindstrom, R., Lynn, M., Mandelbaum, S., McDonald, M., Myers, W.D., Obstbaum, S., Schanzlin, D., Sperduto, R., Waring, G. and the PERK Study Group. (1989) Accuracy and reproductibility of kerascanner analysis in PERK corneal topography. *Current Eye Res.*, **8** (7), 661–74.

Sheridan, M. and Douthwaite, W.A. (1989) Corneal asphericity and refractive error. *Ophthalmol. Physiol. Opt.*, **9**, 235–8.

Sivak, J.G. (1977) A simple photokeratoscope. *Am. J. Optom. Physiol. Opt.*, **54** (4), 241–3.

Smith, T.G. (1977) Corneal topography. *Doc. Ophthalmol.*, **43** (2), 249–76.

Soni, P.S. (1982) Effects of oral contraceptive steroids on corneal curvature. *Am. J. Optom. Physiol. Opt.*, **59**, 199–201.

Stone, J. (1962) The validity of some existing methods of measuring corneal contour compared with suggested new method. *Br. J. Physiol. Opt.*, **19**, 205–30.

Thomas, G.B. (1975) *Calculus and Analytic Geometry* (4th edn), Addison-Wesley, Reading, p. 475.

Tomlinson, A. and Bibby, M.M. (1977) Corneal clearance at the apex and edge of hard corneal lens. *Int. Contact Lens Clin.*, **4** (6), 73–81.

Tomlinson, A. and Schwartz, C. (1979) The position of the corneal apex in the normal eye. *Am. J. Optom. Physiol. Opt.*, **56** (4), 236–40.

Townsley, M.G. (1967) New equipment and methods for determining the contour of the human cornea. *Contacto*, **11** (4), 72–81.

Townsley, M.G. (1970) New knowledge of the corneal contour. *Contacto*, **14** (3), 38–43.

Townsley, M.G. (1974) Controversy on keratoscopy. Comments from MG Townsley. *Aust. J. Optom.*, **57** (4), 118–22.

Vihlen, F.S. and Wilson, G. (1983) The relation between eyelid tension, corneal toricity and age. *Invest. Ophthalmol. Vis. Sci.*, **24**, 1367–73.

Von Fieandt (1964) Keratometry in the fitting of corneal contact lenses. *Acta Ophthalmologica*, **42**, 347–52.

Warnick, J.W., Rehkope, P., Curtin, D., Burns, S.A., Arffa, R.C. and Stuart, J. (1987) Corneal topography using rasterstereography. *Invest. Ophthalmol. Vis. Sci.*, **Suppl. 28**, 223.

Wechsler, S. (1978) Model of the corneal contour. *J. Br. Contact Lens Assoc.*, 18–26.

Wesley, N.K. (1982) The position of the corneal apex in the normal and the keratoconic eye. *Contacto*, **26** (3), 4–7.

Westheimer, G. (1965) A method of photoelectric keratoscopy. *Am. J. Optom. Arch. Am. Acad. Optom.*, **42** (5), 315–20.

Wilms, K.H. (1974) Considerations about the topometry of cornea and contact lens. *Contacto*, **18** (2), 12–21.

Wilms, K.H. (1981) Topometry of the cornea and contact lenses with new equipment. *Ophthalmic Optician*, **21** (16), 516–19.

Wilms, K.H. and Rabbetts, R.B. (1977) Practical concepts of corneal topometry. *The Optician*, **174** (4502), 7–13.

Wittenberg, S. and Ludlam, W.M. (1966) Derivation of a system for analysing the corneal surface from photokeratoscopic data. *J. Opt. Soc. Am.*, **56** (11), 1612–15.

York, M.A. (1969) *A System of Photokeratoscope Calibration and its Application in the Study of Corneal Development*. Master of Science Thesis, University of Berkeley, California.

York, M.A. and Mandell, R.B. (1969) A new calibration system for photokeratoscopy. Part II, Corneal contour measurements. *Am. J. Optom.*, **46**, 818–21.

PART 1 BIOMICROSCOPY

S. Zantos and I. Cox

18.1 INTRODUCTION

The transparent nature of the ocular tissues enables non-invasive examination of the living eye that is unique in clinical work. The slit lamp microscope combines a clever illumination system with a convenient stereomicroscopic viewing system. Its great variety of attachments make it an extremely versatile instrument for examining the human eye.

The first binocular corneal microscope was constructed by H. Aubert in 1891. Improvements were made by S. Czapski, and in particular by Alvar Gullstrand who, in 1911, presented his design of an illumination system that made slit lamp microscopy practical by providing a sufficiently bright and focused beam of light to the eye. A subsequent modification, the so-called Kohler illumination system, served to enhance the homogeneity of the slit beam projected on the eye, enabling optical sectioning of the eye tissues, and it became the basis of today's instruments. Over the next 40 years numerous improvements were made by Henker, Koeppe, Vogt, Koby, Poser, Goldmann, Littman and others, culminating in instrumentation that resembled and operated similarly to today's slit lamps (Fig. 18.1). Concurrently, numerous publications appeared on the subject of biomicroscopy of the eye, the first books being published in the early 1920s by Koby, Vogt and Koeppe. Other noteworthy treatises were later published by Butler (1924), Berliner (1943) and Doggart (1949). This was a period of discovery – the various slit lamp techniques for illuminating and observing the ocular tissues were discussed meticulously, and the normal and abnormal appearances of the eye were beautifully described and illustrated, with detail similar to that seen using modern instrumentation.

A significant advance in slit lamp evolution came in 1965 with the introduction of instrumentation capable of photographing

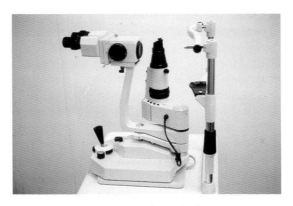

Figure 18.1 A typical modern slit lamp.

Contact Lens Practice. Edited by Montague Ruben and Michel Guillon.
Published in 1994 by Chapman & Hall, London. ISBN 0 412 35120 X

optical sections of the eye. This coupled with the development of numerous attachments (pachometer, goniolens, Hruby fundus lens, applanation tonometer, filters, polarizers, fluorophotometer, endothelial lens, video, etc.), have made the modern slit lamp microscope an extraordinarily useful instrument in research and in clinical practice. Its application to contact lens work is extensive.

With regard to biomicroscopic examination of the eye, it is worth adding that in recent years two new instruments have been investigated in the search for higher magnification and resolution of tissue structures: the specular microscope and the confocal (tandem scanning) microscope. Both instruments can be used for the living eye, though the confocal microscope is presently in the research and development phase, and not yet used in clinical practice. The specular microscope is widely available for clinical work, having been extensively used for evaluation of the corneal endothelium before and after cataract surgery and intra-ocular lens implantation; in contact lens research, the instrument has been used for investigating long-term changes in the endothelium, as well the effects of lens wear on the corneal epithelium. Where the specular microscope reveals cellular patterns only at tissue layers differing in refractive index (e.g. epithelium-to-air; endothelium-to-aqueous), the confocal microscope reveals tissue structure at any layer. Moreover, it does so with considerably more detail, for example, stromal keratocytes and cell nuclei can be seen *in vivo* with the confocal microscope. Numerous fine review articles exist on the optical principles and applications of the specular microscope (Koester & Roberts, 1990; Mayer, 1984) and the confocal microscope (Cavanagh *et al.*, 1990; Masters & Kino, 1990). Still, the slit lamp microscope remains the instrument of choice for clinical practice, and its main features, applications, and procedures will now be discussed.

18.2   INSTRUMENTATION

Many well-designed and well constructed slit lamps are available today. The main features of slit lamps can be seen in Figures 18.2, 18.3 and 18.4. The three essential components of all instruments are the slit illumination system, the stereomicroscope viewing system and the mechanical system for adjusting position and height of the instrument and of the patient. Detailed reviews of these are available in several textbooks (e.g. Brandreth, 1978), and familiarization is best done using the actual instrument. However, in selecting a brand of slit lamp, we recommend that particular attention be given to certain features.

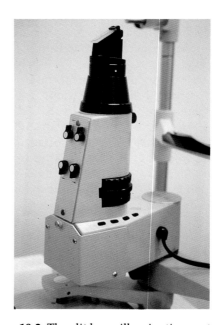

Figure 18.2 The slit lamp illumination system. Slit beam width and height are adjusted by the knurled rings at the front, while the knobs on the rear of the housing allow coloured filters to be introduced into the light beam. The diffusing filter can be seen at the top of the illumination housing ready to be flipped into place in front of the prism. Slit beam offset is adjusted by turning the prism housing laterally.

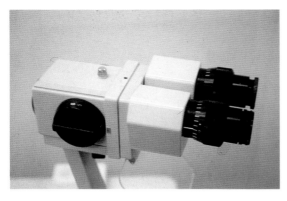

Figure 18.3 The stereomicroscope viewing system. The eyepieces are adjustable to compensate for the viewer's refractive error and pupillary distance. Magnification is adjusted by turning the handle located on either side of the lens housing.

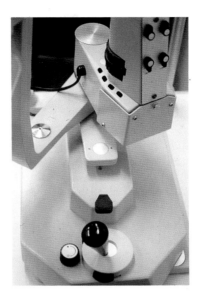

Figure 18.4 The mechanical system. Lateral movements are controlled by the joystick, while vertical adjustments are made with the electric switch located in front of the joystick. This adjustment may be manual on many slit lamps. Illumination intensity can be altered using the rheostat located on the left of the joystick.

18.2.1 THE SLIT LAMP ILLUMINATION SYSTEM

1. High illumination is required to enhance detection of subtle conditions in the eye tissues when using optic section or indirect illumination techniques (e.g. for assessing corneal thickness or for evaluating changes in corneal transparency). A slit illumination up to 600 000 lux is desirable, and a halogen or xenon light source is preferred to a tungsten lamp for reasons of longevity, colour, temperature and low heat generation.

2. The ability to displace (offset) the slit beam sideways is invaluable for performing indirect illumination techniques (e.g. sclerotic scatter, retro-illumination), and it is necessary that a control device for doing this be present, conveniently and finely adjustable, and steady. A click-stop position is useful for re-setting the beam to its normal position.

3. A diffusing filter and a cobalt blue filter should always be incorporated into the instrument, and other filters are desirable, e.g. green (red-free) and polarizer.

18.2.2 THE STEREOMICROSCOPE VIEWING SYSTEM

The optical design of today's slit lamps is quite good, so that the practitioner need not be too concerned with the resolution, brightness, and stereoscopic results. Detailed discussion of these items is given in other books (e.g. Müller; Schmidt, 1975). From a more practical standpoint, the magnification, focus adjustment and parfocality, and the working distance are more important considerations:

1. The magnification should be easily changeable, and it should preferably cover the range approximately 5× to 30× before one has to change eyepieces to achieve higher magnification.

2. It is advisable to check periodically that the object of regard remains in focus as

the magnification is changed through the range available. A well-constructed focusing rod accompanying the slit lamp can be invaluable in checking the parfocality of the slit illumination system and the microscope viewing system. It is also worthwhile to check for absence of vertical prismatic effect between the two eyepiece views as the objective magnification is changed.

3. The working distance of the microscope (from object plane to the front lens of the microscope) should be approximately 110 mm, long enough to allow for manipulation of the eye or of accessory attachments, but not too long so as to require an uncomfortable arm position during such manipulations.

18.2.3 THE MECHANICAL SYSTEM

Accurate and convenient positioning of the instrument in relation to the patient's eyes is vital to efficient biomicroscopy:

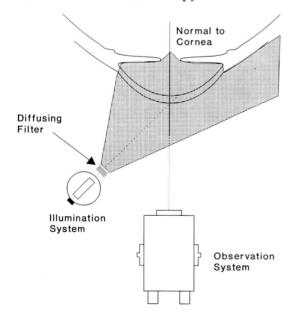

Figure 18.5 Diffuse illumination. The diffusing filter in front of the illumination system spreads a wide beam of unfocused, scattered light uniformly across the field of view.

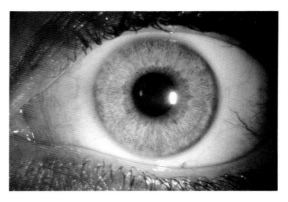

Figure 18.6 Diffuse illumination. Low magnification overview of the whole eye.

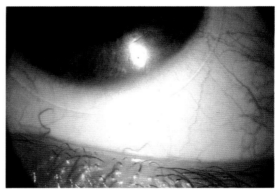

Figure 18.7 Diffuse illumination. Medium magnification view of the edge of a soft lens.

1. It is preferable that the height adjustment of the slit lamp and the joystick for lateral adjustment and focus be combined, or be near enough to each other so that one hand can control all these functions, leaving the other hand free to manipulate the patient's eyelids or an accessory device, or to manoeuvre the illumination system or the microscope.

2. It is important that the friction in the sliding stage be not so loose that slippage occurs as the instrument is moved, and not so tight that the joystick might be jerky or excessively tilted from its

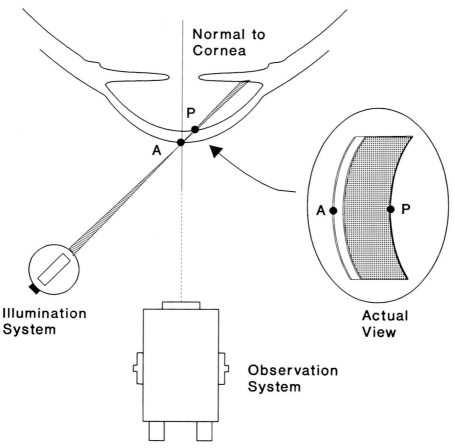

Figure 18.8 Optic section. The illumination system sections the cornea with a thin, beam of light, focused co-incidentally with the axis of the observation system.

vertical position as the instrument is moved during the examination.

3. The well-constructed instrument will have the slit illumination system and microscope system nearly perfectly coaxial, so that as the former is rotated (swung) from one side to the other, the slit beam will not shift significantly sideways in the field of view, and parfocality can be maintained. The focusing rod can be used to check this, but it must be perfectly constructed and positioned in the coaxial slot to be of any value.

In addition to the slit lamp microscope, illumination system and mechanical stage, the construction of the patient's headrest and of the instrument table are obviously important to the ease of performing biomicroscopy. As with other ophthalmic instruments, the comfort and adjustability of these functions should be tried for suitability to the practitioner's personal preference before purchase.

Reviews of the specifications of the various commercially available instruments have been published elsewhere, and the reader is referred to these articles for comparison of

instrument features (Stockwell, 1983 Martonyi, 1989;).

18.3   SLIT LAMP ILLUMINATION AND
OBSERVATION TECHNIQUES

The ability to detect and diagnose the various anterior segment conditions which may
occur depends to a large extent on the ability
of the observer to correctly adjust and position the illumination system of the slit lamp.
In many cases, subtle changes to anterior
segment structures can only be detected and
thoroughly assessed by using a combination
of illumination techniques. Slit lamp illumination can be categorized into four main
groups:

1.   Diffuse illumination.
2.   Direct illumination.
3.   Indirect illumination.
4.   Filtered illumination.

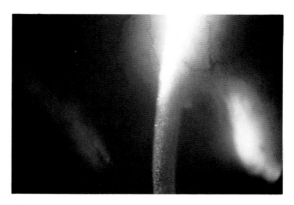

Figure 18.10 Optic section. High magnification
view of infiltrates invading the peripheral cornea.
Note that the optic section reveals the infiltrates to
be concentrated towards the anterior stroma.

Within each of these categories are several
techniques which are defined and described
in the following section according to the
adjustment and positioning of both the illumination and observation systems. This
differentiation is important for the inexperienced observer to ensure that the optimal observation technique is used for
viewing each particular condition or structure. However, it should be understood that,
in reality, several different methods of illumination may be simultaneously present in
the field of view at any one moment during
the slit lamp procedure, providing the experienced observer with the necessary differential information without resorting to several
different physical adjustments of the slit
lamp. This speeds up the slit lamp examination and reduces patient fatigue and discomfort.

18.3.1   DIFFUSE ILLUMINATION

Diffuse illumination is so named because a
ground glass diffusing filter is placed in the
focused light beam of the slit lamp. This
defocuses and scatters the light to give a
broad even illumination over the entire field
of view of the observation system (Fig. 18.5).

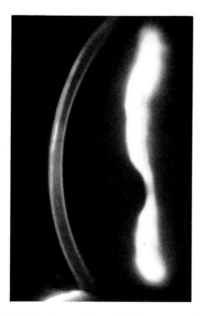

Figure 18.9 Optic section. Medium magnification
view of a central corneal scar. Note that the optic
section allows the depth of the scar to be easily
determined.

The angle of the illumination arm is not critical when the diffuser is in place and can be anywhere from 10 to 70 degrees in relation to the observation arm. Brightness is controlled by both the slit width and the illumination rheostat of the slit lamp.

Diffuse illumination is typically used for low magnification views of the anterior segment, particularly for assessing conjunctival redness, contact lens fitting performance, or for initial gross scanning views of anterior ocular structures (Figs 18.6 and 18.7)

18.3.2 DIRECT ILLUMINATION

Direct illumination describes any illumination technique where the slit beam from the illumination arm and the optics of the observation system are focused co-incidentally on the object or area under view. The following set-ups are considered to be direct illumination techniques:

1. Optic section.
2. Parallelepiped.
3. Broad beam.

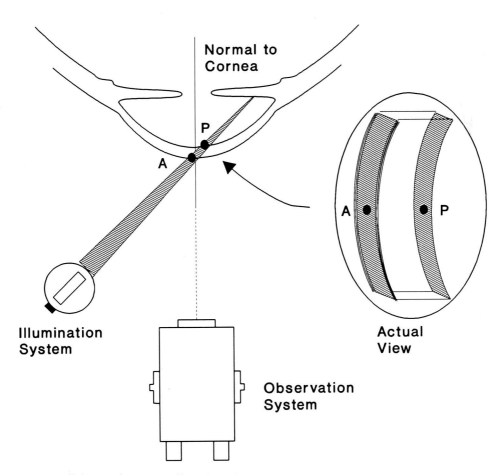

Figure 18.11 Parallelepiped. Essentially a broadened optic section. Note that the size of an object within a parallelepiped can be estimated by comparing the width of the parallelepiped to its depth (which is approximately 500 μm).

4. Conical beam.
5. Specular reflection.
6. Oblique.

Optic Section

Optic section describes an illumination technique which utilizes an extremely thin beam of light (e.g. 0.02–0.1 mm) to 'cross-section' the corneal tissue in much the same way as would be seen with a transverse histological section. This provides the ability to assess the depth of an object within the corneal layers or the depth of the tear film between a rigid lens and the anterior cornea.

To set up an optic section, the illumination arm is positioned on the side of the microscope that corresponds to that section of the cornea to be viewed (i.e. temporal side for temporal cornea) and is set at an angle between 30 and 60 degrees to the observation arm. Increasing the angle creates a wider section but may not allow the intersection of several objects separated by depth (Fig. 18.8).

The illumination rheostat is turned fully on and the slit beam is narrowed as much as possible while still providing sufficient illumination for viewing. The slit width can be

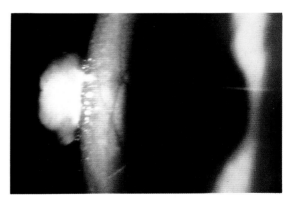

Figure 18.13 Parallelepiped. High magnification view of endothelial folds caused by stromal oedema. Note that the anterior portion of the cornea is out of focus when the plane of focus is at the endothelium. This demonstrates the short depth of field that accompanies higher magnification views.

refined while viewing the cornea through the microscope.

Optic section is used for viewing anything where a sense of depth will enhance the appreciation of the object's size and location, such as a foreign body embedded in the cornea, corneal haziness and oedema, endothelial bedewing or pigment cells, or the clarity of the corneal epithelium (which appears dark when it is clear and grey when it is oedematous) (Figs. 18.9 and 18.10).

Parallelepiped illumination

A parallelepiped is perhaps the most commonly used form of direct illumination used in slit lamp examinations. It is essentially the same in setup as an optic section, except that the slit beam is widened until it is approximately the same width as the apparent corneal depth (e.g. 0.1–0.7 mm) (Fig. 18.11). This view allows an appreciation of an object in true three dimensions, since its width, height and depth can be assessed simultaneously.

Parallelepiped is used to assess the corneal

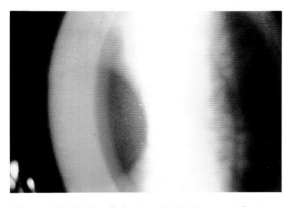

Figure 18.12 Parallelepiped. High magnification view of the central cornea, the parallelepiped being almost twice as wide as it is deep. Note the microcysts seen to the right of the parallelepiped in indirect retro-illumination.

endothelium, corneal scarring, corneal staining, neovascularization, corneal infiltrates, and corneal striae and folds (Figs. 18.12 and 18.13).

Broad beam illumination

Broad beam illumination is the next logical step from the optic section and parallelepiped, and refers to a similar setup, except that the slit beam is now widened to somewhat broader than the apparent corneal depth (e.g. 1–5 mm) (Fig. 18.14). Light intensity should be reduced using the illumination rheostat. The angle between the illumination and observation arms is not critical and should be adjusted to provide the optimum view of the object in question.

Broad beam illumination is particularly useful for viewing corneal nerve fibres, debris trapped beneath soft and rigid lenses, conjunctival abnormalities and pterygia, and larger scars and opacities within the cornea (Figs. 18.15 and 18.16).

Conical beam illumination

Conical beam is useful primarily for observing inflammatory cells and protein in the anterior chamber as a result of a uveal

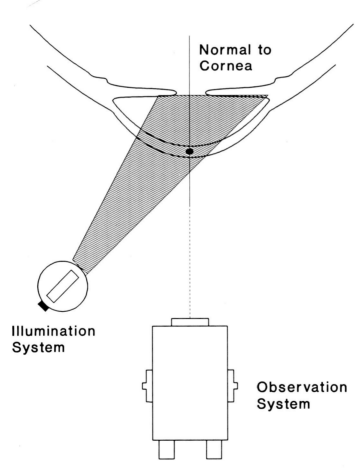

Figure 18.14 Broad beam. An extremely wide parallelepiped, used mostly for looking at large corneal defects.

inflammatory response. The conical beam is formed by setting up an optic section and then reducing the height of the slit beam until it is about 1–2 mm in height. Light intensity should be maximized using the illumination rheostat. Since the illumination intensity of the conical beam is low, observer sensitivity will be increased if the room illumination is turned off. The anterior chamber should then be scanned at low to medium magnification from side to side. Cells (inflammatory cells) will appear as bright, white reflections as they pass through the conical beam, while flare (protein) will appear as yellowish particles. These reflections will be more easily detected if viewed against a dark background, it is therefore best to reduce light scattering by avoiding having the conical beam strike the iris, and by enhancing pupil dilatation by directing the conical beam entering the pupil away from the foveal area. Some observers suggest oscillating the slit beam using the offset control to enhance the visibility of cells and flare (Fig. 18.17).

Specular reflection

Specular reflection is a specific case of the parallelepiped setup where the angle of the incident slit beam to the corneal surface

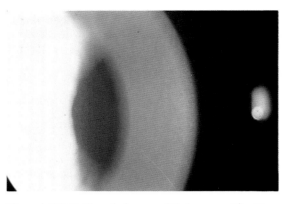

Figure 18.16 Broad beam. High magnification view of corneal nerves.

equals the angle of the observation axis through one of the oculars (Fig. 18.18). At this specific angle the illumination beam is reflected from the smooth surfaces of the anterior segment (tear film, contact lens posterior surface, endothelium and anterior lens capsule) and provides a bright, mirror-like reflection. To achieve specular reflection, set-up the slit lamp to form a parallelepiped. Adjust the magnification to the lowest available setting. Move the observation arm up to 20 degrees away from the illumination arm, and then begin to move the illumination arm in the opposing direction while observing the corneal surface. At the point where specular reflection is achieved, a bright reflex will fill one of the oculars. Note that specular reflection cannot be achieved binocularly. Having located the specular reflex, increase the magnification of the observation system stepwise to its highest setting to provide a clear view of the endothelial mosaic or other object of interest.

Specular reflection is used for observing the quality of the tear layer, since it allows the lipid layer of the tears to be viewed. Obviously, lens front surface wetting can also be observed in this manner. It is also important to note that specular reflection is the only technique which allows observa-

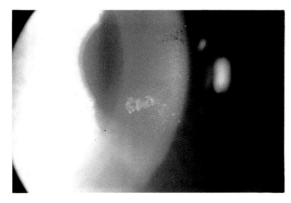

Figure 18.15 Broad beam. High magnification view of debris trapped beneath a soft lens.

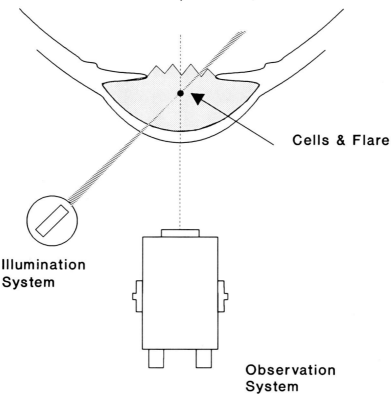

Figure 18.17 Conical beam. A narrow optic section with the height reduced to form a small oval beam. Note that the dilated pupil is used as a dark field background to enhance observation of any cells or flare in the anterior chamber.

tion of the corneal endothelial mosaic *in vivo*, along with guttae, folds and blebs. However, it is often difficult for the inexperienced observer to clearly view the endothelial reflex because the significantly brighter reflex from the tears causes visual distraction. Increasing the overall angle between the two arms of the slit lamp will increase the separation between the two specular reflexes and minimize this interference. For this same reason, viewing the endothelial specular reflex is easier for the peripheral areas of the cornea than for the central region, since the cornea's greatest thickness is in the periphery (Figs. 18.19 and 18.20).

Oblique illumination

Although infrequently used in contact lens practice, oblique illumination provides a unique view of contour changes which would not be visible by other methods of illumination. As the name suggests, oblique illumination is achieved by setting up a parallelepiped and then moving the illumination arm away from the observation system until the angle between them is close to 90 degrees. The illumination arm is adjusted so that the light beam is almost tangential to the object of regard. In this way, very small deviations in the topography of the iris, for example, will cast large areas of shadow,

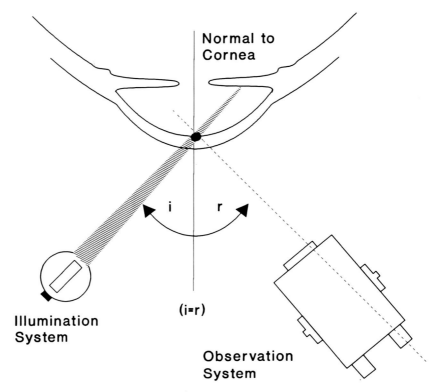

Figure 18.18 Specular reflection. Note that specular reflection can only be achieved when the angle of the incident illumination to the normal of the cornea equals the angle of the observation system, and that specular reflection is viewed through one eyepiece only.

clearly defining the high and low points of a surface which appears to be relatively flat under other more frequently used methods of illumination.

Oblique illumination is used to examine the uniformity of the iris surface, as well as any changes in the corneal structure such as Fleischer's ring, which may otherwise be hard to assess using other methods of direct illumination. In contact lens practice, oblique illumination may also be used to investigate the elevation height of front surface deposits, lens edge lift, and the location of bifocal lens optic zones (Figs. 18.21 and 18.22).

18.3.3 INDIRECT ILLUMINATION

Indirect illumination refers to any technique where the focus of the illumination beam does not coincide with the focal point of the observation system (Fig. 18.23). To achieve this the slit beam must be offset (i.e. displaced sideways). This can be achieved manually by turning the prism or mirror controlling the slit beam away from the axis of the illumination arm, or, as is often done by experienced observers, by achieving direct illumination and focusing the slit beam to one side of the object to be viewed and utilizing a different part of the microscope field of view to observe the object which is now indirectly illuminated (Fig. 18.24).

As with direct illumination, indirect illumination can be divided into several specific illumination techniques. The following set-

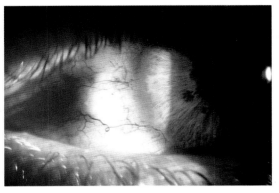

Figure 18.21 Oblique illumination. Medium magnification view of a pinguecula. Note that the shadow cast by the pinguecula when illuminated by oblique illumination provides an indication of the height of the growth.

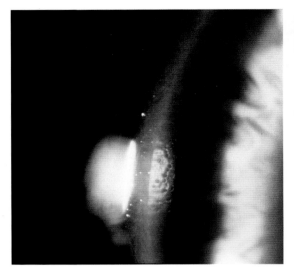

Figure 18.19 Specular reflection. High magnification view of endothelial guttae.

ups are considered indirect illumination techniques:

1. Proximal.
2. Sclerotic scatter.
3. Retro-illumination (direct and indirect).

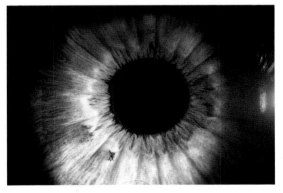

Figure 18.22 Oblique illumination. High magnification view of the iris architecture. The radial folds seen in this photograph were not visible with frontal direct illumination. Note also that the small areas of pigmentation do not cast a shadow, indicating that they are not raised from the surface of the iris.

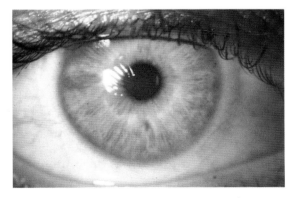

Figure 18.20 Specular reflection. Low magnification view of front surface wrinkling on a soft lens fitted too steeply. Note that the wrinkles are only visible in the area of specular reflection from the tear film.

Proximal

Proximal illumination is very similar to parallelepiped direct illumination, except that the parallelepiped is offset slightly to one side of the object being viewed. This allows the object and its immediate surrounding area to be illuminated by light scattered through the cornea, uncovering subtle

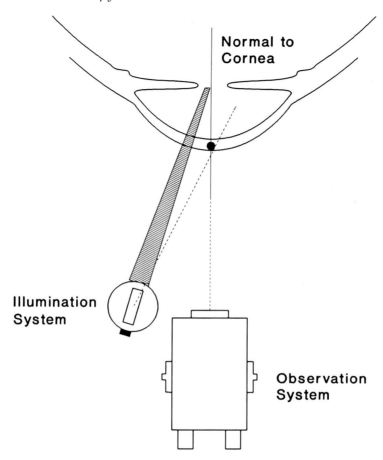

Figure 18.23 Indirect illumination. The illumination and observation system axes do not coincide in indirect illumination. Note that in this case indirect illumination has been achieved by offsetting the slit beam.

changes in the corneal transparency which may not have been visible using direct illumination. One example of this is the observation of the leading edge of a pterygium as it moves onto the cornea. Direct illumination will only display the pterygium itself, while proximal indirect illumination allows the changes in the corneal tissue in advance of the pterygium to be viewed and assessed. Proximal illumination can be used to view all objects and conditions within the cornea which are viewed with direct illumination.

Sclerotic scatter

Sclerotic scatter is a specific case of indirect illumination used to investigate any subtle changes in corneal clarity occurring over a relatively large area, such as the central corneal clouding associated with steeply fitted, low *Dk* rigid lenses. Sclerotic scatter is achieved by setting the slit lamp up for a wide angle (45 to 60 degrees) parallelepiped view of the central cornea, and then manually offsetting the slit beam until it is focused

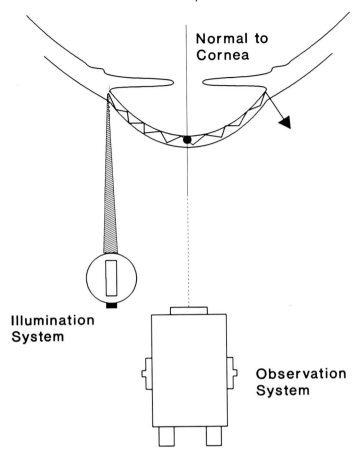

Figure 18.24 Indirect illumination. Note that in this case indirect illumination has been achieved by utilizing the microscope field of view.

on the nasal or temporal limbus (Fig. 18.25). Correct positioning of the slit beam is signalled by a bright glow from the limbal region directly opposite that being illuminated. This glow results from the fact that the light from the slit beam is being totally internally reflected between the epithelial and endothelial layers of the cornea and then scattered as it hits the scleral tissue of the opposing limbus. Obviously any area of the cornea which is altered in such a way as to increase light scatter will interrupt the total internal reflection of the slit beam and can be seen either through the observation system at low magnification or by the naked eye as a grey hazy area within a clear background.

Sclerotic scatter can also be used to observe corneal scars, foreign bodies and deposits within the corneal layers. It should be noted that widespread corneal oedema, such as that seen with soft lenses, will not be detected using sclerotic scatter because there is no portion of non-oedematous cornea with which to compare it (Figs. 18.26 and 18.27).

Retro-illumination (direct and indirect)

Retro-illumination refers to any indirect illumination technique where light is reflected from the iris, anterior lens surface or retina and used to illuminate an object or area in the cornea from behind. It should be noted that in retro-illumination there is no light being reflected directly from the object of regard.

Direct retro-illumination

This is that specific situation where the object of regard is illuminated entirely from behind (by light reflected from a deeper tissue), *and* is viewed against an *illuminated* background, causing the object to be seen in shadow. Therefore, objects seen as white or opaque against a darker background in direct illumination are seen as black or dark objects on a lighter background in direct retro-illumination. Direct retro-illumination is achieved by setting the slit lamp as if forming a direct illumination parallelepiped, then offsetting the slit beam until the reflected light of the slit beam from the surface of the iris is directly behind the object under observation when viewed through the eyepieces (Figs. 18.28, 18.29 and 18.30).

Direct retro-illumination of objects within the central region of the cornea and lens/vitreous can also be achieved by aligning the slit lamp centrally as if forming a direct

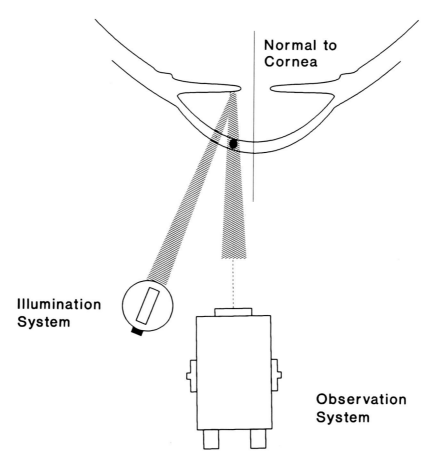

Figure 18.25 Sclerotic scatter. Corneal illumination is achieved by directing the illumination beam to the limbal region of the cornea and creating total internal reflection of the light beam within the cornea.

illumination optic section on the geometric axis of the eye. The slit lamp is focused in the plane of the object under observation and then the slit beam is offset to pass just inside the edge of the pupil. The slit beam will be reflected from the retina/choroid and the object under observation will be seen against the red glow of the fundus. This procedure is more easily performed with large or dilated pupils.

Indirect retro-illumination

Like direct retro-illumination, indirect retro-illumination has the object of regard being illuminated entirely from behind (by light reflected from a deeper tissue) but now it is being viewed against a *dark* background. Indirect retro-illumination can be achieved using a similar setup to that used for direct retro-illumination, except that the illumination system is offset such that the reflected image from the iris is *not* directly behind the object under observation (Fig. 18.31). It is interesting to note that if several objects are viewed in *direct* retro-illumination, such as epithelial microcysts, those to the left and right of the centrally viewed microcysts are seen in *indirect* retro-illumination.

Retro-illumination is used to investigate

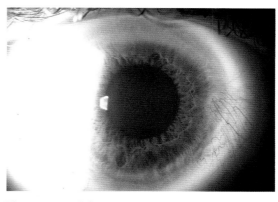

Figure 18.27 Sclerotic scatter. Medium magnification view of a pterygium on the cornea. Note that the full extent of the encroachment of the pterygium is visible under this illumination.

the full extent of changes in the corneal layers, such as epithelial microcysts, vacuoles, scars, degenerations and dystrophies, and trauma. Direct retro-illumination from the retina is also used for estimating the extent of lenticular opacities and changes, and also the location of optic zones in bifocal contact lenses. It should be noted that, even though stereoscopic perception is present, the depth of anomalies or lesions cannot be assessed reliably when only retro-illumination is used; therefore, the optic section technique is used to complement the retro-illumination technique (see Figs. 18.32 and 18.33).

18.3.4 FILTERED ILLUMINATION

Slit lamps are typically fitted with two coloured filters which can be introduced into the light path of the illumination system – a cobalt blue filter to aid in fluorescein observation and a green ('red-free') filter to enhance the contrast of blood vessels.

Fluorescein stain is routinely added to the tear film to aid in the observation of corneal and conjunctival staining, rigid contact lens fittings and qualitative assessment of the tear film itself (soft lenses require the use of special high-molecular-weight fluorescein).

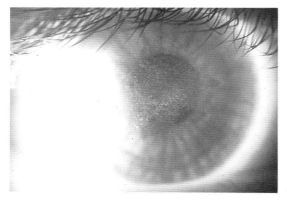

Figure 18.26 Sclerotic scatter. Medium magnification view of cellular debris trapped behind a soft lens.

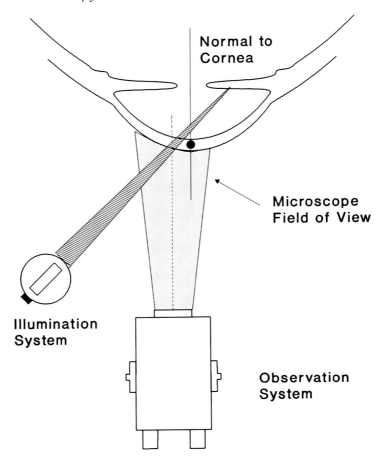

Figure 18.28 Direct retro-illumination. The illumination beam is directed so that the axes of the light reflected from the iris and the observation system coincide.

Following fluorescein instillation, illumination of the tear film with cobalt blue light of about 490 nm maximum causes a greenish light with a maximum of about 520 nm to be emitted by the excited fluorescein molecules. The brightness of the emitted light is an indicator of the amount of fluorescein accumulated in a local area, and hence variations in the brightness of the area under observation can be used as an indication of the relative thickness of the tear film or, in the case of epithelial staining, the severity of the tissue damage, at that location. Addition of a yellow filter in front of the microscope objective (e.g. Kodak Wratten No. 15), which allows transmission of the green light emitted by the fluorescein but blocks most of the blue light reflected from the ocular surface, greatly enhances the contrast between adjacent areas covered by fluorescein (Figs. 18.34 and 18.35). This allows a more accurate assessment of subtle variations in tear film thickness beneath a rigid lens, and areas of corneal staining which would otherwise go undetected. When fluorescein is instilled, the cobalt blue filter is typically used with broad beam illumination and maximum slit lamp intensity since the combination of blue and yellow filters significantly decreases image brightness through the oculars. It should be

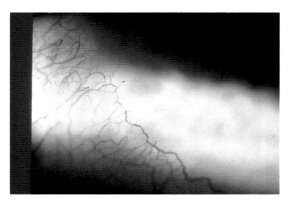

Figure 18.29 Direct retro-illumination. High magnification view of limbal vessel spikes growing towards the centre of the cornea. Note that the looping of the vessels is visible under the direct retro-illumination from the iris.

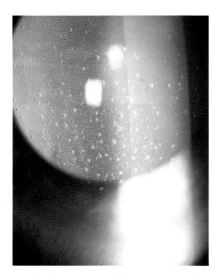

Figure 18.30 Direct retro-illumination. High magnification view of epithelial microcyst seen in direct retro-illumination from the retina.

noted that the majority of cobalt blue filters provided by the slit lamp manufacturer are not ideal in their spectral and overall light transmission characteristics. Typical glass cobalt blue filters transmit unwanted longer wavelengths which are not blocked by the yellow filter, and often transmit less than 50% of the overall available light energy. This can be improved by using long pass interference filters in place of the regular cobalt blue filter (Fig. 18.36). Long pass interference filters typically have an extremely sharp 'cut-off' around the 490 nm region with essentially no transmission above that value. Average light transmission is typically above 75% for the short wavelength region. These characteristics enhance the contrast and brightness of the area under observation above and beyond that seen with the typical cobalt blue filter.

Cobalt blue filters used without fluorescein and the yellow filter can also be used to enhance the view of certain intracorneal anomalies such as Fleischer's ring (sometimes seen in keratoconic patients) and the Hudson–Stahli line.

'Red-free' filters are actually greenish-blue in colour and are so-named because they block all wavelengths of light at the red end of the visible spectrum. Red-free filters enhance the contrast of any structure which is red in colour, such as arteries and veins, or stains such as rose bengal, by displaying them as dark against the lighter green background of the sclera, lids and iris.

18.4 PROCEDURE FOR THE SLIT LAMP EXAMINATION OF THE ANTERIOR SEGMENT

Examination of the anterior segment of the potential contact lens patient with the slit lamp should be done in a systematic and ordered fashion to ensure that all structures are investigated, not just those indicated by the patient's history and symptoms. In the case of the pre-fitting baseline examination, this is especially important, since this information will be the basis for all future decisions regarding patient management and care.

The procedure outlined here is designed to flow smoothly from one group of structures to the next, allowing adequate observation of

Sign/ condition	Grade (0–4)	Description
Epithelial microcysts	0	None. No microcysts seen using retro-illumination.
	1	Trace. Fewer than approximately 50 microcysts over the central or paracentral cornea. No overlying staining or surface anomaly.
	2	Mild. More than approximately 50 microcysts over the central or paracentral cornea. No overlying staining or surface anomaly.
	3	Moderate. More than approximately 50 microcysts, tending to be coalescent. Surface anomaly manifesting itself as faint staining and/or dry spots when fluorescein is used.
	4	Severe. Very numerous, dense, coalescent microcysts, visible using direct and retroillumination, with overlying staining and erosions.
Corneal neovascular- ization	0	None. Normal limbal vessel dilation and advancement.
	1	Trace. Slight dilation and less than 1.5 mm of advancement into the cornea in one quadrant only.
	2	Mild. Slight dilation and less than 1.5 mm of advancement into the cornea in more than one quadrant.
	3	Moderate. 1.5 mm to less than 3.0 mm of advancement in any quadrant.
	4	Severe. More than 3.0 mm of advancement in any quadrant.
Lens deposits	0	No surface deposits.
	1	Presence of 5 or less, small (<0.1 mm) individual deposits.
	2	Presence of more than 5 small, individual deposits and/or one individual deposit 0.1mm to 0.5mm in diameter.
	3	Multiple deposits 0.1mm to 0.5mm in diameter or one individual deposit larger than 0.5mm in diameter.
	4	Multiple deposits of 0.5mm in diameter or larger.

enhanced if the practitioner knows in advance the type of contact lens wear that the patient is using, since there are expected slit lamp findings for the different types of lens wear (Table 18.2).

18.5   SLIT LAMP PHOTOGRAPHY

Since one of the main uses of the slit lamp is to enable assessment of the structures of the anterior segment as an aid to the detection and diagnosis of abnormal conditions, it is beneficial if a photographic record of any abnormalities can be made as an aid to identifying any changes over time.

Ideally, a photographic slit lamp with an inbuilt flash and camera mounts should be used for taking anterior segment photographs (Fig. 18.37). However, a less expensive alternative is to attach a camera and ordinary flash unit to a non-photographic slit lamp (Fig. 18.38) (Khaw & Elkington, 1988). Before describing these two methods of achieving photographic slit lamp records in detail, it is worth introducing a few terms for the photographic neophyte.

Film speed or ASA rating is an indicator of how much light a particular film type needs to provide a correctly exposed image. 'Fast' films are those which need lower amounts of light for correct exposure, while 'slow' films need more light. ASA 1000 or ASA 400 films are considered fast, while ASA 25 or ASA 64 are considered slow. Other typical film speeds are ASA 100 and ASA 200. Fast films usually produce grainier images with lower resolution than do slow films. Since the majority of changes to structures in the anterior segment are subtle, such as endothelial polymegethism or stromal striae, it is best to use the slowest film which still provides the correct exposure.

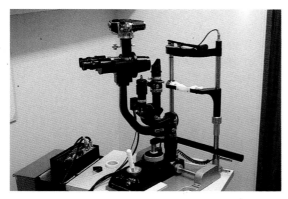

Figure 18.37 A dedicated photo slit lamp. Note the camera attached to the objective housing, and the flash charging unit attached to the table.

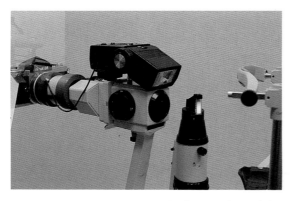

Figure 18.38 A non-photo slit lamp adapted for photographic use. Note that the camera is attached to the eyepiece, and that the flash is positioned to provide additional illumination.

Film colour temperature describes the spectrum of light to which the film was designed to respond. All light sources emit a range of wavelengths described by their colour temperature. All these light sources may be described as 'white' in general terms, but, just as their colour temperatures differ, so does the composition of their emitted spectra. Therefore, there are more blue wavelengths in the apparently 'white' light emitted by a fluorescent light source than in the 'white' light provided by an equivalent halogen light source. Colour films are matched to

the colour temperature of specific light sources. Hence, films may be described as 'daylight' films or 'tungsten' films. Since preferred films are often not matched to the colour temperature of the light source being used, specific filters can be used to compensate for the difference in colour temperature between film and light source and provide a more realistic rendition of the true colour of the subject being photographed. Daylight film should be used with flash photography.

Exposure describes the amount of light which is allowed to fall on the film. Exposure can be controlled by the shutter speed, i.e. the fractions of a second that the camera shutter is open, such as 1/60th or 1/125th. Ideally, exposure times should be kept as short as possible since even the slightest eye movement will cause a blurred photograph. Many of the anterior segment conditions which clinicians would like to photograph at high magnification cannot be correctly exposed using the available illumination of the slit lamp. Therefore, dedicated photographic slit lamps have in-built flash systems which provide sufficient light to enable correct exposure with very short shutter speeds.

Aperture size refers to the size of the iris in the camera lens and, along with the shutter speed, controls the exposure of the film. Aperture sizes are usually described in 'f-stops', where the larger the number, the smaller the aperture size. It is important to note that large apertures also shorten the depth of field. However, in most commercially available photo slit lamps, the camera is used without a lens, so that lens aperture is not a factor. In slit lamps where the camera and lens are positioned behind the eyepiece (e.g. the Holden–Zantos technique, described later), changing the aperture setting on the camera lens changes the size of the field of view but not the brightness. In this situation, film exposure is controlled by camera shutter speed or flash intensity.

18.5.1 DEDICATED SLIT LAMP PHOTOGRAPHY

Slit lamps designed for photography have two additional facilities – an in-built flash system which allows a powerful beam of high intensity light to be generated and flashed through the slit beam as illumination for the photograph, and a camera mount somewhere on the slit lamp microscope.

The flash system usually uses a semi-reflecting mirror in the illumination system of the slit lamp to allow both the regular incandescent/halogen light and the flash tube generated light to follow identical pathways through the slit aperture. Therefore, all structures illuminated by the regular light source will be illuminated in the same pattern by the flash tube. However, the intensity of the flash will be very different, and this is usually controlled by a switch on the flash generator housing. Typically there are four settings for flash intensity, and the best one to use will vary according to the reflectance of the structure being viewed and the slit lamp set-up chosen.

Thus, a photograph of the sclera and bulbar conjunctiva will require a low intensity flash setting, whereas a high magnification shot of an optic section of the cornea will require a high flash intensity. The optimum flash settings for a particular photographic slit lamp are best determined by trial and error, and they will depend on the film ASA rating and the structure being photographed. However, a good starting point is to use 200 ASA film and the lowest intensity flash setting for diffuse and broad beam, low magnification shots; and the highest flash intensity setting for low magnification parallelepiped and optic section photographs, and for all medium to high magnification shots. It should be noted that good fluorescein photographs of corneal staining or rigid lens fitting patterns can only be taken using a slit lamp equipped with a high output flash tube when the cobalt blue and yellow barrier filters are used. Film exposure guidelines for photographic slit lamps have been published elsewhere (Spivak, 1977; Zantos *et al.*, 1980).

The camera mount for most photographic slit lamps is placed between the objective lens and the magnification tumbler of the microscope; a right-angled prism or semi-reflecting mirror is put into the optical pathway of the microscope to divert the images to the camera during photography but not during normal viewing. A bayonet-type mount is usually provided to which the camera body (without lens) is mounted. The mount is designed in such a way that the image seen by the observer in the eyepieces is focused simultaneously on the film plane of the camera, ensuring correct focus if the microscope eyepieces have been correctly adjusted for the observer. Drawbacks to this type of mounting system is that the magnification of the camera image is fixed, and relatively low (approximately 3×), since the light rays from the objective lens are diverted before entering the magnification tumbler of the microscope head. This limitation can be overcome by mounting the camera and lens over the eyepiece of the microscope, as described by Zantos and Holden. This technique takes full advantage of the increased magnification available through the magnification tumbler of the microscope and alternate high powered eyepieces. A special adapter must be fabricated which clamps over the eyepiece and screws into the filter thread of the camera lens to utilize the Holden–Zantos technique, but this inconvenience is far outweighed by the versatility and enhanced convenience that variable magnification and through-the-camera focusing bring to any photographic slit lamp.

18.5.2 PHOTOGRAPHY USING A NON-PHOTOGRAPHIC SLIT LAMP

While a dedicated photo slit lamp is the preferred method of taking photographs of the anterior ocular segment, quite useful photographs can be obtained by using an auto-exposure camera mounted over the eyepiece of a regular non-photographic slit lamp. The 35 mm camera used should have an aperture priority, auto-exposure mode. The major limitation of this method of photography is the lack of flash, and hence a relatively high speed film should be used (e.g. 400 ASA) in conjunction with the highest light settings of the slit lamp. Ideally, the slit lamp should have a halogen or other high output light source, and the film colour temperature should be matched to the light sources. Since the exposure is automatic and controlled by shutter speed, a good estimate of correct exposure can be judged by listening to the shutter open and close. For shutter speeds of slower than 1/8th second, movement of the eye will blur the photograph. Faster shutter speeds can be produced by increasing the light intensity of the slit lamp or by increasing the width of the slit beam.

This technique is limited to white light photographs, and cannot provide high magnification images of optic sections, but it can provide reasonable quality photographs of many features of the anterior segment which are of interest to the contact lens clinician.

18.5.3 VIDEO PHOTOGRAPHY WITH THE SLIT LAMP

The recent availability of relatively inexpensive video cameras and recorders has made the rather appealing concept of recording slit lamp observations on video tape a clinical reality. The major advantage which such a system provides over 35 mm photography is the ability for immediate playback. This is particularly useful in describing the appearance of many conditions such as lens deposits or lens fitting to patients or colleagues.

Video cameras are usually attached to slit lamps using the same beam-splitters incorporated for 35 mm photographic attachments. Ideally the camera should be compact and light-weight to minimize any interference with the balance and normal functioning of the slit lamp. Cameras with remote heads are ideal for this use. Contemporary video cameras have sufficient gain to allow good images to be captured with the incident light from the slit beam, negating the need for additional light sources or low illumination 'surveillance-type' cameras. The other parameter which should be considered is the resolution capabilities of the camera. Black and white cameras generally have higher resolution capabilities than colour cameras but, for the majority of clinical applications, the advantages of a colour image far outweigh the loss of resolution. It should be noted, however, that while the majority of colour cameras have sufficiently high resolution to demonstrate lens fitting performance and front surface deposits, only the most expensive have the capability of capturing high resolution images such as the endothelial mosaic. The interested reader is directed to recent publications regarding clinical videography both with and without slit lamps (Robboy & Hammack, 1987).

REFERENCES

Berliner, M.L. (1943) *Biomicroscopy of the Eye.* Paul B. Hoeber, Inc.

Brandreth, R.H. (1978) *Clinical Slit Lamp Biomicroscopy*, Blaco Printers, Inc.

Butler, T.H. (1924) Focal illumination of the eye. *Br. J. Ophthal.*, **8**(12), 561–90.

Cavanagh, H.D. *et al.* (1990) Confocal microscopy of the living eye. *CLAO J.*, **16**, 65–73.

Doggart, J.H. (1949) *Ocular Signs in Slit Lamp Biomicroscopy.* C. V. Mosby Co., St Louis.

Goldberg J.B. (1984) *Biomicroscopy for Contact Lens Practice: Clinical Procedures.* The Professional Press, Inc.

Holden, B.A., Zantos, S.G. and Jacobs, K.J. (1978) *The Holden–Zantos technique for endothelial and high magnification slit lamp photography.* Bausch & Lomb.

Khaw, P.T. and Elkington, A.R. (1988) Slit-lamp photography made easy by a spot metering system. *Br. J. Ophthalmol.*, **67**, 63–6.

Koester, C.J. and Roberts, C.W. (1990) Wide-field

specular microscopy. In *Non-invasive Diagnostic Techniques in Opthalmology* (ed. B.R. Masters), Springer-Verlag, New York, pp. 91–121.

Long, W.F. (1988) How to choose and use a photoslitlamp. *Review of Optometry*, **September**, 69–73.

Martonyi, C.L. (1989) Photographic slit-lamp biomicroscopes. *Ophthalmology – Instrument and Book Issue*, pp. 6–19.

Masters, B.R. and Kino, G.S. (1990) Confocal microscopy of the eye. *Noninvasive Diagnostic Techniques in Opthalmology* (ed. B.R. Masters), Springer-Verlag, New York, pp. 152–71.

Mayer, D.J. (1984) *Clinical Wide-Field Specular Microscopy*. Balliere Tindall.

Müller, O. *Ocular Examination with the Slit Lamp.* Carl Zeiss Publication K30–115-e.

Norn, M.S. (1983) *External Eye: Methods of Examination*. Scriptor Publisher ApS.

Robboy, M.W. and Hammack, G.G. (1987) Videotape recording system for use with the slitlamp biomicroscope. *J. Am. Optom. Assoc.*, **58**(4), 290–2.

Schmidt, T.A.F. (1975) On slit-lamp microscopy, *Doc. Ophthalmol.*, **39**, 117–53.

Spivak, T.W. (1977) Photography through the Nikon slit lamp biomicroscope. *Rev. Optom.*, **November**, 56–60.

Stockwell, H.J. (1983) Considering the slit lamp and biomicroscope, *The Optician*, **June 10**, 16–20.

Terry, J.E. and Kercheval, D.B. (1979) Interpretive biomicroscopy. *J. Am. Optom. Assoc.*, **50**, 793–803.

Zantos, S. G. (1984) *Slit Lamp Examination of Contact Lens Wearers*. Bausch & Lomb.

Zantos, S.G. and Pye, D.C. (1979) Clinical photography in optometric practice, *Aust. J. Optom.*, **62**, 279–85.

Zantos, S.G., Holden, B.A. and Pye, D.C. (1980) A guide to ocular photography with the Nikon photo slitlamp. *Aust. J. Optom.*, **63**, 26–32.

PART 2 REAL-TIME CONFOCAL MICROSCOPY OF THE *IN VIVO* HUMAN CORNEA

B.R. Masters, A.A. Thaer and O.-C. Geyer

18.6 ABSTRACT

A new, non-applanating, real-time slit scanning confocal microscope is described for the *in vivo* examination of the living human eye. This confocal microscope produces real-time video images of the *in vivo* human cornea. In contrast to other confocal microscopes designed for *in vivo* ocular imaging, which are based on either the Nipkow disk (pinholes) or the modified wide-field specular microscope (a photographic system which is not real-time), this new instrument produces images which are captured as single video frames which have superior contrast. This new real-time slit scanning confocal microscope produces *en face*, high contrast, high resolution, images of superficial epithelial cells, wing cells, epithelial basal cells, corneal innervation, nuclei of stromal keratocytes, and the cell bodies of the stromal keratocytes in the posterior stromal region.

18.7 INTRODUCTION

This chapter presents the principles of *in vivo* confocal microscopy and applications to the observation of the *in vivo* human cornea. A new, real-time, scanning slit confocal microscope is described. Examples are presented of confocal microscopic examination of the normal human cornea which illustrate the resolution and the contrast of single video frames. The photographs are unprocessed and devoid of any digital image processing enhancements.

The primary instrument for the examination of the cornea is the slit lamp. This important instrument was developed in its present form by Gullstrand who developed the system to condense the illumination light into a slit aperture and then project the image of the slit into the eye. The modern slit lamp uses a narrow slit which removes the light scattered from adjacent tissue and provides a degree of optical sectioning. However, the slit lamp provides an oblique view across the cornea and provides limited contrast of cellular components.

A more recent development for imaging the cells of the corneal endothelium is the specular microscope. If the illumination and the observation axes are adjusted correctly, then the specular reflection from the boundary of the corneal endothelium and aqueous humor will show the cell outlines of the endothelial cells. These cells were first observed and described by Vogt who used the modified Gullstrand slit lamp to examine the human corneal endothelium. There are several problems with the specular microscope; the surface reflection from the tear–corneal interface degrades the contrast of the endothelial cells. An edematous stroma will also reduce contrast of the endothelial cells. The field of view is small with the standard specular microscopes. The development of a

Contact Lens Practice. Edited by Montague Ruben and Michel Guillon.
Published in 1994 by Chapman & Hall, London. ISBN 0 412 35120 X

scanning wide-field specular microscope by Koester provided high-contrast, wide-field views of about one square millimeter of corneal endothelium. This microscope scanned a narrow slit over a larger area of the endothelium and recorded the composite image on film.

Both the slit lamp and the specular microscope are limited in their ability to observe cellular and subcellular details throughout the full thickness of the cornea. In this chapter we introduce a new tech-

nique, real-time scanning slit confocal microscopy, with the capability to overcome the limitations of the slit lamp and the specular microscope. *In vivo* real-time scanning slit confocal microscopy provides a new approach to the observation of the human eye.

18.8   CONFOCAL MICROSCOPY

This section provides a brief introduction to the principles of confocal microscopy and

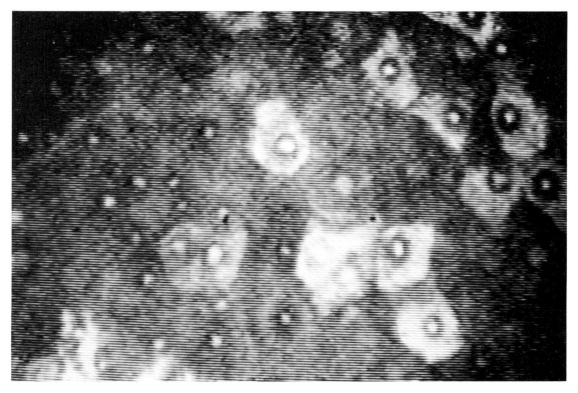

Figure 18.39 *In vivo* confocal microscopic *en face* image of human cornea. The U-matic tape was stopped on a single video frame, using the pause mode, and a 35 mm film camera was used to photograph the television monitor to produce the image. No digital or analog image enhancement or processing was used. There was no frame averaging applied to the video images. The photograph shows the raw data directly photographed from the screen of the television monitor. This figure shows a single video frame of the superficial cells of the corneal epithelium. This cell layer, which is just below the tear film, has the following characteristics: the cell nucleus appears as a highly reflecting bright oval which is surrounded by a darker band; the focal plane is set to optically section the most superficial cells which appear brightest; cells slightly below this focal plane appear darker. Some of these superficial epithelial cells are in the process of desquamation. Objective 25×, NA 0.6.

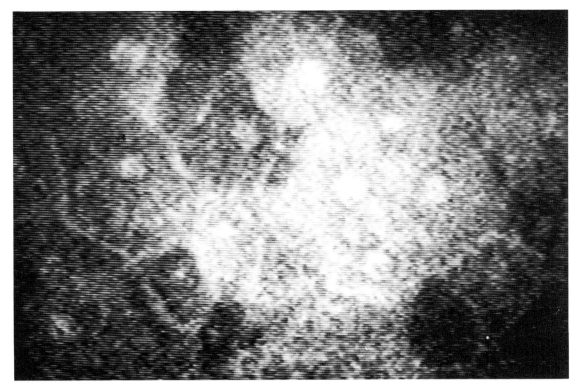

Figure 18.40 *In vivo* confocal microscopic *en face* image of human cornea. This optical section is in the plane of the wing cells which are located between the superficial epithelial cells and the basal epithelial cells of the human cornea. The image of these cells is characterized by the bright cell nuclei which are devoid of the darker band which is observed in the superficial epithelial cells. Objective 50×, NA 1.0.

describes the basic types of confocal microscopes (Wilson, 1990; Pawley, 1990). First we answer the question: What is a confocal microscope?

In 1957 Minsky filed a patent application for a confocal microscope which elucidated the principles of operation upon which today's commercial confocal systems work. A confocal microscope has two sets of pinholes, or apertures, which are arranged in conjugate, or confocal, planes. One pinhole or slit is placed in the illumination path and another set is placed in the detection path. These sets of conjugate apertures only illuminate a narrow field of the specimen and detect the back-scattered and reflected light from the same narrow field of view.

The confocal microscope has a scanning mechanism such that the narrow field of illumination, which is identical to the detection field, is scanned over the specimen to generate a composite image of it. This is the principle of confocal microscopy.

In a standard microscope – which is operated in the epi-illumination mode – the lateral and axial resolutions are functions of the wavelength of the light used for the illumination and of the numerical aperture of the microscope objective. In a confocal microscope there is an increase in both the axial and lateral resolutions of the microscope objective. While the increase in the axial resolution of a confocal micro-

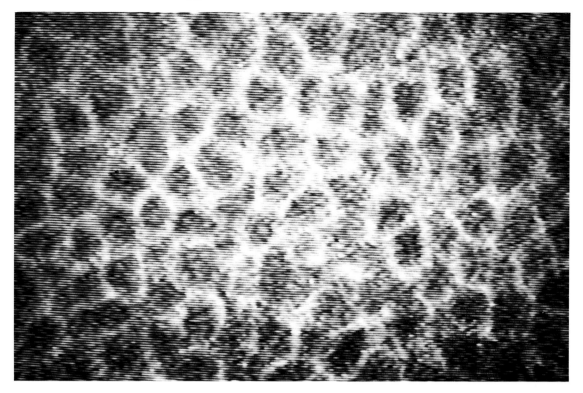

Figure 18.41 *In vivo* confocal microscopic *en face* image of human cornea. The optical section is in the plane of the basal epithelial cells. The image shows the bright cell borders and the darker cell interiors. The cell borders appear thick since there is a high degree of invagination between the adjacent cells. Water immersion microscope objective 50×, NA 1.0.

scope is important, it is the increase in the lateral resolution which is of prime importance for imaging thick specimens. The increased lateral resolution gives the confocal microscope the unique ability to optically section the specimen. It is important to note that the axial resolution is about three times the lateral resolution.

There are several advantages of the optically-sectioning capability of a confocal microscope as compared to the standard microscope. The first advantage is that images are obtained with enhanced contrast; this is because the confocal microscope excludes light scattered from optical sections above and below the section in the focal plane, therefore the focal plane is not degraded in sharpness and contrast as in a standard light microscope. The second advantage is that thick sections of living tissues and cells can be optically sectioned for observation and subsequent three-dimensional reconstruction.

There are several types of confocal microscopes. Some designs are based on a rotating disk which contains many sets of pinholes arranged in a spiral pattern. This design is called a Nipkow disk-based microscope; such designs are further divided into tandem-scanning confocal microscopes and one-sided Nipkow disk-based confocal microscopes.

The tandem-scanning confocal microscope uses two sides of the disk which contains

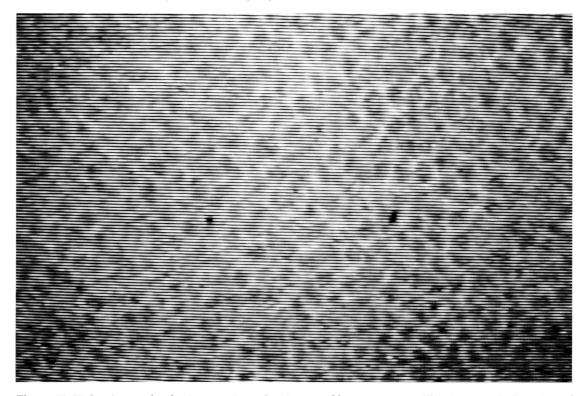

Figure 18.42 *In vivo* confocal microscopic *en face* image of human cornea. This is an optical section of the basal epithelial cells similar to that shown in Figure 18.41. The wider field is obtained with the use of a microscope objective with a lower magnification. Water immersion microscope objective 25×, NA 0.6.

two sets of conjugate pinholes. One set of pinholes is in the illumination path, and the other is in the detection path. As the Nipkow disk rotates, the full field of view is swept out by both the illumination spots of light and the detection spots. Since both sets of pinholes are conjugate to each other the system is a confocal microscope. It is called a tandem-scanning confocal microscope since both sets of pinholes rotate in tandem.

Another type of Nipkow disk-based microscope uses the same set of pinholes on one side of the rotating Nipkow disk for both the illumination path and the detection path. This is the basis of the so-called one-sided, real-time, confocal microscope. Other designs are based on conjugate slits.

They are also real-time confocal systems.

18.9 CONFOCAL MICROSCOPES FOR IN VIVO **CLINICAL EXAMINATION OF THE CORNEA**

The advantages of confocal microscope imaging systems as compared to standard microscopy include enhanced x, y and z resolution and improved contrast of the images. These factors permit the optical sectioning of thick living tissue. The resulting images are sharp and free from significant blur due to contributions of scattered light from adjacent sections. In contrast to slit lamp observations, and other standard imaging techniques, confocal microscopy is

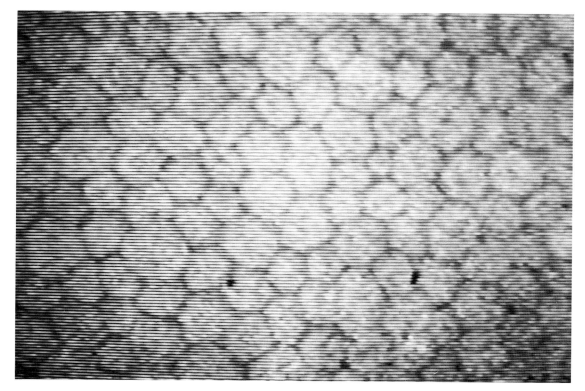

Figure 18.47 *In vivo* confocal microscopic *en face* image of human cornea. This optical section shows the polygonal corneal endothelial cells. This image is 500 microns below the surface of the cornea (Figure 18.39). The focal plane is at the interface between the cornea and the aqueous humor. Objective 25×, NA 0.6.

monitor in order that the operator can observe the confocal images of the subject's eye in real time.

5. Hard copy of individual video frames is obtained immediately with a video printer. Individual video frames can also be digitized. These digital images can be registered and preprocessed by digital image processing techniques for further analysis and quantification. However, in this chapter all the figures are photographs of single video frames of the raw data – no analog or digital enhancements were used.

6. The real-time confocal microscope is mounted on a special ophthalmic head rest (Leitz). The microscope stand pro-

vides three-axis control. Immediately before the corneal examination, the eye was anaesthetized. The subject was seated at the ocular examination table and a drop of methylcellulose gel was applied to the tip of the microscope objective; the microscope was slowly positioned to make contact between the gel and the cornea. The tip of the microscope objective never touches or flattens the corneal surface; a layer of gel is always present between the objective and the eye. The z-axis position of the confocal microscope was controlled by manual movement of the microscope stage with a joystick. Alternatively, a computer-controlled stepping motor

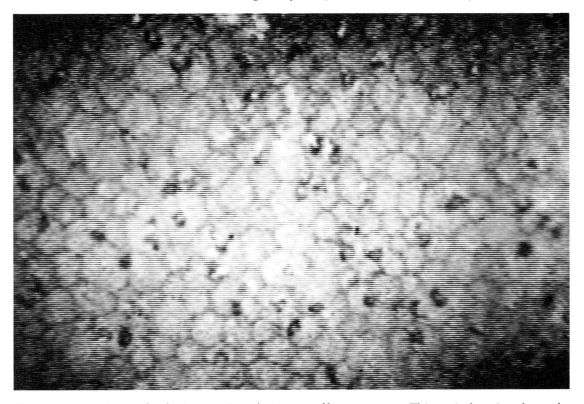

Figure 18.48 *In vivo* confocal microscopic *en face* image of human cornea. This optical section shows the polygonal corneal endothelial cells. This image is 500 microns below the surface of the cornea (Figure 18.39). The numerous small black particles are due to inflammation of the eye. The focal plane is at the interface between the cornea and the aqueous humor. Objective 25×, NA 0.6.

scanned the focal plane of the confocal microscope across the full thickness of the cornea.

7. The microscope is built from a modular system. This design concept permits rapid modification of the system to suit different applications. The confocal microscope can be used in several modes.

The first configuration is capable of obtaining real-time (video rates) *en face* optical sections across the full-thickness of the *in vivo* human cornea. The thickness of the optical section can be modified by adjusting the width of the two confocal slits in the microscope. The depth of the optical section can be manually adjusted, or automatic continuous scanning (Z-Scan attachment) of the depth of the focal plane can be initiated. Both scan time and scan depth can be adjusted.

The second configuration provides a quantitative measure of the reflected and back-scattered light in a given focal plane. This Z-Scan attachment is used for the confocal photometric recording of scattered light and fluorescence intensity profiles through the full thickness of the cornea. The Z-Scan can also be used for quantitative photometric measurements of fluorescence and/or scattering in the anterior chamber.

This configuration can also be used for fluorescence measurements. Both autofluo-

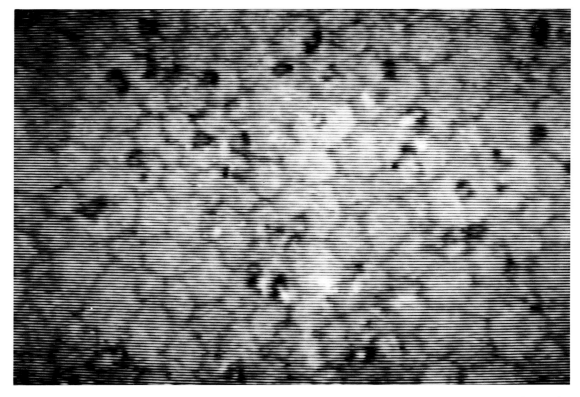

Figure 18.49 *In vivo* confocal microscopic *en face* image of human cornea. This optical section shows the polygonal corneal endothelial cells. This image is 500 microns below the surface of the cornea. The numerous small black particles are due to inflammation of the eye. The focal plane is at the interface between the cornea and the aqueous humor. This image shows a different field of view than in the previous figure. Objective 25×, NA 0.6.

rescence and fluorescence from externally applied fluorescent dyes or fluorogenic substrates can be measured (Thaer *et al.*, 1990). This configuration is suitable for the *in vivo* measurements of cellular metabolism based on the principles of non-invasive redox fluorometry.

18.11 RESULTS

The following *in vivo* human corneal confocal microscopic images were made by photographing the single still video frames on the monitor with a camera. **These figures are photographs of single video frames. There was no image processing or frame averaging.**

The figures are typical raw data. The figures show the superficial cells (Fig. 18.39), the wing cells (Fig. 18.40) and two fields of the normal human basal epithelium (Figs. 18.41 and 18.42). High contrast photographs of corneal nerves are shown in Figs. 18.43–18.46. The corneal endothelium is shown in Figs. 18.47–18.50.

The full three-dimensional reconstruction of the *ex vivo* rabbit cornea is the only figure in this chapter which is not from the *in vivo* human cornea (Fig. 18.51). The optical sections which were used for the reconstruction were obtained with a laser scanning confocal microscope. The inclusion of this figure in the chapter is to present the future of *in vivo*

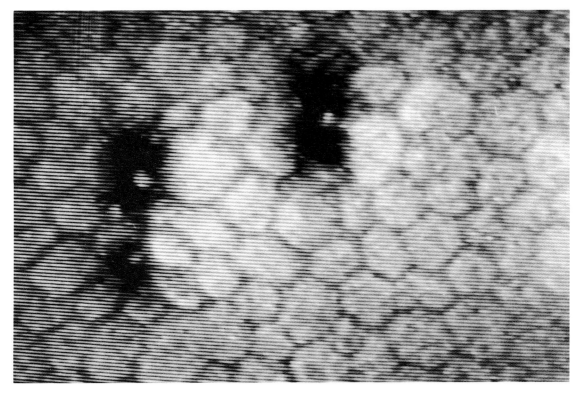

Figure 18.50 *In vivo* confocal microscopic *en face* image of human cornea. The image shows a region of the corneal endothelium with endothelial defects. The three black regions represent endothelial defects.

three-dimensional visualization of ocular imaging.

18.12 DISCUSSION

A new, non-applanating, non-invasive real-time, slit-scanning confocal microscope has been developed for the observation of the *in vivo* human eye. This chapter illustrates the use of the instrument for the observation of the cornea. The high contrast and large light collection efficiency of the microscope are due to the use of confocal slits in conjunction with a high numerical aperture objective.

The microscope does not contact the cornea nor does it applanate the surface of the cornea; a polymer gel is applied in a layer between the ocular surface and the tip of the microscope objective. This instrument has

sufficient light collection efficiency so that single video frames show high contrast, sharp images of the living *in vivo* human eye. There is no need for video frame averaging or digital image processing techniques to enhance the contrast of the single video images. This is not the case for confocal microscopes designed on Nipkow disk (pinhole) configuration – they pass such low light from the eye to the camera that frame averaging and digital image processing enhancements are required.

The light collection efficiency of this flying slit *in vivo* ocular confocal microscope is due to the use of slits (instead of pinholes) and a microscope objective with a numerical aperture of 1.0. These two design implementation results are bright, sharp, high-contrast, high-resolution confocal images of the *in vivo*

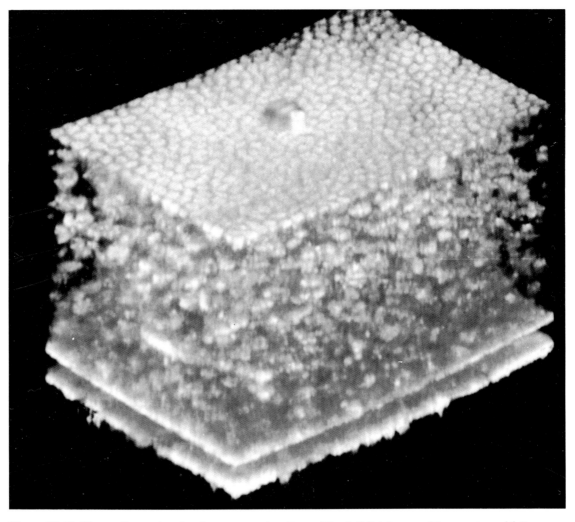

Figure 18.51 Three-dimensional volume reconstruction of the full thickness of the *ex vivo* rabbit cornea shown in an isometric view. The endothelium is on the top of the figure and the epithelium is on the bottom. The linear bright feature on the front face is a nerve fiber. The thickness of the reconstruction is 400 microns and the epithelial thickness is 40 microns. This figure demonstrates that thin optical sections of living cornea can be reconstructed in a computer to yield a three-dimensional volume visualization of the cornea.

human cornea. The images are obtained in real time and are stored on magnetic video tape (Sony U-Matic).

The advantages of slits over confocal microscope systems based on Nipkow disks containing pinholes are the following. Slits have the possibility of continually adjusting the depth of focus on the z-axis. In addition, a slit confocal system passes many times more light from the subject's eye to the detector as compared to pinhole type confocal systems. Another advantage of adjustable slits is that the scanned field of view and the light intensity, incident on the field of view, can be easily varied. Finally, the light intensity incident on the subject's eye is significantly less with a slit confocal microscope as compared to a Nipkow disk pinhole system.

This new *in vivo* confocal instrument has unique advantages over other confocal systems. The bright, high contrast confocal images of the wing cells and the basal cells demonstrate its unique optical characteristics. The low reflectivity of the wing and basal epithelial cells in the normal human cornea presents a low contrast object for confocal microscopy. The high rejection of stray light and narrow depth of field, coupled with the high numerical aperture microscope objective (NA 1.0), results in the ability of the instrument to clearly image these cell layers in the live, normal human cornea.

The clear advantage of slit-scanning confocal microscopes (the new microscope discussed here, and the Koester wide field specular microscope) for ophthalmic diagnostics and basic eye research is best appreciated when imaging the *in vivo* human basal epithelium in the anterior cornea. The real-time confocal microscope described here provides high-contrast, high-resolution images of both the wing and basal epithelial cells in the normal *in vivo* human eye. The modified wide-field specular microscope of Koester has the ability to image basal epithelial cells in the normal *in vivo* human eye. however, the Koester microscope uses a 35 mm film camera as the detector and is therefore not real-time.

Ocular confocal microscopes designed on the slit-scanning principle provide sensitivity and resolution that has not been possible with Nipkow disk based microscopes. The advantages of a slit-scanning confocal system over a Nipkow disk pinhole system are illustrated below.

A Nipkow disk (pinhole) real-time confocal microscope (Tandem Scanning Corporation, Inc.) did not have the capability to image basal epithelial cells *in vivo* in the normal eye; however, in swollen or pathological specimens it was capable of imaging the basal epithelial cells. Jester *et al.* have written several papers in which they categorically state their inability to image basal epithelial cells in the normal *in vivo* cornea (Jester *et al.*, 1990; 1991; 1992). They state, 'Reflections from cells below the surface are not normally resolved but can be imaged in certain disease states.' In another paper Jester *et al.* state, 'By *in vivo* confocal microscopy, only the first layer of superficial cells can normally be imaged in the intact, living eye.' They then state, '*In vivo* confocal optical sections do not detect any reflections from the wing and basal cell layers in the intact, normal living eye.' Finally, in a recent paper published in *Investigative Ophthalmology and Visual Science*, Jester *et al.* wrote on their *in vivo* confocal observations of the normal cornea in the live rabbit, 'Below the superficial epithelium, wing and basal epithelial cells do not appear to reflect light above background levels. Because the cornea is a transparent tissue and optically configured not to scatter light, it is to be expected that some structures of the cornea may not be visualized . . . under pathologic and *ex vivo* conditions, images of the wing and basal epithelial cells can be detected.' Although they averaged video frames they were still unable to image the normal *in vivo* basal epithelial cells. They used a Nipkow disk confocal microscope produced by the Tandem Scanning Corporation, Inc. Furthermore, they 'explain' their inability to image basal epithelial cells in the normal *in vivo* eye by stating that the normal epithelium of the cornea is transparent and should not reflect light. Our results on many human subjects, all made on the normal living cornea, are at variance with the results of Jester *et al.* Koester has also published results indicating the ability of his wide-field specular microscope (slit confocal microscope) to image the basal epithelial cells in the normal *in vivo* eye. Our results, and those of Koester, demonstrate the advantage of a slit-system-based confocal microscope for the *in vivo* examination of the eye.

persistence of corneal damage. Morgan *et al.*, (1987) advanced this idea by showing the mean corneal thickness ratios at day 3 of observation (treated/control eye) were predictive of the irritation at day 21 (correlation co-efficient = 0.98), and of the duration of corneal cloudiness (correlation co-efficient = 0.86). These studies suggest that by utilizing pachometry, the same information as the conventional Draize test measures could be obtained, but require a much shorter period of observation.

Earlier reports utilizing pachometry as an index of irritation utilized optical pachometers mounted on biomicroscopes (Burton, 1972; Ballantyne, 1983–84; Morgan *et al.*, 1987; Kennah *et al.*, 1989). This arrangement had the advantage of concurrent use of the slit lamp for both thickness measurement and assessment of conjunctival, corneal and iris irritation. However, as discussed below, the ultrasonic pachometer is the instrument of choice for monitoring corneal thickness in animals (Chan *et al.*, 1983; Chan-Ling *et al.*, 1985). It is portable, and requires less operator skill and measuring time than optical pachometry. Because of the lower corneal sensitivity of rabbits (Millodot *et al.*, 1978, Chan-Ling *et al.*, 1987) and cats (Chan-Ling, 1989) a corneal anaesthetic is not required for ultrasonic pachometry. Jacobs and Martens (1988; 1989) have shown an excellent correlation between optical and ultrasonic pachometry for assessing eye irritation.

Therefore, by using pachometry as an objective method for assessing eye irritation of most agricultural, industrial and consumer products, the cost of this testing as well as the duration of discomfort to test animals have been effectively reduced. The greater objectivity may also reduce intra-and inter-laboratory variability in the test results and, as a consequence, the number of animals required for evaluation. The use of pachometry in toxicity studies represents the most successful application of pachometry outside visual science.

19.2 TECHNIQUES

The earliest measurement of corneal thickness in the living eye was made by Blix in 1880. His technique involved the observation of the specular reflex from the corneal epithelial and endothelial surfaces. The specular reflex is utilized in modern procedures for corneal thickness measurements, including the specular and confocal microscopes. Since the earliest attempt to measure corneal thickness *in vivo*, many advances have been made. The reader is referred to reviews by von Bahr (1956), Donaldson (1966), Mishima (1968), Ehlers and Hansen (1971) and Molinari (1982) for historical accounts.

19.2.1 OPTICAL PACHOMETRY

The modern optical pachometer usually consists of a Haag–Streit pachometer mounted on a slit lamp biomicroscope (Fig. 19.2). The method uses two glass plates on top of each other. A split image device, designed by Jaeger (1952), is inserted into one eyepiece of the slit-lamp. Rotation of the upper plate displaces the light path and moves the upper half of the image of the cornea in relation to the fixed lower half. The angle of rotation of the upper plate is proportional to the apparent thickness of the cornea. When the endothelium of the upper field is aligned with the epithelium of the lower field, the angle of rotation of the upper plate is read off a scale. The Haag–Streit pachometer has an external scale ranging from 0 to 1.2. This scale is related linearly to the angle of rotation of the glass plates, where 0 corresponds to the position where the plates are parallel and 1.2 corresponds to a rotation of the upper plate by 60°. This scale can be used to obtain a relative value of corneal thickness, as the relationship between displacement of the image and the angle of rotation of the glass plates is linear over a limited thickness range. However, this scale is incapable of the accuracy required for determination of absolute corneal thickness. When accuracy is less critical, true corneal thickness can be determined by means of a conversion graph or table. In the clinical situation, corneal thickness is usually read directly from the top of the pachometer after alignment of the corneal images.

Optimization of performance

The Payor–Holden optical pachometer consists of a Haag–Streit pachometer mounted on to a Rodenstock 2000 biomicroscope, interfaced with an Apple II microcomputer with dual disk drives (Fig. 19.2a). By incorporating a number of modifications the designers have achieved an accuracy of 4–7 μm. First, measurement of the different layers of the cornea is facilitated by increasing the angle between the illumination and observation systems, thereby producing a wider optic section. Second, by decreasing the width of the slit, and increasing the brightness of the illumination, the brightness of the optic section is increased. Third, by aligning the observation tube of the system slightly away from the perpendicular and nearer to the angle of the specular reflex, the anatomical restrictions to peripheral pachometry which are often experienced with a wide angular separation are reduced. The corneal measurement location is maintained by an equal angular shift of the alignment light emitting diodes (LEDs) in the opposite direction. Fourth, a semi-circular arc of fixation lights is also mounted to allow topographical measurement of corneal thickness (Fig. 19.2b). Finally, the Payor–Holden optical pachometer incorporates an improvement made by Mandell and Polse (1969) where the rotation of the glass plate is coupled to a potentiometer (Alsbirk, 1974; Binder *et al.*, 1977; Holden *et al.* 1979; Bonnano & Polse, 1985) (Fig. 19.2b) or shaft encoder. The voltage output can then be input directly into a computer programmed to convert apparent to true corneal thickness,

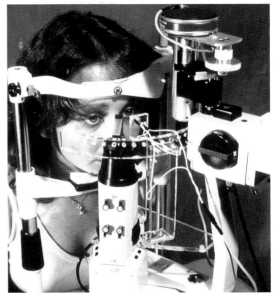

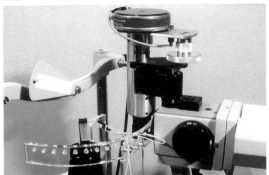

Figure 19.2 (a) The Payor–Holden optical pachometer consists of a Haag–Streit pachometer mounted on to a Rodenstock 2000 biomicroscope. (b) A close up view of the Payor–Holden optical pachometer showing the semi-circular arc of fixation lights for topographical measurement of corneal thickness and the potentiometer which converts the rotation of the glass plate to a voltage output which is input directly into the computer (photographs supplied courtesy of CCLRU).

and to calculate the mean and standard deviation of a number of measurements of corneal thickness. This microcomputer system results in quicker data collection and effective file management (Holden *et al.*, 1979).

Brennan *et al.* (1989) have provided a set of equations relating apparent thickness to true corneal thickness where neither the angle of illumination nor the angle of observation are aligned with, or symmetrical about, the normal to the cornea. As the authors point out, true thickness cannot be expressed explicitly in terms of the apparent thickness and other variables, but an approximate relationship can be used.

The accuracy of an optical pachometer can be increased by making the modifications discussed above. The following sections deal with each of these areas in turn and are only relevant to users who wish to determine absolute corneal thickness measurements with a high level of accuracy.

Angle between the observation and illumination systems

Most pachometers use a system where the illumination slit is directed along the patient's visual axis. The resultant optic section is viewed from approximately 40° and has an apparent width of 0.2 mm. The apparent width of the optic section can be greatly increased by increasing the angular separation of the illumination and viewing systems, thereby also increasing the accuracy. When the angle of incidence is approximately 71°, the apparent thickness equals the true thickness (Ehlers & Hansen, 1971). By setting this angle at 65° (observation = 25° and illumination = 40°) the area of corneal observation is close to the specular reflex, resulting in increased image brightness (Holden *et al.*, 1979). This enables better definition of the layers of the optic section, thus improving accuracy (Olsen, *et al.*, 1980b).

To determine accurately the angular separation between the illumination and observation systems and the normal to the point of focus of the instrument, Zantos (1981) suggested using a graticule when the illumination system is normal to the grati-

cule surface. By measuring the apparent width of the separations, the angle of observation could be calculated. An alternative method utilizes a protractor, focussing rod and needle point (A. Ho, personal communication). Once this angular separation is determined it should not be altered throughout the use of the instrument, as variation in this angular setting will lead to significant variation in the measurements of corneal thickness.

Other changes to improve the accuracy of the optical pachometer include selecting a slit lamp with a quartz halogen light source to achieve maximum beam intensity and a slit width diaphragm system which enables a minimal slit width.

Alignment and fixation LEDs

It is most important to ensure that the microscope is perpendicular to the corneal surface at every measurement position. This has been achieved by Donaldson (1966) and Mandell and Polse (1969), by the placement of two small lights, one above and one below the objective of the microscope. When the images of the bulbs were seen reflected from the epithelium of the corneal sections, the microscope was considered to be normal to the corneal surface.

The Holden–Payor pachometer uses two red LEDs, to ensure horizontal and vertical alignment. The vertical and horizontal alignment LEDs are located in a perspex plate situated between the illumination and observation systems. They are separated by 10 mm horizontally and vertically, the upper one being used for horizontal alignment and the lower for vertical alignment. The observation system and the horizontal alignment LED are separated by equal and opposite angles from the perpendicular to the corneal position being measured. Alignment is obtained when the upper red image coincides with the centre of the corneal section, and the lower red image is bisected by the biprism line

(Fig. 19.3). This allows exact replication of the corneal location being measured on different

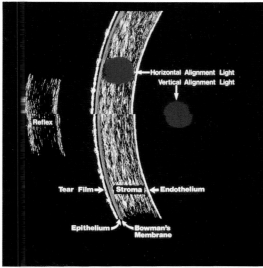

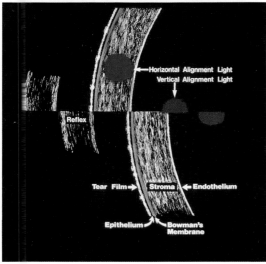

Figure 19.3 Image of the cornea through the Payor–Holden optical pachometer when aligned for measurement of (top) epithelial and (bottom) total corneal thickness. To ensure that the same location is measured between sessions, a measurement is only taken when the upper image of the red LED coincides with the centre of the corneal section and the lower image is bisected by the biprism line (figure supplied courtesy of CCLRU).

measurement sessions.

To facilitate topographical measurement of corneal thickness, the Holden–Payor optical pachometer uses a series of eighteen green LEDs arranged in a horizontal semi-circular arc (see Fig. 19.2 bottom). By asking the patient to fixate each of the LEDs in turn, the cornea can be measured at successive regions from the centre to the limbus along the horizontal meridian.

Stability and linearity of the potentiometer output

As part of the calibration of an optical pachometer, it is necessary to ensure that the attached potentiometer or shaft encoder has a linear output in relation to the pachometer scale. Where this is not linear, allowances have to made when converting apparent to true corneal thickness.

Ray tracing to convert apparent to true corneal thickness

If the illumination system is not normal to the cornea, the von Bahr formula for converting apparent to true corneal thickness can no longer be used (von Bahr, 1956). Zantos (1981) and Brennan *et al.* (1989) have developed ray tracing programs which enable the calculation of true corneal thickness for any corneal location, and for any combination of angles of observation and illumination.

Calibration of the instrument: calibration lenses, ray tracing

Optical pachometers are usually calibrated using a set of hard contact lenses of known thicknesses with a common front surface radius of curvature (Polse & Mandell, 1969). The lenses are mounted in a dial and the operator measures each in turn. A correction is then made for the difference in refractive index between the contact lens material and the cornea. However, as noted previously by

Zantos (1981), the optical quality of the contact lens is inferior to that of the cornea, making alignment of the optic sections more difficult and potential calibration error greater. This procedure has to be carried out only once during the initial calibration of the instrument. The contact lens system enables compensation to be made for slit width, depth of focus and observer bias.

Three series of mathematical computations are then used to obtain true corneal thickness. The first involves trigonometric ray tracing to convert the physical thickness of the contact lens to apparent width of the optic section. A curve of best fit is fitted to the data, from which the apparent width of the section for each calibration lens is derived. Second, the voltage recorded for each lens is plotted against the apparent width of the optic section. Finally, the apparent width of the optic section is converted to true corneal thickness using a ray tracing program. The latter two calibration curves are entered into a microcomputer, to allow rapid calculation of true corneal thickness.

Measurement technique

Before attempting to use an optical pachometer, each user should focus the eyepiece using the focusing rod supplied by the manufacturer. The optic section is brought into view by movement of the slit lamp base and the optic section is viewed, with the dominant eye, through the split image device in the eyepiece. Determination of corneal thickness in the living eye is made more difficult by fixational movements of the eye and light scatter from debris in the tear film. By asking the patient to hold the sides of the chin support on the slit lamp and to make a firm biting action on their jaw, patient movements can be minimized. The patient is asked to fixate one of the green fixation lights on the semi-circular arc. To ensure that the same location is measured between sessions, a measurement is only

taken when the upper image of the red LED coincides with the centre of the corneal section and the lower image is bisected by the biprism line (Fig. 19.3).

A simpler technique suitable for clinical practice has been suggested by Stone (1974). The Haag–Streit pachometer is mounted on a slit lamp and the patient is asked to fixate the light source through the supplied aperture. The first Purkinje image of the slit formed on the front surface of the crystalline lens is used to align the instrument vertically.

Measurement of epithelial thickness

By varying the alignment of the upper to lower image, optical pachometry is adequate for the measurement of total corneal thickness or stromal corneal thickness (Fig. 19.3). However, due to its low magnification and resolution, the accurate determination of the thickness of the corneal epithelium is not possible without large numbers of subjects to enable statistical significance. To overcome this, Wilson and colleagues (1980) developed a micropachometer for the measurement of epithelial thickness in the living eye. This device consisted of a projector, condenser lens, slit, rotatable doubling plate and microscope (see Fig. 1, Wilson *et al.*, 1980). The instrument provides a view similar to that provided by the Haag–Streit pachometer, except that the magnification has been increased to 40×.

Topographical measurement of corneal thickness

In certain applications, such as for keratoconic patients or for monitoring the effects of contact lenses on corneal physiology, it is desirable to measure corneal thickness in different regions over the cornea. The most common technique requires the patient to monocularly fixate each of a number of fixation lights mounted on a semicircular arc. The movement of the eyes to fixate each LED in turn results in a different region of the cornea being measured. This technique is used in the Holden–Payor and Diagnostic Concepts Electronic Pachometers (see Fig. 19.2b above).

El Hage and Leach (1975) suggested that the action of the extra-ocular muscles in extreme positions of fixation may distort corneal thickness measurements. They adopted a second technique where the patient's head and eyes are kept steady while a millimeter rule and magnifier system is used to slide the instrument base 2.5 to 4.0 mm nasally and temporally. The base of the instrument is locked in position while the biomicroscope and slit lamp assembly is rotated about its axis until it is perpendicular to the cornea. The subject maintains a straight ahead fixation by viewing a bull's-eye target.

Most modern research optical pachometers adopt the former technique discussed previously. Mandell and Polse (1969) estimated the peripheral corneal location by assuming the cornea to be spherical. Edmund (1987) and Brennan *et al.* (1989) have described equations which take into account the aspheric nature of the anterior corneal surface, and discuss errors of corneal location introduced by different corneal asphericities.

The determination of corneal location must also include an allowance for angle kappa (the angle between the visual axis and the pupillary axis of the eye measured at the nodal point (Cline *et al.*, 1989). This is discussed by Ehlers and Hansen (1971) and also by Brennan *et al.* (1989). If angle kappa is not considered, Ehlers and Hansen suggest that a small but systematic artefactual difference may result between measurements obtained from the right and left eyes. One may be able to make an allowance for this, prior to performing topographical pachometry, by observing the corneal reflex of the slit source when a number of subjects fixate the various fixation lights in the central area. This will enable the operator to calculate the average corneal position of each eye measured when the subject fixates particular fixation targets. This usually means that a given fixation target, when viewed, will correspond to a different measured location in each eye and a reference table has to be used to determine the approximate corneal location measured.

Possible sources of error

Variations in corneal refractive index and anterior corneal curvature within the population can lead to errors due to the use of standard values in the ray tracing formulae (Arner & Rengstroff, 1972). The error introduced by differences in the anterior curvature of the cornea is negligible, amounting to less than 0.2% of corneal thickness. Differences in the refractive index of the cornea could lead to a change of approximately 3% in the estimate of corneal thickness at the extremes of refractive indices encountered physiologically (1.333 to 1.419). A decrease in refractive index would make the cornea appear thicker, while an increase in refractive index would make the cornea appear thinner. However, Fatt and Harris (1973) and Patel (1987) suggest that the effect of variation in refractive index is negligible.

The adoption of either the touch or overlap technique of optical pachometry can lead to significant differences for the two measurement methods (Molinari & Bonds, 1983). The adoption of the touch method (i.e. endothelium just touching epithelium) produces a thicker corneal measurement than when using the overlap technique (i.e. endothelium overlapping epithelium) (see Figs. 2 and 3 in Molinari & Bonds, 1983). However, for relative thickness changes, this difference is not relevant as long as the operator uses the same criteria between measurements. The problem of measurement of corneal thickness through hydrogel contact lenses has been considered by Snyder (1984) and Mutti and Seger (1986). Snyder compared the magnification effect of pachometry through contact lenses of 0.035 mm centre thickness with a 0.25 mm thick lens and found an over-estimate of 3% in the determination of corneal thickness.

Other possible sources of error include:

1. Angle kappa (Ehlers & Hansen, 1971).
2. Intersession and intrasession precision (Azen *et al.*, 1979).
3. Inter- and intra-observer variation (Olsen *et al.*, 1980b; Binder *et al.*, 1977).
4. Diurnal variation – 6 μm (Edmund & La Cour, 1986).
5. Slit lamp adjustments – 5 μm (Edmund & La Cour, 1986).
6. Adjustment of the pachometer – 13 μm (Edmund & La Cour, 1986).
7. Corneal front surface asphericity (Edmund, 1987; Brennan *et al.*, 1989).
8. Non-linearity of pachometer scale (Olsen *et al.*, 1980a).
9. Pachometry through thick hydrogel lenses may result in an over-estimate of corneal thickness (Snyder, 1984; Mutti & Seger, 1986).
10. Observer experience: standard deviation for a trained observer is 5–6 μm and 32 μm for an inexperienced observer (Chan-Ling, personal observations; Hirji & Larke, 1978).

19.2.2 ULTRASONIC PACHOMETRY

With the increasing application of radial keratotomy and other keratorefractive procedures as a means of correcting refractive error, it is necessary for the surgeon to accurately determine topographical corneal thickness prior to surgery. In this particular application, ultrasonic pachometry has become the method of choice (Unterman & Rowsey, 1984; Villasenor *et al.*, 1986). In addition, ultrasonic pachometers have also become the instrument of choice for studies of corneal physiology involving animals (Chan-Ling *et al.*, 1985; Ling, 1987; McKnight *et al.*, 1988; Ling *et al.*, 1988; Madigan, 1989).

As discussed above, corneal thickness across the cornea is nearly uniform in many animals, including the cat, rabbit and rat, making the placement of the probe less critical. In addition, their portability, ease of use and accuracy have made the use of ultrasonic pachometers widespread in toxicology (Morgan *et al.*, 1987; Jacobs & Martens, 1989; Kennah *et al.*, 1989).

Principle of ultrasonography

High frequency sound waves are propagated through soft tissues and the reflection of these waves by tissues in the path of the beam is recorded. The ultrasonic pachometer is based on traditional A-scan ultrasonography instruments (time–amplitude ultrasound), where the recording is in one dimension, allowing an accurate measurement of tissue dimensions. This contrasts with B-scan instruments, where the recordings give a two-dimensional cross-section of the eye.

Since sound is in the mechanical energy spectrum and travels by alternate compression and rerefraction of molecules, a fluid is necessary to transmit the sound from a transducer to the eye. For pachometric applications, ultrasound is transmitted to the eye from a transducer. The transducer is made of a material with piezo-electric properties, that is when an acoustic wave strikes the material, an electric charge which can be recorded is developed. Consequently, when electric energy is pulsed into a transducer, mechanical waves can be directed into the eye and reflected energy received by the transducer can be displayed on an oscilloscope. Sound is reflected back to the transducer from tissue interfaces which possess different acoustic impedance properties. The boundary between two tissues of different acoustic impedances act as an acoustic reflecting surface, much like a mirror acts as a light reflecting surface. In this way, the cornea–

aqueous interface represents the acoustic reflecting surface for corneal thickness measurements. Other reflecting surfaces such as the anterior lens surface are gated out of the range over which measurements are possible.

A transducer probe emits high frequency sound wave pulses, which are reflected from the anterior and posterior corneal surfaces. The transducer also acts as a sensor to receive the echoes and measures the time difference between the two pulse signals. The corneal thickness is computed as the product of the time delay between the two echoes and the velocity of sound in the corneal tissue. An accurate determination of ultrasound velocity in corneal tissue is thus critical for measurement of absolute corneal thickness.

Determination of the velocity of sound in corneal tissue

True corneal thickness can be determined simply by ultrasonic pachometry if the velocity of ultrasound through the cornea is accurately known. The velocity of sound in human corneal tissue as quoted in the literature varies between 1502 (Nakajima *et al.*, 1967) and 1610 m/s (Nover & Glanscheider, 1965).

Using interferometry, Oksala and Leihtinen (1958) determined the velocity of sound in bovine corneal tissue to be 1550 m/s at 22 °C. Five pieces of excised bovine cornea were placed together inside a container filled with distilled water, and pressure was applied to remove any water between the pieces. The time taken to traverse the test tissue was compared with the time taken to traverse a water column of known height. Since the velocity of sound in water is accurately known at various temperatures, the velocity of sound in a test piece could be determined using the following equations, where t is the time taken for the sound impulse to pass through the water column and test piece.

$$t = \frac{\text{length of test piece}}{\substack{\text{velocity of test piece} \\ \text{at given temperature}}}$$

$$= \frac{\text{length of water}}{\text{velocity of water at given temperature}}$$

Velocity in test piece =

$$\text{velocity of water} \times \frac{\text{length of test piece}}{\text{length of water}}$$

The velocities of ultrasound in cat and rabbit corneal tissue have been reported to be 1590 (Ling *et al.*, 1986) and 1580 (Chan *et al.*, 1983) m/s at 33 °C respectively. These values were determined using a technique which compared *in vivo* thickness measurements with the excised thickness measurements, using an accurate electronic thickness gauge. Corneal thickness was measured using the Cilco 55 Villasenor Ultrasonic Pachometer with a hand-held transducer (No 55–1). The pachometer was adjusted for a velocity of 1550 m/s, which was the manufacturer's recommended setting for absolute determination of corneal thickness in the human. The corneas with a small scleral rim were then immediately excised and placed between two spherical PMMA surfaces – a dome of radius 7.0 mm and a 'foot' of radius 8.5 mm attached to a digital length gauge (Heidenhain MT-10). During 'in situ' measurements, the cornea was compressed by an amount equal to the intra-ocular pressure. Thickness measurements using the electronic gauge on excised tissue were therefore made under a compression pressure of 15 mmHg. The dome on which the excised cornea rested was placed in a water bath and maintained at 33 °C, the temperature at the anterior surface of the cornea (Fig. 19.4). The digital gauge recorded the displacement of the foot to within 1 μm, thus giving an accurate measurement of corneal thickness over the central 4 mm. The velocity that resulted in a match between measurements made using the ultrasonic pachometer and the thickness gauge was calculated using the formula:

Matched velocity =

$$\frac{1550 \times \text{Heidenhain gauge thickness}}{\text{ultrasonic pachometer thickness}}$$

Using this procedure, we determined the velocities of ultrasound in cat and rabbit corneal tissue to be 1590 m/s and 1580 m/s, respectively. This is in close agreement with Yamamoto *et al.* (1961) and Rivara and Sanna (1962), who found the velocity of sound in human corneal tissue to be 1580 and 1588 m/s at 37 °C respectively. Salz *et al.* (1983) also found that by using a velocity in the vicinity of 1590 m/s, the thicknesses obtained were in close agreement with optical pachometry. Therefore 1580–90 m/s appears to be the most accurate velocity of sound in human, cat and rabbit corneal tissue resulting in a true measure of corneal thickness. Since temperature at the anterior surface of the eye is 34.4 °C under open eye conditions and 35.9–36.2 °C under closed eye conditions (Mapstone, 1968; Holden & Sweeney, 1985) and approximately 37 °C at the endothelial–aqueous interface, the velocity of

sound in corneal tissue should also be determined within this temperature range.

A further question remains to be investigated. The refractive index of the cornea is slightly decreased as the tissue swells; is the velocity of sound in corneal tissue affected by corneal swelling? The only clue to this question comes from our earlier work. Using an accurate thickness gauge, the velocity of sound in hydroxyethyl methacrylate (HEMA – 38% water content) lenses was found to be 1740 m/s and 1700 m/s in Snoflex contact lenses (50% water content) (Ling *et al.*, 1986). Assuming insignificant differences in ultrasound velocity due to lens material, a change of 12% water content only altered sound velocity by 2%. Since the velocity decreases with increases in water content, an error would be introduced into these measurements leading to a slight under-estimate of corneal thickness in the hydrated (swollen) cornea. However, at physiological levels of corneal swelling, this error would be insignificant. For studies involving massive corneal swelling, such as may occur in toxicology, post-surgical recovery of corneal thickness, or where the barrier properties of the epithelium or endothelium have been compromised, this under-estimate of corneal swelling may have to be allowed for.

Measurement technique

After setting the velocity of sound at an appropriate value, the instrument is ready for use. A topical anaesthetic is instilled and the patient reclined. The patient is asked to fixate a point in the distance along the central position of gaze. Readings are taken covering the central cornea by placing the probe over the centre of the pupil. The probe is hand held and placed to ensure perpendicular corneal contact, or alternatively, mounted on a slit lamp base. Excessive compression of the cornea should be avoided. The point of perpendicular contact is indicated differently depending on the brand of pachometer used.

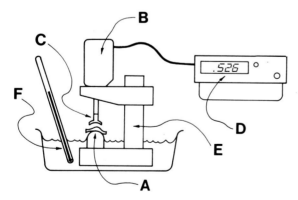

Figure 19.4 Mechanical thickness gauge. The cornea is placed on a perspex dome (A) in line with the gauge head (B) fitted with a concave contact (C). A digital counter (D) receives and displays the reading from the gauge head. This assembly is mounted on a sturdy base (E) that is kept in a water bath (F) at 33 °C (from Ling *et al.*, 1986).

The Acutome® ultrasonic pachometer indicates that the probe is within 10° of the perpendicular with a beep signal. With the KOI® and VIDA® instruments, the readings are taken when the readings seen on the screen are 'locked in' at the one-hundreth decimal point with minimal variation in the thousanth reading. When an ultrasonic pachometer is used on animals, the transducer is well tolerated without a corneal anaesthetic, presumably due to their lower corneal sensitivity (Millodot *et al.*, 1978; Chan-Ling *et al.*, 1987; Madigan *et al.*, 1987; Chan-Ling, 1989) (Figure 19.5).

Topographical corneal thickness measurement

Measurements of the regional variation in corneal thickness can be obtained easily using ultrasonic pachometry. However, due to the significant variation of topographical corneal thickness in the human, repeatability of probe placement and ensuring perpendicular contact of the transducer are more critical. The cornea is anaesthetizied prior to the application of the transducer in human subjects but not in animals. The probe is

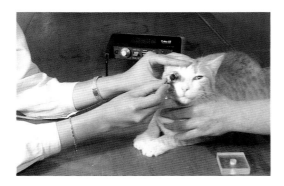

Figure 19.5 Corneal thickness is measured on an adult cat using the VIDA-55 ultrasonic pachometer with hand-held probe. The cat is gently restrained and the upper lid retracted. No corneal anaesthetic is required (photograph from T. Chan-Ling).

hand-held and maintained in an orientation normal to the cornea. Readings are taken at 17 locations covering the central, mid-peripheral and peripheral cornea, as shown in Figure 19.6. Placement of the probe is judged visually by the operator, using the centre of the pupil as a guide to probe placement. A number of readings are taken at each position and the mean and standard deviation are calculated for each position.

Choice of an ultrasonic pachometer

When choosing an ultrasonic pachometer, the scientist/clinician is faced with two main decisions. Should the instrument be a dedicated single use instrument which can only be used for the mesurement of corneal thickness or is the additional capacity of acquisition of axial length data required? An instrument which measures both, such as a combined biometric rule with a pachometer capacity, is usually dearer and bulkier. In addition, there is a trade-off between tissue penetration and resolution. The higher the frequency of the transducer the better the resolution but the signal cannot penetrate deep into the tissue before it is absorbed. Therefore high resolution transducers such as 15–20 MHz are used for anterior segment biometry, while lower frequency transducers of 5–10 MHz are used for ocular and orbital evaluation. An example of a combined ultrasonic pachometer with biometric rule is the Storz Omega biometric ruler as shown in Figure 19.7.

A second decision concerns the transducer type. There are two types of transducers, a soft-tip filled with a liquid medium or a solid cone probe made of a crystal with piezoelectric properties as discussed above. The solid probes are more easily cleaned and do not require re-calibration for each use; whereas the liquid filled probes require regular replenishment of the fluid. However, the solid tip probes could shorten axial length measurement if excess pressure is

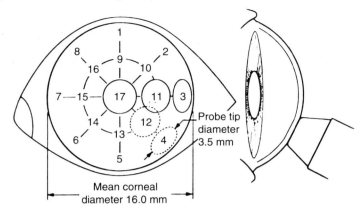

Figure 19.6 Schematic drawing of a rabbit eye showing the 17 locations where corneal thickness was measured. The probe placement areas are drawn to scale for the VIDA-55 Ultrasonic pachometer with hand-held probe (from Ling *et al.*, 1986).

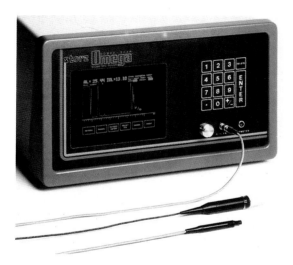

Figure 19.7 Storz biometric ruler with two types of probes, a solid cone probe in the foreground and a soft tip behind. The screen displays a typical output when the instrument is used as a biometric ruler for determination of the power of an intraocular lens.

applied. This potential source of error is only relevant if axial length data is also acquired.

Further considerations when purchasing an ultrasonic pachometer include whether the operation of the instrument requires a second technician to determine the align-

ment of the probe or to record the measurements. Often the convenience of automated recordings and alignment devices is offset by increased cost of the instrument.

19.2.3 COMPARISON WITH OPTICAL PACHOMETRY.

To gain maximum accuracy from optical pachometry substantial instrument modification and operator training are required. This is borne out by the fact that when the Payor-Holden optical pachometer is used by an experienced operator, a standard error of measurement of 5 µm can be achieved (Hirji & Larke, 1978; Ling *et al.*, 1986) compared to 19 µm with an inexperienced operator (Salz *et al.*, 1983). The major advantage of ultrasonic pachometry over optical pachometry is that it requires minimal observer judgement and therefore is consistent and reproducible between observers (Salz *et al.*, 1983; Gordon *et al.*, 1990). An ultrasonic pachometer is also more portable than an optical pachometer, making it suitable for pre-operative measurements in the supine position. In addition, it does not require the patient to be seated at a slit lamp or to have excellent fixation.

Another point of comparison lies in the

relative cost of the two types of pachometers. The basic Haag-Streit optical pachometer, which can be mounted on most conventional slit lamps, costs around £800. This is a modest outlay, but as outlined earlier the modifications required to increase accuracy and speed of use, necessitate extensive workshop modifications to ensure a minimal slit width, accurate fixation LEDs to ensure repeatability of the location of measurement, appropriate software and connection to a microcomputer for ease of analysis of output. These modifications make it difficult to use the slit lamp for other examination purposes. The dedication of a slit lamp for pachometry alone, the cost of a microcomputer, and the workshop modifications make the total cost of an optical pachometer in the vicinity of over £15 000. However, with these modifications optical pachometry can result in an accuracy of 5–10 µm. An optical pachometer is also the instrument of choice where repeated monitoring of corneal thickness is required since ultrasonic pachometry on human subjects requires the use of a corneal anaesthetic. In addition, unlike optical pachometers, ultrasonic pachometers do not have fixation lights for precise control of patient gaze during repeated measurements, allowing for some variation in placement and positioning of the probe on the cornea.

19.2.4 SPECULAR MICROSCOPY

Blix (1880) was the first to utilize the specular reflex for the measurement of corneal thickness. The principle underlying this technique is to focus successively on the specular reflection from the anterior and posterior corneal surfaces and to measure the distance travelled. More recently, corneal thickness has been measured using specular microscopy by a number of investigators (Klyce & Maurice, 1976; Azen *et al.*, 1979; Wilson & Fatt, 1980; Olsen & Ehlers, 1984).

Modern specular microscopes utilize a dipping cone which is applanated on to the

centre of the subject's cornea. The corneal endothelium is then brought sharply into focus by rotating the microscope's dipping cone. Measurements are then read directly from a micrometer gauge, and these readings are then converted to corneal thickness using the following formula (corneal thickness (mm) = $[100 - (x + 30)]/100$ where x = reading from the micrometer gauge) (Azen *et al.*, 1979). When compared to a basic Haag-Streit optical pachometer, with and without the Mishima-Hedbys attachment, the specular microscope showed significantly smaller intrasession variation than the optical pachometer (Azen *et al.*, 1979). This technique offers the advantage that endothelial cell density and morphology can be examined simultaneously. However, its use does require a corneal anaesthetic as well as significant operator skill to avoid epithelial damage. Commercially available units include the Syber, Heyer-Schulte specular microscopes (Medical Optics, Irvine California) and the PRO/Koester wide-field scanning corneal microscope ® (Fig. 19.8).

By increasing the magnification and using a very bright light source, Wilson *et al.* (1980) constructed a specular microscope which could monitor epithelial thickness *in vitro*, with an accuracy of 1–2 µm. This technique is the most precise method of monitoring epithelial swelling at present.

19.2.5 CONFOCAL MICROSCOPY

The image seen through a conventional microscope includes the in-focus image and the out-of-focus image above and below. The blur produced by the out-of-focus image reduces the resolution of the instrument. Confocal microscopy is unlike conventional microscopes in that defocus causes the image to disappear rather than to appear as a blurred image. This feature arises because the confocal instrument selects against features that lie outside the plane of focus, and consequently, it only delivers an optical sec-

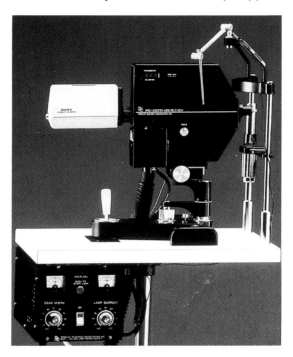

Figure 19.8 PRO/Koester wide-field scanning corneal microscope. A dipping cone is applanated onto the centre of the subject's cornea; the corneal endothelium is then brought sharply into focus by rotating the microscope's dipping cone. Measurements are then read from the micrometer gauge, top left hand corner of the instrument (display = 523 μm).

tion confined within the plane of focus of the object. This feature is achieved by employing a detector in the final image plane, which has a very limited field of view, and by having the point of interest optimally illuminated by light concentrated there into a diffraction-limited spot. An extended view of a thick object is then built up by scanning a succession of points in object space (Wilson & Sheppard, 1984).

With the development of laser scanning confocal instruments, high quality images can be achieved using both reflected and fluorescent emission (Masters, 1984; Jeacocke, 1989). Figure 19.9 shows an optical

section of a mildly oedematous enucleated porcine cornea, obtained using a laser confocal microscope with a water immersion objective lens (Zeiss) with physiological saline as the immersion fluid. The illuminating argon ion laser light was at 488 nm. This image was obtained by scanning the focused laser beam of an MRC500 (Bio-Rad Microscience) scanning system along a selected line in the XY plane and then displacing the fine focus of the microscope, using a stepper motor, in steps between successive scans. With this set-up the resolution in the Z direction is approximately 3–4 μm. The corneal epithelium, the epithelial basement membrane, the keratocytes lying between stromal lamellae, Descemet's membrane and the endothelium are clearly discernable. An accurate determination of corneal thickness is clearly possible using a confocal microscope. However, this complete image took approximately 50 seconds to acquire. The major factor limiting more rapid image acquisition is the time taken to drive the stepping motor to each new focus position. Presently a number of prototype models of confocal microscopes are being developed to overcome eye movements relative to the microscope and to reduce the time taken for a measurement (R. Jeacocke, personal communication). Confocal microscopes hold great promise as an accurate means of determining corneal thickness without requiring corneal contact, but serious limitations remain to be overcome.

19.2.6 FEMTOSECOND OPTICAL RANGING

With the development of argon–fluoride excimer lasers it is possible to remove corneal tissue in submicron increments. Because each laser pulse removes so little tissue, the depth of an incision can be controlled much more precisely than with a diamond knife. However, the precision possible with the laser is of limited value unless the incision depth can be measured accu-

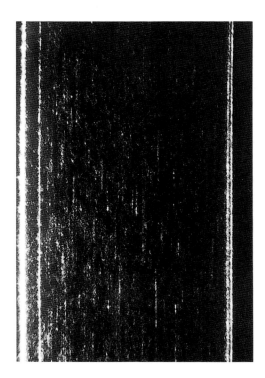

Figure 19.9 Optical section through the full thickness of the central cornea of an intact pig eye imaged by reflected (scattered) light, using an MRC500 (Bio-Rad Microscience) scanning confocal microscope. The horizontal axis represents displacement measured along the optical axis of the eye. From left to right, the nearly continuous bright line corresponds to the outer surface of the cornea, the basement membrane of the epithelium, Descemet's membrane, the basement membrane of the endothelium and finally the boundary between the endothelium and the aqueous. The discontinuous bright streaks within the stroma represent the keratocytes lying between stromal lamellae (figure supplied courtesy of R. Jeacocke).

rately and non-invasively. Because the transverse spatial resolution of ultrasonic pachometry is limited by the size of the ultrasonic probe tip (at least 1 mm in diameter), this technique is not suitable for measurement of corneal incision depth. Femtosecond optical ranging has been suggested as an alternative to ultrasonic pachometry for the determination of corneal incision depth during excimer laser ablation for keratorefractive surgery. This technique is effectively an optical analogue of ultrasonic pachometry (Stern *et al.*, 1989). The time required for a femtosecond laser pulse (10^{-15} s) to make a round trip between the corneal surface and the bottom of the incision is measured. This time can be converted to incision depth by multiplying by the speed of light. Alternatively the corneal thickness can be determined by measuring the time required for the laser pulse to make a round trip between the anterior and posterior surfaces of the cornea (Fujimoto *et al.*, 1986).

The depth resolution of femtosecond ranging is limited by the precision with which the peak position in the cross-correlation traces can be determined. Using 65 fs pulses, the depth resolution is about 5 μm. Despite the apparent accuracy of this technique, its clinical application is still severely limited. If it is to be used for measurement of corneal incision depth, it must be performed on a relatively dry eye. If the corneal surface is moist, the incision gradually fills with tears and the depth of incision is only measured to the surface of the tear film, leading to a significant underestimate. The eye must be positioned carefully so that the probe beam is perpendicular to the corneal surface. In addition, the eye must be stationary during the course of the measurement for maximal accuracy. Therefore, despite its potential, substantial development of its optical and mechanical design is required before this technique can be considered as a viable option.

19.2.7 INTERFEROMETRY

Interferometry can be used to determine central corneal thickness in both transparent and opaque corneal tissue (Green *et al.*, 1975). This technique involves directing a coherent light source at the cornea and, because the cornea has a different refractive index from the surrounding media, light is reflected from the anterior and posterior corneal surfaces. The wave fronts reflected from the two surfaces interfere, forming a pattern of alternating dark and light fringes. By measuring the fringe spacing and performing the relevant calculations, corneal thickness can be determined.

In principle, this technique only requires a laser and a camera (Green *et al.*, 1975) and results agree closely with determinations of corneal thickness using optical pachometry. Despite this potential, interferometry for the measurement of corneal thickness in the clinical environment has not eventuated.

19.2.8 BIOMICROSCOPIC AND VISUAL SIGNS INDICATIVE OF CORNEAL SWELLING

In addition to the pachometric quantification of corneal thickness, a number of biomicroscopic signs are indicative of corneal oedema. When a pachometer is not readily available, these signs can be usefully employed to aid in the detection of corneal swelling. Three biomicroscopic techniques are available to detect different types of corneal oedema. Although the techniques predominantly differentiate between stromal, epithelial and endothelial oedema, it is difficult to isolate the presence of one type of oedema only.

The first technique is the detection of corneal striae or striate lines, which are generally indicative of stromal oedema. Using direct focal illumination (parallelepiped) they appear as greyish thread like lines at low levels of corneal oedema, which become greyer and thicker as the level of oedema increases. The optimal viewing conditions for observing striae is when a wide angle between the microscope and the light source is used. Using retro-illumination, the lines appear dark against the orange retinal reflex (Fig. 19.10a).

Striae are commonly seen in patients wearing extended wear hydrogel contact lenses, in elderly patients, following cataract surgery, and in some corneal pathologies such as bullous keratopathy (Sarver, 1971). Striae are found predominantly in the posterior stroma and usually with a vertical orientation. Polse and Mandell (1976) demonstrated that as corneal swelling increases, striate lines begin to appear at approximately 7% corneal swelling. La Hood and Grant (1990) have extended these observations by quantifying the relationship between corneal oedema and the number of striae and folds present. Hydrogel lenses were worn for 20 hours, including 8 hours sleep. Striae and folds were observed with the biomicroscope, while oedema was quantified using optical pachometry. The numbers of striae and folds were found to be highly correlated with the level of corneal oedema ($r = 0.923$ and $r = 0.874$ respectively, Spearman-Rank). By counting striae and folds, the level of corneal oedema could be predicted to within $\pm 2\%$ for striae and $\pm 3\%$ for folds. A count of 10 striae represents $11\% \pm 2\%$ oedema and a count of ten folds represents $15\% \pm 3\%$ oedema. Corneal folds can be viewed with an optic section or a parallelepiped. They are seen in Figure 19.10b in the posterior one-third of the cornea, forming an oblique cross appearance.

Two biomicroscopic techniques for detecting epithelial oedema utilize retro-illumination. The cornea is illuminated with light reflected from the iris, lens or retina. Using high magnification, the microscope is focused on the cornea. The retro-reflected light makes the swollen epithelial cells appear aberrated. Alternatively, if the epithelial oedema is observed using sclerotic scatter or split limbal types of illumination, it is evident as a hazy, cloudy area against the black background of the pupil. A third method of detecting epithelial oedema is with direct focal illumination. The cornea appears greyer, or

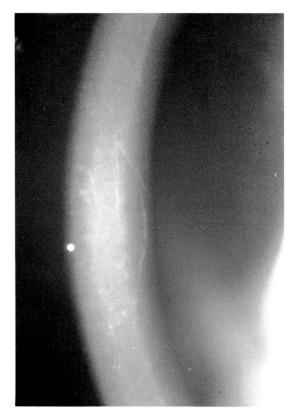

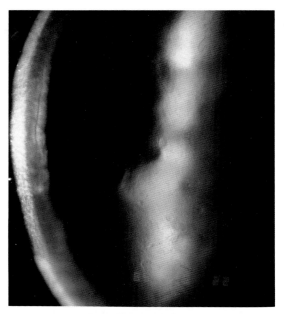

Figure 19.10 (a) Grade 1 vertical corneal striae. Stromal nerve fibres are present at the upper and lower portions of the parallelepiped (photograph supplied courtesy of S. Zantos).

more granular in appearance. However, direct illumination is less sensitive than retro-illumination for detecting small amounts of epithelial oedema.

At the present time there is no widespread agreement that endothelial oedema exists as a clinical entity. However, when the endothelium is examined following trauma or iridocyclitis, corneal guttae are evident. Endothelial oedema, if it exists, is usually associated with epithelial oedema and as a result may be masked by the epithelial oedema. Epithelial oedema may be reduced temporarily by the instillation of a hypertonic salt solution or glycerine on to the

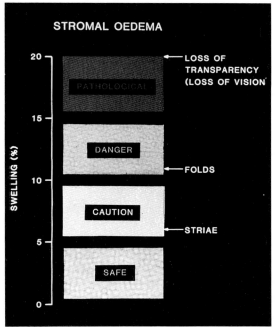

Figure 19.10 (b) Corneal folds intersecting in the posterior one-third of the cornea, forming an oblique cross appearance. Gross stromal oedema due to bullous keratopathy (reprinted from Pye and Collin, 1986). (c) Schematic indicating the levels of stromal oedema associated with striae, folds and loss of transparency.

cornea. The endothelial surface can then be viewed using specular reflex. A transient appearance of corneal guttae, black holes or blebs within the endothelial mosaic is indicative of endothelial oedema. When retro-illumination is used endothelial oedema can manifest as numerous silvery-looking dots, or minute water droplets on the endothelial layer.

In addition to pachometry and biomicroscopic signs of corneal swelling, visual loss can give an indication of the site of corneal oedema. Cox and Holden (1990) induced corneal oedema using both osmotic and anoxic stimuli, and correlated corneal swelling with visual loss as assessed by halometry and contrast sensitivity. Halo brightness was directly affected by the degree of induced epithelial oedema, whereas halo size remained constant. They found a strong relationship ($r = -0.76$, $P < 0.01$) between halo brightness and loss of contrast sensitivity, suggesting that the structural changes within the epithelium that produce physiological haloes are also responsible for the light-scatter-induced visual loss associated with corneal oedema. In contrast, there was no relationship at all between corneal swelling, as assessed with pachometry, and vision loss ($r = -0.22$, $P > 0.10$), suggesting that the cornea can swell considerably without a detectable loss of vision. Therefore, it is clear that the degree of visual loss is directly related to the magnitude of epithelial oedema, but a very poor indicator of stromal swelling.

19.3 DISCUSSION

Pachometry has come a long way since its introduction by Blix in 1880. Experimental techniques, such as confocal microscopy, offer promising alternatives in the near future. At present, however, ultrasonic and optical pachometry are the two most viable techniques for corneal thickness measurement. Using a Haag–Streit optical pachometer, with some instrument modifications or an ultrasonic pachometer with a high frequency transducer, it is possible to measure thickness with 5–6 µm accuracy. This level of accuracy is desirable for applications such as evaluation of contact lens materials and design, studies of corneal physiology, toxicity studies and the measurement of corneal thickness prior to refractive surgery. However, as an aid to diagnosis of certain pathological conditions, such as keratoconus, diabetes and other corneal dystrophies, a basic Haag–Streit optical pachometer mounted on a conventional biomicroscope should achieve an accuracy in the range of 17 µm (Salz *et al.*, 1983).

We have attempted to provide a review of the recent advances in pachometry with the aim of maximizing the accuracy of this technique and to draw the attention of the practitioner to the relevance of corneal thickness measurements in eyecare.

REFERENCES

Alsbirk, P.H. (1974) Optical pachymetry on the anterior chamber. *Acta Ophthalmol. (Copenhagen)*, **52**, 747–58.

Arner, R.S. and Rengstorff, R.H. (1972) Error analysis of corneal thickness measurements. *Am. J. Optom. Arch. Am. Acad. Optom.*, **49**, 862–5.

Azen, S.P., Burg, K.A., Smith, R.E. and Maguen, E. (1979) A comparison of three methods for the measurement of corneal thickness. *Invest. Ophthalmol. Vis. Sci.*, **18**, 535–8.

Ballantyne, B. (1983–84) Local ophthalmic effects of dipropylene glycol monomethyl ether. *J. Toxicol. Cut. Oc. Toxicol.*, **3**, 17–30.

Baum, J.P., Maurice, D.M. and McCarey, B.E. (1984) The active and passive transport of water across the corneal endothelium. *Exp. Eye Res.*, **39**, 335–42.

Bigar, F. and Witner, R. (1982) Corneal endothelial changes in primary acute angle-closure glaucoma. *Ophthalmology*, **89**, 596–9.

Binder, P.S., Kohler, J.A. and Rorabaugh, D.A. (1977) Evaluation of an electronic corneal pachometer. *Invest. Ophthalmol. Vis. Sci.*, **16**, 855–8.

Blix, M. (1880) *Uppsala Läk Fören Förh*, **15**, 349.

(Cited by von Bahr, 1948.)

Bonnano, J.A. and Polse, K.A. (1985) Central and peripheral corneal swelling accompanying soft lens extended wear. *Am. J. Optom. Physiol. Opt.,* **62**, 74–81.

Bowman, K.J., Carney, L.G. and Collin, H.B. (1979) Bilateral keratoconus posticus circumscriptus: a case report. *Am. J. Optom. Physiol. Opt.,* **56**, 435–40.

Brennan, N.A., Efron, N. and Holden, B.A. (1986) Oxygen permeability of hard gas permeable contact lens materials. *Clin. Exp. Optom.,* **69**, 82–9.

Brennan, N.A., Smith G., Macdonald, J.A. and Bruce, A.S. (1989) Theoretical principles of optical pachometry. *Ophthal. Physiol. Opt.,* **9**, 247–54.

Burton, A.B.G. (1972) A model for the objective assessment of eye irritation. *Fd. Cosmet. Toxicol.,* **10**, 209–17.

Busted, N., Olsen, T. and Schmitz, O. (1981) Clinical observations on the corneal thickness and the corneal endothelium in diabetes mellitus. *Brit. J. Ophthalmol.,* **65**, 687–90.

Carney, L.G. (1975) Hydrophilic lens effects on central and peripheral corneal thickness and topography. *Am. J. Optom. Physiol. Opt.,* **52**, 521–3.

Cejkova J., Lojda, Z., Brunova, B. and Michalek, J. (1988) Disturbances in the rabbit cornea after short-term and long-term wear of hydrogel contact lenses. *Histochemistry,* **89**, 91–7.

Chan, R.S. and Mandell, R.B. (1972) Corneal swelling caused by Allum Cepa. *Am. J. Optom. Arch. Am. Acad. Optom.,* **49**, 713–15.

Chan, R.S. and Mandell, R.B. (1975) Corneal thickness changes from bathing solutions. *Am. J. Optom. Physiol. Opt.,* **52**, 465–9.

Chan, T., Payor, S. and Holden, B.A. (1983) Corneal thickness profiles in rabbits using an ultrasonic-pachometer. *Invest. Ophthalmol. Vis. Sci.,* **24**, 1408–10.

Chan-Ling, T. (1989) Sensitivity and neural organisation of the cat cornea. *Invest. Ophthalmol. Vis. Sci.,* **30**, 1075–82.

Chan-Ling, T., Efron N. and Holden, B.A. (1985) Diurnal variation of corneal thickness in the cat. *Invest. Ophthalmol. Vis. Sci.,* **26**, 102–5.

Chan-Ling, T., Tervo, K., Tervo, T. Vannas, A., Holden, B.A. and Eranko, L. (1987) Long-term neural regeneration in the rabbit following 180° limbal incision. *Invest. Ophthalmol. Vis. Sci.,* **28**, 2083–8.

Cline, D., Hofstetter, H.W. and Griffin, J.R. (1989) *Dictionary of Visual Science.* Chilton, Pennsylvania, p. 33.

Cook, C. and Langham, M. (1953) Corneal thickness in interstitial keratitis. *Brit. J. Ophthal.,* **37**, 301–4.

Cox, I. and Holden, B.A. (1990) Can vision be used as a quantitative assessment of corneal edema? *ICLC,* **17**, 176–80.

Donaldson, D.D. (1966) A new instrument for the measurement of corneal thickness. *Arch. Ophthal.,* **76**, 25–31.

Draize, J.H., Woodward, G.C. and Calvery, H.O. (1944) Method for the study of irritation and toxicity of substances applied topically to the skin and mucous membranes. *J. Pharmacol. Exp. Ther.,* **82**, 337–90.

Edmonds, C. and Iwamoto (1972) Electron Microscopy of late interstitial keratitis *Ann. Ophthalmol.,* **6**, 493–6.

Edmund, C. (1987) Determination of the corneal thickness profile by optical pachometry, *Acta Ophthalmol. (Copenhagen),* **65**, 147–52.

Edmund, C. and La Cour, M. (1986) Some components affecting the precision of corneal thickness measurements performed by optical pachometry. *Acta Ophthalmol. (Copenhagen),* **64**, 499–503.

Efron, N. and Carney, L.G. (1979) Oxygen levels beneath the closed lid. *Invest. Ophthalmol.,* **18**, 93–5.

Ehlers, N. and Hansen, F.K. (1971) On the optical measurement of corneal thickness. *Acta Ophthalmol. (Copenhagen),* **49**, 65–81.

El Hage, S.G. and Beaulne, C. (1973) Changes in central and peripheral corneal thickness with menstrual cycle. *Am. J. Optom. Physiol. Opt.,* **50**, 853–71.

El Hage, S. and Leach, N.E. (1975) Central and peripheral corneal thickness changes included by 'on K', steep, and flat contact lens wear. *J. Am. Optom. Assoc.,* **46**, 296–302.

Fatt, I. (1969) Oxygen tension under a contact lens during blinking. *Am. J. Optom.,* **46**, 654–61.

Fatt, I. and Bieber, M.T. (1968) The steady-state distribution of oxygen and carbon dioxide in the in vitro cornea. I. The open eye in air and closed eye. *Exp. Eye Res.,* **7**, 103.

Fatt, I. and Harris, M.G. (1973) Refractive index of the cornea as a function of its thickness. *Am. J. Optom. Arch. Am. Acad. Optom.,* **50**, 383–6.

Fatt, I. and Lin, D. (1976) Oxygen tension under a soft or hard, gas-permeable contact lens in the presence of tear pumping. *Am. J. Optom. Physiol. Opt.*, **53**, 104–11.

Fatt, I. and St Helen, R. (1971) Oxygen tension under an oxygen permeable contact lens. *Am. J. Optom. Physiol. Opt.*, **48**, 545–55.

Fatt, I., Freeman, R.D. and Lin, D. (1974) Oxygen tension distributions in the cornea: a re-examination. *Exp. Eye Res.*, **18**, 357–65.

Fischbarg, J. (1973) Active and passive properties of the rabbit corneal endothelium. *Exp. Eye Res.*, **15**, 615–38.

Fujimoto, J.G., DeSilestri, S., Ippen, E.P., Puliafito, C.A., Margolis, R. and Oseroff, A. (1986) Femtosecond optical ranging in biological systems. *Optics Lett.*, **11**, 150.

Fujita, S. (1980) Diurnal variation in human corneal thickness. *Jap. J. Ophthalmol.*, **24**, 444–56.

Gasset, A.R. (1981) Therapeutic applications. In *Contact Lens Practice*. (ed. R.B. Mandell), Charles C. Thomas, Springfield. IL, pp. 607–18.

Gerstman, D.R. (1972) The biomicroscope and Vickers image splitting eyepiece applied to clinical variation in human central corneal thickness. *J. Microscopy*, **96**, 385–8.

Gordon, A., Boggess, E.A. and Molinari, J.F. (1990) Variability of ultrasonic pachometry. *Optom. Vis. Sci.*, **67**, 162–5.

Green, D.G., Frueh, B.R. and Shapiro, J.M. (1975) Corneal thickness measured by interferometry. *JOSA.*, **65**, 119–23.

Henkind, P. and Wise, G.N. (1961) Descemet's wrinkles in diabetes. *Am. J. Ophthalmol.*, **52**, 371–4.

Hirji, N.K. and Larke, J.R. (1978) Thickness of the human cornea measured by topographic pachometry. *Am. J. Optom. Physiol. Opt.*, **55**, 97–100.

Hodson, S. (1969) Increased intracellular pressure accompanying active transport in corneal endothelium. *Nature (Lond.)*, **222**, 676–7.

Hodson, S. and Miller, F. (1976) The bicarbonate ion pump in the endothelium which regulates the hydration of rabbit cornea. *J. Physiol. (Lond.)*, **283**, 563–77.

Holden, B.A. and Mertz, G. (1984) Critical oxygen levels to avoid corneal oedema for daily and extended wear contact lenses. *Invest. Ophthalmol. Vis. Sci*, **25**, 1161–7.

Holden B.A. and Sweeney, D.S. (1985) The oxygen tension and temperature of the superior palpebral conjunctiva. *Acta Ophthalmol.*, **63**, 100–3.

Holden, B.A., Payor, S. and Mertz, G.W. (1979) Changes in thickness of the corneal layers. *Am. J. Optom. Physiol. Opt.*, **56**, 821.

Holden, B.A., Mertz, G.W. and McNally, J.J. (1983) Corneal swelling response to contact lenses worn under extended wear conditions. *Invest. Ophthalmol. Vis. Sci.*, **25**, 218–26.

Holden, B.A., Sweeney, D.F., Vannas, A., Nilsson, K.T. and Efron, N. (1985), Effects of long-term extended contact lens wear on the human cornea. *Invest. Ophthalmol. Vis. Sci*, **26**, 1489–501.

Huff, J.W. and Green, K. (1981) Demonstration of active sodium transport across the isolated rabbit corneal endothelium. *Curr. Eye Res.*, **1**, 113–14.

Insler, M.S. and Cooper, H.D. (1986) New correlations in keratoconus using pachymetric and keratometric analysis. *CLAO J.*, **12**, 101–5.

Iwamoto, T. and Smelser, G.K. (1965) Electron microscopy of the human corneal endothelium with reference to transport mechanisms. *Invest. Ophthalmol.*, **4**, 270–84.

Jacobs, G.A. and Martens, M.A. (1988) The enucleated eye test: a comparison of the use of ultrasonic and optic pachometers. *Toxic. in Vitro*, **2**, 253–6.

Jacobs, G.A. and Martens, M.A. (1989) An objective method for the evaluation of eye irritation in vivo. *Fd. Chem, Toxic.*, **27**, 255–8.

Jaeger, W. (1952) Tiefen meassung de menschlichen Vorderkammer mit plan parallelen platten (zusatzgerat zur spaltlampe). *Graefes Arch Ophthalmol.*, **153**, 120–1.

Jeacocke, R.E. (1989) *Confocal Microscopy of the Cornea*, Trans. Soc. Prom. Vis. Sci., Churchill College, Cambridge.

Johnson, M.H., Boltz, R.L. and Godio, L.B. (1985) Deswelling of the cornea after hypoxia. *Am. J. Optom. Physiol. Opt.*, **62**, 768–73.

Kaufman, H.E., Capella, J.A. and Robbins, J.E. (1966) The human corneal endothelium. *Am. J. Ophthalmol.*, **61**, 835–41.

Kaye, G.I. and Donn, A. (1965) Studies on the cornea. IV. Some effects of ouabain on pinocytosis and stromal thickness in the rabbit cornea. *Invest. Ophthalmol.*, **4**, 844–52.

Kennah. H.E., Hignet, H., Laux, P.E., Dorko, J.D. and Barrow, C.S. (1989) An objective procedure for quantifying eye irritation based upon changes of corneal thickness. *Fund. Appl. Toxicol.*, **12**, 258–68.

Kikkawa, Y. (1973) Diurnal variation in corneal thickness. *Exp. Eye Res.*, **1**, 46.

Klyce, S.D. and Maurice, D.M. (9176) Automatic recording of corneal thickness. *Invest. Ophthalmol.*, **15**, 550–3.

La Hood, D. and Grant, T. (1990) Striae and folds as indicators of corneal edema. *Optom. Vis. Sci.,* **Suppl. 67**, 196.

La Hood, D., Sweeney, D.F. and Holden, B.A. (1988) Overnight corneal oedema with hydrogel, rigid gas-permeable, and silicone elastomer contact lenses. *ICLC*, **15**, 149–54.

Ling, T. (1987) Osmotically induced central and peripheral corneal swelling in the cat. *Am J. Optom. Physiol. Opt.,* **64**, 674–7.

Ling, T., Ho, A. and Holden, B.A. (1986) Method of evaluating ultrasonic pachometers. *Am. J. Optom. Physiol. Opt.,* **63**, 462–6.

Ling, T., Vannas, A. and Holden, B.A. (1988) Long-term changes in endothelial morphology following wounding in the cat. *Invest. Ophthalmol. Vis. Sci.,* **29**, 1407–12.

Lowe, R.F. (1969) Central corneal thickness. *Brit. J. Ophthal.,* **53**, 824–6.

Madigan, M.C. (1989) *Cat and Monkey Cornea as Models for Extended Hydrogel Contact Lens Wear in Humans.* PhD Thesis, University of New South Wales.

Madigan, M.C., Gillard-Crewther, S., Kiely, P.M., Crewther, D.P., Brennan, N., Efron, N. and Holden, B.A. (1987) Corneal thickness changes following sleep and overnight contact lens wear in the primate (*Macaca fascicularis*). *Curr. Eye Res.,* **6**, 809–16.

Mandell, R.B. and Fatt, I. (1965) Thinning of the human cornea on awakening. *Nature*, **208**, 292–3.

Mandell, R.B. and Polse, K.A. (1969) Keratoconus: spatial variation of corneal thickness as a diagnostic test. *Arch. Ophthal.,* **82**, 182–8.

Mandell, R.B. and Polse K.A. (1971) Corneal thickness changes accompanying central corneal clouding. *Am. J. Optom. Arch. Am. Acad. Optom.,* **48**, 129–32.

Mandell, R.B., Polse, K.A. and Fatt, I. (1970) Corneal swelling caused by contact lens wear. *Arch. Ophthal.,* **83**, 3–9.

Mapstone, R. (1968) Determinants of corneal temperature. *Br. J. Ophthalmol.,* **52**, 729–41.

Martola, E.-L. and Baum, J.L. (1968) Central and peripheral corneal thickness. *Arch. Ophthal.,* **79**, 28–30.

Masters, B.R. (1984) Noninvasive redox fluorometry: How light can be used to monitor alterations of corneal mitochondrial function. *Curr. Eye Res.,* **3**, 23–6.

Mastman, G.J., Baldes, E.J. and Henderson, J.W. (1961) The total osmotic pressure of tears in normal and various pathologic conditons. *Arch. Ophthal.,* **65**, 509–13.

Maurice, D.M. (1969) The cornea and sclera. In *The Eye, Vol. I, Vegetative Physiology and Biochemistry* (ed. H. Davson,), Academic Press, London, pp. 489–600.

Maurice, D.M. (1972) The location of the fluid pump in the cornea. *J. Physiol. (Lond.),* **221**, 43–54.

McKnight, S.J., Fitz, J. and Giancomo, J. (1988) Corneal rupture following radial keratotomy in cats subjected to BB gun injury. *Ophthalmic Res.,* **19**, 165–7.

Mertz, G.W. (1980) Overnight swelling of the living cornea. *J. Am. Optom. Assoc.,* **51**, 211–14.

Millodot, M., Lim, C.H. and Ruskell, G.L. (1978) A comparison of corneal sensitivity and nerve density in albino and pigmented rabbits. *Ophthalmic Res.,* **10**, 307.

Mishima, S. (1968) Corneal thickness. *Surv. Ophthalmol.,* **13**, 57–96.

Mishima, S. and Maurice, D.M. (1961) The effect of normal evaporation on the eye. *Exp. Eye Res.,* **1**, 46–52.

Molinari, J.F. (1982) A review of pachometry. *Am. J. Optom. Physiol. Opt.,* **59**, 912–17.

Molinari, J.F. and Bonds, T. (1983) Pachometry: A comparison between touch and overlap measurement method. *Am. J. Optom. Physiol. Opt.,* **60**, 61–6.

Morgan, R.L., Sorenson, S.S. and Castles, T.R. (1987) Prediction of ocular irritation by corneal pachymetry. *Fd. Chem. Toxic.,* **25**, 609–13.

Mutti, R.O. and Seger R.G. (1986) Artifact in optical pachometry with contact lenses in situ. *Am. J. Optom. Physiol. Opt.,* **763**, 847–52.

Nakajima, A., Kimura, T., and Yamazaki, M. (1967) Applications of ultrasound in biometry of the eye. In *Ultrasonics in Ophthalmology, Diagnostic and Therapeutic Applications.* (eds R.E. Goldberg and L.K. Sarin), W.B. Saunders, Philadelphia, pp. 124–44.

Nover, A. and Glanschneider, D. (1965) Untersuchungen iiber die Gortpflanzungsgeschwindindigkeit und Absorption des Ultraschalls in Gewebe. *Graefew Arch. Ophthal.,* **168**, 304–21.

Oksala, A. and Lehtinen, A. (1958) Measurement of the velocity of sound in some parts of the eye. *Acta Ophthalmologica,* **36**, 633–9.

Olsen, T. and Ehlers, N. (1984) The thickness of the human cornea as determined by a specular method. *Acta Ophthalmol.,* **63**, 859–71.

Olsen, T., Nielsen, C.B. and Ehlers, N. (1980a) On the optical measurement of corneal thickness. I.

Optical principles and sources of error. *Acta Ophthalmol. (Copenhagen)*, **58**, 760–6.

Olsen, T., Nielsen, C.B. and Ehlers, N. (1980b) On the optical measurement of corneal thickness. II. The measuring conditions and sources of error. *Acta Ophthalmol. (Copenhagen)*, **58**, 975–84.

O'Neal, M.R., Polse, K.A. and Sarver, M.D. (1984) Corneal response to rigid and hydrogel lenses during eyelid closure. *Invest. Ophthalmol. Vis. Sci.*, **25**, 837–42.

Parving, H-H, Noer, I., Deckert, T., Evrin, P.-E., Nielsen, S.L., Lyngsoe, J., Mogensen, M., Rorth, M., Svendsen, P.A., Trap-Jensen, J. and Lassen, N.A. (1976) The effect of metabolic regulation on microvascular permeability to small and large molecules in short-term juvenile diabetics. *Diabetologia*, **12**, 161–6.

Patel, S. (1987) Refractive index of the mammalian cornea and its influence during pachometry. *Ophthal. Physiol. Opt.*, **7**, 503–6.

Polse, K.A. (1979) Tear flow under hydrogel contact lenses. *Invest. Ophthalmol. Vis. Sci.*, **18**, 409–13.

Polse, K.A. and Mandell, R.B. (1976) Etiology of corneal striae accompanying hydrogel lens wear. *Invest. Ophthalmol. Vis. Sci.*, **15**, 553–6.

Pye, D.C. and Collin, H.B. (1986) Aphakic bullous keratopathy. *Clin. Exp. Optom.*, **69**, 71–2.

Rao, G.N. and Aquavella, J.V. (1980) *Morphological Pattern of Healing in Human Corneal Endothelium. The Cornea in Health and Disease.* VIth Congress of the European Society of Ophthalmology, Royal Society of Medicine International Congress and Symposium Series No. 40, Academic Press, (Lond), pp. 249–55.

Rivara, A. and Sanna, G. (1962) Determinazione della velocita' degli ultrasuoni nei tessuti oculari di uomo e di maiale. *Annali di Ottalmologia e Clinica Oculisics*, **88**, 675–82.

Roscoe, W.R. and Hill, R.M. (1980) Corneal oxygen demands: a comparison of open and closed-eye environments. *Am. J. Optom. Physiol. Opt.*, **57**, 67–9.

Salz, J.J., Azen, S.P., Berstein, J., Caroline, P. Villasenor, R.A. and Schauzlin, D.J. (1983) Evaluation and comparison of sources of variability in the measurement of corneal thickness with ultrasonic and optical pachymeters. *Ophthalmic Surg.*, **14**, 750–4.

Sanders, T.L., Polse, K.A., Sarver, M.D. and Harris, M.G. (1975) Central and peripheral corneal swelling accompanying the wearing of Bausch & Lomb Soflens contact lenses. *Am. J. Optom. Physiol. Opt.*, **52**, 393–7.

Sarver, M.D. (1971) Striate lines among patients wearing hydrophilic contact lenses. *Am. J. Optom. Physiol. Opt.*, **48**, 762–3.

Schaeffer, A.J. (1950) Osmotic pressure of the extraocular and intraocular fluids. *Arch. Ophthal.*, **43**, 1026–35.

Schnider, C.M., Holden, B.A., Terry, R., Zabkiewicz, K. and La Hood, D. (1988) Effects of rigid gas permeable extended wear on the cornea. In *The Cornea: Transactions of the World Congress on the Cornea III.* (ed. H.D. Cavanagh), Raven Press Ltd, New York, 287–8.

Snyder, A.C. (1984) Optical pachometry measurements: reliability and variability. *Am. J. Optom. Physiol. Opt.*, **61**, 408–13.

Soni, P.S. (1980) Effects of oral contraceptive steroids on the thickness of human cornea. *Am. J. Optom. Physiol. Opt.*, **57**, 825–34.

Stern, D., Lin, W-Z., Puliafito, C.A. and Fujimoto, J. G. (1989) Femtosecond optical ranging of corneal incision depth. *Invest. Ophthalmol. Vis. Sci.*, **30**, 99–104.

Stone, J. (1974) The measurement of corneal thickness. *Contact Lens J.*, **5**, 14–19.

Tomlinson, A. (1972) A clinical study of the central and peripheral thickness and curvature of the human cornea. *Acta Ophthalmol. (Copenhagen)*, **50**, 73–82.

Unterman, S.R. and Rowsey, J.J. (1984) Diamond knife incisions. *Ophthal. Surg.*, **15**, 199–202.

Van Horn, D.A. and Schultz, R.O. (1971) Electron microscopy of syphilitic interstitial keratitis. *Invest. Ophthalmol. Vis. Sci. suppl.*, **10**, 469.

Villasenor, R.A., Santos, V.R., Cox, K.C., Harris, D.F., Lynn, M. and Waring, G.O. (1986) Comparision of ultrasonic corneal thickness measurements before and during surgery in the prospective evaluation of radial keratotomy (PERK) study. *Ophthalmol.*, **93**, 327–30.

Von Bahr, G. (1941) Konnte der Flussigkeitsabgang Durch die cornea von Physiologischer Bedeutung Sein? *Acta Ophth.*, **19**, 125–34.

Von Bahr, G. (1948) Measurements of the thickness of the cornea. *Acta Ophth.*, **26**, 247–66.

Von Bahr, G. (1956) Corneal thickness: its measurement and changes. *Am. J. Ophthalmol.*, **42**, 251–66.

Waring, G.O., Font, R.L. and Rodrigues, M.M. (1976) Alterations of Descemet's membrane in interstitial keratitis. *Am. J. Ophthalmol.*, **81**, 773–85.

Westerhout, D. (1981) The use of soft lenses in ocular pathology. In *Contact Lenses*. (eds J. Stone and A.J. Phillips), Butterworths, London, pp. 604–16.

Wilson, G. and Fatt, I. (1980) Thickness of the corneal epithelium during anoxia. *Am. J. Optom. Physiol. Opt.*, **57**, 409–12.

Wilson, J. and Sheppard, C.J.R. (1984) *Theory and Practice of Scanning Optical Microscopy*. Academic Press, London.

Wilson, G., O'Leary, D.J. and Henson, D. (1980) Micropachometry: A technique for measuring the thickness of the corneal epithelium. *Invest. Ophthalmol. Vis. Sci.*, **19**, 414–17.

Yamamoto, Y., Namiki, R., Baba M. and Kato, M. (1961) A study on the measurement of ocular axial length by ultrasonic echography. *Jap. J. Ophthal.*, **5**, 58–65.

Ytteborg, J. and Dohlman, C. (1965a) Corneal edema and intraocular pressure I. Animal experiments. *Arch. Ophthalmol.*, **74**, 375–81.

Ytteborg, J. and Dohlman, C. (1965b) Corneal edema and intraocular pressure II Clinical results. *Arch. Ophthalmol.*, **74** 477–84.

Zantos S.G. (1981) *The Ocular Response to Continuous Wear of Contact Lenses*. PhD Thesis, University of New South Wales.

tested is small, covering at most a dozen epithelial cells.

Other instruments have, over the years, been built, some of them more advanced and others more accurate than the Cochet–Bonnet aesthesiometer. These instruments are cited in a recent review of corneal sensitivity (Millodot, 1984). None of these has gained wide popularity among clinicians. This may be accounted for by the fact that in corneal aesthesiometry, unlike keratometry or biomicroscopy, the most advanced instrument does not guarantee a better reading. The response is more dependent on the subject's attitude, apprehension and collaboration than on the sophistication of the apparatus.

20.2.1   CLINICAL USE

If the Cochet–Bonnet aesthesiometer is a simple instrument, some precautions still need to be taken in order to obtain accurate readings. It should be mounted in a suitable apparatus (Fig. 20.1) rather than held by hand. The essential feature of this system is the availability of a moveable frame which allows the displacement of the instrument in

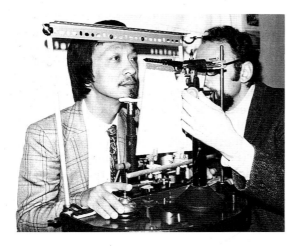

Figure 20.1 The Cochet–Bonnet aesthesiometer mounted in a suitable apparatus allowing it movement in three directions (after Millodot, 1975b).

the x, y and z meridians, thus permitting application of the nylon filament at right angles to a given corneal spot. This apparatus using three knobs also makes it easy to approach the filament to the eye in a carefully controlled way. Because the nylon filament can be affected by humidity (Millodot & Larson, 1967) it is necessary to monitor it, and to obtain measurements when humidity stays within a certain range.

20.2.2   METHOD OF MEASUREMENT

The measurement of corneal touch threshold (CTT) is carried out as follows. Subjects fixate a point situated somewhere in front of them, depending upon which corneal point is to be stimulated. The nylon filament is moved toward the eye perpendicular to the cornea at the point of contact. The cornea is considered to have been touched when the experimenter notices the minimum amount of bending of the nylon filament. The readings are made starting with a low pressure and then increasing by small increments. Starting with a high pressure, on the other hand, would leave an 'after-glow' which persists for some time and tends to elevate the threshold (Millodot, 1974a; Millodot & O'Leary, 1981).

At each length of the nylon filament four to eight measurements are made and the subject is requested to indicate when the probe is felt by pressing a buzzer. A few blanks (that is when the filament is brought to the eye without actually touching it) are also made to test the reliability of the subject. The length of the filament is then decreased (in 0.5 cm steps) until the threshold is encompassed and extrapolated. CTT is defined as the length of the nylon filament at which the subject responds to 50% of the number of stimulations. This length is converted into pressure using the table given with the aesthesiometer or a calibration curve relating length and pressure for the Cochet–Bonnet instrument (Millodot, 1969). Corneal sensitivity is defined as the reciprocal of the CTT.

Alternatively, data can be obtained objectively by monitoring the eye blinks in response to the stimulation. This technique is more fastidious as physiological eye blinks must be distinguished from the actual responses to stimulation. This necessitates many more stimulations. However, the results can yield a high correlation with the subjective measurements, especially for peripheral corneal points (Millodot, 1973). The objective technique is therefore most appropriate with animals, particularly rabbits who blink infrequently (Millodot *et al.*, 1978; Millodot & Vogel, 1981).

Reproducibility of measurements on the same subject is very good. Hirji (1978) found a repeatability of ± 4% with the Cochet–Bonnet aesthesiometer and Millodot and O'Leary (1981) reported a correlation of + 0.99 on the same group of subjects using the same instrument. In another study (unpublished) I found that variations in data did not exceed ± 5% from one time to another. All the above measurements were made on the periphery of the cornea. Measurements on the central part of the cornea do give rise to considerable apprehension, particularly in some subjects (Bonnet & Millodot, 1966). In these conditions the threshold is not only under-estimated but the reproducibility is also much less good than when testing the periphery of the cornea.

20.3 CORNEAL SENSITIVITY IN NON-CONTACT LENS WEARERS

20.3.1 CORNEAL AREA

Corneal sensitivity varies from a maximum at the centre of the cornea to a minimum at the periphery, with least sensitivity at the superior region which is frequently covered by the upper lid (Strughold, 1953; Boberg-Ans, 1955; Cochet & Bonnet, 1960; Kemmetmueller, 1969; Millodot & Larson, 1969; Draeger, 1979). Average central CTT varies

between 10 and 14 mg/mm^2 (Fig. 20.2). The average CTT in the periphery ranges between 20 and 30 mg/mm^2 whereas in the superior periphery it ranges between 30 and 45 mg/mm^2. This corneal area of reduced sensitivity is actually useful in contact lens wear as this is where the contact lens often rests most heavily because of the pressure produced by the upper lid. A considerable drop in sensitivity is found beyond the limbus; but at the lid margin sensitivity has been found to be as high as in the centre of the cornea (Lowther & Hill, 1968).

20.3.2 AGE

Corneal sensitivity remains practically unchanged from about the age of 10 to 50 years. Beyond that age it diminishes, reduc-

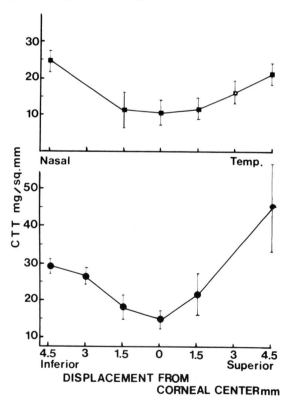

Figure 20.2 Corneal touch threshold as a function of corneal eccentricity (after Millodot & Larson, 1969).

ing to half after 65 years (Jalavisto *et al.*, 1951; Boberg-Ans, 1955; Millodot, 1977a; Draeger, 1979). The data shown in Figure 20.3 are those of Millodot on 205 subjects.

20.3.3 IRIS COLOUR

A striking finding is that people of different iris colour display different corneal sensitivity (Millodot, 1975a; Douthwaite & Kaye, 1980; Tota & la Marca, 1982). People with blue eyes were found, on average, to be much more sensitive than people with brown eyes by about 2:1. And non-white people with dark brown irises have less sensitive corneas than Caucasians with similar eye colour (Fig. 20.4). On the other hand, and seemingly contradictory, albino human corneas are much less sensitive than corneas of pigmented eyes (Millodot, 1978a). This may indicate that some other disturbances besides pigmentation deficiencies exist in albinism. These results found in people with different eye colour are useful in contact lens management.

The reason for this variation in corneal sensitivity still eludes us. Corneal nerve density in pigmented rabbits with dark irises

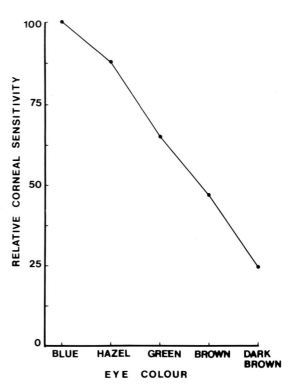

Figure 20.4 Relative corneal sensitivity as a function of eye colour (after Millodot, 1975).

was found to be the same as in albino rabbits with light blue eyes, although their sensitivity was markedly different. As in humans, the cornea was more sensitive in pigmented than in albino rabbits. (Millodot *et al.*, 1978).

20.3.4 MISCELLANEOUS

Corneal sensitivity is usually about the same between the two eyes (Millodot, 1976a) and between the sexes, although at premenstruation, at the onset of menstruation (if no contraceptive pill is used) and in the last few weeks of pregnancy, sensitivity in women was found to be greatly reduced (Millodot & Lamont, 1974; Millodot, 1977b; Riss & Riss, 1981). Surprisingly the decrease in corneal sensitivity prior to menstruation was not observed by Riss *et al.* (1982), yet they found

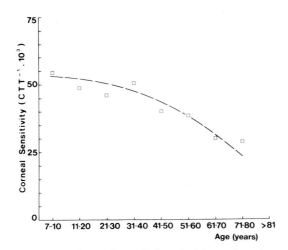

Figure 20.3 Corneal touch threshold as a function of age (after Millodot, 1977).

a change at the end of pregnancy (Riss & Riss, 1981).

Ambient temperature also affects corneal sensitivity. Kolstrad (1970) observed a nine-fold reduction as the outside temperature varied between 22 and − 14 °C. This may explain the relative comfort of contact lens wearers outside when it is cold.

Also of interest to the contact lens practitioner is that in diabetic (Schwartz, 1974; Neilsen, 1978; O'Leary & Millodot, 1981) and in keratoconic eyes (Millodot & Owens, 1983) corneal sensitivity is greatly reduced. Thus contact lens wear is likely to be more comfortable. However, it must also be kept in mind that the fragility of the corneal epithelium is greater in these eyes and contact lens wear must be monitored and limited to shorter periods of time than in normal eyes (O'Leary & Millodot, 1981; Millodot & Owens, 1983).

20.4 SHORT-TERM EFFECT OF CONTACT LENS WEAR

20.4.1 HARD CONTACT LENS (PMMA)

Earlier investigations of the effect of contact lens wear on corneal sensitivity dealt obviously with hard lenses (PMMA) and for short periods of time such as months or up to 3 years of wear. The first such report appears to be that of Boberg-Ans (1955) using his own aesthesiometer. He found a slight reduction in corneal sensitivity after about 2 hours of wear, progressing to a loss of nearly three times throughout the day. This was followed by numerous other investigations using, in most cases, the Cochet-Bonnet aesthesiometer. Unfortunately, not all of these studies controlled the various variables or gave all the information needed. These investigations were made by Cochet and Bonnet (1960), Hamano (1960), Schirmer (1963), Dixon (1964), Gould and Inglima (1964), Edmund (1967), Moore and McCollum (1967), Sabell

(1968), Morganroth & Richman (1969), Larke and Sabell (1971), Millodot (1975b), Millodot (1976b), Polse (1978), Millodot *et al.* (1979), Tanelian & Beuerman (1980), Draeger *et al.* (1980), Gligo *et al.* (1981), Douthwaite and Atkinson (1985) and Lydon (1986).

The unequivocal conclusion from almost all these studies is that corneal sensitivity decreases with hard (PMMA) contact lens wear. One investigator (Millodot, 1976b) obtained data from subjects who had worn their lenses for at least 3 months asymptomatically, prior to inserting their lenses in the morning, after 4 hours of continuous uninterrupted wear, after 8 hours of continuous uninterrupted wear and after 12 hours of continuous uninterrupted wear. These data are shown in Figure 20.5 (labelled hard lenses). We see that on average sensitivity diminishes appreciably after some 3 hours of wear and progressively falls by about a half after 12 hours' wear. It is also worth noting

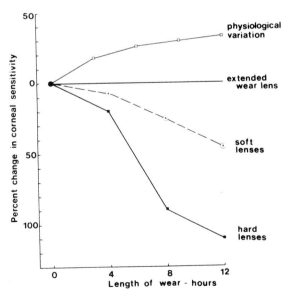

Figure 20.5 The effect of various types of contact lenses on corneal sensitivity. The physiological variation indicates the diurnal change in CTT in non-contact wearers (after Millodot, 1976b).

that there is a physiological diurnal variation in corneal sensitivity (Millodot, 1972) as shown by the curve labelled physiological variation. Therefore the average percentage loss is even slightly greater if that is taken into account.

However, corneal sensitivity does not diminish in all subjects. Some subjects exhibit little or no change in sensitivity. This interindividual subject variation is accounted for by biological differences and also by the fit of the lenses and has been noted by many authors (Dixon, 1964; Gould & Inglima, 1964; Moore & McCollum, 1967; Edmund, 1967; Tanelian & Beuerman, 1980). The quality of the fit of the lenses was

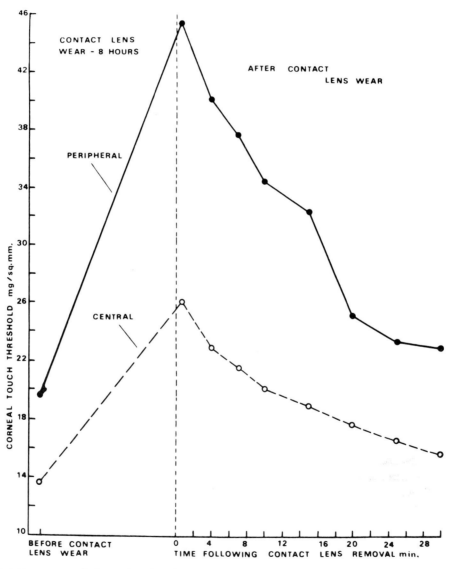

Figure 20.6 Recovery of CTT after hard contact lens wear. Data were obtained in the centre and periphery of the cornea (after Millodot, 1975b).

believed to be mainly responsible for the interindividual variations by Boberg-Ans (1955), Cochet and Bonnet (1960), Moore and McCollum (1967), Sabell (1968), Draeger *et al.* (1980) and Douthwaite & Atkinson (1985). Obviously a well designed and a well fitted lens will enable optimum tear exchange and consequently minimum interference with corneal metabolism.

20.4.2 RECOVERY

Several authors have specifically carried out measurements after removal of the lenses (Boberg-Ans, 1955; Ko & Tomiyama, 1963; Millodot, 1975b; Polse, 1978; Tanelian & Beuerman, 1980; Draeger *et al.*, 1980; Gligo *et al.*, 1981). The recovery of sensitivity was always found. However, the length of time for recovery varies between 20 minutes and 1 week. This variation depends again on biological differences to some extent, but to a large extent on the length of time that the patient has been wearing the lenses and the fit. We shall see that if patients have worn hard lenses for more than 10 years it takes a great deal longer than a week to regain original threshold levels. Figure 20.6 shows the mean data of Millodot (1975b) from 11 subjects who had worn their lenses for 14 months (median). Recovery is not complete in half an hour as CTT should drop to a level below what it was before contact lens wear in the morning due to the diurnal variation. It would take, on average, several hours to reach complete recovery, taking into account the diurnal variation.

20.4.3 SOFT LENSES

The first study of the effect of soft lenses (HEMA) on corneal sensitivity was carried out by Knoll and Williams (1970) and followed by Larke and Sabell (1971). Both investigations concluded that soft lenses gave rise to no statistically significant loss of sensitivity. However, in both instances they were unaware of the existence of a diurnal variation in corneal sensitivity (Millodot, 1972), which should be taken into account. Millodot (1974a, 1976b) measured CTT before and after 4, 8 and 12 hours of continuous, uninterrupted wear of HEMA lenses by 15 subjects. A small but significant increase in CTT was observed after 8 hours of wear, becoming more significant after 12 hours. If the diurnal variation is also taken into account the difference becomes very significant after 8 hours. The data are shown in Figure 20.5 (labelled soft lenses). Similar results were found by Draeger *et al.* (1980) Guillon (1981) and Beuerman and Rozsa (1985). Wide interindividual differences are also noted, which may be due to biological differences and to the fit of the lenses.

Recovery from loss of corneal sensitivity induced by soft lenses is usually more rapid than with hard lenses but also depends upon the nature and duration of wear. Data on recovery have been obtained by Millodot (1974a) and Draeger *et al.* (1980).

High water content soft lenses produce practically no change in corneal sensitivity over a 12-hour period, although different lenses and different fit may cause slightly different results (Millodot, 1976b, 1984; Larke & Hirji, 1979). Data obtained by Millodot (1976b) are also illustrated in Figure 20.5 (labelled extended wear).

20.5 LONG-TERM WEAR

20.5.1 HARD LENSES (PMMA)

Several authors have reported on the effect of wearing of contact lenses on corneal sensitivity after a period of some months, sometimes years of wear. Most of these studies are cross-sectional, while some others are longitudinal in nature.

Cochet and Bonnet (1960) report some longitudinal measurements which were made after 4 hours' wear in 22 myopes over a period of 6 months. It was found that CTT increased rapidly, being highest after 1 month's wear and then decreased progressively in the next few months to regain almost normal threshold level at 6 months. At about the same time, Hamano (1960) reported on a cross-sectional investigation involving four groups of contact lens patients who had worn lenses for different periods of time: 1 month, 2–3 months, 4–8 months and more than 12 months. The greatest change in CTT compared to the control group was found after 1 month's wear and CTT diminished afterwards, although it did not return to normal level. Hamano (1960) did not specify after how many hours of wear he took the measurements. Ko and Tomiyama (1963) also found that subjects who had worn lenses for more than 3 years exhibited marked decrease in corneal sensitivity (by

two or three times) immediately after removing their lenses. Gould and Inglima (1964) observed little change after 10 weeks' wear and 1 year but, again, no reference was made as to how many hours the patient had worn the lenses that day. This is important as measurements made in the morning prior to inserting the lenses would indeed show no change (as there is usually complete recovery) in the first few years of wear. Sabell (1968) mentioned that he found CTT to increase two or three times after adaptation and that in some rare cases which were long term use CTT had increased by some 10-fold. Kemmetmueller (1969) mentioned that contact lens wearers soon have their corneal sensitivity completely restored, although he does not present any data to support his view. Morganroth and Richman (1969) measured two groups; one in

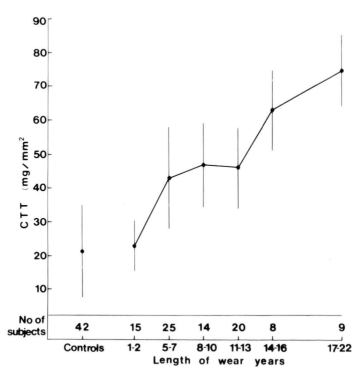

Figure 20.7 Corneal touch threshold as a function of length of wear of hard contact lenses. Controls indicate non-contact lens wearers (after Millodot, 1978c).

which lenses had been worn for no more than 3 months and the other for 5–19 years. Both of these groups showed CTT higher than a third control group and the group wearing lenses for the longest time had a CTT twice as high as the group wearing lenses for a short time.

In a longitudinal investigation lasting 20 weeks Larke and Sabell (1971) observed a progressive and significant reduction in corneal sensitivity. Millodot (1976b) measured the same group of nine subjects 2 years in a row and found a small but not significant difference, as some subjects exhibited an improvement while others showed a degradation. Draeger *et al.* (1980) measured CTT in several groups of subjects who had worn hard lenses for up to 36 months and found a remarkable increase in CTT (more than ten times) up to 2 years, diminishing slightly afterwards. However, with the wear of rigid gas permeable lenses Lydon (1986) obtained a small loss of corneal sensitivity which did not appear to progress over a period of 6 months, while PMMA lenses induced a substantial and progressive loss of sensitivity over the same period of time.

What would happen, though, if lenses were worn for more than, say, 5 years? Morganroth and Richman (1969) already noted a two-fold increase in CTT in their 5–9 years of wear group, compared to their other group of patients (less than 3 months). Millodot (1978b) carried out a systematic cross-sectional investigation of patients wearing their PMMA lenses for up to 22 years. His data obtained in the morning before inserting the lenses showed that after up to 2–3 years of wear recovery was more or less complete overnight. However, after 5 years of wear there was a significant increase in CTT, indicating that recovery was not complete some 12 hours after removal and CTT increased progressively as the number of years of wear increased. The mean data are given in Figure 20.7.

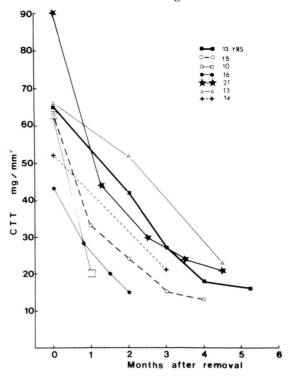

Figure 20.8 Recovery of corneal sensitivity in 7 patients who had worn hard (PMMA) contact lenses for many years (after Millodot, 1978c).

20.5.2 RECOVERY

In view of the dramatic loss of corneal sensitivity accompanying the long-term wear of hard (PMMA) lenses, it was important to establish whether removal of the lenses leads to recovery or whether this loss was irreversible.

Some of the subjects who participated in Millodot's studies (1978b,c) were persuaded to temporarily cease lens wear. In all, seven people, who had worn lenses for 10 to 21 years, obliged. It took between 1 and 4 months to regain normal corneal sensitivity (Fig. 20.8). It also appeared that the longer the initial wear, the longer it took to recover, all other factors (e.g. fit) being the same. Hence long-term wear of hard lenses may induce a greater risk as corneal sensation is chronically depressed.

Therefore, lenses with high oxygen transmissibility such as gas permeable (with high *Dk*) and soft lenses, especially those with high water content, should be the lenses of choice for long-term daily use with respect to corneal sensitivity. However, empirical evidence of very long-term use of these lenses still remains to be presented.

20.5.3   SOFT LENSES

A glimpse of what may happen in the long term to corneal sensitivity with daily wear of soft lenses (HEMA or high water lenses) may be provided by looking at two longitudinal studies with high water extended wear lenses. Larke and Hirji (1979) followed patients who were wearing Sauflon 85 lenses and Millodot (1984) monitored people who were wearing X-Ten lenses for 13 weeks (Fig. 20.9). In both instances corneal sensitivity diminished progressively with the number of weeks of wear reaching about 50% increase in CTT by the end of the 13th week with the X-Ten lens (*Dk* 45). Thus it may be inferred that, even with lenses of high oxygen transmissibility, some loss of corneal sensitivity occurs.

20.6   MECHANISM OF CORNEAL SENSITIVITY LOSS

The dramatic decline and recovery of corneal sensitivity accompanying short- and long-term asymptomatic contact lens wear is perplexing. Sufficient evidence exists to show that it is not a direct consequence of oedema. Indeed, daily wear of lenses for short- and long-term and extended wear lenses can give rise to little or no oedema but large losses of corneal sensitivity. (Hirji, 1978; Millodot, 1978c; Polse, 1978; Millodot, 1984; Lydon, 1986).

The loss could be attributed to sensory adaptation to mechanical stimulation. The

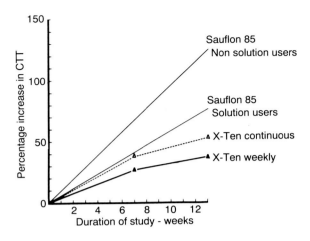

Figure 20.9 Change in corneal touch threshold with two types of high water content soft lenses worn either continuously (Sauflon 85 and X-Ten continuous) or one week at a time (X-Ten weekly), or with a solution of saline water morning and night each day (Sauflon solution users) (after Millodot, 1984).

most obvious support for this view stems from the fact that contact lenses that produce less and less mechanical stimulation (i.e. going from hard to soft to extended wear lenses) give rise to a smaller and smaller decrease in corneal sensitivity. Thus the effect of mechanical stimulation has face validity and could contribute to the reduction in corneal sensitivity when wearing contact lenses. However, this suggestion is irreconcilable with the following two observations. First, when the eyes are closed corneal sensitivity declines dramatically and progressively (Fig. 20.10) as a result of the lower oxygen pressure at the corneal surface and not as a result of mechanical stimulation (Millodot & O'Leary, 1979). Second, exposing the cornea to reduced partial pressure of atmospheric oxygen clearly yields a progressive loss of corneal sensitivity starting 2 or 3 hours after exposure (Fig. 20.11). Yet the cornea is free of any mechanical stimulation.

Fitting gas permeable and PMMA lenses to

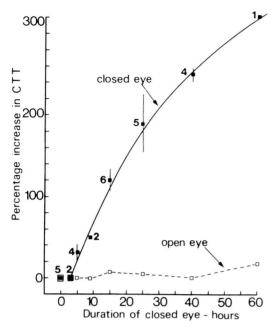

Figure 20.10 Corneal touch threshold as a function of eyelid closure. The open eye served as a control (after Millodot & O'Leary, 1979).

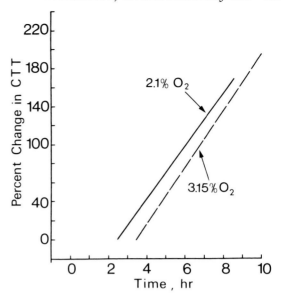

Figure 20.11 Change in CTT as a function of time with exposure to partial oxygen mixtures of 2.1% and 3.15% (after Millodot, 1981).

different groups of people, and also one type of lens to one eye and the other type of lens (of identical design) to the other eye of the same subject led Douthwaite and Connelly (1986) to observe that PMMA lenses led to a greater loss of corneal sensitivity than the gas permeable lenses. Over a 3-month period CTT was not only higher but increased with PMMA lenses, whereas it remained practically the same (or even tended to diminish) with gas permeable lenses. In fact the data obtained for several types of gas permeable lenses tended to show that the greater the Dk the smaller the loss of corneal sensitivity (W.A. Douthwaite, personal communication). In a similar study Lydon (1986) compared the effect of three types of rigid contact lenses and arrived at the same conclusion that epithelial oxygen availability was directly related to changes in corneal sensitivity.

Bergenske and Polse (1987) noted that patients who are refitted with rigid gas permeable lenses after having worn PMMA lenses often regain lens awareness. They substantiated this clinical observation by measuring corneal sensitivity, which they found had returned to almost normal levels, in most subjects of a group of seven, 6 months after refitting.

All the results described above confirm the hypothesis presented by Millodot and O'Leary (1980) that corneal sensitivity is dependent upon the epithelial oxygen level. However, for a given oxygen level (except normal or near normal corneal oxygen pressure) corneal sensitivity does not remain constant. It decreases slowly and progressively. There is a relationship between the time necessary to produce a given loss of corneal sensitivity (say, half the initial value) and epithelial oxygen pressure (Fig. 20.12). Therefore, contact lenses with the greatest possible transmissibility, all other factors being equal, should least affect corneal integrity. For example a daily wear not exceeding

16 hours would require an epithelial oxygen tension of at least 55 mmHg (or an equivalent oxygen pressure of about 8%). Such oxygen tension is easily obtained with material having a permeability of at least 10 and a thickness of no more than 0.1 mm (or any other combination of Dk and t which arrives at the same oxygen transmissibility). However, if tear interchange occurs with each blink the value could be smaller. For continuous wear, or for many years of daily wear, oxygen transmissibility might need to be higher and the lens fitted somewhat loosely to facilitate tear exchange.

20.7 NEUROTRANSMITTER FOR CORNEAL SENSITIVITY

The search for a neurotransmitter to modulate corneal sensitivity is continuing, but evidence is steadily accumulating in favour of acetylcholine. The corneal epithelium is known to possess a high concentration of this substance (von Brucke *et al.*, 1949; Hellauer, 1950; Fitzgerald & Cooper, 1971). Hellauer (1950) suggested that the epithelial cholinergic system was involved in corneal sensitivity, because he found that, by and large, the higher a species' corneal acetylcholine content, the greater the sensitivity. Other evidence for acetylcholine is that the concentration of acetylcholine and corneal sensitivity are greater in the centre than in the periphery of the cornea (Mindel *et al.*, 1979) and that acetylcholine concentration is lower in older animals (Hellauer, 1950), as is corneal sensitivity. Nevertheless, the evidence is not unequivocal and attempts at blocking or enhancing corneal sensitivity with cholinergic drugs have not been one-sided. For example, atropine (a drug that prevents the action of acetylcholine) was found to depress corneal sensitivity in some studies (Umrath & Mussbichler, 1951; von Oer, 1961) but did not affect it in studies by d'Amato (1956) and Tanelian *et al.*, (1982). Similarly with eserine (which neutralizes

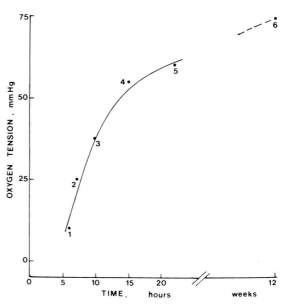

Figure 20.12 Oxygen tension at the corneal surface and time to produce a reduction by half in corneal sensitivity with: 1, 2.1% oxygen mixture (Millodot & O'Leary, 1980); 2, 3.15% oxygen mixture (Millodot & O'Leary, 1980); 3, Hard (PMMA) contact lenses (Millodot & O'Leary, 1980); 4, Eyelid closure (Millodot & O'Leary, 1979); 5, This point is based on some assumptions concerning soft lenses. Soft lenses (HEMA 38%) would produce a loss of a half in sensitivity when extrapolating the data of Millodot (1976). Oxygen transmissibility of such lenses and of that thickness (about 0.18 mm) should lead to an epithelial oxygen tension far lower than the value suggested here and therefore it is hypothesized that appreciable tear exchange with each blink might take place; 6, Extended wear lenses, Sauflon 85 (Larke & Hirji, 1979). Lenses with greater oxygen transmissibility would take longer to induce a reduction by half in corneal sensitivity.

acetylcholinesterase, leaving the action of acetylcholine to continue) was found by von Oer (1961) to enhance sensitivity slightly and by d'Amato (1956) to decrease it.

A controlled study (O'Leary *et al.*, 1986) demonstrated that atropine significantly depresses corneal sensitivity and eserine and pilocarpine significantly increase it. And Tanelian *et al* (1982) found that acetylcholine applied to the corneal epithelium increased action potential frequency. These last two investigations provide strong evidence supporting the hypothesis that epithelial acetylcholine is a neurotransmitter to the corneal nerves. Moreover, indirect evidence was provided several years earlier in an experiment in which the eyelids were closed for various periods of time and corneal sensitivity found to decrease progressively (Millodot & O'Leary, 1979). This was analogous to the observations of Mindel *et al* (1979) who noted that lid closure in rabbits led to a suppression of epithelial acetylcholine.

However, other substances have been considered as possible neurotransmitters such as potassium (Maurice, 1984) or substance P (Tervo *et al.* 1983; Tullo *et al.* 1983) but so far little or no evidence substantiates these suggestions (Tullo *et al.* 1983; Bynke *et al.* 1984). Nevertheless, the ultimate test of acetylcholine as a corneal neurotransmitter will rest on direct evidence obtained by actually measuring this substance in the epithelium under various experimental conditions simultaneously with corneal sensitivity. The mechanism by which stimulation of the corneal epithelium is transduced into a nerve impulse may have to be rethought as there do not seem to be any cholinergic receptors in the epithelium of the rabbit (Olsen & Neufeld, 1979) although more recently Cavanagh & Colley (1981) detected some cholinergic receptors in the rabbit corneal epithelium. It remains to be shown whether such receptors exist in the cornea of man.

20.8 CONCLUSIONS

The utility of testing corneal sensitivity in contact lens practice is becoming apparent. Formerly, it had been thought by many authors that it would serve as a screening device for predicting contact lens tolerance (Berens *et al.*, 1952; Cochet & Bonnet, 1960; Hamano, 1960; Schirmer, 1963; Kraar &

Cummings, 1965; Morganroth & Richman, 1969; Draeger *et al.*, 1980). Hypersensitive people would possibly be unable to endure the lenses. Unfortunately, it was noted that clinical correlation appeared poor as patient motivation is probably more important in adapting to contact lenses. The correlation is in fact more likely to happen with the sensitivity of the eyelids and corneal sensitiveness is not a consideration, *per se*, with soft and ultra-thin soft lenses.

On the other hand, it is useful to detect cases of hypo-aesthesia prior to fitting. These people must be advised to heed the slightest discomfort as failure to act could lead to a corneal infection going unnoticed until quite advanced. Moore and McCollum (1967) reported the case of a patient with a corneal ulcer who was unaware of it and wearing his hard lenses very comfortably.

After fitting, and using the pre-fit CTT as a baseline, the benefit of testing corneal sensitivity is to assess the state of corneal metabolism accompanying the wear of contact lenses. It is a precocious and sensitive indicator of corneal disturbances. For that reason it can help in establishing the optimum fit of a lens (Cochet & Bonnet, 1960; Moore & McCollum, 1967; Sabell, 1968) and whether the lens is being worn properly or overworn. Some diminution of corneal sensitivity will occur in any case with contact lens wear, but the lower the epithelial oxygen pressure, the greater the sensitivity loss. However, it is important to ensure that the amount of hypoaesthesia does not go beyond a given amount (e.g. half its initial value). Otherwise, as corneal sensitivity continues to decline, the cornea deprives itself of its unique alarm signal which normally warns it of something untoward happening to the eye.

The value of corneal sensitivity testing is only lessened by the care that must be taken in measuring CTT. If appropriate precautions are taken, the information supplied can be invaluable to contact lens practice in evaluating the fit of the lenses and the physiological effect of the lens material. Such a suggestion has been made by several authors (Cochet & Bonnet, 1960; Millodot, 1981; Bergenske & Polse, 1987; Douthwaite & Connelly, 1986; Lydon, 1986). In fact, Douthwaite and Connelly (1986) and Lydon (1986) felt that aesthesiometry was the most sensitive test for monitoring the status of the cornea fitted with various types of rigid lenses as compared to refraction, keratometry and pachometry.

REFERENCES

Berens, C., Girard, L. and Foree, K. (1952) Corneal contact lenses. *Trans. Amer. Ophthalmol. Soc.*, **50**, 55–75.

Bergenske, P.D. and Polse, K.A. (1987) The effect of rigid gas permeable lenses on corneal sensitivity. *J. Amer. Optom. Ass.*, **3**, 212–15.

Beuerman, R.W. and Rozsa, A.J. (1985) Threshold and signal detection measurements of the effect of soft contact lenses on corneal sensitivity. *Current Eye Res.*, **4**, 742–4.

Boberg-Ans, J. (1955) Experience in clinical examination of corneal sensitivity. *Br. J. Ophthalmol.*, **39**, 709–26.

Bonnet, R. and Millodot, M. (1966) Corneal aesthesiometry, its measurement in the dark. *Am. J. Optom.*, **43**, 238–43.

von Brucke, H., Hellauer, H.F. and Umrath, K. (1949) Azetylcholin und aneuringehat der hornhaut und seine beziehungen zur nerven versorgung. *Ophthalmalogica*, **117**, 19–35.

Bynke, G., Hakanson, R. and Sundler, F. (1984) Is substance P necessary for corneal nociception? *Eur. J. Pharmacol.*, **101**, 253–8.

Cavanagh, H.D. and Colley, A.M. (1981) Beta-adrenergic and muscarinic binding in corneal epithelium. *Invest. Ophthal.*, **20** (ARVO Suppl.) 37.

Cochet, P. and Bonnet, R. (1960) L'esthésie cornéenne. *Clin. Ophthal.*, **4**, 3–27.

d'Amato, A. (1956) Richerche di estesiometria corneale in condizioni normali, patalogische e dopo instillazione e iniezione sotto-conjiuntivale di colliri. *Gior. Ital. Oftal.*, **9**, 223–34.

Dixon, J.M. (1964) Ocular changes due to contact lenses. *Am. J. Ophthalmol.* **58**, 424–42.

Douthwaite, W.A. and Atkinson, H.L. (1985) The effect of hard (PMMA) contact lens wear on the corneal curvature and sensitivity. *J. Br. Contact Lens Ass.*, **8**, 21–5.

Douthwaite, W.A. and Connelly, A.T. (1986) The effect of hard and gas permeable contact lenses on refractive error, corneal curvature, thickness and sensitivity. *J. Br. Contact Lens Ass.*, **9**, 14–20.

Douthwaite, W.A. and Kaye, N.A. (1980) Is corneal sensitivity related to corneal thickness? *The Ophthal. Optician*, **20**, 753–8.

Draeger, J. (1979) Klinische Ergebnisse der Aesthesiometrie der Hornhaut. *Ber. Dtsch. Ophthal. Ges.*, **76**, 389–95.

Draeger, J., Heid, W. and Luders, M. (1980) L'esthésiometrie chez les porteurs de lentilles de contact. *Contactologia*, **2**, 83–93.

Edmund, J. (1967) The cosmetic indication for using contact lenses. *Acta Ophthalmol.*, **45**, 760–8.

Fitzgerald, G.G. and Cooper, J.R. (1971) Acetylcholine as possible sensory mediator in rabbit corneal epithelium. *Biochem. Pharmacol.*, **20**, 2741–8.

Gligo, D., Vojnikovic, B., Volkoric, A. and Butorac, V. (1981) The effect of hard contact lenses on corneal sensitivity, ocular pressure and coefficient of outflow. In *The Cornea in Health and Disease* (ed. P.D. Trevor Roper), Academic Press, London.

Gould, H.L. and Inglima, R. (1964) Corneal contact lens solutions. *The Eye, Ear, Nose and Throat Monthly*, **43**, 39–49.

Guillon, M. (1981) Long term effects of soft contact lenses. A preliminary report. *J. Br. Contact Lens Ass.*, **4**, 50–8.

Hamano, H. (1960) Topical and systemic influences of wearing contact lenses. *Contacto*, **4**, 41–8.

Hellauer, H.F. (1950) Sensibilitat und acetylcholingehalt der hornhaut verschieder tiere und des menschen. *Z. Verg. Physiol.*, **32**, 303–10.

Hirji, N. (1978) *Some Aspects of the Design and Ocular Response to Synthetic Hydrogel Contact Lenses Intended for Continuous Usage*. PhD dissertation, University of Aston, Birmingham.

Jalavisto, E., Orma, E. and Tawast, M. (1951) Aging and relation between stimulus intensity and duration in corneal sensitivity. *Acta Physiol. Scand.*, **23**, 224–33.

Kemmetmueller, H. (1969) Corneal sensitivity and contact lens fitting. *J. Jap. Contact Lens Soc.*, **20**, 7–12.

Knoll, H.A. and Williams, J. (1970) Effects of

hydrophilic contact lenses on corneal sensitivity. *Am. J. Optom.*, **47**, 561–3.

Ko, L.S. and Tomiyama, S.K. (1963) The influence of contact lens application on the corneal sensitivity. *Trans. Ophthal. Soc. Republic of China.*, **2**, 1–9.

Kolstrad, A. (1970) Corneal sensitivity by low temperatures. *Acta Ophthalmol.*, **48**, 789–93.

Kraar, R.S. and Cummings, C.M. (1965) Lacrimation, corneal sensitivity and corneal abrasive resistance in contact lens wearability. *Optom. Wkly.*, **56**, 25–32.

Larke, J.R. and Hirji, N.K. (1979) Some clinically observed phenomena in extended contact lens wear. *Br. J. Ophthalmol.*, **63**, 475–7.

Larke, J.R. and Sabell, A.G. (1971) A comparative study of the ocular response to two forms of contact lens. *The Optician*, **162** (4187), 8–12.

Lowther, G.E. and Hill, R.M. (1968) Sensibility threshold of the lower lid margin in the course and adaptation to contact lenses. *Am. J. Optom.* **45**, 587–94.

Lydon, D.P.M. (1986) *Effects of Rigid Contact Lens Materials on the Cornea and Tear Film of the Human Eye.* PhD dissertation, University of New South Wales.

Maurice, D.M. (1984) The cornea and sclera. In *The Eye*, Vol. 1 (ed. H. Davson), Academic Press, London.

Millodot, M. (1967) One year after: analysis of a group of contact lens wearers. *The Optician*, **154** (3982), 79–82.

Millodot, M. (1969) Studies on the sensitivity of the cornea. *The Optician*, **157** (4067), 267–71.

Millodot M. (1972) Diurnal variation of corneal sensitivity. *Br. J. Ophthal.*, **56**, 844–7.

Millodot, M. (1973) Objective measurement of corneal sensitivity. *Acta Ophthal. (Kbh)*, **51**, 325–34.

Millodot, M. (1974a) The sensitivity of the cornea. *Atti Fond. Contrti Ist. naz Ottica*, **29**, 889–901.

Millodot, M. (1974b) Effect of soft lenses on corneal sensitivity. *Acta Ophthal. (Kbh)*, **52**, 603–8.

Millodot, M. (1975a) Do blue eyed people have more sensitive corneas than brown eyed people? *Nature (Lond.)*, **255**, 151–2.

Millodot, M. (1975b) Effect of hard contact lenses on corneal sensitivity and thickness. *Acta Ophthal.*, **53**, 576–84.

Millodot, M. (1976a) Corneal sensitivity in people with the same and with different iris colour. *Invest. Ophthal.* **15**, 861–2.

Millodot, M. (1976b) Effect of the length of wear of

contact lenses on corneal sensitivity. *Acta Ophthal.*, **54**, 721–30.

Millodot, M. (1977a) Influence of age on the sensitivity of the cornea. *Invest. Ophthal.*, **16**, 240–2.

Millodot, M. (1977b) The influence of pregnancy on the sensitivity of the cornea. *Br. J. Ophthal.*, **61**, 646–9.

Millodot, M. (1978a) Corneal sensitivity in albinos. *J. Pediat. Ophthal.*, **15**, 300–2.

Millodot, M. (1978b) Effect of long term wear of hard contact lenses on corneal sensitivity. *Arch. Ophthal. N.Y.*, **96**, 1225–7.

Millodot, M. (1978c) Long term wear of hard contact lenses and corneal integrity. *Contacto*, **22**, 7–12.

Millodot, M. (1981) Corneal sensitivity. In 'Complications of contact lenses'. *Int. Ophthalmol. Clin.*, **21**(2), 47–54.

Millodot, M. (1984) Clinical evaluation of an extended wear lens. *Int. Contact Lens Clin.*, **11**, 16–23.

Millodot, M. and Lamont, A. (1974) Influence of menstruation on corneal sensitivity. *Br. J. Ophthal.*, **58**, 49–51.

Millodot, M. and Larson, W. (1967) Effect of bending of the nylon thread of the Cochet-Bonnet aesthesiometer upon recorded pressure. *The Contact Lens*, **1**(3), 5–28.

Millodot, M. and Larson, W. (1969) New measurements of corneal sensitivity: a preliminary report. *Am. J. Optom.*, **46**, 261–5.

Millodot, M. and O'Leary, D.J. (1979) Loss of corneal sensitivity with lid closure in humans. *Exp. Eye Res.*, **29**, 417–21.

Millodot, M. and O'Leary, D.J. (1980) Effect of oxygen deprivation on corneal sensitivity. *Acta Ophthal. (Kbh)*, **58**, 434–9.

Millodot, M. and O'Leary, D.J. (1981) Corneal fragility and its relationship to sensitivity. *Acta Ophthal. (Kbh)*, **59**, 820–6.

Millodot, M. and Owens, H. (1983) Sensitivity and fragility in keratoconus. *Acta Ophthal. (Kbh)*, **61**, 908–17.

Millodot, M. and Vogel, R. (1981) The effect of timolol eye drops on corneal sensitivity in pigmented rabbits. *Res. Clin. Forums*, **3**, 79–83.

Millodot, M., Lim, C.H. and Ruskell, G.L. (1978) A comparison of corneal sensitivity and nerve density in albino and pigmented rabbits. *Ophthal. Res.*, **10**, 7–12.

Millodot, M., Henson, D. and O'Leary, D.J. (1979) Measurement of corneal sensitivity and thickness with PMMA and gas permeable contact lenses. *Am. J. Optom.*, **56**, 628–32.

Mindel, J.S., Szilagyi, P.I.A., Zadunaisky, J.A., Mittag, T. and Orellana, J. (1979) The effects of blepharorrhaphy induced depression of corneal cholinergic activity. *Exp. Eye Res.*, **29**, 463–8.

Moore, C.D. and McCollum, T.H. (1967) Corneal sensitivity and contact lenses. In *Corneal and Scleral Contact Lenses* (ed. L.J. Girard), C V Mosby, Saint Louis, pp. 408–12.

Morganroth, J. and Richman, L. (1969) Changes in the corneal reflex in patients wearing contact lenses. *J. Pediat. Ophthalmol.*, **6**, 207–8.

Neilsen, H.V. (1978) Corneal sensitivity and vibratory perception in diabetes mellitus. *Acta Ophthalmol.*, **56**, 406–12.

O'Leary, D.J. and Millodot, M. (1981) Abnormal epithelial fragility in diabetes and contact lens wear. *Acta Ophthalmol.*, **59**, 827–33.

O'Leary, D.J., Nazarian, J. and Millodot, M. (1986) Which neurotransmitters modulate corneal sensitivity? *Clin. Exp. Optom.*, **69**, 108–11.

Olsen, J.S. and Neufeld, A.H. (1979) The rabbit cornea lacks cholinergic receptors. *Invest. Ophthalmol.*, **18**, 1216–25.

Polse, K.A. (1978) Etiology of corneal sensitivity accompanying contact lens wear. *Invest. Ophthalmol.*, **17**, 1202–6.

Riss, B. and Riss, P. (1981) Corneal sensitivity in pregnancy. *Ophthalmologica*, **183**, 57–62.

Riss, B., Binder, S., Riss, P. and Kemeter, P. (1982) Corneal sensitivity during the menstrual cycle. *Br. J. Ophthalmol.*, **66**, 123–6.

Sabell, A.G. (1968) Ocular changes in contact lens wearers. *The Ophthal. Optician*, **8**, 1051–7.

Schirmer, K.E. (1963) Corneal sensitivity and contact lenses. *Brit. J. Ophthalmol.*, **47**, 493–5.

Schwartz, D.E. (1974) Corneal sensitivity in diabetics. *Arch. Ophthalmol.*, **91**, 174–8.

Strughold, H. (1953) The sensitivity of cornea and conjunctiva of the human eye and the use of contact lenses. *Am. J. Optom.*, **30**, 625–30.

Tanelian, D.L. and Beuerman, R.W. (1980) Recovery of corneal sensation following hard contact lens wear and the implication for adaptation. *Invest. Ophthalmol.*, **19**, 1391–4.

Tanelian, D.L., Beuerman, R.W. and Young, M. (1982) Stimulation of rabbit corneal nerves by acetylcholine and nicotine. *Soc. Neurosci. Abst.*, **8**, 858.

Tervo, T., Tervo, K., Eranko, L., Vannas, A., Eranko, O. and Cuello, A.C. (1983) Substance P immunoreaction and acetylcholinesterase activity in the cornea and gasserian ganglion. *Ophthalmic Res.*, **15**, 280–8.

Tota, G. and Le Marca, F. (1982) Correlazioni tra sensibilita corneale e colore dell'iride. *Atti Fond. Contrti Ist. naz. Ottica.*, **37**, 59–69.

Tullo, A.B., Keen, P., Blyth, W.A., Hill, T.J. and Easty, D.L. (1983) Corneal sensitivity and substance P in experimental herpes simplex keratitis in mice. *Invest. Ophthalmol.*, **24**, 596–8.

Umrath, K. and Mussbichler, H. (1951) Die blockierung der erregring-subertragung von sekundaren sinneszellen auf die herabsetzung der hornhautemfindlichkeit durch atropin. *Z. Vitamin-Hormaon Fermentforsch*, **4**, 182–90.

von Frey, (1894) Cited in Cochet, P. and Bonnet, R. (1960).

von Oer, S. (1961) Uber die beziehung des acetycholins des hornhautepithels zur erregungsubertragung von diesem auf die sensiblen nervenden. *Pflugers Arch. Ges Physiol.*, **273**, 325–34.

J.-P. Guillon and M. Guillon

21.1 INTRODUCTION

Contact lenses do not make direct contact with the ocular tissues but are fully covered by tears. This close interaction between contact lenses and tears impart to tears a particularly important role in achieving successful long-term contact lens wear. This interaction has several disparate aspects. First, contact lenses are very thick, irregular, and permanently moving foreign bodies placed within a much thinner tear film; the net effect of this is to destabilize the tear film. Second, contact lenses selectively attract various components of the tear film. This attraction, which is highly material and lens-type-dependent, imports to contact lenses their on-eye wetting properties. These in turn determine the physical acceptance of contact lenses.

The previous introductory remarks point to a very complex physical and chemical interaction between contact lenses and tears. In order to fully understand this interaction and its evaluation in contact lens practice we will consider both the tear film before the insertion of contact lenses, and during contact lens wear. For the tear film in the absence of contact lenses we refer to the pre-ocular tear film (POTF), and we will briefly summarize its functions, production

formation and drainage with particular reference to contact lenses. We will describe the various techniques available to us to study both the POTF and the pre-lens tear film (PLTF) and evaluate the wettability of contact lenses on the eye. Finally we will describe the interaction between contact lenses and tears by studying the characteristics of the PLTF.

21.2 PRE-OCULAR TEAR FILM CHARACTERISTICS

21.2.1 TEAR FILM FUNCTIONS

Introductory remarks

Maurice (1990) attributes three functions to the tear film; one optical, the second protective and the third lubricative. He argues that the functions of supplying nutrients to the epithelium, which is widely accepted as the fourth function of the tear film, is debatable. These functions and, in particular their relevance to contact lens wear, are summarized below.

Provision of an optical surface

The POTF provides a perfectly smooth optical surface to the strongest refracting component of the eye by forming a continuous film

Contact Lens Practice. Edited by Montague Ruben and Michel Guillon.
Published in 1994 by Chapman & Hall, London. ISBN 0 412 35120 X

that compensates for the micro-irregularities of the anterior epithelial surface (see Chapter 00). The PLTF similarly compensates for the irregularities such as scratches and/or deposits that rapidly appear at the surface of both rigid gas permeable (RGP) (Allary *et al.*, 1989a,b), and hydrophilic contact lenses (Allary *et al.*, 1989b; Guillon *et al.*, 1992) during use.

Protective action

Removal of foreign bodies

There are two aspects to the removal of foreign bodies. First, there is the well known removal of airborne particles and/or chemical irritants that takes place by the flushing of the anterior ocular surfaces via reflex lacrimation, but also as important is the action of the basal lacrimation that removes the necrotic epithelial cells from the anterior ocular surface (Lemp, 1976), via the normal blinking action and the specific role of the mucous component of the tear film (Holly & Lemp, 1977). In fact this latter role is the key to successful contact lens wear, in particular for extended wear. For that modality of wear it has been shown that unless all epithelial metabolic debris, that may be trapped between the contact lens and the cornea, are totally flushed within four hours of eye opening, adverse ocular reactions will most likely take place (Mertz & Holden, 1981).

Antimicrobial activity

Both the basal and reflex tear compositions reveal a wide range of proteins (Fullard & Snyder, 1990). Amongst these, lysozyme gives the tear film its main bacteriolytic activity. This action is enhanced by several other proteins, such as transferrin (Ford *et al.*, 1976), lactotransferrin (Liotet *et al.*, 1980), immunoglobulin (McClellan *et al.*, 1973) and possibly betalysin (Jansen *et al.*, 1984) which are normally found in the tear film. The

second antimicrobial activity is mechanical and associated with the mucus system that forms a strand that traps small particles such as bacteria and eliminates them (Holly & Lemp, 1977).

The presence of a contact lens alters the tears' antibacterial activity. Several studies have shown that the conjunctival flora is altered by the presence of a contact lens (Rehim & Samy, 1988), usually with a reduction in antibacterial activity. Recently, however, studies have suggested no effect (Elander *et al.*, 1992), and at least one study (Boles *et al.*, 1991) has shown that ionic lenses that attract high levels of lysozyme during wear offer an enhanced antibacterial activity.

Lubrication

The presence of relatively large amounts of mucin along the lid margins and the spontaneous mucin spread over the whole corneal surface during blink (Lemp *et al.*, 1970) ensures that no direct solid-to-solid contact takes place during blink. This lubricating action is essential for an efficient, trauma-free blink action. Similarly, when a contact lens is worn the mucin coating contributes to ensuring a trauma-free contact lens movement. In fact, variation in the nature of the lens coating during overnight wear leads to a highly viscous PLTF at waking and reduces contact lens movement at that time of day (Guillon, 1991; Guillon & Guillon, 1991).

Maintenance of ocular integrity

The tears ensure the maintenance of ocular integrity by creating a moist surface at the anterior epithelial surface, any failure leads to keratinization and loss of transparency (Tiffany & Bron, 1978). It is via the tears that the atmospheric oxygen during the day and the palpebral vascular oxygen at night reach the epithelium. It is also via the tears that the carbon dioxide that builds up during the epithelial metabolic activity is eliminated.

The role of the tear film, however, is only a passive one; no effect takes place during either the passage of oxygen or carbon dioxide.

Similarly, whereas one often thinks of the tear film as a source of nutrients for the epithelium, Ehlers (1965) has put forward information suggesting the contrary. He showed that most nutrients, which are hydrophilic components, cannot penetrate the epithelial surface.

21.2.2   TEAR FILM STRUCTURE AND GEOGRAPHIC DISTRIBUTION

Tear film structure

General description

The classic description of the tear film is a basic trilaminar structure (Wolff 1946, 1954), with a basal mucous layer spread over the corneal surface, an intermediate aqueous layer and a superficial lipid layer. That basic structure has been refined to include supplementary aqueous mucous interface and aqueous lipid interface regions with slightly different mixed compositions (Fig. 21.1) (Holly & Lemp, 1971). It is that model that we briefly describe and will use to explain the interaction of contact lenses with the tear film.

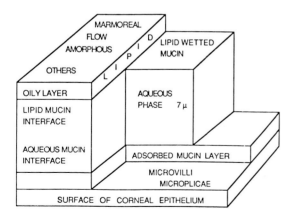

Figure 21.1 Schematic representation of modified trilaminar tear structure.

Mucous layer

The inner mucous layer is thought to be extremely thin (0.02 to 0.04 μm) (Holly, 1973a) and have a complex mucoglycoproteinic structure (Holly 1973a, Greiner *et al.*, 1980, Van Haeringen, 1981). The glycoprotein part of the layer is surface active, producing a hydrophobic segment that attaches to the cornea, and a hydrophilic one on which is formed the aqueous film. That active role explains the extreme importance of this very thin layer in maintaining a stable tear film.

Aqueous layer

The intermediate aqueous layer accounts for over 90% of the tear film thickness and is made of 98% water and of 1.8% solids (Ridley & Sorsby, 1940). The solids present are both organic components, mainly high molecular weight proteins such as lysozyme, albumin and globulin (Fullard & Snyder, 1990) and inorganic electrolytes such as sodium, potassium, calcium, chloride and bicarbonate. These inorganic components give to the tears their chemical characteristics. Sodium (145 mg/ml), potassium (16 to 24 mg/ml) and chloride (128 to 144 mg/ml) regulate the osmotic pressure (Bothelo, 1964; Guilhard *et al.*, 1968). The osmotic pressure of the tears is approximately 305 mosml/kg, equivalent to 0.95% sodium chloride (Guilhard *et al.*, 1968; Terry & Hill, 1978). The tear osmotic pressure varies with the ocular location and is known to be affected by contact lens wear in non-adapted patients. Bicarbonate (26 mg/ml), involved with pH regulation, has a buffering action keeping the pH near tonicity (7.45) with ranges between 7.14 and 7.82 (Carney & Hill, 1976). Both diurnal (Carney & Hill, 1976) and contact-lens-induced variations have been observed. Calcium is found in low concentration (0.4 to 1.1 mg/ml) and seems not to have any particular role.

Lipid layer

The outer lipid layer, which is relatively thin (0.01 to 1.5 µm), is composed mainly of cholesterol esther and other esther waxes, some free cholesterol and very few free fatty acids (Furukawa & Polse, 1978, Nicolaides, 1986). Its main role is to prevent evaporation and, as for the mucous layer, the lipid layer plays a key role in maintaining a stable tear film. Because its structure is highly variable, the lipid layer gives different properties to the tear film. It is those differences in structure that are studied during the clinical evaluation.

Geographic tear distribution

The tear volume that totals approximately 7 µl (Mishima *et al.*, 1966) to 8.5 µl (Furukawa & Polse, 1978) is best described in two parts: the exposed tear volume (ETV), which is in direct contact with the air, and the unexposed tear volume (UTV) (Port & Asaria, 1990). The exposed part of the lacrimal fluid that constitutes just under half the total volume (Mishima *et al.*, 1966) is the most significant one as far as contact lens wear is concerned. The ETV is divided into the preocular part, a thin continuous layer covering the cornea and exposed conjunctiva and a marginal part, called alternatively lid tear meniscus or lid tear prism, situated along the upper and lower lids. It is estimated that between 72.5 and 90% (Mishima *et al.*, 1966; Holly, 1981; Kwok, 1984; Bron, 1985; Guillon & Guillon, 1988a; Port & Asaria, 1990) of the ETV is found within the lid tear meniscus. On average the lid tear meniscus has a volume of 5.25 µl and the pre-ocular part a volume of 1.75 µl (Mishima *et al.*, 1966). The most critical part of the tear film is the junction between the lid tear meniscus and pre-ocular tear. At that point the surface tension forces present make the formation of a continuous film near impossible (Holly, 1978) (Fig. 21.2). The result is a line of minimal thickness, often referred to as

the black line because of its appearance when fluorescein is instilled in the eye (Fig. 21.3). That junction zone of minimal thickness corresponds to the zone of the tear film with the greatest instability. Its effect has been demonstrated in various ways in contact lens practice. Several studies have shown that the film, whether pre-ocular (Guillon & Guillon, 1988a, 1989a), pre-lens soft (Guillon & Guillon, 1988c, 1989b) or RGP (Guillon & Guillon, 1988d) first breaks in that region.

21.2.3   THE LACRIMAL SYSTEM

Introductory comments

The lacrimal system can be divided into three components: secretory, distributional and excretory. The secretory component is made up of a series of glands distributed throughout the anterior ocular surface. The distribution relates to the distribution of tears over the ocular surface. The excretory component refers to the elimination of tears from the eye.

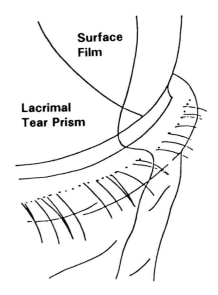

Figure 21.2 Schematic representation of junction between tear meniscus and pre-ocular tear film (by courtesy of McDonald, 1968).

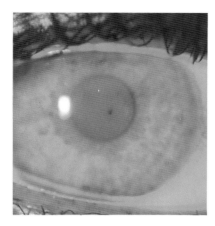

Figure 21.3 Tear fluorescein coloration showing the 'black' junction line of highest tear film instability between the tear meniscus and the pre-ocular tear film.

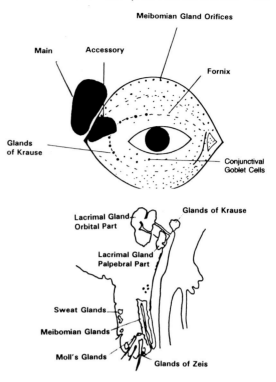

Figure 21.4 Distribution of the various glands producing the lacrimal fluid. (a) frontal view; (b) section through eyelid (by courtesy of Tiffany & Bron, 1978).

Tear production

The secretory component is responsible for both the basal and reflex tear secretions. The various glands responsible for producing the tear film (Adler, 1965) (Fig. 21.4) are:

1. The lacrimal gland proper, located in the upper temporal quadrant of the eye, which is divided into a main and accessory part (Allansmith *et al.*, 1976). Both parts of the lacrimal gland proper are seromucous glands (Ruskell, 1968; Jensen *et al.*, 1969; Allen *et al.*, 1972) and are responsible for producing the basal and reflex aqueous parts of the lacrimal fluid (Jordan & Baum, 1980).
2. The accessory lacrimal glands of Krause, which are situated in both fornices, but mainly in the upper one, and the glands of Wolfring near the tarsus. These glands also contribute in a minor role to the production of the aqueous tears.
3. The goblet cells or Crypts of Henle, found in the fornices, produce the ocular mucus which appears as a complex gel, made up mainly of mucin (Folch *et al.*, 1957). This part of the lacrimal fluid is also produced by the conjunctival epi-

thelial cells (Greiner *et al.*, 1980; Dilly, 1986) and the lacrimal gland proper (Allansmith *et al.*, 1976).

4. The glands of Meibomius, which are numerous and situated within the tarsal plates, with their orifices at the lid margin immediately posterior to the lashes line, are responsible for the lipidic part of the lacrimal fluid.
5. The glands of Zeis and Moll, both with their orifices situated at the lid margin, are also responsible for a minor part of the lipidic component of the lacrimal fluid.

Tear distribution

The tears are redistributed over the ocular surface at every blink, or 5 to 12 times a minute in a normal situation. The formation of the pre-ocular tear film is therefore a very dynamic phenomenon due to the physico-chemical interactions taking place during the blinking process, that lasts on average 0.3 s (Doane, 1980). Holly (1973a) was the first to describe this process fully, and a summary of this description is of help to explain contact lens on-eye wettability and the relevance of the various clinical tests. The closing of the lids has three effects (Forst, 1982):

1. It eliminates the aqueous part of the tears.
2. It redistributes the mucin over the ocular surface, to render it highly wettable.
3. It squashes the lipids between the upper and lower lid edges.

During lid closure the lipids are prevented from migrating under the lids due to the lid edge mucous and form a thick film in the narrow space between the two eyelids (Holly, 1980).

The opening of the eyelids redistributes the aqueous tear immediately, along with a monomolecular lipid layer at its anterior surface (Holly, 1973b). A secondary upper lipid motion accompanied by a slight increase in the aqueous layer follows. The process results in a stable tear film less than 1s after eye opening.

In between blinks, the tear film destabilizes relatively rapidly, leading to the formation of dry spots that trigger the next blink. Dry spots are thought to be due to the migration of the superficial lipids towards the ocular surface, rendering it hydrophobic by contaminating the mucous coating (Fig. 21.5) (Holly 1973a). The rapidity of the contamination is increased by the local thinning of the aqueous tear film when, as during contact lens wear, the overall tear film is thinner than normal. The latter is a very important determining factor in producing a low tear film stability.

In between blinks, a vector flow also exists which is limited to the upper and lower tear prisms (Holly & Lemp, 1977) and does not

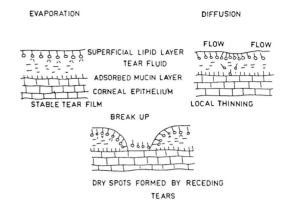

Figure 21.5 Diagrammatic representation of the mechanism of dry spot formation (by courtesy of Holly, 1973a).

affect the pre-ocular tear film (Ehlers, 1965).

Tear Excretion

The tears leave the ocular surface via three mechanisms: (1) the exchange of tears across the conjunctival surface: (2) loss due to evaporation; and (3) tear drainage at the puncti. In humans it has been estimated that between 8% (Schirmer, 1903) and 20% (Maurice, 1973) of the tear film is eliminated each minute by exchange across the conjunctival surface. The amount of tears lost by evaporation depends greatly upon environmental conditions, in particular, relative humidity and turbulent air flow (Holly, 1973b). A decrease of the first and an increase of the second contribute towards increasing the evaporation. A recent study indicates that evaporation could eliminate tears at a rate of 10 to 15% per minute (Tomlinson *et al.*, 1991). Finally during blinking, tears are pushed towards the puncti at the inner canthus, where they are passed in the nasolacrimal duct.

21.3 CLINICAL EVALUATION TECHNIQUES

21.3.1 INTRODUCTORY REMARKS

Numerous routine and/or research clinical techniques have been used to study the tears of the contact lens wearer (Guillon, 1990).

Initially the techniques used were those that had been developed to study patients with pathological dry eye, such as the Schirmer test (Schirmer, 1903). Such tests proved to be of limited use for the evaluation of contact lens wearers. More recently, clinical techniques have been either modified and/or developed with the prime objective the contact lens wearer (Guillon, 1990). Some of the techniques developed are limited to the research environment. In this category are all the techniques that aim to measure tear evaporation, using evaporometers with different levels of invasiveness (Hamano *et al.*, 1981; Cedarstaff & Tomlinson, 1983; Rolando & Refojo, 1983) and techniques to measure tear flow rate using modified fluorophotometers (Benedetto *et al.*, 1984; Occhinpinti *et al.*, 1988). Also in this category are the techniques that use biodifferential interference microscopy (Hamano *et al.*, 1979) to study the structure of the tear film. These techniques will not be discussed in the current chapter.

This chapter is limited to research and/or routine techniques that can be used or easily introduced in general clinical routine. These techniques can be divided into two groups based upon the instrumentation used. The majority are based around the slit lamp biomicroscope and include easier, alternative ways of using the instrument or special attachments. The second group of techniques are those that stand alone (e.g. Schirmer) or use other instruments such as the keratometer. The approach adopted in this chapter has been to group the techniques into three categories according to their aim: (1) evaluation of the tear film structure; (2) evaluation of the tear volume; and (3) evaluation of the tear film stability.

The same techniques are directly applicable to the evaluation of both the pre-ocular and pre-lens tear films, and therefore described as one; when minor differences are present they are highlighted.

21.3.2 EVALUATION OF THE TEAR FILM STRUCTURE AND ADJACENT STRUCTURES

Lid edge anomalies

Introductory remarks

Anomalies of the lid border, where the exposed tear film comes into contact with the complex ocular structures present at the lid edge, must be considered when evaluating the tears of the contact lens wearer (Guillon & Guillon, 1989b). This assessment is carried out under diffuse lighting and involves the assessment of both the upper and lower lid margins. The structures of particular interest are the lashes and meibomian gland orifices.

Observations and classifications

Lashes The lashes are a potential source of contamination of the tear film because of their close proximity to the tear meniscus. Scaly lashes associated with epidermic problems and contamination associated with make-up are often encountered. The level of contamination of both the lower and upper lashes can be classified into five categories:

1. Clean lashes.
2. Scaly lashes.
3. Light make-up contamination.
4. Medium make-up contamination.
5. Heavy make-up contamination.

Any contamination present or scales due to epidermic problems should be eliminated before contact lens fitting is undertaken or during any refitting process. In the latter case, if symptoms are present, elimination of these problems is an essential requirement.

Lid margin

Foam Abnormal meibomian secretion produces bubble-like formations mostly at the canthus and, in more severe cases, along the lid margins. The appearance of these formations, referred to as 'foam' are classified into seven categories according to their location:

0. None.
1. Upper lid.
2. Lower lid.
3. Both lids.
4. Canthus.
5. Canthus and lower lid.
6. Canthus and both lids.

Droplets The lid area within the lashes line becomes wettable only when contamination occurs. This lid edge contamination is revealed by the presence of tear droplets covering the contaminated area. These 'droplets' are classified into five categories according to the number of droplets seen:

1. None.
2. 1 droplet.
3. 2–3 droplets.
4. 4–5 droplets.
5. > 5 droplets.

The presence of 'foam' along the lids, in particular when both are affected and/or the presence of four or more 'droplets', is a source of concern and the underlying cause for these anomalies should be ascertained and remedied before contact lens fitting is undertaken.

Meibomian gland blockage Abnormal meibomian secretions tend to solidify at normal lid temperature and block the meibomian glands, especially when associated with meibomian gland dysfunction. The state of the meibomian glands for each lid is classified into four categories according to the number of glands affected (Fig. 21.6):

1. None.
2. 1–2 glands.
3. 3–5 glands.
4. > 5 glands.

The lid border contamination is more common in females. This is associated with the

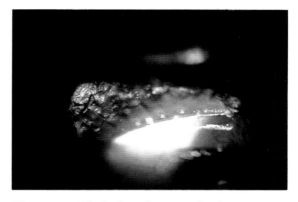

Figure 21.6 Blocked meibomian glands.

use of eyeliner and mascara (Guillon & Guillon, 1988a,b). In that context, the following classification of make-up use is helpful to ascertain the potential risk of contamination:

1. None.
2. Slight make-up.
3. Moderate make-up.
4. Heavy make-up.

It is pertinent to ascertain whether the pencil eyeliner is applied within or outside the line of the lashes. The former practice is always a major source of contamination and potential infection. This practice must be avoided by all contact lens wearers. If the meibomian gland dysfunction is not make-up related, the underlying cause must be determined and remedied. Often a lid scrub treatment is very effective at helping to unblock the meibomian glands.

Palpebral tear menisci

The tear menisci situated along the upper and lower lids, as indicated earlier, hold most of the ETV. Their structure is therefore of great clinical interest (McDonald, 1969; Holly & Lemp, 1977; Taylor, 1980; Guillon & Guillon, 1989a,b; Port & Asaria, 1990). All the techniques mentioned involve the use of the slit lamp biomicroscope. Because of anatomical limitation the lower meniscus is easier to examine and, as similar conclusions are reached following the examination of both the upper and lower tear menisci (Guillon *et al.*, 1988; Guillon & Guillon, 1989a), we suggest limiting the routine clinical evaluation to the latter. Four characteristics of the tear menisci have been evaluated: height, width, regularity and curvature. The latter two parameters are of particular diagnostic interest with regard to the tear meniscus structure.

The regularity of the lower tear menisci is best observed under medium magnification (×20) under diffuse lighting or with a broad (3–4 mm) focal light (Fig. 21.7). Various criteria have been given as to an abnormal tear meniscus:

1. Holly and Lemp (1977) have suggested that a scanty meniscus appearance or the presence of an area of discontinuity were signs of an aqueous tear deficiency and/or lipid abnormality.
2. Taylor (1980) suggests classifying the tear menisci as intact (no zone of irregularity) for a normal patient, as intermittently non-intact (presence of zone(s) of irregularity at times) or permanently non-intact (permanent zones of irregularity) as abnormal menisci.
3. Guillon and Guillon (1988; 1989a) have

described a simple clinical technique (see page 000) and compare the height of the tear prism immediately under the centre of the pupil and both 5 mm nasally and temporally. They suggest that a large difference between the central measurement and either of the peripheral measurements is a sign of irregularity.

The curvature of the tear meniscus is best studied by lighting up the meniscus with a thin vertical slit (McDonald, 1969) and observing it under medium magnification (×20 to ×30). The normal meniscus should be convex near the cornea, concave centrally and convex at its contact with the eyelid.

Pre-ocular tear film structure

General Remarks

The pre-ocular tear film is transparent, which makes the observation of its component structures very difficult. However, basic optics indicate that, at any interface where a difference in refractive index exists, a small percentage of the incident light is specularly reflected. The light reflected at the air lipid interface constitutes the first Purkinje image visible during biomicroscopy (Fig. 21.8). Because the refractive index of the lipid layer is higher than that of the aqueous layer, there is a second interface, between the two layers, which renders that surface visible in specular observation. The reflection taking place between the aqueous layer and the corneal epithelium should be the third interface of relevance. However, we have shown that the surface of the epithelium, due to the presence of microvilli, is highly irregular and does not produce a smooth regular reflecting surface (Guillon, 1986). We know that such a regular surface is neutralized due to its coverage by mucin. When the mucin layer is fully hydrated, the difference in refractive

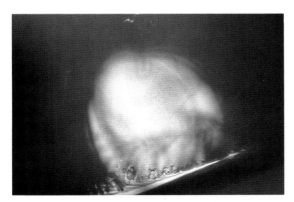

Figure 21.7 Tear prism irregularity observed by slit lamp biomicroscopy under diffuse lighting.

index between the mucin and the aqueous layer is so low that no useful specular reflection takes place. It is the observation and measurement of these specular reflections that permit the evaluation of the pre-ocular tear film structure.

Narrow field slit lamp technique

The observation of the pre-ocular tear film in specular reflection with a biomicroscope is not recent (Marx, 1921; Vogt, 1921; Koby, 1924; Meesman, 1927; Fisher, 1928; Fisher, 1940; Wolff, 1946, Edmund, 1951; Ehlers, 1965; Guillon, 1982; Josephson, 1983; Forst, 1990).

The observation is very easy to carry out. One simply locates the bright reflection produced by the slit beam and focuses the biomicroscope in that region. The observations are usually made at a medium to high magnification (×30 to ×40). The technique has, however, two main drawbacks. First, the light source of the biomicroscope subtends only a small angle. The specular

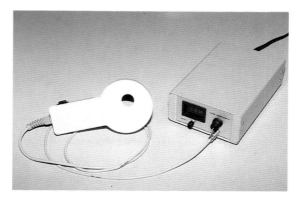

Figure 21.9 Tearscope hand-held cold diffuse light source for biomicroscope.

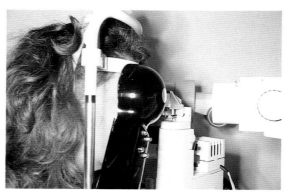

Figure 21.10 Tearscope used in conjunction with biomicroscope.

reflection only allows, at the most, the observation of a 1 mm × 2 mm zone at any one time. Second, because the slit lamp biomicroscope is a heat source, it artificially dries up the tear film and alters its structure in time. Two simple steps to minimize these drawbacks are to use a diffuser in front of the light source to defocalize the light and increase its angular subtend, and to decrease the light output of the slit lamp with the rheostat.

Wide field slit lamp technique

The first solution to the main drawback of the limited field of useful reflection, inherent to the conventional slit lamp technique, was

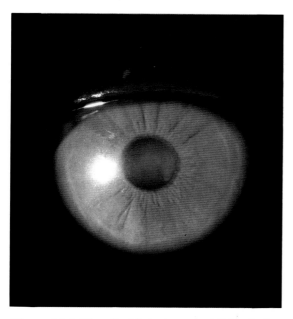

Figure 21.8 First Purkinje image visible during slit lamp biomicroscopy.

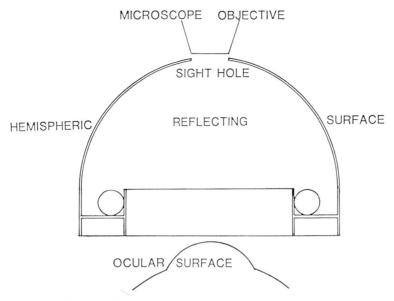

MICROSCOPE   OBJECTIVE

SIGHT HOLE

HEMISPHERIC   REFLECTING   SURFACE

OCULAR / SURFACE

Figure 21.11 Schematic diagram of wide field lighting system for tear film observation.

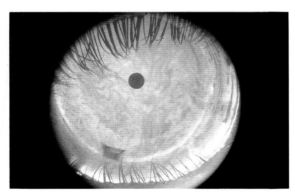

Figure 21.12 Tear film appearance under low magnification when lit up by wide field lighting system.

introduced by McDonald (1968, 1969). He positioned a hemispherical close examination medical lamp in front and slightly to the temporal side of the subject's eye and observed, with the biomicroscope, the large reflection produced by the front surface of the tear film. This led to important new understanding, and inspired various work-

ers to develop different new lighting systems, including a retro-illuminated cone of light (Haberick & Lingelback, 1981), a modification of the standard Bausch and Lomb keratometer to produce a diffuse light source (Knoll & Walters, 1985) and the development of a special hand-held light source for the observation of the tear film with the biomicroscope (Guillon, 1986, 1990). Whereas the former two did not evolve with time, the last one has lead to many publications, the ensuing device being the tearscope.

The tearscope is a hand-held instrument (Fig. 21.9) that is used in conjunction with the biomicroscope (Fig. 21.10). The slit light source of the biomicroscope is positioned nasally to the patient and not switched on. The tearscope acts as the light source for the biomicroscope, which is used at all magnification settings. The tearscope lighting system is a diffuse hemispherical light source with a central hole to allow viewing (Fig. 21.11). The key feature of the system is the use of a cold cathode light source that does not create any artificial drying of the tear film during its examination. One point to remember is that the light source is diffuse and does not have to be in focus with the tear surface to obtain a clear image of the tear film (Fig. 21.12), only the biomicroscope is required to be in focus. The aim is to keep the tearscope as close to the eye as possible to produce the largest illuminated zone possible. The observations of the patterns are made at ×20 to ×40 magnification to study the various details of interest.

General physical interpretation of the observations

The initial observations made revealed the presence of interference fringes (Marx, 1921; Vogt, 1921; Meesman, 1927) and the occasional presence of surface particles (Koby, 1924). These interference fringes were of different colours, due to the light source's wide spectrum; all were from the first order of

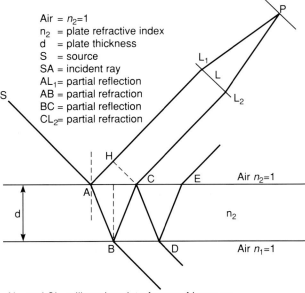

$Air = n_2 = 1$
n_2 = plate refractive index
d = plate thickness
S = source
SA = incident ray
AL_1 = partial reflection
AB = partial refraction
BC = partial reflection
CL_2 = partial refraction

AL_1 and CL_2 will produce interference fringes on plate P after recombination by lens L

At A: there is a change of phase due to reflection at a denser medium

Figure 21.14 Optical diagram depicting the principle of the formation of constructive interference fringes (Guillon, 1989).

interference (Fig. 21.13). The reconstructive interferences observed are produced by the reflected light at the air–lipid and lipid–aqueous interfaces (McDonald, 1969) (Fig. 21.14). For a conventional biomicroscope with non-monochromatic light, the colours most often visible are brown, indigo and blue. These correspond respectively to a lipid layer thickness of 143 nm, 196 nm and 221 nm if we take the average refractive index of lipids to be 1.5. The observation of the tear film by various workers (Hamano *et al.*, 1979, 1980; Norn, 1979; Guillon 1986; Guillon & Guillon, 1988c) have shown that most commonly the lipidic reflection produces a colourless pattern (Fig. 21.15) because its thickness is below the minimal thickness to produce interference fringes. In that case

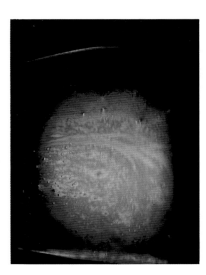

Figure 21.13 First order interference fringes produced by lipid layer and visible within the first Purkinje image.

Norn (1979) has suggested a semi-qualitative technique to estimate the lipid thickness. Norn takes advantage of the phenomenon described earlier, whereby eyelid closure squeezes the lipid layer within the inter-palpebral aperture and thickens it inversely proportionally to the palpebral aperture. The patient is asked to produce a slow voluntary closure, during which it is possible to observe the position when the first fringes appear. The ratio between the full aperture and the aperture when the first fringes appear enables us to estimate the thickness of the lipid layer for that subject.

Early on, during the study of these fringes, it was noticed (McDonald, 1969) that these fringes broke and that, at times, particularly in front of the contact lens, a second series of interferences became visible; these interference fringes, contrary to the lipid fringes, were of increasing order (Fig. 21.16). The thickness involved led to the conclusion that those were produced within the thinning aqueous layer (McDonald, 1969; Guillon, 1990).

The aqueous pattern is, however, not visible most of the time. This is due to the fact that the lipid layer is totally reflective in specular reflection, and hence hides the underlying pattern. The aqueous pattern is

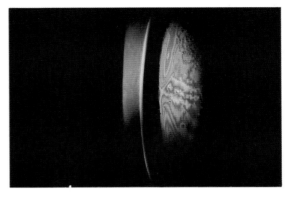

Figure 21.16 Increasing order interference fringes produced by thinning aqueous layer and visible within the first Purkinje image.

therefore most visible when the lipid layer is very thin and semi-transparent

Clinical classifications and interpretation

Lipid layer patterns Three aspects of the lipid layer have been classified: its pattern, thickness and contamination by particles.

Forst (1990) proposes a simple three category classification (Table 21.1):

1. *Grainy, flowing pattern.* This pattern is considered as the normal pattern, present in approximately 70% of the population.
2. *Irregular, yellow-brown pattern.* This pattern is considered to be transitional between the physiological and pathological patterns and encountered in approximately 27% of the population.
3. *Highly coloured pattern.* This pattern is

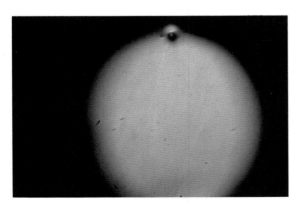

Figure 21.15 Colourless pattern produced by the lipid layer and visible within the first Purkinje image.

Table 21.1 Lipid pattern classification (after Forst, 1990)

Description	Incidence (%)
Grainy/flowing	70
Irregular/yellow–brown	27
Highly coloured	3

thought to be pathological, affecting approximately 3% of the population.

Guillon and co-workers (Guillon, 1986; Guillon & Guillon, 1988b), basing their investigations upon the work of several groups (McDonald, 1969; Hamano *et al.*, 1979, 1980), arrived at a six-category classification (Table 21.2). These patterns are listed in order of increasing thickness:

1. *Open meshwork (open marmoreal).* Appearance: the grey, marble-like pattern is due to thicker local lipid areas found over a thin, lighter colour main layer. The pattern or meshwork is open and fairly sparse (Fig. 21.17). This pattern corresponds to the thinnest lipid layer visible.

    Clinical implications: the main clinical implications are possible contact lens drying problems due to high evaporation rate associated with very thin lipid layer.

2. *Closed meshwork (closed marmoreal).* Appearance (Fig. 21.8): it is a grey, marble-like pattern, as previously described, but with closed meshwork and tight pattern. The pattern corresponds to a thicker, more stable, more visible layer than the open meshwork.

    Clinical implications: this pattern corresponds to a stable POTF and those subjects are good candidates for both rigid and soft contact lenses.

3. *Flow pattern (Wave pattern).* Appearance (Fig. 21.19): it is a wavy, constantly

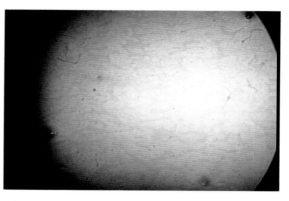

Figure 21.17 Open meshwork (open marmoreal) lipid pattern.

changing pattern during the interblink period; the most commonly encountered pattern. The cause of this pattern is poor mixing of lipids of varying classes. The differential diagnosis from a marmoreal pattern is the constantly changing aspect of the flow pattern and its more round shape.

    Clinical implications: it is generally a stable tear film, contact lens fitting is possible with these subjects. One should however, be aware of the possibility of occasional excess lipid deposition.

4. *Amorphous pattern.* Appearance (Fig. 21.20): the pattern has a blue/whitish appearance due to a thick, well mixed lipid layer. It is the normal lipid pattern amongst non-contact lens wearers.

    Clinical implications: it is a highly

Table 21.2 Lipid pattern classification

Description	Incidence(%)	Estimated thickness (nm)
Open meshwork	21	≈15
Closed meshwork	10	≈30
Flow	23	30 to 80
Amorphous	24	=80
Colour	15	80 to 370
Other	7	variable

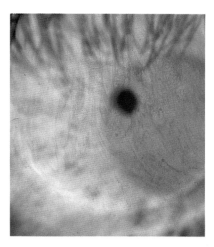

Figure 21.18 Closed meshwork (closed marmoreal) lipid pattern.

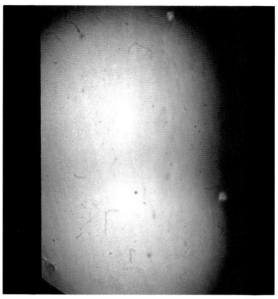

Figure 21.20 Amorphous lipid pattern.

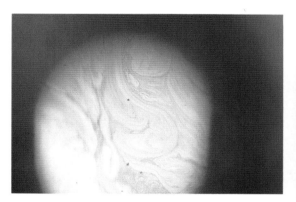

Figure 21.19 Flow (wave) lipid pattern.

stable tear film, usually good for contact lens wear with very occasional greasing problem due to the high volume of lipid present.

5. *Colour fringe pattern.* Appearance (Fig. 21.21): the pattern is formed of interference colours that spread over different discrete areas and are confined to yellow, brown, blue and purple. These coloured parts are the thickest zones of the lipid layer with the grey background being slightly thinner and not producing an interference pattern.

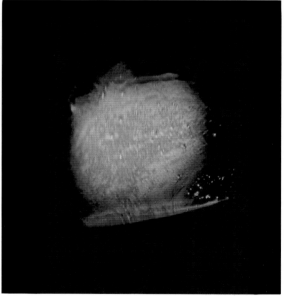

Figure 21.21 Colour fringe lipid pattern.

Clinical implications: it is a very thick stable lipid pattern, contact lens wear is possible. However, contamination of the contact lens surface by the large amount of lipids may lead to a destabilization of the PLTF.

6. *Other patterns.* Lipid patterns that are difficult to classify are also encountered. Usually highly variable coloured patterns (Fig. 21.22) with possible mixing of mucous strands. These patterns can be considered as pathological and a contraindication to contact lens fitting.

Often at low magnification, when the whole cornea is viewed at once, more than one pattern is visible. A particularly common combination is a main closed meshwork pattern combined with areas of flow pattern (Fig. 21.23). Another combination that is often found is that of an amorphous pattern and a coloured fringe pattern (Fig. 21.24). Here the interference colours are of first order yellow and brown and occasionally blue, which correspond to lipid layer thicknesses of 90, 140 and 220 nn, respectively.

The properties of any combination lipid layer are a combination of its two components.

Lipid layer thickness evaluation The lipid layer pattern appearance and visibility give some indication as to its thickness. The open meshwork marmoreal pattern is usually associated with a thin lipid layer, which can be as thin as 15 nm. Its visibility under ×20 to ×30 magnification is very poor and is usually recognizable only by its post-blink movement. As the lipid layer thickness increases, the meshwork becomes denser, changing successively to a closed meshwork and to a wave pattern for thickness approximating 80 nm. Above that thickness an amphorous pattern appears with no distinguishable details, followed by colour fringe pattern indicating usual thicknesses from 90 to 220 nm. Occasionally this layer is much thicker, exhibiting interference fringes corresponding to a lipid layer thickness of 600 nm.

If one wishes to evaluate the thickness more precisely, the technique first described by Norn (1979) is recommended. The thickness can be estimated as:

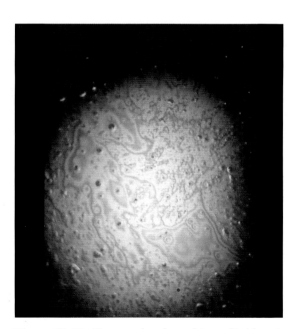

Figure 21.22 Abnormal colour fringe lipid pattern.

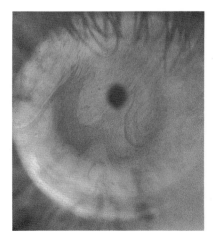

Figure 21.23 Meshwork/flow combination pattern visible at low magnification.

implications of moderate or severe contamination depends upon the types of contaminants.

Regardless of the lipid pattern present it is essential to assess the level of the tear surface contamination by mucus strands, epithelial or atmospheric debris and make-up.

1. Mucus and other surface debris create localized tear film instabilities, which reduce the break-up time and favour deposit formation. Great care should be taken in fitting those patients and the use of in-eye rewetting agents is recommended. Daily wear soft contact lenses should be changed regularly, possibly every month as part of a planned replacement programme. Extended wear should be avoided unless a regular replacement programme is implemented or a disposable lens system (e.g. Acuvue) is used. Rigid lenses should be changed regularly, preferably every six months.

2. Contamination by make-up products such as oily removers or creams completely destabilizes the lipid layer (Fig. 21.25) and produces areas of non-wetting at the contact lens surface. Patient habits and make-up products must be changed before contact lens fitting is undertaken.

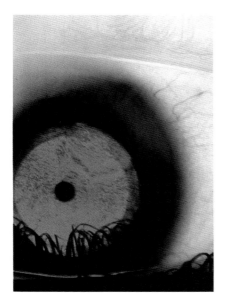

Figure 21.24 Amorphous/coloured fringe pattern visible at low magnification.

Lipid layer thickness (nm) =

$$200 \text{ nm} \times \frac{\text{Palpebral aperture at appearance of first red colour fringe (mm)}}{\text{Normal palpebral aperture (mm)}}$$

Lipid layer contamination classification The contamination of the superficial lipid layer must be assessed regardless of the pattern observed. The presence of contaminants within the lipid layer always destabilizes the tear film. The classification of lipid contamination should be carried out according to the types of contaminants and their severity. One such classification (Table 21.3) has proved useful. The clinical

Aqueous layer The aqueous layer is only visible in the pre-lens tear film. Two aspects of the aqueous layer have been evaluated, its visibility and estimated thickness.

1. Aqueous layer visibility. The visibility

Table 21.3 Lipid layer contamination classification

Type	Severity
1 = Epithelial/atmospheric debris	0 = Absent
2 = Mucous strands	1 = Scant
3 = Make-up	2 = Moderate
	3 = Heavy

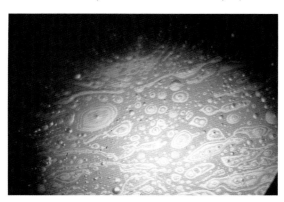

Figure 21.25 Heavy lipid layer contamination by make-up.

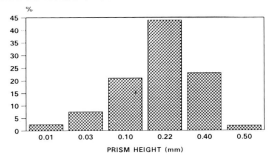

Figure 21.27 Lower tear prism height distribution (by courtesy of Guillon & Guillon, 1989).

of the aqueous layer, especially the interference fringes that form within it, depends upon the reflectivity of the lipid layer as indicated earlier. The rating of the visibility of the aqueous layer (Table 21.4) is therefore an assessment of the lipid layer. The less visible the aqueous layer, the more reflective, hence the thicker the lipid layer.

2. Aqueous layer thickness. When visible, the fringes formed within the aqueous layer (Fig. 21.26) are simply counted or their number estimated. This enables us, assuming a refractive index of 1.337 for

the aqueous layer, to estimate its thickness (Table 21.4).

21.3.3   TEAR FILM VOLUME EVALUATION

General remarks

The investigators that have attempted the assessment of the human tear volume in clinical practice have all opted for the measurement of the tear prism height (Wolff, 1946; Holly & Lemp, 1977; Lamberts *et al.*, 1979; Terry, 1984; Guillon & Guillon, 1988a; Port & Asaria, 1990). The techniques used vary and influence the results obtained. Port and Asaria (1990), for example, have described the most sophisticated technique. They modified a corneal pachometer to carry out accurate measurements of the tear prism height. However, they obtained the lowest values of all investigators; it is thought that this was due to the relative drying of the tear prism height by the slit lamp light.

Proposed clinical technique

We have used a very simple clinical technique to assess the tear prism height, while avoiding artificial drying up of the tear prism. Using the slit lamp biomicroscope, one sets the slit vertically, in alignment with the lid margin immediately adjacent

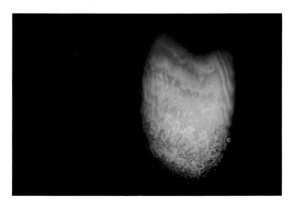

Figure 21.26 Interference fringes formed with the aqueous layer.

Table 21.4 Aqueous layer property classification

(A) Visibility

Classification	Implication
High	Very thin/absent lipid layer
Moderate	Thin lipid layer
Poor	Normal
Not visible	Normal to thick lipid layer

(B) Fringe number

Classification	Estimated thickness(μm)
Less than 5 fringes	< 1.0
5–10 fringes	1.0–1.8
More than 10 fringes	1.8–3.5
Present, not visible fringes	> 3.5

to the tear prism, and alters the slit width until it apparently matches the height of the tear prism. In order to obtain a value in millimetres, it is only necessary to calibrate once the rotation of the knob that controls the slit width using a microscope scale.

In the proposed routine the tear prism height is measured in three positions: (1) immediately below the pupil centre; (2) 5 mm nasally; and (3) temporally. This approach enables us not only to evaluate the tear volume, but also to quantify the regularity of the tear prism. The results obtained on a unselected population of 121 patients aged 17 to 82 years show the lower tear prism height to be normally distributed (Fig. 21.27), peaking at 0.22 mm and giving widely ranging values from a minimum of 0.1 mm to a maximum of 0.8 mm. The evaluation also shows that, overall, men had a greater tear prism height than women and that, in both cases, the tear prism height decreased with age.

21.3.4   EVALUATION OF THE TEAR FILM STABILITY

General remarks

The evaluation of the stability of the tear film is possibly the most important test to evaluate tears *in vivo*. Whereas the test does not identify the origin of any anomaly that may affect the tears, it is the single quantitative evaluation that indicates whether or not the tears are maintaining an efficacious wettability, with or without contact lenses. The conventional way of measuring tear film stability has been to measure the tear film break-up time (BUT). The BUT is defined as the elapsed time in seconds between eye opening following a full blink and the appearance of the first break within the tear film.

The tear film is not normally visible; traditionally the BUT has been measured after the instillation of fluorescein. Fluorescein stains the tears green; the breaks within this film appear as black spots. However, as pointed out by authors who have used the technique recently (Hamano *et al.*, 1982; Mengher *et al.*, 1985a; Patel *et al.*, 1985; Guillon & Guillon, 1989a), the results obtained are not reliable. The main drawback of the technique is its invasive nature. A drop of 1 or 2% fluorescein is instilled in the lower canthus generally, or impregnated paper is applied to the bulbar conjunctiva.

In order to colour the tears, the fluorescein must break through the lipid layer and totally disrupt that layer, with the tendency of destabilizing the tear film. At the same time, the instilled fluorescein introduces a large volume of liquid in relation to the pre-ocular tear volume, and has the tendency momentarily to increase the stability of the tear film. Because the relative influence of the two effects is highly variable from patient to patient, and even from time to time, the results obtained with the technique are unreliable. The values obtained are not well correlated with the BUT measured by non-invasive techniques (Mengher *et al.*, 1985a; Patel *et al.*, 1985; Guillon & Guillon, 1989b). The fluorescein BUT therefore cannot be used, even as a challenge test, and has the further drawback of being unsuitable for use while hydrogel lenses are being worn.

The tests of interest are therefore the available non-invasive tests. The following is a description of these tests.

Non-invasive break-up time measurements

Introductory remarks

The instruments used to measure the non-invasive break-up are, to our knowledge, seven in total. They fall into two categories; those with a small measurement field and those with a wide measurement field (Table 21.5).

The narrow field techniques are of limited use as they involve only a small part of the cornea. In general, the smaller the field, the lower the correlation with the full field measurements. A recent study involving the non-invasive break-up time (NIBUT) measurements by conventional slit lamp specular reflection, keratometry and hand-held keratoscopy, and with the Tearscope (Guillon *et al.*, 1992), showed that the best prediction of the wide angle measurements was with the hand-held keratoscope. Hence this instrument and the modification to the keratometer target designed by Hirji and Callender, and known as the IR-CAL modicication (Hirji *et al.*, 1989), are the most useful of the narrow field instruments.

The NIBUT instruments, both narrow and wide field, also differ according to the nature of the target. Some have a dark background

Table 21.5 Non-invasive instruments used to measure the break-up time

Name	Comment	Reference
Narrow field instruments		
Keratometer		Patel *et al.*, 1985 Guillon *et al.*, 1992
Hand-held keratoscope		Guillon *et al.*, 1992
Slit lamp specular reflection	Measurement in three positions (central, nasal, inferior)	Guillon *et al.*, 1992
IR-CAL modified keratometer	Modified, enlarged keratometric mires	Hirji *et al.*, 1989
Wide field instruments		
Modified bowl perimeter	Modified lighting system and additional target	Lamble *et al.*, 1976 Mengher *et al.*, 1985b
External illuminator	External bilateral illuminator used with slit lamp biomicroscope	Young & Efron, 1991
Tearscope	External monocular illuminator for slit lamp biomicroscope	Guillon, 1986

with a bright grid (keratometer, hand-held keratoscope, IR-CAL modified keratometer, bowl perimeter), while others have a white background (slit lamp specular reflection, external illuminator, tearscope). Not surprisingly, the results obtained vary with the different techniques. In fact, it has been argued that the dark-field instruments do not measure the break-up time at all, but the time when the tear film starts to destabilize or thin down (Patel *et al.*, 1985; Hirji *et al.*, 1989). Also, the problem with the dark-field systems is that they allow only BUT measurements, and not evaluation of the tear film structure.

Measurement techniques

The measurement techniques fall into two categories, depending upon the type of target used. For the dark-field background instruments, the practitioner observes the appearance of any deformation of the target or grid. The time measured has been referred to as the non-invasive tear thinning time (NITTT); this is the elapsed time recorded between a full blink and the appearance of any distortion of the target or grid. For the white background instrument and the slit lamp, the practitioner observes the apparition of any black spots within the tear pattern. The time measured in seconds between a full blink and the apparition of a dark spot is the NIBUT. All the techniques mentioned can be used with and without contact lenses. The white background instruments have the further advantage of enabling the observation of the aqueous thinning up to the apparition of the contact lens surface. The measurement, in seconds, of the time elapsed between a full blink and the appearance of the dried contact lens surface, for RGP lenses, is called the non-invasive drying-up time (NIDUT).

Measurement values

The intrinsic values obtained by any practitioner is technique-dependent, as indicated earlier, but even for a given technique, there may be variations due to differences in environmental conditions in the consulting room, such as heat, humidity and air flow, that offset the results. For this reason we suggest that, whichever technique is used, records of the first 50 or so patients tested should be kept and the practitioner should establish his/her own mean value and distribution. With the two wide-field techniques most commonly used the results are as follows:

1. The modified bowl perimeter (Mengher *et al.*, 1985b) records, for a normal population, a mean value of 47.9 s with a standard deviation of 5.3 (range 4–214 s) for the right eye, and 35.1 ± 3.3 s (range 4–150 s) for the left eye. When comparing normal patients and patients with dry eye symptoms, Mengher *et al.* found that 67% of the normal patients, versus only 37% of the patients in the dry eye group, had a NIBUT greater than 20 s.

2. For the tearscope, Guillon and Guillon (1989b) advise stopping any measurement after 45 s of the eye opening, even if no break-up takes place, in order to avoid undue discomfort. Studying a group of 121 subjects (Guillon & Guillon, 1988a) they found that 28.6% had a break-up time at least equal to 45 s (Fig. 21.28). They also found that the distribution had another peak at 15 s. This led them to conclude that a NIBUT of the pre-ocular tear film of at least 20 s should be taken as a minimum for problem-free contact lens fitting. In this study they also demonstrated that a shorter NIBUT was associated with a greater incidence of staining.

21.4 EFFECTS OF CONTACT LENS WEAR

21.4.1 INTRODUCTION

Very few studies have considered in detail the effect of contact lenses on the structure and stability of the tear film. It is our recom-

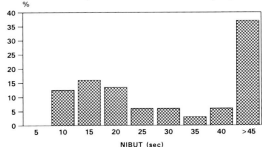

Figure 21.28 Non-invasive break-up time distribution (by courtesy of Guillon & Guillon, 1989).

mendation that the pre-lens tear film should be evaluated carefully for all contact lens patients both at the time of fitting and during aftercare. The interaction is complex and the evaluation of the pre-ocular tear film alone is not sufficient to predict contact lens wettability for individual subjects. Also, the pre-lens tear film (PLTF) changes are precursor to other contact lens surface changes, that lead to adverse effects such as decrease in comfort and tear related problems. Monitoring the PLTF during aftercare permits us to decide whether a conventional soft or rigid contact lens, or a regularly replaced contact lens, needs to be changed (Guillon *et al.*, 1992).

21.4.2   SOFT LENSES

Pre-lens tear film structure

The structure of the PLTF is different to that of the pre-ocular tear film (POTF) for the same group of patients, and also differs with different lens types and wear situations. Whereas one would like to generalize from simple short-term experiments as to the effect of the various parameters, such an approach is not possible. In particular, the suggestion that the thickness of the lipid and aqueous layers are greater with high water content materials (Young & Efron, 1991), is too simplistic.

For daytime measurements, a recent study

carried out with hyperthin (0.035 mm), 38% HEMA lenses (O_3, O_4) (Guillon *et al.*, 1989; Guillon *et al.*, 1992) shows that, both at issue and after one week of extended wear, the PLTF lipid layer is most commonly absent or very thin (Fig. 21.29); this is a marked contrast to the POTF lipid layer, which most commonly has a thicker flow or amorphous pattern. Another study has shown that with new, high water content lenses of conventional thickness, Prima from Igel (67%) and Bausch & Lomb 70 (70%), the PLTF lipid layer is predominantly a wave pattern (Fig. 21.30), and hence only marginally thinner than the POTF lipid layer. It would be easy to conclude from these two studies that a high water content contact lens has a thicker lipid layer. We prefer to limit our conclusions to the fact that thick high water content contact lenses hold a thicker lipid layer than hyperthin, low water content contact lenses.

The visibility of the aqueous fringes is regulated by the relative intensity of the light reflected at the interfaces of that layer. This is influenced by a combination of factors, mainly the lens surface refractive index, the thickness of the aqueous phase, and the presence and thickness of a superficial lipid layer. The visibility of these interference fringes is at its lowest when a thick, highly reflective lipid layer is present (as in the pre-ocular tear film), thus limiting the amount of transmitted light available for interference fringe formation in the aqueous layer. The visibility of the interference colours produced by the aqueous layer will also be low when the aqueous layer present is thick, thereby inducing a further decrease in the visibility of its fringes by spatial narrowing and by intensity loss through successive reflections and by destructive recombination of successive orders of interference. When the surface refractive index of the contact lens material is near to that of water, such as in high water content contact lenses, the visibility is also low (Fig. 21.31). The visibility of the underlying interference

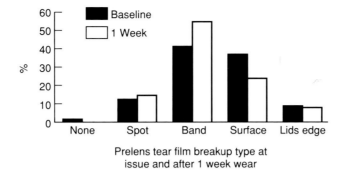

Figure 21.29 Pre-lens tear film lipid layer distribution with hyperthin low water content contact lenses (Bausch & Lomb 03,04) by courtesy of Guillon *et al.*, 1992).

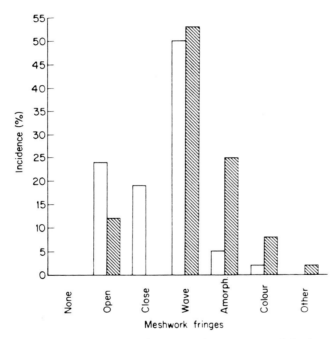

Figure 21.30 Pre-lens tear film lipid layer distribution with conventional thickness high water content contact lenses (Igel Prima and Bausch & Lomb 70) for both open eye wear □ and immediately (3 min) following overnight closed eye wear ▧ (by courtesy of Guillon & Guillon, 1989b).

fringes will be maximized when the water content is low, such as in HEMA lenses. The surface also plays a part; when of poor quality the interference fringes will be minimal.

Because of the relative visibility, the thickness of the aqueous fringes can be assessed principally with low water content contact lenses (Fig. 31.32), where a thick, invisible aqueous layer is still the most common feature.

A significant change in contact lens wettability takes place during overnight wear. In an early study with high water content lenses (Igel, Prima, and Bausch & Lomb 70) (Guillon

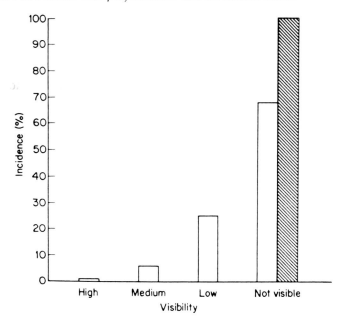

Figure 21.31 Pre-lens tear film aqueous layer visibility distribution with conventional thickness high water content contact lenses (Igel Prima and Bausch & Lomb 70) for both open eye wear □ and wear immediately (3 min) following overnight closed eye wear ▧ (by courtesy of Guillon & Guillon, 1989b).

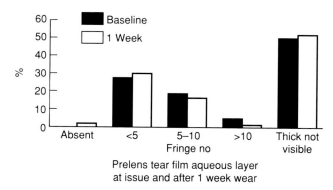

Figure 21.32 Pre-lens tear film aqueous layer fringe distribution with hyperthin low water content contact lenses (Bausch & Lomb 03,04) (by courtesy of Guillon *et al.*, 1992).

& Guillon, 1989c), we have shown that approximately 3 min after eye opening, a thicker lipid (Fig. 21.30) was present than during open eye wear; at that time the aqueous layer was essentially invisible (Fig. 21.31). In addition, soon after eye opening, a much thicker mucous coating was also visible. A recent study (Guillon & Guillon, 1991), with disposable lenses (Acuvue and NewVues) involving both the evaluation of the PLTF immediately upon eye opening and 3 min later, has greatly increased our understanding of the change in wettability during overnight wear. Immediately upon eye opening the aqueous layer is usually absent and the tear film is a very thick, lipid-coated mucin layer. With the initiation of reflex blinking, the aqueous part of the tear film quickly reforms but, because the mucous coating was better than normal, a thick aqueous layer forms within a few blinks, hence the observations made in the first study were confirmed in the second, more extensive study. A clinical implication of those findings is the reduced contact lens movement present at waking compared to pre-closed eye wear. This phenomenon is due to the viscous tear film that reduces movement and not to the physical tightening of the lens fit due to water loss and lens steepening.

Pre-lens tear film stability

Young and Efron (1991), in addition to finding a change in PLTF structure associated with lens water content, also found a connec-

tion between water content and PLTF stability. This study, however, did not consider other factors, such as contact lens thickness and the nature of lens surface characteristics.

Our studies have shown that the PLTF stability measured by the NIBUT with the tearscope is lower than that of the POTF, before contact lens insertion, for the same group of patients (Guillon & Guillon, 1988c). In this investigation the difference was highly significant, with only 2% of eyes with a PLTF NIBUT of 45 s or more versus 60% for the POTF NIBUT. Also, the PLTF NIBUT, both with conventional thickness high water content lenses (Guillon & Guillon, 1988c) and with low water content lenses (Guillon *et al.*, 1992), peaked between 5 and 10 s. The lens geometry also affects the PLTF for HEMA lenses. Lenses with a standard thickness and the ultra-thin lenses such as Z6 (Hydron) and U3 (Bausch & Lomb) have a thicker, more stable PLTF than the hyperthin lenses such as Z4 (Hydron) and 03–04 (Bausch & Lomb), where the lipid layer at times may become

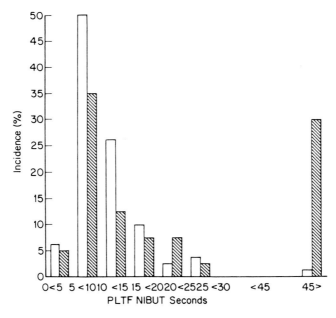

Figure 21.33 Pre-lens tear film non invasive break-up time distribution (□ open eye; ▧ closed eye) (by courtesy of Guillon & Guillon, 1989b).

invisible. In association with the changes in tear film structure that take place overnight, the PLTF stability is greatly altered. Immediately upon eye opening the PLTF NIBUT is, in the majority of cases, extremely short (less than 1 s), but, within a few minutes, becomes longer than the PLTF found during normal open eye wear (Fig. 21.33).

An important aspect of the measurement of the break-up time is the classification of the position and type of breaks that take place within the tear film. We classified the types of break in five categories: none, spot, band, surface and lid edge breaks. Spot, band and surface breaks are increasing levels of break severity. Most commonly a 'band' or 'surface' break takes place (Fig. 21.34); a high incidence of the latter is an indication of poor *in vivo* wettability, whereas a high incidence of spot break is usually associated with a stable pre-lens tear film.

The location of the initial break is an important piece of clinical information. Most often the initial break takes place in the upper and/or lower quadrants, and very rarely in the nasal and temporal quadrants (Fig. 21.35). The reason for this is the destabilization of the tear film at the junction between the lid tear meniscus and the pre-

ocular tear film. This factor has been shown to be associated with corneal desiccation (Guillon *et al.*, 1990). Another aspect of the location of the initial break is its rarity in the central part of the contact lens (approximately 5%). The implication is that all the narrow field instruments will fail to detect the initial break, and hence fail to measure the true NIBUT, in the majority of cases.

Finally, with regard to hydrogel lenses, we have shown (Guillon *et al.*, 1992) using the NIBUT measurement as a means of determining when a lens needs to be changed, a phenomenon that is highly patient-dependent. Our recommendation is to change a contact lens if the NIBUT is decreased by > 25% lower than the base line value and is less than 10 s.

21.4.3   RIGID LENSES

Pre-lens tear film structure

Lipid layer

Contrary to the hydrogel lenses, the characteristics of the PLTF over rigid contact lenses are more affected by the lens geometry and associated lens movements than by the

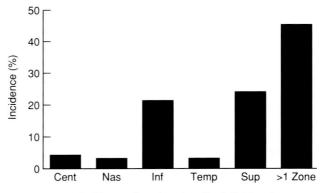

Incidence of pre-lens tear film initial break
position appearance for overall study

Figure 21.34 Distribution of different types of break that take place at the front of hyperthin low water content contact lenses (Bausch & Lomb 03,04) (by courtesy of Guillon *et al.*, 1992).

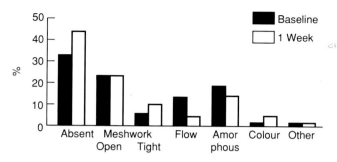

Figure 21.35 Location of initial PLTF break for high water content contact lenses (Igel 77) (by courtesy of Guillon *et al.*, 1990).

nature of the material (Madigan & Holden, 1986). This, however, does not imply that material differences have no influence on wettability (Benjamin, 1987). Typically, in front of PMMA or RGP lenses, the lipid layer is absent or so thin that it is neither visible nor effective in preventing rapid destabilization of the PLTF. Therefore, in addition to classifying the lipid pattern when visible, we rate the amount of the lens surface covered by lipids (Guillon *et al.*, 1989):

0. Lipid coverage absent.
1. Lipid coverage > 0% and ≤ 25%.
2. Lipid coverage > 25% and ≤ 50%.
3. Lipid coverage > 50% and ≤ 75%.
4. Lipid coverage > 75% and ≤ 100%.

Typically the pre-lens lipid layer on poly-(methyl methacrylate) (PMMA) lenses is invisible and the aqueous layer forms a continuously thinning wedge, the thickness of which can be measured by the photography of the interference fringe pattern and the determination of the orders of interference. In the case of PMMA lenses, the intensity of the coloured fringes formed within the aqueous phase is at its maximum due to the absence of lipid layer interference, the thinness of the aqueous layer, and the high refractive index of the contact lens material.

The lipid layer is either totally absent or only partially covers the PLTF of rigid contact lenses. This absence of lipid seems to be independent of the material used, as it has been observed in approximately the same percentage (45%) of new lenses with materials as different as PMMA, silicon acrylates and fluorosilicon acrylates. Furthermore, as these lenses are worn, the incidence of cases showing no lipid coverage increases, suggesting a more abnormal pre-lens tear film with long-term wear. When present, the lipid layer is always thin, as demonstrated by the observed PLTF lipid patterns.

With RGP contact lens wearers, the ocular surface away from the lens is covered by a normal POTF with the superficial lipid layer visible. We believe that the edge of the contact lens acts as a barrier to the propagation of the superficial lipid layer over the surface of the thin, unstable, aqueous pre-lens tear film.

Aqueous layer

PLTF aqueous thicknesses of up to 2.5 μm have been measured in front of PMMA corneal lenses. These thicknesses increase to up to 3.5 μm with the administration of one drop of wetting solution containing 5% polyvinyl pyrrolidine. However, even over this aqueous film of increased thickness, no visible lipid layer has been observed.

The aqueous layer in front of RGP lenses is also thin, and has been estimated to be between 1 and 4 μm, most commonly 2 to 3 μm with silicon acrylates and fluorosilicon acrylates. The aqueous layer thickness seems to be patient-dependent but not material-, lens-care- or time-dependent over a six-month investigation. The mucous coating found on the lens front surface of lenses that show good aqueous coverage and good wettability is always slight to moderate.

Two studies have recently confirmed the above statement: (1) in a daily wear study of six-months duration with Boston IV, Paraperm EW and Equalens I, the lipid layer was absent in 44% of cases and covered the whole contact lens surface in 22% of cases. The mean aqueous thickness was estimated at approximately 2 μm in that study; (2) in an extended wear study with Equalens 2 and Fluoroperm, also of a six-month duration, the lenses generally supported a thin lipid layer and aqueous layer of approximately 4 μm.

Tear film stability

The tear film stability is indicated by the break-up time of the tear film at the front surface of the contact lens recorded by the non-invasive technique (PLTF NIBUT).

PLTIF NIBUT measurements for rigid lenses show that the pre-rigid lens film is far more unstable than the pre-ocular tear film. For example, a group of subjects with a POTF NIBUT of 26.3 s had a PLTF NIBUT of 4.7 s with Excel 02 lenses (Guillon & Guillon, 1988b), which are reported to have good wetting characteristics and a zero degree wetting angle. In fact the average PLTF NIBUT of rigid lenses is approximately 4 to 6 s, hence even shorter than that of hydrogel lenses (Guillon & Guillon, 1988c). Small material differences have been reported. A significantly longer PLTF NIBUT was observed with modified PMMA and a low

Dk RGP materials, with similar *in vitro* wetting angle, than with conventional PMMA lenses (Lydon & Guillon, 1986). Similarly the PLTF NIBUT of fluorosilicon acrylate (Equalens 1) has been reported to be longer than the PLTF NIBUT of two silicon acrylate materials (Boston IV and Paraperm EW) (Guillon & Guillon, 1988d). The latter confirms a previous report indicating also a low incidence of deposits with fluorinated polymers (Feldman *et al.*, 1987). However, more importantly than the average response, it is interesting to note that some individuals do perform better with certain RGP materials, and therefore an extended trial fitting with different materials is useful in problem cases.

REFERENCES

Adler, F.H. (1965) The cornea. In *Physiology of the eye* (4th edn), CV Mosby, St Louis.

Allansmith, M.R., Kajiyama, G., Abelson, M.B. and Simon, M.A. (1976) Plasma cell content of main and accessory lacrimal glands and conjunctiva. *Am. J. Ophthalmol.*, **82**, 819–26.

Allary, J.C., Mapstone, V., Guillon, J.P. and Guillon, M. (1989a) Rigid gas permeable lens surface evaluation. *J. Br. Contact Lens Assoc. Trans. Ann. Clin. Conf.*, 18–19.

Allary, J.C., Mapstone, V., Guillon, J.P. and Guillon, M. (1989b) Dark field examination of rigid gas permeable and hydrogel lenses. *Optom. Vis. Sci.*, **66**, 89.

Allen, M., Wright, P. and Reid, L. (1972) The human lacrimal gland. A histochemical and organ culture study of the secretory cells. *Arch. Ophthalmol.*, **88**, 493–7.

Benedetto, D.A., Clinch, T.E. and Laibson, P.R. (1984) In vivo observation of tear dynamics during fluorophotometry. *Arch. Ophthalmol.*, **102**, 410–12.

Benjamin, W.J. (1987) Care regimen and initial wetting of silicone acrylate surfaces in in vivo. *Trans. Br. Contact Lens Assoc. Conf.*, 55–6.

Boles, S.F., Refojo, M.F. and Leong, F.-L. (1991) Attachment of *Pseudomonas aeruginosa* to human-worn disposable Etafilcon A contact lenses. *Invest. Opthalmol. Vis. Sci.*, **32**, (Suppl. 4), 729.

Bothelo, S.Y. (1964) Tears and the lacrimal gland. *Sci. Am.*, **211**, 78–86.

Bron, A.J. (1985) Prospects for the dry eye. *Trans. Ophthalmol. Soc. UK.*, **104**, 801–26.

Carney, L.G. and Hill, R.M. (1976) Human tear pH. Diurnal variations. *Arch. Ophthalmol.*, **94**, 821–4.

Cedarstaff, T.H. and Tomlinson, A. (1983) Tear volume, quality and evaporation: a comparison of Schirmer, break-up time and resistance hygrometry techniques. *Ophthal. Physiol. Opt.*, **3**, 239–45.

Dilly, P.N. (1986) Conjunctival cells, subsurface vesicles, and tear film mucus. In *The Preocular Tear Film in Health, Disease, and Contact Lens Wear* (ed. F.J. Holly), Dry Eye Institute, Lubbock, Texas, pp. 677–87.

Doane, M.G. (1980) Interaction of eyelids and tears in corneal wetting and the dynamics of human eyeblink. *Am. J. Ophthalmol.*, **89**, 507–16.

Edmund, J. (1951) *The Corneal Gloss*. Thesis, Danish Science Press, Copenhagen.

Ehlers, N. (1965) The pre-corneal tear film. Biomicroscopical, histological and chemical investigations. *Acta Ophthalmol.* **Suppl. 81**, 5–136.

Elander, T.R., Goldberg, M.A., Salinger, C.L., Tan, J.R., Levy, B. and Abbott, R.L. (1992) Microbiological changes in the ocular environment with contact lens wear. *Contact Lens Assoc. Ophthalmol. J.*, **18**(1), 53–5.

Feldman, G., Yamane, S.J. and Herskowitz, R. (1987) *Fluorinated materials and the Boston Equalens*. Contact Lens Forum.

Fischer, F.P. (1928) Uber die Darstellung der Hornhaut – Oberflache und ihrer Veranderung im Reflexbild. *Arch. Augenheilk.*, **98**, Erganzungheft 1–84.

Fischer, F.P. (1940) In *Modern trend in ophthalmology*. (eds. F. Ridley and A. Sorsby), Butterworth and Co Ltd, London.

Folch, J., Lees, M. and Sloane Stanley, G.H. (1957) A simple method for isolation and purification of total lipids from animal lipids. *J. Biol. Chem.*, **226**, 497–509.

Ford, L.C., Delange, R.J. and Petty, R.W. (1976) Identification of a non lysosomal bactericidal factor (beta lysin) in human tears and aqueous humour. *Am. J. Ophthalmol.*, **81**, 30–3.

Forst, G. (1982) Structure of the tear film during the blinking process. *Ophthal. Physiol. Opt.* **7**, 81–3.

Forst, G. (1990) Assessment of the stability of the preocular tear film with the interference method. *Contact Lens J.*, **18**(7), 185–90.

Fullard, R.J. and Snyder, C. (1990) Protein levels in non stimulated and stimulated tears of normal subjects. *Invest. Opthalmol. Vis. Sci.*, **31**, 1119–26.

Furukawa R.R. and Polse, K.A. (1978) Changes in tear flow accompanying aging. *Am. J. Optom. Physiol. Opt.*, **55**(2), 69–74.

Greiner, J.V. Kenyon, K.R., Henriquez, A.S., Korb, O.R., Weidman, T.A. and Allansmith, M.R. (1980) Mucus secretory vesicles in conjunctival epithelial cells of wearers of contact lenses. *Arch. Ophthalmol.*, **98**, 1843–6.

Guillon, J.P. (1982) Tear film photography and contact lens wear. *J. Br. Contact Lens Assoc.*, **5**, 84–7.

Guillon, J.P. (1986) Tear film structure and contact lenses. In *The Pre-Ocular Tear Film in Health, Disease and Contact Lens Wear* (ed. F.J. Holly), Dry Eye Institute, Lubbock, Texas, pp. 914–39.

Guillon, J.P. (1990) *Tear Film Structure of the Contact Lens Wearer*. PhD thesis, The City University, London.

Guillon, M. (1991) Acuvue clinical research update. *The Optician*, **202** (5317), 13–15.

Guillon, J.P. and Guillon, M. (1988a) *Lid Hygiene for Prospective and Current Contact Lens Wearers*. Bausch and Lomb European Research Symposium, Berlin.

Guillon, J.P. and Guillon, M. (1988b) Tear film examination of the contact lens patient. *Contax*, **May**, 14–18.

Guillon, M. and Guillon, J.P. (1988c) The status of the pre soft lens tear film during overnight wear. *Am. J. Optom. Physiol. Opt.*, **65**, 40.

Guillon, M. and Guillon, J.P. (1988d) Pre-lens tear film characteristics of high Dk rigid gas permeable lenses. *Am. J. Optom. Physiol. Opt.*, **65**, 73.

Guillon, J.P. and Guillon, M. (1989a) *How to Predict Tear Related Contact Lens Problems*. Poster presented at the British Contact Lens Association International Contact Lens Conference, London, May 1989.

Guillon, J.P. and Guillon, M. (1989b) How to predict tear related contact lens problems. *Trans. Br. Contact Lens Assoc. Int. Contact Lens Conf.*, 33–5.

Guillon, M. and Guillon, J.P. (1989c) Hydrogel lens wettability during overnight wear. *Ophthal. Physiol. Opt.*, **9**, 355–9.

Guillon, M. and Guillon, J.P. (1991) Disposable contact lenses. Contact lens and tear film interactions. *Invest. Ophthalmol. Vis. Sci.*, **32** (Suppl), 114.

Guillon, M., Guillon, J.P., Mapstone, V. and Dwyer, S. (1989) Rigid gas permeable lenses in vivo wettability. *Trans. Br. Contact Lens Assoc. Conf.*, 24–6.

Guillon, J.P., Guillon, M. and Malgourges, S. (1990) Desiccation staining with hydrogel lenses: tear film and contact lens factors. *Ophthal. Physiol. Opt.*, **10**, 343–50.

Guillon, M., Allary, J.C., Guillon, J.P. and Orsborn, G. (1992) Clinical management of regular replacement. Part 1 – Selection of replacement frequency. *Int. Contact Lens Clin.*, **19** (5 and 6), 104–20.

Haberick, F.J. and Lingelbach, B. (1981) Eine optishe methode zur darstellung von inhomogenitaten des Tranenfilms mit demonstration des verwendeten Schlierenopticschen Verfahrens. Vortrag 14 Aschaffenburger Kontaktlinsen Tatung.

Hamano, H., Hori, M., Kawabe, H., Umeno, M. and Mitsunaga, S. (1979) Bio differential interference microscopic observations on anterior segment of eye. Third report: Observation of surface states of contact lenses on the eye. *J. Japan. Contact Lens Soc.*, **21**, 264–70.

Hamano, H. Hori, M., Kawabe, H. Umeno, M. Mitsunaga, S. Omnishi, Y. and Koma, I. (1980) Change of surface patterns of precorneal tear film due to secretion of meibomian gland. *Folia Ophthalmol. Jpn.*, **31**, 353–5.

Hamano, H., Hori, M. and Mitsunaga, S. (1981) Measurement of evaporation rate from the pre corneal tear film and contact lenses. *Contacto*, **25**(2), 4–14.

Hamano, H., Hori, M. and Mitsunaga, S. (1982) Clinical examinations and research on tears. In *Menicon 30th Anniversary Special Compilation of Research Reports* (eds. K. Tanaka, N. Anan and M. Mikami), Tokyo Contact Lens Company, Tokyo, Japan.

Hirji, N., Patel, S. and Callender, M. (1989) Human tear film pre rupture phase time (TP-RPT). A non invasive technique for evaluating the pre corneal tear film using a novel keratometer mire. *Ophthal. Physiol. Opt.*, 9:139–142.

Holly, F.J. (1973a) Formation and rupture of the tear film. *Exp. Eye. Res.*, **15**, 515–25.

Holly, F.J. (1973b) Formation and stability of the tear film. In *The Preocular Tear Film and Dry Eye Syndrome* (eds. F.J. Holly and M.A. Lemp), *Int. Ophthalmol. Clin.*, **13**(1), 73–96.

Holly, F.J. (1978) Surface chemical evaluation of artificial tears and their ingredients. I. Interfacial activity. *Contact Lens and Intraocular Lens Med J.*, **4**(2), 14–31.

Holly, F.J. (1980) Tear film physiology and contact lens wear I. Pertinent aspects of tear film physiology. *Am. J. Optom. Physiol. Opt.*, **57**(4), 252–7.

Holly, F.J. (1981) Tear film physiology and contact lens wear. I – pertinent aspects of tear film physiology. *Am. J. Optom. Physiol. Opt.*, **58**, 330–42.

Holly, F.J. and Lemp, M.A. (1971) Surface chemistry of the tear film: implications for dry eye syndromes, contact lenses and ophthalmic polymers. *J. Am. Con. Lens Soc.*, **5**, 12–19.

Holly, F.J. and Lemp, M.A. (1977) Tear physiology and dry eyes. *Surv. Ophthalmol.*, **22**, 69–87.

Jansen, P.T., Muytjens, H.L. and Van Bijsterveld, O.P. (1984) Non lysozyme antibacterial factors in human tears (fact or fiction)? *Invest. Ophthalmol. Vis. Sci.*, **25**, 1156–60.

Jensen, O.A., Falbe-Hansen, I., Jacobsen, T. and Michelsen, A. (1969) Mucosubstances of the acini of the human lacrimal gland (orbital part). I. Histochemical identification. *Acta Ophthalmologica*, **47**, 605–19.

Jordan, A. and Baum, J. (1980) Basic tear flow: does it exist? *Ophthalmology (Rochester)*, **87**, 920–30.

Josephson, J.E. (1983) Appearance of the preocular tear film lipid layer. *Am. J. Optom. Physiol. Opt.*, **60**, 883–7.

Knoll, H. and Walters, H. (1985) Pre-lens tear film specular microscopy. *Int. Contact Lens Clin.*, **12**(1), 30.

Koby, F.E. (1924) *Microscopie de l'oeil vivant*. Masson et Cie, Paris.

Kwok, L.S. (1984) Calculation and application of the anterior surface area of a human model cornea. *Theor. Biol.*, **108**, 295–313.

Lamberts, D.W., Foster, C. and Perry, H.P. (1979) Schirmer test after topical anaesthesia and the tear meniscus height in normal eyes. *Arch. Ophthalmol.*, **97**, 1082–5.

Lemp, M.A. (1976) Cornea and sclera. *Arch. Ophthalmol.*, **94**(3), 473–90.

Lemp, M.A., Holly, F.J., Iwata, S. and Dohlman, C.H. (1970) The pre-corneal tear film. I. factors in spreading and maintaining a continuous tear film over the corneal surface. *Arch. Opthalmol.*, **83**, 89–94.

Liotet, S. Cohen, M. and Sainte-Laudy, J. (1980) Un antibiotique naturel des larmes la lactotransferrine. *Journal Francais d'Ophthalmologie*, **3**(3), 159–63.

Lydon, D.P.M. and Guillon, J.P. (1984) The integrity of the pre-lens tear film. In *The Frontiers of Optometry. Transactions of the First International*

Congress. British College of Optometrists, London, pp. 106–35.

Lydon, D.P.M. and Guillon, J.P. (1986) The integrity of the pre-lens tear film. *Transactions of the First International Congress, Vol.2* (ed W.M. Charman) British College of Ophthalmic Optometrists, London.

Madigan, M. and Holden, B.A. (1986) Preliminary report, lens wear and its effects on wetting angle. *Int. Eyecare* 2, 36–44.

Marx, E. (1921) De la sensibilite et du dessechement de la cornee. *Ann. Oculist.*, **158**, 774–89.

Maurice, D.M. (1973) The dynamics and drainage of tears. *Int. Opthalmol. Clin.*, **13**, 103–11.

Maurice, D. (1990) The Charles Prentice award lecture 1989. The physiology of tears. *Optom. Vis. Sci.*, **67**, 391–9.

McClellan, B.H., Whitney, C.R., Newmand, P.C. and Allansmith, M.R. (1973) Immunoglobulins in tears. *Am. J. Ophthalmol.*, **76** 89–101.

McDonald, J.E. (1968) Surface phenomena of tear films. *Trans. Am. Opthalmol. Soc.*, **66**, 905–39.

McDonald, J.E. (1969) Surface phenomena of the tear film. *Am. J. Ophthalmol.*, **67**(1), 56–64.

Meesman, A. (1927) *Die mikroskopie des lebenden Auges an der gullstrandschen Spaltlampe mit Atlas typischer Befunde.* Urban and Schwarzenberg Berlin and Weimar, 33–7.

Mengher, L.S., Bron, A.J., Tonge, S.R. and Gilber, D.J. (1985a) Effect of fluorescein instillation on the pre corneal tear film stability. *Curr. Eye Res.*, **4**, 9–12.

Mengher, L.S., Bron, A.J., Tonge, S.R. and Gilberts, D.J. (1985b) A non invasive instrument for clinical assessment of the pre corneal tear film stability. *Curr. Eye Res.*, **4**, 1–7.

Mertz, G.W. and Holden, B.A. (1981) Clinical implications of extended wear research. *Can. J. Optom.*, **43**, 203–5.

Mishima, S., Gasset, A., Klyce, S.D. and Baum, J.L. (1966) Determination of tear volume and tear flow. *Invest. Ophthalmol. Vis. Sci.*, **5**, 264–76.

Nicolaides, N. (1986) Recent findings on the chemical composition of the lipids of steer and human meibomian glands. In *The Preocular Tear Film in Health, Disease and Contact Lens Wear* (ed. F.J. Holly), Dry Eye Institute, Lubbock, Texas, pp. 570–96.

Norn, M.S. (1979) Semi quantitative interference study of fatty layer of pre-corneal film. *Acta. Ophthalmol. (Kbh).*, **57**, 766–74.

Occhipinti, J.R., Mosier, M.A., La Motte, J. and Monji, G.T. (1988) Fluorophotometric measurements of human tear turnover rate. *Curr. Eye Res.*, **7**, 995–1000.

Patel, S., Murray, D., McKenzie, A, Shearer, D.S. and McGrath, B.D. (1985) Effects of fluorescein on tear break-up time and on tear thinning time. *Am. J. Optom. Physiol. Opt.*, **62**, 188–90.

Port, M.J.A. and Asaria, T.S. (1990) The assessment of human tear volume. *J. Br. Contact Lens Assoc.*, **13**(1), 76–82.

Rehim, M.H.A. and Samy, M. (1988) Effects of different types of contact lenses on fungal flora or healthy eyes. *Contact Lens J.*, **16**, 237–40.

Ridley, F. and Sorsby, A. (1940) *Modern Trends in Ophthalmology* (eds F. Ridley & A. Sorsby), Hoeber Inc., New York.

Rolando, M. and Refojo, M. (1983) Tear evaporimeter for measuring water evaporation from the tear film under controlled conditions in humans. *Exp. Eye Res.*, **36**, 25–33.

Ruskell, G.L. (1968) The fine structure of nerve terminations in the lacrimal glands of monkeys. *J. Anat.*, **103**, 65–76.

Schirmer, O. (1903) Studien zur Physiologie und Pathologie der Tranenabsonderung und Tranenabfuhr. *Graefes Arch. Ophthalmol.*, **56**, 197–291.

Taylor, H.R. (1980) Studies on tear film in climatic droplet keratopathy and pterygium. *Arch. Ophthalmol.*, **98**, 86–8.

Terry, J.E. (1984) Eye diseases in the elderly. *J. Am. Optom. Assoc.*, **55**, 23–9.

Terry, J.E. and Hill, R.M. (1978) Human tear osmotic pressure: diurnal variation and the closed eye. *Arch. Ophthalmol.*, **96**, 120–2.

Tiffany, J.M. and Bron, A.J. (1978) Role of tears in maintaining corneal integrity. *Trans. Opthalmol. Soc. UK.*, **98**, 335–8.

Tomlinson, A., Trees, G.R. and Occhipinti, J.R. (1991) Tear production and evaporation in the normal eye. *Ophthal. Physiol. Opt.*, **11**, 44–7.

Van Haeringen, N.J. (1981) Clinical biochemistry of tears. *Surv. Ophthalmol.*, **26**(2), 84–95.

Vogt, A. (1921) *Atlas der Spaltlampenmikroskopie des lebenden Auges*, Springer Verlag, Berlin, pp. 26–31.

Wolff, E. (1946) The muco-cutaneous junction of the lid margin and the distribution of the tear fluid. *Trans. Ophthalmol. Soc. UK.*, **66**, 291–308.

Wolff, E. (1954) *Anatomy of Eye and Orbit* (4th edn), Blakiston Co, New York, pp. 207–9.

Young, G. and Efron, N. (1991) Characteristics of the pre lens tear film during contact lens wear. *Ophthal. Physiol. Opt.*, **11**, 53–8.

OXYGEN CONSUMPTION AND MEASUREMENT

22

R.M. Hill

22.1 EARLY CLUES

A jungle fighter under compromising conditions, a street trader with keratoconus and a high myope given to an optimistic indifference . . . all shared one thing in common: gross degrees of *overwear syndrome* (Dallos, 1946). When described by Dallos in the 1940s, such examples were still fairly common, even though the origins of such stress were already being explored. Indeed, clinical experiments with lens apertures and tear exchange by Dallos himself were pointing ever more convincingly towards *hypoxia* as a principal cause.

On even cursory review, of course, the earliest literature too was rife with clues of an oxygen starvation problem. Such phenomena as the gradual development of a 'slight bluish haze in daylight and colored halos around lights in the dark' were described as early as 1889 by A. Muller, a response later designated 'Sattler's veil', after Professor C.H. Sattler of Koeningsberg.

By 1934, Dallos and Sattler, through personal communications, had even reached the shared opinion that oedema was the physical cause and the epithelium the site of that veiling effect. It was however, left to Finkelstein (1952), through his elegant observations and mathematical analyses, to relate the two directly.

Other investigators, both earlier and later, such as Fick, Pannus, Muller-Gladbach, Fischer, Duane, de Roetth and Smelser contributed basic pieces to the mosaic as well, firmly linking adequate oxygen to normal corneal physiology, and hypoxia to a catalogue of dysfunctions (Hill & Cuklanz, 1967), ranging from the most subtle fading of sensation as described by Millodot and O'Leary (1980), to frank loss of the epithelium.

22.2 HOW MUCH?

By the early 1960s, the first measurements of corneal oxygen uptake directly on the living human eye were achieved. These observations were made by Hill and Fatt (1963) using several reservoir and contact chamber combinations. Retrospectively, it was a minimum clearance scleral lens design having no membrane, but using balanced saline as a reservoir, which provided the most consistent (and generally median) data. Although cumbersome, and lacking substantially in comfort over the period the subject was required to wear it (the better portion of an hour), this saline medium technique did carry with it the inherent advantage of known gas constants. The parallel constants for a series of membrane reservoirs now commonly used have, however, not been so universally agreed upon, often making their

Contact Lens Practice. Edited by Montague Ruben and Michel Guillon.
Published in 1994 by Chapman & Hall, London. ISBN 0 412 35120 X

associated results difficult to interpret in absolute units.

The average corneal uptake value published by Hill and Fatt for the human cornea, based on their saline reservoir observations, was 4.8 microlitres per square centimetre of corneal surface per hour. There was however another less widely recognized, but perhaps even more important observation given in that report, i.e. that the uptake rates measured where found to slow to as little as 1.5 $\mu l/cm^2/h$, when the reservoir oxygen tension fell to 50 mmHg. Such reduced oxygen conditions may exist (on average) chronically under a contact lens with varying consequences ranging from the clinically undetectable (at very low levels and for extended periods) to the extreme responses reported by those early investigators listed above.

22.3 NORMAL DIFFERENCE

While the earliest figure for human corneal oxygen uptake cited by Hill and Fatt (1963) was a mid-range value, i.e. 4.8 $\mu l/cm^2/h$ from a span of 3.2 to 7.2 $\mu l/cm^2/h$ measured for near ambient (open eye conditions). Larke *et al.* (1981) more recently, on studying 68 male Caucasians, found an even broader range among individuals of that population: some 3 to 9 $\mu l/cm^2/h$.

This three-fold variation among subjects (Larke *et al.*, 1981) was well above the instrumental variation (i.e. error threshold) of their systems (8.1%). Also, when sequences of measurements were done on a given eye, no progressive shift occurred, indicating that irritation or debilitation due to repeated probe contact was not the basis of such differences; neither was the time of day (between 9.00 a.m. and 9.00 p.m.) found to make a significant difference for any particular eye.

Differences in the number of epithelial cell layers among corneas may however be one basis for that population range. Larke *et al.*, (1981) also point out that such natural differ-

ences in corneal oxygen demand 'may provide part of the explanation of the generally observed differences in the manner in which patients respond to contact lens wear.'

22.4 OPEN VERSUS CLOSED EYE

Among the more difficult of the natural corneal factors to analyse is the closed eye condition. The difficulty in part lies in what constitutes a state of 'closure.' If, for example, the lids are held tightly closed by clips, then oxygen levels of 5% or lower (on a scale where 21% = air) may occur, as reported by Roscoe and Hill (1980). Natural closure, i.e. with the lid musculature more relaxed and with a less perfect seal, may result in higher values (e.g 7% by Benjamin (1982) or even 11% by Efron and Carney (1979).

Even under those more physiological conditions, however, Benjamin (1982) found that the new closed-eye oxygen level was established in little more than 3 min, and that 'fluttering' of the eyelids could raise that level measurably. For the average patient, however, such reduced levels over night appear to be less than optimum, as 2 to 4% swelling of the cornea is common on awakening (Mandell & Fatt, 1965; Fatt & Deutsch, 1981)

22.5 THE BLINK

The blink, in the context of corneal oxygenation assumes a special significance of course with the presence of a contact lens. But the efficiency of the lid–lens tear pump resulting can differ markedly between rigid and soft (hydrophilic) lens types. As shown by Polse (1979), very little dependence for oxygen should be placed on the pump in hydrophilic lens cases, as a 1% exchange of tears per blink is about the most to be expected. This is not to say, however, that such a pump is entirely without value. It may in fact be very significant in the clearance of both molecular level and grosser particles (e.g. desquamated cells) from under the lens.

In contrast to the soft lens, when acting in conjunction with a rigid lens the blink can form, with appropriate design, a highly effective tear (oxygen) pump system. The efficiencies of such systems were calculated by Cuklanz and Hill (1969) by loading the bowl of a contact lens with a known concentration of sodium ions and then measuring their progressive escape into the outside tear pool on successive blinks. The four eye–lens systems studies were all fitted parallel to the flattest meridian of the cornea, and using a first order model (i.e. one that did not compensate for small amounts of backflow), the proportion of the post-lens tear pool replaced per blink was found to range from 10 to 17%. This exchange rate is on the average some 13 times more efficient than for the soft lens systems described earlier, and is, of course, the physiological key to those many thousands of oxygen impermeable PMMA lenses that were fitted with reasonable success over several decades.

By the end of the 1960s, it was possible to observe the blink-driven lens–tear pump directly. This was done by Hill and Schoessler (1969) by building a sensor right into a corneal contact lens in such a way that the oxygen level of the post-lens tear pool could be continuously monitored. This experiment revealed a 'saw-toothed' cycle, composed of a slow 'down-drift' segment (as the cornea drew oxygen from the post-lens tear pools during the interval between blinks), followed by a rapid up stroke (as the blink action brought freshly oxygenated tears into the pool again). For any particular blink frequency, an average oxygen level would eventually be established. The faster the blink rate, the higher that average would be. In certain systems however, if the blink rate became very slow, the post-lens tear pool could become entirely depleted of oxygen over the latter portion of the inter-blink interval (Cuklanz & Hill, 1969; Fatt & Hill, 1970).

22.6 THE EQUIVALENT OXYGEN PERCENTAGE (EOP)

Although *leading* estimates of how a lens might influence or impair oxygen availability at the corneal surface have long been possible (i.e. by advance physical testing, such as Dk/L measurements), as have *trailing* assessments (e.g. pachometry of a resulting oedematous state), a rapid response, minimum stress observation involving a particular lens on a particular eye could be very useful as well.

Further, such a test should be non-invasive and its results should be directly and quantitatively comparable to common standards and reproducible conditions, such as a no lens state (i.e. the open eye in air), an impermeable lens state (e.g. a thick PMMA lens under non-blink conditions) or to the response of a reference lens with an oxygen transmissivity between those two extremes.

Also, such a test of corneal oxygen demand should lend itself to assessing a closed eye history, as well as the steady open eye state, or any blink rate (i.e. lid–lens tear pump) combination of frequency and gaze positions. The influences of temperature, humidity, pH, tear osmolality and other environmental factors affecting corneal metabolism and lens status should be detectable and assessable through such a procedure.

A technique called the equivalent oxygen percentage (EOP) method was developed in the late 1960s to approach these requirements and needs for contact lens and corneal studies (Hill, 1977). The rationale for the method is reflected in the four effects shown schematically in Figure 22.1. In Frame (a), an oxygen probe and reservoir are placed down onto the surface of a cornea that has been freely exposed to air. The emptying time of oxygen from the probe reservoir in this case is relatively slow, as indicated by the gentle slope of the graphical trace.

In Frame (b), the same procedure is repeated except that the cornea in this

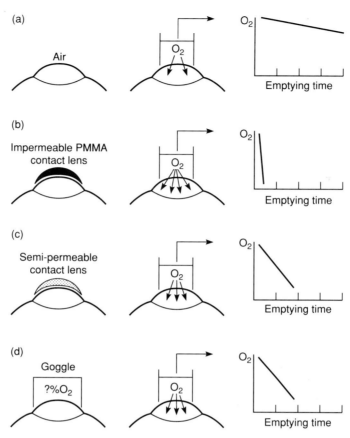

Figure 22.1 Corneal responses to four oxygen conditions. (a) Just following a prolonged period in air; note the slow emptying rate of the measuring probe's oxygen reservoir. (b) Just following a prolonged period under an impermeable PMMA contact lens; note the very rapid reservoir emptying rate. (c) Just following a prolonged period under a semi-permeable contact lens. (d) Just following prolonged exposure to an oxygen percentage (contained by a goggle over the eye), which produces immediately afterwards, a reservoir emptying rate equal ('equivalent') to that caused by the semi-permeable contact lens.

instance has an immediate past history of oxygen impermeability (e.g. thick PMMA contact lens wear). The reservoir exhaustion rate here is very rapid, indicating that the cornea during that period of wear had fallen to, and had been maintained at, some very much lower oxygen level. The steepness of the graphical slope (in mmHg/s units) is directly related to the relative severity of that hypoxic condition. In Frame (c), the reservoir exhaustion rate following semi-gas permeable lens wear is somewhere between those two extreme conditions in Frames (a) and (b).

A means of calibrating the oxygen passing performance of that semi-permeable lens is shown in Frame (d), wherein a series of known oxygen percentages are maintained in a goggle over the cornea, until that particular percentage is identified which produces the identical reservoir exhaustion rate (graphical slope) as did the semi-permeable contact lens being tested. Once that slope match is made, the test lens can then be said to have caused the cornea to behave as if it had been living in an atmosphere *equivalent* to that percentage of oxygen which mimicked it in the goggle experiments – hence the equivalent oxygen percentage (EOP) designation. Standard calibration curves based on statistically constructed goggle experiments have been generated, originally for rabbit, and now for the human cornea as well (Benjamin, 1982; Roscoe & Wilson, 1984).

The 'air' experiment in Frame (a) is of course a kind of 'natural' (i.e. open eye, best oxygen condition) control, against which the performances of test lenses can be directly compared. However only certain flexible 'pure' silicon rubber lenses have approached that level of oxygen passage (Hill, 1977).

Another control, in diametric contrast to the 'air' condition, is the tight impermeable (e.g. a thick PMMA) lens condition. Under static circumstances, such a lens fitted 'parallel' to the eye surface can produce a state of near maximum hypoxia within 120 s. A nitrogen filled goggle can be used to create this extreme condition as well, but may differ slightly in the final steady state level of oxygen achieved, as the two methods vary in several fundamental ways. For example, a 100% nitrogen atmosphere may actually drain oxygen from the eye, acting like an infinite sink for that gas; carbon dioxide may be vented in an unusually efficient way for the same reason. A gas impermeable (contact lens) shell, on the other hand, would not draw oxygen from the eye by such an aqueous to atmosphere gradient, and would tend as well to block carbon dioxide escape by containing it in the post-lens tear pool. For contact lens testing, then, the impermeable plastic control rather than the 'infinite' nitrogen sink would seem to be the more appropriate model to use for lens testing.

It should be noted that the fundamental steps for determining an EOP value, as described above, related to how the cornea responds to a test lens under 'static' or 'steady state' conditions, i.e. *without* a lid–lens pump acting, and following the establishment of a steady flow of oxygen into the cornea based on the tension gradient across it, the associated tear and tissue resistances, and the on-going oxygen demands of the cornea. The 'static' EOP, then, should be reflective of (or related to) the *transmissivity* properties of a test lens only. As the lid–lens pump is unique for each lens–eye examination, the 'static' EOP offers the unique advantage of 'factoring out' the pump variable.

Should it be desirable, however, to know for a given eye the summed effects of pump and transmissivity, a 'dynamic' EOP can be measured, i.e. following a sufficient sequence of blinks for the regular oscillations of oxygen within the tear pool to remain about a stable average. Efron and Carney (1981) have demonstrated for example, using the dynamic EOP, the very small oxygen contribution made by the lid–lens pump in hydrophilic lens systems. Their measurements directly confirm the fluorescein observations described by Polse (1979), who found very little tear exchange per blink under hydrophilic lenses as well. Although Efron and Carney did not include rigid lenses directly in their study, the dynamic EOP for these lens types based on the earlier ion tracking measurements of Cuklanz and Hill (1969) might be predicted to be substantially higher, most particularly, however, because the success of earlier impermeable (i.e. PMMA) lens systems relied entirely on tear pump exchange for corneal oxygen.

While determination of oxygen passage through a given lens and at a particular site (e.g. the centre) would be the most fundamental yield of the static procedures above, an EOP evaluation over a *range* of material thicknesses can be very useful to the manufacturer and practitioner alike – to the former, for determining the thinnest warp-free dimension for a test material while achieving the highest oxygen throughout.

For the practitioner, knowing the oxygen limitations of materials helps in the choice of the most effective trade-offs between that property and others of special importance in the ultimate choice of lenses. An 'EOP curve' is such a summary of 'static' condition oxygen performances across the lens thickness spectrum, and can be used to determine oxygen availability at local sites under a lens or, knowing its average thickness, the average EOP performance for the entire lens.

EOP values generated in this laboratory have three inherent characteristics: (1) they are relative to an altitude of 235 metres above sea level, thus approximating the tension environments of a large proportion of the contact lens wearing population; (2) being done on a living eye, EOP values relate only to eye temperature conditions; and (3) in the case of hydrophilic lenses, the water level of the tested lens is set to approximately 90% of the label value in order to reside within the hydration range characteristic of most ambient wearing conditions.

22.7   OTHER OXYGEN ESTIMATES

The Dk/L estimate of lens performance differs from the *in vivo* method above in that it does not involve an eye in its measurement process. It is, rather, a physical or 'bench' measurement of oxygen passage, and as such serves as a predictor of what a lens may provide on the eye (i.e. its 'static' or non-lid – lens pump contribution). Reference to Fatt (1978) is recommended for a detailed description of the Dk/L method.

Being a physical test which can be done under carefully controlled and replicated conditions, the Dk/L estimate does have the potential for good accuracy and repeatability. As with all such critical testing procedures, however, best absolute (and comparative, i.e. between lenses) results can be expected only when samples are measured within the same laboratory.

Initially the most popular index (or refer-

ence value) taken from that physical testing procedure was the Dk, or oxygen *permeability* value, of the material from which a test lens was to be made (obtained by multiplying the Dk/L of a lens or flat which was actually measured by L, the thickness of the tested specimen in centimetres). Two problems chronically resulted however from using the Dk value alone as a performance index: (1) deriving the Dk is dependent on knowing the exact thickness at the site(s) of measurement of a test lens (or better, a uniform thickness flat). Maintaining a constant thickness in hydrophilic cases and then measuring it accurately remains a challenge; and (2) as lenses or flats (of the same material) are made progressively thinner (particularly in the range of common myopia prescriptions), the calculated Dk, may not be constant throughout (i.e. the ratings for thinner samples tend to be relatively poorer than their performances should actually merit (Fatt & Chaston, 1982).

Use of a directly measured Dk/L, i.e. lens or flat *transmissivity*, combined with the application of a carefully calibrated system for determining thickness (or better average thickness for the whole lens), should provide a more reliable measure of oxygen passage than a Dk (i.e. material permeability) for a particular polymer being studied.

Also, as the performance of an ophthalmic plastic must ultimately be judged under 'in the eye' conditions, the convention of measuring all Dk/L values at eye temperature should be encouraged. Such a convention would (1) eliminate different Dk/L values being cited for the same specimen due to different testing temperatures; and (2) make comparisons with EOP findings (which are only made at eye temperature) legitimate then in all cases.

Can reasonable agreement be found among predictors of oxygen performance? As the EOP and Dk/L procedures can both be done without the presence of the lid–lens tear pump, a comparison of their results should be possible. The more fundamental question then becomes: How well does each predict the other?

Several sets of independent observations and assessments have been made upon which equations containing these two predictors have been based. Three of the more recent analyses are:

1. Fatt and Chaston's (1982) model fitted to the data of Novicky and Hill (1981). Their equation for relating those two numbers is:

$$EOP = 2.06 \times 10^8 \, (Dk/L) -0.07$$

The correlation coefficient of the two based on the original data was found to be +0.94.

2. Holden and Mertz's (1984) model fitted to EOP data from Hill's laboratory for various lens types during the period of 1975 to 1980 for which Dk/L values could be obtained. Their equation for relating these two measures is:

$$EOP \, (\%) = 6.915 \times \ln (Dk/L \times 10^9) -9.778$$

The correlation coefficient of the two from that database was found to be +0.995.

3. Roscoe's (1984) model derived from his own EOP and Dk/L data base on the same lenses yielding the equation:

$$EOP \, (\%) = 7.2 \times 10^8 \, Dk/L - 0.50$$

The correlation coefficient for those two measures for the open eye was found to be +0.96.

For the closed eye, the relationship found was:

$$EOP \, (\%) = 1.4 \times 10^8 \, Dk/L - 0.27$$

with a correlation coefficient of +0.99.

Similarly, relationships between corneal swelling (pachometry) due to lens induced hypoxia and lens Dk/L have now been demonstrated by Holden and Mertz (1984) with correlation coefficient values for 'Day 1 maximum' swelling responses, and the 'first

overnight' swelling response with lens transmissivity, being − 0.96 and − 0.92, respectively.

The EOP and Dk/L procedures might be classed as 'leading indicators' (i.e. by having early feasibility and by being immediate in outcome) of long-term wear results to be expected from an experimental material. Corneal enzyme analyses, e.g SDH and LDH/MDH determinations under laboratory conditions may prove to be useful advance (pre-human trial) estimates of material performance as well (Rengstorff & Hill, 1974; Fullard & Carney, 1984).

Pachometry, for the purpose of monitoring corneal swelling, lends itself very well to the tracking of those changes over extended periods in the daily or extended wear. Particularly where weeks or months may be involved, pachometry can be considered a highly useful, non-invasive 'intermediate indicator' of hypoxic responses (Holden *et al.*, 1983).

One example of a promising 'following indicator' may be endothelial polymegathism. Although this long-term result of lens wear may have multiple bases (e.g. pH, enzyme or waste disturbances), its relatively greater prominence in association with impermeable (e.g. PMMA) materials, versus its lesser development or near absence in association with progressively more permeable materials, suggest oxygen deprivation to be a primary aetiological factor (Schoessler, 1983).

22.8 SOME EXCEPTIONAL SUBJECTS AND CIRCUMSTANCES

Apart from normal variations of corneal demand and the superimposed effects of environment e.g. blink rates (Carney & Hill, 1982), closed eye periods (Efron & Carney, 1979), altitude (Hill, 1981), several other factors may influence the oxygen demand of the cornea. Just four examples will be mentioned here:

immediately following lid closure, and the degree of relief associated with lid 'flutter' (Benjamin & Hill, 1986); and (3) the individuality of oxygen demand among normal, healthy corneas, and the implications of those differences (Benjamin & Hill, 1988b). In many areas, the more subtle, but in the long-term most critical, thresholds and tolerances associated with corneal oxygen demand may just now be coming into view.

REFERENCES

Andrasko, G. and Schoessler, J.P. (1980) The effect of humidity on dehydration of soft lenses on the eye. *Int. Contact Lens Clin.*, **7**, 210–22.

Arey, L.B. and Corode, W.M. (1943) The method of repair in epithelial wounds of the cornea. *Anat. Rec.*, **86**, 75–86.

Augsburger, A.R. and Hill, R.M. (1972) Corneal anesthetics and epithelial oxygen flux. *Arch. Ophthalmol.*, **88**, 305–7.

Benjamin, W.J. (1982) *Corneal physiology under the closed eyelid of humans*. PhD dissertation, The Ohio State University Libraries, Columbus, Ohio.

Benjamin, W.J. and Hill, R.M. (1985) Human cornea: oxygen uptake immediately following graded deprivation. *Graefe's Arch. Clin. Exp. Ophthalmol.*, **223**, 47–9.

Benjamin, W.J. and Hill, R.M. (1986) Human corneal oxygen demand: The closed-eye interval, *Graefe's Arch. Clin. Exp. Ophthalmol.*, **224**, 291–4.

Benjamin, W.J. and Hill, R.M. (1988a) Human cornea: superior and central oxygen demands, *Graefe's Arch. Clin. Exp. Ophthalmol.*, **226**, 41–4.

Benjamin, W.J. and Hill, R.M. (1988b) Human cornea: individual responses to hypoxic environments, *Graefe's Arch. Clin. Exp. Ophthalmol.*, **226**, 45–8.

Carney, L.G. and Hill, R.M. (1982) The nature of normal blinking patterns. *Acta Ophthalmol.*, **60**, 427–33.

Cuklanz, H.D. and Hill, R.M. (1969a) Oxygen requirements of the contact lens system. *Am. J. Optom.*, **46**, 228–30.

Cuklanz, H.D. and Hill, R.M. (1969b) Oxygen requirements of contact lens systems: I. comparison of mathematical predictions with physiological measurements. *Am. J. Optom.*, **46**, 662–5.

Dallos, J. (1946) Sattler's veil. *Br. J. Ophthalmol.*, **300**, 607–14.

Efron, N. and Carney, L.G. (1979) Oxygen levels beneath the closed eyelid. *Invest. Ophthalmol. Vis. Res.*, **18**, 93–5.

Efron, N. and Carney, L.G. (1981) Models of oxygen performance for the static, dynamic and closed-lid wearer of hydrogel contact lenses. *Aust. J. Optom.*, **64**, 223–33.

Fatt, I. (1978) Gas transmission properties of soft contact lenses. In *Soft Contact Lenses: Clinical and Applied Technology* (ed. M. Ruben), John Wiley & Sons, New York, p. 83.

Fatt, I. and Chaston, J. (1982a), Measurement of oxygen transmissivity and permeability of hydrogel lenses and materials. *Int. Contact Lens Clin.*, **9**, 76–88.

Fatt, I. and Chaston, J. (1982b) Relation of oxygen transmissibility to oxygen tension or EOP under the lens. *Int. Contact Lens Clin.*, **9**, 119–20.

Fatt, I. and Deutsch, T.A. (1981) The relationship of conjunctival PO_2 to capillary bed PO_2. *Crit. Care Med.*, **11**, 445–8.

Fatt, I. and Hill, R.M. (1970) Oxygen tension under a contact lens during blinking – a comparison of theory and experimental observations. *Am. J. Optom.*, **47**, 50–5.

Finkelstein, I.S. (1952) Biophysics of corneal scatter and diffraction of light induced by contact lenses. *Am. J. Optom.*, **29**, 185–208.

Fullard, R.J. and Carney, L.G. (1984) Diurnal variation in human tear enzymes. *Exp. Eye Res.*, **38**, 15–26.

Hill, R.M. (1977) Oxygen permeable contact lenses: how convinced is the cornea? *Int. Contact Lens Clin.*, **4**, 34–6.

Hill, R.M. (1981) Perils of the pump. In *Curiosities of the Contact Lens*. Professional Press, Inc., Chicago, IL, p. 32.

Hill, R.M. and Cuklanz, H. (1967) Oxygen transmissivity of membranes in contact with the cornea: physiological observation. *Br. J. Physiol. Optics*, **24**, 206–16.

Hill, R.M. and Fatt, I. (1963) Oxygen uptake from a reservoir of limited volume by the human cornea *in vivo*. *Science*, **142**, 1295–7.

Hill, R.M. and Keates, R.H. (1969) Quantifying epithelial healing of the cornea, *in vivo*. *Arch. Ophthalmol.*, **82**, 675–80.

Hill. R.M. and Schoessler, J.P. (1969) Tear pumps: reservoir oxygen measurements in situ. *J. Am. Optom. Assoc.*, **40** 1102–5.

Holden, B.A. and Mertz, G.W. (1984) Critical oxygen levels to avoid corneal edema for daily and extended wear contact lenses. *Invest. Ophthalmol. Vis. Sci.* **25**, 1161–7.

Holden, B.A., Mertz, G.W. and McNally, J.J. (1983) Corneal swelling response to contact lenses worn under extended wear conditions. *Invest. Ophthalmol. Vis. Sci.*, **24**, 218–26.

Kuwabara, T., Perkins, D.G. and Cogan, D.G. (1976) Sliding of the epithelium in experimental corneal wounds. *Invest. Ophthalmol. Vis. Sci.* **15**, 4–10.

Larke, J.R., Parrish, S.T. and Wigham, C.G. (1981) Apparent human corneal oxygen uptake. *Am. J. Optom.* **58**, 803–5.

Mandell, R.B. and Farrell, R. (1980) Corneal swelling at low atmospheric oxygen pressure. *Invest. Ophthalmol. Vis. Sci.*, **19**, 697–702.

Mandell, R.B. and Fatt, I. (1965) Thinning of the human cornea on awakening. *Nature*, **208**, 292.

Mauger, T.F. and Hill, R.M. (1985) Epithelial healing: quantitative monitoring of the cornea following alkali burn. *Acta. Ophthalmol.*, **63**, 264–7.

Millodot, M. and O'Leary, D.J. (1980) Effect of oxygen deprivation on corneal sensitivity. *Acta Ophthalmol.*, **58**, 434–9.

Novicky, N.N. and Hill, R.M. (1981) Oxygen measurements: Dk's and EOP's. *Int. Contact Lens Clin.*, **8** 41–3.

Polse, K.A. (1979) Tear flow under hydrogel contact lenses. *Invest. Ophthalmol. Vis. Sci.*, **18**, 409–13.

Polse, K.A. and Mandell, R.B. (1970) Critical oxygen tension at the corneal surface. *Arch. Ophthalmol.*, **84**, 505–8.

Polse, K.A., Holden, B.A. and Sweeney, D. (1983) Corneal edema accompanying extended lens wear. *Arch. Ophthalmol.*, **101**, 1038–41.

Rengstorff, R.H. and Hill, R.M. (1974) The corneal epithelium: effects of anoxia on Kreb's cycle activity. *Arch. Ophthalmol. (Paris)*, **34**, 615–20.

Roscoe, W.R. (1984) *Comparative polarographic investigation of the human cornea.* PhD dissertation, University of Alabama at Birmingham Libraries.

Roscoe, W.R. and Hill, R.M. (1980) Corneal oxygen demands: a comparison of open and closed eye environments. *Am. J. Optom.*, **57**, 67–9.

Roscoe, W.R. and Wilson, G. (1983) Effects of a topical anesthetic on human equivalent percentages (EOP) and corneal oxygen flux values. *Am. J. Optom. Physiol. Optics*, **60**, 879–82.

Roscoe, W.R. and Wilson, G.S. (1984) Equivalent oxygen percentage (EOP) technique: a standard calibration curve. *Am. J. Optom.* **61**, 601–4.

Schoessler, J.P. (1983) Corneal endothelial polymegathism associated with extended wear. *Int. Contact Lens Clin.*, **10**, 148–55.

PART SIX

Practical Routine

INTRODUCTION

This section of the book deals with the detailed clinical routines essential in achieving successful, long-term contact lens wear. They are set in a logical order. First, the indications and contraindications for contact lens wear are highlighted. Such chapters sometimes give advice that may appear dogmatic, but these are based upon past contact lens experience and research information reported in other sections of the text. The basis for the advice given is, in particular, based upon considerations of the optical and physiological aspects of contact lens performance. The preliminary examination is closely related to the indications and contraindications for contact lens wear and aims at identifying the criteria that will lead the practitioner to decide upon whether or not to fit a patient with contact lenses and, in the former case, what type of contact lens to use. Contact lens dispensing involves both the clinical measurement carried out at that time and the advice given to patients to ensure successful wear. In this way, it is closely linked with Chapter 25, dealing with care systems. Chapter 25 reviews the products available from the aspect of pharmaceutical performance and routine use, and is closely associated with Chapter 26, on aftercare and symptomology, which discusses the routine to follow, precautions to take and, amongst others, differentiates between contact lens and care solution-related problems.

M. Ruben

23.1 INTRODUCTION

There are many diverse indications for contact lens wear and, for the purposes of this chapter, they will be dealt with in the following order:

1. Visual indications:
   for cosmetic use and essentially low refractive errors;
   to improve acuity;
   to maintain and/or obtain binocular vision.
2. For use during sport and in the armed services.
3. Therapeutic indications:
   in eye disease and trauma;
   with surgical procedures;
   postoperatively;
   chemotherapeutic.
4. Diagnositc indications:
   electrodiagnostic techniques;
   radiography.

23.2 VISUAL INDICATIONS

23.2.1 COSMETIC USES AND CORRECTION OF LOW REFRACTIVE ERRORS

The meaning of the term 'cosmesis' is to enhance beauty. Spectacles used to correct low refractive errors may, in the opinion of the wearer produce an abnormal appearance, but the alternative of contact lens wear will enhance their appearance. The corollary is that if the spectacle wearer has abnormalities of the face around the eyes, such as wrinkles, or if the eyes have an abnormal appearance, such as undue prominence or congenital deformities, then the use of spectacles with suitable tints may be preferred because they mask the unwelcome appearance.

Low refractive errors account for well over 90% of all refractive errors (below 5 dioptres) and therefore the vast majority of wearers are to be found in this group.

The motivation to wear contact lenses instead of spectacles is highest in women, and the age when there is a desire to wear lenses is related directly to the degree of sophistication in the particular society and the economic status of the individuals in that society. At one extreme are those who refuse to wear spectacles and can even exhibit obsessional symptoms that require referral to a psychiatrist. This may occur even when good vision is dependent upon wearing an optical correction.

The use of spectacles in the young has limiting factors on the normal development

Contact Lens Practice. Edited by Montague Ruben and Michel Guillon.
Published in 1994 by Chapman & Hall, London. ISBN 0 412 35120 X

of the child and young adult. The recession of the psyche, particularly the ability to communicate with others, a partial withdrawal from society and a preference for indoor activities, often characterize myopes. Myopia from 1 to 6 dioptres is the usual visual defect in young patients in populations. The onset of myopia is chiefly in the 7–10 and 14–18 age groups. In both these groups there are often excessive demands on performance, both academic and social, and a physical defect such as poor vision that has need for correction becomes a source of irritation to the developing individual. Adolescence has many problems and the onset of a visual error can prove sufficient to cause behavioural problems in some young people. Contact lenses can therefore be advised, even at a young age, the proviso being that the parents and child can manage the lenses according to the instructions of the practitioner.

It has been noted that successful wear of contact lenses in children and young people leads to a more outgoing personality, less introspection and a slight delay in the progression of myopia (see Chapter 37; Polse, 1977).

There are many people who, because of their occupation, wish to avoid the use of spectacles, including theatrical and film artistes, dancers, acrobats and politicians. The acuity obtained by this group with contact lenses may not be any better than with spectacles; in some instances it is less. There are several reasons for this. For example, the wearer may have an insufficiency of tears, corneal oedema, or induced or residual astigmatism but is prepared to have a visual disadvantage, for cosmetic reasons, rather than wear spectacles (see Chapter 41).

Presbyopia is a problem in older age groups. Many practitioners find that presbyopia cannot be corrected satisfactorily by contact lenses (Maltzman *et al.*, 1985; Chapter 33 covers this subject in detail). When measured in the consulting room, the practitioner may find some of these visual defects

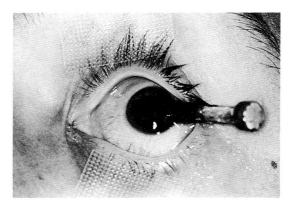

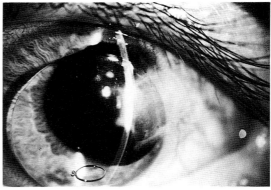

Figure 23.1 These two photographs show the eye of a young man presenting (a) with a penetrating ocular wound from job-related trauma and (b) the same eye some months later. Removal of the embedded metal nail, cataract extraction, retinal repair and patch corneal graft have resulted in an eye which has a potential of 20/30 vision, but which is so topographically distorted that a rigid lens will not remain on the eye and a hydrogel will not provide vision better than 20/200. Vision was eventually restored by use of a piggyback contact lens system: high plus-powered, large diameter hydrogel, and top low minus-powered rigid (gas permeable) contact lens, as shown in photograph (b), to 20/30 (photograph (a) courtesy of Y Sidikaro).

with contact lenses relatively minor in degree. Yet to some sensitive individuals, or to those with poor motivation, they are insurmountable and the lenses, whilst they can be worn for long periods, are abandoned.

In this major group of low refractive error patients, whilst the practitioner may not find any of the contraindications that are to be described later in the chapter, there is a failure rate with contact lenses. Contact lenses are therefore not the ultimate cosmetic optical correction for low refractive vision errors; this is especially true of errors below 1 dioptre.

23.2.2 IMPROVEMENT OF VISION

There are many conditions where spectacles do not fully correct the vision and there is a demand for better acuity because it is known that the posterior segment of the eye has no functional abnormality. For example:

1. High refractive errors, e.g. myopia, hyperopia, aphakia and astigmatism.
2. Irregular astigmatism, e.g. post-operation or as a result of trauma to the cornea (Fig. 23.1).
3. Keratodystrophies, such as keratoconus.
4. Hereditary keratodystrophies (Fig. 23.6).

In those conditions where there is both a refractive error and a macular pathology, and the basic problem is hyperopia, the use of spectacles may be preferred to obtain a magnification effect. In high myopia associated with a macular pathology, contact lenses will result in a larger image than spectacle lenses (see Chapter 7) and in a fuller field of vision.

In high degrees of congenital hyperopia there may be a disfiguring microcornea and a combined optical and cosmetic effect can be obtained by the use of thick, soft lenses (Fig. 23.3). In such cases the practitioner must

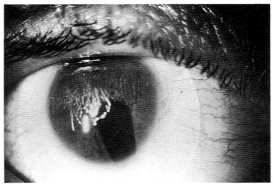

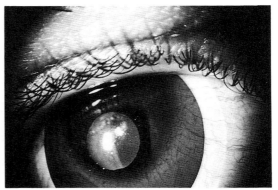

Figure 23.3 The right eye of a hyperopic patient with microcornea is shown wearing a clear hydrogel lens (a) and a tinted hydrogel lens (b) designed to 'reconstruct' the anterior segment cosmetically. Her original horizontal visible iris diameter (HVID) is 6.5 mm; the lens has a pupil diameter of 4.0 mm and an artificial iris diameter of 11.0 mm.

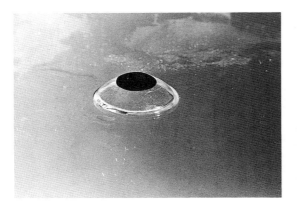

Figure 23.2 Photograph of a hydrogel contact lens with a black 7 mm diameter occluder central zone. Such a lens might be used for ambylopia therapy (although usually larger opaque optic zones are needed), to eliminate uncorrectable diplopia from, for example, macular trauma to one eye, or to cosmetically mask an unsightly inoperable cataract or corneal scar.

ascertain the best appliance (by using trial lenses) and proceed accordingly.

It has to be noted that full myopic contact lens corrections can induce a state of pseudopresbyopia, which can be corrected satisfactorily only by the addition of spectacles to the contact lense prescription. Such spectacle addition can also be used to correct the residual astigmatism (see Chapter 33).

Regular astigmatism may present fitting and acuity problems but, with sophisticated lens design, these may be overcome (Weissman & Chun, 1987; and see Chapters 28 and 29).

Aphakia

The use of contact lenses for the correction of aphakia is today limited to those patients who, for one reason or another, cannot be fitted with an intraocular implant or where an intraocular implant has been removed as a secondary procedure. Infants and children are rarely fitted with pseudoaphakic implants.

There remains a group of patients in whom, as a result of trauma, aphakia results. A secondary insertion of an implant is not advised in such patients.

In an ageing population, where cataract is a not uncommon condition and surgery is now improved to such an extent that in many clinics it is a day procedure, there are a number of individuals requiring a contact lens either because they have no implant or because they have an induced irregular astigmatism or a large degree of regular astigmatism. There are instances of large iridectomies following trauma or with aphakia, and artificial iris lenses can give good results (Allerger, 1971; Tomlinson, 1972) (Figs 23.4 and 23.5).

The entire range of contact lenses and materials is available in high plus powers and the practitioner can therefore decide which is the correct lens for the aphakic eye and what are the specific differences between this and the normal eye. Some of the indications will now be considered.

Cataracts can be removed from the eye by several techniques. The final optical result depends upon the surgical technology and the degree of trauma suffered by the cornea, the vitreous, and the iris, and on the healing of these tissues. Scleral incisions open the eye external to the limbus; corneal incisions open it within the limbus. Suturing will affect the rate of healing and the degree of stress upon the corneal curvature. In general, when healed, a scleral incision will tend to displace the apex of the cornea superiorly and therefore produce a variable degree of astigmatism; the axis of flatness may be horizontal, but is more usually oblique. A corneal incision should not alter the original curves of the cornea but there is a tendency to produce astigmatism, with the flatter corneal axis vertically. In the majority of patients the astigmatism is usually within 2 dioptres. However, cornea with greater degrees of astigmatism can occur; in such cases vision can be corrected fully by a contact lens.

Large incisions produce a degree of desensitization of the cornea, which is beneficial to initial contact lens wear and tolerance (see Chapter 20); this loss of sensitivity is also present after keratoplasty procedures. It is

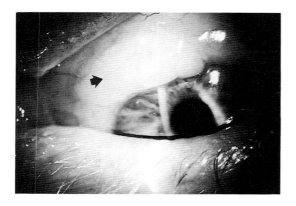

Figure 23.4 Photograph of a large unplanned filtering bleb (at arrow) following cataract surgery (courtesy of T.H. Pettit).

also possible that the metabolism of the cornea is affected by the operation, and the endothelium requires less oxygen than usual. Both these factors, and the likelihood of astigmatism, favour the use of a hard, gas permeable contact lens, rather than a soft lens. Lenses of 9–10 mm can be used to obtain good centration and a good visual result. Lenses with reduced optics and plus power configuration edge design result in a stable lid-held lens. If the corneal astigmatism tends to lead to a misfit then toric back curves and compensatory front curves can be utilized (see Chapters 28 and 29).

Other, more modern, procedures for cataract extraction use small limbal incisions and irrigation and/or ultrasound technology, which do not affect the original corneal curvatures. In such cases, steep corneas can be fitted with single cut design, thin, small corneal lenses. At the other extreme, flat but regularly curved corneas will require larger lenses of a more complicated design (see Chapter 5). However, the corneal surface may have retained its original sensitivity, in which case a soft lens would be the lens of choice (see Chapter 27). The choice of a soft lens to obtain immediate tolerance has to be considered and the better acuity, which may be possible with a hard lens, must be sacrificed. A spectacle lens in addition to the soft lens will correct the residual astigmatism and the reading vision (multifocals).

In children and infants, the early fitting of the eye, even at the end of the cataract extraction, has to be considered. Higher powers and steeper curved soft lenses are required in the form of fitting sets (see Chapter 34).

In those instances where the shape of the eye obviates the use of a normal sized corneal hard lens, or where soft lenses are of no value because of poor acuity, then the practitioner has to consider a form of scleral lens (see Chapter 31).

The miniscleral lenses are the easiest for a practitioner to fit because they are available in trial sets (see Chapter 31). Scleral hard lenses can be fitted and are especially useful when the lens has to be combined with prosthetic effects as well as optical power (Ruben, 1989). Centration of the optic is not a problem with the scleral lens, but corneal metabolism tolerance and fitting difficulties often negate the theoretical advantages.

Irregular astigmatism

The correction of this indication is covered in Chapter 35. The most common corneal conditions showing an irregular astigmatism are:

1. Aphakia (Fig. 23.5).
2. Keratoconus.
3. Corneal scarring, trauma and disease (Fig. 23.6).
4. Infective ulcers.
5. Postoperative corneal procedures, e.g. keratoplasty, glaucoma drainage, refractive surgery (Shivitz *et al.*, 1987).

Keratoconus

Keratoconus can be diagnosed early in the condition if the practitioner uses a keratometer and if retinoscopy is carried out by an

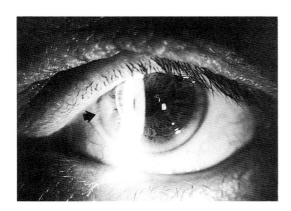

Figure 23.5 Photograph of an eye wearing a bitoric lenticular cut rigid contact lens for optical correction of aphakia. This lens was designed specifically as a bitoric to centre the lens and allow wear concomitant with the large pterygium shown nasally (at arrow). No staining of the pterygium was observed with full time wear.

expert. A remarkable benefit can be obtained in visual acuity by the use of contact lenses.

In the early stages, small corneal hard lenses are preferable and, as the condition progresses there is a need for larger sized lenses, until in the late stages of the condition, if keratoplasty is not possible, then scleral lenses are required to give improved acuity. However, in most eyes with advanced irregular astigmatism, the cornea suffers central scarring, which reduces the acuity. There are different approaches to fitting keratoconus and even the most experienced fitters have been known to say 'I fit them any way I can' (see Chapter 35).

Overwear of lenses on a thin cornea, as may be evident in keratoconus, can produce a rupture of the endothelium and acute hyrops can result. The vision can also be variable, as a result of recurrent corneal oedema. The only type of soft lens likely to give improved acuity in keratoconus is a specially prescribed high gas permeable material with a central thickness of between 0.2 and 0.3 mm. However, successful results are likely to be limited. Soft peripheral lenses combined with hard centres are more successful but are difficult to obtain in steep fittings; they are also more easily broken. The combination of a soft, large thin lens with a large corneal lens superimposed (piggy back lens) is possible but, again, management can be difficult. Low concentration steroid eye drops (0.1%) can be used to maintain good tolerance, but this requires close supervision (see Chapters 5 and 35).

If the sutures prove troublesome, a soft therapeutic lens can alleviate pain and blepharospasm (see Chapter 38). Hard lenses can be fitted with the sutures *in situ*, providing that the knots are buried. In all these conditions of epithelial debridement due to operative technique the risk of infection due to contact lens wear must be noted and sometimes prophylactic antibiotics will be required.

Contact lenses may be required to correct the vision after radiokeratometry (see Chapter 36) and some practitioners believe that they can also be beneficial to the cornea (Shivitz *et al.*, 1987). Because patients who obtain marked visual gain wear contact lenses for long periods, the complications of corneal vascularisation and infiltrates of an inflammatory nature can occur (see Chapters 45 and 46).

23.2.3 BINOCULAR VISION INDICATIONS

Binocular vision indications include:

1. The phorias.
2. The tropias.
3. Anisometropia and aniseikonia.
4. Amblyopia.
5. Nystagmus.

Most of these conditions affect children and therefore the indications for children (apart from refractive errors including aphakia) are given now.

Phorias

Esophoria and hyperopia

With spectacles it is possible to overcorrect the power and obtain satisfactory control of the defect; bifocals will also reduce conver-

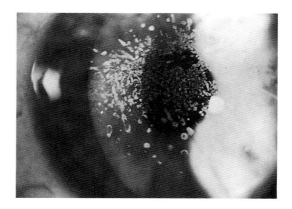

Figure 23.6 Corneal lesions in the eye of a young man with the diagnosis of anterior stromal granular dystrophy. Both eyes are similar. Maximum visual acuity with spectacles is 20/40; this improves with a simple rigid lens design to 20/25.

gence excess problems. Contact lenses can do exactly the same as spectacles, with the advantage that power changes can be altered with greater facility than with spectacles. Furthermore, unequal corrections permitting good distance correction with one eye and near for the other will often control low degrees of esophoria.

Exophoria and myopia

Overcorrection will control small degrees of exophoria but, unless bifocals are used, reading vision can suffer. Contact lenses can also be used in overcorrection, and also in one eye only, as suggested for the correction of esophoria.

Anisometropia and anisiekonia

These conditions become a problem if one eye deteriorates more rapidly than the other and a 4 dioptre or more difference results. Contact lens correction reduces the retinal image difference magnification and maintains binocularity. Anisometropia induced by keratoplasty or unilateral aphakia are other examples of large differences in power between the two eyes that, if present in young people or infants, lead rapidly to irremediable amblyopia (see Chapter 34).

The widespread use of intraocular implants in the treatment of cataract has resulted in problems of induced anisiekonia (Bradley *et al.*, 1983), although the symptoms of this condition can, if slight, resolve in time. Contact lenses to correct residual ametropia can help in place of spectacles. In cases where the degree of anisometropia is larger, a combination of powered contact lens and correcting spectacle lenses to produce a magnification or minification effect can be tried.

Amblyopia

Contact lenses can be used as occluders (see Fig. 23.2) and can be made in various degrees of light transmission occlusion and with coloured irises. For children, soft materials are best. For cosmesis, the other eye should be fitted with an iris tinted lens with a clear optic. Good centration is essential. Total occlusion by this method is very difficult to achieve (Grayson & Boling, 1961; Sellers, 1971; Weissman & Donzis, 1990). Optical occlusion can be achieved by making a high plus or high minus lens for the good eye; this gives only a degree of macular confusion but is effective in low degrees of amblyopia.

Nystagmus

It is thought that fine congenital nystagmoid movements can be decreased by the use of hard contact lenses, even if the child is emmetropic. Whilst there is no good objective evidence for this, individual cases are reported in the early literature. Those with albinism associated with refractive errors and nystagmus are often fitted with tinted lenses, with variable results. Desperate conditions often require experimental treatments that require objectivity in assessment.

23.3 SPORTS AND ARMED SERVICES

The use of contact lenses in sports and in the armed services overlaps, as they are both concerned with physical tasks where spectacle wear can be either impossible or a hindrance to performance. Training begins at a very young age in sports such as swimming and, in general, the ability to play ball games, shoot and/or take part in field athletics or horse riding makes varying demands upon the acuity of the individual. Many of these events can put the individual with myopia at a severe disadvantage, and contact lenses are often advised, even if worn only for sporting activities.

The type of lens fitted will depend upon many factors (see Chapters 39 and 40). Specifically, the type of material, lens size and fit will have to ensure greater stability than if the lens was to be used solely for cosmetic purposes. The centration and acuity, and therefore quality, of the optic are of special concern, and adverse binocular vision effects from contact lens wear must be avoided.

There are alternatives for water sports and swimming for pleasure. Watertight goggles can be fitted with prescription lenses powered for air correction and, if required only for underwater vision, the power can be modified for the water-to-lens refractive difference. Contact lenses can be worn under the watertight goggles, in which case the lenses of the goggles are plano, as for emmetropic use. The only contact lens advisable if goggles are not allowed in a water sport is a scleral hard lens.

The armed services will allow contact lenses only if the wearer is proven to be a habitual and successful user of lenses. For certain missions it would even be necessary to prove a few days of continuous wear with suitable lenses. The use of contact lenses in aeroplanes and fighter aircraft can pose several problems, which depend upon whether the cabins are pressurized, on the use of helmets and on the type and effectiveness of the ventilation – its humidity and oxygen pressure. There is a decrease in oxygen pressure at high altitudes and therefore a lens in balance with the corneal oxygen demands at sea level may not be so efficient at high altitudes, with resultant corneal oedema (Weissman, 1980; Fig. 23.7).

However, by fitting contact lenses, it is possible to retain the services of a pilot who has developed myopia; the loss of such a person would not be advised unless absolutely necessary. The possible use of contact lenses as protectives against chemicals is another area where research is needed, to evaluate the likely chemicals and their interaction with contact lens materials (see Chapter 39).

23.4 THERAPEUTIC INDICATIONS

The use of scleral glass shells filled with medication to treat severe eye disease was considered in the late nineteenth century. In the 1930s, isolated examples of the use of contact lenses for retaining conjunctival grafts were cited and, much later, when corneal plastic lenses became available, they were used to retain corneal penetrating and lamellar grafts *in situ* with overlay sutures.

The concept of protective moulded flush fitting shells of PMMA material was introduced in the 1950s (see Chapter 31). They were used to alleviate pain from corneal ulcers, bullous keratopathy, failed keratoplasty or lid surgery, or to apply radiation. In the form of lead shells, they are used to protect the eye from radiation. There are many other indications specific to the individual case (see Chapter 31).

In the early 1960s the therapeutic indications were, to a certain extent, reduced by progress in surgical technology for keratoplasty and cataract extraction and implantation (of the pseudoaphakic lens). However, hydrophilic soft lenses became available at this time and were used in preference to the hard scleral lenses (Gassett & Kaufman, 1970). Hydrophilic soft lenses are most useful when they are large and thin (see Chapter 38). The therapeutic soft lens is now used in high gas permeable material and even in material that dissolves slowly whilst in use (the B & L Federov Therapeutic lens is an example), although abbreviated forms of the hard scleral lens are still indicated for certain surgical procedures. These take the form of tints and are used for symblepharon prevention in burn treatments and after the division of such adhesions (see Chapter 31).

23.4.1 DRY EYE

The only type of lens advised for this type of condition, and then not without reservation, is the scleral hard lens (Gould, 1970). Minor degrees of dry eye can be fitted with soft hydrophilic lenses but require wetting drops almost every few minutes to give good vision and avoid serious complications.

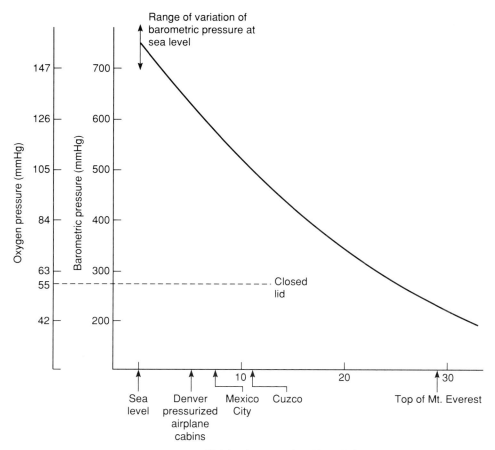

Height above sea level (×1000 feet)

Figure 23.7 Change in barometric and oxygen tension with altitude above sea level. Range at sea level is shown at upper left (reprinted, with permission, from Weissman, 1980).

23.4.2 CORNEAL ANAESTHESIA AND HYPOSENSITIVITY

Some causes of corneal loss of sensation should be considered as indications for contact lens wear; there are also definite contraindications unless management is correct. Here, expert judgement and medical supervision are essential before fitting any type of lens.

23.4.3 POST-HERPETIC OPHTHALMICUS EYE

The eye surface is often hyposensitive after resolution of the disease. This can result in complications such as corneal scarring and the absence of reflex lacrimation. It is essentially a dry eye problem, although, to a lesser degree, the mucoid content of the tears is abnormal. Conventional contact lens wear to correct irregular astigmatism and/or other refractive errors is therefore fraught with problems, such as corneal vascularization and infection. Where contact lens wear is imperative for a vision gain not otherwise possible, a large scleral worn for limited periods is advised. Soft lenses should be considered only with frequent instillation of artificial tear drops, and then only for limited periods.

23.4.4   FIFTH AND SEVENTH CRANIAL NERVE LESIONS

Treatment of brain tumours, tic doloreux and head trauma can result in complete corneal anaesthesia. In those patients when the corneal integrity is at risk, only a tarsorrhaphy provides protection.

23.4.5   CHEMOTHERAPEUTIC USES

Hydrophilic material readily adsorbs small molecules held in solution by water. It is therefore possible to charge a hydrophilic lens with high concentrations of drugs, such as antibiotics, steroids, pilocarpine and atropine; the correct concentration is important if corneal epithelial damage is to be avoided. The medication is released slowly over several hours. Indications for use include corneal suppurative infections, acute angle closure glaucoma and anterior uveitis.

23.5   DIAGNOSTIC INDICATIONS

Most practitioners keep sets of hard and soft lenses, of a range of powers, to assess acuity, binocularity (for example unilateral aphakia) and even tolerance (Korb, 1984). There are also special electrodiagnostic lenses with small insertions of conduction terminals. These, when they are made in the form of hard scleral PMMA, are useful for repetitive use and can be sterilized easily between patients. They are also available as disposable soft lenses.

Scleral hard lenses with four or more lead inserts at the limbal zone can also be used on eyes that have suspected intraocular foreign bodies. X-rays of the eye with the lens *in situ* taken from the front and side will permit accurate localization where more advanced radiographic equipment is not available.

23.5.1   PROSTHETIC USES

This chapter will not deal with ocular prosthetics, but there are many instances where the initial fitting and manufacture is dependent upon conventional contact lens practice.

There are many indications for the use of such appliances: disfigured eyes as a result of injury or disease account for most (Fig. 23.3), but there are many congenital abnormalities that cannot be treated surgically and that are helped by the use of contact lens prostheses. Most of these conditions are associated with poor sight or no useful vision; this makes the task of the fitter easier. Prostheses cannot promise the patient normality but only an approach to normality. In some instances it is necessary to fit the other eye, which may be normal, with a partial prosthesis to obtain a balanced appearance. It must be noted that the contact lens prosthesis carries the iris coloration in a more anterior plane than normal and this in itself can be a disfigurement to the critical viewer.

Partial prostheses are available in all contact lenses and are useful to mask partial scarring of the cornea or large iridectomies, especially when they occur inferiorly and affect vision (Ruben, 1989). Photophobia of any aetiology can be helped with tinted lenses.

23.5.2   EPILEPSY

Individuals who need to wear spectacles and who have major attacks uncontrolled by medication might be considered for contact lenses.

23.5.3   INFANTS AND CHILDREN

In general, fitting cannot be undertaken without the full co-operation and understanding of the parent or guardian. The type of lens most readily tolerated and managed is advised so that treatment can be commenced immediately and the confidence and trust of the child is obtained.

With careful handling, infants can tolerate hard corneal lenses, although insertion and removal is difficult; long periods of wear of soft materials is the easiest management.

Where lens wear is considered essential for the development of vision (such as in aphakia), the fitting can best be done using sedation or general anaesthesia. Once contact lens wear has been established, a change to a more complicated lens to give better acuity can be performed, i.e. changing from soft to hard lenses (see Chapter 34).

23.5.4 LOW VISION AID

A combination of high power minus contact lenses neutralized by spectacle plus lenses at a sufficiently long distance from the eye (about 20 mm) will give a magnification effect in the region of ×2, but the field is usually restrictive (Ruben, 1975; Mandell, 1981).

23.6 CONTRAINDICATIONS

It may seem paradoxical that many conditions of the cornea and lid are suitable for treatment with contact lenses, yet at the same time lenses can, occasionally, cause diseases of the cornea with the same pathology (see Chapters 45 and 46).

This section is therefore not concerned with eye diseases requiring contact lenses as treatment but with all eye conditions that require a contact lens for the correction of a refractive error. However, such eyes may have had previous eye disease that has been treated, or is in a latent or subclinical phase of an eye disease and therefore asymptomatic at the time of fitting a contact lens. A full ophthalmological examination is always essential before proceeding to fit contact lenses (see Chapter 24).

The contraindications to fitting contact lenses will be dealt with under the relevant headings. It should follow that, if the practitioner has eliminated all the contraindications for a particular patient then the failure rate after fitting should be reduced to a minimum. Sadly, this is not the case. There are many patients who, theoretically, should not be fitted but who, for one reason or another, are fitted and succeed beyond all expectation; the converse is also true. In such cases a patient can succeed initially but fail later, due to a contraindication that becomes evident some time after fitting. The practitioner should therefore be wary and always on the look-out for new contraindications. At the same time, with the advances in new materials and lens design, the reasons for intolerance will decrease.

There will always be a small group of patients not fitted for fear of complications, or who have failed to wear lenses successfully, and who return to practitioners time and again for refitting in the hope of becoming a contact lens wearer.

23.6.1 INDIVIDUAL CONTRAINDICATIONS

Age

Providing the patient is physically able to manage a lens-care programme there is no upper age limit. Infants and children have been mentioned and need special treatment. In all age groups, lack of motivation or inability to learn procedures must be considered a contraindication.

Intelligence, behaviour and toilet

Practitioners often see patients who desire contact lenses, whose initial motivation may be high, but whose personal toilet and elemental hygiene makes the use of contact lenses a hazard. In most instances instruction in hygiene will overcome the problem. However, inability to comply with the practitioner's instructions can lead to failure and possibly more serious consequences (Wilson *et al.*, 1981b; Mondino *et al.*, 1986; Chun & Weismann, 1987; Donzis *et al.*, 1987).

Touch sensitivity

Most humans have two levels of sensitivity:

1. Cerebral sensitivity – the fear of any-

thing entering the eye, even eye drops. On examination, such patients can go into blepharospasm, and even opisthotonus; extreme cases may use their hands to fight the practitioner. Use of local anaesthetic drops does not always help; hypnosis could be tried by a qualified practitioner.

2. Peripheral sensitivity – this is much more common and is often associated with excessive histamine reaction to the contact lens or solutions; even after the usual periods of adaptation for the particular lens there is no improvement. After lens insertion the conjunctival tissues become oedematous and the conjunctival vessels dilate; there is little to no adaptation with time. Peripheral sensitivity may be related to a history of allergy, such as hay fever and house-dust sensitivity (an allergist may advise the exact causology and treatment).

Allergy and hypersensitivity

The allergic sensitivity mentioned above, whilst not a serious eye disease, is a nuisance to contact lens wearers because, if they have an allergy to pollen they may be unable to tolerate lenses when the pollen count is high, even with antihistamine-type eye drops (Pederson, 1976).

Evidence of chronic allergic conjunctivitis affecting the palpebral conjunctivae and resulting in papillae, and/or follicles (and, in the severe cases, with old keratoconjunctivitis corneal scarring) should not be fitted without due caution and warnings to the patient.

Preservative in contact lens preparations

Many of the techniques used to clean, disinfect and store contact lenses use bacteriocidal chemicals as active agents. Two well-known examples for use with soft lenses are chlorhexidine and thimersal (an organic mercury compound); benzyl chloride is used for hard lenses (Gasset, 1974 and 1978). It is not always possible to foresee complications arising from the use of such preparations, as many of the signs and symptoms are delayed in time of onset.

The chemical compounds are thought to bind selectively to proteins and to hydrophilic lens materials. Binding to human tissue can initiate an allergic-type response in the conjunctival tissues (Pederson, 1976), with corneal infiltration of inflammatory cells. This is possibly the mechanism for chlorhexidine (Gasset & Ishi, 1975; Hubbard, 1975; Refojo, 1976; Ruben, 1980). There is also evidence that other chemicals used as disinfectants have a cytotoxic effect (Burstein, 1980; Mondino & Groden, 1980).

Thimersal is not a stable compound and the mercury contained in it can come out of solution. This has led to reports of mercury depositions in the contact lens and in the corneal and conjunctival tissues (Wilson *et al.*, 1981a; Zadnic, 1984). If used in high concentrations, the mercury can penetrate the cornea and enter the inner eye (Abrams, 1963, Winder *et al.*, 1980). There is therefore the possibility of cytotoxicity and allergic responses in hypersensitive patients.

At initial consultations a history of allergy and of contact dermatitis should make the practitioner wary of using preparations likely to have a cytotoxic reaction (Rudner, 1972).

Aphakia

Contact lens fitting is contraindicated if blebs in the incision area are continuous with the anterior chamber fluid (see Fig. 23.4; Bellows & McCulley, 1981). If conjunctivitis is induced by contact lens wear then there is a real danger of panophthalmitis. Exposed suture knots should be removed to reduce the risk of tarsal papillitis and excessive mucous formation. If the eye has hypotony and the vision is fluctuating then the advice of the physician managing the patient should be sought before proceeding with the fitting.

When there is evidence of endothelial trauma and loss, and/or Descemet's ruptures, lenses that are likely to cause stromal oedema should be avoided.

In the elderly aphakic or in any patient with a low general resistance to infection, the use of extended wear lenses should be approached with caution or not at all. This applies particularly to diabetes mellitus (see Chapters 45 and 46).

Glaucoma

There is no contraindication to fitting small, hard gas permeable lenses, except in eyes where a filtrating bleb is present and is continuous with the fluid of the anterior chamber. Furthermore, if soft lenses are fitted to an eye being treated with local hypotensive drugs the lens may prevent the drug from entering the anterior chamber. The lens must therefore be removed and the prescribed treatment inserted onto the eye surface. Even soft lenses have been reported as inducing angle closure glaucoma (Krefman & Wilensky, 1982). Scleral hard lenses are contraindicated in glaucoma because they can cause an increase in pressure (Huggert, 1951).

Lacrimal apparatus and glands

Contact lens fitting should be carried out only if tear secretion and drainage are normal. If there are diseases that affect tear formation then the problem of dry eye must be considered from the therapeutic aspect (see Chapter 21). Many forms of contact lenses exacerbate dryness, with resultant epithelial desiccation, erosion and corneal infiltration if not treated (see Chapter 43).

When the problem is excessive tear formation (either reflex in origin or due to lid and lacrimal drainage anomalies), the fitting of

corneal hard lenses may prove impossible, and even soft lenses will not provide good vision.

Lids and secretory glands

The apposition of the lids to the eye surface, and the intervening tear film suction, is a finely balanced mechanism permitting rapid eye movement and a healthy transparent cornea. All contact lenses interfere to a degree with this balance, perfected by nature to cope with all habitable environments. Diseases of the lids affecting the meibomian secretion will adversely affect the tear film and contact lens surface, and lead to rapid drying of the lens and the corneal surface. Meibomianitis of bacterial origin with soapy secretions is particularly suspect and seen in all the drug sensitivity syndromes, such as Stevens–Johnson's syndrome.

Dry eye

Any history of drug sensitivity or medication for vascular hypertensive disorders, cardiac dysrhythmia or anxiety states may suggest induced dry eye problems, which do not auger well for successful wear.

The late signs of pathological dry eye are obvious but the early signs, which have diverse aetiologies and periodic symptoms, are very troublesome to the contact lens practitioner and are difficult to assess. Early signs and symptoms include chronic superficial keratitis in the lower third of the cornea, symblepharon in its most early phase, irritation and redness of the eyes.

A dry eye is particularly prone to infection and this, combined with contact lens wear, can lead to serious complications and even loss of the eye (Seal *et al.*, 1986).

Anterior uveitis

A history of anterior uveitis and evidence of past attacks may be part of the postoperative picture following cataract extraction. Treatment should be completed before proceeding to a fitting. It is important to note that the excessive use of steroids can lead to a fragile epithelium.

Young people may show some idiopathic recurrent types of anterior uveitis and, if treatment is in process, fitting must be delayed until the condition resolves.

In older age groups, association of urinary infection with uveitis may require postponement of the lens fitting or wear.

Infections

All infections of the external eye are a contraindication to contact lens wear, particularly if the cornea is in any way involved or if a viral aetiology is suspected. After treatment and complete healing, wear can recommence with caution.

Hormonal imbalance

The menstrual cycle can affect the rate and/or amount of body secretions, including tears. Changes in the hormonal balance can therefore lead to periods of lens intolerance. Practitioners should avoid trial fittings if there are dry eye problems related to a particular part of the menstrual cycle.

Premenstrual stress and menopausal hormonal deficiency also make it difficult for women to start wearing, or to have trials of, contact lenses. However, with suitable treatment by a physician, contact lens wear can be contemplated. The use of contraceptive pills containing excessive oestrogen can cause dryness of the eyes, although these symptoms should no longer be a problem as most preparations now contain little or none of this hormone.

Thyroid dysfunction

Hypothyroidism can result in dryness of the skin and in tear deficiency and, unless treated by a physician, contact lens fitting is not advised.

Hyperthyroidism can have a degree of exophthalmos, with exposure drying of the cornea; hydrophilic lenses are therefore problematic in the advanced states. The upper lid may not retain corneal lenses of rigid design, and these are therefore impossible to fit. If contact lenses are essential then hard scleral lenses can be considered.

Pancreatic dysfunction

Diabetes mellitus affects glucose metabolism. The corneal epithelial cells can show abnormal fragility and contact lens fitting can therefore be associated with desiccation and even erosions. Infection is a problem in advanced states of diabetes and hard gas permeable lenses, worn for limited periods, are advised (O'Leary & Millidot, 1981).

Skin disorders

As the external eye is part of the outer teguement of the body, any neurodermal disease can affect the eye. Some examples are atopic eczema, psoriasis and acne rosaea. It is wise in all such instances to consider the contact lens as a therapeutic device only, although in most instances there may well be an increase in acuity.

Human immune virus

There is no contraindication to fitting lenses for patients who are HIV-positive, providing the eye tissues are healthy. Practitioners should wear protective gloves if they have open skin lesions and a protective shield for their eyes if there is any risk of the patient's tear fluid contacting their own eyes. The risks are minimal but the usual care with disinfection procedures is required.

Contact lens wear is not advised if the patient has progressed to AIDS, unless this is supervised closely, as such patients are prone to secondary infections from opportunist organisms.

References 515

23.6.2 ENVIRONMENTAL FACTORS

The air temperature, oxygen pressure, humidity, contamination and air speed are all part of our daily environment. There can be large variations in each element but, given time and a healthy constitution, humans can adapt to these variations. However, certain extremes of environmental conditions can cause problems for contact lens wearers. Normal ranges of temperature are no contraindication but excessive infrared radiation is a potent drier of the lens surface and permits transmission of heat to the eye. Excessive doses of ultraviolet radiation will injure the eye tissues and cause inflammation and keratitis. The human crystalline lens can absorb most normal exposure doses but in aphakia the protection is absent and the contact lens material must have an ultraviolet blocking agent in the material, or tinted glasses should be worn in the sun.

At work, industrial processes have a range of pollutants from irritating chemicals to dust particles and even flash exposure. Most Western communities have developed regulations to protect workers from injury and to negate the harmful effects of some industrial processes. If there is any doubt, and the safety officer, insurance officers or union officials cannot give an all clear for contact lens wear at work, then wear should be considered contraindicated (see Chapter 39).

ACKNOWLEDGEMENT

The author wishes to thank Dr Barry Weissman for supplying the illustrations for this chapter.

REFERENCES

Alleger, C. (1971) The case of the artificial iris. *Optom. Weekly*, **62**, 55–7.

Abrams, J.D. (1963) Mercurial preservatives in eye drops. *Trans. Ophth. Soc. UK*, **83**, 263.

Bellows, A.R. and McCulley, J.P. (1981) Endophthalmitis in aphakic patients with unplanned filtering blebs wearing contact lenses. *Ophthalmology*, **88**, 839–43.

Bradley, A., Rubin, J. and Freeman, R.D. (1983) Nonoptical determinants of aniseikonia. *Invest. Opthalmol. Vis. Sci.*, **24**, 507–12.

Burstein, N.L. (1980) Corneal cytotoxicity of topically applied drugs. *Surv. Ophth.*, **25**, 15–30.

Chun, M.W. and Weissman, B.A. (1987) Compliance in contact lens care. *Am. J. Optom. Physiol. Opt.*, **64**, 274–6.

Donzis, P.B., Mondino, B.J., Weissman, B.A. and Bruckner, D.A. (1987) Microbial contamination of contact lens care systems. *Am. J. Ophthalmol.*, **104**, 325–33.

Gassett, A.R., *et al.* (1974) Cytotoxicity of opthalmic preservatives. *Am. J. Opthalmol.*, **78**, 98–105.

Gassett, A.R. and Ishi, Y. (1975) Cytotoxicity of chlorhexidine. *Can. J. Opthalmol.*, **10**, 98–100.

Gassett, A.R. and Kaufman, H.E. (1970) Therapeutic uses of hyrophilic contact lenses. *Am. J. Opthalmol.*, **69**, 252–9.

Grayson, M. and Boling, R. (1961) Clinical application of contact lenses. *Int. Ophthalmol. Clin.*, **1**, 327–36.

Gould, H.L. (1970) The dry eye and scleral contact lenses. *Am. J. Ophthalmol.*, **70**, 37–41.

Hubbard, W.L. (1975) Chlorhexidene uptake and release. *Contact Lens J.*, **9**.

Huggert, A. (1951) Increase of the intraocular pressure when using contact glasses. *Acta Ophthalmol.*, **29**, 475–81.

Korb, D.R. (1984) Predicting the successful patient; clinical and diagnostic tests. *J. Am. Optom. Assoc.*, **55**, 191–3.

Krefman, R.A. and Wilensky, J.T. (1982) Case report: angle-closure attach with hydrogel lens wear. *Int. Cont. Lens Clin.*, **9**, 366–8.

Maltzman, B.A., Harris, M. and Espy, J. (1985) Experience with soft bifocal contact lenses. *CLAO J.*, **11**, 73–7.

Mandell, R.B. (1981) *Contact Lens Practice*. CC Thomas, Springfield IL, USA.

Mondino, B.J. and Groden, L.R. (1990) Conjunctival hyperemia and corneal infiltrates with chemically disinfected soft contact lenses. *Arch. Opthalmol.*, **98**, 1767–70.

Mondino, B.J., Weissman, B.A., Farb, M.D. and Pettit, T.H. (1986) Corneal ulcers associated with daily wear and extended wear contact lenses. *Am. J. Ophthalmol.*, **102**, 58–65.

O'Leary, D.J. and Millidot, M. (1981) Abnormal epithelial fragility in diabetes and contact lens wear. *Acta Ophthalmol.*, **59**, 827–33.

Pederson, N.B. (1976) Allergy to chemical solutions for soft lenses. *Lancet*, **ii**, 1363.

Polse, K.A. (1977) Orthokeratology as a clinical procedure. *Am. J. Optom. Physiol. Opt.*, **54**, 345–6.

Refojo, M.F. (1976) Reversible binding of chlorhexidine gluconate. *Contact and Intra-Ocular Lens J.*, **2**, 47–56.

Ruben, M. (1975) *Contact Lens Practice*. London: Bailliere Tyndall.

Ruben, M. (1980) Chlorhexidine and the poly-Hema soft lens. *Contact Lens J.*, **9**.

Ruben, M. (1989) *Color Atlas of Contact Lenses* (2nd ed). Wolfe Medical Publications, London.

Rudner, E.J. *et al.* (1973) Epidemiology of contact lens dermatitis in North America (1972). *Arch. Dermatol.*, **537**.

Seal, D.V. *et al.* (1986) Bacteriology and tear protein profiles of the dry eye. *Br. J. Ophthalmol.*, **70**, 122–5.

Sellers, E. (1971) The restoration of visual function in cases of amblyopia utilizing contact lenses. *Br. J. Physiol. Opt.*, **26**, 130–42.

Shivitz, I.A. *et al.* (1987) Contact lenses in the treatment of patients with overcorrected radial veratotomy. *Opthalology.* **94**, 899–903.

Tomlinson, K. (1972) The therapeutic value of contact lenses in cases of ocular abnormalities. *The Optician*, **163**, 8–11.

Weissman, B.A. (1980) Predicted changes in tear layer oxygen. *Int. Cont. Lens Clin.*, **7**, 41–4.

Weissman, B.A. and Chun, M.W. (1987) The use of spherical power effect bitoric rigid contact lenses in hospital practice. *J. Am. Optom. Assoc.*, **58**, 626–30.

Weissman, B.A. and Donzis, P.B. (1990) Contact lenses. In Morgan, M.M. and Rosenbloom, A.A. (eds), *Pediatric Optometry*. JB Lippincott, Philadelphia, USA.

Wilson, L.A., McNatt, J. and Reitschel, R. (1981) Hypersensitivity to thimersal in C.L. wearers. *Ophthalmology*, **88**, 804–9.

Wilson, L.A., Schlitze,r R.L. and Ahearn, D.G. (1981b) Pseudomonas corneal ulcers associated with soft contact lens wear. *Am. J. Ophthalmol.*, **92**, 546–54.

Winder, A.F., Ruben, M. and Astbury, N.J. (1980) Penetration of mercury into the eye. *Lancet*, 237–9.

Zadnik, K. (1984) Severe allergic reactions to thimersal *J. Am. Optom. Assoc.*, **55**, 507–9.

M. Guillon and B.A Weissman

24.1 INTRODUCTION

The preliminary examination is defined as the series of tests and discussions which allow the clinician to decide whether the patient is suitable for contact lens wear and, if so, lead to the selection of the first trial contact lens. This selection is the subject of the chapters on basic and specialized contact lens fittings (Chapters 27, 28, 29 and 33). The preliminary examination of a patient attending for contact lenses follows the same principles as the entry level ophthalmic examination, however, due to specific requirements of contact lens fitting the examination requires some additional procedures.

The preliminary examination can be divided into three parts: (1) a complete ophthalmic examination to determine patient suitability for contact lenses; (2) once suitability is established, a series of preliminary specialized measurements; and (3) consultation with the patient to discuss the type of contact lens best suited to the needs of the patient.

Details of the procedures used in the first two parts of this examination are covered in other chapters of this textbook, in particular biomicroscopy (Chapter 18), keratometry (Chapter 16), photokeratoscopy (Chapter 17), tear evaluation (Chapter 21), aesthesiometry (Chapter 20), oxygen uptake (Chapter 22) and pachometry (Chapter 19), as well as other textbook references. This chapter will limit itself to discussing procedures in terms of their implications to contact lens fitting.

Consultation with the patient is a most essential part of the preliminary examination. It allows the practitioner to ascertain whether the expectations of the patient of the contact lenses are unrealistic and, if so, to either abandon lens fitting or counsel the patient on the limitations of the chosen modality and also to explain the requirements for successful lens wear.

The procedures making up the preliminary examination are usually carried out in sequence during a single visit. The subsequent trial lens fitting is then carried out either immediately following the preliminary examination or at a subsequent visit depending on the time needed to fit the chosen modality and/or the practice organizational set up.

24.2 OPHTHALMIC EXAMINATION

The ophthalmic examination is divided into its conventional components of: (1) patient history; (2) refractive evaluation (Borish, 1975; Edwards & Llewellyn, 1988); and (3) binocular evaluation (Borish, 1975; Reading, 1983).

24.2.1 PATIENT HISTORY

The main aim of patient history taking is to gather general information which will help the practitioner determine the suitability of

Contact Lens Practice. Edited by Montague Ruben and Michel Guillon.
Published in 1994 by Chapman & Hall, London. ISBN 0 412 35120 X

the patient for contact lenses and select the most suitable lens type and modality of wear. Patient history is usually conducted by the practitioner asking a series of open questions. However, as some standard information is always required, it is often beneficial to have an assistant administer a standard questionnaire prior to the patient seeing the practitioner. Such an approach saves the practitioner time while ensuring collection of relevant information, which allows for immediate in depth questioning by the practitioner on the most critical points.

Patient history can be divided into three parts: (1) patient details; (2) general history; and (3) ocular history.

Patient details

Patient details which need to be identified include those necessary for identification and correspondence, such as full name, address and telephone numbers (daytime and evening). It is essential for good patient care that such information is checked regularly to ensure current validity so that contact with the patient is always easily obtained. Details of patient age, sex, occupation and hobbies can assist the practitioner in many ways. The first two may point to specific problems (see Chapter 23), such as the possibility of dry eye in older patients (Guillon & Guillon, 1992) in particular women (McMonnies & Ho, 1987). Details of occupation and hobbies will greatly influence the lens type and modality chosen for the patient. Certain occupations and hobbies will have special requirements from contact lens wear (see Chapters 39 and 40). For example, soft contact lenses are recommended for most sports, but special attention needs to be paid to swimming to avoid losing contact lenses or creating adverse effects. Some outdoor hobbies, such as camping or mountaineering, where lens care is difficult, may influence the modality of wear, for example, flexible wear

and/or disposable contact lenses. Another important activity to assess is driving habits. For those people involved with significant night driving, particular attention should be paid to ensure that the lenses have a sufficiently large optical zone, particularly if RGP lenses are chosen (Chissadon *et al.*, 1992).

General History

Detailed general history will help identify any contraindications (see Chapter 23) to contact lens wear. This history is taken in three broad sections: (1) past or active systemic diseases; (2) familial conditions; and (3) medications. The presence of any systemic disease must be identified. In particular, it is important to identify any allergy (see Chapter 23) that will make tolerance to contact lens wear more difficult and indicate the need for careful patient management. Familial conditions may not contraindicate lens wear (with the exception of certain corneal dystrophies), however, they may have an impact on the type of lens chosen and on patient management strategies, e.g. keratoconus. Knowledge of the medications being used by the patient is essential. In most countries, the national pharmaceutical society publishes a book listing all drugs commercially available, along with any known side effects. It is essential, when a medication is not known to the practitioner, that he/she obtains such information in order to be aware of any possible problem with contact lens fitting. Medications which induce or exacerbate dry eyes are the most common sources of complaints relating to the use of prescribed or over-the-counter drugs.

A final aspect that should be investigated is the patient dietary regime, especially when obesity is indicated. Excessive cholesterol intake (Hill & Terry, 1976) has been shown to be associated with increased greasing problems of the contact lens surfaces, and high alcohol intake is often associated with dry eye problems.

Ocular history

The following aspects of the patient's ocular history need to be reviewed: (1) the patient's past and current correction modalities; (2) any past history of eye diseases; and (3) any unusual eye problems.

Knowledge of the patient's past and present correction modalities are essential. This information should include:

1. Date of last examination and the refractive findings.
2. Date of the current correction.
3. Details of previous contact lens wear and solutions.

A standard questionnaire such as that in Appendix 24.A is often useful in gathering this information. If the information given by the patient is sparse or vague, it is recommended that, if known, the patient's previous practitioner should be contacted to obtain any missing information.

Any previous or current eye disease, surgery and/or associated eye drop usage that may contraindicate contact lens wear and/or put restrictions on the type of contact lenses to be used (see Chapter 23) should be investigated.

Identification of any ocular problems, in particular dryness or irritation problems should be made. Questionnaires such as that developed by McMonnies (McMonnies & Ho, 1987) for non-contact-lens wearers enables the detection of any dry eye problem and quantification of its severity. The presence of a contact lens may destabilize the tear film, and exacerbate the problem. A modified version of the McMonnies questionnaire has been developed for contact lens wearers (Guillon *et al.*, 1992). A positive answer to this questionnaire indicates the need for greater care in clinical management. For example, those patients screening positively on the modified McMonnies questionnaire will need to use shorter replacement frequencies than asymptomatic patients.

24.2.2 REFRACTIVE AND BINOCULAR VISION EVALUATIONS

The refractive evaluation must begin with a full sphero-cylindrical refraction (Borish, 1975; Edwards & Llewellyn, 1988) and the measurement of visual acuity (Guillon & Sayer, 1988). Some practitioners tend to limit their examination to the best spherical refraction when intending to fit a spherical soft contact lens. Such an approach is unacceptable, as it does not allow the assessment of the full visual potential of the patient from which to compare the contact lens performance. Further, for all refractive errors greater than ±4.00 D, the refractive information must include the measurement of the back vertex distance.

The evaluation of binocular vision is too often neglected when contact lens fitting is undertaken. Because contact lenses present a different binocular situation to spectacles, in particular to the high ametrope, it is essential to evaluate binocular vision (Borish, 1975; Reading, 1983) before any contact lens fitting is undertaken.

24.3 PRELIMINARY MEASUREMENTS

24.3.1 INTRODUCTORY REMARKS

The preliminary measurements to contact lens fitting are all described in detail in other chapters. The purpose of this section is to list the various tests that are available according to their use and relevance to routine and/or specialized contact lens fitting. The tests can be divided into three general groups: (1) measurements of the anterior segment; (2) examination of the ocular tissues; and (3) assessment of corneal functions.

24.3.2 MEASUREMENTS OF THE ANTERIOR SEGMENT

The main four parameters measured prior to contact lens fitting are corneal curvature, corneal diameter, palpebral aperture and pupil size.

Corneal curvature

The anterior corneal surface is the most powerful refractive surface of the eye and the ocular structure upon which contact lenses rest. The measurement of corneal curvature is therefore nearly universal in contact lens fitting. Most often the measurements are limited to the evaluation of the curvature at the corneal apex. Recently, however, with advanced modern information, the corneal curvature is determined for the whole cornea. The two techniques used are keratometry (see Chapter 16) and photo- or video-keratoscopy (see Chapter 17). The keratometer, which is the instrument most commonly used in the clinic, is principally used to measure accurately the central corneal curvature. Certain authors (Wilms, 1981) have suggested using the keratometer to measure peripheral corneal curvature, but the accuracy of such a technique is poor and of limited clinical value. Wherever peripheral corneal curvature measurements are necessary, photo- or video-keratoscopy is the technique to choose, as it enables an overall mapping of the cornea.

The measurement of corneal curvature is made with the following aims:

1. To monitor the effects of contact lens wear by recording a baseline value prior to contact lens fitting.
2. To select the first trial contact lens for RGP fitting.

For soft contact lenses, in particular modern thin lenses, these measurements are of lesser importance as the mechanical performance of those lenses is not closely linked to the corneal shape.

Corneal diameter

The cornea is not circular but oval in shape, with its longest dimension along the horizontal meridian, the average difference between horizontal and vertical dimensions being approximately 0.5 mm. The usual measurement technique does not measure the true corneal diameter but estimates its value by measuring the horizontal visible iris diameter (HVID) and occasionally the vertical visible iris diameter (VVID). The instrumentation used for that varies in sophistication and includes:

1. A millimetre ruler (Fig. 24.1) and a comparator (Fig. 24.2), most commonly used in practice with the naked eye or with a low power magnifier such as a Burton lamp.
2. A graticule attachment to the biomicroscope, usually situated in the eye piece and projected onto the cornea.
3. A macro video or photographic system that produces an image later captured and analysed, with a digitizer, after image filtering (Fig. 24.3), which permits more accurate measurement in clinical research practice.

The true corneal diameter, defined as the continuous zone of regular surface terminating at the limbus, can be directly measured by using the image of two strips of light (Holden & Martin, 1982). This measurement indicates that the visible iris diameter does not reflect accurately the true corneal diameter but tends to under-estimate it by approximately 0.9 mm.

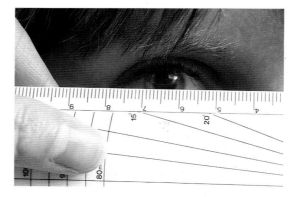

Figure 24.1 Measurement of horizontal visible iris diameter (HVID) with millimetre ruler.

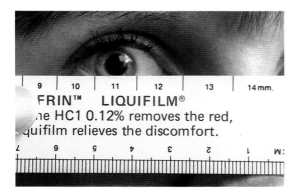

Figure 24.2 Measurement of horizontal visible iris diameter (HVID) with comparator ruler.

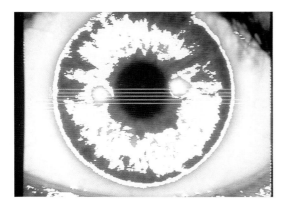

Figure 24.3 Measurement of horizontal visible iris diameter (HVID) from filtered macrophotographic image analyzer with image digitizer.

The measurement of corneal diameter is not habitually used in routine contact lens practice as it is not the major factor determining the parameters of the contact lens to be fitted. For RGP lenses, the contact lens diameter is chosen with reference to the lid cornea interaction. For most soft contact lenses, the diameter is usually standard and should provide ample limbal coverage. The measurement of corneal diameter is left to exceptional cases involving a micro or macro cornea, or when fitting cosmetic contact lenses. In the latter case, it is essential to ensure full corneal

coverage by the tinted part of the lens to obtain a good cosmetic effect when lenses are fitted bilaterally to patients wishing to alter the colour of their eyes. Similarly, when a lens is fitted unilaterally to mask a corneal or iris defect, the corneal diameter must be measured to ensure a good match with the fellow eye. In fact, with cosmetic contact lenses, the relevant measurement is not the true corneal diameter but the visible iris diameter, hence the current techniques used in practice are suitable.

Palpebral aperture

The measurement of the vertical palpebral aperture is carried out with the same instruments as the visible iris diameter, the millimetre ruler (Fig. 24.4) being the most common method. This measurement is, however, not common in routine practice. For soft contact lenses, the size of the palpebral aperture does not play a significant role in lens selection and performance. For RGP contact lenses, the interaction between the contact lenses and the lids is a critical factor controlling the lens' mechanical performance. However, in that context the relative position of the lids with regard to the limbus is more important than the size of the palpebral aperture (see Chapter 27). The size of the palpebral aperture is, at times, measured by the practitioner before fitting RGP lenses for extended wear, as it has been shown that these lenses create a small relative ptosis (Fonn & Holden, 1988).

Pupil size

The pupil diameter is not often measured in contact lens practice because it is a difficult measurement to carry out accurately. The techniques used are similar to those described for the visible iris diameter (Figs. 24.5 and 24.6). For this measurement, however, it is essential in addition to control the lighting level, and accommodation and con-

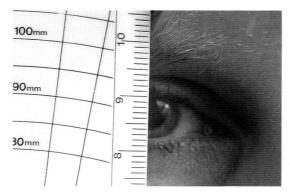

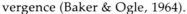

Figure 24.4 Measurement of vertical palpebral aperture with millimetre ruler.

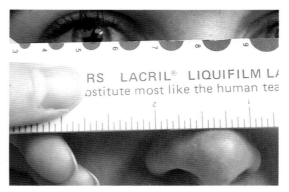

Figure 24.6 Measurement of pupil diameter with comparator ruler.

vergence (Baker & Ogle, 1964).

The measurement of the visible iris diameter is, however, important. For some contact lens application as large inter-patient variations have been demonstrated (Chissadon *et al.*, 1992). The pupil size should be measured under low luminance (1–5 cd/m^2) to mimic night driving light conditions when an RGP contact lens is fitted to young myopes involved in extensive night driving. Young myopes (Chissadon *et al.*, 1992) have been shown to have particularly large pupils, which could be problematic with RGP lenses, which are usually slightly off-centred in normal use. The measurement of pupil size should also be considered for all bifocal contact lens fitting, where small differences in optic zone size have important implications for the overall performance. The measurement in these cases should be made at least in average indoor light conditions (approximately 50 cd/m^2) and possibly under bright day time conditions ($\geq$ 250 cd/m^2).

24.3.3 EXAMINATION OF THE OCULAR TISSUES

The slit lamp biomicroscope is the instrument Brandreth, (1978) used to evaluate the ocular tissues before contact lens fitting and at subsequent visits. The slit lamp biomicroscope, combining a sophisticated focalized lighting system with a range of magnifications (see Chapter 18), permits an in-depth examination of the different structures. The examination begins with a low magnification ($\times$10) observation using a diffuser for an even lighting of the structures observed. The examination then continues by altering both the lighting techniques and observation magnifications. The usual approach is to begin by observing the outer structures, lid, conjunctiva and tears and the cornea, beginning with the epithelium and progressing to the endothelium. A number of attachments to the slit lamp biomicroscope enable more

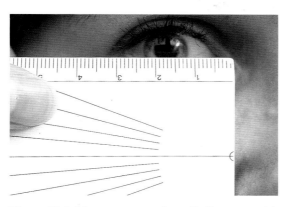

Figure 24.5 Measurement of pupil diameter with millimetre ruler.

detailed examination. Of particular relevance to the examination of the potential contact lens wearer are:

The tearscope

A broad diffuse light source that replaces the lighting system of the biomicroscope and allows the examination of the undisturbed tear film under variable magnification (see Chapter 21). This technique allows detection of those patients for whom contact lens wear is contraindicated due to abnormal tears. It also helps to identify border line cases, for whom particular attention must be paid as to possible tear-related contact lens problems.

Optical pachometer

The pachometer is composed of a modified eye piece and a beam splitter that divides the view into two vertical halves. The device permits the measuring of the overall corneal thickness or, under special circumstances, the epithelial thickness alone (see Chapter 19). The pachometer is rarely used during routine examination of the potential contact lens wearer. Its main application is to obtain baseline measurements before prescribing soft extended wear lenses that are known to produce long-term corneal thinning (Holden *et al.*, 1985). It can also be used to measure the corneal thickness profile when fitting a keratoconic patient.

24.3.4 ASSESSMENT OF CORNEAL FUNCTIONS

The assessment of corneal function is rarely carried out prior to contact lens fitting. The main reason is that the techniques available are usually complex and time consuming. The most common functions evaluated are as follows:

Corneal sensitivity

Corneal sensitivity is measured using an aesthesiometer, a hand-held device that is best used as an attachment to the biomicro-scope (see Chapter 20). The measurement of corneal sensitivity is indicative of the state of epithelial physiology.

Corneal oxygen uptake

The measurement of corneal oxygen uptake is also an indication of epithelial physiology. It indicates the amount of oxygen required by the corneal epithelium and anterior stroma, to maintain its normal metabolic rate. The technique is particularly complex and the equipment expensive, so that its use prior to contact lens wear is limited to specialist research clinics (see Chapter 22).

Endothelial function

The endothelial function is assessed by measuring the capacity of the cornea to deswell from induced corneal swelling. To that effect, corneal swelling is induced by either passing gases with reduced concentration of oxygen for a period of a few minutes or by closing the eye over a thick (0.40 mm) low water content contact lens for two hours. The endothelial function is then measured by assessing the rate of corneal thinning by pachometer following discontinuation of the hypoxic stress (by return to normal environmental removal of the contact lens). The technique requires the use of a sophisticated pachometer and is therefore limited to research clinics prior to contact lens wear.

24.4 PATIENT CONSULTATION

Armed with the data from the physical examination of the patient, the patient's previous experience and future needs and the results of the diagnostic evaluation, the clinician must spend time with the patient discussing the pros and cons, the benefits and risks, and the likely expectations of contact lens wear with a specific design and material.

No way of assuring any patient of contact

lens 'success' has yet been found. First one must define 'success' – as Sarver and Harris (1971) have done (Fig. 24.7).

One must then allow each patient to modify their criteria to his/her particular situation: one patient, knowing his/her own motivation and availability, might consider 4 hours a day during the weekend of comfortable wear and good vision to be a total success. Another might be unhappy with less than comfortable continuous wear for three months at a stretch. True success, unfortunately, can only be determined after the best contact lens prescription has been dispensed and worn for some period of time.

Financial considerations should not be ignored. Some patients are very concerned about their investment, and the unpredictability of the outcome. Others express no concern at all. The careful practitioner should be pessimistic prior to the decision to order lenses, and then optimistic afterwards. The practitioner should also be careful to fully discuss with the patient the financial responsibility involved both in ordering and in continuing to use contact lenses.

Physical risks to corneal health and benefits must be additionally weighed. All contact lens wear carries with it some physical risk. Most clinicians and researchers agree risks are greater with extended wear than with daily wear contact lenses; with adequate hygiene, common sense and compliance, use of contact lenses on a daily wear schedule really appears to involve minimal risk (Mondino *et al.*, 1986) of serious, sight threatening complications. Informed consent is nonetheless helpful in this regard and probably should be used for all contact lens applications (Fig. 24.8).

Beyond such generalities, special considerations occasionally must be made: a 20-year-old 3 dioptre myope should not continue extended contact lens wear, in my opinion, in the face of 2 mm of 360° neovascularization; daily wear might still be appropriate. A unilateral 60-year-old aphake, however, with an identical biomicroscopic appearance, might be allowed to continue wear with a gentle discussion and photodocumentation of the physical appearance of the cornea so that the changes may be accurately monitored.

24.5 CONCLUSION

Modern contact lens practice has opened up excellent potential for both patients and clinicians. We are able to help patients today as never before. The combination of advanced

1.	Wearing time:	The patient must be able to wear his lenses regularly and continously for a minimum period of eight hours.
2.	Comfort:	The patient may experience no more than a slight lens awareness, slight photophobia in sunlight, and/or an occasional foreign body sensation.
3.	Vision:	The patient must report no significant blur, flare, or edge reflections, and his visual acuity must be within one Snellen line of the visual acuity achieved with his best spectacle lens correction. He must report no significant spectacle blur following lens removal.
4.	Ocular tissue changes:	The cornea (and other ocular tissues) must be free of any significant disturbances. Only slight peripheral corneal staining, faint central corneal clouding immediately upon removing the lenses, and corneal curvature changes not exceeding ± 0.75 DK are acceptable.
5.	Normal appearance of the patient:	There must be no squinting or significant alteration in either head posture, blinking pattern, or eye injection.

Figure 24.7 Criteria for a successful patient response (reprinted, with permission, from Sarver & Harris, 1971).

Contact lens wear has some associated risks. Contact lenses may cause pain, irritation, watering of the eyes, red eyes, allergies, blood vessel growth, sensitivity to light, and infection – which if in the cornea can lead to scarring and perhaps loss of vision. Daily wear contact lenses offer minimal risk to the patient, provided that conscientious and hygienic care is used, the lenses are not overworn or slept (or napped) in, and the patient returns at indicated intervals for continuing professional care. Extended wear contact lenses have been shown to offer somewhat greater risks of ocular infection and both personal and professional care is additionally important.

Certain conditions may increase the risk of infection even when lenses are only used for daily wear such as (circle one if appropriate):

- having only one good eye and wearing a contact lens on it
- using steroid drops while wearing a contact lens
- wearing a contact lens after corneal surgery (i.e., corneal transplants, RK)
- wearing a contact lens on an eye with a filtering bleb (for glaucoma)

It may still be in your overall best interest to wear a lens if one of these conditions applies to you, but you should consider your options and discuss your individual situation with your doctor(s).

Alternatives to contact lens wear include spectacles and perhaps surgery, but these also have associated risks and benefits. My contact lenses are intended for (circle one) DAILY WEAR   EXTENDED WEAR. I understand that if I develop any eye pain, discomfort, redness, tearing, severe sensivity to light or foggy vision I will remove all contact lenses IMMEDIATELY and report to my eye doctor.

This is to acknowledge that I have read the information contained herein and recognize that it is my responsibility to follow all instructions, to care for my contact lenses conscientiously and hygienically, and to report for office visits as requested.

PLEASE TAKE A MOMENT AND BE CERTAIN THAT YOU HAVE ASKED YOUR DOCTOR OR THE STAFF ANY QUESTIONS YOU MAY HAVE AT THIS TIME REGARDING THE ABOVE INFORMATION.

Signature   Date

Witness/Parent   Date
(if necessary)

Figure 24.8 Informed consent.

materials and improved contact lens design, in skilled hands, allows a much higher potential for successful application. Many more patients, responding to these advances, are wearing contact lenses today than ever before, perhaps in excess of 40 million worldwide. It is the responsibility of the ophthalmic professions to do their work wisely and well, and minimize the risks while maximizing the benefits: clear and comfortable vision without spectacles.

REFERENCES

Baker, W.D. and Ogle, L.N. (1964) Papillary response to fusional eye movements. *Am. J. Ophthalmol.*, **4**(58), 743–56.

Borish, I.M. (1975) *Clinical Refraction, Vol 1* (3rd ed), Professional Press.

Brandreth, R. (1978) *Clinical Slit Lamp Biomicroscopy*. Multimedia Communications, University of California School of Optometry, Berkeley, California.

Chissadon, M.L., Guillon, M., Shah, D. and Guillon, J.P. (1992) Pupil dimension age related changes and their implications for contact lens design. *Optom. Vis. Sci.*, **Suppl. 69** (12s), 134.

Edwards, K. and Llewellyn, R. (1988) *Optometry*. Butterworths.

Fonn, D and Holden, B.A. (1988) Rigid gas permeable versus hydrogel contact lenses for extended wear. *Am. J. Optom. Physiol. Opt.*, **65**(7), 536–44.

Guillon, J.P. and Guillon, M. (1992) Preocular tear

film normative data. *Optom. Vis. Sci,* **Suppl. 69** (12s), 132.

Guillon, M, and Sayer, G. (1988) Critical assessment of visual performance in contact lens practice. *Contax,* **May,** 8–10.

Guillon, M.G., Allary, J.C., Guillon, J.P. and Orsborn, G. (1992) Clinical management of regular replacement: Part I. Selection of replacement frequency. *ICLC,* **19**, May/June.

Hill, R.M. and Terry, J.E. (1976) Human tear cholesterol levels. *Arch. Ophthal. (Paris),* **36**, 155–60.

Holden, B.A. and Martin, D.K. (1982) A new method for measuring the diameter of the in vivo human cornea. *Am. J. Optom. Physiol. Opt.,* **59**(5), 436–41.

Holden, B.A., Sweeney, D.F., Vannas, A., Nilsson, K.T. and Efron, N. (1985) Effects of long term extended contact lens wear on the human cornea. *Invest. Ophthalmol. Vis. Sci.,* **26**, 1489–501.

McMonnies, C.W. and Ho, A. (1987) Responses to a dry eye questionnaire from a normal population. *J. Am. Opt. Assoc.,* **58** (7), 588–91.

McMonnies, C.W. and Ho, A. (19XX) Marginal dry eye diagnosis: History versus Biomicroscopy. In *The Pre-Ocular Tear Film in Health, Disease and Contact Lens Wear* (ed. F.J. Holly) Dry Eye Institute, Lubbock, TX, pp. 32–40.

Mondino, B.J., Weissman, B.A., Farb, M.D. and Pettit, T.H. (1986) Corneal ulcers associated with daily wear and extended wear contact lenses. *Am. J. Ophthalmol.,* **102**, 58–65.

Reading, R.W. (1983) *Binocular Vision: Foundations and Applications.* Butterworths.

Sarver, M.D. and Harris, M.G. (1971) A standard for success in wearing contact lenses. *Am. J. Optom. Physiol. Opt.,* **48**, 382–5.

Wilms, K.H. (1981) Topometry of the cornea and contact lenses with new equipment. *Ophthalmic Optician,* **21**(16), 516–19.

APPENDIX 24.A

Please answer the following questions by ticking the appropriate responses. (Tick one, or more if appropriate). The information gathered in this questionnaire will remain confidential and help us to ascertain your suitability to wear contact lenses. Please omit any questions you do not understand.

1.   When did you have your last eye examination?

1.   ( ) Less than 6 months ago
2.   ( ) 1 year ago
3.   ( ) 2 years ago
4.   ( ) 2–5 years ago
5.   ( ) More than 5 years ago: specify . . . years

2.   Do you wear glasses or contact lenses at present? (Tick one, or more if appropriate).

1.   ( ) No
2.   ( ) Yes, glasses
3.   ( ) Yes, contact lenses

If NO, go to question 5

3.   If you answered *Yes, glasses* to Question 2, please answer Question 3, otherwise go to Question 4.

a.   What type of glasses do you have and when do you wear them? (Tick one or more if appropriate).

1.   ( ) General use, worn most of the time
2.   ( ) Worn when not wearing my contact lenses
3.   ( ) For distance vision only
4.   ( ) For near vision only
5.   ( ) Two pairs, one for distance and one for near
6.   ( ) Bifocals
7.   ( ) Multifocals (e.g. Varilux, Progressive lenses, Trifocals)
8.   ( ) Other please specify. . .

b.   Were your glasses changed at your last examination?

1.   ( ) Yes
2.   ( ) No

If NO, how old are your present glasses?

1.   ( ) Less than 6 months old
2.   ( ) 1 year old
3.   ( ) 2 years old
4.   ( ) 2–5 years old
5.   ( ) More than 5 years old, specify . . . years

c.   Are you happy with your present glasses?

1. ( ) Yes
2. ( ) No

If NO specify why. . .

4. If you have answered *Yes, contact lenses,* to Question 2, please answer Question 4, otherwise go to Question 5.

a. What type of contact lenses do you wear now?

   1. ( ) Soft lenses
   2. ( ) Soft disposable lenses. You replace them every . . . days/weeks.
   3. ( ) Hard lenses
   4. ( ) Gas permeable lenses
   5. ( ) Others, please specify. . .

b. When did you start wearing those contact lenses?

   1. ( ) Less than 6 months ago
   2. ( ) 1 year ago
   3. ( ) 2 years ago
   4. ( ) 2–5 years ago
   5. ( ) More than 5 years ago, specify . . . years

c. How old are your present contact lenses?
   Right lens:. . .
   Left lens:. . .

d. Do you wear your contact lenses?

   1. ( ) Daily wear (remove lenses every night)
   2. ( ) Extended wear (sleep with lenses in)

   If *Daily wear*, how long do you wear your contact lenses? (on average)
   i. Hours per day. . .
   ii. Days per week. . .

   If *Extended wear*, how many days and nights without taking the lenses out? (on average). . .

e. Do you use a contact lens cleaner?

   1. ( ) No
   2. ( ) Not sure
   3. ( ) Yes, Which cleaner?. . .

If Yes, do you use the cleaner each time you remove your lenses overnight?
( ) Yes ( ) No

f. Do you disinfect your lenses?

   1. ( ) No
   2. ( ) Not sure
   3. ( ) Yes, which solutions?. . .

If Yes, do you disinfect your lenses each time you remove them overnight?
( ) Yes ( ) No

g. Do you use protein removal tablets (enzyme tablets)

   1. ( ) No
   2. ( ) Not sure
   3. ( ) Yes   How often?. . .
                Which tablets?. . .

h. Have your eyes ever had any adverse reactions to contact lens wear?

   1. ( ) No
   2. ( ) Not sure
   3. ( ) Yes, please specify. . .

i. Have your eyes ever had any adverse reactions to contact lens solutions?

   1. ( ) No
   2. ( ) Not sure
   3. ( ) Yes, please specify. . .

j. Are you happy with your present contact lenses?

   1. ( ) Yes
   2. ( ) No
      If *NO*, why. . .

Go to Question 6

5. Have you worn other types of contact lenses or tried contact lenses before?

   1. ( ) Yes. If Yes, answer Question 5
   2. ( ) No. If No, go to Question 6

a. What type of contact lenses were they?

   1. ( ) Soft lenses
   2. ( ) Hard lenses
   3. ( ) Gas permeable lenses
   4. ( ) Others, please specify. . .

b. How long did you try or wear those contact lenses for?

1. ( ) Less than 6 months
2. ( ) 1 year or less
3. ( ) 2 years or less
4. ( ) 2–5 years
5. ( ) More than 5 years, specify . . . years

c. Did you wear those contact lenses?

1. ( ) Daily wear (removed lenses every night)
2. ( ) Extended wear (slept with lenses in)
3. ( ) Not applicable, I only tried them for a very short time.

d. Why did you stop wearing those contact lenses?. . .

CONTACT LENS CARE SYSTEMS AND SOLUTIONS USED BY THE PRACTITIONER

Fiona Stapleton and Judith Stechler

25.1 INTRODUCTION

The purpose of a contact lens care system is to maintain lenses clean, free of microbial contamination and wettable in the eye.

Lens cleaning is necessary to remove surface debris and to prevent the formation of surface deposits. Deposition may reduce acuity, alter lens performance by changing the lens fitting and movement, cause allergic responses such as giant papillary conjunctivitis, cause corneal oedema, discomfort, lens related red eye and reduce lens life (see Tripathi & Tripathi, 1984, for a review).

Maintaining a lens free of microbial contamination is an important consideration in the prevention of ocular infection. It has been established that lens wearers are at a significantly higher risk of microbial keratitis compared with non-lens wearers (Dart *et al.*, 1991), although the relationship between lens wear and microbial conjunctivitis has not been well established. Microbial keratitis requires corneal epithelial damage and an inoculum of organisms. Contact lenses may increase the susceptibility of the cornea to infection in several ways. Epithelial barrier function may be reduced as a result of impaired corneal metabolism or mechanical stress causing microtrauma (Holden *et al.*, 1985), tear flow dynamics and normal tear resurfacing mechanisms are altered during lens wear; toxic or hypersensitivity responses may arise from the carry over of lens care solutions to the eye (Wilson *et al.*, 1981a) and raised temperature behind a lens may encourage bacterial proliferation (Martin & Fatt, 1986).

Pseudomonas aeruginosa, a ubiquitous environmental Gram-negative rod, is frequently associated with soft contact lens related infections (Weissman *et al.*, 1984; Ormerod & Smith, 1986), although other Gram-negative rods, such as *Serratia* species (Lass *et al.*, 1981), *Proteus* species (Alfonso *et al.*, 1984) and other *Pseudomonas* species (Wilson *et al.*, 1981b), have been reported. Of the Gram-positive organisms, *Staphylococcus* species are the most prevalent (Galentine *et al.*, 1984; Ormerod & Smith, 1986). Much less commonly, other micro-organisms such as filamentous fungi (Wilhelmus *et al.*, 1988) and protozoans such as *Acanthamoeba* species (Stehr-Green *et al.*, 1989) have been associated with lens related keratis.

Contact lens wear alone is thought not to modify the spectrum of organisms which can

Contact Lens Practice. Edited by Montague Ruben and Michel Guillon.
Published in 1994 by Chapman & Hall, London. ISBN 0 412 35120 X

be recovered from the normal non-lens wearing conjunctiva (Tregakis *et al.*, 1973a; Rauschl & Rogers, 1978; Smolin *et al.*, 1979; Callender *et al.*, 1986a; Larkin & Leeming, 1991). Common conjunctival organisms rarely cause infection in normal eyes. Gram-negative pathogens are rarely isolated from the conjunctiva of asymptomatic wearers, hence other sources of organisms are likely. Bacteria may be spread from other regions in the body, such as the upper respiratory tract, the skin or gastro-intestinal tract, or from exogenous environmental sources. The external environment may cause micro-organism contamination, via the lens care materials (Cooper & Constable, 1977; Galentine *et al.*, 1984; Mayo *et al.*, 1987), eye drops or make-up (Wilson & Ahern, 1977). Most lens case contamination is thought to arise from the fingers when inserting and removing the contact lens from the storage case. Other routes for environmental contamination arise from the fingers when inserting the lenses (Cooper & Constable, 1977; Wilson *et al.*, 1981b; Adams *et al.*, 1983; Hart & Shih, 1987), by rubbing the eyes or from airborne contaminants. Lens disinfection aims to reduce the potential for microbial inoculation to the cornea.

Lens surface wettability is an important consideration for the maintenance of good lens comfort and optical properties. Poor lens wetting may lead to tear resurfacing disorders, reduced acuity, irritation and corneal surface abnormalities.

25.2 LENS CARE SYSTEMS

The licensing of all contact lens solutions is regulated in the UK and in the USA. To gain a product licence, manufacturers must provide information on the quality, including stability, efficacy and safety of the product. This must also include data on toxicity of the product, its compatibility with lenses, other solutions and solution containers, and its microbiological efficacy (see Meakin, 1984,

for review and history of licensing in the UK).

Desirable properties of contact lens care solutions include:

1. The solution should be manufactured sterile with means of minimizing chance microbial contamination when in use.
2. It should cause minimal effect on the ocular tissues.
3. There should be compatibility with lens materials, inducing no significant lens parameter changes.
4. There should be compatibility with other solutions used.
5. The solution must have a product licence, and be labelled with an expiry date two years from the date of manufacture.

25.2.1 CLEANING SYSTEMS

During wear and handling, lenses are subject to the accumulation of mucus, protein, lipid and inorganic salts from the tear film, and exogenous debris such as nicotine, cosmetics, micro-organisms and atmospheric pollutants. Hydrophobic surfaces on lenses tend to attract debris. Daily cleaning of lenses prior to lens disinfection removes organic debris likely to inactivate antimicrobials (see Martindale, 1989a, for a review), and has been shown to reduce the numbers of viable organisms recoverable from a lens (Shih *et al.*, 1985). Routine daily cleaning is a prophylactic measure for all types of lenses and does not restore lenses to their original unworn state (Fowler & Allansmith, 1981).

Daily cleaners

Cleaning solutions may include surfactants, preservatives, chelating agents, buffering agents, purified water and sodium chloride.

Surfactants are surface active detergents which solubilize debris and emulsify lipids. Surfactants lower the interfacial tension between two immiscible phases. Molecules contain two localized regions, one hydrophilic in nature and the other hydrophobic. Surfactants form a surface monolayer with the hydrophobic region of the molecule orientated towards the surface of the lipid (Phillips, 1980). Since the hydrophilic region is water soluble, lipids may be emulsified.

Surfactants used for their cleaning capability, may be non-ionic, anionic or amphoteric. Non-ionic molecules have no charge or ionization of the molecule, and are generally compatible with anionic and cationic substances. Surfactants for use with hydrogel lenses are generally non-ionic to reduce interaction with lens polymers. Non-ionic and some amphoteric surfactants also have low ocular irritancy. Anionic surfactants dissociate in aqueous solution, to form an anion, which is responsible for the surface activity and a cation, devoid of surface properties. Conversely, cationic dissociate to form a surface active cation and non-active anion. Amphoteric surfactants contain anionic and cationic groups on the molecule, and can behave with anionic, non-ionic or cationic properties depending on the pH of the solution. Cationic surfactants such as benzalkonium chloride, which are used only as antimicrobial agents and not for cleaning purposes, may become bound to ionic components of lens materials.

Preservatives are incorporated to prevent chance contamination of the solution once opened. Rigid lens cleaners may contain benzalkonium chloride at a concentration between 0.004 and 0.02%. Both rigid and soft lens cleaners use thiomersal at a concentration of 0.001–0.004% and chlorhexidine at 0.002–0.006%. Sorbic acid or potassium sorbate may be used in hydrogel lens cleaners at a concentration of 0.1–0.25%, as an alternative to thiomersal and chlorhexidine. Alcohols such as isopropyl alcohol (20%) may be incorporated as preservatives in hydrogel lens cleaners. These have an additional action as lipid solvents.

Chelating agents, usually ethylene diamine tetra-acetic acid (EDTA) or its salts, are incorporated to bind divalent metal ions such as calcium or magnesium. Removal of such divalent ions from solutions prevents their use in intracellular and cell wall metabolism by micro-organisms.

Phosphate or borate buffers are incorporated to maintain pH less than 7.4 since certain formulations become less stable above pH 8.

Sodium or potassium chloride is incorporated to maintain the tonicity of the solution. Certain daily cleaners or multipurpose solutions are formulated hypertonic to enhance their cleaning action.

Rigid lens cleaners have also been formulated containing 10% sodium tridecylether sulphate and silicon or polymeric beads as friction agents to enhance the cleaning activity. It is thought that the surfactant emulsifies deposits, reduces surface tension, and subsequently the polymeric beads serve to shear the protein build up and lipid complexes from the lens surface. This type of formulation is not suitable for surface coated lenses or silicon rubber lenses.

Cleaning solutions are generally used with manual rubbing of the lens followed by rinsing with sterile saline or the disinfecting solution. Mechanical devices such as sponges or turbulent cleaning and storing cases may be used when the wearer has poor lens handling or poor manual dexterity.

Enzyme treatments

Tear film proteins are derived mainly from the lacrimal gland and include albumin, globulin and lysozyme. Proteinaceous deposits on contact lenses are predominantly lysozyme (Sack *et al.*, 1987), which is selectively adsorbed to the lens surface. The protein layer formed on ionic hydrogel lenses has been shown to be thicker compared with that formed on non-ionic lenses (Sack *et al.*, 1987). Bound protein is not removed by daily surfactant cleaning (Kleist & Thorson, 1978) and is thought to contribute to allergic and inflammatory conditions in hydrogel lens wearers (Allansmith *et al.*, 1977) and in rigid lens wearers (Allansmith *et al.*, 1978). The removal of protein is an important step in contact lens care regimes, and has been shown to reduce or alleviate symptoms of lens associated papillary conjunctivitis (Korb *et al.*, 1983). Protein removal is usually performed using enzyme treatment. Enzymes are biochemical catalysts which are usually specific for single chemical reactions. Proteases hydrolyse proteolytic deposits to soluble peptide residues. Contact lens care systems require broad spectrum proteases, which cleave protein molecules at multiple sites, for more effective protein removal, and which ideally act rapidly without interacting with lens polymers.

Proteases fall into two main groups (Huth, 1987).

1. Sulphydryl proteases. These are based on the amino acid cystein, and are deactivated by heat or hydrogen peroxide, for example papain.

2. Serine proteases. These are based on the amino acid serine, and maintain their proteolytic activity in heat or hydrogen peroxide, for example subtilisin or subtilisin A. Maintaining proteolytic activity in hydrogen peroxide enables simultaneous disinfection and protein removal for hydrogel lenses. It has been suggested that combination of protease and peroxide increases disinfection efficacy over peroxide alone, and improved protein removal compared with protease alone.

These two types of protease have been compared in a clinical study (Larcabal *et al.*, 1989). Subtilisin A was found to be more effective at removing light deposits, whereas papain was more effective for medium to heavy deposits.

Multiple enzyme treatments may also be used. These generally contain a protease, lipase (for the hydrolysis of lipids) and an amylase (for the hydrolysis of polysaccharides). Multiple enzymes such as pancreatin or pronase, are useful where lens wearers are sensitive to papain (Carmichael, 1983; Davis, 1983). The effectiveness of papain for the removal of protein was compared with pancreatin in a clinical study (Kurashige *et al.*, 1987). Papain was found to be more effective in the removal of heavy proteinaceous deposits, although both treatments were equally effective at removing light deposits. Similar results were shown for heavily deposited lenses in a laboratory study (Kjellsen *et al.*, 1984).

In summary, it appears that papain is a more effective means of protein removal for moderate to heavy protein deposition on hydrogel lenses, but that subtilisin A and pancreatin are more effective at removing light to moderate protein deposition. Pancreatin is a useful choice where lens wearers are sensitive to papain, and subtilisin A gives effective protein removal when combined with peroxide. This simultaneous action may encourage patient compliance. Regular use of enzyme treatment appears to reduce the build-up of proteinaceous deposits on both rigid and hydrogel lenses.

Professional cleaners

These are intensive oxidative cleaners for professional use only. Sodium perborate may be used in conjunction with heat (50–60 °C) and agitation for 2–4 hours, evolving reactive oxygen. In addition to the cleaning effect, sodium perborate has limited antimicrobial activity, due to the generation of hydrogen peroxide. This type of aggressive lens cleaning is now less frequently carried out due to the current use of disposable or frequently replaced lenses.

25.2.2 DISINFECTION SYSTEMS

All micro-organisms can exist as viable vegetative cells; in some cases they are able to form dormant spore forms, which are much more resistant to the lethal effect of heat and chemicals. Sterilization is the destruction of all viable forms including spores. Disinfection processes will destroy vegetative cells, but spores frequently survive. Contact lens care systems aim for disinfection of lenses and not sterilization, so all spores are unlikely to be destroyed.

Disinfection systems can be divided into physical and chemical agents:

Physical agents

These depend upon generating sufficient energy to cause lethal protein denaturation and cell changes.

Heat

Disinfection of vegetative organisms requires heating in the presence of water at 80 °C for 10 min. Disinfection may also be achieved with heating between 60–80 °C for longer periods of time, for those lens materials which are unstable at higher temperatures. However, effective disinfection of *Acanthamoeba* cysts has been shown to require temperatures above 65 °C (Kilvington, 1989). Sterilization for complete removal of viable organisms requires autoclaving at 121 °C for 15 min. Moist heat is effective at lower temperatures than dry heat, and destroys organisms by coagulating and denaturing cell protein.

Thermal disinfection correctly performed, is an effective method of disinfection against the majority of micro-organisms (Tregakis *et al.*, 1973b; Busschaert *et al.*, 1978; Ludwig *et al.*, 1986a). Repeated exposure of high water content hydrogel lenses to thermal disinfection is thought to damage lens materials, however low water content lenses have shown little change in lens parameters (Reidhammer & Falcetta, 1980). Heat denatures tear protein, and results in increased deposition and reduced lens life. Another consideration is that the lens storage case must also be able to withstand the thermal process (Amos & Ward, 1988).

Ultraviolet radiation

The emission spectrum from ultraviolet (UV) radiation from low pressure UV lamps, typically used for sterilization, has a peak at 260 nm, which is close to the absorption maximum of DNA and RNA. Airborne organisms are very susceptible to destruction by UV radiation. However the efficacy of UV radiation in destroying organisms on dirty surfaces is questionable. One study performed in the USA has found that ultraviolet disinfection of lenses contaminated with a small range of pathogens, was able to rapidly reduce the concentration of viable organisms (Dolman & Dobrogowski, 1989), and that lenses were able to survive up to 8 h of exposure. Recent studies however, have been unable to demonstrate satisfactory contact lens disinfection with devices currently available (Palmer *et al.*, 1991).

Microwave radiation

Microwave disinfection of contact lenses has been suggested as a rapid, effective, inexpensive and convenient method for hydrogel lenses (Rohrer *et al.*, 1986). Microwave radiation produces an antimicrobial effect due to destruction of cellular constituents, and may achieve this with both thermal and nonthermal effects (see Harris *et al.*, 1989a for a review). Rohrer *et al.*, (1986) evaluated a 700 W microwave against an inoculum of 10^6 organisms/ml for seven common bacterial pathogens, two fungi and two viruses. Complete sterilization was achieved in 8 min, however lenses were dehydrated during this procedure and needed to be subsequently rehydrated. Harris *et al.*, (1989a) showed that 90 s of exposure in a 600 W microwave was effective for disinfection of a limited range of organisms. Microwave disinfection may prove to be an effective future means for the disinfection of hydrogel trial lenses. A further study by Harris *et al.*, (1990) demonstrated rapid kill times for contaminated lens storage cases. However, there have been few controlled studies to determine optimal exposure times for a range of organisms and the long-term effects on lens polymers are unknown. A preliminary study performed on 32 hydrogel lenses exposed to one microwave disinfection cycle (Hatch & Paramore, 1990) showed no significant change in lens parameters measured.

Ultrasound radiation

Ultrasound refers to sound waves with a frequency higher than 16–20 Hz. It is an effective means of surface disinfection, and this may make it suitable as a contact lens cleaning and disinfection system. Ultrasound cleans by cavitation, whereby sound waves produce frictional forces in the liquid medium, which generates heat and bubble formation. The bubbles then dissolve almost immediately, causing implosion or cavitation. The disinfection ability of ultrasound is partly due to cavitation within bacterial cells, mechanical pressure generated on the cell walls and as a result of the heat generated. There is limited information on the use of ultrasound with deposited or contaminated lenses, but one study evaluating a single unit with a small number of patients has shown that ultrasound has limited antimicrobial activity (Phillips *et al.*, 1989). Fatt (1991) evaluated the physical limitations of ultrasonic cleaning and has shown that effective cleaning of high water content hydrogel lenses requires high levels of sonic energy. Although units could be designed with such a high output, this level of surface energy dissipation would damage low water content hydrogel or gas permeable lenses. Efron *et al.*, (1991) demonstrated similar results for an ultrasonic cleaning unit, which was effective for cleaning soiled low water content hydrogels, but was less effective for gas permeable or high water content hydrogel lenses.

Chemical agents

Chemical disinfection systems must be sufficiently cytotoxic to eliminate viable microorganisms, but must have minimum toxicity to ocular tissues. This often requires removal of active components from the lens prior to lens insertion, either by degradation, rinsing or neutralization. Solution formulation has an important role in the antimicrobial efficacy and human cytotoxicity. Consequently, increasing the concentration of the active agent will not necessarily increase the antimicrobial efficacy or toxicity.

Fresh disinfecting solutions should be used each time lenses are returned to the storage case.

Chemical systems may be divided into two groups:

Preserved systems

These contain active antimicrobial agents (which also act as preservatives), a chelating agent, buffering agent, purified water and sodium chloride, with or without potassium chloride.

Antimicrobials Antimicrobials in rigid lens disinfection systems are often the same as in the respective cleaning solution. However, concentrations are higher in disinfection solutions as the major function is not to deal with chance contamination but to destroy organisms on lenses. In rigid lens systems, benzalkonium chloride, (usually at a concentration of 0.004–0.02%), and chlorhexidine gluconate (0.006%) dissolve lipid from the cell membrane of bacteria and fungi. Preservatives such as organic mercurials bind to enzyme groups and denature proteins. Antimicrobials such as benzalkonium chloride and chlorhexidine gluconate show reduced antimicrobial activity in the presence of ionic molecules. Non-ionic agents such as glycerol or propylene glycol may be incorporated to increase the antimicrobial efficacy (Meakin, 1989).

Combinations of chlorhexidine gluconate (0.002–0.006%), thiomersal (0.001–0.0025%) and EDTA (0.1–0.128%) are commonly used for the disinfection of hydrogel lenses. The bactericidal strength of these solutions tends to be lower compared with those for rigid lenses as hydrogel lenses may act as a reservoir for solutions which elute from the lens onto the eye (Refojo, 1976). Antimicrobials may be absorbed by or adsorbed onto lenses, which may act as haptens, causing a local delayed hypersensitivity response (Wilson *et al.*, 1981c). Interactions between these compounds, the contact lens surface and adsorbed surface mucoproteins may contribute to toxic and hypersensitivity responses (Binder *et al.*, 1981; Mondino *et al.*, 1987). Partly reversible binding of chlorhexidine gluconate to hydrogel lenses has been reported (Plant *et al.*, 1981). This preservative binding is thought to be enhanced by protein deposition on lenses (Kaspar, 1976) and an animal model has demonstrated toxic epithelial responses associated with chlorhexidine gluconate (Green *et al.*, 1980). There is less binding of preservatives to rigid lenses and solution related disorders are less common. Interactions between rigid lens materials and benzalkonium chloride have been reported, although there have been considerable differences in the reported levels of preservative adsorption. Using fluorescence spectroscopy, laboratory studies have suggested that benzalkonium chloride uptake occurs with silicone/acrylate molecules as a result of charged binding of the preservative with the lens surface (Rosenthal *et al.*, 1986). In one clinical study, using similar methodology, attributed to electrostatic interaction of the molecule with silicone acrylate copolymers (Herskowitz, 1987). However, this methodology has been criticized, and using an alternative assay, minimal uptake ot benzalkonium chloride with CAB (Richardson *et*

al., 1980) and silicone acrylate materials (Wong *et al.*, 1986) has been shown. Using a radioactive tracer technique, adsorption and release of benzalkonium chloride has been demonstrated for both rigid and hydrogel materials (Chapman *et al.*, 1990). In this recent comparative study of rigid lens materials, greatest uptake and release of benzalkonium chloride was found to occur for fluorosilicone acrylate polymers (Chapman *et al.*, 1990).

Other combinations of antimicrobials and preservatives in hydrogel lens disinfection systems include:

1. Alkyltriethanol ammonium chloride (0.013%), which is chemically similar to benzalkonium chloride, but is less cytotoxic to both micro-organisms and human cells, is used in conjunction with thiomersal (0.002%).
2. Chlorhexidine-based tablet, containing 0.4 mg of chlorhexidine gluconate, for use with 10 ml of potable tap water, resulting in a chlorhexidine concentration of 0.004%. The resulting solution contains a sequestering agent to remove polyvalent metal ions which may be present in tap water, and is buffered with malic acid (Davies *et al.*, 1990a). The formulation of this tablet purifies the tap water in the lens storage case (Anthony *et al.*, 1991). As the antimicrobial efficacy of chlorhexidine is reduced in the presence of ionic molecules, this system is contraindicated for use with Type IV hydrogel lenses.

Chelating agents These are incorporated to enhance the antimicrobial activity of certain disinfectants, such as EDTA, which enhances the activity of benzalkonium chloride (see page 000).

Buffering agents Buffering agents are incorporated to maintain optimal solution pH for enhanced antimicrobial efficacy.

Sodium chloride, with or without potassium chloride is incorporated into solutions intended for carry over to the eye. This maintains the solution tonicity equivalent to that of tears, at 0.9% sodium chloride.

Antimicrobial activity Solution formulations which are highly toxic to microorganism cells are also toxic to human cells. Less toxic formulations may be offset by a longer recommended disinfection period. The benefits of faster kill rates must be balanced against the incidence of toxic or allergic responses.

Cleaning solutions and those for rinsing or wetting lenses are formulated to deal only with chance contamination. It has been well established that cleaning and rinsing lenses reduces the microbial load on lenses. Using an initial inoculum of 10^6, cleaning and rinsing lenses is found achieve an 3.7 log unit reduction in the number of organisms recoverable. Individually cleaning and rinsing reduce by 1.9 log units each (Houlsby *et al.*, 1984).

All available solutions have passed licensing requirements for antimicrobial efficacy, however, under current UK regulations, contact lens disinfecting *units* do not require a product license from the Medicines Control Agency. Microbiological efficacy of disinfection systems can be compared by using D values (Decimal reduction time), which is the time taken to achieve a 1 log cycle reduction in the inoculum. Where the destruction rates are non-linear, plots of the log survivors against time gives the total log reduction achieved during the disinfection period, following a fixed challenge.

Studies using different testing procedures have compared the efficacy of different disinfecting solutions (Penley *et al.*, 1981a,b; Houlsby *et al.*, 1984; Reinhart *et al.*, 1990). The antimicrobial activity of solutions can be very dependent on several formulation factors, such as pH, the presence of ionic molecules, temperature and whether lenses have

been cleaned and rinsed prior to disinfection. Chemically preserved solutions appear to show good antimicrobial activity against bacteria under laboratory conditions, but appear to be less good against fungi. Houlsby *et al*, (1984), have demonstrated slow kill rates for chemically preserved solutions using a sensitive recovery test for viable organisms. This study concluded that solutions containing chlorhexidine (0.005%) and thiomersal (0.001%) provide effective disinfection of bacteria, but not for yeast and fungi. A solution containing quaternary ammonium chloride (0.013%) and thiomersal (0.002%) was not found to provide effective disinfection for any test organisms.

There has recently been concern for disinfection ability against *Acanthamoeba* species and several studies have demonstrated inadequate kill times for either trophozoites or cysts using disinfection systems containing either quaternary ammonium compounds (Lindquist *et al.*, 1988; Brandt *et al.*, 1989; Penley *et al.*, 1989) chlorhexidine/thiomersal (Ludwig *et al.*, 1986b; Brandt *et al.*, 1989), benzalkonium chloride (Penley *et al.*, 1989) and sorbate (Sylvany *et al.*, 1990). However, other studies using different methodologies, have demonstrated effective antiacanthamoeba activity with systems containing chlorhexidine alone (Anthony *et al.*, 1991) or in combination with thiomersal (Sylvany *et al.*, 1990). Rigid lens disinfection systems containing benzalkonium chloride were found to be effective (Sylvany *et al.*, 1990).

Unpreserved systems

Oxidative systems are frequently used to eliminate toxic and hypersensitivity disorders resulting from the carry over of preservatives and antimicrobial agents to the eye. Oxidative systems break peptide links in proteins and reduce them to soluble amino acid products. These depend on the chemical breakdown of an active toxic agent to a non-toxic product at physiological pH.

epithelium and endothelium. *Arch. Ophthalmol.*, **98**, 1273–8.

Gyulai, P., Dziabo, A., Kelly, W., Kiral, R. and Powell, C.H. (1987) Relative neutralisation ability of six hydrogen peroxide disinfection systems. *Contact Lens Spectrum*, **2**, 61–8.

Gyulai, P. *et al.* (1989) Lens plus Oxysept 2 neutralising tablets. *Contact Lens Forum*, **14** (12), 38.

Harris, M.G., Torres, J. and Tracewell, L. (1988) pH and H_2O_2 concentration of hydrogen peroxide disinfection systems. *Am. J. Optom. Physiol. Optics*, **65**, 527–35.

Harris, M.G., Kirby, J.E. Tornatore, C.W. and Wrightnour, J.A. (1989a) Microwave disinfection of soft contact lenses. *Optom. Vis. Sci.*, **66**(2), 82–6.

Harris, M.G., Brennan, N.A., Lowe, R.L. and Efron, N. (1989b) Hydration changes of Acuvue disposable lenses during disinfection. *Clin. Exp. Optom.*, **72**(5), 159–62.

Harris, M.G., Rechberger, J., Grant, T. and Holden, B.A. (1990) In-office microwave disinfection of soft contact lenses. *Optom. Vis. Sci.*, **67**(2), 129–32.

Hart, D.E. and Shih, K.C. (1987) Surface interactions on hydrogel extended wear lenses: microflora and microfauna. *Am. J. Optom. Physiol. Optics*, **64**(10), 739–48.

Hatch, S.W. and Paramore, J.E. (1990) Effects of microwave disinfection on hydrogel contact lenses. *Int. Contact Lens Clin.*, **17**, 264–70.

Herskowitz, R. (1987) Solution interaction and gas permeable lens performance. *Contact Lens J.* **15**(2), 3–8.

Holden, B.A. Sweeney, D.F., Vannas, A., Nilsson, K.T. and Efron, H. (1985). Effects of long-term extended contact lens wear on the human cornea. *Invest. Ophthalmol. Vis. Sci*, **26**, 1489–1501.

Houlsby, R.D., Gajar, M. and Chavez, G. (1984) Microbiological evaluation of soft contact lens disinfecting solutions. *J. Am. Optom. Assoc.*, **55**, 205–11.

Huth, S.W. (1987) Protein deposits and removal with modern hydrogel contact lenses. *Die Kontactlinse*, **21**(2), 17–18.

Janoff, L.E. (1984) The Septicon system: A review of pertinent scientific data. *Int. Contact Lens Clin.*, **11**(5), 275–9.

Josephson, J.E. and Caffery, B. (1986) Sorbic acid revisited. *J. Am. Optom. Assoc.*, **57**(3), 188–9.

Kaspar, H. (1976) Binding characteristics and microbiological effectiveness of preservatives. *Aust. J. Optom.*, **59**, 4–9.

Kelly, W.S., Ward, G., Williams, W. and Dziabo, A. (1990) Eliminating hydrogen peroxide residuals in solutions and contact lenses. *Contact Lens Spectrum*, **5**(1), 41–4.

Kilvington, S. (1989) Moist heat disinfection of pathogenic *Acanthamoeba* cysts. *Applied Microbiol.*, **9**, 187–9.

Kjellsen, T., Kiral, R. and Eriksen, S.P. (1984) Single-enzyme versus multi-enzyme contact lens cleaning system: Speed and efficiency in removing deposits from hydrogel lenses. *Int. Contact Lens Clin.*, **11**(11), 660–7.

Kleist, F.D. and Thorson, J.C. (1978) How effective are soft lens cleaners? *Rev. Optom.*, **115**(4), 43–9.

Korb, D.R., Greiner, J.V., Finnemore, V.M. and Allansmith, M.R. (1983) Treatment of contact lenses with papain. *Arch. Ophthalmol.*, **101**, 48–50.

Kurashige, L.T., Kataoka, J.E., Edrington, T. and Vehige, J.G. (1987) Protein deposition on hydrogel contact lenses: A comparison study of enzymatic cleaners. *Int. Contact Lens Clin.*, **14**(4), 150–9.

Larcabal, J.E., Hinrichs, C.A., Edrington, T.B. and Kurishige, L.T. (1989) A comparison study of enzymatic cleaners: Papain versus Subtilisin A. *Int. Contact Lens Clin.*, **16**(11), 318–21.

Larkin, D.F.P. and Leeming, J.P. (1991) Quantitative alterations of the commensal eye bacteria in contact lens wear. *Eye*, **5**, 70–4.

Larkin, D.F.P., Kilvington, S. and Easty, D.L. (1990) Contamination of contact lens storage cases by *Acanthamoeba* and bacteria. *Br. J. Ophthalmol.*, **74**, 133–5.

Lass, J.H., Haaf, J., Foster, C.S. and Belcher, C. (1981) Visual outcome in eight cases of *Serratia marcescens* keratitis. *Am. J. Ophthalmol.* **92** (3), 384–90.

Levy, B. and Gross, M.L. (1988) Clinical evaluation of a chlorine based disinfection system for soft contact lenses. *Can. J. Optom.*, **50**(1), 16.

Lindquist, T.D., Doughman, D.J., Rubenstein, J.B., Moore, J.W. and Campbell, R.C. (1988) Acanthamoeba-contaminated hydrogel contact lenses. *Cornea*. **7**(4), 300–3.

Lowe, R. and Brennan, N.A. (1987) Hydrogen peroxide disinfection of hydrogel contact lenses: An overview. *Clin. Exp. Optom.*, **70**(6), 190–7.

Ludwig, I.H., Meisler, D.M., Rutherford, I. Bican, F.E., Langston, R.H.S. and Visvesvara, G.S. (1986a) Susceptibility of Acanthamoeba to soft contact lens disinfection systems. *Invest. Ophthalmol. Vis. Sci.*, **27**(4), 626–8.

Ludwig, I.H., Meisler, D.M., Rutherford, I., Bican, F.E., Lanston, R.H.S. and Visvesvara, G.S. (1986b) Susceptibility of Acanthamoeba to soft contact lens disinfection systems. *Invest. Ophthalmol. Vis. Sci.*, 27(4), 626–8.

Martin, D.K. and Fatt, I. (1986) The presence of a contact lens induces a very small increase in the anterior corneal surface temperature. *Acta Ophthalmol.*, 64, 512–18.

Martindale (1989a) *The Extra Pharmacopoeia* (29th edn), (ed. J.E.F. Reynolds), Pharmaceutical Press, London, Part 1, pp. 949–72.

Martindale (1989b) *The Extra Pharmacopoeia* (29th ed), (ed. J.E.F. Reynolds), Pharmaceutical Press, London, Part 1, 94–186.

Martindale (1989c) *The Extra Pharmacopoeia* (29th ed), (Ed. J.E.F. Reynolds), Pharmaceutical Press, London, Part 111, 1419–22.

Mayo, D.S., Schlitzer, R.L., Ward, M.A., Wilson, L.A. and Ahern, D.G. (1987) Association of *Pseudomonas* and *Serratia* corneal ulcers with use of contaminated solutions. *J. Clin. Microbiol.*, 25(8), 1398–400.

McCulloch, R.R., Torres, J.G., Wilhelmus, K.R. and Osato, M.S. (1988) Biofilm on contaminated hydrogel contact lenses protects adherent *Pseudomonas aeruginosa* from antibacterial therapy. *ARVO Abstracts* (supplment to *Invest. Ophthalmol. Vis. Sci.*) 12, 228.

McKenney, C. (1990) *The effect of pH on hydrogel lens parameters and fitting characteristics after hydrogen peroxide disinfection.* Transactions of the British Contact Lenses Association Annual Clinical Conference, Glasgow, pp. 46–51.

McNally, J.J. (1990) Clinical aspects of topical application of dilute hydrogen peroxide solutions. *C.L.A.O.J.*, 16(1), S46–S51.

Meakin, B.J. (1984) Contact lens solutions in the United Kingdom. *J. Br. Contact Lens Assoc.*, 7(4), 192–202.

Meakin, B.J. (1989) Contact lens care systems: An update. *J.B.C.L.A.*, 12, 26–31.

Mondino, B.J., Brawman-Mintzer, O. and Boothe, W.A. (1987) Immunological complications of soft contact lenses. *J. Am. Optom. Assoc.*, 58(10), 832–5.

Moore, K. (1987) Necessity and methods of HTLV-III inactivation in contact lens practice. *J. Am. Optom. Assoc.*, 58 (3), 180–6.

Moore, M.B., McCulley, J.P., Newton, C., Cobo, L.M. Foulks, G.N., O'Day, D.M., Johns, K.J., Driebe, W.T. Wilson, L.A. Epstein, R.J. and Doughman, D.J. (1987) *Acanthamoeba* keratitis:

A growing problem in soft and hard contact lens wearers. *Am. J. Ophthalmol.*, 103 (6), 1654–61.

O'Connor-Davies, P.H., Hopkins, G.A. and Pearson RM (1989) *The actions and uses of ophthalmic drugs* (3rd ed.), Butterworths, London, 14–18.

Ogunbiyi, L. (1986). The use of sodium thiosulfate for inactivating residual hydrogen peroxide on contact lenses after disinfection. *Clin. Exp. Optom.*, 69(1), 16–21.

Ormerod, L.D. and Smith, R.E. (1986) Contact lens-associated microbial keratitis. *Arch. Ophthalmol.*, 104, 79–83.

Palmer, W., Scanlon, P. and McNulty, C. (1991) Efficacy of an ultraviolet light contact lens disinfection unit against microbial pathogenic organisms. *J. Br. Contact Lens Assoc.*, 14(1), 13–16.

Paugh, J.R., Brennan, N.A. and Efron, N. (1987) Ocular response to hydrogen peroxide. *Am. J. Optom. Physiol. Optics*, 65, 91–8.

Penley, C.A., Ahern, D.G., Schlitzer, R.L. and Wilson, L.A. (1981a) Laboratory evaluation of chemical disinfection of soft contact lenses. Part I. *Contact and Intraocular Lens Med. J.*, 7, 101–10.

Penley, C.A., Ahern, D.G., Schlitzer, R.L. and Wilson, L.A. (1981b) Laboratory evaluation of chemical disinfection of soft contact lenses. Part II. Fungi as challenge organisms. *Contact and Intraocular Lens Med. J.*, 7, 196–204.

Penley, C.A., Liabres, C., Wilson, L.A. and Ahern, D.G. (1985) Efficacy of hydrogen peroxide systems for soft contact lenses contaminated with fungi. *C.L.A.O.J.*, 11(1), 65–8.

Penley, C.A., Willis, and Sickler, S.G. (1989) Comparative antimicrobial activity of soft and rigid gas permeable contact lens solutions against *Acanthamoeba*. *C.L.A.O.J.*, 15(4), 257–60.

Phillips, A.J. (1980) The cleaning of hydrogel contact lenses. Contact lens review. *Ophthalmic Optician*, 20, 375–88.

Phillips, A.J., Badenoch, P. and Copley, C. (1989) Ultrasound cleaning and disinfection of contact lenses: A preliminary report. *J. Br. Contact Lens Assoc.*, 12(6), 20–3.

Pitts, R.E. and Krachmer, J.H. (1979) Evaluation of soft contact lens contamination in the home environment. *Arch. Ophthalmol.* 97, 470–2.

Plaut, B.S., Davies, D.J.G., Meakin, B.J. and Richardson, N.E. (1981) The mechanism of interaction between chlorhexidine digluconate and poly (2-Hydroxyethylmethacrylate). *J. Pharm. Pharmacol.*, 33, 82–8.

Rauschl, R.T. and Rogers, J.J. (1978) The effect of hydrophilic lens wear on the bacterial flora of the human conjunctiva. *Int. Contact Lens Clin.*, 5, 37–43.

Refojo, M.F. (1976) Reversible binding of chlorhexidine gluconate to hydrogel contact lenses. *Contact Intraocular Lens Med. J.*, 2, 47–56.

Reidhammer, T.M. and Falcetta, J.J. (1980) Effects of long term heat disinfection on Soflens (Polymacon) contact lenses. *J. Am. Optom. Assoc.*, 51, 287–9.

Reinhart, D.J., Kaylor, B., Prescott, D. and Sapp, C.S. (1990) Rapid and simplified comparative evaluation of contact lens disinfection solutions. *Int. Contact Lens Clin.*, 17, 9–12.

Richardson, N.E., Gee, H.G. and Meakin, B.J. (1980) The compatibility of benzalkonium chloride with a C.A.B. lens material. *J. Br. Contact Lens Assoc.*, 3, 120–4.

Rohrer, M.D., Terry, M.A., Bulard, R.A., Graves, D.C. and Taylor, E.M. (1986) Microwave sterilisation of hydrophilic contact lenses. *Am. J. Ophthalmol.*, 101, 49–57.

Rosenthal, P., Chan, M.H., Salamore, J.C. and Israel, S.C. (1986) Quantitative analysis of chlorhexidine gluconate and benzalkonium chloride adsorption on silicone/acrylate polymers. *C.L.A.O.J.*, 12(1), 43–50.

Rosenthal, R.A., McNamee, L.S. and Schlech, B.A. (1988) Continuous antimicrobial activity of contact lens disinfectants. *Contact Lens Forum*, 13 (11), 72–5.

Sack, R.A. Jones, B. Antignani, A. Libow, R. and Harvey, H. (1987) Specificity and biological activity of the protein deposited on the hydrogel surface. *Invest. Ophthalmol. Vis. Sci.* 28, 842–9.

Sack, R.A., Harvey, H. and Nunnes, I. (1989) Disinfection associated spoilage of high water content ionic matrix hydrogels. *C.L.A.O.J.*, 15(2), 138–45.

Shih, K.L. Hu, J. and Sibley, M. (1985) The microbiological benefit of cleaning and rinsing contact lenses. Int Contact Lens Clin 12(4): 235–242.

Shih, K.L., Raad, M.K. Hu, J.C., Gresh, W.J., Jones, S.I., Caldwell, L.J. and Bergamini, M.V.W. (1991) Disinfecting activities of non-peroxide soft contact lens cold disinfection solutions. *C.L.A.O.J.*, 17 (3), 165–8.

Sibley, M.J. (1984) Contact lens solution incompatibilities. *Contact Lens Forum*, 9 (5), 67–71.

Smolin, G., Okumoto, M. and Nosik, R.A. (1979) The microbial flora in extended wear soft contact-lens wearers. *Am. J. Ophthalmol.*, 88, 543–47.

Snyder, C., Daum, K.M. and Campbell, J.B. (1990) Rigid contact lens base curve constancy between wet and dry lens storage conditions. *J. Am. Optom. Assoc.*, 61 (3), 184–7.

Sokol, J.L., Mier, M.G., Bloom, S. and Aspell, P.A. (1990) A study of patient compliance in a contact lens wearing population. *C.L.A.O.J.*, 16 (3), 209–13.

Stehr-Green, J.K., Bailey, T.M. and Visvesvara, G.S. (1989) The epidemiology of *Acanthamoeba* keratitis in the United States. *Am. J. Ophthalmol.*, 107, 331–6.

Stewart-Jones, J.H., Hopkins, G.A. and Phillips, A.J. (1990) Drugs and solutions in contact lens practice and related microbiology. In *Contact Lenses* (eds. Phillips and Stone) pp. 125–185.

Sylvany, R.E., Dougherty, J.M., McCulley, J.P., Wood, T.S., Bowman, R.W. and Moore, M.B. (1990) The effect of currently available contact lens disinfection systems on *Acanthamoeba castellanii* and *Acanthamoeba polyphaga*. *Ophthalmology*, 97, 286–90.

Tregakis, M.P., Brown, S.I. and Pearce, D.B. (1973a) Bacteriologic studies of contamination associated with soft contact lenses. *Am. J. Ophthalmol.*, 73, 496–9.

Tregakis, M.P., Brown, S.I. and Pearce, D.E. (1973b) Bacteriological studies of contamination associated with soft contact lenses. *Am. J. Ophthalmol.*, 75, 496–9.

Tripathi, R.C. and Tripathi, B.J. (1984). Lens spoilage. In *Contact Lenses: The CLAO Guide to Basic Science and Clinical Practice* (2nd edn) (ed. O.H. Dabezies), Little, Brown & Co, Boston, MA, pp. 299–334.

Tse, L.S., Callender, M.G. and Charles, A.M. (1987) Antimicrobial effectiveness of some soft contact lens care systems. *Am. J. Optom. Physiol. Optics*, 64 (11), 824–8.

Walker, P.J. (1981) Do storage solutions affect soft lens parameters? Contact Lens Review. *The Ophthalmic Optician*, 21 (8), 240–2.

Weissman, B.A., Mondino, B.J., Pettit, T.H. and Hofbauer, J.D. (1984) Corneal ulcers associated with extended wear soft contact lenses. *Am. J. Ophthalmol.*, 97, 467–81.

Wilhelmus, K.R., Robinson, N.M., Font, R.A., Hamill, M.B. and Jones, D.B. (1988) Fungal keratitis in lens wearers. *Am. J. Ophthalmol.*, 106, 708–14.

Wilson, L.A. and Ahern, D.G. (1977) *Pseudomonas*

induced corneal ulcers associated with contaminated eye mascaras. *Am. J. Ophthalmol.*, **84**(1), 112–19.

Wilson, L.A. and Ahern, D.G. (1986) Association of fungi with extended wear soft contact lenses. *Am. J. Ophthalmol.*, **101**, 434–6.

Wilson, L.A., McNatt, J. and Reitschel, R. (1981a) Delayed hypersensitivity to thimerosal in soft contact lens wearers. *Ophthalmology*, **88**, 804–9.

Wilson, L.A., Schlitzer, R.L. and Ahern, D.G. (1981b) *Pseudomonas* corneal ulcers associated with soft contact lens wear. *Am. J. Ophthalmol.* **92**, 546–54.

Wilson, C.R., Woodward, E.G. and Stapleton, F. (1993) Contact lens compliance in a university population. *J. Br. Contact Lens Assoc.*, in press.

Wolff, E. (1976) *Anatomy of the eye and orbit* (7th ed), Lewis, London, p. 226.

Wong, M.P., Dziabo, A.J. and Kiral, R.M. (1986) Adsorption of benzalkonium chloride by rigid gas permeable lenses. *Contact Lens Forum*, **11**(5), 25–32.

Wright, P., Warhurst, D. and Jones, B.R. (1985) Acanthamoeba keratitis successfully treated medically. *Br. J. Ophthalmol.*, **69**, 778–82.

APPENDIX 25.A: CARE PRODUCTS CURRENTLY AVAILABLE

Solution (Manufacturer)	Suitability		Active ingredients	Comments
	Rigid	Hydrogel		
Cleaning				
Boston Cleaner (Polymer technology)	Y	N	Sodium tridecylether sulphate 10% w/v Polymeric beads (as friction enhancing agent)	Not suitable with surface coated lenses
Cleaner No 4 (Pilkington Barnes-Hind)	N	Y	Octylphenoxy ethanol 1.0% w/v Thiomersal 0.004% w/v Disodium edetate 0.2% w/v	Contains a non-ionic surfactant Alkaline pH
Clens (Alcon)	Y	N	Tergitol TMN 0.1% w/v Tyloxapol 0.1% w/v Benzalkonium chloride 0.02% w/v Disodium edetate 0.1% w/v	
Contactaclean (Ciba Vision)	Y	N	Chlorhexidine gluconate 0.006% w/v Benzalkonium chloride 0.004% w/v Disodium edetate 0.128% w/v Non-ionic surfactant	
Daily cleaner (Bausch & Lomb)	N	Y	Sorbic acid 0.25% w/v Disodium edetate 0.5% w/v	
Hydroclean (Ciba Vision)	N	Y	Chlorhexidine gluconate 0.0025% w/v Thiomersal 0.0025% w/v Disodium edetate 0.128% w/v Non-ionic surfactant	
Hydron Cleaning (Allergan)	Y	Y	Chlorhexidine gluconate 0.002% w/v	
Intensive Cleaner (Pilkington Barnes-Hind)	Y	N	Alkyl imidazoline dicarboxylate Alkyl carboxylic acid amine Polyoxyalkylene dimethylpolysiloxane Thiomersal 0.001% w/v Disodium edetate 0.1% w/v	Weekly intensive cleaner, containing a high concentration of surfactant cleaners For use with turbulent Hydra-Mat cleaning case

Solution (Manufacturer)	Suitability		Active ingredients	Comments
	Rigid	Hydrogel		
LC65 (Allergan)	Y	Y	Miranol 2% w/v Disodium edate 0.127% w/v	New formulation – preservative free
Liprofin (Alcon)	N	Y	Sodium perborate 2g	Not for use by patient Regular use with high water content lenses may cause altered parameters
Miraflow (Ciba Vision)	Y	Y	Isopropyl alcohol 20% w/v Poloxamer 407 Miranol H2M	Preservative free
02 Care (Ciba Vision)	Y	N	Benzalkonium chloride 0.005% w/v Disodium edetate 0.128% w/v	Recommended for Menicon 02 RGP lenses
Pliagel (Alcon)	Y	Y	Poloxamer 407 15% w/v Sorbic acid 0.1% w/v Trisodium edetate 0.50% w/v	Not for use with Menicon 02 RGP lenses Care with CAB lenses
Preflex (Alcon)	Y	Y	Thiomersal 0.004% w/v Disodium edetate 0.2% w/v	
Prymeclean (Smith & Nephew)	Y	Y	Pluronic L64 0.5% w/v Chlorhexidine gluconate 0.002% w/v	
RGP Cleaner (Bausch & Lomb)	Y	N	Sodium tridecylether sulphate 10% Polymeric beads (as friction enhancing agent)	Not suitable with surface coated lenses
Soft lens daily cleaner (Sauflon)	Y	Y	Thiomersal 0.004% w/v Disodium edetate 0.1% w/v	
Steri-clens (Sauflon)	Y	Y	Thiomersal 0.004% w/v Disodium edetate 0.1% w/v	
Titan (Pilkington Barnes-Hind)	Y	N	Ethoxylated polypropylene glycol Benzalkonium chloride 0.02% w/v Hydroxyethyl cellulose Disodium edetate 2.0% w/v	Contains a non-ionic surfactant
Transclean (Smith & Nephew)	Y	N	Pluronic 64 0.5% w/v Benzalkonium chloride 0.01% w/v Disodium edetate 0.1% w/v	
Soaking				
Ami-10 (Abatron)	Y	Y	Thiomersal 0.001% w/v Chlorhexidine gluconate 0.005% w/v Disodium edetate	New formulation
Contactasoak (Ciba Vision)	Y	N	Chlorhexidine gluconate 0.006% w/v Benzalkonium chloride 0.004% w/v Disodium edetate 0.128% w/v Non-ionic surfactant	

Solution	Suitability		Active ingredients	Comments
(Manufacturer)	Rigid	Hydrogel		
Flexcare (Alcon)	N	Y	Chlorhexidine gluconate 0.005% w/v Thiomersal 0.001% w/v Disodium edetate 0.1% w/v	Disinfection and rinsing solution High water content lenses may have increased CHX uptake
Flexsol (Alcon)	N	Y	Chlorhexidine gluconate 0.005% w/v Thiomersal 0.001% w/v Disodium edetate 0.1% w/v	Disinfection solution; lenses must be rinsed with saline subsequently
Hexidin (Pilkington Barnes-Hind)	N	Y	Povidone Octylphenoxy ethanols Chlorhexidine gluconate 0.003% w/v Thiomersal 0.002% w/v Disodium edetate 0.1% w/v	Disinfection and rinsing solution
Hydrocare Cleaning and Soaking (Allergan)	N	Y	Alkyl triethanol ammonium chloride 0.03% w/v Thiomersal 0.002% w/v	Cleaning and disinfection solution
Hydron Soaking (Allergan)	N	Y	Chlorhexidine gluconate 0.002% w/v	Rinsing and disinfection solution
Hydrosoak (Ciba Vision)	N	Y	Chlorhexidine gluconate 0.0025% w/v Thiomersal 0.0025% w/v Disodium edetate 0.128% w/v	Disinfection and storage
Normol (Alcon)	N	Y	Chlorhexidine gluconate 0.005% w/v Thiomersal 0.001% w/v Disodium edetate 0.2% w/v	Rinsing and storage solution; buffered multidose saline
OptimEyes Disinfection Tablet (Bausch & Lomb	N	Y	Chlorhexidine gluconate 0.004% w/v	Tablet containing 0.4 mg chlorhexidine, soluble in 10 ml tap water Contraindicated for class IV lenses
Prymesoak (Smith & Nephew)	N	Y	Chlorhexidine gluconate 0.002% w/v	
Softlens Soaking (Bausch & Lomb)	N	Y	Alkyl triethanol ammonium chloride 0.03% w/v Thiomersal 0.002% w/v	Disinfection solution
Soquette (Pilkington Barnes-Hind)	Y	N	Polyvinyl alcohol Benzalkonium chloride 0.01% w/v Disodium edetate 0.2% w/v	
Steri-Sal 2 (Sauflon)	N	Y	Thiomersal 0.002% w/v Chlorhexidine gluconate 0.002% w/v/ Disodium edetate 0.1% w/v	

Solution	Suitability		Active ingredients	Comments
(Manufacturer)	Rigid	Hydrogel		
Sterisoak (Sauflon)	Y	N	Chlorbutol 0.4% w/v Benzalkonium chloride 0.002% w/v Disodium edetate 0.1% w/v	
Transoak (Smith & Nephew)	Y	N	Benzalonium chloride 0.02% w/v Disodium edetate 0.2% w/v	

Wetting solutions and re-wetting solutions

Clerz (Ciba Vision)	Y	Y	Poloxamer 407 Hydroxyethylcellulose	Preservative and enzyme free. Unit dose
Contactasol (Ciba Vision)	Y	N	Chlorhexidine gluconate 0.006% w/v Benzalkonium chloride 0.004% w/v Wetting agents Disodium edetate 0.128% w/v	Contains non-ionic surfactant
Hydron Comfort (Allergan)	N	Y	Chlorhexidine glucontae 0.0025% w/v Thiomersal 0.0025% w/v Disodium edetate 0.1% w/v	
Hydrosol (Ciba Vision)	N	Y	Chlorhexidine gluconate 0.0025% w/v Thiomersal 0.0025% w/v Wetting agents Disodium edetate 0.128% w/v	
Liquifilm (Allergan)	Y	N	Polyvinyl alcohol 2% w/v Methyl cellulose 0.35% w/v Benzalkonium chloride 0.004% w/v Disodium edetate 0.127% w/v	
Transdrop (Smith & Nephew)	Y	N	Polyvinyl alcohol 1.4% w/v Hydroxyethyl cellulose Benzalkonium chloride 0.004% w/v	Comfort drop
Transol (Smith & Nephew)	Y	N	Polyvinyl alcohol 2% w/v Benzalkonium chloride 0.004% w/v Hydroxyethyl cellulose Disodium edetate 0.02% w/v	
Wetting Solution (Pilkington Barnes-Hind)	Y	N	Polyvinyl alcohol 2% w/v Benzalkonium chloride 0.004% w/v Disodium edetate 0.02% w/v	

Combined solutions

Boston Wetting & Soaking (Polymer Technology)	Y	N	Chlorhexidine gluconate 0.006% w/v Disodium edetate 0.05% w/v	Disinfection and wetting
Cleaning & Soaking (Pilkington Barnes-Hind)	Y	N	Benzalkonium chloride 0.01% w/v Disodium edetate 0.2% w/v	Cleaning and disinfection
Clean-N-Soak (Allergan)	Y	N	Phenylmercuric nitrate 0.004% w/v Disodium edetate 0.127% w/v	Cleaning and disinfection

Solution (Manufacturer)	Suitability		Active ingredients	Comments
	Rigid	Hydrogel		
Complete Care	Y	Y	Benzalkonium chloride 0.1% w/v Disodium edetate 0.05% w/v Poloxamer 407 Lipid solubilizer	
One solution (Pilkington Barnes-Hind)	Y	N	Ethanol 0.035% w/v Polyvinyl alcohol 0.5% w/v Benzalkonium chloride 0.01% w/v Disodium edetate 0.1% w/v	Cleaning, disinfection and wetting
RGP Wetting & Soaking (Bausch & Lomb)	Y	N	Chlorhexidine gluconate 0.006% w/v Disodium edetate 0.05% w/v	Disinfection and wetting
Soaclens (Alcon)	Y	N	Polysorbate 80 0.005% w/v Benzalkonium chloride 0.01% w/v Disodium edetate 0.1% w/v	Disinfection and wetting
Total (Allergan)	Y	N	Polyvinyl alcohol 2.5% w/v Benzalkonium chloride 0.004% w/v Disodium edetate 0.127% w/v	Cleaning, disinfection and wetting
Wetting and Soaking (Pilkington Barnes-Hind)	Y	N	Oxyphenoxy ethanols Polyvinyl alcohol Benzalkonium chloride 0.005% w/v Disodium edetate 0.1% w/v	Contains non-ionic surfactant
Salines				
Aerosol Salette (Alcon)	Y	Y	Sodium chloride 0.9% w/v Phosphate buffer	Unpreserved Use with Softab
Aerosol Saline (Alcon)	Y	Y	Sodium chloride 0.9% w/v	Unbuffered unpreserved Use with Softab
Aerosol Saline (Bausch & Lomb)	Y	Y	Sodium chloride 0.9% w/v	Unbuffered unpreserved
Aerosol Saline (Sauflon)	Y	Y	Sodium chloride 0.9% w/v Phosphate buffer	Unpreserved Use with Aerotab
Amidose saline (Abatron)	Y	Y	Sodium chloride 0.9% w/v	Unit dose unpreserved
Hydron Saline B (Allergan)	Y	Y	Sodium chloride 0.762% w/v Sodium phosphate 0.22% w/v	Unpreserved
Hydron Solusal (Allergan)	Y	Y	Sodium chloride 0.9% w/v Sodium phosphate 0.22% w/v	Unbuffered unpreserved
Lens Plus (Allergan)	Y	Y	Sodium chloride 0.9% w/v	Unbuffered unpreserved
Lensrins (Ciba Vision)	Y	Y	Sodium chloride 0.85% w/v Thiomersal 0.001% w/v Disodium edetate 0.1% w/v Buffers	Neutralization stage for Septicon peroxide system
Softmate Saline (Alcon)	Y	Y	Sodium chloride 0.4% w/v Borate buffer	Unpreserved
Solar Saline (Ciba Vision)	Y	Y	Sodium chloride 0.66% w/v Borate buffer	Unpreserved

Solution	Suitability		Active ingredients	Comments
(Manufacturer)	Rigid	Hydrogel		
Oxidative systems **Peroxide**				
Oxysept System (Allergan)	N	Y	Disinfection; 3% w/v hydrogen peroxide stablizer Neutralization; Catalase Miranol 2% w/v Disodium edetate 0.127% w/v	Catalytic decomposition of peroxide Vented storage case
Oxysept One Step (Allergen)	N	Y	Disinfection; 3% w/v hydrogen peroxide stabilizer Neutralization; Catalase 0.1 mg/tablet	Coated catalase tablet added to peroxide
10–10 Cleaning & Disinfection (Ciba Vision)	N	Y	Disinfection; 3% w/v hydrogen peroxide stablizer Neutralization; Sodium pyruvate 0.5% w/v Disodium edetate 0.1% w/v Sodium chloride Buffers	Chemical decomposition of peroxide
Lensept/Lensrins (Ciba Vision)	N	Y	Disinfection; 3% w/v hydrogen peroxide stablizer Neutralization; Sodium chloride 0.85% w/v Thiomersal 0.001% w/v Disodium edetate 0.1% w/v	Catalytic decomposition using Septicon disc
Perform System (Pilkington Barnes-Hind) case	N	Y	Disinfection; 3% w/v hydrogen peroxide stablizer Neutralization; Sodium thiosulphate 0.5% w/v Sodium chloride Borate buffer	Use with Hydromat Chemical decomposition of peroxide
Chlorine release				
Aerotab System (Sauflon)	N	Y	Halozone (Dichlorosuphamoyl benzoic acid) 0.16 mg tablet	Use with unpreserved saline, produces 8 ppm of available chlorine
Softab System (Alcon)	N	Y	Di-isochlorocyanurate 0.065 mg effervescent tablet	Dissolve in 10 ml unpreserved saline, produces 4 ppm of free chlorine

Solution (Manufacturer)	Suitability		Active ingredients	Comments
	Rigid	Hydrogel		
Enzyme cleaners				
Amiclair Triple Enzyme (Abatron)	Y	Y	Protease Lipase Pronase Disodium edetate	Removal of protein, lipid mucin and calcium Does not contain papain
Clen-Zym (Alcon)	N	Y	Pancreatin BP 2.5 mg	Multiple enzyme treatment Not licensed for GP CL
Fizzy Protein Tablets (Bausch & Lomb)	Y	Y	Stabilized papain	
Hydrocare Fizzy (Allergan)	Y	Y	Stabilized papain 10 mg	15 min exposure for high water content lenses
Protein Remover Tablets (Sauflon)	Y	Y	Stabilized papain	
Prymecare (Smith & Nephew)	Y	Y	Stabilized papain	
Ultrazyme (Allergan)	N	Y	Subtilisin A 0.4 mg	Serine protease use with Oxysept 1

J.E. Josephson, Barbara E. Caffery, P. Rosenthal, A. Slonovic and S. Zantos

26.1 INTRODUCTION: THE AFTERCARE CONCEPT

Routine aftercare is the major factor in continuing good contact lens performance and patient satisfaction. Typically, aftercare consists of periodic routine visits to assess both the patient's ocular response to contact lenses and the condition of the lenses. Patient orientation during the fitting and dispensing process is an essential aspect of patient management that positively prepares the patient for the process of routine aftercare. Further verbal reinforcement during aftercare visits strengthens the concept of routine continuing aftercare and is important in the maintenance of optimal contact lens performance.

McMonnies (1987) has reported that aftercare consumes the greatest proportion of the contact lens fitter's time. He demonstrated that in 81% of aftercare visits, although symptoms were virtually absent, there were adverse clinical signs (conjunctival hyperaemia, surface deposits, oedema, epitheleopathy, etc.). These clinical signs required remedial action to be taken.

McMonnies' investigation also confirmed that aftercare management is an important problem-preventing mode of practice. He found that in the years following the time when the first pair of contact lenses were prescribed, 67% of aftercare management was concerned with areas other than the technical aspects of lens and fit modification. For example, additional instruction and counselling were major areas of management, accounting for 36% of all remedial and prophylactic actions. McMonnies further emphasized the importance of long-term control of patient compliance with proper lens care.

26.2 INITIAL PATIENT ORIENTATION

Patients should be made aware of the importance of periodic and routine aftercare visits. When patients are trained in the use and care of their contact lenses, they should also be made aware of any ocular symptoms that require prompt contact lens removal. If the symptoms do not resolve immediately, or should they reoccur, patients should know the importance of seeking an immediate (unscheduled) aftercare appointment.

26.3 THE REASSESSMENT EXAMINATION

The skilled reassessment of the patient's response to contact lens wear, during the aftercare visit, requires knowledge based on the details recorded of the prefitting ocular assessment. This, together with careful observation, enables the practitioner to detect subtle contact-lens-induced changes

Contact Lens Practice. Edited by Montague Ruben and Michel Guillon.
Published in 1994 by Chapman & Hall, London. ISBN 0 412 35120 X

in tissue appearance and to determine whether they are pathological or physiological responses. If practitioners are not aware of these potential subtle changes and their implications, they will often be overlooked and management of the contact lens patient will be inefficient. The following points summarize the complete reassessment examination:

1. History taking: a review of the patient's previous experience with contact lens wear and analysis of their symptoms (for full discussion of symptoms see page 000).
2. Procedural review: a review of the proper hygiene and lens handling methodologies and of the solutions used. This should be followed by reinforcement of the correct techniques.
3. Monocular visual acuities and refraction over the contact lenses.
4. Biomicroscopy: an *in situ* assessment of the lens condition and fit.
5. Biomicroscopy after contact lens removal.
6. Keratometry.
7. Lens inspection off the eye.
8. Supplementary tests.
9. Summary and advice to the patient.

26.3.1 RECENT HISTORY AND EXPERIENCE WITH CONTACT LENS WEAR

A personal history should be taken after a written questionnaire has been answered. The purpose of this interview procedure is to help the practitioner focus on the areas that require attention. Leading questions should be avoided. Practitioners should be good listeners and leave the answering of questions open to the patient, without constant prompting or leading the patient's replies. Interviewing skills which take into account the patient's personality and mood are essential to the process of defining specific problems. In addition, it is important to earn the patient's trust by demonstrating an interest in all of the patient's concerns, even if they appear trivial. If there is no obvious problem to address, a general opening question such as 'Do you enjoy wearing your lenses?' can begin the interview.

The history should document the patient's recent experience with contact lens use, including the average number of hours that the lenses are worn each day, the usual time of insertion and removal and the consistency of the wearing schedule. Any recent and unusual limitations in wearing time should be noted during this interview. If the patient relates any symptoms, they should be thoroughly analysed in regard to when they occur, how long they last during and after lens wear, if they are associated with any activity or environment, how often they have occurred and how many days that they have occurred during the wearing cycle since the previous visit. Any change in general health or medications should be noted (for full analysis of symptoms see page 000).

26.3.2 REVIEW OF HANDLING, HYGIENE AND SOLUTIONS

At each successive routine aftercare visit, the nurse, technician or practitioner should ask the patient briefly to review their methods of handling contact lenses (without regard for their years of contact lens wearing experience). This follow-up procedure can help to reduce patient errors in lens care and also can reinforce compliance.

Some of the questions that practitioners should address are as follows: What does the patient do if the lens suddenly pops out? The patient should describe this occurrence in detail, step by step, from the time the lens pops out to the time that it is re-inserted, i.e. does the patient clean and rinse the lens or simply wet it with saliva and reinsert it? In addition, when the patient re-inserts the lenses, do they first wash their hands?

Our approach is to ask patients to describe their contact lens handling regimen, step by step, from the time prior to inserting their lenses to the actual insertion. We encourage the patient to take the time to describe each procedure in detail, as if they were actually going through the motions. If we suspect that the patient is not following a recommended procedure, such as washing their hands, this is carefully noted on the chart and the correct procedures of routine contact lens care are emphasized at the conclusion of the visit. Specific procedures that were reviewed and corrected should be documented. Thus, the procedures necessary for maintaining good quality long term patient care are periodically reinforced.

26.3.3 MONOCULAR VISUAL ACUITIES WITH CONTACT LENSES AND OVER-REFRACTION

Routine assessment of visual performance with contact lenses is important to confirm that the patient's vision is satisfactory. This documentation is also valuable for medical–legal reasons. The visual acuity of each eye should be assessed (monocular acuities) and a careful over-refraction should be performed. For this procedure, we recommend using hand held trial lenses rather than a phoropter. In complex refractive cases an optometer is a useful device for obtaining objective refractive information.

26.3.4 BIOMICROSCOPY: *IN SITU* ASSESSMENT OF THE LENS CONDITION AND FIT

Assessing the fit of a hydrogel lens

The assessment of a hydrogel lens fit can be accomplished by means of a biomicroscopic examination with white light. The fitting characteristics considered include lens centration, movement and edge tightness. Lens centration should typically be concentric with the limbus. Lens movement is a function of the lens design. The amount of movement should follow the manufacturer's recommendations. Edge tightness can be assessed by evaluating the edge lift effect (Josephson, 1977, 1978) to determine the potential for compression of the bulbar conjunctiva by the lens periphery. Any compression of the conjunctiva may reduce or obstruct local blood flow and cause conjunctival vascular hyperaemia and some conjunctival chemosis. A marginally tight fit will usually cause the patient to have slightly reduced visual acuity or to report that their vision fluctuates with blinking. A marginally tight lens can be diagnosed by assessing the fundus reflex with a retinoscope. The retinoscopy reflex will appear to be irregular or keratoconus-like between blinks.

Assessing the fit of a rigid lens

The fitting relationship of a rigid lens is assessed with the biomicroscope after the instillation of fluorescein. The light should be passed through a cobalt blue filter and a wratten #12 filter should be placed in front of the biomicroscope. Lens centration, lens movement between blinks and lens movement during blinking should be evaluated. In addition, the circulation of the pre-ocular tear film under the lens during blink induced lens motion must be assessed to determine whether the lens is fitting steeply, approximately in parallel or flat relative to the cornea.

The condition of the anterior and posterior surfaces of rigid and hydrogel lenses should be examined with white light for debris, scratches and coatings. This should be done while the lens is on the eye (Josephson & Caffery, 1989a; Shiobara *et al.*, 1989), as well as after removal and cleaning (Rudko & Proby, 1974; Wedler, 1977; Kleist, 1979; Hart, 1984; Gudmundsson *et al.*, 1985; Hart *et al.*,

1986; Fowler *et al.*, 1987; Le Naour & Day, 1987).

Lens surface quality

Reduced surface wettability is a problem often associated with rigid contact lenses. This problem may be related directly to the material from which the lens is made, or to the presence of deposits on the lens surface. A lens that wets poorly reduces the stability of the tear film. This can cause reduced vision and may also be associated with symptoms of discomfort. Assessing the surface characteristics of a contact lens *in situ* after it has interacted with the eye and preocular tear film is invaluable because it better reflects tear chemistry, surface dehydration, and other factors that may affect the actual surface wettability (Josephson & Caffery, 1989a).

Since patients will continue to experience blurring from poorly wetting lenses, one must be able to diagnose and manage the problem. A history of constant or intermittent foggy or blurry vision is an important clue. The patient will often complain that careful cleaning does not relieve the problem – or does so only a very short period. The slit lamp observation of the lens on the eye will demonstrate dry spots or areas that will only wet briefly between blinks. A filmy coating may also be seen on the lens surface. Patients presenting these problems should again be advised to wash their hands well with a pure soap. Female patients should be cautioned to apply make-up only after lens insertion. If the problem persists despite optimal care, polishing the lens surfaces may help. If not, the lens should be replaced.

If these changes do not help, consider selecting a different lens material, whether it is a hydrogel or an RGP lens. If the latter, consider one with less siloxane, or one that incorporates a fluoropolymer. One may also consider changing the patient's cleaning, soaking and/or wetting solutions.

26.3.5 BIOMICROSCOPY AFTER LENS REMOVAL

Biomicroscopy should include an assessment of each of the following tissues:

1. Cornea:
   i. epithelium;
   ii. stroma;
   iii. endothelium.
2. Limbal area.
3. Bulbar conjunctiva.
4. Palpebral conjunctiva:
   i. superior;
   ii. inferior.
5. Lid margins.

Assessment of the anterior segment must be made with maximum illumination and low magnification (5–10×). Then, with the biomicroscope slit width set approximately 2–4 mm wide, the magnification should be increased to moderate (15–20×) and then to high (25–35×), during which an assessment of the corneal epithelium, stroma and posterior cornea is made, while the angle of the light source and the light source arm are varied to aid observations. These observations should be followed by an assessment of the limbal region, including the condition of the blood vessels and the determination of the presence of vascular ingrowth, of the corneal tissue immediately inside the limbus and of the adjacent bulbar conjunctival area immediately outside the limbal region. The entire circumference of the cornea must be assessed in this way, with particular attention given to the nasal and superior regions. The upper and lower lids should be everted for examination of the inferior and superior palpebral conjunctivae.

Following the examination of these tissues with white light, fluorescein staining observations should be made with the biomicroscope using a cobalt blue filter. A Kodak #12 wratten filter placed over the microscope will enhance the observation of fluorescence. We suggest that fluorescein should be instilled twice, with a 2-min interval between instillations. Multiple instillations of fluorescein can be more revealing than a single instillation (Norn, 1969). During this procedure, patients should be encouraged to blink normally. It is preferable to use 2% liquid sodium fluorescein in unit dose vials, however, if that is unavailable, we recommend Ayerst Fluor-i-strips® (Ayerst Laboratories, New York) which should be saturated with preservative-free saline solution to instil an adequate volume of fluorescein. One minute after the second instillation, the second observation should be made. Examine the surface of the bulbar conjunctiva, the limbal region, as well as the cornea. Then, the lids should be everted and the surfaces of the inferior and superior palpebral conjunctivae should be assessed for any local regions of staining pooling patterns that may highlight papillary hyperplasia or accumulations of fluorescein absorbed by mucous sheets or strands.

26.3.6 KERATOMETRY

In aftercare, keratometry is used to identify and assess contact lens induced changes in the corneal curvature. Keratometry is also a measure of the integrity of the corneal surface. Keratometry does not have to be performed at every visit if there are no suspicious observations such as a change in non-contact lens refraction or pertinent symptoms. However, this procedure should be performed routinely at least once a year. If the refraction or the fit appears to have changed, keratometry helps to determine if they are the result of changes that have been induced in the anterior surface of the cornea. Normal (permanent) or contact lens induced (transient) changes in refraction can be thus differentiated and appropriately managed.

26.3.7 LENS INSPECTION OFF THE EYE

To thoroughly inspect the surfaces of a hydrogel lens, the lens should be placed in the palm with some normal saline and rinsed

well. To document surface deposits, the lens is held with tweezers and examined with the biomicroscope, against a dark background, using maximum illumination. The power of the lens should also be measured.

Prior to examination, a rigid lens should be cleaned with a surfactant cleaner while being gently massaged between thumb and finger, rinsed thoroughly and then wiped dry with a lint-free tissue. The lens surfaces and base curve are then inspected. Assessment by means of the radiuscope allows the practitioner to confirm that the base curve is unchanged and that there is no significant lens warpage. The edges should also be inspected (McMonnies, 1986).

26.3.8 SUPPLEMENTARY TESTING

Ophthalmoscopy, colour vision and visual field testing may be necessary to rule out certain pathological conditions, such as an unexplained reduction in vision.

26.3.9 SUMMARY AND ADVICE TO THE PATIENT

After completing the examination, the practitioner should summarize his observations, giving special emphasis to any noteworthy observations. Advice should then be given about routine wearing time and its limits, until the next routine follow-up examination. Any special changes recommended in hygiene, solution care or wearing time should also be noted in the record.

26.4 ANALYSIS OF SYMPTOMS AND SIGNS

Common contact-lens-related symptoms are listed below:

1. Blurry/hazy vision.
2. Ghost imagery.
3. '3-D' imagery.
4. Shadow images.
5. Burning.

6. Itching.
7. Dryness.
8. Pain.
9. A scratchy sensation.
10. Headache.
11. Deep eye ache.
12. Tearing.
13. Discharge, 'sleep'.
14. Nose 'runs'/drips.
15. Lid swelling: unilateral or bilateral.
16. Redness.

Common contact-lens-related clinical signs are:

1. Conjunctival injection.
2. Chemosis of the conjunctiva.
3. Corneal oedema, microcysts, tissue haze, striae or folds.
4. Infiltrates: epithelial and/or stromal.
5. Corneal vascularization.
6. Endothelial polymegathism and pleomorphism.
7. Limbal follicles.
8. Palpebral conjunctival papilli.
9. Conjunctival compresion associated with hydrogel lens wear or corneal compression associated with hard lens wear.
10. Rigid gas permeable lens binding (adhesion) to the corneal epithelium.
11. Hydrogel lens binding (adhesion) to the ocular surface
12. Giant capillary conjunctivitis (GPC):
    i. RGP related;
    ii. hydrogel lens related.

26.4.1 VISUAL SYMTOMS

The following is a discussion of the most frequently encountered complications that are associated with visual symptoms in contact lens wearers.

Visual symtoms in rigid lens wearers

1. Early onset of presbyopia.
2. *Ghosts or shadow images caused by: lens warpage, residual astigmatism, keratoconus, lens deposits, the optical zone border crossing the entrance pupil.
3. Normal refractive changes.
4. Oedema.
5. Lens coating.
6. Scratches.
7. Flare.
8. *Lens inside-out.
9. *Lens warpage.
10. Superficial punctuate keratitis.
11. Trapped bubbles or debris.
12. *Unexpected change in the lens base curve.
13. *Lenses inadvertently switched between the right and left eye
14. Inappropriate lens positioning.
15. Insufficient quality control or power and/or base curve.
16. Pathological change in the cornea (i.e. keratoconus).
17. Off-centre lens binding to the corneal surface.

Refractive changes

Any patient can have refractive changes in the course of wearing contact lenses. This is typically diagnosed by an over-refraction of both spherical and cylindrical components while the lenses are being worn. A confirmation that this is a true refractive change and not the result of corneal warpage can be accomplished by removing the lenses, taking keratometric measurements, performing a refraction without contact lenses and comparing the data to previous findings. The optics of RGP lenses must also be reassessed by cleaning the lens, wiping it dry with a soft lint-free tissue and mounting it on a 3 mm aperture stop of a projection lensometer. The power of the lens should then be accurately recorded and compared to the prescribed contact lens power. The lens should then be mounted on a larger aperture stop (5 mm

---

* The visual symptoms related to these causes may have a sudden onset.

diameter) and the quality of the optics evaluated by considering the sharpness of the lensometer mires. Finally, the lens base curve should be measured with a radiuscope and compared to the prescribed base curve. In addition, the radiuscope mires should be assessed to identify and measure warpage.

Fit-induced visual symptoms

Flare This problem may arise in rigid lens wearers and results from the prismatic displacement of light passing through the peripheral curves and edge of the lens, into the pupil. Light interaction at the optic zone/peripheral curve junction, if it is within the pupillary zone, can also cause optical aberration.

Patients presenting flare may report a variety of symptoms, such as blurry vision, flashing or streaking lights, fringing, glare, ghost images and halos. These symptoms are often observed when looking at point light sources, such as the head or tail lights of a car.

To diagnose flare, first carefully over-refract to rule out prescription under-correction as a cause of the visual disturbance. Then, dim the lights and hold a white light circle target in front of the patient. Ask the patient to draw or describe the light they see. Often, the direction of the doubling or streaking of light will indicate whether better lens centration by changing the design will help to reduce flare.

Next, using the slit lamp with dim illumination, determine the position of optical zone border in relation to the pupillary margin. After the instillation of sodium fluorescein, one may be able to determine the relative position of the inside portion of the peripheral curve relative to the pupillary area. As described above, to enhance the dye's fluorescence, place a Kodak #12 wratten filter in front of the microscope.

Finally, remove and inspect the lens and confirm that the optic zone diameter matches the ordered specifications and assess the quality of the contact lens optics using the previously described procedure. Once this information is collected and the situation assessed, the value of changing the lens design can be determined.

Blurring/ghosting Blurred vision may result from uncorrected ametropia, residual refractive error induced by lens flexure or a lens that is decentred so that the optic zone does not completely cover the pupil. A spherocylindrical over-refraction can uncover any significant residual astigmatism (against the rule) (at least 0.50 D) as the cause.

A good patient history can pinpoint the cause of a patient's blurred vision. For example, immediate and persistant symptoms suggest a residual refractive error. Fluctuating vision suggests an eccentric lens position, an excessively small optical zone or non-wetting areas on the lens surface. A gradual reduction in vision may indicate increasing ametropia.

If the reduced vision is experienced at night and associated with glare, the optical zone may be too small. If the patient tells you that the symptoms only occur later in the day, one should suspect corneal oedema or a deposit build-up on the front surface of the lens as often occurs with incomplete blinkers.

Visual symptoms in hydrogel lens wearers
The causes of visual symptoms in wearers of hydrogel contact lenses are listed below:

1. Early onset of presbyopia.
2. Ghost or shadows caused by keratoconus, residual astigmatism, a marginally steep fitting lens.
3. Normal refractive changes.
4. Oedema.
5. *Lenses switched between the right and left eyes.
6. Lens coating.

7. Lens scratches.
8. *Lens inside-out.
9. *Lens warpage as occurs with long-term lens use, coating and discoloration producing edge curl.
10. Absorption of toxic environmental vapours causing subsequent corneal changes that produce slow but insidious changes in patient refraction.

Hydrogel lenses that have become dehydrated, or have aged, acquire permanent surface deposits and can also become warped. These changes in parameters may cause visual disturbances. Lens surfaces should be first inspected on the eye (Josephson & Caffery, 1989a). Surface deposits of various types can be identified as well by the rapidity of disruption of the prelens tear layer. Next, the lens should be removed, cleaned and placed in a buffered saline solution for 5 min to become adequately rehydrated. Then, it should be removed from the solution, quickly blotted and the shape of the lens assessed. Any abnormal curling may mean that the lens may have extensive deposits. The lens power should then be assessed after the lens is mounted on the aperture of a projection lensometer. Then, the quality of the optics may be assessed by placing the lens in a wet cell, mounting the cell over a 5 mm diameter aperture stop affixed to the projection lensometer, and after focusing for the correct power, assessing the quality of the mires. However, a simpler method of evaluating the level of a trial performance of a soft lens is to compare the quality of its vision correction with that of a new diagnostic lens. The following discussion of the differential diagnosis will help in the analysis and management of this presenting symptom:

1. *Sudden reduction of visual acuity*:
   Differential diagnosis
   i. inverted (inside-out)lens, lost or displaced lens;

   ii. a non-contact lens related pathology;
   iii. lenses switched.

2. *Rapid reduction in visual acuity*:
   Differential diagnosis
   i. hypoxic induced keratometric changes in a soft contact lens wearer that cause either increased myopia and/or astigmatism;
   ii. rapid lens coating (such as occurs with giant papillary conjunctivitis – GPC);
   iii. non-related contact lens pathology.

3. *Gradual reduction of visual acuity*:
   Differential diagnosis
   i. normal hypoxia induced refractive changes;
   ii. lens coating;
   iii. corneal changes caused by hydrogel lens contamination by some toxic environmental or chemical vapours.

26.4.2 SYMPTOMS OF 'RED EYES'

Of all of the presenting symptoms of lens wearers the red eye should alert both practitioner and patient to potentially serious complications. The following discussion of the differential diagnosis will help in the analysis and management of the presenting symptom or sign:

1. *Sudden onset with pain, photophobia, with or without discharge that does not resolve rapidly and completely after lens removal*:
   Differential diagnosis
   i. corneal ulcer;
   ii. corneal infiltrates;
   iii. acute red eye syndrome;
   iv. recurrent erosions;
   v. iritis.

2. *Onset of pain with lens insertion, with or without photophobia, which resolves quickly and completely after lens removal*:
   Differential diagnosis
   i. posterior lens surface defects or deposits;
   ii. contact lens edge defects;

    iii. incomplete neutralization of hydrogen peroxide;

    iv. non-contact lens related corneal pathology.

3. *Gradual onset of discomfort and infection without discharge, which does not resolve after lens removal.*
SLK syndrome (superior limbal kerato-conjunctivitis).

4. *Gradual onset of injection without pain, with rapid resolution after contact lens removal:*
Differential diagnosis
    i. preservative sensitivity;
    ii. giant papillary conjunctivitis (GPC).

5. *Gradual onset of injection with discomfort and rapid resolution after lens removal:*
Differential diagnosis
    i. poor *in vivo* lens lubrication
    ii. giant papillary conjunctivitis (GPC);
    iii. lens deposits.

6. *Gradual onset of injection, with or without discomfort which slowly resolves after contact lens removal:*
Differential diagnosis
    i. 3–9 staining;
    ii. preservative sensitivity.

7. *Discharge with (or without) injection:*
Differential diagnosis
    i. *Serratia marscesens* contamination of the solutions in an RGP lens wearer;
    ii. giant papillary conjunctivitis.

26.4.3 SYMPTOMS OF DISCOMFORT

Rigid lens related

1. Discomfort associated with lens motion (or a lack thereof).
2. Discomfort associated with an ocular surface condition.
3. Discomfort associated with the incompatibility of a contact lens solution.
4. Discomfort associated with improper rinsing of a cleaning solution.
5. Discomfort associated with improperly finished contact lens edges and inadequately blended peripheral curves.
6. Discomfort associated with a damaged edge or a crack in a lens.
7. Discomfort associated with lens warpage.
8. Discomfort associated with anterior surface deposits.

Discomfort may be an isolated symptom or may be associated with other symptoms such as redness, visual changes, discharge, itching, etc. One should note the severity of discomfort, whether it is constant or intermittent, whether or not it occurs during lens wear and/or after lens removal, the nature of the discomfort, i.e. stinging, burning, gritty, foreign body, dryness, hot, etc. Is the discomfort present after sleeping overnight without the lenses and on waking the following day?

It is important to assess the contact lens itself. What is the condition of the lens? Are the front or back surfaces marred by cracks, scratches, coatings or deposits of any kind? Is the soft lens being worn inside-out? If it is a hard contact lens, it is also possible for a lens to be turned inside-out if it is of a softer variety such as some RGP lenses. Although this is a rare occurrence, this has occurred with some lenses and the lens should be carefully checked with a radius-cope. Lens inversion can also be assessed by holding the lens between the fingers or with tweezers under moderate magnification with a biomicroscope. A rigid lens that is pushed inside-out will often be seen to have parallel striations visible in the matrix of the lens material that radiate from near the centre and outward toward the circumference.

The hard lens posterior surface transitions at the peripheral curve junction should be assessed, particularly near the edge. This examination is made with a 20× magnifying lens using a method described by McMonnies (1986). The lens should be inspected with a radiuscope to make sure that the radius of curvature has not changed. If the lens appearance seems to be satisfactory, the parameters are found to be within tolerances and the ocular surface looks to be healthy, the lenses should be inserted and the fit evaluated for any excessive looseness, tightness or heavy bearing areas.

The comfort of a soft lens depends on many factors. Centration, edge thickness and edge configuration are parameters that can affect comfort. If previously comfortable lenses have become uncomfortable, lens damage, surface coatings or other surface defects should be ruled out. Lens replacement is the obvious action to take in this situation.

26.4.4   SYMPTOMS OF DISCHARGE

Patients may present with a complaint of tearing, excess mucus or pus-like discharge. As with all symptoms, it is important to understand the degree of the problem, time of onset and any associated ocular or systemic condition that the patient has experienced.

Differential diagnosis

1.   Watery discharge:
     i.   solution related adverse response (Josephson & Caffery, 1981);
     ii. some types of keratoconjunctivitis;
     iii. corneal abrasion;
     iv. tight-fitting lenses.
2.   Mucuous discharge:
     i.   allergy,
     ii. giant papillary conjunctivitis (GPC);
     iii. various types of conjunctivitis.
3.   Purulent discharge:
     i.   bacterial infection.

26.4.5   CORNEAL SIGNS

The corneal epithelium undergoes a number of changes during lens wear. Fortunately, almost all the epithelial changes are transient and reversible because of the regenerative properties of the corneal epithelium.

The observation and identification of some of the epithelial changes can be difficult in practice because of the minute size and refractile nature of these lesions. However, detection and differentiation of these epithelial changes is important in determining the prognosis and management of the contact lens patient.

Most of the transparent refractile lesions in the cornea are best observed by using the technique of marginal retro-illumination with the slit lamp microscope (Brown, 1971). The authors' procedure is to scan the cornea from temporal limbus to nasal limbus using a 3–4 mm wide slit beam (Humphreys *et al.*, 1980). For initial observation, a magnification of 15× is recommended. The slit beam arm should be separated by an angle of approximately 45° from the microscope axis. The slit lamp mirror should be rotated horizontally relative to the slit lamp beam arm by ± 7°, as required during scanning examination of the cornea. The illumination should be set at maximum intensity. In this way refractile lesions in the cornea can best be detected.

Once observed, the lesion is centred in the field of view of the microscope while the slit beam is narrowed to a width of 2–3 mm and is displaced 5–10° laterally by rotating the slit lamp mirror from its click-stop position. This creates an alternate light/dark background on the iris for marginal retro-illumination. The iris/pupil border can be used to create the light/dark background. The optical appearance of the refractive lesion can now be studied at 20× to 40× magnification.

An object of higher refractive index than the surrounding corneal tissue will act as a converging refracting lens, resulting in a 'reversed' appearance (Fig. 26.1). Conversely, an object of lower refractive index than the surrounding tissue will act as a diverging lens, resulting in an 'unreversed' appearance (Fig. 26.1) (Brown, 1971). Intra-

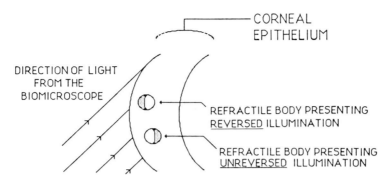

Figure 26.1 Marginal retro-illumination technique illustrating reversed and unreversed illumination of a refractile body.

corneal lesions that are not refractile will reflect the light and will have a white, buff or grey appearance.

26.4.6 DESCRIPTION OF CONTACT-LENS-RELATED CORNEAL PATHOLOGY

Striae or folds

Contact lens induced corneal striae are a clinical sign of corneal hypoxia (Sarver, 1975) that can only be observed when corneal swelling is greater than 6% (Kearn, 1974). With swelling beyond that level, the prominance and number of striate lines increase. Folds are observed when corneal swelling approaches 12% (Kame, 1976). These clinical signs are primarily observed as a hypoxic response to hydrogel lens wear. Corneal hypoxia secondary to rigid lens wear typically manifests as corneal haze, referred to as central corneal clouding (CCC).

Epithelial microcysts

Epithelial microcysts are most commonly associated with extended wear of hydrogel contact lenses and tend to appear after the first few weeks of lens wear (Zantos, 1983, 1984a). Epithelial microcysts are associated with a depressed corneal metabolism sustained over

Figure 26.2 Microcysts under high magnification.

a period of weeks to months (Hamano & Hori, 1983; Holden *et al.*, 1985). The microcysts appear as minute, translucent dots toward the centre or mid-periphery of the cornea (Fig 26.2 and 26.3). Typically they are irregular in shape and vary in size from 15 to 50 μm. Their refractive nature indicates that they have a generally higher refractive index than the surrounding tissue. Often, microcysts may show a mixture of reversed or unreversed illumination, indicating that they have a variable optical density (Fig. 26.3). In this respect they differ from epithelial vacuoles and bullae, which always show unreversed illumination. Microcysts may be present anywhere in the epithelium, from the deep layers to the most superficial layers. They do not stain with fluorescein provided that the anterior corneal surface is intact. In advanced cases, the cysts represented pockets of cellular debris and disorganized cell growth. These pockets of debris migrate anteriorly to the corneal surface where they will present as punctate staining after fluorescein is instilled.

Epithelial vacuoles

Epithelial vacuoles are transparent, round, small formations usually occurring toward the mid-periphery of the cornea. They resemble the tiny air bubbles sometimes seem in glassware. These vacuoles are typically observed when contact lenses are worn on an extended wear basis. They can easily be distinguished from microcysts as they almost always have a perfectly round shape, distinct edges and show unreversed illumination, indicating that they are of lower refractive index than the surrounding corneal tissue. Typically, they vary in size from 20 to 50 μm (Fig. 26.4).

Epithelial vacuoles usually appear any time after 1 week of wear. Usually there are just a few vacuoles present, sometimes in clusters of two to four. In contact lens wearers, vacuoles sometimes occur concurrently with microcysts. When viewed using retro-illumination, epithelial vacuoles show a close resemblance to epithelial dimpling (i.e. 'dimple veiling' or depressions in the epithelial surface), particularly if the contact lens is still on the eye. However, when fluorescein is used, areas of dimpling will fill with fluorescein while vacuoles will not stain, as they are intra-epithelial (Fig. 26.3).

Epithelial bullae

Epithelial bullae are transparent, flattened, irregularly shaped, cobblestone-like forma-

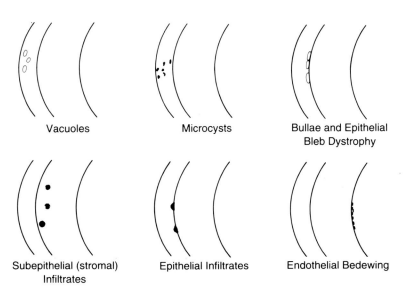

Vacuoles

Microcysts

Bullae and Epithelial
Bleb Dystrophy

Subepithelial (stromal)
Infiltrates

Epithelial Infiltrates

Endothelial Bedewing

Figure 26.3 Optic section of different corneal complications.

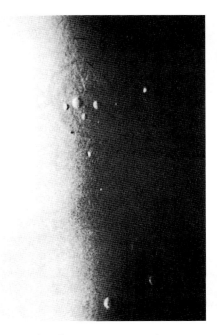

Figure 26.4 Vacuoles (from Zantos, 1983).

Figure 26.5 Bullae (from Zantos, 1983).

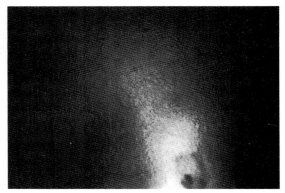

Figure 26.6 Epithelial bleb dystrophy (from Zantos, 1983).

tions that tend to vary in size and are fairly large (i.e. 40 μm and larger). They are observed in the deep epithelial region. They do not stain with fluorescein or rose bengal. They present an unreversed illumination appearance and, therefore, are of lower refractive index than the surrounding tissue (Zantos, 1984a). Epithelial bullae occur infrequently in contact lens wearers and tend to be associated with advanced and persistent stromal oedema. Epithelial bullae are differentiated from vacuoles by their somewhat oval shape, their larger size, their less distinct borders and their tendency to coalesce into clusters containing many bullae (Fig 26.3, 26.5 and 26.6).

Epithelial bleb dystrophy

Epithelial bleb dystrophy is a benign condition and does not affect vision (Bron & Brown, 1971). These lesions are typically observed just below the corneal centre as regular, refractile, small, flat, pebble-like shapes of fairly uniform size, seen at the level of the basement membrane of the epithelium (Fig. 26.6).

This condition may be confused with the appearance of epithelial bullae, which are often larger, less regular in shape and are usually not limited to appearing in the basal epithelial layer.

Corneal infiltrates

Corneal infiltrates represent one of the most common adverse reactions of both daily and extended contact lens wear (Litvin, 1978; Josephson & Caffery, 1979; Zantos, 1984b).

They may occur in a white and quiet eye (Fig. 26.7) or in a red eye (Fig. 26.8). They may also be observed in a white and quiet eye of patients who do not wear contact lenses (Hamano & Hori, 1983). The appearance of contact lens-induced corneal infiltrates is typically associated with tight fitting contact lenses, extended wear lenses and allergic or toxic reactions to contact lens solution preservatives. They also occur in association with adenoviral infections, chlamydial (TRIC) infection and staphylococcal exotoxin hypersensitivity.

A red eye with corneal infiltrates represents an inflammatory response, whereas the previously described cystic formations (microcysts, vacuoles and bullae) are responses of the epithelium to chronic hypoxia and/or mechanical effects of contact lens wear. The differential diagnosis between the two types of epithelial responses, when the eye appears white and quiet, can be difficult in clinical practice because of similarities in appearance. Patient management is quite different for the acute and the chronic inflammatory responses and the chronic non-inflammatory responses.

Corneal infiltrates can occur in the epithelium (Fig 26.3, 26.9 and 26.10), in the stroma (Figs 26.3, 26.8, 26.11 and 26.12) or in both layers simultaneously (Fig. 26.7). Infiltrates

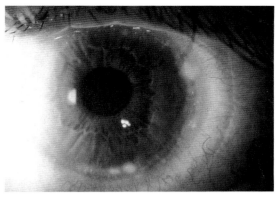

Figure 26.8 Limbal corneal infiltrates (marginal infiltrates) in 'red' eye.

are formations that are composed of the chemical mediators of inflammation, inflammatory cells and debris. In the centre of the infiltrate, the inflammatory cells are densely packed and become less packed toward the periphery. Localized mild oedema and the aggregation of the inflammatory cells give infiltrates in the corneal epithelium a translucent appearance.

Stromal infiltrates (Figs 26.3, 26.8, 26.11 and 26.12) are seen to be snowball-like in appearance, quite round, densely white or buff-coloured in the centre, with a diaphanous border. This formation is associated

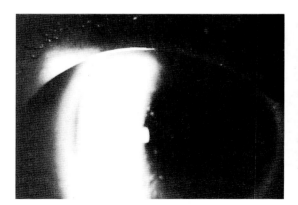

Figure 26.7 Corneal infiltrates in a 'white' eye (no apparent injection).

Figure 26.9 Epithelial corneal infiltrate observed at high magnification with marginal retro-illumination.

Figure 26.10 Epithelial corneal infiltrate observed with high magnification and marginal retro-illumination (from Josephson & Caffery, 1979).

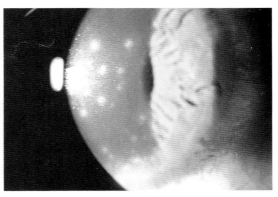

Figure 26.12 Stromal infiltrates (Courtesy Dr Barry Weiner).

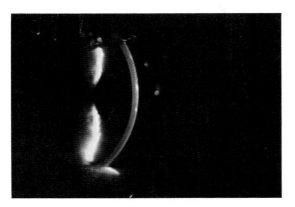

Figure 26.11 Stromal infiltrates seen in optic section (courtesy Dr Barry Weiner).

radiating around the entire central core (Fig. 26.13).

Epithelial infiltrates often occur in the form of single or multiple small grey or whitish clusters (Fig 26.7 and 26.10) and reflect light when viewed with direct focal illumination. When epithelial corneal infiltrates are viewed using high intensity marginal retro-illumination, and high magnification, it is possible to observe minute refractile or grey bodies (Fig 26.7, 26.10 and 26.14) within the infiltrate patch. Diagrams of a cross-sectional view of the cornea and a

with moderate to severe forms of corneal inflammation.

Corneal infiltrates can be viewed by using either direct illumination, including the optic section technique or indirect retro-illumination. However, the epithelial cystic formations can usually only be viewed using retro-illumination. When viewed with direct illumination, infiltrates appear nummular, cloudy and somewhat amorphous in appearance with a slightly denser centre. They may also look like ice crystals, presenting a somewhat solid centre with arm-like projections

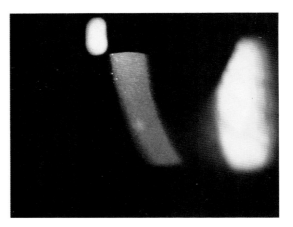

Figure 26.13 Corneal infiltrate with a stellate appearance (courtesy Dr Ian Lane).

hypothetical epithelial infiltrate can be seen in Figures 26.3 and 26.13. When stromal infiltrates are observed in this way, no similar defined bodies can be observed within the infiltrate.

Infiltrates appear different from epithelial microcysts when maximum illumination and magnification are used. Unlike infiltrates, microcysts do not occur in discrete patches, but tend to be more uniformly scattered.

Infiltrates can also be differentiated from vacuoles as vacuoles do not significantly reflect light and therefore are almost invisible when direct focal illumination is used. Vacuoles also have relatively smooth, sharply defined borders.

The limbus is a key area for observing corneal infiltrates that may be very small and subtle in presentation (Fig. 26.16). They are typically seen overlying limbal vessels, or may occur as band infiltrates grouped along the limbus (see Fig. 26.8). Serum leakage around terminal limbal vessels that project into the normally transparent cornea causes the immediate area surrounding these vessels to appear somewhat cloudy. Very small epithelial infiltrates are sometimes observed with this presentation, located near the ter-

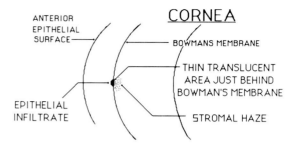

Figure 26.15 Corneal epithelial infiltrate.

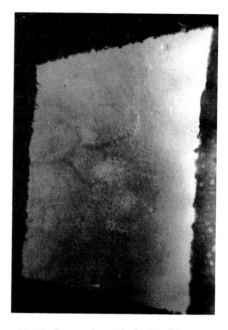

Figure 26.16 Corneal epithelial infiltrate overlying the vessels in the limbal region observed with high magnification and indirect retro-illumination (from Josephson & Caffery, 1979).

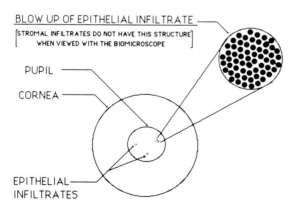

Figure 26.14 Magnified view of an epithelial infiltrate (diagram rendered from observations using a Rodenstock 2002 biomicroscope utilizing a quartz halogen light source at maximum illumination and viewed at maximum magnification).

minal ends of these vessels. They are frequently overlooked in many examinations and may be the forerunner of many corneal inflammatory episodes experienced by soft lens wearers. The stromal opacities seen as band infiltrates may have a rather lacy, ill-defined border and a relatively dense buff-coloured centre, or may appear dense and ball-like, with a white or buff-coloured appearance. These infiltrates can be easily differentiated from epithelial infiltrates when viewed with the slit lamp using an optic section (see Figs 26.3 and 26.11).

If a very thin optic section is used to observe deep epithelial infiltrates, a haze can sometimes be observed just posterior to Bowman's membrane (see Fig 26.29 and 26.13). This haze may be composed of the substances of inflammation and associated oedema, and could also be associated with the agglomeration of leukocytes in the adjacent deepest layers of the epithelium (Josephson & Caffery, 1989b). Because of the occasional presence of substantial subepithelial haze adjacent to an epithelial infiltrate, this formation can easily be misdiagnosed as a subepithelial (stromal) infiltrate when it is viewed with the slit lamp using conventional direct illumination.

26.4.7 MANAGEMENT OF CONTACT LENS-INDUCED CORNEAL PATHOLOGY

Microcysts, vacuoles and bullae

Patients presenting with these contact lens-induced lesions should be refitted with contact lenses that transmit significantly more oxygen. Microcysts may also be caused by a toxic reaction to preservatives in contact lens care solutions. These microcysts can be treated by having the patient switch to preservative free disinfecting and soaking solutions.

Epithelial infiltrates

Contact lens wear should be discontinued until the infiltrates have completely resolved. If symptoms persist after discontinuing contact lens wear for several days, a short course of topical steroids might be indicated. Contact lens wear should only be resumed if the cornea remains clear for at least 2 weeks after discontinuing medication. It is important that the lenses to be worn are in excellent

condition and that the patient's care system should be free of preservatives. The use of frequent and regular lens replacement programmes, or disposable lenses have been shown to significantly reduce the likelihood of occurrence.

Stromal infiltrates

Lens wear should be discontinued until the infiltrates are completely resolved. After a quiet period of 3–4 weeks where the cornea remains clear without medication and lens wear, lens wear can be continued. We suggest that preservative-free disinfection and soaking solutions be prescribed.

26.4.8 CONJUNCTIVAL SIGNS

The conjunctiva is a potentially reactive mucous membrane that is constantly exposed to the environment and to the solutions and plastics used in contact lenses. It must be monitored closely when caring for contact lens wearers.

Conjunctivitis

Bacterial conjunctivitis can occur during contact lens wear. In the acute form it usually begins unilaterally but may become bilateral quite quickly. Although pain is not a common feature the patient may report non-specific irritation. Most patients will report a history of one to two days of increasing intensity of signs and symptoms. Patients will report that their lashes mat or are crusty in the morning and that their eyes have become red.

Injection of the bulbar and tarsal conjunctiva is usually significant. The involved vessels are superficial. It is important to check at this point that the cornea is clear. The palpebral conjunctiva may show papillary hyperplasia. There will often be an associated discharge that is most noticeable on awakening. The usual aetiology of bacterial conjunctivitis is staphylococcal. However, streptococcus and *Haemophilus influenzae* can also cause this condition. *Pseudomonas* is a hyperacute and rapidly advancing infection and must be treated immediately to reduce any serious corneal complications. In almost all instances, appropriate medication must be applied topically and the patient should be monitored closely. Culture and scrapings should be taken in cases of corneal involvement. No lenses should be worn and lenses should be replaced prior to rewearing.

Patients may also present with viral conjunctivitis. The most common aetiology is adenovirus. These patients often do not seek care because of the frequently mild and short acute phase. It is usually unilateral and 3–5 days later presents in the other eye. Patients sometimes report a previous medical history of upper respiratory tract infection, low grade fever, etc. These patients present with a purplish-pink hypaeremic bulbar conjunctiva. There is often an associated diffuse secondary superficial punctate keratitis. The palpebral conjunctiva almost always shows follicular changes. Preauricular lymphadenopathy may be present. It is important that the practitioner rule out epidemic keratoconjunctivitis (EKC) in its early stages as this may lead to the contamination of other patients. Herpes simplex virus must also be ruled out (the condition is almost always unilateral). The treatment of this condition depends on its aetiology. Discontinuing lens wear is mandatory until all signs and symptoms disappear and remain absent without medication.

Allergy is a frequent seasonal cause of conjunctivitis. The most common presenting symptom is bilateral itching. A history of allergies, eczema or asthma and its reoccurrence on a seasonal basis is suggested evidence for this diagnosis. The bulbar conjunctiva may or may not be injected or chemotic. There may be a mucous or stringy whitish discharge. The palpebral conjunctiva can show velvety or hypaeremic changes (Spring, 1974; Friedlaender *et*

Table 26.1 Monitoring the limbus (from Davies, 1989)

	SEALS*	SLK**	Infiltrates	Vascularization
Symptoms	Visually asymptomatic	Reduced lens tolerance, irritation worse on lens removal.	Irritation, photophobia, lacrimation	Asymptomatic
Onset	Chronic	Chronic	Acute	Chronic
Binoc/monoc	Either	Binocular	Monocular	Either
Injection	None	Superior bulbar conjunctival/tarsal conjunctiva	Bulbar/limbal quadrant	Chronic around limbal capillaries
Staining	Accurate punctate	Dense superior ⅓ of cornea	Rarely	No
Site	Superior	Superior	Any quadrant	Any quadrant
Depth	Epithelial	Epithelial	Anterior/stromal posterior/epithelial	Any

* SEALS, superior (corneal) epithelial arcuate lesions.
** SLK, superior limbal keratitis (Sendele *et al.*, 1983; Abel *et al.*, 1985).

al., 1984). Contact lens wearing may be continued if the symptoms are mild and discharge is absent.

Toxic and irritative conjunctivitis may also occur in the contact lens practice. These patients present as a red eye situation but it is difficult to establish the primary aetiology. Their onset is usually insidious and there is an associated history of chronic exposure to an irritating or toxic substance that is an air-borne pollutant. Some of the possible toxic substances include chemical vapours either in the air or by contact. Sometimes patients are affected by systemic medications, or an auto-immune response. The situation may present as unilateral or bilateral, depending on the primary cause. There is mild to moderate bulbar conjunctival hypaeremia, often greater inferiorly. There is a mixed papillary and follicular palpebral conjunctival response, usually of only a mild to moderate degree. There is rarely a pronounced discharge or exudate.

The practitioner should beware of such aetiologies as dry eye conditions, outdoor exposure, dry environments, incorrect use of cosmetics, etc. The obvious treatment is to remove the offending agent if one can be found.

26.4.9 LIMBAL SIGNS

A summary of limbal pathology related to contact lens wear can be found in Table 26.1.

26.5 COMMON CLINICAL SYNDROMES

There are certain syndromes that reoccur in every contact lens practice and should be recognized by the practitioner. The following discussion outlines their presentation and management.

26.5.1 GIANT PAPILLARY CONJUNCTIVITIS

Giant papillary conjunctivitis (GPC) (Spring, 1974; Allansmith *et al.*, 1977; Greiner *et al.*, 1984) is one of the more common complications of contact lens wear. It may be a result of a mechanical irritation especially in hard lens wearers or of an immunological nature in hydrogel lens wearers whose lenses have become coated with deposits. The patient presents with symptoms of itching, mucous discharge, foreign body sensation and blurred vision. They may also report that their lenses tend to move more than usual with blinking.

Objective signs include protein coating on contact lenses and mucous discharge. After everting the upper lid, one will observe the presence of giant papillae and mucous sheets or strands in between the papillae. The instillation of fluorescein will stain these mucous sheets.

The papillae associated with hydrogel lens wear are usually a reaction to protein build-up on the lens surfaces. They are located higher on the upper palpebral conjunctiva than those caused by rigid contact lenses. The rigid lens induces GPC by mechanical means.

26.5.2 ACUTE RED EYE

This condition occurs most often in patients wearing contact lenses on an extended wear basis. The patient often wakes up in the morning with a painful, red eye and blurred vision. When extended wear patients report a red eye, it must be considered an ocular emergency and they must be seen promptly. The lenses should be removed immediately. When the patient presents in the office, the visual acuities of each eye should be documented and each eye examined with the slit lamp. There will often be limbal vessel dilation as well as limbal conjunctival chemosis. The cornea will often present infiltrates and there will be hypaeremia of the bulbar conjunctiva. The crucial decision at this point is to determine whether this ocular condition is sterile or a result of significant bacterial infection. The instillation of fluorescein

INTRODUCTION

This part of the text presents the fitting methods applicable to the normal eye that has a refractive error. But it will be evident that many of the principles that are described also apply to the abnormal eye (Part 8). Therefore we find in this section scleral lens fitting (Chapters 31 and 32), which are in fact mostly, if not always, applicable to the abnormal state, albeit historically, were used to fit the normal eye.

Those who seek contact lenses do so mainly for cosmetic reasons. They are the young patients who are aged up to 25 years and who are mostly myopic; a small proportion are hyperopic, who elect to wear contact lenses as a cosmetic device rather than spectacles or have refractive surgery. Then there is another group of patients who become hyperopic with reading problems later in life and are in the 30 to 40 age group and the presbyopes of all refractive errors who wish to be corrected with contact lenses, sometimes combined with spectacles (Chapter 33).

Children requiring contact lenses usually have abnormal eye conditions (Chapter 34) but it is not uncommon for children of 10 to 16 years of age to wear contact lenses for sports activities so that their vision problems do not detract from their co-ordination and prowess in the development of ball games or athletic activities.

The development of normal binocular vision is in many instances both a motility and a refractive error problem and not an abnormal eye condition and contact lenses can play a role in preference to spectacles (Chapter 34). In this particular group of chil-dren the wearing of high powered spectacle lenses and the use of occlusion can affect the sensitive child and lead to withdrawal symptoms and even abnormal behaviour patterns.

There are some general principles (Chapter 27) in the fit of a lens that apply to all lens designs and materials. For example, the optimal vision correction that is related to the lens design and the position of the lens about the eye's visual line. Whilst this may appear axiomatic the forces that tend to decentre and destabilize lenses of all materials and sizes means the eye being fitted has an individual identity. This individuality is mostly concerned with measurement but, since eyes and lid motility enter into the problem, with other factors such as tears and environment, the total presents a complex evaluation of fit required even for the normal shaped eye. It will be understood from Chapter 27 that a hemispherical shape placed upon a tilted ellipsoid can result in only three basic fits, the lens being the regular hemispherical shape and the anterior surface of the eye being the irregular ellipsoid.

This is the problem stated in its simplest form. Initially contact is made over three, or more areas between the two shapes (eye and lens), thereby achieving stability. Further, zones of contact occur if the lens moulds by virtue of material plasticity and in the instance of a very soft thin lens complete conformity to the eye ellipsoid then occurs. But in those instances where rigidity is maintained then, depending upon the degree of variance that exists between the two shapes, three fits can result. When only peripheral contact occurs then a steep fit results, with central clearance. With overall contact there is a parallel fit and if only central contact then an open fit or flat fit occurs. With each of these fits a dynamic situation arises from eye and lens movement often in contra directions. Chapters 27 and 31 will illustrate some of the principles for the large scleral lens and the small corneal lens. A degree of misfit is always present to permit function for the tear flow and gaseous exchanges. Thus there are many factors, some often discovered by the complications that occur after fitting and wearing the lenses.

The fit is also concerned with achieving rapid tolerance – both sensory and visual. The optimal size of any optic for the specific power and the back surface lens design are one aspect concerned with vision correction and lens design (Chapters 5 and 7) which has to consider the thickness distribution over the whole lens that will be complementary to the particular material. This means consideration of factors such as gas transference and maintenance of lens form to obtain a fit and yet for rigid lenses avoiding thickness that will cause flexion astigmatism and, in the case of soft lenses, irregular astigmatism (Chapters 28 and 29). Some of the theoretical considerations of soft lens kinetics (Chapter 6) permit the use of scientific formulation to the problems of tear movement and retrolens pressures that determine stability of fit and centration.

The problem of astigmatism correction (Chapters 28 and 29) is in some ways peculiar to contact lens wear. This is because the astigmatism can be induced by the contact lens if the lens (rigid) flexes on the eye or the optics have toric surfaces or the spherical soft contact lens can completely copy the corneal astigmatism. The tear lens between a rigid lens has a refractive index very similar to the cornea and thus the anterior corneal astigmatism is negated. There remain posterior corneal astigmatism and lenticular astigmatism

to consider. The physiological cornea rarely has a posterior corneal astigmatism greater than 0.75 D, and this much is tolerated by the visual acuity sensory mechanisms. But if internal astigmatism is revealed by the wear of the contact lens it can be intolerable to a patient used to obtaining normal acuity by a spectacle lens. In addition to this corneal astigmatism there is lenticular astigmatism, which would normally be corrected by the spectacle lens but not the contact lens. How these refractive errors can be corrected is described in the chapters on hard and soft fits for astigmatic patients (Chapters 28 and 29). It must be stated that in the majority of patients with anterior corneal astigmatism the rigid corneal lens does provide a good acuity correction, albeit the fit may be more difficult to achieve.

The use of toric contact lenses does bring to the fore the whole problem of lens manufacturing standards especially when applied to soft lenses. Even when high tolerances of manufactured perfection as to power and image quality are possible it may not be possible to have a fit that is stable during the whole period of wear. This part of contact lens practice can be the cause of many disappointments for the practitioner.

The fitting of coloured or tinted lenses can best be categorized as to function, although it is possible to classify the different types of coloured lenses available (Chapter 30). The chief use of a tinted contact lens will be as a cosmetic device and intended to beautify or, put another way, to attract attention to a face that has enhanced normality or beauty. Tints are available in several colours and since they are transparent they will affect the iris colour of those with lightly pigmented irises. To change the colour of a darkly pigmented iris would require an opaque coloured contact lens. The opaque colours can be patterned to simulate the iris, with and without a black pupil. The latter will be only of use for occlusion (Chapter 34) or as a prosthesis for masking an ugly eye deformity.

It must be appreciated that there are limitations to the perfection attainable with all coloured devices. The colour is at the corneal surface whereas the normal iris colour is a few millimetres from the posterior cornea and seen through a convex powered corneal lens, thus reducing and intensifying the true state. Also, the light reflections from the cornea may be different to those from the contact lens. The combined abnormal optical effects can detract from the cosmetic value of such devices. Certainly abnormal colours will result in a 'dolls eye' effect. It is important with all coloured and tinted lenses that the manufacturer conforms to standards with regard to toxicity of coloured additives and that the oxygen transmission is not obstructed in opaque soft lenses.

The use of the scleral contact lens is today only applicable to certain special cases (Chapters 31 and 32), and these indications are chiefly those of the abnormal eye and, rarely, the normal eye when it is used in special circumstances such as sport or prosthesis. Therefore, the rigid scleral technology as applied to the normal eye to obtain a fit belongs to history (Chapter 1) rather than every-day practice. There are lessons to be learnt from this technology that are applicable to other modern lens forms and their fit. Chapter 31, whilst giving the theory of the preformed scleral rigid lens, does emphasize how objective data can be applied for a lens to be manufactured to give an initial fit.

It must be admitted that the use of scleral lens trial fitting sets, unless very large and therefore prohibitively expensive, are not practical. Therefore, the chapter describes the preferred procedure of manufacture and fit of the eye impression lens, the impression of the eye shape being the best basis for a good fit for both the normal and abnormal eye shape.

It would seem that better results are to be obtained by the use of gas permeable rigid materials. It remains to be seen how these materials can best be used, either as thermo-labile or thermosetting and, to this end, how thickness of a scleral lens will affect the flow of gases even coupled with the other methods of ventilation such as fenestration. For the fitter who has no means of fitting rigid scleral lenses there are mini-scleral gas permeable rigid lenses, which are preformed and available in trial sets, which can be fitted to abnormal eyes especially those with decreased corneal sensitivity (Chapter 31).

The corneal rigid lens introduced in the 1950s (Chapter 1) very rapidly made practitioners aware that a greater percentage of patients could become successful wearers with very little fitting or manufacturing problems as compared with the scleral rigid contact lens. Therefore much thought and experiment was given, and is still ongoing (for example in the design of multifocal contact lenses for the presbyopic patient) to this problem.

The simplest solution of presbyopia still remains the uncomplicated (Chapter 33) use of supplementary reading spectacles or the provision of a contact lens for either eye with a plus power add to give monocular reading vision. The latter works well for many patients, especially if the refractive error is hyperopic. However, there are many lens designs, which copy in minuscule the bifocal and multifocal spectacle lens design, that have to be accompanied by stabilizing mechanisms to function well. On the other hand, the use of concentric design for the distribution of power using solely refractive technology or combined with diffraction bands has, for some patients, achieved a successful outcome. The availability of more than one image with the lens in one position relative to the vision line has brought into discussion whether the visual mechanism can alternate or whether translation from one to the other portion of the lens occurs. The ultimate successful correction for the contact lens wearing presbyope has yet to come.

Binocular vision problems can arise because of contact lens wear which, on the other hand, can be used in specific instances to alleviate or treat anomalies of binocular vision.

In the adult myope the wearing of contact lenses, and especially if these give full or over-correction, can cause a breakdown in binocular vision. The use of spectacle lenses for myopia has a prism base in effect for near fixation tasks. Thus the need to converge decreases as the power of correction increases. At the same time, accommodation power may also decrease, and therefore the patient has a latent convergence accommodation deficiency. The effective power of the spectacle-lens-wearing myope at near fixation in the plane of the crystalline lens is less than in emmetropia and hypermetropia, and therefore the accommodation has fewer demands made of it when reading. This state of affairs is upset when the patient starts to wear contact lenses, and a condition of pre-presbyopia occurs. Another example is the contact lens fit that is not centred and which produces a prismatic effect that can cause binocular vision distress, especially if a latent disorder is already present. Small degrees of binocular vision imbalance can be corrected by incorporating prism in the contact lens but this is limited even at the higher powers because of the small size of the optic. Even so, the lens must be a stable fit, which for smaller lenses involves the use of ballast-

ing and the consequent loss of tolerance. In induced anisometropia corrected by the contact lens, a residual aniseikonia can cause binocular vision problems. The general treatment principles to correct binocular vision problems include contact lens occlusion; prisms are not used unless there is a good reason for contact lens wear for the basic refractive disorder, the exceptions being the use of a cosmetic occlusive pupil lens for insuperable diplopia or in the instance of congenital nystagmus where there is good near vision present and contact lenses reduce nystagnus for distance fixation.

The use of contact lenses in infants and children (Chapter 34) presents problems in fitting and in management. Because of difficulties in the estimation of acuity there is always some doubt as to the measurable value of wearing contact lenses in such conditions as congenital cataract and the subsequent induced aphakic state. Certainly in high myopia of congenital refractive aetiology they have a value. Eye disfigurement requires prosthetic devices to help both the child and the parents.

This part of the text, entitled Fitting Technology, refers mainly to the normal eye but certain references to the abnormal eye are made and more extensive details are to be found in Part 9.

M. Guillon

27.1 INTRODUCTION

The scope of this chapter is to describe the basic fitting procedure for both soft and rigid contact lenses. It assumes that the patients are suitable candidates for contact lens wear and that all preliminary measurements have been taken. The objectives are to give the reader a general approach to the evaluation of lens fitting and provide guidelines for choosing and/or altering lens parameters in order to achieve an optimal fit. The chapter deals with basic fitting principles and does not concern itself with specific products.

27.2 FITTING CRITERIA

The criteria on which both rigid and soft lenses are fitted are identical: comfortable wear, clear stable vision and a respect for ocular metabolism and tissue integrity.

27.2.1 COMFORTABLE WEAR

Comfort is essential if successful lens wear is to be achieved. Comfort is gained by mechanical performance with adequate lens movement, lens design without brusque discontinuity, smooth clean surfaces and suitably formed edges.

27.2.2 CLEAR STABLE VISION

Clear stable vision is the key functional requirement of a contact lens. It is achieved by a well centred lens with controlled movements. The lens must be of good optical quality in order to fully correct ametropia, if present.

27.2.3 RESPECT OF CORNEAL METABOLISM AND TISSUE INTEGRITY

The most common metabolic requirement for contact lenses is that they supply sufficient oxygen for maintenance of corneal metabolism during the period of lens wear. The lens must also respect the corneal tissue by avoiding any adverse mechanical effect on either corneal or palpebral tissues, in particular excessive pressure with rigid lenses (Kenyon *et al.*, 1989) or excessive dehydration with soft contact lenses (Orsborn & Zantos, 1988).

27.3 SOFT CONTACT LENS FITTING

27.3.1 BASIC FITTING CRITERIA

Soft contact lens fittings are judged using both static and dynamic criteria. The static criteria include lens centration and corneal coverage, and the dynamic criteria include lens movement, in particular movement in response to the reflex blinking action.

Lens centration is necessary for clear vision. Full corneal coverage at all times is also essential. The lens edge must never encroach over the limbal region, as this is likely to result in poor comfort, destabilized tear film in that region and associated cor-

Contact Lens Practice. Edited by Montague Ruben and Michel Guillon.
Published in 1994 by Chapman & Hall, London. ISBN 0 412 35120 X

neal staining. Poor centration is often but not always related to incomplete corneal coverage. For example, lenses that are too small but tight fitting usually achieve good centration but can often give incomplete corneal coverage.

Conversely, lenses that are of a sufficient diameter, but fitted too loosely may achieve full corneal coverage yet exhibit marked vertical decentration due to the effect of the upper lid.

Soft contact lens movement is often limited and does not contribute significantly to the supply of oxygen via tear exchange (tear pump) during blink. In the best case, that is, with thick low water content soft lenses, the lens movement at blink produces only a 1% tear exchange (Polse, 1979). The key role of soft lens movement is to provide sufficient tear exchange under the lens in order to eliminate metabolic by-products and epithelial waste products (desquamated epithelial cells) which build up between the cornea and the back surface of the contact lens. This clearance avoids adverse mechanical and/or toxic effects of such debris (Mertz & Holden, 1981; Weissman, 1982). This is particularly important for extended wear, when lenses remain on the eye for periods of up to one week. This time is estimated to correspond to the normal turnover time of the full epithelium (Hanna *et al.*, 1961). For extended wear, it has been suggested that the debris that has accumulated over the closed eye period must be eliminated within a maximum of four hours after eye opening in order to minimize these adverse effects (Mertz & Holden, 1981).

27.3.2   BASIC PRINCIPLES OF LENS MECHANICAL PERFORMANCE CONTROL

The mechanical performance of soft contact lenses is dictated by the interaction of several forces, whose relative magnitudes combine to give the overall lens fitting. These forces are dependent upon lens material characteristics as well as ocular and lens parameters.

Understanding the interaction of these forces enables the practitioner to evaluate the performance of all types of soft contact lenses, and to identify the key parameters involved in the lens fit and make the relevant lens parameter alterations if required. Several systems have been proposed to summarize the forces involved in soft lens fitting (Kikkawa, 1979; Jenkins & Shimbo, 1985; Martin & Holden, 1986; Martin *et al.* 1989).

The simplified clinical model proposed here aims to help practitioners to understand the forces involved in lens fitting and their relative action and importance. The model incorporates four major forces (Fig. 27.1): eyelid force (ELF), tear fluid squeeze pressure (TFSP), tear fluid force (TFF) and contact lens stress force (CLSF).

Eyelid force (ELF)

The eyelid force is divided into a normal component and a tangential component. Between blinks, the normal component forces the lens periphery onto the eye helping to maintain the lens in stable equilibrium position and at the same time distorting the lens periphery. During blinks

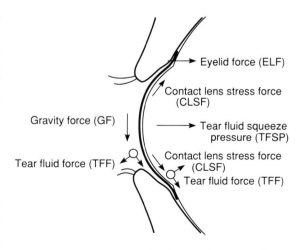

Figure 27.1 Forces involved in soft contact lens fitting.

the eyelid force is the main force which displaces the contact lens from its equilibrium position. Tight eyelids, found in oriental races and children, will therefore have a relatively greater effect than loose eyelids (often found in older patients). Eyelid action is made more efficient if the contact lens is thick and/or if the front surface design is uneven (e.g. high positive and negative lenses).

The tear fluid squeeze pressure (TFSP)

The tear fluid squeeze pressure is that pressure which develops within the post-lens tear film. Its amplitude is associated with the relationship between the saggita of the contact lens back surface and the corneal front surface over the lens diameter:

1. When the contact lens sagitta is greater than the ocular sagitta, TFSP is negative and helps to maintain the lens in a centred position between blinks. It resists the eyelid force (ELF) and the contact lens stress forces (CLSF) during blink.
2. When the contact lens sagitta is equal to or less than that of the ocular surface, TFSP contributes little to maintaining

the lens in a centred position between blinks and produces no opposition to the eyelid force during blink. Such lenses are usually loose fitting.

In general, all other parameters being equal, tight lenses create higher TFSP and smaller diameter and/or thinner lenses and more elastic materials create lower TFSP. An investigation using a range of lenses covering different water contents and lens thicknesses has shown that the TFSP is not linear (Martin *et al.* 1989). An optimal lens movement is achieved with a TFSP of −7.00 mm of water. Virtually no lens movement is seen with a TFSP greater than −14.00 mm of water.

The tear fluid force (TFF)

The tear fluid, both pre-and post-lens, has a lubricating role during lens movement. Its relative efficiency depends upon the viscosity of the tear fluid. The more viscous the tear fluid the lower the relative lens movement. A recent study (Guillon & Guillon, 1990) evaluating lens *in vivo* wettability and mechanical performance of soft lenses worn overnight, has shown that tear film viscosity has a significant effect on lens movement. At wak-

Table 27.1 Ocular parameters, anomalies and remedial actions

Force involved	Abnormal action	Effect	Remedial action if effect is excessive
Eyelid force	Tight eyelid	High ELF excessive lens movement	(i) use thin overall and edge lens design (ii) use regular/even front surface periphery (iii) tighten fit by increasing back surface sagitta and/or increasing lens diameter
	Loose eyelid	Low ELF insufficient movement	(i) use thick lens overall design (ii) use special front surface design with uneven thick mid-periphery (iii) loosen fit by decreasing back surface sagitta
Tear fluid force	Excessive viscosity	High TFF insufficient lens movement	(i) use low viscosity in-eye rewetting eyedrop (e.g. normal saline)

ing the viscosity of the tear film is much higher than during open eye wear and lens movement is reduced.

The contact lens stress force (CLSF)

The effect of external forces on the contact lens acts to deform the lens and create internal stress forces which can be divided into normal and tangential components. These stress forces help to maintain the lens in position between blinks and to recentre the lens immediately after a blink. These forces are dependent upon the elastic modulus (Young's modulus) of the lens material and the local lens thickness. The higher the modulus and the greater the lens thickness the greater the stress and recentration forces.

Our simplified model summarizes the effects of ocular and lens characteristics on lens fitting. An optimal fit can therefore be achieved by altering the contact lens parameters (Tables 27.1 and 27.2).

Table 27.2 Lens fitting anomalies and remedial actions

Abnormal action	Force involved	Remedial action
Insufficient movement	Excessive squeeze pressure	(i) decrease back surface sagitta (ii) thin contact lens periphery (iii) decrease lens diameter

	Excessive lens stress forces	(i) flatten peripheral radii
		(ii) decrease local lens rigidity:
		      (a) material with lower Young's modulus
		      (b) thin peripheral lens geometry

Excessive movement	Insufficient squeeze pressure	(i) increase back surface sagitta (ii) increase lens diameter (iii) thickness contact lens periphery

	Insufficient lens stress forces	(i) steepen peripheral radii
		(ii) increase local lens rigidity:
		      (a) material with higher Young's modulus
		      (b) thick peripheral lens geometry

Poor centration with full corneal coverage		**Normal Eyelid:** (i) decrease back surface sagitta (steepen BOR (and BPR)) (ii) increase lens flexibility (thin down lens design/change material) (iii) increase lens diameter **Excessive Eyelid Action:** (i) increase lens flexibility (thin down lens design) (ii) decrease back surface sagitta (steepen BOR (and BPR))
Incomplete corneal coverage with acceptable centration		(i) increase lens diameter
Incomplete corneal coverage with unacceptable centration		(i) increase lens diameter (ii) decrease back surface sagitta (Steepen BOR (and BPR)) (iii) increase lens flexibility (thin down lens design)

27.3.3 FITTING TECHNIQUE

Overall routine

The flexibility of soft contact lenses is such that a small range of lens parameters often suffice to adequately fit a large percentage of the population. This explains why no strict guidelines exist for choosing the contact lens parameters that will give an optimal fit, based on the anterior ocular parameters. Ocular parameters can therefore only be used as initial broad guidelines in selecting the first trial contact lens for a given lens type. The evaluation of the trial lens fit is the key to the final lens choice. We therefore propose the following routine:

1. Selection of lens type and material.
2. Selection of first trial lens based upon preliminary measurements and observations:
     i. keratometric readings;
     ii. horizontal visible iris diameter;
     iii. lid position;
     iv. spectacle refraction.
3. Lens fit evaluation:
     i. initial precaution;
     ii. general remarks;
     iii. evaluation by biomicroscopy;
     iv. evaluation by additional techniques.
4. Choice of additional contact lenses.
5. Over refraction and visual performance evaluation.
6. Order of final contact lens.

Detailed fitting routine

Selection of lens type and material

Soft contact lens materials have major inherent properties regardless of the parameters available in any specific lens design. This is true whether a standard design, as is usually the case in present day practice, or one's own design is used. In both cases it is necessary to decide on the lens material and type before choosing the lens parameters.

The choice of lens type is based upon several factors, primarily the intended lens wear modality with special considerations to be given to refractive errors and special ocular or general patient features.

Effect of lens wear modality

The practitioner must first consider the intended modality of wear:

1. Daily wear defined as the wearing of lenses during waking hours only.
2. Extended wear defined as the wearing of lenses up to seven days and six nights without removal.
3. Flexible wear defined as the wearing of lenses on a daily wear modality with intermittent overnight wear (usually up to two nights per week).

The key requirements for daily wear are to supply sufficient oxygen to the cornea for maintenance of normal corneal physiology and sufficient lens rigidity for good handling characteristics. This is possible with several lens types. The following alternative combinations have all been successfully fitted:

1. Ultrathin (0.06 to 0.07 mm) low water content (38%) lenses.
2. Ultrathin (0.05 to 0.07 mm) mid-water content (45%–55%) lenses.
3. Conventional thickness (0.12 to 0.15 mm) high water content (65%) lenses.

Recent studies suggest that the thin low water content lenses mentioned above may not supply enough oxygen to avoid hypoxic corneal changes. In the absence of other special requirements it is this author's preference for daily wear to fit thin mid-water content lenses as it is felt that they offer better comfort than thicker designs. For extended wear, the key requirement is to achieve as high an oxygen supply to the cornea as possible. The oxygen supply to the cornea can be increased by decreasing the lens thickness and/or increasing the lens water content.

To that effect the following combinations have been suggested:

1. Hyperthin (0.035 to 0.04 mm) low water content (38%) lenses.
2. Ultrathin (0.055 to 0.07 mm) mid-water content (45%–55%) lenses.
3. Conventional thickness (0.12 to 0.15 mm) high water content (> 65%) lenses.

For long-term extended wear, it is the author's preference to fit the latter two types rather than hyperthin low water content lenses. As previously shown, the oxygen transmissibility at the central point of the lens over-estimates its performance and a more functional approach is to consider the average transmissibility over the central 6 mm diameter area of the contact lens (Holden & Mertz, 1984). The very large relative difference in thickness between central and average values for the hyperthin lenses suggests that whereas those lenses have similar central transmissibility than higher water content lenses they have comparatively low oxygen supply as shown by *in vitro* oxygen transmission measurements (Winterton *et al.*, 1988). For −3.00 D contact lens the oxygen flux for Bausch and Lomb O_4^{TM} (low water, hyperthin) is 0.13 µl O_2 cm^2/min and 0.29 µl O_2/cm^2/min for Acuvue (mid-water, ultrathin) and 0.24 µl O_2/cm^2/min for Permaflex^{TM} (high water, conventional thickness).

We feel that the choice between mid- and high water contact lenses is a matter of personal preference, keeping in mind that if comfort is a problem the thinner mid-water content lenses should be chosen, and if insufficient movement is a problem the conventional thickness high water content lenses should be considered first.

For flexible wear the requirements are similar to those for extended wear as the lenses are worn overnight on a regular basis. A further point to consider with this modal-ity is that the handling characteristics of the lenses must allow for daily manipulation.

Effect of refractive error

Once the wear modality has been established, an important secondary consideration is refractive error. The previous suggested modalities refer to myopic patients with low refractive errors (up to −6.00 D). Considerations of other spherical and astigmatic refractive errors are as follows:

Hyperopia It is obvious that for positive lenses, ultrathin designs are not possible. Also, as the central part of the lens corresponds to the area of lowest oxygen transmissibility and highest corneal oedema (Guillon, 1982), it is important to maximize the oxygen transmissibility by using mid- or high water content lenses for hyperopic correction. Such an approach is valid even for daily wear lenses where it has been shown (La Hood & Holden, 1989) that low water content lenses create significant daytime cornea oedema because of the thickness required to achieve plus lens power.

Aphakia From the viewpoint of refractive error correction, aphakia is an extreme case of hyperopia, with refractive errors of the order of +15.00 D. From a physiological viewpoint, however, the cornea post-aphakic surgery is very different to that of a normal non-operated eye. The cornea of an aphakic eye swells significantly less than the non-operated eye (Holden *et al.*, 1980; Guillon & Morris, 1981) following the wearing of a thick soft contact lens. This reduced swelling response takes place in the presence of apparently similar oxygen uptake rate in both corneas (Guillon & Morris, 1981; Guillon & Morris, 1982), but reduced corneal sensitivity and endothelial cell density (Guillon & Morris, 1982) in the aphakic eye.

The previous considerations make it mandatory to opt for high water content lenses as any design, including special front aspheric designs (Guillon & Bleshoy, 1983), will result in a thick lens. The reduced sensitivity of the cornea, and usually loose lids of the aphakic patient, however, ensure that a thick lens is normally well tolerated and fits in a good central position as the eyelid force is weak, and hence does not adversely affect the lens fit.

High myopia For mid- to high myopic refractive errors (> 6.00 D) it is important to consider carefully the overall and mid-peripheral oxygen transmissibility of the lenses. Consideration should be given to high water content lenses, whose oxygen transmissibilities are adequate, special thin peripheral designs (Guillon, 1988) and reduced front optic zone diameter lenses.

Astigmatism The ability to correct low degrees of astigmatism (≤ 0.50 DC) with any spherical soft contact lens is similar. Slightly higher degrees of astigmatism (0.75 DC) are better corrected by more rigid materials or thicker lenses, as they have a tendency to mask some of the astigmatism and afford a better visual performance. Oxygen transmissibility of the thicker lenses should, however, be considered in these cases.

For astigmatism ≥ 1.00 DC, spherical soft contact lenses do not give satisfactory visual performance. In these cases it is necessary to fit lenses with a special design to correct astigmatism. The most commonly prescribed are toric lenses, but as suggested recently special aspheric designs may also be of use (Lydon, 1990).

Tear-related problems

Tear-related problems are treated in more detail in Chapter 21, however, one should keep in mind the following simple rules when choosing a specific lens type:

1. Patients being exposed to relatively dry environmental conditions for significant periods of time (e.g. long-haul airline personnel) should be fitted with conventional thickness lenses (>0.10 mm) rather than hyperthin lenses, to avoid the corneal staining associated with the latter lenses (Orsborn & Zantos, 1988). The restriction with such lenses is that they must supply sufficient oxygen to the cornea for a normal metabolism.

2. Patients with tear-related contact lens problems, such as poor comfort due to a rapidly breaking pre-lens tear film, should be fitted with conventional high water content contact lenses (these hold a more stable tear film) rather than hyperthin low water content lenses (Guillon *et al.*, 1989). When poor comfort is progressive, regular replacing of contact lenses has been shown to be an advantage (Ames & Cameron, 1989).

Selection of first trial contact lens

Once the practitioner has chosen a lens type based on the criteria described earlier, the choice of the first trial lens is straightforward and depends on the alternative parameters available for that lens design.

In the simplest case, the lens design is a 'one-fit' system and the only parameter to select is the lens power. This is often the case for very thin lens designs, where the lens is highly flexible and conforms to the anterior ocular surface of the majority of a normal population. The trial lens power should be as close as possible to the final power and must not under any circumstances differ by more than ± 4.00 D from that power.

For designs where alternative fittings are available parameter variations can be usually be made on the back optic radius and/or diameter. In these cases there are general guidelines based upon the patient central corneal curvature (Table 27.3) for the choice of back optic radius and upon the patient's visible iris diameter for the choice of diameter (Table 27.4). Patients with very small palpebral aperture are often best fitted with small diameter lenses. Patients with high refractive errors should not be fitted with small diameter lenses as problems with centration and corneal coverage can be encountered.

Lens fit evaluation

Initial precautions

Several precautions must be taken to ensure a reliable lens evaluation. The trial lens should be rinsed with unpreserved, buffered, sterile saline after removal from the vial prior to insertion. Buffering is particularly important for high water content ionic lenses, which have parameters that are highly pH dependent (McKenney, 1990). Lens rinsing often improves lens wettability and also helps to unfold very thin lenses without tearing them.

Before insertion, the trial lens should be checked for correct inversion. This is done by gently squeezing the lens and observing the behaviour of the lens edges. If the lens is correctly inverted, the lens edge will not curl (Fig. 27.2a). If the lens is incorrectly inverted, the edges tend to curl and appear like a hat rim (Fig. 27.2b). This test is at times inconclusive for thin lenses. In such cases, the lens should be left to dry on the finger for approximately 30 seconds and the test repeated.

Finally, one must make sure that the lens surface wettability is good. It is not uncommon to find lens surfaces to be hydrophobic

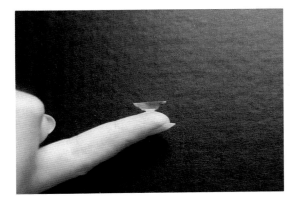

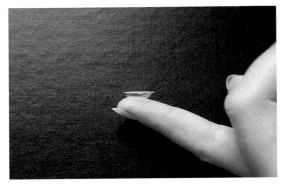

Figure 27.2 Method to identify the lens front and back surfaces. (a) Correct contact lens; (b) inverted contact lens.

when removed from their vial for the first time. The exact cause of this phenomenon is unknown but it is believed to be due to lens manufacturing and has been observed at different times with all three manufacturing processes of lathing, spin casting and cast moulding for both low and high water content lenses. If poor surface wettability is

Table 27.3 General guideline for choice of first trial contact lenses based upon the mean keratometric values.

Mean keratometric reading	Back lens sagitta	Back optic care radius
K < 7.50 mm	High	Steep
7.50 ≤ K ≤ 8.10 mm	Average	Average
K > 8.10 mm	Low	Flat

Table 27.4 General guideline for choice of first trial contact lens based upon the measured horizontal visible iris diameter.

Horizontal visible iris diameter (mm)	Lens diameter
HVID < 10.50 mm	Small
10.50 mm ≤ HVID ≤ 12.50 mm	Average
HVID > 12.50 mm	Large

observed the lens should not be inserted, as it may be uncomfortable, creating reflex lacrimation and mild blepharospasm. These symptoms will not allow a true evaluation of the lens fit. The poor surface wettability problem is most commonly solved by a saline rinse but, if this fails, the lens should be rubbed with saline. In the event that wettability is still unimproved, the lens should be rubbed with a surfactant and rinsed in saline.

After the lens has been inserted it is necessary for the lens to settle and for the initial reflex lacrimation, if any, to subside.

The main environmental difference between the vial and the eye is an increase in temperature from room temperature to between 32.5 and 35.5 °C for the open eye environment and 35.6 and 36.5 °C for the closed eye (Fatt & Chaston, 1980). Such a temperature change creates a decrease in the lens water content (Fatt & Chaston, 1980) and a steepening of the lens fit with the lens on the eye having a slightly smaller diameter and steeper back optic radius (BOR) than in the vial. This effect, which is particularly marked for high water content lenses (approximately 6% for a 70% water content lenses versus 1% for a 38% water content lens is quite rapid and a settling time of 30 minutes is ample (Wechsler *et al.*, 1983; Efron *et al.*, 1987). A longer settling time may be necessary if the patient produces marked lacrimation.

Lens fit evaluation general remarks

A number of techniques have been proposed and used to evaluate the fit of soft contact lenses including retinoscopy (Mandell, 1974a,b; Gasson, 1980) front surface keratometry (Mandell, 1974c; Bier & Lowther, 1977; Ruben, 1978; Gasson, 1980), keratoscopy (Gasson & Stone, 1977; Ruben, 1978) and photokeratoscopy. All these techniques have some use and will be described briefly, however, biomicroscopy is the main technique and suffices to assess the fit of soft contact lenses. (In order to achieve a similar on eye lens diameter it is necessary to choose lenses with a greater label diameter for the high water content than for the low water content lens materials.)

Lens fit evaluation by biomicroscopy

The overall lens fitting characteristics are best judged with the biomicroscope initially under ×20 magnification. More specific details of fit can then be assessed under ×30 to ×40 magnification. Diffuse lighting is the preferred to observe the lens fitting characteristics (Brandreth, 1978). This is produced by the addition of a diffuser in front of the focal lighting source giving an even distribution of light which is not excessive. Excessive lighting can lead to patient discomfort due to the drying out of the lens on the eye.

The lens fitting characteristics are judged in chronological order in terms of static and dynamic performance. Lens centration and corneal coverage are indicative of the lens static performance and lens movements following a blink, during eye version and upgaze, and following the 'digital push-up', are indicative of the lens dynamic performance. It is nowadays possible to measure with accuracy these fitting characteristics by using a projection graticule attachment to the slit lamp biomicroscope or by video-taping the lens fit. Video-taping the lens fit, however, is often time consuming and is of more relevance to a clinical research practice.

To gain repeatability in lens fit evaluation it is best to adopt a forced choice classification system for each parameter observed. We find that such a classification system gives a more structured approach to clinical judgement and facilitates comparisons between visits and/or practitioners. Our system of choice is described in detail below.

Evaluation of static fitting performance

Lens centration Lens centration is the main indicator of the lens static fitting characteristics. Centration is judged when the lens has reached equilibrium after a blink with the patient comfortably set up at the biomicroscope and looking straight ahead (primary gaze).

Lens centration is judged on a three-point scale by comparing the position of the lens edge and the apparent visible iris:

0   = Optimal.
1   = Acceptable decentration
2   = Unacceptable decentration

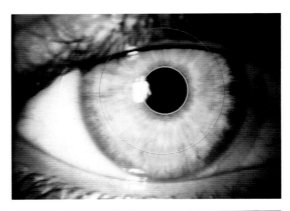

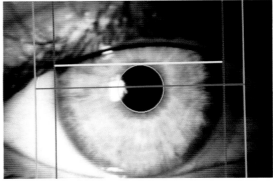

Figure 27.4 Evaluation of soft contact lens vertical centration. (a) By comparison of front optic zone and pupil position; (b) by comparison of contact lens and visible iris vertical tangent positions.

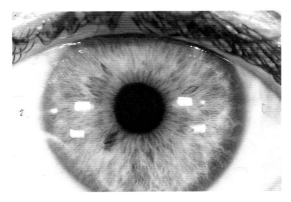

Figure 27.3 Soft contact lens optimal centration.

An optimal centration (Fig. 27.3) is achieved when a lens demonstrates similar nasal and temporal conjunctival overlap and appears vertically centred. The comparison of the vertical overlap is at times difficult because the superior part of the lens is covered by the upper lid. Despite this, one can usually assess the vertical centration without referring to an alternative method. One way is to compare the vertical position of the front optic zone and pupil (Fig. 27.4a) or the vertical position of the imaginary vertical tangent to the iris and the lens (Fig. 27.4b).

An acceptable decentration (Fig. 27.5) is one where the amount of decentration is in the order of 0.50 mm. An easy way to quantify the amount of decentration is to compare it to the amount of limbal overlap. For a typical lens of diameter 14.00 mm and an average horizontal visible iris of 11.50 mm, a perfectly centred lens will have both a nasal and temporal overlap of 1.25 mm, whereas a lens with 0.50 mm decentration will have one overlap of 0.75 mm and another of 1.75 mm.

An unacceptably decentred lens (Fig. 27.6) is one exhibiting a difference in nasal and temporal conjunctival overlaps or vertical misaligment of 0.75 mm or more.

The direction of decentration (nasal, temporal, superior and inferior) should be recorded, as well as its classification which has been described earlier (e.g. 1 (N) for acceptable nasal decentration).

Corneal coverage Corneal coverage is judged both in primary gaze, upgaze and during nasal and temporal versions. Corneal coverage is primarily an evaluation of the static fitting characteristics when judged in primary position after the lens has reached its equilibrium position following a blink. It is also an indication of the lens dynamic characteristics associated with eye movements.

Corneal coverage is rated on a three-point scale:

0 = Full corneal coverage at all times.
1 = Partial corneal exposure with extreme eye movements.
2 = Partial corneal exposure in primary gaze.

Full corneal coverage, at all times, indicates an optimal fit where the edge of the lens never appears to encroach over the cornea and always appears in apposition to the conjunctiva. Partial corneal exposure with extreme eye movements is borderline acceptable if it produces no undue discomfort. Partial corneal exposure in primary gaze is totally unacceptable as it will certainly produce corneal staining in the area of exposure (Fig. 27.7).

The direction of gaze creating corneal

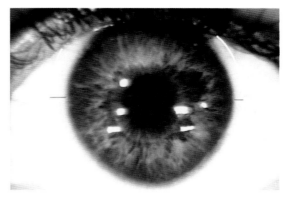

Figure 27.5 Soft contact lens exhibiting acceptable decentration.

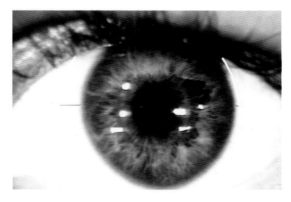

Figure 27.6 Soft contact lens exhibiting unacceptable decentration.

exposure or the region of the cornea exposed in primary gaze should always be indicated (e.g. 1 (V) for partial exposure on extreme upgaze or 2 (T) for temporal corneal exposure in primary gaze).

Lens centration and corneal coverage Lens centration and corneal coverage are two different evaluations of the lens static fit. Both can be at fault at the same time (Fig. 27.7) but often only one is unacceptable. Poor lens centration on its own is mainly indicative of an excessive decentration force, for example, excessive interaction of the upper lid on a thick contact lens or an insufficient centra-

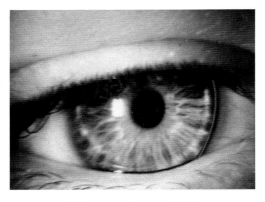

Figure 27.7 Soft contact lens exhibiting unacceptable decentration and partial corneal exposure in primary gaze.

tion force. Incomplete corneal coverage alone, in particular in primary gaze, is indicative of an insufficient lens diameter.

Evaluation of lens dynamic performance

The lens dynamic performance is judged in terms of lens movement observed under five different conditions: (1) during blink in primary position; (2) during version; (3) during upgaze; (4) during blink in an upgaze position; and (5) following digital push-up.

In each case the movement is rated on a five-point scale:

−2 = Insufficient, unacceptable movement.
−1 = Acceptable but less than optimal movement.
0 = Optimal movement.
+1 = Acceptable but more than optimal movement.
+2 = Excessive, unacceptably movement.

In several textbooks (Mandell, 1974b; Gasson, 1980) values quoted for lens movement have been of the order of 1 to 2 mm. Such a magnitude is much greater than the lens movement typically encountered with current soft contact lenses. Our unpublished data indicate that the average movement achieved with highly flexible lenses, such as hyperthin low water content or ultrathin mid-water content lenses, is of the order of 0.25 to 0.75 mm versus 1.00 to 1.25 mm for more rigid conventional thickness high water content lenses. The small movements encountered with modern soft contact lenses contribute to their comfort. This amount of movement is usually sufficient to clear debris that forms between the cornea and contact lens back surface.

Movement after a blink in primary position

The movement after a blink in primary position is the recentring movement that takes place upon eye opening at the end of the normal blink while the patient looks straight ahead. This movement is often reduced, particularly with thin and very flexible contact lenses. It is best observed under ×30 magnification. When in doubt with regard to this movement, it may be useful to ask the patient to blink and observe the recentring movement following this voluntary forced blink. An optimal recentration movement after a normal blink is a small, smooth movement from a slightly decentred position (<1.00 mm) to a centred position.

An unacceptable insufficient movement is when no recentration movement, even after a forced blink, is shown.

A less than optimal recentration but acceptable movement at blink, is one that is of limited magnitude (<0.50 mm) and of a 'jerky' nature. It shows a brisk return to the centred position. On the contrary, a greater than optimal movement after a blink is one of large magnitude (more than 1.00 mm for ultrathin contact lenses and more than 1.50 mm for conventional thickness contact lenses). Such movement is often associated with an overshoot of the original lens preblink position before recentration.

An excessive movement after a blink can be as large as that indicated above and is also associated with a lack of recentration, i.e. the lens fails to reach an equilibrium position and remains in a decentred position between blinks.

Movement at nasal, temporal versions and at upgaze The movement on nasal and temporal versions and upgaze are the relative lag of movements that take place as the lens does not follow exactly the eye but is being held by the lid and orbital structures. The lens shows greater conjunctival overlap in that direction than during primary gaze. The amplitude of the average lens movements encountered during nasal and temporal versions and upgaze is similar to that observed at blink (0.50 to 1.00 mm).

The lens movements observed at versions and at upgaze can only be a definitive diagnostic sign of insufficient lens movement. They cannot easily differentiate between normal and excessively moving lenses. No observable lag is unacceptable and lag less than 0.5 mm can be considered less than optimal but acceptable.

The lens movement at upgaze similarly indicates an unacceptable tight contact lens when no lag is seen and a less than optimal movement when less than 0.50 mm lag is observed. In addition, under the influence of gravity, the lens movement at upgaze is excessive if a lag of 2.00 mm or more is encountered. In these cases, the lenses are often uncomfortable during upgaze and the patient produces rapid reflex blinking in order to maintain the lens centred over the cornea.

Movement at blink in upgaze The lens movement after a blink in upgaze follows the same rules as the lens movement after a blink in primary gaze. However, because the lower edge of the lens is not covered by the lower lid, the magnitude of the lens movement obtained is slightly larger and also much easier to detect.

Lens movement at digital push-up The lens movement following digital push-up is the most important dynamic diagnostic fitting test for thin soft contact lenses. It indicates the level of adherence of the contact lens to the anterior ocular surface and is therefore a direct indication of the ease with which debris that has built up between the cornea and the contact lens can be eliminated. The test is carried out in primary gaze. The practitioner decentres the lens vertically by pushing it with the edge of the lower lid (Fig. 27.8). The recentration movement is then observed.

An optimally fitted contact lens is one that can be easily dislodged and returns to its initial centred equilibrium position in a rapid and smooth manner. A tight lens is one which resists decentration and returns to its equilibrium position in a fast 'jerky' manner. A loose lens is one that is easily decentred but demonstrates a sluggish movement on return to its equilibrium position. Occasionally, a loose lens overshoots this equilibrium position when the lower lid is held away from the eye.

Lens fit evaluation by additional techniques

Keratometry Front surface keratometry has been used to evaluate soft lens fitting characteristics. This method is based on the observation of the quality of the keratometric mire image formed at the lens front surface and its variations with a blink. This technique was

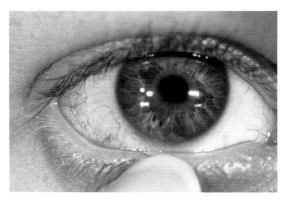

Figure 27.8 Vertical decentration with lower lid during 'push-up' test.

used extensively in the early days of soft contact lens fitting. The assessment of lens fitting with the biomicroscope was not well established at that time and the keratometric technique offered simple observation of gross defects.

The technique is based on the effects transmitted to the contact lens front surface of variations in the conformity of the contact lens back surface to the corneal front surface. Those variations are seen with relatively rigid contact lenses, such as standard thickness low water content soft lenses, but not with highly flexible soft contact lenses where the technique is not useful. The technique involves the focusing of the keratometric mires on the contact lens front surface once the lens has reached its equilibrium position between blinks. The mire quality is observed before the blink and immediately following a forced blink.

The appearance of the mires and diagnosis of lens fitting are given below:

1. With an optimal fit, where the lens back surface conforms to the corneal front surface, the keratometric mires are clear both at equilibrium and immediately following a blink.
2. With a tight fit, where the lens back surface saggita is significantly larger than the corneal sagitta, there is a clearance between the contact lens and the cornea at equilibrium between blinks. The tangential component of the eyelid force makes the lens conform to the corneal surface. The mires, which are slightly distorted at equilibrium, become clear immediately upon eye opening.
3. With a loose fit, the lens back surface saggita is smaller than the corneal front surface sagitta. At equilibrium, the contact lens back surface is in contact with the cornea and the mires are clear. The eyelid force, however, displaces the lens and the lack of recentration forces result

in a distorted keratometric mire image.

Front surface keratometry has other applications. It gives an indication of the stability of the pre-lens tear film (see Chapter 21). It also permits the measurement of any residual front surface cylinder. The difference between the keratometric values in the two principal meridians is a direct measurement of the residual astigmatism. (Most keratometers have both milimetric and dioptric graduations. For those where only milimetric graduations exist, 0.1 mm radius is equivalant to 0.50 D of astigmatism.) The difference between the corneal front surface astigmatism and contact lens front surface cylinder is a measurement of the astigmatism masked by the contact lens.

Keratoscopy The hand-held keratoscope (Gasson & Stone, 1977) has also been used to assess the lens fitting characteristics in a similar manner to the keratometer.

The keratoscope gives an indication of the overall fit rather than only the central fit of the lens. However, interpretation is often more difficult because of distortions of the keratoscopic mires present at the edge of the front surface optic zone due to the brusque discontinuity. This difficulty has limited the popularity to this technique.

Retinoscopy The quality of the retinoscopic reflex has been used to judge the fit of soft contact lenses. (Mandell, 1974c; Gasson 1980).

1. With an optimal fit, the retinoscopic reflex appears clear and undistorted at all times.
2. With a tight fit, the retinoscopic reflex has a black, distorted shadow in the central area, similar to the shadow observed in early keratoconic patients. Distortion and the shadow disappear momentarily immediately after the blink.

3. With a loose fit the retinoscopic reflex has a peripheral distorted shadow that tends to worsen immediately after the blink.

27.3.4 CHOICE OF ADDITIONAL CONTACT LENSES

If the trial lens fitting is acceptable, we proceed to an over-refraction in order to determine the final lens power. If the fitting is not acceptable a second trial contact lens needs to be chosen.

A new trial contact lens can be chosen by referring to Tables 27.1 and 27.2 once the reasons for failure of the first trial lens have been established. In these tables, the remedial actions are described in order of importance to facilitate the practitioner's next choice of lens. In many cases, the available lens parameters are limited and a change in lens type may be needed.

27.3.5 OVER-REFRACTION AND VISUAL PERFORMANCE

Once the ideal fit has been achieved, the practitioner should use a conventional refractive technique to determine both the full sphero-cylindrical and best sphere over-correction.

The investigation may involve objective evaluation by retinoscopy or automated refractometry or subjectively by conventional refraction.

Automated refractometers are very useful in these cases as they enable a rapid routine measurement of the full over-refraction. It is essential to measure the full sphero-cylindrical over-refraction. As shown in Chapter 41, conventional evaluation of the visual performance with a high contrast letter chart under normal room illumination on its own is not a good indication of the true contact lens performance. A 6/6 acuity may correspond to a significant loss in performance under different conditions, in particu-

lar, during night time wear. Whenever the cylindrical over-correction is > 0.50 D, we recommend the use of a full visual performance evaluation (see Chapter 41) to ensure that the lens functional performance is adequate.

Finally, as we indicated, it is essential to use trial lenses within ± 4.00 D of the final lens power, in order to evaluate the true lens mechanical performance. However, if for any reason the trial contact lens is more than ± 4.00 D from the final lens power, it is necessary to adjust for the back vertex distance of the over correcting lens (see Chapter 7).

27.3.6 FINAL CONTACT LENS ORDER

In order to avoid misinterpretation when ordering the final lens from the contact lens laboratory, it is essential to ensure that the lens order is complete and easily understood. Also, that the same information is given to the patient at lens delivery, as a record of the lens he/she is wearing should any urgent replacement be required. For this reason, a prescription must be easily understood world-wide. We recommend use of the International Standards (ISO) classification system which has been standardized by

the EEC standards organization or Comité Européen de Normalisation (CEN). That committee has considered that in many cases, standard soft contact lens design details are unknown and in these cases a simplified method can be used as an alternative to the full specification (see Chapter 11). That method will indicate the name of the lens design and all necessary parameters to identify that lens within the design chosen:

e.g. 1. Hydron Zero6
   BOZR 8.70
   BVP −3.00
2. Acuvue
   BVP −3.00

27.4 RIGID GAS PERMEABLE LENS FITTING

27.4.1 BASIC FITTING CRITERIA

The fitting criteria for rigid gas permeable (RGP) contact lenses are both static and dynamic. The static performance includes lens position between blinks and the lens/cornea relationship. The dynamic performance includes lens movement during and following the reflex blink action.

The lens position at equilibrium between blinks is a key criterion for a successful fit. The eyelid force is greater than for soft contact lenses and strongly influences the position of the RGP lens. In an optimal RGP fit the lens is positioned slightly superiorly because of this eyelid force. Another key aspect of the static fit is the relationship between the contact lens back surface and the corneal front surface. The aim is to achieve slight central clearance, intermediate contact between the lens and the cornea and little edge clearance. For extended wear, the optimal fitting relationship is central alignment or slight central touch with greater edge clearance than for daily wear.

Lens movement is a key characteristic of an ideal rigid lens fitting. The lens should move to a decentred position with little resistance to the eyelid force. It should recentre smoothly and rapidly on eye opening to a stable equilibrium position with no further movement until the next blink.

Lens movement occurs either as a response to the eyelid force or attached to the upper lid.

27.4.2 BASIC PRINCIPLES OF LENS MECHANICAL PERFORMANCE CONTROL

In a manner similar to soft contact lenses, the mechanical performance of RGP lenses is also dictated by the relative magnitude of several forces. For RGP lenses, as for soft contact lenses, these forces are dependent on the lens geometry, material characteristics and ocular parameters. However, because of the very different lens characteristics, the relative effect of the forces is different than for soft contact lenses. The proposed model incorporates five forces (Fig. 27.9) – three identical to the soft lens model: eyelid force (ELF), tear fluid squeeze pressure (TFSP), tear fluid force (TFF) and two further forces – edge tension force (ETF) and gravity force (GF).

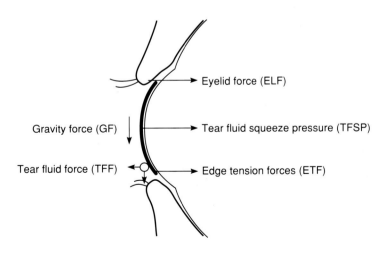

Figure 27.9 Forces involved in extrapalpebral RGP lens fitting.

Eyelid force (ELF)

The ELF plays a principal role in the RGP lens mechanical performance.

First, during lid closure at blink the tangential component to the cornea displaces the contact lens by 2 to 3 mm with the bottom of the lens saddling the lower limbus and contacting the lower bulbar conjunctiva.

Between blinks the ELF plays a variable role, from no action to being the major force determining the lens equilibrium position. The ELF acts whenever it contacts the lens. Also, the greater the contact, the greater the effect. In this sense, two types of RGP lens fittings should be considered – the intrapalpebral and extrapalpebral fit. In the intrapalpebral fit, the lens is located completely within the palpebral aperture and the eyelid force has no action on the fitting characteristics between blinks (Fig 27.10). In the extrapalpebral fit, the eyelid force normal to the contact lens acts to hold the lens against the cornea (Fig. 27.9) counteracting the gravity force which tends to force the lens to ride low. This results in negative pressure, which tends to keep the lens in a centred position. In a normal fit, the eyelid force tends to over-compensate the gravity force and nega-

tive pressure maintains the lens in a slightly superior position.

The action of the upper eyelid depends on the eyelid characteristics, particularly position and tonus.

A high riding lid which covers only a small area of the upper cornea or is tangential to it will have little action on rigid contact lens centration. A low riding lid, which can be as low as the upper edge of the pupil, will have a significant effect on maintaining the lens in a superior position.

The action of the upper eyelid can be altered by modifying the lens parameters, in particular the lens diameter and peripheral geometry. For example, the centration of a low riding lens can be improved by increasing the lens diameter, hence, increasing the zone of contact between the eyelid and the lens. Also, if the contact lens is sufficiently covered by the upper lid, centration can be altered by varying the peripheral lens geometry. One approach is to create a thickness differential at the lens edge. This is referred to as a negative carrier as it has the shape of a negative powered lens (Fig. 27.11a). This method increases the effectiveness of the eyelid, hooking the contact lens under the upper lid. Conversely, when a lens rides too

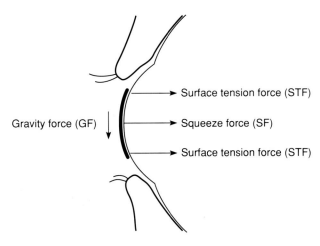

Figure 27.10 Forces involved in intrapalpebral RGP lens fitting.

high due to excessive eyelid action, particularly for high negative lenses, the lens peripheral geometry can be altered using a positive carrier (Fig. 27.11b), decreasing the action of the eyelid.

The tear fluid squeeze pressure (TFSP)

The TFSP is the pressure that is developed in the post-lens tear film situated behind the optic zone of the contact lens. This force maintains the contact lens in a central position by opposing the gravity force that acts to decentre the contact lens inferiorly and the eyelid force that acts to decentre the lens superiorly at equilibrium. Also, during blink it is the main recentration force as its dynamic action creates a symmetrical force on the contact lens.

This force is proportional to the irregularity of the post lens tear layer in that region; it is directly proportional to the tear layer thickness (TLT) at the apex of the contact lens (Fig. 27.12). The greater the TLT the greater the TFSP.

It is, in fact, this concept which is used by the practitioner when judging the fluores-

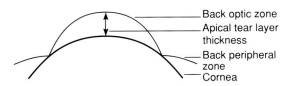

Figure 27.12 Tear layer thickness diagram.

cein fitting pattern. Assessment is made on the position of the zones (black areas) of contact and clearance (green areas), and the magnitude of the clearance by assessing the brightness of the green area. It has been shown that a central 'alignment' to slight central clearance corresponds to a TLT of 10 to 25 µm (Fig. 27.13), whereas a steep fit corresponds to a TLT of 35 µm or more (Fig. 27.14). The TFSP in a flat fit (Fig. 27.15) corresponds to a central TLT of zero and plays no part in maintaining lens centration.

The TFSP is influenced by altering the back optic radius (BOR) and the back optic diameter (BOD). A change as low as 0.05 mm in BOR creates a significant change in lens fitting. A change of at least 0.2 mm in BOD is necessary to significantly change the lens clinical fit. However, there are limitations to altering the BOD. If the BOD becomes too small (< 7.40 mm) visual problems are created. If the BOD is too large, intermediate

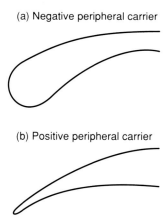

Figure 27.11 RGP lens peripheral lid controlled peripheral designs. (a) Negative carrier to maximize eyelid effect; (b) positive carrier to minimize eyelid effect.

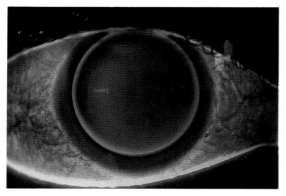

Figure 27.13 Fluorescein picture of a centrally aligned RGP lens.

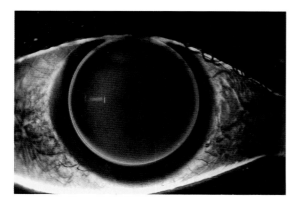

Figure 27.14 Fluorescein picture of a steep fitting RGP lens.

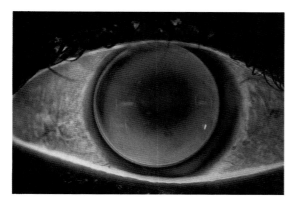

Figure 27.15 Fluorescein picture of a flat fitting RGP lens.

touch cannot be achieved. In general, a minimum peripheral width of 0.6 mm should be present.

Corneal topography significantly affects the TLT. For example, if we fit a population that has the same central corneal curvatures but different corneal rates of flattening with lenses of the same design, a wide range of BOR and fitting increments will be necessary to achieve a similar fit (Table 27.5). If details of the peripheral corneal topography are unknown, selection of the first trial lens is often only an approximation.

Tear fluid force (TFF)

The tear fluid force, as for soft contact lenses, has a lubricating role during lens movement (see Fig 27.9 and 27.10). Its efficiency also depends on the viscosity of the tear film. The TFF is of minor importance for RGP lens fitting in most modalities of wear. During overnight wear of RGP lenses, however, we believe that the lack of a front and back surface aqueous tear film phase and an increase in the tear film viscosity contribute to the lens adherence syndrome.

Edge tension force (ETF)

The edge tension force acts to hold the RGP lens against the cornea. This force operates at the lens edge whenever it is not covered by the upper or lower lids and where a tear meniscus is present (see Fig 27.9 and 27.10). This force varies according to the radius of the tear meniscus observed, ie. the smaller

Table 27.5 Back optic radius selection to achieve similar tear layer thickness for 95% of the population with same central corneal radius but with different rates of peripheral corneal flattening

Corneal model[1]	R_o for TLT = 15μm[2]	Fitting increment
Steep p = 1.15	7.67	$R_o = K_f - 0.20$ mm
Average p = 0.85	7.84	$R_o = K_f$
Flat p = 0.55	7.99	$R_o = K_f + 0.15$ mm

[1] Corneal model (Guillon *et al.*, 1986). Central corneal radius K_f 7.85 mm. Peripheral corneal flattening p = 0.85 ± 0.15 (0 < p < 1 flattening ellipse/p = 1 esphere/p steepening ellipse).
[2] Contact lens BOD = 8.00 mm. Spherical BOR

Table 27.6 RGP material *Dk* requirements as per Holden corneal physiological requirements for the average subject and 95% of subjects (Holden & Mertz, 1984) for contact lenses of average thickness (Avt) 0.15 mm and 0.20 mm

Contact lens *Dk/L* physiological criteria	Contact lens *Dk/L* requirements $(\times 10^{-9}(\text{cm} \times \text{ml O}_2)/ (\text{s} \times \text{ml} \times \text{mm/Hg})$	Material *Dk* requirement $(\times 10^{-11}\text{ml O}_2)/ (\text{s} \times \text{ml} \times \text{mm/Hg})$	
		Avt 0.15 mm	Avt 0.20 mm
0% daily wear swelling			
Average subject	24.1	36.1	48.2
95% Population	29.5	44.3	59.0
0 % residual extended wear swelling			
Average subject	34.3	51.5	68.6
95% Population	44.7	67.1	89.4
4% overnight extended wear swelling			
Average subject	87.3	131.0	174.5
95% Population	93.6	140.0	187.2

back vertex power (BVP) of the trial lens should be close to the refractive error of the patient in order to avoid large over-corrections, which are sometimes more difficult to determine.

Astigmatism For any given material the amount of astigmatism influences the choice of the lens minimal thickness. In a thin design, the RGP materials usually correct less corneal astigmatism than thicker designs. It is therefore common practice to order thicker lenses for patients with higher levels of astigmatism. In cases of very high degrees of astigmatism, a rigid toric contact lens may be required, as the lens thickness needed for correction with a spherical lens may compromise corneal metabolism (see earlier notes). Various formulae have been suggested but a useful rule is to add 0.02 mm to the recommended minimal thickness for every dioptre of astigmatism over 1.00 DC.

Previous contact lens wear

The most common problematic situation when refitting established wearers arises when refitting long-term PMMA wearers. The corneas of these patients show all the adverse mechanical effects of rigid contact lenses fitted to an oedematous cornea, principally distorted and fluctuating corneal shape and reduced corneal sensitivity. When these patients are taken out of PMMA lenses, the cornea, over a period of a few days to a few months (depending upon the length of PMMA wear and the severity of the distortions present), returns to its original undistorted shape.

Our clinical experience suggests that the rate at which corneal changes take place is influenced by the oxygen availability to the corneal front surface. Spectacle use during the recovery phase leads to erratic vision changes and major intermittent visual problems. We therefore suggest refitting these patients initially with low to medium oxygen transmissibility daily wear RGP lenses during the recovery phase. On a number of occasions, we have refitted current PMMA wearers with high *Dk* daily wear lenses. This has led to clinical failure in the majority of cases, as the patients experience fluctuating vision due to the rapidity of recovery of the cornea and the rapid return of corneal sensitivity. We therefore advise changing the PMMA wearer to a high *Dk* daily wear material only after a period of recovery (three to six months) with a low to medium *Dk* material.

Our second approach is to transfer these patients directly to RGP extended wear with high *Dk* materials. This approach has shown good patient acceptance and none of the initial problems associated with high *Dk* daily wear as mentioned previously. Many of these long-term PMMA wearers are asymptomatic and are happy with their PMMA lenses, which require little maintenance and few replacements. Because it is difficult to convince successful PMMA patients to be refitted with RGP lenses, the convenience of extended wear often helps them to accept refitting.

Selection of first trial contact lenses

Initial remarks

Once the lens material and lens design have been chosen, the next step is to select the first trial lens. The selection of the first trial lens will be based on the ocular parameters, the modality of wear and the range of parameters available for that design. To describe the fitting principles, we will use for simplicity the example of a multicurve contact lens, available both in a range of back surface geometries and diameters. The basic fitting principles are applicable to all lens types, including aspheric designs, and are explained in Chapter 5. Two general lens designs will be used as examples – one for daily wear and one for extended wear. Details of these designs are given in Appendices 27.A and 27.B. A single trial set suffices for each lens design. Any alterations in the final lens choice can be made from extrapolation of observations of the fitting of trial lenses from these sets.

Preliminary measurements

The ocular parameters to consider are corneal contour, corneal diameter, lid characteristics, pupil diameter and spectacle refraction.

Corneal contour Information regarding corneal contour, at this stage, is limited to the central corneal curvature which is given as keratometric readings in millimetres of the flattest (Kf) and steepest (Ks) meridians. The quality of the keratometric mires should also be assessed, e.g.:

7.85 mm at 180
7.70 mm at 90
Regular mires

The peripheral corneal contour is evaluated indirectly by assessing the contact lens peripheral fluorescein fit.

Corneal diameter The true corneal diameter is not usually measured by the clinician – the horizontal visible iris diameter (HVID), in millimetres, is routinely measured (Martin & Holden, 1982) and under-estimates the true corneal diameter by 1.1 mm, on average.

Lid characteristics In many cases, the sole lid characteristic measured is the vertical palpebral aperture (VPA), in millimetres. It is, however, often difficult to measure the habitual palpebral aperture because any technique tends to stimulate a reflex blink and/or partial lid closure. Our clinical experience has shown that it is preferable to estimate the position of the lid margin versus the upper and lower limbus (Fig. 27.16) and to classify the lids as either loose, average or tight according to their resistance to pull.

Pupil diameter The measurement of the pupil diameter, which is difficult in routine practice, is a parameter of secondary interest with RGP lenses. Most designs incorporate large optic zones, which should avoid problems of flare. However, in cases where the practitioner notices an unusually large pupil, it is necessary to measure, with a comparator, the pupil diameter under low room illu-

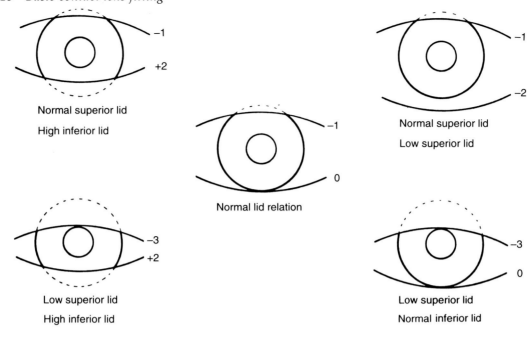

Figure 27.16 Classification of eyelid position with reference to superior and inferior limbus.

mination. In such cases it is essential to ensure that the visual performance achieved with the lenses is also adequate under reduced luminance.

Spectacle refraction The spectacle refraction must be given in full sphero-cylindrical form, including the back vertex distance for any meridional power greater than +4.00 D, e.g. –5.00/–1.00 × 180 BVD = 14 mm; mean sphere equivalent = –5.50 D. The full spectacle refraction is used to deduct the mean sphere equivalent, which will help select a trial contact lens of appropriate power. The spectacle refraction also permits comparison of the corneal and refractive cylinders. It is necessary to avoid trial fitting with a spherical RGP lens when it is predicted that the lens type will not be suitable. An example of this is where there is significant lenticular astigmatism that is not corrected by the corneal astigmatism (Table 27.7). In these instances one should fit either toric or spherical soft contact lenses, as applicable, before choosing a complex bi-toric RGP design. A second example concerns the presence of high levels of astigmatism. In such cases one should choose a toric RGP lens (see Chapter 28), but not without previously attempting a spherical RGP trial fit.

Lens parameter selection

Lens diameter The first parameter to be selected is the lens diameter. The selection of the lens diameter is identical for both daily and extended wear. This selection is based primarily on the position of the lid margin versus the limbus.

The first fitting principle is to aim for a large total diameter achieving an extra palpebral fit. Interpalpebral fits were popular with PMMA lenses as they resulted in small diameter lenses giving minimum corneal coverage, which led to minimal corneal

Table 27.7 Typical cases where RGP lenses are contra indicated due to the residual astigmatism induced

---

Near spherical spectacle refraction and significant corneal astigmatism

Keratometry	Spectacle refraction
7.70 mm al 180	−2.00/−0.25 × 180
7.45 mm al 90	

Regular corneal astigmatism −1.25 × 180
Residual/lenticular astigmatism −1.00 × 180
Fit spherical soft contact lens

Significant spectacle astigmatism with near spherical cornea

Keratometry	Spectacle refraction
7.70 mm al 180	−2.00/−1.75 × 180
7.60 mm al 90	

Regular corneal astigmatism −0.50 × 180
Residual/lenticular astigmatism −1.25 × 180
Fit toric soft contact lens

Spectacle and corneal astigmatism at different angle (opposite or obique)

Keratometry	Spectacle refraction
7.70 mm al 180	−2.00/−0.50 × 90
7.45 mm al 90	

Regular corneal astigmatism −1.00 × 180
Residual/lenticular astigmatism −1.50 × 90
Fit spherical soft contact lens

---

physiological disturbances. The corresponding absence of the eyelid force led to the use of excessively tight fits in order to maintain lens centration. This resulted in poor comfort with the lid bridging the upper lens edge at each blink and the lens resisting the blink force.

On average, a total diameter of 9.50 to 9.70 mm enabling ample contact with the upper lid and good control of the lens lid interaction is recommended. The total diameter should be altered by at least 0.4 mm in order to change the lens fitting characteristics. Our clinical experience indicates that smaller changes are ineffective in achieving a significant change in fitting characteristics.

The general guidelines for selection of the lens diameter (Fig. 27.17) are as follows:

1. If there is a normal lid position, select an average lens diameter (e.g. 9.60 mm).
2. If there is a superior lid position tangential to the superior limbus or inferior lid position with inferior conjunctival exposure, select a large lens diameter (e.g. 10.0 mm).
3. If there is a low superior lid associated with a high lower lid, select a small lens diameter (e.g. 9.20 mm).

There are a number of supplementary factors to consider when selecting the trial contact lens diameter. These factors are concerned with further ocular characteristics that may play a part in some cases.

The selection of a large diameter is recommended in the presence of loose lids, large HVID (> 12 mm), in the absence of corneal astigmatism or the presence of a high spherical refractive error (> ±8.00 D).

In the case of loose lids, the eyelid force normal to the cornea is reduced. By increasing the lens diameter, and hence the zone of contact between the eyelid and the lens, we increase the effectiveness of that force in maintaining the lens in position. In such a case, it is essential to use a lenticular contact lens design to avoid increasing the lens

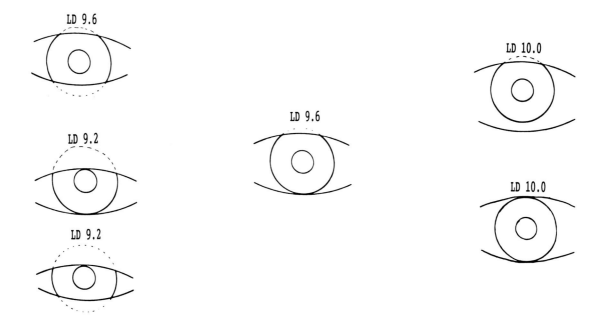

Figure 27.17 RGP lens diameter selection in function of eyelid position.

weight which would neutralize the action of the upper eyelid force.

In cases of large HVID (> 12 mm) a larger lens diameter is necessary to achieve an extra palpebral fit.

In the absence of corneal astigmatism, the tear fluid squeeze force obtained with a conventional fit is often limited in its capacity to maintain the lens centred between blinks. Rather than decreasing lens mass, thus creating possible lens adherences, it is best to increase the effectiveness of the eyelid force by increasing the lens diameter.

High power lenses tend to be heavy resulting in a low riding lens. It is therefore useful to use a large diameter with a lenticular design. This creates a more efficient eyelid force without significantly increasing the lens weight.

The selection of small diameter lenses is recommended for tight lids, small HVID (>

11 mm) and high corneal astigmatism (> 2.00 D). Patients with high degrees of corneal astigmatism may have acceptable central lens fits but unacceptable peripheral fits because of the large discrepancies between the principal meridians. In such cases, it is possible to achieve an acceptable fit with a spherical contact lens of smaller diameter.

Back surface geometry The trial contact lens is chosen by selecting the back optic radius for the appropriate lens diameter. In all cases, the lens periphery will be that of the selected design. The selection of an alternative periphery will only be made after the evaluation of the trial contact lens fitting characteristics. These parameters are chosen after consideration of the central keratometric measurements. The lens/cornea relationship will differ for each lens design and lens wear modality as discussed previously. Daily wear lenses should show minimal central clearance and alignment to mild central touch for extended wear. Excessive central clearance must be avoided for extended wear as it has been reported to induce lens adherence during overnight wear (Kenyon *et al.*, 1989). As a guideline, (Table 27.8), we present the recommended BOR fitting increment for both daily wear and extended wear, based upon the flattest keratometric reading (K_f) and the amount of corneal toricity ($K_f - K_s$).

Power The power of the trial contact lenses should be within $\pm$ 4.00 D of the anticipated final lens power. This ensures that the trial lens and final lens geometries are similar and that the clinical observations made with the trial-contact lens will be applicable to the final contact lens. Also, it facilitates ease at over-refraction.

Lens fit assessment

General remarks

As indicated earlier, the two main aspects to be evaluated for RGP lenses are the lens fitting characteristics and the patient's subjective tolerance. An unadapted rigid contact lens wearer may require a local anaesthetic to avoid excessive lacrimation which may prevent the accurate evaluation of the true lens fitting characteristics.

Dynamic fit assessment

General remarks The dynamic fit assessment is the evaluation of the lens position at equilibrium between blinks and the nature and magnitude of the blink induced lens movement. The tear fluid squeeze pressure and tear film force have significant effects on the lens dynamic fit, so it is therefore essential not to disturb these forces. To this effect, we evaluate the dynamic fit using white light before inserting any fluorescein which will affect both the tear volume and tear viscosity. Also, because the eyelid force plays a major role in RGP fitting, it is essential to ensure normal head and lid posture. For this reason we prefer to initially judge the lens dynamic fit with a hand-held Burton lamp before

Table 27.8 Guideline for selection of BOR for first trial contact lenses for both daily and extended wear RGP lenses

Lens type		Target central TLT (µm)	Corneal astigmatism < 2.00 D or K_f-K_s < 0.40 mm	Corneal astigmatism > 2.00 D or K_f-K_s > 0.40 mm
Lens TD mm	BOD			
DW				
9.20	7.80	≈ 15	BOR (mm) = K_f (mm) −0.05 mm	Decrease BOR by 0.05 mm for any amount of corneal astigmatism equal to 0.50 D above 2.00 D or 0.10 mm above 0.40 mm
9.60	8.20	≈ 15	BOR (mm) = K_f (mm)	
10.00	8.20	≈ 15	BOR (mm) = K_f (mm)	
EW				
9.20	7.80	0	BOR (mm) = K_f (mm) + 0.05 mm	Decrease BOR by 0.05 mm for any amount of corneal astigmatism equal to 0.50 D above 2.00 D or 0.10 mm above 0.40 mm
9.60	8.20	0	BOR (mm) = K_f (mm) + 0.10 mm	
10.00	8.20	0	BOR (mm) = K_f (mm) + 0.10 mm 0.10 mm above 0.40 mm	

evaluating the fit with the slit lamp biomicroscope under ×20 magnification.

Position at equilibrium between blinks The lens position at equilibrium is judged by the magnitude of any decentration and the stability of the habitual position.

The magnitude of decentration is measured by a three-point classification:

0   = Centred over cornea.
1   = Slightly decentred.
2   = Excessively decentred.

The direction of decentration is recorded as superior, inferior, nasal or temporal.

The stability of the equilibrium position is rated as either:

1   = Stable.
2   = Unstable.

Blink-induced   movement The   blink-induced movement is fairly complex and is evaluated from the post-lens lag.

During a blink the lens movement occurs in several stages (Hayashi, 1977) (Fig. 27.18):

1.   During the lid closing phase under the effect of the eyelid force, the lens is pushed downwards to a position arching the lower cornea and limbal conjunctiva in the lower canthus.
2.   When the lids are closed, under the recentration action exerted by the tear fluid squeeze force, the lens moves spontaneously upwards towards a centred or slightly superior position.
3.   Finally, on eye opening, the tear fluid squeeze force returns the lens to its equilibrium position.

This final recentration movement is the only one easily visible and it is the entity we clinically evaluate. It is often referred to as the blink lag. The speed of the recentration movement is rated on a three-point scale:

1   = Fast.
2   = Average.
3   = Slow.

A fast movement indicates a large tear fluid squeeze recentration force due to an excessively tight fit. The slow movement indicates a low tear fluid squeeze recentration force due to a flat central fit.

The type of the recentration movement observed is classified into four groups:

1   = Rocky.
2   = Smooth.
3   = Apical rotation.
4   = Lid attachment.

A rocky movement is often rapid movement produced by a high tear fluid squeeze force due to a tight fit.

A smooth movement is that corresponding to a well fitting lens.

Apical rotation describes a lens that remains in slow rotation over the corneal apex. It corresponds to a low tear fluid squeeze force due to a relatively flat fit where the lid force fails to play a significant role.

Lid attachment describes a lens that is kept

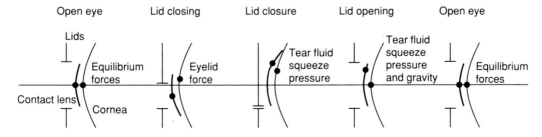

Figure 27.18 Schematic representation of RGP lens movement at blink.

in a superior position by the lid and accurately follows any lid movement. It corresponds to a low tear fluid squeeze force due to a flat fit. Some clinicians suggest that a lid attachment fit produces a better acceptance to comfort because of the total absence of a relative movement between the contact lens and the lid.

Static fit

General remarks The evaluation of the static fit is the evaluation using fluorescein of the tear layer thickness between the back surface of the contact lens and front surface of the cornea (see Fig. 27.14). The dark areas correspond to zones where the tear layer is extremely thin and does not produce any visible fluorescence. They are usually referred to as 'contact zones' or 'zones of touch', although a true contact between the contact lens and lens/corneal epithelium may not exist, that zone corresponding rather to an area of minimal tear layer thickness not providing any fluorescence. The brightness of the green zones is proportional to the tear layer thickness in that zone; the brighter the area, the thicker the tear layer.

The proper instillation of fluorescein is essential for correct evaluation of the lens fitting characteristics. Because fluid is inserted into the eye the technique is invasive, the aim should, however, be to create minimal disturbance to the normal situation. Fluorescein is available as a fully prepared eyedrop or a sterile strip (Fig. 27.19) that needs to be hydrated.

The fluorescein eyedrop is preferred as it permits instillation of a known concentration of fluorescein. The recommended method is to instil one drop of 1% concentration into the lower cul de sac. The use of preserved multidose solutions is not recommended because of the potential risk of *Pseudomonas aeruginosa* infections associated with contaminated fluorescein (Chatoo, 1963; Doris,

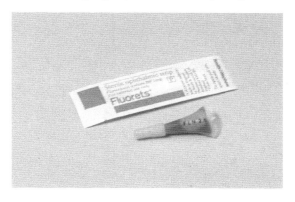

Figure 27.19 Fluorescein recommended dispensers: sterile strip and single dose solution.

1964). Fluorescein strips are also suitable and are most commonly encountered in routine clinical practice. The strips must not be hydrated with rewetting eyedrops, which are highly viscous and will alter the tear film characteristics, which in turn affects the fit.

Because of the concern with *Pseudomonas aeruginosa*, unpreserved single dose or multidose spray-can saline is recommended to wet the flourescine strip. The preferred technique is to gently touch either the upper or lower bulbar conjunctiva with the hydrated strip. Another essential precaution when assessing the fluorescein pattern is to wait for the excessive fluorescein on the lens front surface to dissipate, as it makes it difficult to judge the post lens tear film. This is best achieved by instilling a low volume of fluorescein.

The evaluation of the static lens fit assumes the lens is centred over the corneal apex. In those cases where the equilibrium position is not over the corneal apex, the lens must be centred manually with the help of the lids (Fig. 27.20).

The fluorescein fit evaluation is best carried out with the slip lamp biomicroscope at ×20 to ×30 magnification. A diffusing glass and blue filter in front of the lighting system is recommended. The diffusing glass produces an even light and the blue filter stimulates the tear fluorescence. In addition, to

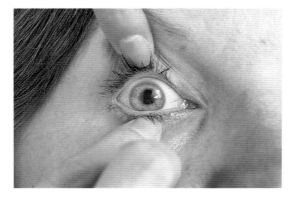

Figure 27.20 RGP lens held centrally over the corneal apex with help of lower lid to evaluate fluorescein pattern.

maximize contrast, a yellow filter should be added to the viewing system. Some practitioners prefer to use the Burton lamp in evaluation of the fluorescein fit. This technique is also acceptable, but it should be remembered that this lamp mainly produces UV, rather than short visible light, to stimulate fluorescence and cannot be used with some modern RGP lenses, which incorporate a UV blocker.

Fitting evaluation The fluorescein evaluation must be systematic and judged in terms of the central, intermediate and peripheral fit.

Central fit The central fit is rated on a five-point scale:

+2 = Excessively steep.
+1 = Slightly steep.
0 = Alignment.
−1 = Slightly flat.
−2 = Excessively flat.

An alignment fit (see Fig. 27.13) is represented by an even, light-green zone over the central area. It corresponds to a minimal visible central clearance of 10 to 20 μm at the apex.

A steep fit is one with a bright green central pool of tears. A classification of slightly steep (Fig. 27.21a) corresponds to an apical clearance of approximately 30 μm. An excessively steep fit (Fig. 27.21b) corresponds to an apical clearance of 40 μm or more, which is sometimes associated with the presence of a trapped air bubble.

A flat fit reveals a dark zone at the central area of the lens. For a slightly flat fit (Fig. 27.22a) the central 'zone of contact' reveals only a mild dark area whereas an excessively flat fit (Fig. 27.22b) reveals a marked area of contact.

Intermediate fit The nature and size of the contact lens corneal 'contact' is recorded. The nature of the contact is recorded on a three-point scale:

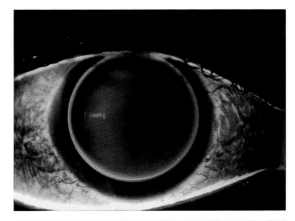

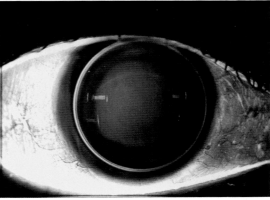

Figure 27.21 Fluorescein pictures of steep fitting RGP lenses. (a) Acceptable steep fit; (b) excessively unacceptable steep fit.

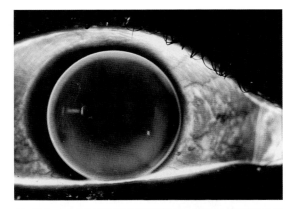

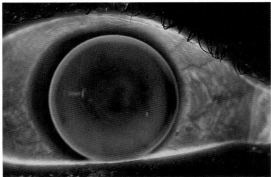

Figure 27.22 Fluorescein pictures of flat fitting RGP lenses. (a) Acceptable flat fit; (b) excessively unacceptable flat fit.

0 = No contact.
1 = Poorly defined contact.
2 = Hard, well defined contact.

In addition, when present, the width of the contact zone will be evaluated in millimetres. No contact is illustrated by a green pool in the intermediate zone (Fig. 27.22b). It is usually associated with a flat central fit where the contact lens touches the cornea at its apex.

A poorly defined zone of contact (see Fig. 27.13) is illustrated by an unevenly dark mid-peripheral area whose limits are not well defined. It corresponds to a zone of light, well distributed pressure and an even, thin TLT.

A well defined zone of contact (Fig. 27.21a) is illustrated by a very dark, well delimited mid-peripheral band. It corresponds to a

zone of heavy localized pressure and an extremely thin TLT.

Peripheral fit The peripheral fit is evaluated by classifying both the width of the peripheral band and the magnitude of the edge clearance. The width of the edge clearance is recorded on a five-point scale:

−2 = Extremely narrow (< 0.1 mm)
−1 = Slightly narrow (0.10 to 0.2 mm)
0 = Optimal (0.2 to 0.3 mm)
+1 = Slightly wide (0.3 to 0.4 mm)
+2 = Extremely wide (> 0.4 mm)

The magnitude of the clearance is also recorded on a five point scale (Fig. 27.23):

−2 = Insufficient ($\leqslant 40\ \mu m$)
−1 = Less than optimal ($\approx 60\ \mu m$)
0 = Optimal ($\approx 80\ \mu m$)
+1 = More than optimal ($\approx 100\ \mu m$)
+2 = Excessive ($\geqslant 120\ \mu m$)

Lens classification

Optimal fit The characteristics of an optimal fit differ for daily and extended wear, as mentioned previously. The fitting characteristics will be described independently.

Optimal daily wear fit The general description of an optimal lens fit for daily wear is one that achieves controlled smooth movement at blink with good recentration at eye opening and good centration over the corneal apex. This is associated with minimal central clearance, intermediate touch and small edge clearance.

The detailed fitting characteristics are as follows:

1. Position at equilibrium. The position at equilibrium is central to superiorly decentred by ~ 1 mm.
2. Movement at blink. The recentration movement at blink should be smooth and of the order of 1.5 mm from a superior position at eye opening to the

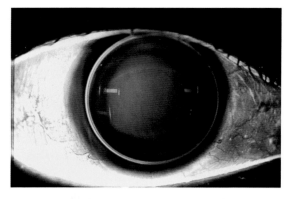

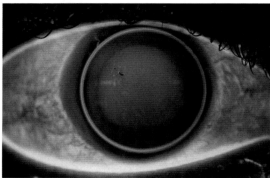

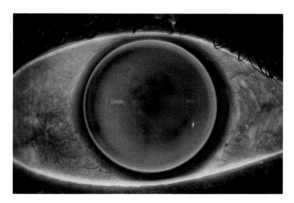

Figure 27.23 Peripheral clearance. (a) Slightly insufficient clearance ≈ 260 μm; (b) optimal clearance, ≈ 80 μm; (c) slightly excessive clearance, ≈ 0 μm.

equilibrium position. The duration of the recentration movement is of the order of 0.5 to 1 second (Hayashi, 1977).

3. Fluorescein pattern. The optimal fluorescein pattern reveals a green central zone

corresponding to a zone of slight corneal clearance to corneal alignment. This central zone is associated with an intermediate even 'zone of contact' with poorly defined limits. The peripheral zone of clearance should be narrow (∼ 0.30 mm) and of the order of 80 μm.

Optimal extended wear fit An optimal extended wear fit shows more movement than the optimal daily wear fit – frequently a lid attachment type movement. The corresponding fluorescein pattern indicates a flat fit with large edge clearance. The details of the fit are as follows:

1. Position at equilibrium. The position at equilibrium is superior, with the lens being held by the upper lid. The equilibrium position is stable and mimics the upper lid movements.
2. Movement at blink. During the blink action the movement is large with a poor tendency to recentre. Between blinks, the lens usually adopts a lid attachment fit and faithfully follows any eyelid movement. This phenomenon is due to the lack of recentration tear fluid squeeze force.
3. Fluorescein pattern. The fluorescein pattern reveals a dark central area corresponding to a zone of contact, increasing in the intermediate zone. Towards the lens periphery there is a wider zone of clearance (∼ 0.5 mm) with a greater edge clearance than for daily wear (∼ 120 μm).

Loose fit A loose fit is defined as being more mobile than the optimal fit, which is applicable to both daily and extended wear. Because a mobile lens lacks recentration forces, a loose fit is often associated with a decentred lens. The acceptability of such a fit depends on the magnitude of the decentration. The major characteristics of a loose fit are detailed below:

1. Position at equilibrium. At equilibrium, the lenses are usually decentred and sit superiorly and/or temporally due to the

unopposed action of the upper lid or, alternatively, decentred inferiorly when the upper lid fails to achieve sufficient contact.

2. Movement at blink. The upper lid force usually creates excessive lens movement during lid closure. This is followed, on eye opening, by the absence of a recentration movement. The lens adopts one of two behaviours. If the eyelid action is sufficient, the lens follows any eyelid movement (lid attachment fit). Alternatively, when the lid action is minimal, the lens rotates over the corneal apex as the tear fluid squeeze force is insufficient to achieve a stable centration.

3. Fluorescein pattern. The central fluorescein pattern reveals a marked central dark area indicating a zone of heavy central contact. The intermediate zone shows significant corneal clearance, which results in an excessively wide peripheral band of clearance.

Tight fit A tight fit is less mobile than the optimal fit. As for a loose fit, the acceptability of a tight fit depends on the relative magnitude of the difference from the optimal fit.

1. Position at equilibrium. The equilibrium position of a tight fitting lens is often not a differentiating diagnosis. Typically, the lens is well centred, indicative of the effect of the tear fluid squeeze force.

2. Movement at blink. The lens has a tendency to resist the action of the upper lid during the eye closing force. This produces a delayed movement of minimal amplitude. After eye opening, the effect is opposite. The lens recentres in a fast, rocky movement of short duration.

3. Fluorescein pattern. The fluorescein pattern is the main diagnostic feature. It reveals a marked central green zone corresponding to an excessive apical corneal clearance. This is associated with a well defined intermediate zone of mini-

mal corneal clearance appearing as dark band. The edge clearance is usually, but not always, insufficient.

Astigmatic fit In some cases, the tear fluorescein pattern is significantly different along the two principal meridians. This lens fit is considered astigmatic.

In such a case one should apply an analytic approach in assessing the fluorescein pattern in each meridian. If the subsequent lens fit alterations do not resolve the lens fitting problems, a toric RGP contact lens should be considered (see Chapter 18). With regard to the dynamic fitting characteristics of an RGP lens on a toric cornea, the movement observed is often rocky over the astigmatic corneal surface.

Choice of additional lenses

When the fit is less than optimal, it is necessary to use additional trial contact lenses to achieve an acceptable fit. The selection of these additional lenses will be based on determining the lens characteristics that need to be altered. Returning to first principles and considering the forces involved in the fitting behaviour, the remedial actions are as follows:

Loose high-riding contact lens Several remedial actions can be taken.

The primary actions are:

1. Increasing the tear fluid squeeze force. This is achieved by increasing the tear layer thickness by reducing the lens BOR and/or increasing the lens BOD.

2. Decreasing the effectiveness of the lid force. This is achieved by reducing the lens diameter and/or thinning the lens edge thickness by producing a design that does not interact with the upper lid (positive carrier).

The secondary actions are:

1. To increase the peripheral force by decreasing the width and magnitude of the edge clearance.

2. To increase the gravity force by increasing the lens weight. This is achieved by making the lens thicker or by using a material of higher specific weight. The former approach is not favoured as any increase in lens thickness is potentially detrimental to the lens oxygen transmissibility.

Loose low-riding rigid contact lenses The remedial actions are more limited than those for tight high-riding RGP lenses.

The primary action is to make the eyelid force more effective. This is achieved by increasing the lens diameter and incorporating a thick lenticular periphery.

Secondary actions are:

1. To increase the tear fluid squeeze pressure to help the recentration movement.
2. To decrease the gravity force. This is achieved by decreasing the lens mass by incorporating a smaller front optic diameter and/or decreasing the central thickness.

Tight, well centred fit The primary action is to decrease the tear fluid squeeze force by flattening the BOR. The secondary action is to increase the lid force by altering the lens lid relationship.

27.4.4 OVER-REFRACTION AND VISUAL PERFORMANCE EVALUATION

Full sphero-cylindrical over-refractions are needed. The best spherical over-refraction determines the final lens power, whereas the cylindrical element of the refraction indicates whether or not a more sophisticated RGP lens design is required. It is then essential to evaluate carefully the visual performance. In particular, as RGP lenses may take a slightly decentred position, it is essential to evaluate the visual performance under low luminance conditions when the pupil is dilated.

27.4.5 TOLERANCE TRIAL

For those patients requiring a local anaesthetic, a longer tolerance trial should be carried out on a separate visit before ordering the contact lens. The tolerance trial should last one or two hours to ascertain whether the patient will tolerate RGP lenses.

27.4.6 FINAL CONTACT LENS ORDER

The final lens should be ordered according to the recommended ISO terminology, e.g.:

Tricurate Contact Lens
BOR BOD/BPR1 BPD1/BPR2 TD
7.80:7.80/8.60:8.60/9.20:10.50 mm
BVD – 2.50 D
ct 0.15 et 0.14 mm
FOD 8.00 mm

REFERENCES

Ames, K. and Cameron M. (1989) The efficacy of regular lens replacement in extended wear. *Int. Contact Lens Clin.*, **16**, 104–11.
Bier, N. and Lowther, G.E. (1977) Flexible lens fitting. In *Contact Lens Correction* (ed. N. Bier and G.E. Lowther), Butterworths, London.
Brandreth, R.H. (1978) Use of the slit lamp biomicroscope in a contact lens examination. In *Clinical Slit Lamp Biomicroscopy* (ed. R.H. Brandreth) Multimedia Communications, University of California School of Optometry, Berkley, CA.
Chatoo, B.A. (1963) Fluorescein in ophthalmic practice: *Ophthal. Optician*, **8**, 723–35.
Doris, J.A. (1964) Maintenance of sterility of eyedrops in ophthalmic practice. *Ophthal. Optician*, **4**, 12–14; 19.
Efron, N., Brennan, M.A., Bruce, A.S., Duldig, D.I. and Russo, N.S. (1987) Dehydration of hydrogel lenses under normal wearing conditions. *Contact Lens Assoc. Ophthalmol. J.*, **13**, 152–6.
Fatt. I. and Chaston, J. (1980) The effect of temperature on refractive index, water content and central thickness of hydrogel contact lenses. *Int. Contact Lens Clin.*, **7**, 250–5.
Fatt, I. and Hill, R.M. (1970) Oxygen tension under a contact lens during blinking: a comparison of theory and experimental observation. *Am. J. Optom.*, **47**, 50–5.
Gasson, A.P. (1980) Soft lens fitting. In *Contact Lenses. A textbook for practitioner and student* (2nd ed) (eds. J. Stone and A.J. Phillip), Butterworths, London.

Gasson, A.P. and Stone, J. (1977) The Placido disk in soft lens fitting. *The Optician*, **173** 4482, 9–10.

Guillon, M. (1982) Topographical study of corneal swelling for lenses of identical oxygen transmissibility. *J. Br. Contact Lens Assoc.*, **5**(4), 130–40.

Guillon, M. (1988) *Modern concepts in soft contact lens design*. Association of Contact Lens Manufacture Contact Lens, Convention, June 22, London.

Guillon, M. and Bleshoy, H. (1983) Comparative study of the visual performance of various aphakic corrections. *Acta Ophthalmologica*, **61**, 851–9.

Guillon, J.P. and Guillon, M. (1988) Tear film examination of the contact lens patient. *Contax*, **May**, 14–18.

Guillon, J.P. and Guillon, M. (1990) Hydrogel lens *in vivo* wettability during sleep. *Optom. Vis. Sci.*, **67**, 170.

Guillon, M. and Morris, J.A. (1981) Corneal response to a provocative test in aphakia. *J. Contact Lens Assoc.*, **4**, 162–7.

Guillon, M. and Morris, J.A. (1982) Corneal evaluation of prospective aphakic wearers of contact lenses. *Br. J. Ophthalmol.*, **66**, 520–3.

Guillon, M., Lydon, D.P.M. and Wilson, C. (1986) Corneal Topography: a clinical model. *Ophthal. Physiol. Opt.*, **6**, 47–56.

Guillon, J.P., Guillon, M., Dwyer, S. and Mapstone, V. (1989) Hydrogel lens in vivo wettability. *Trans. Br. Contact Lens Assoc.*, **12**, 144–5.

Hanna, C., Bicknell, D.S. and O'Brien, J.E. (1961) Cell turn over in the adult human eye. *Arch. Ophthalmol.*, **65**, 695–8.

Hayashi, T.T. (1977) *Mechanics of Contact Lens Motion*. PhD dissertation, University of California, Berkeley.

Holden, B.A. and Mertz, G.W. (1984) Critical oxygen levels to avoid corneal oedema for daily and extended wear contact lenses. *Invest. Opthalmol. Vis. Sci.*, **25**, 1161–7.

Holden, B.A., Mertz, G.W. and Guillon, M. (1980) Corneal swelling response of the aphakic eye. *Invest. Ophthalmol. Vis. Sci.*, **19**, 1394–7.

Jenkins, J.T. and Shimbo, M. (1985) The distribution of pressure behind a soft contact lens. *J. Biomech. Eng.*, **106**, 62–5.

Kenyon, E., Mandell, R.B. and Polse, K.A. (1989) Lens design effects on rigid lens adherence. *J. Br. Contact Lens Assoc.*, **12**(2), 32–6.

Kikkawa, Y. (1979) Kinetics of soft contact lens fitting. *Contact*, **23**(4), 10–17.

La Hood, D. and Holden B.A. (1989) Daytime oedema level with high and low water content plus hydrogel contact lens. *Optom. Vis. Sci.*, **66**, 234.

Lydon, D. (1990) Improved optics and control of astigmatism without cylinders. *Trans. Br. Contact Lens Assoc.*, **12**, 41–3.

Mandell, R.B. (1974a) Spin-cast hydrogel lenses. In *Contact Lens Practice – hard and flexible lenses* (2nd ed) (ed. R.B. Mandell), Charles C. Thomas, Springfield, Il.

Mandell, R.B. (1974b) Lathe out hydrogel lenses. In *Contact Lens Practice – hard and flexible lenses* (2nd ed) (ed. R.B. Mandell), Charles C. Thomas, Springfield, Il.

Mandell, R.B. (1974c) Basic principles of corneal lenses. In *Contact Lens Practice – hard and flexible lenses* (2nd edn) (ed. R.B. Mandell), Charles C. Thomas, Springfield, Il.

Martin, D.K. and Holden, B.A. (1982) A new method for measuring the diameter of in vivo human cornea. *Am. J. Optom. Physiol. Opt.*, **59**, 436–41.

Martin, D.K. and Holden, B.A. (1986) Forces developed beneath hydrogel contact lenses due to squeeze pressure. *Phys. Med. Bid.*, **30**, 635–49.

Martin, D.K., Boulos, J., Gan, J., Gauriel, K. and Harvey, R. (1989) A unifying parameter to describe the clinical mechanics of hydrogel contact lenses. *Optom. Vis. Sci.*, **66**, 87–91.

McKenney, C. (1990). The effect of pH on hydrogel lens parameters and fitting characteristics after hydrogel peroxide disinfection. *Transactions of the British Contact Lens Association Annual Clinical Conference*, pp. 46–51.

Mertz, G.W. and Holden, B.A. (1981) Clinical implications of extended wear research. *Can. J. Optom.*, **43**, 203–5.

Orsborn, G.A. and Zantos, S.G. (1988) Corneal desiccation staining with thin high water contact lenses. *Contact Lens Assoc. Ophthalmol. J.*, **14**, 81–5.

Polse, K.A. (1979) Tear flow under hydrogel contact lenses. *Invest. Ophthalmol. Vis. Sci.*, **18**, 409–13.

Ruben, M. (1978) Fitting principles. In *Soft Contact Lenses – Clinical and applied technology* (ed. M. Ruben), Bailliere Tindall, London.

Wechsler, S., Johnson, M. and Businger, V. (1983) *In vivo* hydration of hydrogel lenses – the first hour. *Int. Contact Lens Clin.*, **10**, 349–52.

Weissman, B.A. (1982) An introduction to extended wear contact lenses. *J. Am. Optom. Assoc.*, **53**, 193–6.

Winterton, L.C., White, J.C. and Su, K.C. (1988) Coulometrically determined oxygen flux and resultant Dk of commercially available contact lenses. *Invest. Opthalmol. Vis. Sci.*, **25**, 1161–7.

APPENDIX 27.A: DAILY YEAR DIAGNOSTIC SET

BOZR	BOZD	BPR	BPD	PR^2	LD
7.20	8.2	7.75	9.0	9.00	9.6
7.30	8.2	7.90	9.0	9.20	9.6
7.40	8.2	8.00	9.0	9.40	9.6
7.50	8.2	8.10	9.0	9.55	9.6
7.60	8.2	8.25	9.0	9.75	9.6
7.70	8.2	8.35	9.0	9.95	9.6
7.80	8.2	8.45	9.0	10.20	9.6
7.90	8.2	8.60	9.0	10.40	9.6
8.00	8.2	8.70	9.0	10.60	9.6
8.10	8.2	8.80	9.0	10.80	9.6
8.20	8.2	8.95	9.0	11.00	9.6
8.30	8.2	9.05	9.0	11.25	9.6
8.40	8.2	9.20	9.0	11.45	9.6

APPENDIX 27.B EXTENDED WEAR DIAGNOSTIC SET

BOZR	BOZD	BPR	BPD	PR^2	LD
7.20	8.2	8.00	9.0	9.40	9.6
7.30	8.2	8.10	9.0	9.60	9.6
7.40	8.2	8.25	9.0	9.80	9.6
7.50	8.2	8.35	9.0	10.05	9.6
7.60	8.2	8.50	9.0	10.25	9.6
7.70	8.2	8.60	9.0	10.50	9.6
7.80	8.2	8.75	9.0	10.75	9.6
7.90	8.2	8.85	9.0	11.00	9.6
8.00	8.2	9.00	9.0	11.20	9.6
8.10	8.2	9.25	9.0	11.70	9.6
8.20	8.2	9.35	9.0	12.50	9.6
8.30	8.2	9.40	9.0	12.00	9.6
8.40	8.2	9.55	9.0	12.25	9.6

T. Chan-Ling and D.C. Pye

19.1 INTRODUCTION

Pachometry/pachymetry is the measurment of corneal thickness in the living eye. The word is derived from the Greek words *pachys*, meaning thick, and *metry*, the process of measuring. Since the first attempt to measure corneal thickness in the living eye, by Blix in 1880, improvements in measurement now make it possible to determine corneal thickness to an accuracy of 5–6 μm. The scientist or practitioner has available a range of techniques for quantifying corneal thickness. The aims of this chapter are: (1) to discuss the application of pachometry in contact lens practice, monitoring of corneal pathology and in corneal research; (2) to describe the principles and techniques of pachometry; and (3) to evaluate the relative merits of the several techniques available. Detailed information is provided on instrument modifications to increase accuracy and to allow for special applications, such as the measurement of regional variations in corneal thickness, calibration of the instrument and sources of error. Recent, still experimental techniques of corneal thickness measurement, such as femtosecond optical ranging, interferometry and confocal microscopy, are also discussed.

19.1.1 APPLICATIONS OF PACHOMETRY

Topographical, individual and diurnal variation of normal corneal thickness

The thickness of the normal human cornea varies dramatically across the cornea. Corneal thickness in the central 3 mm is 520 μm (Mishima, 1968), increasing to 630 (Martola & Baum, 1968) to 660 um (Tomlinson, 1972) 2 mm from the limbus. This topographical variation in corneal thickness means that for measurements of thickness to be comparable, their location of measurement must be consistent. In contrast, in non-primates such as rabbits (Chan *et al.*, 1983) and cats (Ling, 1987), the thickness of the cornea is more uniform and the location of measurement less critical. Within a normal human population central corneal thickness was found to vary between 430 and 560 μm (Mandell & Polse, 1969). As a result, detection of corneal oedema must rely on changes relative to an individual's baseline thickness, and corneal swelling is usually expressed as a percentage increase in corneal thickness.

Previous workers have noted a significant diurnal variation in corneal thickness in the human (Mandell & Fatt, 1965; Fujita, 1980; Holden *et al.*, 1983), primate (Madigan *et al.*, 1987), cat (Chan-Ling *et al.*, 1985) and rabbit (Mishima & Maurice, 1961; Kikkawa, 1973). It

Contact Lens Practice. Edited by Montague Ruben and Michel Guillon.
Published in 1994 by Chapman & Hall, London. ISBN 0 412 35120 X

28.2.1 CORNEAL TORICITY

The term 'corneal toricity' refers to the *physical* contour of the anterior surface of the cornea, expressed in terms of both the amount of toricity and the orientation of the flattest corneal meridian. As measured by means of a keratometer, corneal toricity can be expressed in terms of either the difference in the radii of curvature or the difference in the dioptric powers of the two principal meridians.

28.2.2 CORNEAL ASTIGMATISM

The term 'corneal astigmatism' refers to the *optical* (rather than the physical) effect of corneal toricity; it is the astigmatism, as determined by the use of a keratometer, expressed in terms of the power of the lens required for its correction. For example, if the keratometer finding is 42.00 D at 180/43.00 D at 90, the corneal astigmatism is expressed as −1.00 D axis 180.

It is convenient to think of the keratometer as measuring the refracting power (and the toricity) of the *air/tear interface*, rather than that of the cornea: this is because the keratometer is calibrated for an index of refraction of 1.3375 (taking into consideration the refraction at the back surface of the cornea), which is very close to the index of the tear layer (1.336). If a spherical contact lens is sufficiently rigid so that it maintains its shape while on the cornea, it will provide the tear layer (behind the lens) with a spherical anterior surface, therefore eliminating this surface as a source of astigmatism. The toric refraction between the tear layer and the cornea is very small, due to a change in index of only 0.40 (from 1.336 to 1.376), and can be neglected. Internal astigmatism (defined below) will, however, remain uncorrected.

28.2.3 INTERNAL ASTIGMATISM

The term 'internal astigmatism' refers to astigmatism other than that measured by the keratometer. The main source of internal astigmatism (Bailey, 1961), is the obliquity of incidence of light entering the eye with respect to the optic axis of the cornea: an obliquity of 5 degrees could account for 0.50 to 0.75 D of against-the-rule astigmatism. Other possible causes are toricity of the back surface of the cornea, a tilting of the lens, and the shape of the surface of the retina. The use of the old term 'physiological astigmatism' should be discouraged, since this term implies that this form of astigmatism is not anatomically based.

28.2.4 REFRACTIVE ASTIGMATISM

The term 'refractive astigmatism' refers to the total astigmatism of the eye, as determined by objective or subjective refraction. It is made up of corneal astigmatism and internal astigmatism, as shown by the relationship:

Refractive astigmatism = corneal astigmatism + internal astigmatism

When a significant amount of refractive astigmatism is present, *corneal* astigmatism is almost always responsible. Internal astigmatism has been found to have a narrow, leptokurtic (peaked) distribution, the great majority of eyes falling between zero and 1.00 D against-the-rule. Although corneal astigmatism also has a relatively narrow distribution, it is much broader than that of internal astigmatism. Lyle (1971) plotted the distribution of corneal astigmatism for 1208 eyes of patients seen in his optometric practice. As shown in Figure 28.1, the majority of eyes have with-the-rule corneal astigmatism between zero and about 1.50 D, but some eyes have as much as 7.00 D of with-the-rule astigmatism, 2.25 D of against-the-rule astigmatism, or 2.50 D of oblique astigmatism.

28.2.5 UNCORRECTED ASTIGMATISM

The term 'uncorrected astigmatism' refers to the astigmatism that remains uncorrected when a contact lens is worn. This is the

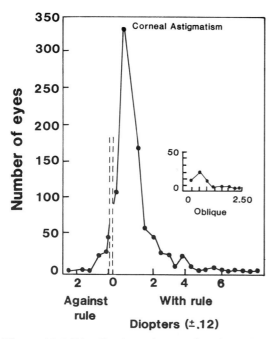

Figure 28.1 Distribution of corneal astigmatism, for 1208 eyes of patients of various ages (from Lyle, 1971).

astigmatism that one would expect to find by objective or subjective over-refraction. For a spherical lens that is sufficiently rigid to maintain its shape while on the cornea, the uncorrected astigmatism is equal to the internal astigmatism; but if a lens tilts with respect to the optic axis of the cornea, or if it *flexes* on the cornea (see 'lens flexure', below) the amount of uncorrected astigmatism may be either more or less than the internal astigmatism.

28.2.6   RESIDUAL ASTIGMATISM

The term 'residual astigmatism', although normally used to designate the uncorrected astigmatism present when a contact lens is worn (Grosvenor, 1963) has been used by some authors as a synonym for *internal* astigmatism. In the present chapter, it will be considered to have the same meaning as the

term 'uncorrected astigmatism'; however, the latter term is to be preferred, since its meaning is not open to question.

28.2.7   LENS FLEXURE

The term 'lens flexure' refers to the tendency for a spherical rigid lens to fail to maintain its spherical curvature while on a toric cornea, assuming a portion of the cornea's toricity, with the result that not all of the corneal astigmatism is eliminated.

28.3   PREDICTION AND MEASUREMENT OF UNCORRECTED ASTIGMATISM

When a patient is to be fitted with rigid lenses, the practitioner must first determine whether the patient's astigmatism will be adequately corrected with spherical lenses, or whether toric lenses should be considered. It is a simple matter to predict the amount of uncorrected astigmatism that will be present if a spherical lens is fitted, and then to measure the amount of uncorrected astigmatism by performing an over-refraction while a well-fitting spherical lens is worn.

28.3.1   PREDICTING UNCORRECTED ASTIGMATISM

For patients having no more than about 3 or 4 D of myopia or hyperopia, internal astigmtism is very nearly equal to the difference between the corneal and refractive astigmatism (Bailey, 1961). The astigmatism that will be uncorrected when a spherical contact lens is worn (neglecting any effects of lens tilt or flexure) can therefore be predicted by comparing the corneal and refractive astigmatism, using the formula:

Uncorrected astigmatism = refractive astigmatism − corneal astigmatism

The use of this formula will be illustrated by the following examples:

Example 1

A patient's keratometer finding is 41.00 D at 180/41.75 D at 90, and the subjective refraction is –3.00 DS. What is the predicted amount and axis of uncorrected astigmatism if a spherical rigid lens is fitted?

The corneal astigmatism could be corrected by a lens whose power is –0.75 DC axis 180. The amount of uncorrected astigmatism, therefore, is:

$$0.00 - (-0.75 \, DC \times 180) = +0.75 \, DC \times 180, \text{ or } -0.75 \, DC \times 90$$

It should be noted that transposition from the plus cylinder form to the minus cylinder form would normally bring about a residual sphere (+0.75 DS, in this case). However, this can safely be neglected, since, in this situation, we are interested only in astigmatism.

Example 2

A patient's keratometer finding is 43.00 D at 180/44.00 D at 90, and the subjective refraction is –4.00 DS – 0.50 DC axis 180. What is the predicted amount and axis of uncorrected astigmatism if a spherical rigid lens is fitted?

The corneal astigmatism could be corrected by a lens whose power is –1.00 DC axis 180. The amount of uncorrected astigmatism is therefore:

$$-0.50 \, DC \times 180 - (-1.00 \, DC \times 180) = +0.50 \, DC \times 180, \text{ or } -0.50 \times 90$$

28.3.2 MEASUREMENT OF UNCORRECTED ASTIGMATISM

If comparison of keratometer and the subjective refraction findings indicates a significant amount of uncorrected astigmatism, the recommended procedure is to perform retinoscopy and subjective over-refraction while the best fitting trial lenses are worn (making use of both spheres and cylinders), and then to do a 'best sphere' (spherical equivalent)

subjective over-refraction: the spherocylindrical over-refraction will determine the amount of uncorrected astigmatism; while the best sphere refraction will determine the best attainable visual acuity *in spite of* any uncorrected astigmatism.

If internal astigmatism is the only source of uncorrected astigmatism, the cylindrical component of the retinoscopy finding should be identical to the predicted residual astigmatism (within the experimental error of obtaining keratometer and refractive findings, of about ±0.25 D). If there is a significant difference between the predicted and measured amounts of uncorrected astigmatism, it is most likely due to lens flexure.

28.3.3 USE OF THE KERATOMETER TO DETERMINE LENS FLEXURE

Whether or not a spherical rigid lens flexes on a toric cornea may be determined by taking a keratometer reading while the patient wears the lens. Once the mire images have been brought into opposition in the usual manner, they should be carefully watched during a complete blink cycle. In extreme cases, the 'minus signs' in the vertical meridian of the keratometer mire image may appear to separate and then come back together, with each blink; this may be an indication of an extreme amount of flexure or, in some cases, may only indicate a large amount of blink lag which may settle down with time. In any event, the keratometric astigmatism with the lens in place should be compared to that found when no lens was worn. The analysis of 'over-k' findings will be illustrated by the following examples:

Example 1

A patient's keratometer finding (without a lens) is 42.50 D at 180/44.50 D at 90. While wearing a spherical rigid lens, the keratometer finding is 39.00 D at 180/39.00 D at 90. What is the amount and axis of the astigmatism created by lens flexure?

The corneal astigmatism (without a lens) would require a correction of –2.00 DC axis 180, but with the lens in place there is no astigmatism. Therefore, the contact lens completely eliminates the corneal astigmatism, so there is no uncorrected astigmatism due to lens flexure. In this case, the amount of uncorrected astigmatism measured by retinoscopy should equal the predicted amount.

Example 2

A patient's keratometer finding (without a lens) is 42.00 D at 180/44.00 D at 90. While wearing a spherical rigid lens, the keratometer finding is 40.00 D at 180/40.75 D at 90. What is the amount and axis of the astigmatism created by lens flexure?

The corneal astigmatism would require a correction of –2.00 DC axis 180, and the astigmatism while wearing the lens would require a correction of –0.75 DC axis 180. Therefore, the contact lens has eliminated only 1.25 D of the corneal astigmatism, leaving 0.75 D uncorrected. Because of this uncorrected astigmatism, due to lens flexure, the astigmatism measured by retinoscopy should differ from the predicted amount by approximately –0.75 D axis 180.

28.4 FACTORS INFLUENCING LENS FLEXURE

It is fortunate that any uncorrected with-the-rule astigmatism due to lens flexure usually serves to compensate for against-the-rule internal astigmatism, with the result that the amount of uncorrected astigmatism is often *less* than if there were no lens flexure. This is shown by Example 2 in the previous section, in which the lens flexed sufficiently to fail to correct –0.75 D of with-the-rule corneal astigmatism: if the patient had –0.75 D of against-the-rule internal astigmatism, the two sources of uncorrected astigmatism would cancel each other, with the result that an

over-refraction should indicated no astigmatism at all! However, in those cases where the astigmatism induced by lens flexure proves to be *greater* than the amount of internal astigmatism, a significant amount of uncorrected astigmatism may result.

Bailey (1961d) first pointed out the effects of lens flexure, commenting that a 'markedly thin lens will sometimes produce a variable astigmatic effect due to warping'. In a study involving 204 patients fitted with PMMA lenses, Sarver (1969) found that the although the mean predicted residual astigmatism was 0. 51 D, the mean residual astigmatism found by over-refraction was only 0.30 D. He suggested that this difference may have been due to lens flexure. The effect of lens flexure was also noted by Dellande (1970a), who predicted that 33 of 100 eyes fitted with PMMA lenses would have against-the-rule residual astigmatism of 0.75 D or more but found, on over-refraction, that only 7 eyes had that amount.

28.4.1 THE EFFECTS OF LENS DIAMETER, THICKNESS AND POWER

Bailey (1961d) reported that he attempted to alter the residual astigmatism by fitting lenses in diameters from as small as 8.5 to as large as 12.0 mm, with almost no effect. Harris (1970) quantified the effects of flexure by fitting both a spherical cornea and one having 3.00 D of toricity with PMMA lenses having diameters of 8.0, 8.5, and 9.4 mm and centre thicknesses from 0.08 mm to 0.20 mm, and measuring flexure by taking keratometer readings while the lenses were being worn. He found no significant flexure when lenses were fitted on the spherical cornea; but for the toric cornea he reported a mean flexure of 0.50 D for lenses having centre thicknesses less than 0.12 mm, with lens diameter having no effect on lens flexure.

Harris and Chu (1972) continued to study the effects of flexure of PMMA lenses on corneas having with-the-rule toricity, and found that lenses having a centre thickness less than 0.13 mm flexed in a predictable manner: for a lens having a centre thickness of 0.8 mm, the flexure amounted to almost one-half of the corneal toricity; but for a lens having a centre thickness of 0.12 mm the flexure amounted to only about one-eight of the corneal toricity. In a later study of lens flexure on toric corneas, Harris and Applequist (1974) found that the amount of lens flexure decreased with increasing minus power. They attributed the decreased flexure to the increased edge thickness of a high minus lens. Commenting on the Harris and Chu results, Weschler (1979) suggested that in order to minimize the effects of lens flexure, centre thicknesses of 0.12 mm or greater should be used. He also suggested that flexure may be a greater problem with gas permeable lenses than with PMMA lenses, because of their greater flexibility.

28.4.2 THE EFFECT OF CORNEAL TORICITY

As stated above, Harris & Chu (1972) found no significant flexure when lenses of various centre thicknesses were fitted on a spherical cornea. Dellande (1970b) fitted PMMA lenses greater than 0.12 mm thick on patients with various amounts of corneal toricity, and found that the measured amount of residual astigmatism was less than the predicted amount, i.e. there was lens flexure, only when the amount of corneal toricity was 0.75 D or more, in the with-the-rule direction. No significant difference (flexure) was found for against-the-rule astigmatism.

28.4.3 FLEXURE WITH RIGID GAS PERMEABLE LENSES

Williams (1979) reported that when Polycon silicone–acrylate lenses having centre thicknesses of 0.10 mm were fitted on corneas having up to 2.00 D of toricity, the resulting flexure was 20 to 30% of the corneal toricity. Harris *et al.*, (1982a) fitted both PMMA and Polycon lenses (9.5 mm in diameter with centre thicknesses ranging from 0.07 to 0.16 mm) on corneas with toricities from 1.25 to 4.25 D, and found that the Polycon lenses flexed significantly more than the PMMA lenses. Data plotted on their graph show that for an equivalent amount of flexure, a Polycon lens must be about 0.03 mm thicker than a PMMA lens. In a later study, Harris *et al.*, (1982b) fitted Cabcurve cellulose acetate butyrate (CAB) lenses on toric corneas and compared the results to those for PMMA and Polycon lenses. Their data (reproduced here as Fig. 28.2) show that for an equivalent amount of flexure, a CAB lens must be about 0.03 mm thicker than a Polycon lens or about 0.06 mm thicker than a PMMA lens.

Herman (1984) reported that when Polycon and PMMA lenses of identical design were fitted (apparently on corneas having with-the-rule toricity) Polycon lenses flexed 'slightly more on an individual cornea, but not by a significant amount'. However, Holden (1984) reported that when he applied a known pressure to the edge of a contact lens, he found that flexibility increased with decreasing thickness and increased with increasing silicone content. He commented that whereas the 'critical thickness' for

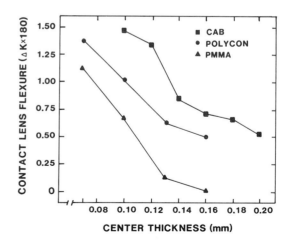

Figure 28.2 Flexure of PMMA, Polycon and CAB lenses on a toric cornea (from Harris *et al.*, 1982b).

PMMA lenses is about 0.12 mm, flexure for many gas permeable lenses was still obvious at 0.15 mm centre thickness.

On the basis of the above findings, the following 'rule-of thumb' is proposed: when fitting a rigid gas-permeable lens on a cornea having a toricity of 1.00 D or more, in order to obtain an amount of flexure roughly equal to that of a PMMA lens, the lens should be 0.03 to 0.04 mm *thicker* than a PMMA lens for the same eye.

The effect of optic zone diameter on flexure of 9.5 mm diameter Paraperm O_2 lenses was investigated by Brown *et al.* (1984), who found that lenses having small optic zone diameters (7.2 mm) flexed significantly less than those having optic zone diameters of 7.8 or 8.4 mm. Herman, in the paper already cited (1984), found that the flexure of 9.0 and 9.5 mm Polycon lenses varied significantly as the base curve of the lens was changed: flexure on a cornea having 3.50 D of with-the-rule toricity was at a maximum when the base curve was fitted 0.30 mm steeper than the flattest corneal meridian, and at a mini-

mum (and even in the against-the-rule direction) when the base curve was fitted 0.30 mm flatter than the flattest corneal meridian. Since most practitioners would routinely fit a spherical lens on a cornea having 3.50 D of toricity with a lens somewhat steeper than the flattest meridian, an unfavourable effect of the base curve on lens flexure would normally be expected.

The somewhat confusing findings concerning the factors having an influence on the amount of flexure of a rigid lens on a cornea having with-the-rule toricity, for PMMA and rigid gas-permeable lenses, are summarized in Table 28.1.

The tendency for a rigid lens to flex on a toric cornea undoubtedly depends not only on the amount of corneal toricity and the parameters of the lens but on a number of factors which vary from one patient to another and are difficult to quantify. These include the positions of the upper and lower lid margins in relation to the cornea, the pressure exerted on the lens by the eyelids (particularly by the upper tarsal plate), the

Table 28.1 Factors having an influence on the amount of flexure of rigid lens on a cornea having with-the-rule toricity, for PMMA and rigid gas-permeable (RGP) lenses

	Factors causing an increase in lens flexure	Factors causing a decrease in lens flexure
Corneal toricity	Increase in toricity	Decrease in toricity
Material	Increased silicone content*	Decreased silicone content*
Center thickness	Decreased thickness (PMMA 0.12 mm or less) (RGP 0.15 mm or less)	Increased thickness (PMMA 0.13 mm or more) (RGP 0.16 mm or more)
Optic zone diameter	Increased OZ diameter (RGP 7.8 or more)	Decreased OZ diameter (RGP 7.2 mm)
Lens–cornea relationship	Steeper than flat meridian (RGP 0.30 steeper 3.50 D toric cornea)	Flatter than flat meridian (RGP 0.30 mm flatter on 3.50 D toric cornea)
Minus sphere power	Low spherical power	High spherical power

* Although little data on flexure of the lenses made of the second and third generation rigid gas permeable lenses are available, these lens materials would be expected to flex considerably more than those of the earlier lenses such as Polycon I and Paraperm O_2.

corneal rigidity and the topography of the peripheral cornea. Consequently the best procedure, when dealing with a given patient, is to determine the effects of lens flexure by doing both keratometry and a sphero-cylinder over-refrction while the lenses are being worn.

28.4.4 HOW MUCH UNCORRECTED ASTIGMATISM CAN BE TOLERATED?

The amount of uncorrected astigmatism that a patient can tolerate varies widely from one person to another: an individual who spends a good bit of time out-of-doors during the daytime hours (with small pupils) may have sufficient depth of focus so that uncorrected astigmatism of 1.00 D or more can easily be tolerated; but one who must do a large amount of reading or other close work may have difficulty tolerating even 0.50 D of uncorrected astigmatism. However, it is generally agreed that if astigmatism of about 0.75 D or more is not corrected, most patients will experience poor visual acuity or asthenopia, or both. Fortunately, the majority of rigid lens candidates will be found to have no more than 0.50 D of uncorrected astigmatism with spherical lenses, so the fitting of toric lenses is seldom necessary.

28.5 FITTING SPHERICAL RIGID LENSES FOR ASTIGMATISM

The following discussion applies to the fitting of both PMMA lenses and rigid gas-permeable lenses, bearing in mind the fact that gas permeable rigid lenses tend to exhibit more flexure than PMMA lenses.

28.5.1 INDICATIONS

When a patient having astigmatism is fitted with spherical lenses, it is normally because the practitioner has come to the conclusion that the fitting of toric lens for the patient is *not* indicated. There are two basic reasons for

fitting contact lenses having toric surfaces:

1. A toric *front* surface lens may be required when an excessive amount of uncorrected astigmatism would be present if a spherical lens were fitted.
2. A toric *back* surface lens may be required when the amount of corneal toricity is sufficient to prevent a comfortable fit with a spherical back surface lens.

Determining whether or not a prospective rigid contact lens wearer can be fitted with spherical lenses must, therefore, be based upon the practitioner's judgement as to whether or not: (1) the patient will be able to tolerate the uncorrected astigmatism that will result if spherical lenses are fitted; and (2) the patient's corneal toricity is sufficiently low for a spherical lens to be worn with comfort. Experience has shown that many patients can wear spherical lenses comfortably in the presence of as much as 3.00 D. of corneal toricity.

28.5.2 FITTING PROCEDURES

The first decision to be made when fitting an astigmatic patient with rigid lenses is whether to use PMMA lenses or lenses made of one of the gas permeable materials. The advantage of lenses made of gas permeable materials is obvious: the fact that the material is oxygen permeable means that corneal oedema is less likely to occur than with PMMA lenses. However, this advantage is to some extent offset by a number of disadvantages, which include: (1) greater initial expense; (2) an increased tendency to become coated with protein materials from the tears; and (3) an increased tendency to accumulate scratches with daily use. The fact that gas permeable lenses are more flexible than PMMA lenses can, as already pointed out, be either an advantage or a disadvantage in terms of the correction of astigmatism. In general, for small to moderate amounts of with-the-rule corneal astigmatism, lens flexure reduces the amount of uncorrected astigmatism.

Many hard lens candidates are long-term wearers of PMMA lenses who have begun to have problems with their lenses after wearing them successfully for as long as 10 or 15 years. The intolerence to the lenses is often due to anoxia and, unless sufficient oxygen can be obtained by 'tear pumping' with a PMMA lens, a gas permeable rigid lens is the lens of choice. Furthermore, many long-term PMMA lens wearers have developed a large amount (3 dioptres or more) of with-the-rule corneal toricity, and for these patients the greater flexibility of a gas permeable lens often provides a more comfortable fit.

Diagnostic lens procedures

Prior to beginning the diagnostic lens fitting, the amount and axis of the uncorrected astigmtism should be predicted for each eye by comparing the keratometer finding and the subjective refraction. This will then be confirmed by over-refraction while wearing the best fitting diagnostic lenses. If over-refraction shows an excessive amount of uncorrected astigmatism or if a comfortable physical fit cannot be obtained with spherical lenses, the fitting of toric rigid gas permeable lenses or toric hydrogel lenses should be considered.

The recommended method of fitting is usually referred to as the 'on K', or 'alignment' method. Ideally, diagnostic lenses should be available in an overall diameter of 9.0 mm with an optic zone width of 7.6 mm, and in an overall diameter of 8.6 mm with an optic zone diameter of 7.2 mm. A 9.0 mm diameter lens is normally used as the starting lens, unless the patient has an unusually small palpebral fissure or a steep cornea (or both), in which case the 8.6 mm lens is used. The use of lenses having diameters in the neighbourhood of 9.5 mm is not recommended, since the fitting of such a lens is usually successful only if the lens moves with

the upper eyelid (as described by Korb & Korb, 1970) and such a fit is difficult to achieve in the presence of significant corneal toricity.

Diagnostic lenses should be of the same diameter, optic zone width and centre thickness as the lenses to be ordered, in addition to being made from the same material. For a patient who has a more than 1 D of corneal astigmatism, a good rule of thumb is to begin with a lens that is steeper than the flattest corneal meridian by approximately one-third of the corneal toricity: for example, if the keratometer finding of 42.00 D at 180/45.00 D at 90 (or 8.04 mm at 180/7.50 mm at 90), the first diagnostic lens should have a radius of curvature corresponding to 43.00 D (7.85 mm).

The lens should centre well on the cornea, it should lag from 2 to 3 mm after each blink, and the fluorescein pattern should show a 'dog-bone' area of touch, with the axis of the 'dog-bone' corresponding to the flattest corneal meridian. In with-the-rule corneal astigmastism (particularly if the patient is a long-term PMMA lens wearer) the lens may tend to ride high. If this occurs, a lens having a slightly steeper base curve may be tried; but if the steeper lens proves to have inadequate movement, the high-riding lens may have to be fitted. This often presents no problem, as long as the optical zone is sufficiently large so that the transition zone or the lens edge does not cause the appearance of 'flare' in low illumination.

Once the best fitting lens has been decided upon, both sphero-cylindrical and 'best sphere' over-refractions should be done. The predicted and measured amounts of uncorrected astigmatism should be compared: any difference between the predicted and measured amounts can be assumed to be due to lens flexure. In order to evaluate lens flexure, a keratometer finding can be taken while the lens is being worn. It should be understood that if *no* lens flexure takes place, the amount of corneal astigmatism found while wearing the lens will be the same (within an experimental error of ±0.25 D) as that found when no lens is worn.

If more than 0.50 D of astigmatism is found to be uncorrected while the lens is worn, or if the corrected visual acuity is significantly less than that with glasses (i.e. by one line or more), the use of a toric rigid or hydrogel lens should be considered. If the diagnostic lens is a gas permeable lens, it is sometimes possible to reduce the amount of uncorrected astigmatism by trying a thicker gas permeable lens (of the order of 0.04 mm thicker than the diagnostic lens) or by fitting a PMMA lens. If a thicker gas permeable lens is to be tried, it must usually be ordered from the laboratory: this has the disadvantage of delaying the fitting procedure, with a possible loss of patient motivation. For this reason it is a good idea to keep on hand a good selection of PMMA lenses in 'standard' thicknesses, since a PMMA lens will provide a good idea of the maximum reduction in flexure that can be obtained by use of an extra-thick gas permeable lens.

28.5.3 ORDERING AND VERIFYING LENSES

The procedures for ordering and verifying the lenses will, of course, be no different than those for any patient requiring spherical rigid lenses. The following parameters should be specified in the lens order:

1. Base curve radius.
2. Secondary curve radius.
3. Peripherial curve radius and width.
4. Overall diameter.
5. Optic zone diameter.
6. Refractive power.
7. Centre thickness.
8. Material.
9. Tint.

Upon receipt of the lenses from the laboratory, base curve radius is verified by means of a radiuscope; refracting power is verified by means of a lensometer; overall diameter,

optic zone width and the width of the peripheral curve are verified by means of a measuring magnifier; and the tint is verified by inspection. Radii of secondary and peripheral curves cannot be verified.

28.5.4 FOLLOW-UP CARE

Procedures for follow-up care are identical to those used whenever spherical rigid lenses are fitted. If the lenses tend to ride high, the patient should be questioned concerning the possibility of 'flare' in low illumination. In cases of high corneal toricity, the tendency for the lenses to lag excessively with each blink, bumping the lids in the process, may add to the difficulty of adaptation.

28.5.5 PROBLEMS TO BE ANTICIPATED

The problems the practitioner should anticipate will depend upon whether the patient is a new contact lens wearer or is an adapted wearer (i.e. a former PMMA lens wearer who is being refitted). For the new wearer, wearing time will have to be built up (as with any new hard lens wearer) and, in cases of high corneal toricity, the tendency for the lenses to rock on the flattest corneal meridian may make adaptation more difficult than it would be otherwise. The patient should therefore be monitored closely during the adaptation period, and the practitioner should make every effort to assist the patient in maintaining his or her motivation.

The uncorrected astigmatism, the corrected visual acuity and the physical fit of the lenses should be monitored during the follow-up visits. Normally, if there are no problems during the first two or three visits (or, for the new wearer, by the time full wearing time has been attained) none should be anticipated. The anticipated problems fall into two categories: (1) problems to do with uncorrected astigmatism, i.e. poor visual acuity or complaints of eyestrain; (2) problems to do with physical fit, i.e. discomfort due to the rocking of the lenses. If problems in either of these categories prove to be insurmountable, the option of fitting toric lenses (either rigid or hydrogel) remains.

28.6 FITTING TORIC FRONT SURFACE LENSES

28.6.1 INDICATIONS

Toric front surface lenses are indicated for those patients who would have an excessive amount of uncorrected astigmatism – due to internal astigmatism – if fitted with spherical rigid lenses. The practitioner should first predict the amount of astigmatism that will remain uncorrected with a spherical lens by comparing the keratometric astigmatism and the astigmatism found by subjective refraction; and should then measure the uncorrected astigmatism by performing a spherocylindrical over-refraction with a well-fitting spherical lens. In addition, the amount of uncorrected astigmatism due to lens flexure can be found by taking a keratometer finding while the spherical lens is worn: any keratometric astigmatism present will be due to lens flexure.

Even in those instances in which the amount of uncorrected astigmatism with a spherical rigid lens – due to excessive lens flexure – appears to be sufficient to require the fitting of a front surface toric lens, it is often advisable to avoid the fitting of a toric lens by making use of a thicker lens of the same material, or by fitting a lens made of a more rigid material. If a thicker lens is to be used, a good starting point is to try a lens having a centre thickness approximately 0.04 mm greater than that of the diagnostic lens that resulted in excessive flexure. And, of course, there remains the possibility of fitting a PMMA lens.

An additional method of fitting a patient having internal astigmatism has been suggested, which involves the use of a lens having an *aspheric* front surface. The use of such a lens has been suggested, not only for internal astigmatism but also for presbyopia, but just *how* the lens corrects for astigmatism or presbyopia has been poorly understood. Kerns (1974) fitted ten subjects having from 0.50 D to 1.75 D of residual astigmatism with both spherical lenses and Panofocal aspheric front surface lenses, and found that mean visual acuity was significantly better with the Panofocal lenses than with the spherical lenses. However, since there was no difference in the mean amount of residual astigmatism for Panofocal and spherical lenses, Kerns concluded that the improvement in visual acuity may have been due to a reduction in spherical aberration by the aspheric lens.

28.6.2 METHODS OF ACHIEVING MERIDIONAL ORIENTATION

An ordinary rigid contact lens tends to rotate on the eye, rotating upward and temporally with each blink. This does not represent a problem as long as the lens is a spherical lens: however, a toric lens must be manufactured in such a way that the meridional orientation of the lens can be maintained in a predictable manner. Numerous methods of achieving meridional orientation have been attempted, the most successful of which have been the use of prism ballast (Fig. 28.3) and the use of a lower truncation (Fig. 28.4). In the case of a highly toric cornea, a toric back surface can be utilized to stabilize the lens so that a toric front surface can be provided for the correction of internal astigmatism, resulting in a bi-toric lens. However, this is seldom done.

Borish (1961, 1963) has developed a method of fitting toric front surface PMMA lenses which makes use of 0.75 to 1 prism dioptre of prism ballast. He uses lower truncation (along with the prism ballast) for plus lenses, but not for minus lenses: the reason for this (Fig. 28.5) is that when a plus lens is truncated the amount of ballast is increased;

28.6.9 ORDERING THE TORIC FRONT SURFACE

When the lenses are returned to the laboratory for incorporation of the toric front surface, it is necessary only to specify any residual spherical power along with the cylinder power and axis (as related to the base–apex meridian). The procedure will be illustrated by the following example:

Example

A patient has been wearing a prism ballasted lens with 1 prism dioptre of prism power and with a refractive power of –3.00 DS. After adaptation to the lens, the over-refraction is found to be +1.00 DS –1.00 DC axis 95. The lens orientates on the eye in such a manner that the base–apex meridian, indicated by the line at the bottom of the lens, is located at 80 degrees. What information should the practitioner forward to the laboratory concerning the required change in the power of the front surface of the lens?

As shown in Figure 28.9, the base–apex meridian is displaced 10 degrees *clockwise* from the vertical meridian. The procedure, therefore, is to *add* 10 degrees to the cylinder axis. The necessary change in the power of the front surface of the lens will therefore be:

+1.00 –1.00 axis 105

or, specifying the change in power in the plus cylinder form:

plano +1.00 axis 15

When the finished lens assumes its position with the base at 80 degrees, the minus cylinder axis will be 95 degrees with respect to the eye.

28.6.10 VERIFICATION AND DISPENSING THE TORIC FRONT SURFACE LENS

Verification of any toric lens is difficult since modern lensometers, even though having lens stops designed to accommodate a con-

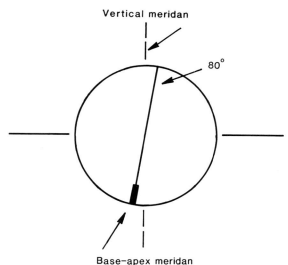

Figure 28.9 The base–apex meridian is displaced 10 degrees from the vertical meridian, in the clockwise direction, so 10 degrees must be added to the cylinder axis. Since the desired axis is 95 degrees, the axis to be ordered from the laboratory is 105 degrees. When the lens orientates on the eye with the base–apex meridian at 80 degrees, the cylinder axis will be 95 degrees.

tact lens, have no satisfactory method of orientating a contact lens so that the cylinder axis (in relation to the base–apex meridian) can be determined with certainty. The accuracy with which the procedures, to be described below, can be carried out will depend both on the particular type of lensometer used and the practitioner's experience in verifying toric lenses.

Verification of the lens will require a method of orientating the lens in the base–apex meridian (which, of course, is the reference meridian for the cylinder axis). The first procedure, therefore, is to place the lens on the lensometer stop and to locate the base–apex meridian of the prism, and then to mark this meridian with a felt pen. Once this has been done, the lens is placed on the lensometer stop in such a manner that the target is centred on the amount and direction of the prism component incorporated into the lens (in our example, 1 prism dioptre base down at 80 degrees, as shown in Figure 28.10). With the lens orientated in this position, the lens should be found to have the following power (remembering that the power prior to modification was –3.00 DS):

–2.00 –1.00 × 105

or, in the plus cylinder form:

–3.00 +1.00 axis 15

When the lens is dispensed to the patient, visual acuity, refraction and lens fit should be checked in the usual manner, and the position of the base–apex meridian should be verified, using the same procedure as that used originally (slit lamp protractor or trial lens and trial frame).

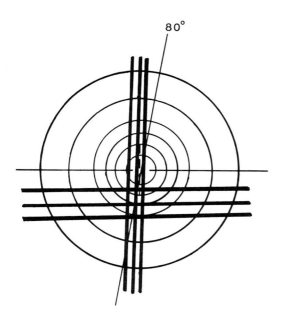

Figure 28.10 Toric front surface lens placed in the lensometer stop so that the target is centred on the amount and direction of the prism component in the lens (1 prism dioptre base down at 80 degrees). If not measured in this manner, the cylinder power and axis may be incorrect because of radial astigmatism.

28.6.11 PROBLEMS TO BE ANTICIPATED

If all of the problems, such as adaptation to the lenses, lens position and lag, and orientation of the base–apex meridian, were solved while the spherical lenses were being worn, a minimum of follow-up care would be required and few, if any, problems should be anticipated. The great advantage of beginning the procedure by fitting the patient with spherical prism-ballasted lenses is that success is practically assured by the time the toric front surface is ordered from the laboratory. If the patient were to be fitted with toric front surface prism-ballasted lenses at the outset, the possibility of success would not be nearly as great.

28.7 FITTING TORIC BASE CURVE AND BI-TORIC LENSES

Toric back surface lenses and bi-toric lenses, although not often fitted, have been available for many years from a large number of PMMA lens laboratories and are currently available from at least one of the manufacturers of silicone–acrylate lenses.

28.7.1 INDICATIONS

A comfortable fit can almost always be obtained with a spherical base curve lens when the corneal toricity is no more than about 2.50 to 3.00 D, but many patients having more than this amount of toricity will find spherical rigid lenses uncomfortable, and may therefore be candidates for toric back surface lenses. The percentage of patients having this amount of astigmatism is rather small: Lyle (1971) found that only 68 of 1288 eyes, or 5.5%, had corneal astigmatism of 2.75 D or more. However, this percentage may be augmented to some extent by long-term wearers of PMMA lenses who have developed significant with-the-rule corneal toricity while wearing the lenses, who are often potential candidates for toric back surface lenses. In any case, toric lenses should not be fitted without a trial session with spherical base curve lenses: lenses made of some of the newer high-permeability materials may flex sufficiently on a highly toric cornea to provide a comfortable fit.

Unfortunately a toric base curve lens, even though providing a comfortable physical fit, induces astigmatism whose axis is *opposite* that of the axis of the corneal astigmatism. Consequently for an eye having with-the-rule corneal astigmatism and against-the-rule internal astigmatism (the ususal situation), the induced astigmatism will *add* to the internal astigmatism. Therefore, with few exceptions, the fitting of a toric base curve necessitates the use of a toric front surface for the correction of this astigmatism, resulting in the fitting of a *bi-toric* lens.

28.7.2   ACHIEVING MERIDIONAL ORIENTATION

With sufficient corneal toricity, the toric back surface alone is sufficient to achieve meridional orientation. However, the fact that the lens fails to rotate on the eye has the disadvantage that the lens may tend to fit *too tightly*, causing oedema and often limiting wearing time. This is a greater problem with PMMA lenses than with gas permeable rigid lenses, since the entire oxygen supply to the cornea must be supplied by tear pumping when a PMMA lens is worn: indeed, only limited success was achieved with toric base curve lenses until gas permeable materials became available.

An alternative method of achieving meridional orientation on a toric cornea involves the use of a *toric secondary curve*. This procedure has the advantage that a spherical (rather than toric) base curve can be used, so no additional astigmatism is induced. The overall diameter of such a lens must be quite large, in order to achieve meridional orientation, with the result that

the lenses tend to fit so tightly that oedema and other problems tend to occur. Since the results obtained with these lenses have not, on the whole, been satisfactory, they will not be discussed here.

28.7.3   OPTICAL PRINCIPLES

The optical principles of toric base curve and bi-toric lenses lenses are, unfortunately, more complicated than those of toric front surface lenses. The first step in understanding these principles involves the use of three conversion factors. In deriving these conversion factors, the following refractive indices will be used:

Keratometer calibration	1.3375
Tears	1.336
Silicone–acrylate	1.480

Since the conversion factors will be calculated only for silicone–acrylate lenses, the index of refraction of PMMA, 1.490, will not be used. Note that these conversion factors apply (to the finished lens) only to toric base curve lenses. They are, however, useful for calculating the parameters for a bi-toric lens.

Conversion factors for toric base curve lenses

The first conversion factor is used to convert the 'keratometer value' of a lens surface (the power that would be found by the use of a keratometer, indicated, as suggested by Sarver (1970), by the symbol Dk) to the *actual* refracting power of the lens surface, in air. This factor is derived by finding the ratio of the refraction at the interface between air and the contact lens to the refraction measured by the keratometer:

$$\frac{1.480 - 1}{1.3375 - 1} = 1.422, \text{ or approximately } 3/2$$

This conversion factor is used when a toric base curve lens, received from the laboratory, is verified by the use of a lensometer. For example, in verifying a lens having a base curve with a toricity of 3.00 Dk (e.g. 42.00 Dk at 180/45.00 Dk at 90, or 8.04 mm at 180/7.50 mm at 90), the cylinder as indicated by the lensometer should be:

$$1.422 \, (-3.00 \, DC \times 180) = -4.27 \, DC \times 180$$

The second conversion factor converts the astigmatism measured by the keratometer for a rigid gas-permeable toric base curve lens to the astigmatism induced at the plastic-to-tears interface. This factor is derived by finding the ratio of the refraction between the contact lens and the tear layer to the refraction measured by the Keratometer:

$$\frac{1.336 - 1.480}{1.3375 - 1} = -0.427, \text{ or approximately } 1/2$$

This conversion factor tells us how much induced astigmatism will have to be corrected by a toric front surface, when a toric base curve is used. For example, for the base curve 42.00 Dk at 180/45.00 Dk at 90, the amount of induced astigmatism will be

$$-0.427 \, (-3.00) = +1.28 \, D$$

and the axis of the plus cylinder required to correct the induced astigmatism will be 90 degrees from that of the lens required to correct the corneal astigmatism.

The third conversion factor is used to convert the astigmatism caused by the toric base curve lens, in air, to the astigmatism induced when the lens is on the eye. This factor is derived by finding the ratio of the refraction between the contact lens and the tear layer to the refraction between the contact lens and air:

$$\frac{1.336 - 1.480}{1.480 - 1} = 0.300, \text{ or approximately } 1/3$$

This conversion factor tells us that the amount of astigmatism induced by a toric back surface lens, while on the eye, is 0.300 (or approximately one-third) of that measured by the lensometer. Therefore, for the 42.00 Dk at 180/45.00 Dk at 90 lens, which resulted in astigmatism of −4.27 Dk × 180 when measured on the lensometer, the induced astigmatism while on the eye will be:

$$0.30 \, (-4.27) = -1.28 \, D$$

which is equal to the amount of astigmatism determined (above) by multiplying the conversion factor −0.422 by the keratometer value of the toricity of the back surface of the lens.

28.7.4 BI-TORIC LENS DESIGN

The point has been made that the astigmatism induced by a toric base curve is almost always of sufficient amount to require the use of a toric front surface for its correction, resulting in a bi-toric lens. The best way to visualize the optics of a bi-toric lens is to consider each of the two meridians separately, just as if lenses for two separate eyes were being considered. By doing so, it is possible to consider the refraction taking place at an interface (air-to-plastic and plastic-to-tears) in each meridian, using the appropriate indices of refraction.

The problem that must be addressed is twofold: (1) determining the amount of astigmatism that will be induced by the use of a toric base curve; and (2) determining the power of the toric front surface necessary to correct this astigmatism. This problem, and its solution, will be illustrated by the following example:

Example

An eye having the keratometric findings 42.00 D at 180/45.00 D at 90 is to be fitted with a silicone–acrylate lens having a toric base curve. The lens will be designed in such a way that the radii of curvature of the back toric surface are identical to those of the cornea, in each of the principal meridians.

(1) What will be the amount of the induced astigmatism? Will it be with-the-rule or against-the-rule astigmatism?

For the *horizontal* meridian, the first step is to determine the radius of curvature for the 42.00 Dk finding. This can be done by calculation or by reference to a table. The radius is found to be 8.04 mm. The next step is to find the dioptric value of the plastic-to-tears refraction:

$$F_{2h} = \frac{1.336 - 1.480}{0.00804} = -17.91 \text{ D}$$

For the *vertical* meridian, the radius of curvature corresponding to the 45.00 Dk finding is 7.50 mm. The plastic-to-tears refraction is therefore:

$$F_{2v} = \frac{1.336 - 1.480}{0.00750} = -19.20 \text{ D}$$

The astigmatism induced by the toric base curve is therefore equal to:

$$-19.20 \text{ D} - (-17.91 \text{ D}) = -1.29 \text{ D}$$

and since the negative vergence is greater in the vertical meridian than in the horizontal meridian (or positive vergence is greater in the horizontal meridian), the induced astigmatism is in the *against-the-rule* direction.

(Note that the refractive values, −17.91 D and −19.20 D, for the horizontal and vertical meridians, could have been obtained by multiplying the keratometer values (42.00 Dk and 45.00 Dk) by the conversion factor −0.427; and the amount of induced astigmatism, 1.29 D, could have been obtained by multiplying the difference in the Dk values for the two meridians (−3.00) by −0.427.)

(2) If the refractive error for the eye in the above example is −2.00 DS −3.00 DC × 180, what front surface curves would be required, in designing a bi-toric lens, to eliminate the astigmatism induced by the toric base curve?

For the *horizontal* meridian, the first step is to find the refractive power, in air, of the back surface of the lens. The next step will be

to combine this with −2.00 D (the refractive error correction in the horizontal meridian), to find the refracting power of the front surface of the lens in that meridian. The refracting power of the back surface is:

$$F_{2h} = \frac{1 - 1.480}{0.00804} = -59.70 \text{ D}$$

The refractive power of the front surface (assuming the lens to be infinitely thin) in the horizontal meridian is found by the expression:

$$
\begin{aligned}
F &= F_{1h} + F_{2h}, \text{ or} \\
F_{1h} &= F - F_2 \\
&= -2.00 - (-59.70) = +57.70 \text{ D}
\end{aligned}
$$

For the *vertical* meridian, the refracting power of the back surface, in air, is:

$$F_{2v} = \frac{1 - 1.480}{0.00750} = -64.00 \text{ D}$$

In order to correct the astigmatism induced by the back surface, the front surface must incorporate the cylinder, +1.29 DC × 180. In order to do this, the vertical meridian must have a refracting power 1.29 D greater than that of the horizontal meridian, or:

$$F_{1v} = +57.7 + 1.29 = +58.99 \text{ D}$$

In order to verify the fact that this lens accurately corrects the eye's ametropia, we must find the refracting power of the lens in each of the two principal meridians. For the horizontal meridian:

$$F_{1h} + F_{2h} = +57.70 + (-59.70) = -2.00 \text{ D}$$

while for the vertical meridian:

$$F_{1v} + F_{2v} = +58.99 + (-64.00) = -5.01 \text{ D}$$

The lens, therefore, satisfactorily corrects the refractive error:

−2.00 DS − 3.00 DC × 180.

Note that the values for refracting power in air of the back surface in the two principal meridians, −59.70 D and −64.00 D, could have been obtained by multiplying the keratometric values (42.00 Dk and 45.00 Dk) by the conversion factor 1.422.)

The resulting bi-toric lens, as shown in Figure 28.11, corrects the eye's refractive error in both principal meridians, therefore behaving as if it were a *spherical* lens. Such a bi-toric lens has been described by Sarver (1963) as having a 'spherical power effect'.

28.7.5 FITTING PROCEDURES

Fitting procedures will be discussed only for bi-toric lenses, since the fitting of a toric base curve lens without the inclusion of a toric front surface will almost never result in satisfactory optical performance. An exception to this general rule could apply to the fitting of a toric base curve on an eye having against-the-rule corneal toricity, in which case the induced astigmatism would be in the with-the-rule direction and would be expected to compensate for any against-the-rule internal astigmatism. However, such a situation is very unlikely: in the distribution of corneal astigmatism for 1208 eyes reported by Lyle (1971), there were *no* eyes having more than 2.25 D of against-the-rule astigmatism.

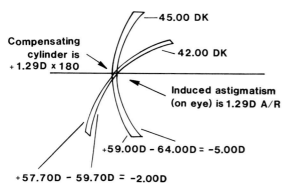

Figure 28.11 Bitoric lens having a spherical power effect. The astigmatism induced by the back surface cylinder is corrected by a front surface cylinder, with the result that the lens acts as a spherical lens and can rotate on the eye and still correct the eye's refractive error.

Any method of fitting a bi-toric lens that does not include a trial with a toric base curve lens tends to be a risky undertaking, since the practitioner has no method of assuring (before ordering the patient's lens) that the lens will provide a satisfactory lens–cornea relationship. If bi-toric lens fitting is done without the aid of base curve diagnostic lenses, the practitioner may wish to consider the initial bi-toric lens ordered for the patient as a trial lens, which (if not satisfactory) can later be used in fitting other patients.

28.7.6 FITTING WITH TORIC BASE CURVE DIAGNOSTIC LENSES

Sarver (1963) outlined a method of fitting a bi-toric PMMA lens having a spherical power effect, based on the use of both spherical and toric diagnostic lenses. The procedure will be illustrated by making use of Sarver's example, which follows:

Example

For a given eye, a spherical contact lens having a base curve of 42.00 Dk and a power of –2.00 DS is found to adequately correct the refractive error; and a toric base curve, 42.00 Dk/45.00 Dk, is found to provide an optimum lens–cornea relationship. The patient's refractive error is –2.00 DS –3.00 DC ×180 (i.e. –2.00 DS in the 42.00 Dk meridian and –5.00 DS in the 45.00 Dk meridian). A bi-toric lens with the following parameters is ordered:

Flattest meridian: 42.00 Dk, –2.00 D
Steepest meridian: 45.00 Dk, –5.00 D

When this lens is verified by means of a lensometer, the reading will be –2.00 D in the flattest meridian and –5.00 D in the steepest meridian. Sarver (1963) made the point that a spherical power effect lens will continue to correct the eye's ametropia even if it rotates on the eye.

Even though a bi-toric lens having a

spherical power effect compensates for the astigmatism induced by the toric back surface, it should be understood that it does not correct for internal astigmatism. If a significant amount of internal astigmatism is present, it can be corrected by increasing the amount of front surface cylinder.

As the reader will understand, the value in using this procedure to fit a bi-toric lens is that it does not involve the use of mathematical formulae: once the toric lens providing the desired lens–cornea relationship is obtained, the power in the flattest meridian is found by using the refraction through a spherical trial lens, and the power in the steepest meridian is found by adding to this the power of the minus cylinder in the refractive correction.

An alternative method of determining the power of the lens (not suggested by Sarver) would be to base it on an over-refraction through the best-fitting trial lens. If this were done, both the astigmatism induced by the toric back surface and the internal astigmatism would be corrected.

28.7.7 FITTING WITH BI-TORIC DIAGNOSTIC LENSES

A 36-lens set of Polycon II bi-toric lenses is currently available. This set consists of three series of 12 lenses each, base curves for each series ranging from 39.00 Dk to 44.50 Dk in the flattest meridian, the three series having 2.00 Dk, 3.00 Dk and 4.00 Dk of toricity. The lenses are 'spherical power effect lenses', designed so that the toric front surface compensates for the astigmatism induced by the toric back surface. All lenses have an overall diameter of 9.0 mm.

Using this trial set, the optimum lens–cornea relationship can be obtained by selecting a trial lens whose toricity is equal to or slightly *less* than that of the cornea, and whose curvature in the flattest meridian is equal to or somewhat flatter than that of the flattest corneal meridian. For the eye used in the example, having a keratometer find-ing of 42.00 D at 180/45.00 D at 90, a good starting lens would be one having a base curve of 42.00 Dk/45.00 Dk (paralleling both principal meridians of the cornea).

The position of the lens, the blink lag and the fluorescein pattern should be evaluated, just as they would be evaluated for a spherical lens. The fluorescein pattern will not have the 'dog-bone' area of touch typical of a spherical lens on a highly toric cornea, but will look very much like the pattern of a spherical lens on a spherical cornea. Since the lens will not rotate on the cornea as a spherical lens does, care must be taken to make sure that the lens does not fit too tightly. As when fitting a spherical lens, if the lens is fitting too tightly (insufficient lens movement or a 'steep' fluorescein pattern) a lens having a flatter base curve should be tried; whereas if a lens is fitting too loosely (excessive lens movement or a 'flat' fluorescein pattern) a lens with a steeper base curve should be tried.

28.7.8 DETERMINING LENS POWER

Once the lens that provides the best physical fit has been selected, both a spherocylindrical and a best sphere over-refraction should be done. When toric base curve diagnostic lenses are used, any cylinder found in the over-refraction will compensate for the astigmatism induced by the toric back surface as well as for internal astigmatism. However when bi-toric 'spherical power effect' lenses are used, any uncorrected astigmatism found in the sphero-cylindrical over-refraction will compensate only for internal astigmatism: uncorrected astigmatism of 0.25 D or 0.50 D can be ignored, but astigmatism of 0.75 D or more should be corrected by specifying additional cylinder power, which will be incorporated in the front surface toric curve.

28.7.9 ORDERING LENSES

In the order for a bi-toric lens, the practitioner must specify the base curve radii (or Dk values) in each of the two principal meridians, in addition to the required spherical and cylindrical powers. The manner in which the power is specified will depend upon the type of diagnostic lenses used. When toric base curve lenses are used as diagnostic lenses, the power of the lens to be ordered will be the power of the best-fitting diagnostic lens combined with the over-refraction, very much the same as would be the case in ordering spherical base curve lenses.

For example, assume that the toric base curve diagnostic lens has the following parameters:

Base curve: 42.00 Dk at 180/45.00 Dk at 90
Power in horizontal meridian: −2.00 D

and that the result of the over-refraction is:

−0.25 −1.00 × 90

The required lens power will therefore be:

−2.25 −1.00 × 90

Since the cylinder resulting from the over-refraction will be incorporated in the lens as a front surface cylinder, the lens formula should be given in the plus cylinder form:

−3.25 +1.00 × 180

When spherical power effect lenses are used as diagnostic lenses, the lens power ordered will, in most cases, not require the specification of a cylindrical component. It will, however, be necessary to specify to the laboratory the base curve of the spherical power effect lens used.

For example, assume that a spherical power effect lens has the following parameters:

Base curve: 42.00 Dk at 180/45.00 Dk at 90
Power in horizontal meridian: −2.00 D

and that the result of the over-refraction is:

−0.50 DS

The simplest way to order the lens, in this case, would be to specify a spherical power effect lens having the base curve:

42.00 Dk/45.00 Dk

with the power:

−2.50 D in the 42.00 Dk meridian

An alternative method would be to use a lensometer to determine the power of the diagnostic lens in both the horizontal and vertical meridians, and then to add −0.50 D (the spherical over-refraction) to both meridians in specifying the lens power to the laboratory.

28.7.10 VERIFICATION OF LENSES

In verifying a bi-toric lens that is designed to provide a spherical power effect, the base curve radii are verified in the two principal meridians, using a radiuscope; and the refracting power is verified, again in the two principal meridians, by the use of a lensometer. The findings should, of course, be exactly as ordered. Since the base curve and refracting power are ordered separately for each meridian, no conversion factors are needed. For example, if the lens order was specified as given in the example by Sarver (1963), namely:

Flattest meridian: 42.00 Dk, −2.00 D
Steepest meridian: 45.00 Dk, −5.00 D

verification should result in the radii and powers, as ordered.

28.7.11 FOLLOW-UP CARE

Since a toric back surface lens does not rotate on the eye as a spherical lens does, the practitioner should be on the look-out, as wearing time is built up, for indications (both symptoms and findings) that the lenses may be too tight. Should the lenses prove to fit too tightly, they can be loosened by any of the usual procedures, including reducing optic zone diameter, flattening the secondary and/or peripheral curve or reducing the overall diameter.

28.8 CLINICAL EVALUATION OF SPHERICAL POWER EFFECT LENSES

In a report involving the use of the Polycon II bi-toric lens on 50 patients, Sarver *et al.* (1985) stated that the mean base curve in the flattest meridian was 0.45 D flatter than the flattest corneal meridian, and that the mean base curve was fitted with 0.50 D less toricity than the corneal toricity. However, they found a considerable amount of variation in the lens–cornea bearing relationship, many eyes being fitted with lenses having toricities as much as 1.00 or even 2.00 D less than that of the cornea, and a few eyes being fitted with toricities slightly greater than that of the cornea. They reported that 36 of the 50 patients were fitted with spherical power effect lenses, while 14 were fitted with cylindrical power effect lenses (having an additional cylindrical component for the correction of internal astigmatism).

Sarver *et al.* judged patient response on the basis of the following criteria: comfort, vision, wearing time and corneal changes, with the following results: Comfort was good to excellent for 84% of the sample. Vision was good to excellent for 91%, vision problems being caused by five lenses that flexed because they were too thin and by nine lenses that had to be made larger than the standard 9.0 mm diameter in order to improve lens centration. Wearing time was limited for ten patients (20% of the sample) for various reasons including discomfort, dry eyes, corneal staining and poor motivation. Corneal response was good to excellent for 91% of the sample, with two eyes showing moderate corneal staining and none showing corneal oedema.

28.9 SUMMARY: MANAGEMENT OF ASTIGMATISM WITH RIGID LENSES

Rigid lenses provide the following fitting modalities for patients having astigmatism:

1. Spherical rigid lenses are indicated for those patients: (1) not having significant uncorrected (residual) astigmatism when wearing spherical lenses; and (2) not having sufficient corneal toricity to make spherical rigid lenses uncomfortable. For moderate amounts of corneal toricity, the astigmatism induced by the flexure of a gas permeable rigid lens will often compensate for any internal astigmatism; for larger amounts of corneal toricity, the astigmatism induced by flexure will often serve as a source of uncorrected astigmatism. In the latter case the flexure can often be controlled by fitting a somewhat thicker lens.

2. Toric front surface lenses are indicated for those patients who would have a significant amount of uncorrected astigmatism if spherical rigid lenses were worn. The method of fitting described by Borish (1961, 1963, 1974, 1986) is recommended: the patient is first fitted with a spherical prism ballasted lens, and after adaptation has occurred the lens is returned to the laboratory for the working of the toric front surface.

3. Bi-toric lenses are recommended for those patients having sufficient corneal toricity to make the wearing of a spherical rigid lens uncomfortable. The toric back surface is for the purpose of providing a comfortable fit, and the toric front surface is for the purpose of compensating for the astigmatism induced by the toric back surface. The method of fitting described by Sarver (1963) and by Sarver *et al.* (1985) is recommended. Either toric base curve or bi-toric lenses having a spherical power effect may be used as diagnostic lenses.

REFERENCES

Bailey, N.J. (1961a) Residual astigmatism with contact lenses. I – Incidence. *Opt. J. Rev. Optom.*, **98**, 30–1.

Bailey, N.J. (1961b) Residual astigmatism with

contact lenses. II – Predictability. *Opt. J. Rev. Optom.*, **98**, 40–5.

Bailey, N.J. (1961c) Residual astigmatism with contact lenses. III – Possible sites. *Opt. J. Rev. Optom.*, **98**, 31–2.

Bailey, N.J. (1961d) Residual astigmatism with contact lenses IV – Corrective techniques. *Opt. J. Rev. Optom.*, **98**, 43–4.

Boltz, R. (1982) *Continuing education lecture.* University of Houston, Houston, Texas.

Borish, I.M. (1961) *Report on 500 cases of residual astigmatism corrected with ballasted contact lenses.* 1st AOA Contact Lens Symposium. Ohio State University, Columbus, Ohio.

Borish, I.M. (1963) Procedure for fitting ballasted cylinder lenses and high-riding bifocals. *J. Ill. Optom. Assoc.*, **Sept**, 15–16; **Oct** 24–30.

Borish, I.M. (1974) Specialized procedure for fitting ballasted corneal contact lenses. *Contact Lens Clin.*, **1** (4), 56–64.

Borish, I.M. (1986) *Fitting toric front surface hard contact lenses* [ecture]. University of Houston, Houston, Texas.

Brown, S., Baldwin, M. and Pole J. (1984) Effect of the optic zone diameter on lens flexure and residual astigmatism. *Int. Contact Lens Clin.*, **11**, 759–63.

Dellande, W.D. (1970a) A comparison of predicted and measured residual astigmatism in corneal contact lens wearers. *Am. J. Optom. Arch. Am. Acad. Optom.*, **47**, 459–63.

Dellande, W.D. (1970b) Corneal toricity and predicted residual astigmatism. *Am. J. Optom. Arch. Am. Acad. Optom.*, **47**, 739–40.

Grosvenor, T. (1963) *Contact Lens Theory and Practice.* Professional Press, Chicago.

Harris, M.G. (1970) The effect of contact lens thickness and diameter on residual astigmatism: a preliminary study. *Am. J. Optom. Arch. Am. Acad. Optom.*, **47**, 442–63.

Harris, M.G. and Appelquist, T.D. (1974) The effects of contact lens diameter and power on flexure and residual astigmatism. *Am. J. Optom. Physiol. Opt.*, **51**, 266–70.

Harris, M.G. and Chu, C.S. (1972) The effect of contact lens thickness and corneal toricity on flexure and residual astigmatism. *Am. J. Optom. Arch. Am. Acad. Optom.*, **49**, 304–7.

Harris, M.G., Kadoya, J., Nomura, J. and Wong, V. (1982a) Flexure and residual astigmatism with Polycon and polymethyl methacrylate lenses on toric corneas. *Am. J. Optom. Physiol. Opt.*, **59**, 263–6.

Harris, M.G., Sweeney, K.E., Rocchi, S. and Pettit, D. (1982b) Flexure and residual astigmatism with cellulose acetate butyrate (CAB) contact lenses on toric corneas. *Am. J. Optom. Physiol. Opt.*, **59**, 858–62.

Herman, J.P. (1984) Lens flexure: clinical rules. *J. Am. Optom. Assoc.*, **55**, 169–71.

Holden, B.A. (1984) Predicting contact lens flexure from *in vitro* tests. *J. Am. Optom. Assoc.*, **55**, 171.

Kerns, R.L. (1974) Clinical evaluation of the merits of aspheric front surface contact lenses for patients manifesting residual astigmatism. *Am. J. Optom. Physiol. Opt.*, **51**, 750–7.

Korb, D.R. and Korb, J.M. (1970) A new concept in contact lens design. *J. Am. Optom. Assoc.*, **41**, 1023–4.

Lyle, W.M. (1971) Changes in corneal astigmatism with age. *Am. J. Optom. Physiol. Opt.*, **48**, 467–78.

Sarver, M.D. (1963) A toric base curve corneal contact lens with spherical power effect. *J. Am. Optom. Assoc.*, **34**, 1136–7.

Sarver, M.D. (1969) A study of residual astigmatism. *Am. J. Optom. Physiol. Opt.*, **46**, 578–82.

Sarver, M.D. (1970) Visual correction with contact lenses. In *Clinical Refraction* (3rd edn) (ed. I.M. Borish), Professional Press, Chicago.

Sarver, M.D., Kame, R.T. and William, C.E. (1985) A bitoric gas permeable hard contact lens with spherical power effect. *J. Am. Optom. Assoc.*, **56**, 184–9.

Wechsler, S. (1979) Effects of rigid lens flexure on vision. *J. Am. Optom. Assoc.*, **50**, 327–9.

Williams, C.E. (1979) New design concepts for permeable rigid contact lenses. *J. Am. Optom. Assoc.*, **50**, 331–6.

N.F. Burnett Hodd and J.E. Josephson

29.1 INTRODUCTION

It has been estimated that 45% of individuals who wish to wear soft contact lenses have significant astigmatism (0.75 D or more) (Holden, 1975), a condition for which toric hydrogel contact lenses are required for proper visual correction. The flexure of thin hydrogel lenses, 'wrapping' toward the shape of the host cornea affects the expected power effect of the lens (Josephson, 1973; Sarver *et al.*, 1974; Strachan, 1975; Bennett, 1976; Weissman, 1984a) and may inadvertently increase or decrease the total ocular refractive astigmatism. Thus, the distortion of the contact lens shape that affects the curvature of the anterior contact lens surface can result in a different refracting power of the lens than the intended design. Even corneal surfaces with a slight toricity have been known to cause significant residual astigmatism with the wearing of hydrogel contact lenses.

Since hydrogel lenses were first commercially introduced by Griffin Laboratories in 1969, early manufacturers of these lenses often claimed that astigmatism from 0.50 D to 2.00 D could be masked by their 'proprietary' spherical power contact lens products, with special claims being made for their lens materials or designs. These claims were often supported by the results from the field, in the form of publications by clinicians (Isen, 1972; Gasson, 1973; Burnett Hodd, 1980/1). Further attempts at 'masking' with thick lenses have not proven to be predictable. In addition, the effect of masking has been shown to be not greater than 0.30 D (Lee & Sarver, 1972; Bennett, 1976; Weissman, 1984a, b; Wechsler *et al.*, 1986; Snyder & Talley, 1989).

It has been our experience that spectacles with an astigmatic component require very accurate prescribing to avoid patient intolerance. A prescribing error of ±0.25 D in the cylinder power or a mislocation of the axis of only a few degrees can cause asthenopia in some individuals. Yet, with the prescribing of toric hydrogel contact lenses, there has been a tendency for practitioners to be more flexible in their concern for the accuracy of the cylindrical power or axis components of the prescription. This is because the manufacturing tolerances for toric hydrogel contact lenses are greater than those for spectacle lenses. When one also considers the difficulty that the practitioner has in the precise quality control of hydrogel contact lenses that are received from a laboratory, the slight 'play' in lens rotation that sometimes occurs with patient blinking and the practitioner difficulty in accurately assessing the axis alignment of the lens *in situ*, it is understandable that these factors have led to reduced practitioner concern for accuracy, particularly if any reduced vision did not cause the patient concern (Burnett Hodd, 1976a; Hallak, 1982; Hanks & Weisbarth, 1983; Ivins, 1984; Levin, 1977; Lieblein, 1980; McMon-

Contact Lens Practice. Edited by Montague Ruben and Michel Guillon.
Published in 1994 by Chapman & Hall, London. ISBN 0 412 35120 X

nies & Parker, 1977; Myers, 1985; Remba, 1979, 1981a,b; Young, 1982). Furthermore, it has been demonstrated that when patients have ocular requirements necessitating a toric hydrogel lens in one eye and a spherical lens for the contralateral eye, good vision from the spherical eye can compensate for the slightly diminished acuity in the astigmatic eye thus creating a situation in which binocular acuity was acceptable (Attridge, 1979).

Some patients are critical observers who demand good vision. Certain patients may have occupational requirements that require excellent acuity and visual efficiency. Both of these groups of patients may be quite unhappy with residual astigmatism of 0.50 D (Brungardt, 1972; Remba, 1981b). From our experience, this is especially true if the uncorrected negative cylinder was against-the-rule (X090). In the past, because of the conditions imposed on the practitioner, the fitting of these visually critical patients has been a chancy and somewhat inaccurate process of repetitive trial and error.

It is now becoming evident that new contact lens manufacturing technologies, such as moulding, dual axis lathing, laser interferometry quality control devices and more precise methodologies for controlling material quality are producing more precisely made products. This makes the fitting of hydrogel toric lenses more accurate, efficient and less time-consuming. Better methods for in-practice quality control of toric lenses and for *in situ* assessment of toric lenses have also improved fitting accuracy. The fitter must decide whether a particular product will work well for their patient. If lens performance is not consistently predictable during the diagnostic lens trial fitting period, there are many different designs (or better manufacturers) to choose from in selecting an alternative toric contact lens product.

The astigmatic component of the prescription imposes a challenging set of conditions for the fitter. Skilled fitters must not only consider the ocular characteristics, but also the personality of the patient. To be efficient and to achieve a high rate of success the fitter also needs to be familiar with all the various forms of stock and custom designs of toric hydrogel lenses.

29.2 USEFUL DEFINITIONS

29.2.1 SPECTACLE ASTIGMATISM

The cylindrical portion of the refractive error manifested in the sphero-cylindrical refraction.

29.2.2 CORNEAL ASTIGMATISM

The dioptric or metric difference between the major and minor meridians of the cornea, measured by ophthalmometry.

29.2.3 RESIDUAL ASTIGMATISM

The astigmatism manifested while any contact lens is worn. This may be caused by ocular components (internal astigmatism), by certain aspects of the contact lens or by some combination of these two factors.

29.2.4 MASKING ASTIGMATISM

The reputed ability of certain designs, materials or thicknesses of hydrogel lenses to minimize or to eliminate refractive astigmatism. Alternatively, the acceptance by the patient of 'comfortably' blurred vision, seemingly precluding the need for toric hydrogel lenses.

29.3 THE CORRECTION POTENTIAL OF TORIC HYDROGEL CONTACT LENSES

Most manufacturers of stock toric lenses make available a maximum cylinder power of 2.25 D. However, custom lens manufacturers offer significantly higher powers. Clinicians have reported success in correcting astigmats with over 5.00 D of astigmatism (Lebuisson &

LeRoy, 1979; Egan & Streiter, 1985).

One must consider the overall expectations for success. In our experience, given an adequate and sufficiently varied inventory and range of diagnostic trial lens designs, with enough patience, care and perseverance, we believe it is possible to achieve at least an 85% success rate. Even before today's more efficient, better quality-controlled lens designs became available, investigators had reported a high success rate. In 1981, Remba reported a 90% success rate if one persevered with a large and varied inventory with at least three manufacturers' diagnostic trial sets. Interestingly, in 1985 when better quality control was possible, Remba reported an average 77% success rate after a maximum of three lens changes with six manufacturers diagnostic trial lenses available, a lower rate of success than in 1981, presumably because his expectations for success increased.

29.4 THE SPECIAL DESIGN CHARACTERISTICS OF A TORIC HYDROGEL LENS

There are five basic designs used either individually or in combination, to stabilize lens rotation. These are:

1. Inferior truncation.
2. Double truncation (i.e. superior and inferior).
3. Thin zones (also known as 'dynamic stabilization' or 'double slab-off').
4. Back surface toricity.
5. Wedge profile (prism).

Most manufacturers prefer to combine more than one of the above mentioned design features into their proprietary design. The wedge profile design (prism) seems to be the most frequently chosen stabilizing feature. Examples of combinations of design features used in proprietary products are prism with inferior truncation, thin zones with back surface toricity, prism with back surface toricity, etc. The success of these design features first depends on the production skills of the manufacturer. Precision in manufacturing and quality-controlling the design features of a lens are most important factors in efficient and successful toric lens fitting. Accurate reproducibility of the design and the dynamic function of the lens are also important elements in the fitting process. Remba (1981a) conducted a retrospective investigation of 100 patients. He used in office quality control tolerances of ±0.25 D from nominal spherical power and such generous tolerances as ±0.50 from nominal cylinder power and ±5° from cylinder axis. He found that lens quality and inaccurate labelling accounted for 27% of failed fits.

29.4.1 TRUNCATION DESIGNS

Truncations help to stabilize the meridional orientation of a toric lens. This stabilization is affected by the distance of the upper and lower lid margin positions relative to the lens periphery, the angles of the lid margins and by the pressure of the lids, especially the upper lid (Holden, 1975; Burnett Hodd, 1976a; Tomlinson *et al.*, 1978; Grant, 1986; Snyder & Talley, 1989). Truncations also serve as easily visible references for assessing the meridional orientation of the lens. Truncations may allow for better local tear movement as a marginally tightly fitting lens will usually be seen to be tight around the lateral circumference, even when the truncated areas cause no local conjunctival compression and resultant compression ring. A truncation will typically reduce the vertical lens diameter by 0.5 mm to 1.5 mm. Proper edge finishing of the truncation is critical in preventing mechanical insult to the cornea and/or limbal region.

Inferior truncation (single truncation) (Fig. 29.1)

Tomlinson and Bibby (1982) investigated the effect of a single truncation (in a design that did not incorporate a prism) on the rotational

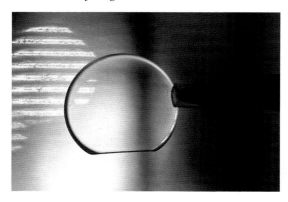

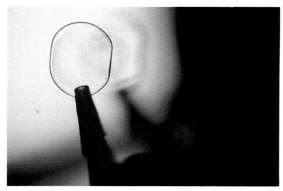

Figure 29.1 A toric lens with an inferior trunca-tion (single truncation).

Figure 29.2 A double truncated toric lens design.

performance of toric lenses having cylinders varying from 1.00 D to 4.00 D with axes of 90° and 180°. They found that a single truncation was an effective aid for stabilizing the orien-tation (rotation) of toric hydrogel lenses. These results supported the similar conclu-sions of their earlier work (Tomlinson *et al.,* 1978). They also observed that for astigmats ⩾ 1.00 D and <2.00 D fitted with a Durasoft® lens having a single truncation but no prism, the lens rotated significantly less than a double truncation design made in the same material. Typically, the single truncation design is rarely used alone – it is used in combination with a wedge construction (prism). The combination of a single trunca-tion with prism is one of the two designs preferred by the authors and by others (Burnett-Hodd, 1976a; Davy, 1976) and will be discussed later in the chapter (see pages 640–4).

Double truncation (Fig. 29.2)

Lens performance

Bayshore (1975, 1977) and Strachan (1975) and, more recently Cheshire (1980), reported an 80% success rate with two different double truncated lens designs. However,

double truncations are not always effective in stabilizing lens rotation. For example, they were found to be inadequate for stabilizing spherical Durasoft® hydrogel lenses (Tomlin-son *et al.,* 1978).

Fitting

The use of a trial lens set manufactured with this design feature is essential (Bayshore, 1975). Custom-made torics can be designed with non-parallel truncations to take advan-tage of atypical lid angles in meridional alignment (Bennett, 1976) (see pages 643, 647). Most manufacturers do not offer this custom design service. In fact, because of the difficulties in precisely finishing the edges of the truncation and controlling the reproduc-ibility of lens performance, this design has proven to be unpopular with most manufac-turers and some clinicians.

Each truncation reduces the effective sagit-tal value, equivalent to a 0.20 mm flattening of the base curve. Therefore one should 'think' 0.40 mm steeper to compensate in fitting a double truncated lens. Ideally, for optimal fitting efficiency (only practical in a large specialized contact lens practice) we sug-gest a 42 lens trial fitting set with powers of plano/–1.50 × 090; plano/–1.50 × 180; +3.00/–1.50 × 180; +3.00/–1.50 × 090; –3.00/–1.50 × 180; –3.00/–1.50 × 090. The base curves should range from 7.60 mm to 8.80 mm, in 0.2 mm steps, for each power. We do not suggest a spherical power fitting set (although it would be a much smaller investment) because of our experience with inconsistent lens rotation between the spherical trial lens and the toric lens recieved. Cheshire (1980) suggested that even the spherical double truncated trial lenses may assume a different meridional orientation than lenses of the same design that incorporate a cylinder on the front surface. Thus, predicting lens rotation with a spherical trial set or even a small double truncated spherical power fitting set would be difficult.

We have observed that this lens design does not stabilize consistently because of the thicker centre (and thinner periphery) and steeper front surface curve required for the hyperopic lens. One blink and the higher plus powered lens may rotate 90 degrees off axis.

The typical total diameter is 13.70/11.80 mm. Occasionally, a larger lens is needed and a total diameter of 14.50/12.70 mm may be employed. We have observed that these lenses work best for myopes and low hyperopes with a prescription less than +2.00 D. In order for the truncations to effectively stabilize the lens orientation, it is necessary to make the lens thicker than a typical spherical lens design. In our experience, a thin lens made in this design rarely works adequately. Perhaps because of the necessary increased thickness, it has been customary for this design to be manufactured in a high water content material (70% or greater), to maximize the oxygen permeability of the material in an attempt to increase the oxygen transmission through the thick lens.

Method of fitting

The first lens selected for fitting the patient should be 0.4 mm flatter than flattest K. If the base curve of the lens is too steep and/or the diameter too large, causing the lens to be too tight, it will move very little. The retinoscopic reflex may also appear distorted. If the base curve of the lens is too flat and/or the diameter of the lens too small, the loosely fitting lens will move excessively with blinking and the patient will experience excessive awareness. A lens that fits well will show 0.50 mm to 0.75 mm of vertical movement with blinking and will centre relatively well (minimal lag) with ocular versions. It should provide good consistent vision between blinks. The retinoscopic reflex should appear clear and undistorted.

Once the lens has settled, record the orientation of the optimal fitting lens design diagrammatically *as part of the prescription*. Future reference to this diagram will simplify fitting and problem-solving at future visits. In addition, this diagrammatic information will help in confirming the consistency of the meridional orientation of duplicate lenses or new prescriptions.

Precautions about truncations

It is very important when using truncations to be careful that the lens fits so that it completely covers the cornea. This avoidance of corneal exposure will minimize the incidence of corneal epithelial desiccation. Such exposure, when it occurs, is typically observed in the inferior limbal region. It is important not to truncate excessively or to use lens diameters that are too small. Consider figures 29.3a and 29.3b, a fit that is too small, and 29.3c, a fit that is too loose and probably too flat. If the lens is fitted too tightly it will cause hyperaemia and if too loose or too flat, the lens orientation will be very unstable and the lens will be uncomfortable (Fig. 29.3d).

Disadvantages of truncations

1. An excessively thick or poorly finished edge may lead to patient failure because of excessive lower lid sensation.
2. The squared-off edges of an improperly finished edge of the truncation may

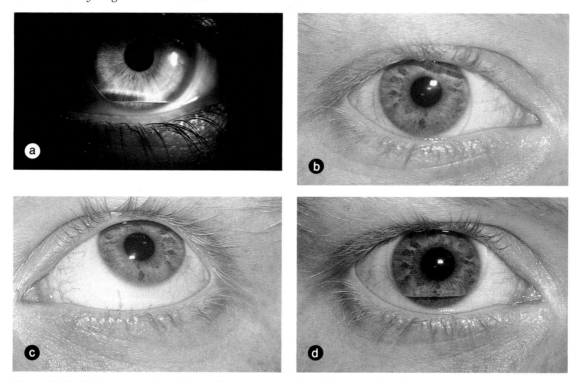

Figure 29.3 (a) A truncated toric lens that is too small and that is riding (positioning) slightly high and temporal; (b) a truncated toric lens that is fitting too flat and that is riding (positioning) slightly high; (c) a truncated toric lens that is fitted slightly too loose and that lags excessively during up gaze; (d) a loosely fitting toric lens exhibiting unstable orientation.

cause abrasion in the limbal region. This will present as corneal epithelial staining after fluorescein is instilled, and local conjunctival injection.

3. Insufficient contact lens coverage of the cornea can result in local corneal epithelial desiccation and, in some rare cases, if the condition is not resolved, this can eventually result in local corneal vascularization and opacification.

4. There have been difficulties in producing consistently good, precisely defined truncation edges.

5. There have been difficulties in manufacturing the lens dimensions in a consistent fashion from lens to lens so that visual performance is consistently achieved when lens parameters are duplicated.

29.4.2 THIN ZONES DESIGNS

Fanti (1975) first reported using the thin zones design. The superior and inferior anterior peripheral portions are slabbed off to thin them down relative to the lateral lens portions that are exposed in the interpalpebral fissure (Figs 29.4, 29.5). This thickness differential causes the lens to be aligned in the interpalpebral fissure by the angle and squeezing pressure of the eyelids (mostly the upper lid), in an attempt to control and limit the meridional orientation of the lens (Hanks, 1983). The thin zone wedge shape

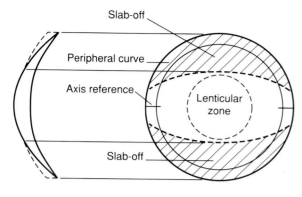

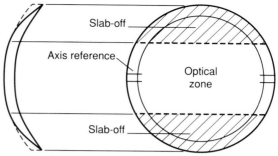

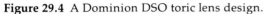

Figure 29.4 A Dominion DSO toric lens design.

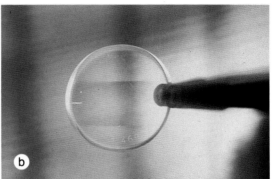

Figure 29.5 (a) The cross-section and frontal view of a thin zone toric lens; (b) the Titmus Eurocon Weicon T Design.

(apex superior, base inferior) of the superior section of the lens interacts with the upper lid in a similar way to a prism wedge. The lower thin zone (base superior, apex inferior) helps the lens align with the lower lid margin in a manner of action somewhat similar to that of a truncation (Grant, 1986). If plus power lenses are to be prescribed, the lens periphery needs to be lenticularized. This is because the relatively uniform, increased thinness of the periphery of the plus lens configuration makes lens orientation unstable (Burnett Hodd, 1976a). With thin zone torics, scribe lines are typically placed at the 0 and 180° positions of the lens, to aid in the assessment of lens orientation. The lens orientation reference line was originally referred to as the dynamic stabilization axis (DS axis) (Fanti, 1975). This is an imaginary line, which if drawn, would join the two scribe marks at the 3 and 9 o'clock positions of the lens.

Tomlinson and Bibby (1982) confirmed that the thin zone lens design concept was an acceptable mechanism for achieving a stable meridional orientation of toric hydrogel lenses. The cylinder power (typically produced within the central 8 mm portion of a lens) has been reported to have little effect on the meridional orientation of the lens (Jurkus & Tomlinson, 1979; Tomlinson & Bibby, 1982; Castellano *et al.*, 1990), although this

hypothesis has been controversial (Grant, 1986; Wechsler *et al.*, 1986).

Attridge (1979) reported difficulty in achieving stable meridional orientation with a thin zones lens design known as the Dominion DSO (see Fig. 29.4), a 'cat's-eye'-shaped version of the original thin zones design.

Lens construction

Toric hydrogel lenses with thin zones were historically constructed with a spherical back surface and with the cylinder on the front surface. Custom lens manufacturers and one large 'stock lens' manufacturer have very recently made available back toric designs with the thin zone construction.

Another proprietary version of the thin zones design reportedly achieves increased stabilization of the meridional orientation of the lens by the additional help of two toric back surfaces (a central toric zone and a different peripheral toric zone). The central zone is for correction and the peripheral zone is for stabilization (Ott, 1978). For with-the-rule astigmatism, the longer meridians of these two surface intersect at 90°, whereas with against-the-rule astigmatism, they are parallel.

Lens performance

An investigator of the DSO thin zones design observed that although only 43% of subjects achieved visual acuity of 20/20 or better, 90% of subjects enjoyed wearing the lens, even with reduced acuity in one eye (Attridge, 1979). This type of result is typical of the evidence of patient acceptance of comfortably blurred vision caused by incompletely or improperly corrected astigmatism. Levin (1977) reported 71% success with the Weicon T lens, the precursor of the Ciba Torisoft lens. No hyperopes were fitted in his study. He also reported better success with his more highly myopic subjects with corrections of −6.00 D than those subjects with corrections of − 1.75 D (Levin, 1977). This observation was later confirmed by other investigators (Castellano *et al.*, 1990). Maltzman and Rengel (1989) reported 70% success with the Ciba Torisoft. In a prospective comparison study by Remba (1985), with several toric lens designs, the success rate achieved with the Ciba Torisoft was found to be similar to the other designs tested. A success rate of 77% was achieved with an average of 1.8 lenses used to successfully fit each eye. Remba also scored and graded lens performance. The ratings were graded out of 10. The Ciba lens was graded as follows (the range of grades for all lenses assessed in the study is the second bracketed figure): performance consistency between the diagnostic lens and the ordered lens 6(5–7); subjective comfort 9(6–9); axis location consistency 6(6–7); stability of orientation 8(7–8); achievable acu-

ity 8(7–8); physiological performance 8(6–9); overall quality 8(6–8); reproducibility 7(5–8). From his data, Remba reported that the thin zones toric design seemed to be the most comfortable when compared to the other designs in the study.

Peripheral prismatic zones ('reverse prism' designs)

This design incorporates two peripheral prism sections joined together at their base (Fig. 29.6). The line of contact with the two bases, is decentred inferiorly, taking into account the more important action of the upper lid. The peripheral superior and inferior portions of the lens are the apices of the two prism sections. We have classified this design as a 'thin zone' because the superior and inferior aspects of the lens are thinner than the central section of the lens. The meridional orientation of the lens is dependent on the actions of both the upper and lower lids in a similar manner to conventional thin zones toric lenses. The central optic zone has no net optical prism effect. The centre of the optic zone is somewhat decentred from the imaginary central line that joins the base of these two 'prisms'.

Custom-made thin zones toric lenses

If ordering the thin zones design from a custom lens manufacturer, we suggest that the fitting set has a 14.5 mm or 15.0 mm

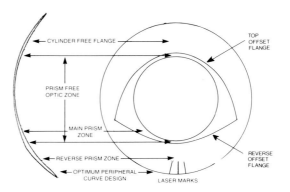

Figure 29.6 The Hydron R-P Design.

diameter, as suggested by most toric lens manufacturers. Larger diameter lenses take better advantage of lid pressure and contour and still maintain good comfort (Bennett, 1976). However, for patients with smaller palpebral fissures, since the lid pressure against the globe is greatest near the lid margins, it is best to also have available a 13.5 mm diameter trial lens set. This diameter is especially valuable in avoiding the tight lens fit characteristics if an excessively large lens design is used on a cornea with a small horizontal visible iris diameter (HVID). We recommend that this smaller lens diameter set should not be used where the HVID exceeds 11.5 mm. The base curves of the smaller diameter fitting set should range from 7.8 mm to 8.8 mm in 0.2 mm steps. The base curve range for the larger diameter set should range from 8.1 mm to 9.4 mm. Ideally, one should also have available two fitting sets for each diameter – one for hyperopes, where the arbitrary power of each lens is +3.50 D, and one for myopes with an approximate power of –3.50 D. The specialized fitter with a large contact lens practice may also wish to have a plano power fitting set.

Advantages of thin zone torics

1. The uniformly round lens design, combined with the peripheral thinness of the lens periphery makes this a relatively comfortable lens design.
2. Because this lens does not incorporate a prism, patients with significant unilateral astigmatism can be fitted with a thin zone toric design in that eye and a spherical lens in the other eye, without inducing any unwanted vertical prism imbalance.

Disadvantages of thin zone torics

1. Most manufacturers only make stock designs in one relatively large diameter. If smaller diameters are required, these designs must be made by a lens manufacturer that will make custom lens designs. Today, extremely few major manufacturers will make custom-ordered lenses.
2. In our experience with thin zones designs, when this controlling feature is used alone, they are less orientationally stable than front toric wedge profile construction lenses which are truncated or back toric wedge constructed designs. Recently, a proprietary back surface toric, thin zones design has been made available. Independent assessments of the stabilizing performance of this new lens design as compared to others have not yet been published.

Method of fitting

1. Fit a spherical lens from a thin zones design fitting set (or use a toric lens selected from a thin zones design lens inventory). Use the lens nearest to the correct spherical power. The initial base curve selected should be 1.0 mm flatter than the flattest K reading of the cornea.
2. Perform an over-refraction over the optimal fitting lens to ascertain: vertex distance corrected spherical power; vertex distance corrected astigmatic error; axis of astigmatism and visual acuity compared to spectacles.
3. Note the comfort and the initial DS axis observed by using slit lamp or retinoscope light and trial frame (as with back surface torics). Diagrammatically record the position of the DS axis. Then, check the DS axis after 10 minutes, after 20 minutes and then confirm the final DS axis, if it remains stable.
4. Record the final lens orientation diagrammatically *as a part of the prescription*. At future visits, reference to this diagram will simplify fitting and prob-

lem solving and help in confirming the consistency of the meridional orientation of duplicate lenses or new prescriptions.

5. Order the final toric lens. For example:

Refraction:	−3.50/−2.25 × 140 VA 6/5 vertex distance 10 mm
'K' readings:	7.80 mm spherical
Visible iris diameter:	12.50 mm
Best fit spherical diagnostic trial lens:	BCOR 9.00; TD 15mm −4.00D
Initial over-refraction:	+0.75/−2.25 × 140 VA 6/5
Over-refraction after 30 minutes:	Same
Trial assessment with thin zones diagnostic lens:	good comfort; initial DS axis 180; DS after 10 minutes 170; DS after 20 minutes ×170; conclusion for order: ×170
Final lens order is:	9.00 × 15.00−3.25/ −2.00 axis 150

Occasionally, one may accidentally order the astigmatic axis at the wrong angle.

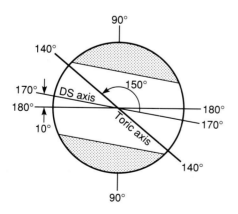

Figure 29.7 Diagram to show the correct axis and angle.

Consideration of Figures 29.7 and 29.8 helps to minimize errors in ordering the final axis specification. Sometimes, the thin zones toric will not stabilize. If this is the case such a lens design is useless. One can juggle around with the fitting to try to correct the situation, but this usually leads to fitting and/or visual complications.

In situ assessment of lens performance is important. The lens may move (mislocate, mal-orientate) through an angle of 30 degrees when the patient looks to the left and then to the right. The lens may even stabilize with its axis at 90 degrees, after heavy blinking. Clearly, one wants to be sure before ordering. It is noteworthy that the Ciba Torisoft was found to have the least rotational instability for oblique astigmatism (±6.2°). With-the-rule astigmatism showed the most rotational instability (±12.7°) and against-the-rule astigmatism showed rotational variability of ±8.2° (Castellano *et al.*, 1990). Very recently an American manufacturer (Sola Barnes Hind, Sunnyvale, California) made a back toric lens available with stabilization being achieved by the combination of back surface toricity and thin zones.

29.4.3 BACK SURFACE TORICS

Back surface toric lenses are typically made in combination with a wedge profile construction for additional orientational stability. One manufacturer uses the added stabilizing factor of a toric periphery (Ott, 1978). Maltzman and Rengel (1989) and Remba (1985) reported that they were able to achieve a significantly greater rate of success with back toric designs that front toric designs. The back surface toric wedge profile hydrogel lens design is presently one of our two most preferred toric lens designs.

Back toric contact lenses can only correct corneal astigmatism. Therefore, careful analysis is necessary to predict the pres-

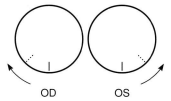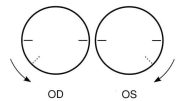

For lenses with scribe marks at the bottom of the lens, if the mark drifts to the left (clockwise), the degrees of rotation from the 6 o'clock* position are *added* to the patient's refractive axis. If the mark drifts counter clockwise, *subtract* the degrees of rotation from the patient's refractive axis.

For lenses with scribe marks at the medial and lateral sections of the lens (3 and 9 o'clock), if the markings rotate clockwise, *add* the degrees of rotation away from the 3 and 9 o'clock* positions to the patient's refractive axis. If the lens rotates in a counter clockwise direction, *subtract* the degrees or rotation from the patient's refractive axis.

*A useful guide is 30° = 1 clock hour.

Figure 29.8 How to order the toric lens cylinder axis from observations made in a trial lens fitting.

ence of any astigmatism not caused by the anterior corneal surface. More than 0.25 D of 'internal' astigmatism may contra-indicate the use of this design, unless by trial fitting and over-refraction analysis, residual astigmatism of 0.25 D or less is found (Burnett Hodd, 1976b, 1977; Gasson, 1977).

Fitting

An empirical method of ordering a custom back toric design

Empirically fitting a custom design is eco-nomically risky and very time-consuming and should only be a last resort; however, it is possible (Edwards, 1982). The laboratory will need to know the two curves and the axis of the cylinder in relation to the prism axis. You will need to do a simple calculation from effectivity tables. Let us take an example:

Refraction: R +12.00/−1.75 × 130
L −3.00/−4.00 × 28
Vertex distance 10 mm

VID: R 12.00 mm
L 12.50 mm

K readings: R 8.44 mm along 130
8.08 mm along 40
L 7.94 mm along 28
7.34 mm along 118

Best fitting
spherical lens: R 8.70 mm/12.50 mm
L 8.00 mm/13.00 mm

Using effectivity tables and rounding off to the nearest 0.25 D (note one has to take each meridian separately and take the difference to get the effective cylinder), ocular refraction is:

R +13.64/−2.22 × 130
L −3.00/−3.63 × 28

From Table 29.1:

Surface power for radius 8.70 mm is   51.13 D
Add ocular cylinder   2.22 D
                                       ───────
                                        53.35 D

The nearest value from Table 29.1 is 8.30 mm.

Table 29.1 Surface powers for refraction index ($n = 1.4448$)

Radius (mm)	Surface power (d)	Radius (mm)	Surface power (d)
6.0	74.13	8.0	55.60
6.1	72.92	8.1	54.91
6.2	71.74	8.2	54.24
6.3	70.60	8.3	53.59
6.4	69.50	8.4	52.95
6.5	68.43	8.5	52.33
6.6	67.39	8.6	51.72
6.7	66.39	8.7	51.13
6.8	65.41	8.8	50.55
6.9	64.46	8.9	49.48
7.0	63.54	9.0	49.42
7.1	62.65	9.1	48.88
7.2	61.78	9.2	48.35
7.3	60.93	9.3	47.83
7.4	60.11	9.4	47.32
7.5	59.31	9.5	46.82
7.6	58.53	9.6	46.33
7.7	57.77	9.7	45.86
7.8	57.03	9.8	45.39
7.9	56.30	9.9	44.93

From Table 29.1:

Surface power for radius 8.00 mm is   55.60 D
Add ocular cylinder   3.63 D
                                      59.23 D

The nearest value from Table 29.1 is 7.50 mm.

So we need to order the following back surface torics:

R 8.70 × 12.50/+13.75 T130
   8.30

L 8.00 × 13.00/−3.00 T 28
   7.50

The T line (toric axis) is the negative axis or the flattest corneal meridian. Both lenses should be made with the prism base 270° (manufacturers generally recommend from 0.75 to 2 prism dioptres; we typically prefer to start with 1.5 prism dioptres).

The finished lenses are inscribed with a horizontal line on the front surface near the edges at the 'true 180° axis' of the lens. Unfortunately, the lens does not always settle with these lines orientated along the 180 degree meridian of the eye. There are various reasons for this, such as the angle of the lid margins, lid pressure and unforeseen differences in peripheral corneal topography. When the lens aligns at the incorrect angle, the visual acuity is affected.

Table 29.2 will not be helpful if the lens is wrongly engraved so that the true 180° line engraving is misaligned. The major problem with back surface torics, particularly with those that are custom made, is in the accuracy of manufacture. The practitioner can only base his decisions on an existing lens when trying to determine the next lens in the sequence of fitting. If, from our example, the left lens (cyl −3.63) settled at 10 degrees then, from Table 29.2, the resultant cylinder would be:

Table 29.2 Residual refractive error induced by mislocation of toric lenses of various cylindrical powers (after Holden and Frauenfelder, 1973)

Mislocation (degrees)	−1.00 DC	−2.00 DC (×2)
5	+0.08 −0.16 × 42.5	+0.17 −0.34 × 42.5
10	+0.17 −0.34 × 40.0	+0.35 −0.69 × 40.0
15	+0.26 −0.52 × 37.5	+0.52 −1.04 × 37.5
20	+0.34 −0.69 × 35.0	+0.68 −1.37 × 35.0
25	+0.43 −0.85 × 32.5	+0.85 −1.69 × 32.5
30	+0.50 −1.00 × 30.0	+1.00 −2.00 × 30.0
35	+0.57 −1.14 × 27.5	+1.14 −2.29 × 27.5
40	+0.64 −1.28 × 25.0	+1.29 −2.57 × 25.0
45	+0.71 −1.42 × 22.5	+1.41 −2.83 × 22.5
50	+0.76 −1.53 × 20.0	+1.53 −3.06 × 20.0
55	+0.82 −1.64 × 17.5	+1.64 −3.28 × 17.5
60	+0.87 −1.73 × 15.0	+1.73 −3.46 × 15.0
65	+0.90 −1.82 × 12.5	+1.81 −3.63 × 12.5
70	+0.94 −1.88 × 10.0	+1.88 −3.76 × 10.0
75	+0.96 −1.93 × 7.5	+1.93 −3.85 × 7.5
80	+0.98 −1.97 × 5.0	+1.97 −3.94 × 5.0
85	+0.99 −1.99 × 2.5	+1.99 −3.98 × 2.5
90	+1.00 −2.00 × 180	+2.00 −4.00 × 180

Counter-clockwise mislocation (+); clockwise mislocation (−).

(+0.17/−0.34 × 40) × 3 axis 40 + 28
= +0.51/−1.02 axis 68
≈ +0.50/−1.00 axis 70

In the hydrated state, it is very difficult to measure the back surface radii or the relationship of the axis of astigmatism to the prism ballast with the accuracy that is required. This is best accomplished by using a 'wet cell' to hold the lens. This is why it is so important when the lenses are made that they be very carefully inspected in the dry state prior to hydration. If the lens settled at 170 degrees the resultant cylinder would be:

= +0.51/−1.02 axis (−40 +28)
≈ +0.50/−1.00 axis 170

As the cylinder rotates off the axis clockwise then, using Table 29.2, the axis should be added negatively. As the cylinder is off axis counter-clockwise, then the axis should be added positively.

To re-order the lens we change the T axis. So, if the left lens aligned at 10 degrees then

we should need to re-order:

$$\frac{8.00 \times 13.00 -3.00 \text{ T18}}{7.50}$$

If the lens is aligned at 170 degrees then we should need T38.

When the remade lens arrives, one would hope that the desired amount of rotation will be achieved so that the lens markings should again align at 10 degrees or 170 (these markings are set perpendicularly to the base–apex line). If this does not occur, there will be an unpredictable result. Then, all one can do is to re-inspect the powers, axis, prism alignment and inscribed orientation marks of the lenses supplied and try to find the error either in manufacture or in calculation. Because one is relying on the back surface toricity and the prism wedge–lid interaction to align the lens, altering the back surface toricity in relation to the prism may not produce the expected 10 degree swing. Thus, we may find that it is not always possible to correct the corneal astigmatism with a back surface toric. If success is not possible after one logical remake, then our advice is to try a front surface toric design, as making a third lens out of sheer desperation is rarely successful.

Back surface toric with prism ballast and a single truncation

To fit this type of lens one uses the same fitting method as previously discussed for back torics and for fitting thin zone toric lenses. The use of the larger lens and the truncation may create better stability and better vision.

Lens performance

Levin (1977) reported a 92.75% success rate on a group of 69 subjects, having first tried a thin zone toric and where that was not successful, trying a wedge design back toric and a wedge design front toric with truncation. Ivins (1984) reported 85% objective success and 71% subjective success with a randomly selected population of subjects fitted with a wedge construction back toric lens. Furthermore, with a group of problem patients who had previously failed with other types of contact lenses for various reasons (discomfort, vision, physiology, etc.) Ivins reported 46% objective success and 63% subjective success. Egan and Streiter (1985) achieved over 85% success with a randomly selected

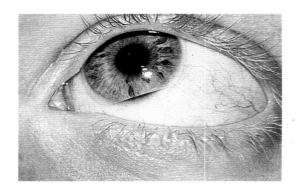
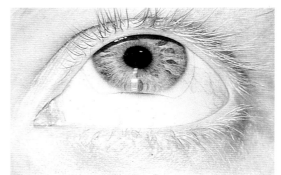
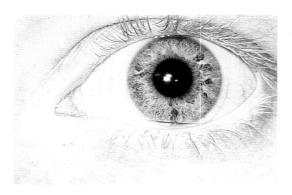
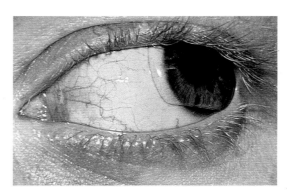

Figure 29.9 The Hydron wedge profile, truncated front toric lens, seen to be stable when the patient is looking in different positions of gaze.

group of subjects with from 1.00 D to 6.00 D of refractive astigmatism, using a back toric, wedge construction lens design with a relatively small diameter (14.0 mm). Maltzman and Rengel (1989) reported a success rate of 93% using 2 brands of back toric lenses as compared to a success rate of 78% achieved with a combination of 4 different front toric lenses. Remba (1985) reported a success rate of 83% with a wedge construction back toric, using 1.7 lenses per eye. In this study, he assessed the quality of the Hydrocurve II toric and graded lens performance out of 10 (the range of grades of all lenses assessed in the study is given in brackets): trial lens ordered agreement 5(5–7); subjective comfort 9(6–9); axis location 7(6–7); stability of orientation 8(7–8); achievable acuity 8(7–8); physiological performance 9(6–9); overall quality 7(6–8); reproducibility 6(5–8).

29.4.4 WEDGE PROFILE DESIGNS (PRISM)

The single truncation, wedge profile, front surface toric was one of the first designs manufactured to stabilize a toric soft lens (Figs 29.9, 29.10 and 29.11). This design, used since the early 1950s for rigid corneal lenses, was expected to work equally well with soft lenses.

In 1969, Gene Hirst's laboratories in New Zealand and Australia were first able to suc-

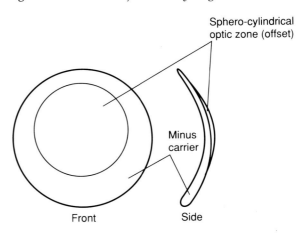

Figure 29.11 A peri-ballast lens design (front and side view) (courtesy of *International Contact Lens Clinic Journal*).

cessfully manufacture soft torics using this principle. Since then, the design has been refined. Lenses are now typically made with 0.75 mm to 1.50 mm inferior truncation and with a wedge of 0.75 to 2 prism dioptres.

Comments about the wedge profile design

The wedge profile design increases the thickness of the inferior portion or the lens. It is the combination of this wedge profile and lid pressure (Forst, 1984, 1987; Hanks, 1983; Josephson & Caffery, 1990; Kilpatrick, 1983), not the weighting some authors have attributed to prism 'ballast' and the effect of gravity (Cohen, 1976; Grant, 1986; Holden, 1975, 1976; Maltzman, 1983; Ott, 1978; Snyder & Talley, 1989; Van Wauwe, 1977; Weissman, 1984b; Westerhout, 1981), that causes the design to orientate in a stable fashion. Gravity has virtually no role in wedge profile (prism) design lens rotational stability and alignment. Thus, the term 'prism ballast' is a misnomer when used in this context; the wedge profile design is thinnest at the top (apex).

With very thin construction toric designs, any uneven thickness across the lens can lead

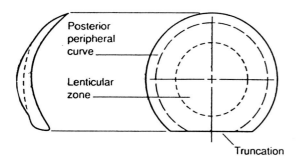

Figure 29.10 A wedge profile design toric hydrogel lens with a single truncation (front and cross-section view).

to problems of asymmetric changes in lens parameter as the thinner portions of the lens dries. The drying effect on the lens can have an exaggerated effect on the lens shape in areas where there may be abrupt changes of corneal contour, such as in the limbal region. In particular, some buckling of the inferior-nasal truncation corner is often seen to occur. This is both uncomfortable and may affect vision. It may also affect the meridional orientation stability of the lens. When this occurs it may be necessary to increase the amount of prism or to increase the overall thickness of the lens. Alternatively, but less successfully, if the lens is truncated, the truncation diameter may be decreased. Care is required in this modification so that the cornea does not become significantly exposed.

The disadvantages of the wedge design

1. Increased lens awareness at the lower lid margin.
2. The increased thickness of some wedge designs can cause reduced oxygen transmission in the region of the cornea covered by the base of the lens. Sometimes this may be clinically unacceptable, particularly if the eventual result is local vascularization.
3. There will be a prismatic imbalance between the two eyes if only one eye requires a toric lens. Although the deviation of light by prism when looking at a distance object is exactly the same on the eye as it is in air, when looking at a near object, the prism effect is reduced, depending on the amount of vergence of light from the near object and the position of the line of sight relative to the optical centre of the lens. The result at near is that the overall prism effect is usually half of what it would be expected to be when measured on the eye (Mandell, 1967 and personal communication, 1990). A prism-corrected

spherical lens may be required to correct the other eye if the measured imbalance is determined to be clinically significant. However, in practice, this is seldom necessary and a spherical lens without prism may be used (Gasson, 1980). Adaptation to vertical prism appears to be rapid. Investigators have reported that it may be complete within 3 minutes when using 2▲ of vertical prism (Ellerbrock, 1950; Henson & North, 1980). A more recent study indicated that most patients typically adapt during the first hour (Eskridge, 1988). In addition, although adaptation does occur, it is rarely complete (Rustein & Eskridge, 1985).

4. The thicker lower edge may attract deposits which may lead to irritation of the lower lid and more frequent lens replacements.
5. A higher incidence of vascularization in the inferior section of the cornea (Solomon, 1987). Vascularization may be caused by a contact lens related factor other than hypoxia (Josephson & Caffery, 1987).

The peri-ballast design

This design confines the wedge profile to the lens carrier (it has an offset lenticular construction). Although prism is not incorpo-

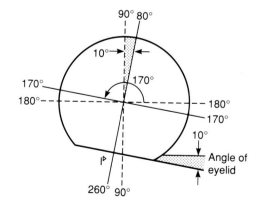

Figure 29.12 A schematic diagram example of a truncated toric lens *in situ*.

rated in the optical zone area (Fig 29.11), the construction is based on the wedge design.

A front surface toric design with prism ballast and a single truncation

Let us take an example (shown diagrammatically in Fig. 29.12):

Refraction:	$-10.00/-4.00 \times 80$; VA 6/6; vertex distance 10 mm
K readings:	7.80 mm along the 80° meridian
	7.50 mm along the 165° meridian
Visible iris diameter:	11.75 mm
Best fitting spherical diagnostic lens:	$8.20 \times 14.00 -3.00$ D
Over-refraction:	$-7.00/-4.00 \times 80$; VA 6/6
Power required allowing for effectivity:	$-8.89/-2.83 \times 080$

The truncation position aligns at the 170° meridian and is also in alignment with the lower eyelid.

Final order:
8.20 × 14.50 –8.75/–2.75 × 090
          13.00

Single inferior truncation at 180 degrees
1 ▲ axis 090°

(Note. The toric lens ordered is 0.50 mm larger in diameter than the best fitting spherical lens because the truncation effectively loosens the fit. The increased diameter compensates the fit for the reduced sagittal value in the meridians of the truncation.)

Aligning the truncation with the lower eyelid will make it more stable between blinks. In a custom design, one can adjust the angle of truncation to try to increase rotational stability. If, in our example, the truncation had not aligned at 180° but at an angle of 10° in relation to the lower eyelid, then the truncation would have needed to be reordered at 170 degrees. The order would then become:

8.20 × 14.50 –8.75/–2.75 axis 080
          13.00

Single inferior truncation at 170 degrees
1▲ axis 090

Similarly, if the eyelid was horizontal (aligned with the true 180° meridian) and the truncation aligned as per Figure 29.12, then the truncation would be at an angle of 170° in relation to it. To compensate for this rotational tendency, the truncation would need to be ordered at an angle of 10 degrees.

Most times, one finds that the lens is quite stable even though the truncation does not align with the lower eyelid. If this is the case, then one need not change the truncation angle. It is simpler if one does not have to bother with the extra calculation.

Sometimes, it may be that the final lens will still align incorrectly. In this case another lens has to be ordered with a change in the axis in relation to the prism base–apex line.

With a custom design, it is better initially to err the fit on the tight side because it is possible to loosen the fit by decreasing the truncation diameter. The angle of truncation can also be adjusted to achieve better alignment with the lower eyelid. The custom manufacturer has to carefully dehydrate the lens before carrying out these adjustments.

Performance of wedge construction, front toric hydrogel lenses with truncation

Lebuisson and LeRoy (1979) in a prospective investigation of 62 patients (105 eyes) with from 2.00 D to 5.00 D of spectacle astigmatism, fitted with a wedge profile, front toric, truncated hydrogel lens design, achieved 68% success for 72 eyes with the first lens fitted, 91% success for 91 eyes after one exchange and 95% success with 100 eyes, after the second exchange. However, in a later report, Remba (1985), working with more than one type of lens, including the lens design above, reported 48% success rate with the first lens ordered.

Van Wauwe (1977) reported an 81.5% overall success rate. Maltzman and Rengel (1989) reported an overall average success rate with three different hydrogel torics (including the one discussed above) of 82%. Remba (1985), using four different manufacturers' wedge profile, front toric designs, two of which were truncated, achieved an average overall success rate of 76%. Interestingly the average success rate for the two truncated designs was the same (76%) as the non-truncated designs. The moulded toric design was found to be the most reproducible.

29.5   SMALL DIAMETER LENS DESIGNS

Small diameter toric lens designs, typically less than 14.0 mm in diameter, are infrequently used today. Strategically, this design is best used for eyes in which the horizontal visible iris diameter is less than 11 mm. The characteristics of lenses that are fitted too steep or too flat are the same as for those characteristics of the large lens design.

29.6   THE EFFECT OF CORNEAL SHAPE ON LENS ROTATION

Corneal shape has been reported to affect hydrogel lens rotation (Harris *et al.*, 1975, 1976). However, these conclusions have been inconsistent and have been disputed (Tomlinson *et al.*, 1978).

29.7   THE EFFECT OF 'SETTLING TIME' ON THE STABILIZATION OF LENS ROTATION

Investigators have demonstrated that measurements of lens rotation at 30-minute intervals were consistent over a 4-hour period (Tomlinson *et al.*, 1978). Thus, during a fitting, it is unnecessary for lenses to settle for more than 30 minutes (Pennington, 1977). In our experience, and that of others (Scarborough & Lopanick, 1979), 20 minutes is a practical settling time.

29.8   FITTING TORIC HYDROGEL CONTACT LENSES

29.8.1   SELECTING THE APPROPRIATE DESIGN AND PARAMETERS: SCREENING PROSPECTIVE PATIENTS

The following observations and ocular measurements may be used in selecting the most appropriate contact lens design and parameters:

K readings and the contour angle

K readings, in particular 'flattest K', are used as a starting point in selecting the base curve and the lens diameter. The fitting increment chosen (the difference between the flattest 'K' reading and the selected base curve) is dependent on the lens design chosen and the overall lens diameter initially selected. The contour angle is the angle bound by sclera and cornea and with the limbus as apex of the angle. It has been our experience that flat corneas (flattest K ≤41.00 D) seem to have relatively large HVIDs (≥11.75 mm) and relatively obtuse contour angles (Fig. 29.13). For this ocular profile, we typically select relatively large diameter lenses (15.0 mm) and use a relatively small 'fitting increment' (the difference between the base curve selected and the flattest K reading). Conversely, steep cornea (K ≥45.00 D) would seem to have smaller HVIDs (≤11.50 mm) and more acute contour angles (Fig. 29.14).

We prefer to concern ourselves with refractive cylinder rather than corneal cylinder in determining when a toric hydrogel lens is required.

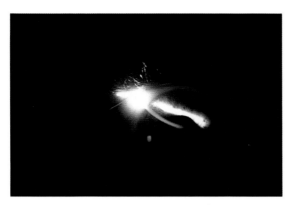

Figure 29.13 An obtuse contour angle.

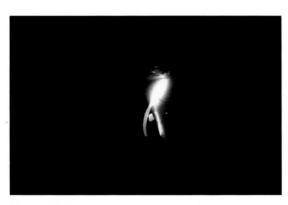

Figure 29.14 An acute contour angle.

The effect of the contour angle and the selection of lens base curve and diameter

The fitting increment for flatter corneas (flattest K ≤41.00 D) is usually less than for steeper corneas (flattest K ≥44.50 D). Thus, one might select a base curve only 2.00 D (1.0 mm) flatter than the flattest K for a cornea that has a flat K of 39.50 D and 4.00 D flatter than a flattest K reading of 45.00 D, for a steeper cornea. It is best to use a trial lens of known parameters to make this assessment. With very acute contour angles, we prefer to use a relatively small lens diameter. If the contour angle of the inferior nasal cornea is particularly acute relative to the inferior-temporal contour angle, it is best to use a lens

diameter that is so large that the differences in curvature are minimal between the nasal and temporal areas where the edges lay on the bulbar conjunctiva, and thus would have very little effect on the fitting performance of the lens.

Horizontal visible iris diameter (HVID)

Our rule of thumb for corneas with HVIDs ≥11.5 mm is to initially select a lens with an overall diameter ≥14.5 mm. For HVIDs <11.5 mm, we initially select a lens with an overall diameter of 14.0 mm.

The prescription

The spectacle prescription can be an aid to selecting the most appropriate toric lens design. In our experience, patients with a spherical component that is nearly emmetropic, can be the most difficult to satisfy visually, especially if the cylindrical component is relatively high (Remba, 1979; Hanks & Weisbarth, 1983). In the first place, those individuals who are nearly emmetropic when fitted with a contact lens, in our experience, tend to be very critical of their visual quality. Those individuals with higher cylindrical components and nearly emmetropic spherical components are very critical of the visual effects produced by any axis misalignment of the lens (Hanks & Weisbarth, 1983). Another concern with these patients is that the manufacturer's power tolerance is ±0.25 D. With an *Rx* that has a spherical component of either plano, –0.25 D or +0.25 D, the visual effects of that tolerance factor in proportion to the overall prescription is substantial. Moreover, when these patients with nearly emmetropic spherical components have a cylinder *Rx* of 0.50 D to 1.00 D, a 0.25 D difference in cylindrical power due to the manufacturer's power tolerances of ±0.25 D has a significant effect on the patients subjective assessment of vision. The adverse effect of all of these factors is compounded when both the spherical and cylindrical components are off 0.25 D in the same direction.

Thus, one must cautiously accept prospective patients with these refractive characteristics. It is best to avoid those nearly emmetropic individuals who are obviously most critical as they are almost impossible to satisfy.

If one must fit these types of patients, it is best to try to use lenses that are inventoried in the office so that a few lenses in the required power range are immediately available. It is always necessary to carefully verify the power and axis of an inventoried lens before insertion. If the patient cannot be fitted from inventory, we prefer to fit a custom-made wedge profile, truncated toric lens to obtain optimal meridional orientation stability and reduced effects of lens drying (which we have found to be less of a problem with thicker lenses).

The spherical spectacle *Rx*

For prescriptions greater than –9.00 D, unless the HVID is less than 11 mm, we will initially select a lens diameter of 14.5 mm for HVIDs of 11.0 mm to 11.5 mm. For HVIDs greater than 11.5 mm but less than 12.5 mm we select a 15.0 mm diameter lens.

The cylindrical *Rx*

Initially we prefer to select lenses with a diameter of at least 14.5 mm for all toric lenses. For cylinders of 2.50 D or greater we prefer to use lens diameters of at least 15.0 mm. For these higher cylindrical power lenses, we also prefer to use wedge construction designs that use one or more other stabilizing design features.

Some investigators have reported that toric lenses requiring an oblique cylinder, have a less stable meridional orientation because of the effects of lid pressure on the thickness differentials of the lens (Holden, 1976;

McMonnies & Parker, 1977). However, with more recent designs, investigational results have not completely supported this concept (Tomlinson & Bibby, 1982; Young, 1982; Castellano *et al.*, 1990).

It is important to remember that with higher cylinder powers, the axis alignment is much more critical and small mislocations in axis alignment will have a much greater effect on vision, visual comfort and visual acuity. With higher spherical powers and cylindrical powers less than 1.50 diopters, axis misalignment of up to 9 degrees may be tolerated by some patients.

The effect of the amount of cylinder and cylinder axis position on lens orientation

Anecdotal comments have been made by some clinicians that the lens power and axis orientation affect the lens orientation and blink initiated rotation of the soft toric lens. Tomlinson and Bibby (1982) investigated toric lenses with axes at 90° and 180° and with cylinder powers ranging from 1.00 D to 4.00 D in 0.25 D steps. Cylinder power was found not to affect blink initiated rotation for any of the power comparisons tested. However, their stability tolerances of meridional orientation for the truncated lens would not be considered acceptably consistent for today's clinical expectations.

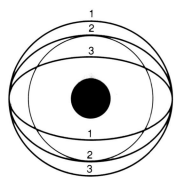

Figure 29.15 Positions of upper and lower lids.

The positions of upper and lower lids (Fig. 29.15)

Common Upper Lid (UL) Positions (P)

1. Above the superior limbus.
2. Tangent to the superior limbus.
3. Below the superior limbus.

Common lower lid (LL) positions (P)

1. Above the inferior limbus.
2. Tangent to the inferior limbus.
3. Below the inferior limbus.

The importance of lid position in lens selection

When the UL lies in P1, and the LL lies in P3, thin zones and truncations, design features which are reliant on lid margin pressure and tension for orientational stabilization, are less efficient. Wedge designs (prism) and/or a back toric design are more efficient stabilizing parameters for controlling lens orientation. The wedge design is strongly affected by the upper lid tension during blinking. When considering the use of the wedge design in this situation, it is necessary to ensure that the patient blinks with more than 50% lid closure for the wedge design to work efficiently. Blink training (Korb & Korb, 1970; Mackie, 1970; Korb, 1974) is recommended for those patients who blink inefficiently.

When the UL lies in position 2 and/or the LL lies in position 2, there is some freedom of choice in considering which orientation parameters would be preferred.

When the UL lies in position 3 and/or the LL lies in position 1, 'total diameter' wedge design lenses are contraindicated. However, lenticularized wedge designs that only occupy a central lenticular zone are acceptable. Truncation designs, back toric and thin zones are also indicated. Perhaps a thin zone design incorporating a back toric construction may be ideal.

Examples of lid angles that can affect lens orientation

These examples of lid angles (Figs 29.16 and 29.17) can affect the orients of thin zone and truncated (especially double truncated) lens designs.

29.8.2 THE IMPORTANCE OF ACCURATE BASELINE DATA

The accuracy of your baseline data is critical for efficient, economical and accurate end results. Thus, it is not only important to be certain of the spectacle prescription and the over-refraction results with the contact lens *in situ*, but also of the lens fit and meridional orientation alignment of the lens. In addition, it is critical that one is certain of the specifications of the lens that is being worked with, whether it is the diagnostic trial lens or the patient lens that was ordered. In order to know the optical characteristics of the lens, careful lens inspection techniques are required.

29.8.3 MEASURING AND INSPECTING SOFT TORIC CONTACT LENSES

Perhaps one of the most difficult tasks besetting the practice is checking the parameters of soft toric lenses. This is especially important when using custom manufactured toric lenses. Practitioners and technicians have to develop skills to detect inaccuracies or inconsistencies so that when a lens does not work

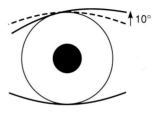

Figure 29.16 Examples of lid angles – lower lid at 180 °; upper lid at 10 °.

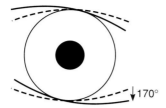

Figure 29.17 Examples of lid angles – lower lid at 170 °; upper lid at 170 °.

as expected it can be returned to the manufacturer with instructions to produce a lens that should work. It is important that both the manufacturer and the practitioner be able to measure the lenses accurately and that they can agree on their findings.

Basic equipment

A refractometer is required to measure the water content, a wet cell for holding the contact lens in a saline bath, a soft lens radiuscope to measure radius, a projection system with a wet cell to assess the diameter and central thickness, a microfilm reader or projection device for assessing lens diameter, surface and edge examination (Fig. 29.18), and a focimeter to measure the power.

A new device is also available that is pertinent to toric evaluation in particular. It is called the Tori-Check®, developed by a US company called General Ophthalmics. The device is a very helpful aid for power and axis measurement and is used in conjunction with a focimeter that has an aperture stop platform.

The following is a brief summary of how to use the Tori-Check®. By using the device the reader can fully appreciate its simplicity and effectiveness:

Step 1: pick up the blotted toric lens with the Tori-Check® (Fig. 29.19). The lens will adhere to the rotatable disc. Two discs are supplied, one for back and one for front vertex measurement.

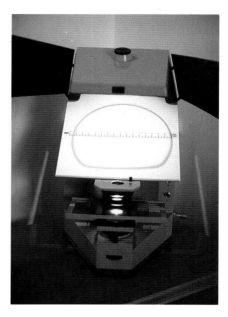

Figure 29.18 A projection device for lens inspection of diameter, surface and edge.

Step 2: rotate the disc into the proper position for toric lens measurement (Fig. 29.20). Use the markings on the lens to achieve correct alignment. Watch out for incorrectly engraved lenses. Clues to correct alignment may be in the thin zone areas or the thickness of the prism wedge.

Step 3: measure the lens power on a focimeter. The speed of measurement is important as the blotted lens will quickly dry. The inspector has to develop skill at the task and be willing to rewet, reblot and remeasure several times to confirm the result.

Step 4: measure mis-marked torics on the special protractor (Fig. 29.21). This protractor will help you to add or subtract the correct number of degrees off axis before ordering the next lens.

Inspection (verification) of lens optics

To begin, first inspect the optics of the lens; we prefer to use a vertical projection vertometer. This unit utilizes a vertically positioned

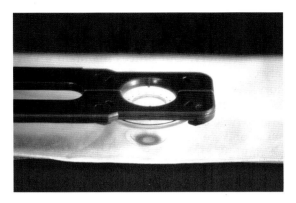

Figure 29.19 Picking up the lens with the Tori-Check® device.

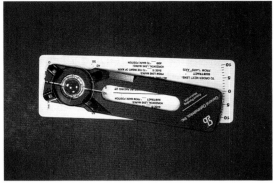

Figure 29.21 The Tori-Check® with protractor.

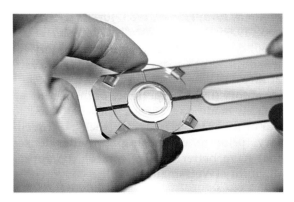

Figure 29.20 Rotation of the lens with the Tori-Check® device.

stage for the aperture. The following discussions will be based on the use of this type of power inspection device.

Typically, a stage aperture stop with a 5 mm diameter is used in conventional power measurements. However, a 7 mm diameter stage aperture stop is also provided by most manufacturers. Clean the lens with a surfactant, rinse it well and then place the lens in a wet cell filled with normal saline. Mount the wet cell on the 7 mm aperture stop. Focus the mires as well as possible. If the mires cannot be focused and appear slightly doubled, this distortion is probably caused by reduced optical quality. When the

optics are good, the mires will appear sharp and clearly defined.

After inspecting the optics, remove the lens from the wet cell, quickly blot it on an unused portion of a blotting surface and properly position it on the 7 mm aperture stop. For those manufacturers that label their lenses with the front vertex power, measure the power with the concave side up. For those manufacturers that use back vertex power, measure the power with the lens mounted over the aperture stop with the concave side down. The manufacturer will indicate which measuring standard that they prefer.

A thin zones toric lens design is more difficult to accurately ascertain whether the cylinder axis is properly aligned with 'true 180°' meridian marked on the lens (marked by scribe marks) (Fig. 29.22: the example shown has three reference lines). It is also difficult to ascertain that the scribe marks are positioned properly relative to the thin zones. Here, the Tori-Check® device is helpful. If correctly placed, the scribe marks should be located near the lens periphery at the mid-point of the thicker zone.

If the toric lens has a truncation but no prism, the truncation can be aligned to be parallel with an imaginary line that would be tangent to the 6 o'clock position of the stage aperture stop. The cylinder axis can be

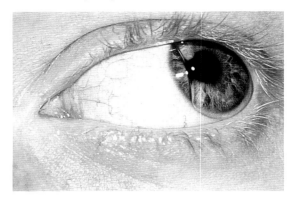

Figure 29.26 A tight fitting lens 'locked on' to an incorrect meridional orientation.

similar spherical and cylindrical powers (Ames *et al.*, 1989; Cheshire, 1980; Egan & Streiter, 1985; Gasson, 1980; Hanks, 1983; Jurkus & Tomlinson, 1979). Some fitters believe that a spherical (non-toric) trial set possessing the same design as the toric lens to be ordered, is adequate (Jurkus & Tomlinson, 1979). This is not our preference.

2.   Measure the horizontal visible iris diameter (HVID) and add 3.0 mm to select the initial overall lens diameter.

3.   Start with a base curve radius 1.2 mm flatter than 'K'.

4.   Use the flattest radius that allows the lens to centre well with no peripheral edge lift off such as seen in Fig. 29.25a (typically observed at the inferior-nasal section, immediately after a blink).

5.   Once the optimal fit is selected, allow this lens to 'settle' on the eye for 10 minutes, observe the lens orientation and then allow the lens to 'settle' further for an additional 10 minutes. Again, assess the orientation position. If it is unchanged at the second observation, then confirm by observation that the lens is moving freely with blink induced lens motion.

6.   Over-refract and combine the resultant prescription with the confirmed refrac-

tive power of the lens.

7.   Note the position of the scribe marks and the lens orientation and then record this information diagrammatically *as part of the prescription*. Make certain that the axis orientation correlates with the lens orientation, or compensate for any difference in the meridional orientation for the cylinder axis to be ordered. If the orientation of the scribed line(s) have drifted (rotated) clockwise from the true 180° meridian (or true 270° meridian, depending on where the scribe marks are placed on the lens) then add the angular difference between the position of the scribe mark and the 'true' 180° or 270° meridian to the spectacle prescription axis in order to arrive at the axis to be ordered (see Fig. 29.7). If the scribe mark drifts counter clockwise from the 'true meridian', then the angular difference must be subtracted from the spectacle prescription axis to arrive at the axis to be ordered. If the lens is truncated, the truncation rotation may be used in the same way as the 3–9 o'clock position scribe marks to arrive at the axis to be ordered.

29.14   A SUMMARY OF THE CHARACTERISTICS OF A WELL FITTING LENS

1.   Good centration: the lens should be centred relative to the cornea. It may sag slightly in the primary position of gaze on depression of the lower eyelid.

2.   Acceptable movement: there should be a movement of 0.50 mm to 1.5 mm on blinking. On upward or lateral gaze, the lens should lag from 0.75 mm to 1.50 mm, but recentre quickly.

3.   Meridional orientation should be stable.

4.   A clear, uniform retinoscopic reflex that does not significantly fluctuate with blinking, should be demonstrated.

5.   Good, non-fluctuating visual acuity.

6. An over-refraction with a definite (clear) end point should be demonstrable.

7. The fit should not cause constriction of the perilimbal conjunctival blood vessels.

8. The fit should not cause any significant visible conjunctival compression mark to be observed immediately after lens removal.

9. The lens should demonstrate a good 'edge lift' with the push up test (Josephson, 1977, 1978) (Fig. 29.27). The observers thumb is used to push the patient's lower lid against the inferior-nasal edge of the contact lens and in an upward and slightly temporal direction. The lower edge will be seen to slightly lift away from the conjunctiva or to show a slight rippling while the lens is digitally moved approximately 2–3 mm.

29.15 THE MARGINALLY STEEP (TIGHT) FITTING LENS

Because a toric contact lens needs to be fitted to achieve stability, there is a tendency to fit too tightly or with too little movement. A lens that is only slightly steep (or tight) is the hardest to detect, especially if the practitioner is not watching for it. It is also potentially the most insidious fit as it can result in

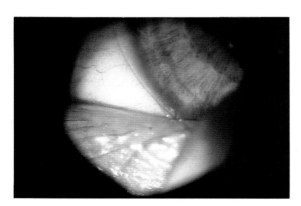

Figure 29.27 Inferior nasal edge lift off produced by using the push up edge lift test.

slightly reduced and/or fluctuating vision and some mild corneal and/or conjunctival complication when the practitioner or patient is least expecting it. It may even cause the patient to fail with their toric lenses 'for no apparent reason'. Thus, fitters must always be alert for the potential of the marginally tight or steeply fitted hydrogel contact lens.

29.15.1 CHARACTERISTICS OF A MARGINALLY TIGHT LENS

1. Good comfort and an apparently good fit with seemingly adequate movement and no obvious impingement on the perilimbal conjunctival vessels.

2. Immediately after lens insertion, small air bubbles may be observed under the lens, especially in mid-periphery, which may clear over time (after about 20 minutes), rather than after several hard, fast blinks performed immediately after lens insertion.

3. If the lens orientation is not correct immediately after contact lens insertion or is disturbed during wear, it may only return to the correct meridional location very slowly, or less frequently; the lens may lock on to the new and incorrect orientation position (Bennett, 1976).

4. Within 2–5 minutes after lens insertion, vision may appear 'quite good'. Visual acuity in each eye may initially be as good as with spectacles. However, over time, especially after one or more hours of wear, visual quality will seem very slightly reduced and may appear to fluctuate immediately after a firm blink. The patient will report that the letters of a visual acuity chart appear sharper for a split second immediately after a hard blink. As the patient continues to stare before the next blink, the letters will gradually appear to become less clear or to fade completely. With continued staring, the bottom one or two lines of the

chart may become completely unreadable.

5. If the patient is asked to blink hard several times, the retinoscopic reflex may appear uniform and sharp for a few seconds, and as the patient stares for a few more seconds, the reflex will gradually appear slightly distorted.

6. When the contact lens is inspected on the eye with the keratometer, slightly distorted keratometric mires may be seen between blinks, especially after staring for 20 seconds.

7. Perilimbal hyperaemia may present towards the end of a day of wear or after several days or weeks of all day contact lens wear.

29.15.2 ASSESSING LENS MISALIGNMENT (MALORIENTATION)

Table 29.2, taken from figures published by Holden and Frauenfelder (1973), shows theoretical residual errors produced by a misalignment of the lens. Dain (1979) also published tables relating the spherocylindrical over-refraction axis to the mislocation, assuming that the lens power was labelled correctly. If an accurate over-refraction can be taken, then this table, in theory, should indicate the axis compensation required. However, we prefer to pre-inspect the exact power and axis of the lens relative to the scribe marks. If there is prism incorporated, we compare the axis of the prism alignment with the scribe marks or truncation, if present, to make sure that both are correctly placed. Then, having assessed the rotation of the lens relative to the true 180° meridian of the eye, we compensate the spectacle cylinder axis for the relative rotation of the lens *in situ* (adding the difference if counter-clockwise or subtracting the difference, if clockwise) (see Fig. 29.7 and Fig. 29.28).

The axis compensation required can also be measured using the graticules of the slit

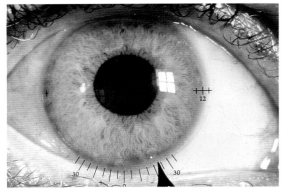

Figure 29.28 Measuring lens rotation *in situ* with a calibrated slit lamp eye piece (courtesy Sola/ Barnes Hind).

lamp or with the slit lamp eyepiece, if it has a graticule. Another method, suggested by Yvonne Schwegler, is to use high molecular weight fluorescein to make the engravings stand out. A trial frame with a single graticule (e.g. a thin wire) is placed on the patient. The trial holder is turned and the graticule aligned with the engravings using either the slit lamp, retinoscope or ophthalmoscope (approximately +10.00 D). Other methods use estimation from multiple markings on the lens as compared to the markings of a clock (i.e. each hour on a clock corresponds to 30°) (Bennett, 1976).

Most toric lens designs will orient with some up-nasal rotation. That is, if the lens is perfectly placed on the eye with the 'true' 0/180° meridian of the lens aligned with the 0/180° meridian of the cornea, the lens will, over a period of about 10 minutes, rotate to a position such that the 0/180° meridian located by noting the scribe marks at the lens periphery, is more upwards and nasal, and will stabilize in that up-nasal position from 4° to 15° from the 0/180° meridian of the cornea (Hanks & Weisbarth, 1983; Castellano *et al.* 1990).

It is best to check the rotational stability of the diagnostic trial lens or the lens to be dispensed, after it has settled (approximately

20 minutes). The stability should be assessed after several firm blinks while the patient looks in the primary position of gaze. One should also assess the stability, with blinking, while the patient looks up, down, and with upward and downward versions. The lens orientation alignment should not vary by more than ±7° with this rather extreme ocular motion. If it does, try another diagnostic lens of similar power and with the same base curve, diameter and design. If the second lens is stable, then one must assume that there may be a quality control problem with the original lens and that it should be reordered or another lens tried with the same characteristics in order to see which action it will mimic, the action of the first lens or the second. This will allow one to make a final decision as to the cause. If the second lens demonstrates the same instability, the patient should be refitted with another toric design.

29.15.3 PRECAUTIONS ABOUT PATIENTS REPORTING READING DIFFICULTIES

If reading difficulties are experienced with an apparently correct fitting lens, one that also manifests no significant over-refraction at distance, one must consider three possible causes: age, increased accommodative demand and fit. The answer that the patient is an early presbyope and having difficulties is an easy one. Also, when a myope is switched to contact lenses, there is an increased accommodative demand induced. More subtle concerns are slight axis misalignment with down gaze, or the effect of a marginally steep fitting lens.

29.15.4 WEARING TIMES

Naturally, one would hope to adapt a patient to all day wear, as with a spherical soft lens. However, it is not always possible because toric lenses are typically thicker than spherical lenses and can have reduced oxygen transmission especially in some of the lower water content designs. It is important to caution the patient before fitting, that a reduced wearing time may be necessary to ensure the long term health of the cornea. The toric soft lens patient who only wants lenses for sport and social uses, is ideal. Discretion in clinical judgement is necessary.

29.15.5 PHYSIOLOGICAL CONCERNS SECONDARY TO TORIC HYDROGEL LENS WEAR

The main complication of toric hydrogel wear that has visual implications and thus may obscure correct fitting diagnosis in follow-up examinations, is hypoxia and the subsequent corneal clouding that can cause reduced visual quality and acuity. This condition may be observed with the slit lamp, evident by observing corneal striae or folds and/or generalized epithelial haze. Scattered epithelial microcysts may also be seen. Corneal vascularization, typically seen in the inferior corneal region with wedge construction designs, especially those with a relatively low water content, may be seen after more than 6 months of continuous daily wear.

Superficial punctate epithelial keratitis may be observed with the slit lamp, using intense white light direct illumination. After lens removal, the lesion may be seen to stain with fluorescein. Typically, the area affected is slightly below the geometric centre of the cornea and often takes a 'smile' like pattern. Because of this, this presentation is sometimes described as 'smile keratitis' (Josephson, 1976). It is thought to be caused by epithelial desiccation caused by pervaporation (Zantos *et al.*, 1986; Orsborn & Zantos, 1988). Unless the central corneal region is obscured by this lesion, vision usually remains unaffected. In our experience, using a lens with a moderate water content material (if a higher water content material was previously used) or increasing the thickness of the lens (consider the implications of possible hypoxia and corneal oedema) may eliminate this complication. Otherwise try reducing the wearing time or consider refitting the patient with a rigid oxygen permeable contact lens.

Hyperaemia, occasionally accompanied by chemosis adjacent to the limbus, typically in the temporal or inferior region, may occur secondary to wearing a lens that is fitting too tightly (assuming that an adverse reaction to a solution preservative is not a factor). Sometimes this tightness is difficult to detect (see previous comments about marginally tight fitting lenses) and at other times more obvious (see comments about tight fitting lenses).

29.15.6   TORIC HYDROGEL LENSES FOR SPORTS

One fitter, with a special interest in fitting athletes with contact lenses has suggested large, thin and tight fitting lenses. He also anecdotally reported subjective visual improvement if a yellow tint is incorporated in the lens (Johnson, 1990). Personally, we agree with the large lens philosophy, we are neutral about lens thinness but disagree with the concept of prescribing tight fitting lenses. We are unable to comment on the effectiveness of the yellow tint.

29.15.7   ASPHERIC LENSES FOR THE 'CONTROL' OF ASTIGMATISM

Over the past few years, there have been anecdotal reports about the astigmatic correcting effects of special designs incorporating aspheric front surfaces. It has been claimed that astigmats with less than 1.5 D of astigmatism benefit from this lens design and do not require a toric hydrogel correction. In fact, claims have even been made for its superiority over toric lens correction (Lydon, 1990).

Beyond quoting the observations and results of this investigator's work, we must concern ourselves with the scientific methodology. The conclusions reached are questionable. First, the author claims that the lens is aberration-free but has provided no evidence for this claim. Second, although the author showed commercial advantages to this product, he provided no data to show that the advantage was statistically significant. His observations that the aspheric lens was noticeably superior is biased as his study was not conducted in a masked fashion. Furthermore, in the toric lens wearing group considered, there was no mention that they were either initially successful or that the subjects had no over-refraction (i.e. that they were fitted and properly corrected).

Thus, although the authors were able to demonstrate that these subjects were able to achieve satisfactory visual acuity under different light conditions, they failed to scientifically demonstrate a statistically significant advantage of this lens. In fact, there have been no controlled studies performed with this lens that have been published in any noteworthy peer reviewed journals.

29.15.8   SUCCESS VERSUS FAILURE

In papers published in the literature, varying degrees of success in toric soft lens fittings have been recorded with numerous definitions of success. There are many factors cited in the literature which affect hydrogel toric lens stability and rotation, such as lens thickness, adherence between the lens and eye, lens hydration, toricity, pH, humidity, temperature, lid contour motion, tightness, the direction of blinking, the location of the lens centre of gravity and the position of the cylinder axis (Holden, 1975; McMonnies & Parker, 1977; Remba, 1979; Stone & Phillips, 1981) and different methods of screening subjects or patients for suitability, if any.

We have tried to attend to the practical parameters that one may consider and utilize in practice, such as length of wear (Forgacs & Dudak, 1975; Henson & North, 1980), lens curvature (Henson & North, 1980; Eskridge, 1988), fit (McMonnies & Parker, 1977; Eskridge, 1988) palpebral fissure size (McMonnies & Parker, 1977; Henson & North, 1980; Eskridge, 1988), corneal diameter (Henson & North, 1980; Eskridge, 1988), curvature, overall lens diameter and prism in the lens (Forgacs & Dudak, 1975; Harris *et al.*, 1977), and direction of gaze (Remba, 1979). Many difficult cases can almost always be solved with patience, perseverance, the use of multiple trial sets, attention to detail and the availability and assurance of quality custom lenses.

REFERENCES

Ames, K.S., Erickson, P. and Medici, L. (1989) Factors influencing hydrogel toric lens rotation. *ICLC*, **16**(78), 221–4.

Attridge, J.G. (1979) Dominion double slab-off front surface toric contact lens. *Aust. J. Optom.*, **62**(4), 147–51.

Bayshore, C.A. (1975) Astigmatic soft contact lenses: A report on 88 patients. *Int. Contact Lens Clin.*, **2**(1), 69–72.

Bayshore, A. (1977) Astigmatic soft contact lenses: A report on 88 patients. *Int. Contact Lens Clin.*, **4**(1), 56–9.

Bennett, A.G. (1976) Power changes in soft contact lenses due to bending. *Ophthal. Optician.*, **16**, 939–45.

Brungardt, T. (1972) The flexible contact lens. *Optom Weekly*, **March 9**, 34; 35; 36.

Burnett Hodd, N.F. (1976a) Clinical appraisal of toric soft lenses. *Optician*, **172**, 8; 11; 13.

Burnett Hodd, N.F. (1976b) How to fit soft lenses – 5 (Wolhk contact lenses: Hydroflex). *The Optician*, **July 2**.

Burnett Hodd, N.F. (1977) Toric soft lenses (Part 2). *The Optician*, **May 6**.

Burnett Hodd, N.F. (1980/81) Contact lens fitting. *International Contact Lens Yearbook*, pp. 23–31.

Castellano, C.F., Myers, R.I., Becherer, P.D. and Walter, D.E. (1990) Rotational characteristics and stabilized soft toric lenses. *J. Am. Optom. Assoc.* **61**(3), 167–70.

Cheshire, R. (1980) Double truncated soft toric contact lenses. *J. Br. Contact Lens Assoc.*, **3**(2), 56–63.

Cohen, A.L. (1976) Role of gravity in prism balasting. *Am. J. Optom. Physiol. Opt.*, **53**(6), 229–31.

Dain, S.J. (1979) Over-refraction and axis mislocation of toric lenses. *Int. Contact Lens Clin.*, **6**(2), 250–3.

Davy, M.W. (1976) Success for toric soft lenses. Letter. *The Optician*, **172**(4451), 33.

Edwards, K.H. (1982) The calculation and fitting of toric lenses. *Ophthal. Optician*, **February 13**, 106; 112; 114.

Egan, D.J. and Streiter, J.F. (1985) A clinical evaluation of the Accugel-it toric soft contact lens. *Int. Eyecare*, **1**(6), 450–3.

Ellerbrock, V.J. (1950) Toricity induced by fusional movements. *Am. J. Optom. Arch. Am. Acad. Optom.*, **27**, 8–20.

Eskridge, J.B. (1988) Adaptation to vertical prism. *Am. J. Optom. Physiol. Opt.*, **65**, 371–6.

Fanti, P. (1975) The fitting of soft torical contact lenses. *The Optician*, **169**(4376), 8; 9; 13; 15; 16.

Forgacs, L.S. and Dudak, M.G. (1975) Rotational characteristics of the Warner Lambert Softcon hydrophilic contact lens. *J. Am. Optom. Assoc.*, **4698**, 807–11.

Forst, G. (1984) Untersuchung zur stabilisierung von kontaktlinsen. 60mm colour film. Staatlitat Sathschule Fur Optik Und Fototechnik, Berlin, 1984.

Forst, G. (1987) Investigations into the stabilization of bifocal contact lenses. *Int. Contact Lens Clin.*, **14** (2), 68–75.

Gasson, A. (1973) Clinical experiences with the Bausch and Lomb lens. *Ophthal. Optician*, **Jan 20**, 6; 8; 11.

Gasson, A. (1977) Back surface toric soft lenses. *The Optician*, **174** (4491), 6; 7; 9; 11.

Gasson, A. (1980) The correction of astigmatism and hydroflex toric soft lenses. *Contact Lens J.*, **June**, 3–12.

Grant, R. (1986) Mechanics of toric soft lens stabilization. *Trans. BCLA Conf.*, 44–7.

Hallak, J. (1982) Standard soft toric lenses: A problem of orientation. *Int. Contact Lens Clin.*, **9** (4), 250–5.

Hanks, A.J. (1983) The watermelon seed principle. *Contact Lens Forum*, **819**, 31–5.

Hanks, A.J. and Weisbarth, R.E. (1983) Troubleshooting soft toric contact lenses. *Int. Contact Lens Clin.*, **10** (5), 305–15.

Harris, M.G., Rich, J. and Tandrow, T. (1975) Rotation of spin cast hydrogel lenses. *Am. J. Optom. Physiol. Opt.*, **52** (1), 22–30.

Harris, M.G., Harris, K.L., Ruddell, D. (1976) Rotation of lathe cut hydrogel lenses on the eye. *Am. J. Optom. Physiol. Opt.*, **53** (1), 20–6.

Harris, M.G., Decker, M.R. and Furnell, J.W. (1977) Rotation of spherical non-prism and prism ballast hydrogel contact lenses on toric corneas. *Am. J. Optom. Physiol. Opt.*, **54** (3), 149–52.

Henson, D.B. and North, R. (1980) Adaptation to prism induced heterophoria. *Am. J. Optom. Physiol. Opt.*, **57**, 129–37.

Holden, B.A. (1975) The principles and practice of correcting astigmatism with soft contact lenses. *Aust. J. Optom.*, **58** (8), 279–99.

Holden, B.A. (1976) Correcting astigmatism with toric soft lenses – An overview. *Int. Contact Lens Clin.*, **Spring**, 59–61.

Holden, B.A. and Frauenfelder, G. (1973) The principles and practice of correcting astigmatism with soft contact lenses. *Aust. J. Optom.*, **58**, 279–99.

Isen, A.A. (1972) The Griffen lens. *J. Am. Optom. Assoc.*, **43**, 275–86.

Ivins, P.G. (1984) Clinical evaluation of the Hydrocurve II 55 toric contact lens. *Optician*, 11–17.

Johnson, S.C. (1990) Custom lens design and sport fitting gets results for athletes. *Contact Lens Forum*, **15** (10), 17; 20; 23.

Josephson, J.E. (1973) A report on the refitting of successful Griffin Naturalens wearers with Bausch & Lomb Softlens contact lenses (Polymacon). *Am. J. Optom. Arch. Am. Acad. Optom.* **50** (5), 416.

Josephson, J.E. (1976) Hydrophilic lens case report. *Int. Contact Lens Clin.*, **3** (4), 54.

Josephson, J.E. (1977) Techniques for determining lens fit acceptability prior to dispensing hydrophilic semi-scleral lathed lenses. *Int. Contact Lens Clin.*, **4** (4), 52.

Josephson, J.E. (1978) Fitting semi-scleral lenses. *Optician*, **176**, 34.

Josephson, J.E. and Caffery, B.E. (1987) Case report: progressive corneal vascularization in a patient wearing a silicone elastomer contact lens on an extended wear basis. *Am. J. Optom. Physiol. Opt.*, **64**, 12.

Josephson, J.E. and Caffery, B.E. (1990) How prism 'ballast' helps bifocal contact lenses work. *Contact Lens Forum*, **March**, 44–6.

Jurkus, J.M. and Tomlinson, A. (1979) Prism ballasted and truncated spherical trial lenses as indicators of toric soft lens rotation. *Am. J. Optom. Physiol. Opt.*, **56**(1) 16–17.

Kilpatrick, M. (1983) Apples, space-time and the watermelon seed. *Ophthal. Optician*, **December 17**, 801–2.

Kleinstein, R.N. Simplified fitting techniques for toric soft contact lenses *JAOA*, **56**(10), 777–8.

Korb, D.R. (1974) The role of blinking in successful contact lens wear; interview. *Int. Contact Lens Clin.*, **Summer**, 52–63.

Korb, D.R. and Korb, J. (1970) A new concept in contact lens design – Parts I and II. *J. Am. Optom. Assoc.*, **41**(12), 96–108.

Lebuisson, D. and LeRoy, L. (1979) Hydron toric soft contact lenses. *Contact Lens Forum*, **April**, 49–53.

Lee, A. and Sarver, D. (1972) The gel lens transferred corneal toricity as a function of lens thickness. *Am. J. Optom.*, **49**, 35–40.

Levin, B.J. (1977) Toric soft lenses. *Contacto*, **July**, 8–12.

Lieblein, J.S. (1980) A study of the Durasoft toric contact lens for astigmatism and a fitting rationale. *Int. Contact Lens Clin.*, **Jan/Feb**, 21–5.

Lydon, D. (1990) Astigmatism control without cylinder. *Optom. Today*, **October 22**, 10; 11.

Mackie, I. (1970) *Blinking mechanisms in relationship to the development of lesions at the corneal limbus at 3 o'clock and 9 o'clock with contact lens wear.* Contact Lens Symposium, XXI International Congress of Ophthalmology, Mexico City, 1970. Karger, Basle.

Maltzman, B.A. (1983) Management of astigmatism with toric soft lenses. *Int. Ophthalmol. Clin.*, 33–56.

Maltzman, B.A. and Rengel, A. (1989) Soft toric lenses: Correcting cylinder greater than sphere. *CLAO J.*, **15**(3), 196–8.

Mandell, R.B. (1967) Prism power in contact lenses. *Am. J. Optom. Arch. Am. Acad. Optom*, **9**, 573–80.

McMonnies, C.W. and Parker, D.P. (1977) Predicting the rotational performance of toric soft lenses. *Aust. J. Optom.*, **April**, 130–8.

Muckenhirn, D. (1978) A new type of soft toric lens. *Int. Contact Lens Clin.*, **5**(6), 51–64.

Myers, R.I. (1985) Off axis fitting of soft toric contact lenses. *Int. Eyecare*, **1**(7), 486–8.

Orsborn, G. and Zantos, S. (1988) Corneal desiccation staining with thin high water content contact lenses. *CLAO J.* **14**(2), 81–5.

Ott, W. (1978) Soft toric contact lenses. *The Optician*, **175** (4534), 29; 32; 33.

Pennington, N. (1977) Toric soft lenses. *The Optician*, **October 7**.

Remba, M.J. (1979) Clinical evaluation of FDA approved toric hydrophilic soft contact lenses (Part I). *J. Am. Optom. Assoc.*, **50**(3), 289–93.

Remba, M.J. (1981a) Clinical efficacy of toric soft lenses. *Int. Contact Lens Clin.*, **Nov/Dec**, 26–9.

Remba, M.J. (1981b) Clinical evaluation of toric hydrophilic contact lenses (Part II) *J. Am. Optom. Assoc.*, **52**(3), 211–21.

Remba, M.J. (1981c) Soft toric lenses. In *Complication of Contact Lenses* (eds. D. Miller and P. White), Little Brown and Co, Inc, Boston, MA, pp. 113–21.

Remba, M.J. (1985) Clinical evaluation of contemporary soft toric lenses. *Int. Contact Lens Clin.*, **12**(5), 294–303.

Rutstein, R.P. and Eskridge, J.B. (1985) Clinical evaluation of vertical fixation disparity. Part III. Adaptation to vertical prism. *Am. J. Optom. Physiol. Opt.*, **62**, 585–90.

Sarver, M.D., Ashley, D., Van Every, J. (1974) Supplemental power effects of Bausch & Lomb Soflens contact lenses. *Int. Contact Lens Clin.*, **1**, 100–9.

Scarborough, S.T. and Lopanick, R.W. (1979) Simplified computer fitting of toric hydrophilic contact lenses. *Rev. Optom.*, **116**(4), 52–4.

Snyder, C. and Talley, D.K. (1989) Masking of astigmatism with selected spherical soft contact lenses. *J. Am. Optom. Assoc.*, **60**(10), 728–31.

Solomon, J. (1987) Cited in Weisbarth, R.E., Clutterbuck, T.A. and Shannon, B.J. (1987) Comparison of toric hydrogel contact lens designs. *Int. Contact Lens Clin.*, **14**(6), 227.

Stone, J. and Phillips, A.J. (eds) (1981) Contact Lenses: A textbook for practitioners and students, Vol. 2, Butterworth, Boston, MA, pp. 555–70.

Strachan, J.P.F. (1975) Correction of astigmatism with hydrogel lenses. *Optician*, **170** (4402), 8–11.

Tomlinson, A., and Bibby, M.M. (1982) Lid interaction and toric soft lens axis location. *Am. J. Optom. Physiol. Opt.*, **59**(3), 228–33)

Tomlinson, A., Jurkus, J. and Bibby, M.M. (1978) Evaluation and control of Durasoft lens rotation. *Am. J. Optom. Physiol. Opt.*, **55**(6), 365–70.

Van Wauwe, L. (1977) The aspheric toric Hydron lens. *Optician*, **October 7**, 893–5.

Wechsler, S., Ingram, T. and Sherill, D. (1986) Masking astigmatism with spherical soft contact lenses. *Contact Lens Forum*, **11**(9), 42–5.

Weissman, B.A. (1984a) A general relation between changing surface radii of flexing soft contact lenses. *Am. J. Optom. Physiol. Opt.*, **61**, 651–3.

Weissman, B. (1984b) Clinical soft lens power changes. *Int. Contact Lens Clin.*, **11** 342–6.

Westerhout, D.M. (1981) Toric soft lenses. In: *Contact Lenses (II)* (eds. J., Stone and A Phillips), Butterworths, London.

White, P. and Scott, C. (1982) Update: toric soft contact lenses. *Contemporary Optom.*, **1**(1), 19–24.

Young, G. (1982) Bausch & Lomb toric soft lenses. *Optician*, 14–24.

Zantos, S., Orsborn, G., Walter, H. and Knoll, H. (1986) Studies in corneal staining with thin hydrogel lenses. *J. Br. Contact Lens Assoc.*, **9**(2), 61–4.

Richard E. Weisbarth

Over the last several years, the 'focus' on contact lenses has been on colour. As a result, tinted contact lenses have become a very common lens modality. Major advantages of tinted hydrogel contact lenses include improved lens visibility for handling purposes, the option to enhance or change eye colour, and the ability to absorb specific wavelengths of light.

30.1 APPLICATIONS OF TINTED LENSES

30.1.1 LENS VISIBILITY

Lens tints provide the advantage of better lens visibility for handling, thereby reducing damage or loss. A tinted lens is easier to see on the finger, in the lens case, on the eye or when dropped (Fig. 30.1). Also in the event a lens becomes decentered, a tint makes it much easier to locate when under the lid.

'Handling tints', usually light blue in colour (number 1 intensity), are a common feature offered by most lens manufacturers and account for the largest proportion of tinted hydrogels prescribed (Fig. 30.2). Table 30.1 lists visibility tinted soft lenses which are currently available from the major lens manufacturers.

Since coloured lenses are rated as easier to handle than clear counterparts, they are extremely useful for first-time lens wearers. Additional candidates would include children, the elderly, presbyopes, hyperopes,

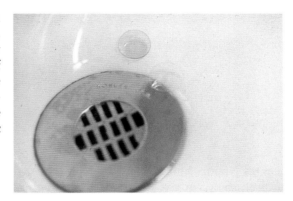

Figure 30.1 Ease of locating a visibility tinted soft lens compared to a clear lens.

low vision patients, patients with previous handling difficulties and patients with a tear or loss history.

30.1.2 COSMETIC USE

Cosmetic beautification of the eyes has been popular for thousands of years. The advent of cosmetic tinted soft contact lenses has allowed contact lenses to be a fun and fashionable vision correction alternative.

In the patient's 'eyes', cosmetic tinted contact lenses are regarded as a 'beauty accessory'. Since the tinted portion of a soft lens covers the entire iris, an extremely natural cosmetic appearance is provided. Therefore, these lenses are worn not only for the correc-

Contact Lens Practice. Edited by Montague Ruben and Michel Guillon.
Published in 1994 by Chapman & Hall, London. ISBN 0 412 35120 X

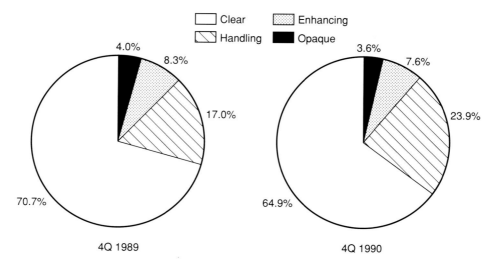

Figure 30.2 Proportions of clear and tinted soft lenses prescribed (courtesy of A. Hanks).

tion of vision ametropias but also by the emmetropic patient. Marketing data has shown that up to 30% of tinted lens wearers do not require vision correction (Golightly, 1990). It is often a difficult decision whether or not to fit the 'plano' patient with contact lenses (Jurkus, 1986b). The perception of the contact lens as a fashion accessory rather than a medical device must be approached with caution. The possible risks with a cosmetic tinted lens are the same as with any lens (Johns & O'Day, 1988).

Available in enhancing or colour-changing varieties, the lenses serve to brighten or dramatically change the colour of the eyes. This occurs because the tinted contact lens absorbs different wavelengths of light (Davies, 1989).

Most patients do not seek a dramatic change in eye colour but rather an enhancement of their existing shade (Davies, 1989). Clinical experience has shown that blue and aqua tints are used most often. Usage of different colours in a typical North American practice has been reported as aquamarine 43%, blue 32%, green 17% and amber 8% (Hanks, 1984).

Lens tints have also tended to disguise corneal arcus, producing a brighter and younger-looking eye. This is especially true of a green, amber or brown tint on a brown iris (Fig. 30.3). This effect increases the interest of the older patient in tinted lenses (Josephson *et al.*, 1985).

30.1.3   THERAPEUTIC USE

Tinted soft contact lenses can also be utilized as prosthetic devices to improve the appearance or visual function of a diseased, damaged or disfigured eye (Spinell & Bernitt 1985; Oleszewski & Wood, 1986; Key & Mobley, 1987; Comstock, 1988; Meshel, 1988; Cuttler & Sando, 1989; Shovlin, 1989).

Translucent lenses are particularly useful in cosmetically changing the appearance of corneal leukomas (Fig. 30.4), but opaque lenses are typically required for all other indications.

Lenses can be manufactured in a variety of patterns with either a clear pupil for sighted eyes or with an opaque black pupil for non-seeing eyes (Fig. 30.5). A list of prosthetic indications includes:

Table 30.1 Visibility tinted soft lenses

Manufacturer/brand	Material (H$_2$O%)	Production method	Base curve	Diameter	Powers	Colors
Allergan Optical						
Hydron Zero 4 Softblue	Polymacon (38)	Cast-molded	8.6	13.8	plano to –10.00	Soft blue
Hydron Zero 6 Softblue	Polymacon (38)	Lathe-cut	8.4, 8.7, 9.0	14.0	+10.00 to –10.00	Soft blue
Omniflex	PVP/MMA Co-polymer (70)	Lathe-cut	8.4	14.3	+6.00 to –8.00	Light blue
American Contract Lens, Inc.						
ACL 38(PES) Practice enhancement series	Polymacon (38)	Lathe-cut	8.4, 8.7	14.0	+5.00 to –8.00	Light blue
Bausch & Lomb						
Optima FW Visibility Tint	Polymacon (38)	Spun front surface, lathed back	8.7 (sag 1)	14.0	+4.00 to –9.00	Light blue
Optima 38 Visibility Tint	Polymacon (38)	Spun front surface, lathed back	8.7 (sag I), 8.4 (sag II)	14.0	+5.00 to –12.00	Light blue
Sequence Disposable Lens	Polymacon (38)	Spun-cast	Varies with power	14.0	+4.00 to –9.00	Light blue
CIBA Vision						
Spectrum Visitint	Vifilcon A (55)	Cast-molded	8.3, 8.6, 8.9 8.9, 9.2	14.0 14.5	+9.50 to –8.00 plano to –8.00	Light blue
Cibasoft Visitint	Tefilcon (37.5)	Lathe-cut	8.3, 8.6, 8.9 8.6, 8.9, 9.2	13.8 14.5	+6.00 to –10.00 plano to –10.00	Light blue
STD Visitint	Tefilcon (37.5)	Lathe-cut	8.3, 8.6, 8.9	13.8	+6.00 to –6.00	Light blue
Contact Lens (Mfg) Ltd.						
Sci-Fi	Co-polymer (77)	Lathe-cut	8.1, 8.4 8.4	13.7 14.4	+3.50 to –7.00	Light blue
Cooper Vision						
Vantage Lens	Tetrafilcon A (43)	Lathe-cut	8.7 8.3, 8.6, 8.9 8.3, 8.6	14.4 14.0 14.0	+6.00 to –10.00 plano to –10.00 +6.00 to plano	Light blue

continued

Product	Material	Type	Base curve	Diameter	Power	Color
Vantage Thin	Tetrafilcon A (43)	Lathe-cut	8.4 8.7	14.0 14.4	plano to −10.00	Light blue
Cooper Classic	Tetrafilcon A (43)	Lathe-cut	8.6, 8.9 8.7 8.6, 8.9	14.0 14.4 14.0	−0.25 to −10.00 +6.00 to −10.00 +6.00 to plano	Light blue
Menicon Menicon Soft MA	Hema (38)	Lathe-cut	7.5 to 9.0 (0.30 steps)	12.5 to 14.0 (0.50 steps)	+25.00 to −25.00	Light blue
Metro Optics Metrolite	Polymacon (38)	Lathe-cut	8.7 8.6	14.0 13.5	plano to −7.00 +20.00 to −20.00	Light blue
Sola/Barnes-Hind CSI Locator Tint	Crofilcon A (38.5)	Lathe-cut	8.0, 8.3, 8.6	13.8	+8.00 to −6.00	Light blue
Custom-Eyes 38-Lite	Polymacon (38)	Lathe-cut	8.4, 8.7	14.0	+5.00 to −8.00	Light blue
Wesley-Jessen Durasoft 3 Litetint (D3●LT)	Phemfilcon A (55)	Lathe-cut	8.3, 8.6, 9.0	14.5	+6.00 to −8.00	Light blue
Durasoft 2 Litetint (D2●LT)	Phemfilcon A (38)	Lathe-cut	8.3, 8.6, 9.0 8.0, 8.3, 8.6	14.5 13.8	+6.00 to −8.00	Light blue
Durasoft 4 Litetint	Ofilcon A (74)	Lathe-cut	8.6, 9.0	14.5	+6.00 to −8.00	Light blue

Products listed represent a range offered by a given manufacturer. Since regulatory policies and market conditions vary, not all products or parameters are available in all countries.

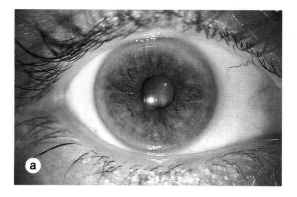

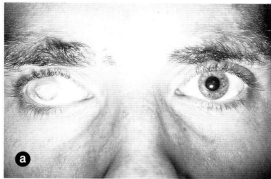

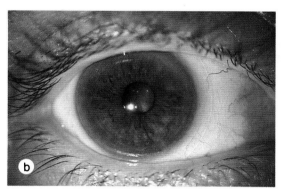

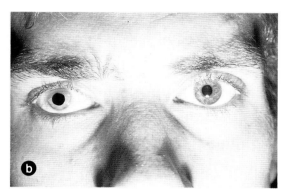

Figure 30.3 Corneal arcus. (a) Appearance of brown eye with corneal arcus; (b) same eye with a green tinted lens in place (courtesy of J. Brackbill).

Figure 30.4 Corneal leukoma. (a) Appearance of corneal leukoma secondary to trauma; (b) same patient with an ocular masking lens in place (courtesy of D. Hansen).

1. *Abnormalities of the globe*:
    i. buphthalmos.
2. *Abnormalities of the cornea*:
    i. leukoma;
    ii. bullous keratopathy;
    iii. traumatic corneal scarring;
    iv. band keratopathy;
    v. congenital anomalies;
    vi. arcus senilis.
3. *Abnormalities of the iris*:
    i. disfigured pupil;
    ii. coloboma;
    iii. aniridia;
    iv. traumatic or neurological iridoplegia;
    v. heterochromia;
    vi. secluded or occluded pupils;
    vii. inadvertent or planned iridectomies.

4. *Abnormalities of the crystalline lens*:
    i. disguising lens cataracts;
    ii. inoperable cataracts;
    iii. aphakia or pseudoaphakia;
    iv. induced photophobia;
    v. subluxated lens.
5. *Vitreoretinal abnormalities*:
    i. vitreal bleeding;
    ii. vitreous or retinal associated photophobia.
6. *Extra-ocular muscle disorders*:
    i. diplopia;
    ii. strabismus;
    iii. amblyopia;
    iv. deutranopia.

Appendix 30.A lists some of the main suppli-

Patterns available:

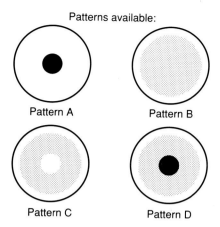

Pattern A   Pattern B

Pattern C   Pattern D

Figure 30.5 Tinted lens patterns available.

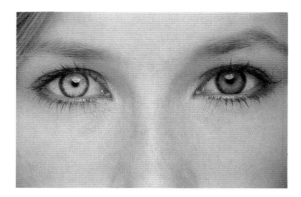

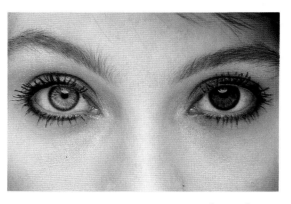

Figure 30.6 Cosmetic appearance of translucent tinted lenses. (a) Right eye – natural eye colour, left eye with an aqua CIBA Vision SOFTCOLORS lens; (b) right eye – natural eye colour, left eye with a green CIBA Vision SOFTCOLORS lens (courtesy of CIBA Vision Corporation).

ers of lenses for ocular masking/prosthetic applications.

30.2 TYPES OF TINTED LENSES

Three different types of tinted lenses are available. These are translucent lenses, opaque lenses and UV absorbing lenses.

30.2.1 TRANSLUCENT LENSES

A translucent lens is transparent, allowing light to pass through, however the tint modifies the colour of light transmitted. Depending on the tint intensity, these lenses can be used strictly for handling purposes ('light'/number 1 intensity) or for enhancing or changing eye colour ('medium'/number 2 and 'dark'/number 3 intensities).

Translucent lenses achieve a cosmetic effect by colour mixing the natural iris colour with the colour of the contact lens. The end result is an enhancement or saturation of iris colour (Fig. 30.6). This effect is most pronounced for patients with light eye colours, such as blue and grey. The effect can be quite different from one patient to another, even though the iris colour may appear similar. Predicting the approximate outcome for any

individual patient is relatively easy based upon a knowledge of the colours resulting from the additive combinations. However, diagnostic tinted lenses should be utilized at the time of fitting in order to determine the actual effect achieved (Hanks, 1984).

In addition to iris colour enhancement, translucent lenses are also effective in masking corneal leukomas and arcus senilis (Lowther, 1987).

Table 30.2 lists translucent tinted lenses offered by the major manufacturers.

Individuals with darker irises do not achieve much of an effect with translucent lenses, since the colour of the iris predomi-

Table 30.2 Translucent tinted soft lenses

Manufacturer/ brand	Material (H$_2$O%)	Production method	Base curve	Diameter	Powers	Pupil sizes(s)	Colors
Allergan Optical							
Hydron Mini Tinted	Polymacon (38)	Lathe-cut	8.1 to 9.1 (0.20D steps)	13.0	+20.00 to −20.00	4.0 4.5 5.0	Aqua, Sapphire, Emerald, Smokey quartz, Amber, Amethyst, Coral
Hydron Z4 Tinted	Polymacon (38)	Cast-molded	8.3	13.8	−0.50 to −7.50	4.0 4.5 5.0	Aqua, Sapphire, Emerald, Smokey quartz, Amber, Amethyst, Coral
Hydron Z6 Tinted	Polymacon (38)	Lathe-cut	8.4, 8.7 9.0, 9.3	14.0	+20.00 to −20.00	4.0 4.5 5.0	Aqua, Sapphire, Emerald, Smokey quartz, Amber, Amethyst, Coral
Hydron SC Tinted	Polymacon (38)	Spin-cast	Varies with power	13.5, 14.5	plano to −8.00	4.0 4.5 5.0	Aqua, Sapphire, Emerald, Smokey quartz, Amber, Amethyst, Coral
Hydron H67 Tinted	Co-polymer (67)	Lathe-cut	8.4,8.8,9.2	14.0	+20.00 to −20.00	4.0 4.5 5.0	Aqua, Sapphire, Emerald, Smokey quartz, Amber, Amethyst, Coral
Bausch & Lomb							
Natural Tint-03 Natural Tint-04	Polymacon (38)	Spin-cast	Varies with power	13.5 14.5	plano to −5.50	full iris	Crystal blue, Aqua, Jade green, Sable brown
Optima FW Natural Tint	Polymacon (38)	Spun front surf acelathed back	8.7	14.0	−0.25 to −9.00	full iris	Crystal blue, Aqua, Jade green
Optima 38 Natural Tint	Polymacon (38)	Spun front surf acelathed back	8.7 (sag I), 8.4 (sag II)	14.0	+5.00 to −9.00	full iris	Aqua, Crystal blue, Green
Natural Tint-B3	Polymacon (38)	Spin-cast	Varies with power	13.5	−0.25 to −6.00	full iris	Crystal blue, Aqua, Jade green, Sable brown.

continued

	Material	Method	Base curve	Diameter	Power	Tint	Colours
Natural Tint-U3	Polymacon (38)	Spin-cast	Varies with power	13.5	plano to –6.00	full iris	Crystal blue, Aqua, Jade green, Sable brown
Natural Tint-U4	Polymacon (38)	Spin-cast	Varies with power	14.5	–0.25 to –6.00	full iris	Crystal blue, Aqua, Jade green, Sable brown
Cantor & Silver Ltd.							
Imago	Co-polymer(72)	Lathe-cut	8.4, 8.8	13.75, 14.5	+30.00 to –30.00	to order	Blue, Green
Translucent Tinted Lens	Hema (38)	Lathe-cut	to order	to order	to order	full iris	Blue (3 Shades), Aqua green, Green, Aqua, Violet, Brown (2 shades of each)
CIBA Vision							
Cibathin Softcolors	Tefilcon (37.5)	Lathe-cut	8.6,8.9	13.8	plano to –6.00	full iris	Aqua, Blue, Green, Amber, Royal blue
Cibasoft Softcolors	Tefilcon (37.5)	Lathe-cut	8.3,8.6,8.9 8.6,8.9,9.2	13.8 14.5	+6.00 to –10.00 plano to –10.00	full iris	Aqua, Blue, Evergreen, Green Amber, Royal blue
STD Softcolors	Tefilcon (37.5)	Lathe-cut	8.3,8.6,8.9	13.8	+6.00 to –6.00	full iris	Royal blue, Evergreen, Aqua
Weicon 38E Bi-colors	Tefilcon (37.5)	Lathe-cut	Flat or Steep	13.0,13.8, 14.6	+25.00 to –25.00	full iris	Green, Blue, Aqua, Amber
Contact Lens (Mfg) Ltd.							
Aquarius Iris Tints	Co-polymer (77)	Lathe-cut	8.1,8.4 8.4	13.7 14.4	+3.50 to –7.00	3.5 4.5 5.0	Unlimited colour/pattern combinations
Cooper Vision							
Vantage Thin Accents	Tetrafilcon A(43)	Lathe-cut	8.4 8.7	14.0 14.4	plano to –6.50	4.9	Sky blue, Auburn, Violet blue, Turquoise, Spring green, Misty brown

continued

Permaflex Thin Color Collection	Tetrafilcon A(43)	Lathe-cut	8.4 8.9	13.8 14.4	plano to −6.00 plano to −6.00	4.9 4.9	Spring green, Sky blue, Violet blue, Turquoise
Vantage Accents DW	Tetrafilcon A(43)	Lathe-cut	8.3,8.6,8.9 8.7	14.0 14.4	plano to −6.50	4.9	Sky blue, Auburn, Violet blue, Turquoise, Spring green, Misty brown
Igel							
Igel CD HI-Tints (with UV inhibitor)	Hema (38)	Lathe-cut	8.3,8.5,8.7,8.9	14.0	+20.00 to −20.00	2.0 3.0 4.0 5.0 6.0	Aqua, Smokey brown, Emerald, Sapphire blue, Violet
Igel 58 Presto HI-Tints (with UV inhibitor)	Co-polymer (58)	Lathe-cut	8.4,8.8	14.5	+10.00 to −20.00	2.0 3.0 4.0 5.0 6.0	Aqua, Smokey brown, Emerald, Sapphire blue, Violet
Igel 77 HI-Tints	Co-polymer (76)	Lathe-cut	8.4,8.8,9.2	14.0	to order	2.0 3.0 4.0 5.0 6.0	Aqua, Smokey brown, Emerald, Sapphire blue, Violet
Lunelle	Co-polymer (70)	Lathe-cut	8.0,8.3,8.6, 8.9,9.2	14.0	+20.00 to −20.00	full iris	Lagon (blue), Menthe (green) Lemon (yellow), Ambre (brown)
Metro Optics							
Metrotint	Polymacon (38)	Lathe-cut	8.7 8.3,8.6,8.9	14.0 13.5	−0.25 to −7.00 +20.00 to −20.00	full iris full iris	Blue, Aqua, Green
Narcisus Contact Lens							
Red Pupil Lens (for color defect)	Ocufilcon B (53)	Lathe-cut	to order	12.0–16.0	+35.00 to −35.00	to order	Red tint to practitioner's specifications

continued

Product	Material	Method	Base curve	Diameter	Power	Pupil/iris	Colours
Ocular Sciences							
Edge II Tint	Polymacon (38)	Spin-cast	varies with power	14.0	plano to −6.00	full iris	Aqua, Blue, Green
Pilkington Barnes-Hind							
Soft Mate I Custom Eyes	Bufilcon A (45)	Lathe-cut FS Molded BS	9.0	14.8	plano to −6.00	4.5	Aqua, Green, Sapphire
Permaflex 74 Tints	Surfilcon A (74)	Cast-molded	8.7	14.4	plano to −6.00	5.0	Violet blue, Sky blue, Golden, Spring green, Turquoise
Sola Barnes-Hind							
Soft Mate Custom Eyes	Bufilcon A(55)	Lathe-cut	9.0 / 8.7	14.8 / 14.3	+6.00 to −6.00 / plano to −6.00	4.0	Aqua, Blue, Green
CSI Colours	Crofilcon A(38.5)	Lathe-cut	8.3, 8.6	13.8	plano to −6.00	4.0	Aqua, Blue, Green, Violet blue
Custom-Eyes 38L	Polymacon (38)	Lathe-cut	8.4, 8.7	14.0	+5.00 to −8.00	4.5	Aquamarine, Coca, Emerald, Sapphire
CTL-M Masking Lens	Polymacon (38)	Lathe-cut	to order	to order	to order	to order	Black pupil with tinted iris
Quadrant Contract Lenses Ltd							
Qsoft Tinted	Hema (38)	Lathe-cut	8.5, 8.7, 8.9	14.0	plano to 8.00	4.0	Sky blue, Denim blue, Garden green, Brown, Canary yellow, Sunburst orange
Thompson Contract Lenses Ltd							
Tintagel	Hema (38)	Lathe-cut	8.3, 8.6	13.8	+25.00 to −25.00	5.0	Aqua blue, Royal blue, Canary yellow, Sunburst orange, Lime green, Jade green

continued

	Material	Type	Base Curve	Diameter	Power	Tint diameter	Colours
Wesley-Jessen							
Durasoft 2 Colors D2LE	Phemfilcon A(38)	Lathe-cut	8.6 8.3, 9.0	14.5 14.5	+4.00 to –8.00 planto to –4.00	5.0 5.0	Sky blue, Jade green, Aquamarine, Violet blue
Wohlk Contact Lenses							
Hydroflex Colour Tinted	Hema(38)	Lathe-cut	8.3 to 9.7 (0.1 steps)	13.5 to 16.0	+20.00 to –20.00	full iris	Light grey, Grey green, Med. grey, Violet brown, Turquoise blue, Blue green, Brown
Hydroflex Mini Colour Tinted	Hema (38)	Lathe-cut	7.1 to 9.1 (0.1 steps)	12.0 to 13.5 (0.5 steps)	–20.00 to –20.00	3.0 4.0 5.0 6.0 7.0 or full iris	Light grey, Grey green, Med. grey, Violet brown, Turquoise blue, Blue, Green, Brown
Weflex Colour Tinted	Co-polymer (55)	Lathe-cut	8.1, 8.4, 8.7, 9.0, 9.3 8.4, 8.7, 9.0, 9.3, 9.6	13.7 14.3	+20.00 to –20.00 +10.00 to –20.00	4.0 or full iris	Green, Turquoise, Blue, Brown

Products listed represent a range offered by a given manufacturer. Since regulatory policies and market conditions vary, not all products or parameters are available in all countries.

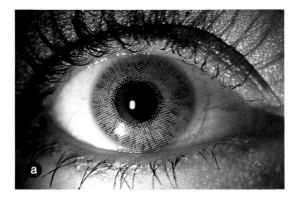

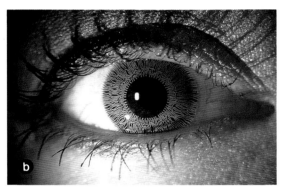

Figure 30.7 Cosmetic appearance of opaque tinted lenses. (a) ILLUSIONS lens (CIBA Vision); (b) COMPLEMENTS lens (Wesley–Jessen) (courtesy of A. Thompson).

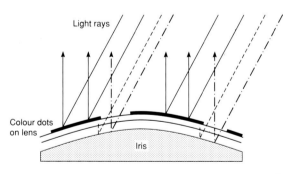

Figure 30.8 Optical principle of opaque tinted lenses (courtesy of Wesley–Jessen Corporation).

nates and cancels the desired result. This occurs because the iris stromal chromato-phores absorb the incident light. Consequently, there is very little light reflected back through the contact lens, which further darkens the eye rather than changing its colour (Davies, 1989). In order to change dark iris colours, an opaque contact lens is required.

30.2.2 OPAQUE TINTED LENSES

The second main type of tinted lens is the opaque lens, also known as 'tinted lenses for dark eye colours'. These lenses are responsible for creating a complete eye colour change, allowing a patient with brown eye colour to change to blue, green, grey or any other colour. (Fig. 30.7). Opaque lenses 'hide' the natural iris colour by totally or partially blocking the passage of light except in a central clear pupillary area. Lenses are usually created by applying an opaque agent across the iris portion of the lens. A natural or pseudo-iris pattern is then dyed or printed in or over the top of the lens using any variety of dye colors. The desired effect is achieved since light passes through the tint and is reflected back from the opacifying agent (Davies, 1989) (Fig. 30.8).

Opaque lenses available are presented in Table 30.3.

30.2.3 ULTRAVIOLET (UV) ABSORBING TINTED LENSES

Ultraviolet (UV) radiation is ever-present in our environment. It is an invisible portion of the same spectrum of energy rays that produces visible light and colours. The UV range consists of wavelengths between 200 and 400 nm, and is usually subdivided into three bands or regions: UV-C, 200–290 nm; UV-B, 290–320 nm; UV-A 320–380 nm (Pitts, 1981).

Standard non-tinted hydrogel lenses absorb little UV radiation, and the addition of a cosmetic tint still allows significant amounts of UV radiation to reach the eye (Bruce & Dain, 1988).

Table 30.3 Opaque tinted soft lenses

Manufacturer/ brand	Material (H$_2$O%)	Production method	Base curve	Diameter	Powers	Pupil size(s)	Colors
Bausch & Lomb Optima Colors	Polymacon (38)	Lathe-cut	sag I, II	14.0	plano to –6.00	5.0	Light green, Green, Blue, Hazel brown, Gray
Cantor & Silver Ltd. Imago	Co-polymer (72)	Lathe-cut	8.4 8.8	13.7 14.5	to order	to order	Blue, Green
Contact Lens (Mfg) Ltd. Aquaris Iris Tints	Co-polymer (77)	Lathe-cut	8.1, 8.4 8.4	13.7 14.4	+3.50 to –7.00	3.5 4.5 5.0	Unlimited color pattern combinations.
Aquarius	Co-polymer (77)	Lathe-cut	to order	to order	to order	to order	Hand painted iris with optional black pupil
Prosthetic Lenses	Co-polymer (79)	Lathe-cut					
CIBA Vision Illusions	Tefilcon (37.5)	Lathe-cut	8.3, 8.6, 8.9	13.8	+4.00 to –6.00	5.2	Blue, Deep blue, Green Deep green, Grey
Weicon Iris Print	Tefilcon (37.5)	Lathe-cut	8.4 to 9.6 (in 0.2 D steps)	15.0	+20.00 to –20.00	to order	Grey, Green, Blue
Weicon Iris Handpainted	Tefilcon (37.5)	Lathe-cut	8.4 to 9.6 (in 0.2 D steps)	15.0	+20.00 to –20.00	to order	Matched according to sample.
Cooper Vision Mystique Opaque Colors	Polymacon (38)	Lathe-cut	8.4, 8.7	14.2	plano to –6.00	4.75	Sapphire blue, Crystal blue, Jade green, Willow green, Pearl grey, Honey brown, Cappuccino

continued

	Material (%)	Construction	Base curve	Diameter	Power		Colours
IGEL							
Igel 58 Presto Hi-Colours (with UV Inhibitors)	Co-polymer (58)	Lathe-cut	8.4, 8.8	14.5	+10.00 to −20.00	2.0, 3.0, 4.0, 5.0, 6.0	Aquamarine, Pacific blue, Lavender, Jade, Honey brown
Igel 77 Hi-Colours	Co-polymer (76)	Lathe-cut	8.4, 8.8, 9.2	14.0	to order	2.0, 3.0, 4.0, 5.0, 6.0	Aquamarine, Pacific blue, Lavender, Jade, Honey brown
Igel 67 Hi-Colours (with UV Inhibitor)	Co-polymer (67)	Lathe-cut	8.3, 8.7	14.5	+10.00 to −20.00	2.0, 3.0, 4.0, 5.0, 6.0	Aquamarine, Pacific blue, Lavender, Jade, Honey brown
Narcisus							
Narcisus	Ocufilcon B (48)	Lathe-cut	to order	15.0	to order	to order	to order
Pilkington Barnes-Hind Ltd.							
Mystique	Polymacon (38)	Lathe-cut	8.7	14.2	plano to −6.00	4.5	Sapphire, Crystal, Jade, Willow
Wesley-Jessen							
Durasoft 3 Complements (D3●CO)	Phemfilcon (55)	Lathe-cut	8.6	14.5	+6.00 to −8.00, plano to −4.00	5.0	Blue green, Brown, Blue violet, Shadow grey
Durasoft 3 Colors (D3●OP)	Phemfilcon (55)	Lathe-cut	8.3, 8.6; 9.0	14.5, 14.5	+6.00 to −8.00, plano to −4.00	5.0	Baby blue, Sapphire blue, Emerald green, Jade green, Aqua, Hazel, Misty grey, Violet
			8.6	14.5	plano to −4.00		Chestnut brown

Products listed represent a range offered by a given manufacturer. Since regulatory policies and market conditions vary, not all products or parameters are available in all countries.

Throughout life, an individual is exposed to UV radiation from a variety of different sources. Although most of the UV radiation comes from the sun, there are also other sources. These include: welding equipment, dental equipment (denture curing), computer terminal screens, fluorescent lighting, ground reflectance from snow, sand, concrete and water (Nash, 1983).

UV radiation under various conditions of exposure has been reported to affect different structures of the eye (Pitts & Lattimore, 1987). Some of the effects are well documented, others are just beginning to be researched. Believed consequences of too much ultraviolet radiation include photokeratitis, cataract formation, uveitis and retinal problems. Ocular tissue damage occurs when UV wavelengths are absorbed and then concentrated in the eye. Research has implied that even low level UV exposure over time may have a harmful cumulative effect (Cullen, 1980). However, specific portions of the UV range are filtered out and never reach internal structures. For example, UV-C is absorbed by the ozone layer protecting the earth and does not reach the eye or the skin, UV-B is absorbed by the cornea and is responsible for skin tanning and burning effects and UV-A is the region responsible for ocular and skin damage.

Normally, the crystalline lens serves as an excellent filter and protects the retina against damaging UV radiation. However, cataract formation may still occur. Then the removal of the crystalline lens during cataract surgery leaves the retina of aphakic individuals susceptible to damage from increased admittance of UV radiation (Pitts & Lattimore, 1987).

Ocular protection from UV radiation has commonly taken the form of spectacles, goggles or shields, which use absorptive tints or filters to selectively eliminate or block the UV rays. Consequently, these are referred to as either UV-absorbing or UV-blocking lenses. A common belief is that tinted lenses (spectacle or contact lens) adequately protect against ultraviolet radiation. This is simply not true. Although some tinted lenses may block out certain UV rays, they are generally ineffective in blocking out the harmful UV-A light rays. A regular sunglass lens also does not properly absorb ultraviolet radiation and can be deceptive by providing a false sense of security (Nash, 1983). Because the sunglass lens is dark, the pupil dilates and the amount of UV radiation transmitted into the ocular media is then increased.

Recently, contact lenses have been developed which also serve to absorb UV radiation. These UV-absorbing soft contact lenses are listed in Table 30.4.

Recommended candidates for UV lenses would be patients who are prone to excessive UV exposure. Persons who may be at risk from UV exposure include:

1. Those who have had cataract surgery.
2. Those who are exposed to excessive reflections from the sun, sand, snow, concrete and water, for example, lifeguards, ski-instructors and construction workers.
3. Those on photosensitizing drugs (drugs which create reactions when individuals are exposed to sun). Examples include oral contraceptives, antibiotics, tranquillizers, sulfa-drugs and medications for acne, psoriasis and other skin problems.
4. Those exposed to artificial UV sources in their occupational environment, for example, computer terminal operators and people working under fluorescent lighting.

Since the complete ocular effects of UV are not totally understood, prescribing UV-absorbing contact lenses is currently considered to be a type of 'preventive medicine'. Conscientious contact lens practitioners use UV-absorbing lenses to protect aphakic patients and those at risk from the harmful rays of the sun. Further research

Table 30.4 UV-absorbing soft contact lenses

Manufacturer/ brand	Material (H$_2$O%)	Production method	Base curve	Diameter	Powers	Colors
Clearview Contact Lens Co.						
Clearview UV	Co-polymer (60)	Lathe-cut	to order	to order	to order	Clear
Cooper Vision						
Permaflex UV Natural	Vasurfilcon A(74)	Cast-molded	8.7	14.4	+6.00 to −10.00	Clear
IGEL International						
Igel CD	Hema (38)	Lathe-cut	8.3, 8.5, 8.7, 8.9	14.0	+20.00 to −20.00	(Translucent) Aqua, Smokey brown, Emerald Sapphire blue, Violet
Igel 58 Presto	Co-polymer (58)	Lathe-cut	8.4, 8.8	14.5	+10.00 to −20.00	Clear (Translucent) Aqua, Smokey brown Emerald, Sapphire blue, Violet (Opaque) Aquamarine, Pacific blue Lavender, Jade, Honey brown
Igel 67 Prima	Co-polymer (67)	Lathe-cut	8.3, 8.7 9.1	14.5 14.5	+10.00 to −20.00 plano to +10.00	Clear (Translucent) Aqua, Smokey brown Emerald, Sapphire blue, Violet (Opaque) Aquamarine, Pacific blue, Lavender, Jade, Honey brown

continued

Lunelle						
Lunelle ES70 UV Inhibitor	Co-polymer (70)	Lathe-cut	8.0, 8.3, 8.6, 8.9, 9.2	14.0	+20.00 to −20.00	Clear
Lunelle Aphakic UV Inhibitor	Co-polymer (70)	Lathe-cut	7.7, 8.0, 8.3 8.0, 8.3, 8.6, 8.9, 9.2	13.0 14.0	+5.00 to −12.00 +10.00 to +20.00	Clear
Lunelle Solaire (UV Inhibitor and sun filter)	Co-polymer (70)	Lathe-cut	8.0, 8.3, 8.6, 8.9	14.0	+10.00 to −10.00	Brown
Pilkington Barnes–Hind						
Permaflex 74 UV	Vasurfilcon A (74)	Cast-molded	8.7	14.4	+6.00 to −10.00	Clear
Vistakon						
UV Bloc	Etafilcon A (58)	Lathe-cut	8.4, 8.7 8.8	14.0 14.5	+4.00 to −6.00	Clear

Products listed represent a range offered by a given manufacturer. Since regulatory policies and market conditions vary, not all products or parameters are available in all countries.

relating to the effects of UV radiation will help shed more light on this complex issue.

30.3 TECHNICAL ASPECTS OF TINTED SOFT CONTACT LENSES

30.3.1 TINT CHEMISTRY

Numerous different technologies have been used to tint hydrogel lenses. Typically, lenses are tinted directly by the manufacturer. However, American Hydron (Ackerman, 1986) and Softchrome have developed and marketed systems which allow an 'in-office' tinting procedure to be used.

Translucent lenses

Dye dispersion

Dye dispersion is a process in which the dye is mixed with the chemical monomers (Maund, 1989). This allows for a uniform distribution of dye in the polymer matrix. However, one difficulty with this technique is that the dye can diffuse from the lens matrix if the lens is placed in a solution which causes the matrix to expand. Since the tint extends across the entire lens, no clear periphery is possible. In addition, there is a lens thickness effect as a result of the dye extending through the entire lens matrix. Currently, there are no major manufacturers which use this technology.

Vat dye/dispersive dyes

In this tinting process, a water soluble dye is permeated into a swollen hydrogel lens. The dye is then chemically converted into a water-insoluble form. This reaction causes the dye molecules to crystallize or aggregate together and become trapped in the matrix or pores of the lens. Under very high magnification the dye particles are visible (Lowther, 1987). The tint is normally placed on the front surface of the lens and affects only the first

few microns of the lens surface (Lowther, 1987) (Fig. 30.9) Since the vat dye is held in place by strong adsorptive forces it can only be extracted by the use of strong solvents (Maund, 1989). Examples of lenses which are tinted with this technology are the CUSTOM TINT (SOLA/Barnes-Hind/Pilkington), NATURAL TINT (Bausch & Lomb), CUSTOM-EYES (SOLA/Barnes-Hind/Pilkington), CSI-COLOURS (SOLA/Barnes-Hind), HI-TINTS (Igel) and HYDRON In-Office tinted lenses (American Hydron).

Covalent bond/reactive dyes

With the covalent bonding process, a reactive dye is exposed to a fully hydrated hydrogel contact lens for a specific period of time at a specific temperature and concentration in the presence of a catalyst. Then, through a chemical reaction, the dye is chemically bonded to the lens and becomes a permanent part of the lens material. The dye permeates only several microns into the surface of the lens (Fig. 30.10). As a result, the colour intensity does not vary with power or thickness of the lens.

Since the dyes are chemically bound to the lens polymer, they cannot migrate from or be leached from the lens. The tints can only be altered by bleaching of the dye molecule, as

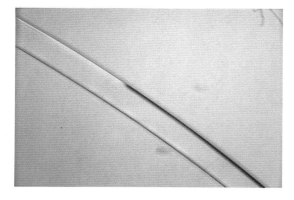

Figure 30.9 Cross-section of lens tinted with a vat dye.

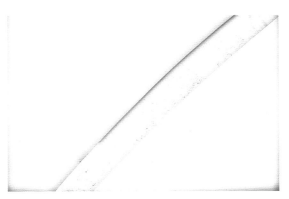

Figure 30.10 Cross-section of lens tinted with a reactive dye.

removal of the dye molecule would require destruction of the lens (Payor, 1984). Research has shown that lenses can be bleached by either strong reducing or oxidizing agents (Payor, 1984), therefore these chemicals should be avoided. Lenses which utilize covalent bonding include VISITINT & SOFTCOLORS (CIBA Vision), VANTAGE ACCENTS & PERMAFLEX THIN COLOR-COLLECTION (Cooper Vision) and SOFT-CHROME custom tinted soft contact lenses (Softchrome Inc.).

Print process

Using this technology, dye is placed on the surface of the contact lens much like ink is transferred to paper during a printing process. Therefore, the dye is concentrated on the surface of the lens. The DURASOFT 2 COLORS lens (Wesley-Jessen) utilizes this technology.

Opaque lenses

Laminate construction

Lenses of this type are produced in three stages (Wodak, 1977; Davies, 1989). First, a button is lathe cut with an annulus on the front surface. This is followed by the iris pattern being painted on with opaque paints/dyes.

Once the paint/dye has dried, additional HEMA is poured over the lens and polymerized. Finally, the material is lathe cut, leaving the iris pattern in the centre of the lens (Fig. 30.11). The disadvantage of this technology is that the oxygen transmissibility across the tinted portion of the lens is decreased. Also, the thickness of the laminate alters the lens fitting characteristics. Examples include the TITMUS EUROCON IRIS PRINT AND HAND-PAINTED lenses (CIBA Vision).

Sandwich technology

Several different methods of 'sandwich' technology can be utilized.

In one method, a three-layered button is produced which consists of top and bottom layers of clear HEMA co-polymerized with non-toxic pigments (Kerr, 1987). The button is then lathed into an ultrathin lens design. This technique is used with the MYSTIQUE lens (Cooper Vision).

Another process involves incorporating opaque pigments, carmine mica and titanium dioxide, in an iris-like pattern between two layers of HEMA. Then the desired colour is tinted on the front surface of the lens (CIBA Vision Corporation, 1991). The ILLU-

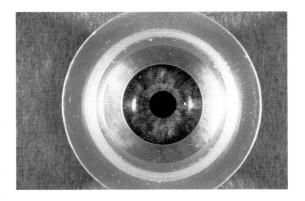

Figure 30.11 Iris print contact lens with iris and pupil imagery between two layers of HEMA (courtesy of Timus-Eurocon).

SIONS lenses (CIBA Vision) are produced in this manner.

Opaque backing

Opacifying agents can be used to block out the normal iris colour and details. Superimposed on top of this are normal tinting dyes. Light that passes through the lens is reflected by the opaque layer through the tinted layer and thus the desired iris colour is produced (Bruce & Dain, 1988; Davies, 1989). Lenses produced in this manner include the HYDRON COLORS (Hydron), HI-COLOURS (Igel) and CLM (Aquaris).

Dot matrix pattern

This technology involves printing dyes on the front surface of a hydrogel lens (Tomlinson, 1987; Golightly, 1990). A dot pattern is utilized which contains a colour, as well as an opacifying agent (Fig. 30.12). The spacing between the dots allow some of the wearer's natural iris detail to show through while at the same time the coloured dots reflect light to produce the lighter iris colour. Lenses produced with this technology include the DURASOFT 3 COLORS (Wesley-Jessen) and COMPLEMENTS (Wesley-Jessen).

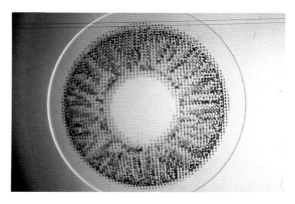

Figure 30.12 Dot matrix pattern of Wesley–Jessen DURASOFT 3 COLORS lens (as viewed from posterior side) (courtesy of J. Brackbill).

Photo-etching process

The NARCISSUS lens (Narcissus Medical Foundation) uses imagery which is similar to a photo-etching process and is stable and non-toxic (Key & Mobley, 1987).

UV lenses

Typically, the UV-absorbing agent is incorporated into the chemical formula for a given hydrogel material. Specific details are not available since this information is considered to be proprietary.

30.3.2 OXYGEN TRANSMISSION

Oxygen transmission of tinted hydrogel lenses appears to be unaffected by the addition of the dye. Studies on the major brands have shown that there is no significant difference in the oxygen transmissibility of hydrogel tinted lenses versus clear counterparts (Hanks, 1984; Kerr, 1987; Melton, 1987; Maund, 1989). Additional research has shown that equivalent oxygen percentage (EOP) remains unchanged after the addition of a lens tint (Benjamin & Rasmussen, 1986).

Hanks (1984) has reported on a pachometry study undertaken to compare corneal swelling response for clear and tinted lenses. Blue (38% H_2O content) lenses were tested against a clear counterpart of identical parameters. Lenses were worn for 4 hours and corneal thickness was measured using a Holden–Payor micropachometer. Average corneal swelling was not significantly different for the clear lenses (1.28%) versus the tinted lenses (1.13%).

30.3.3 TINT DESIGN

A feature of number 2 or 3 intensity transparent, and of all opaque lenses, is a clear peripheral band approximately 1.5 mm wide at the lens periphery. Without the clear area,

"FULL TINT"   "CLEAR PUPIL"

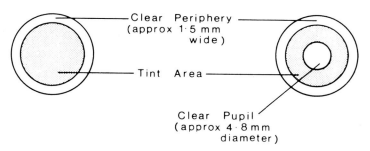

Figure 30.13 Lens design of full iris tint versus clear pupil (courtesy of A. Hanks).

tint overlap at the limbus onto the sclera would be noticeable.

Full iris tint versus clear pupil

Translucent cosmetic tinted soft contact lenses are available in two different varieties. These are full iris tint and iris tint with a clear pupil (Fig. 30.13).

The full iris tint has the advantage of completely covering the iris and pupillary area of the eye, which tends to provide a much more normal cosmetic appearance. The disadvantage of a full iris tint is a slight reduction in light transmission, since the tint occupies the pupillary area. The light transmission of a cosmetic tinted soft contact lens of 'medium' number 2 intensity is approximately 80–85%, which is similar to the transmission of a fashion tinted spectacle lens (Mandell, 1988) or unexposed photosensitive lens. Clinical experience has shown that this minor reduction tends to be of minimal concern (Hanks, 1984).

A clear pupil lens offers the benefit of allowing complete normal transmission of light through pupillary area. However, the disadvantage of a clear pupil lens is that the pupillary diameter will never completely equal the pupil size of the eye, since the normal human pupil varies in diameter,

depending upon different lighting conditions (Fig. 30.14). With a clear pupil lens, the clear pupil may often reveal portions of natural iris colour or be decentred relative to the natural pupil (Fig. 30.15). Either of these situations tends to create cosmetic and/or visual complications.

30.3.4   LIGHT TRANSMISSION

Cosmetic lenses

The amount of light transmitted through a tinted contact lens is equal to the total amount of light available minus the percent-

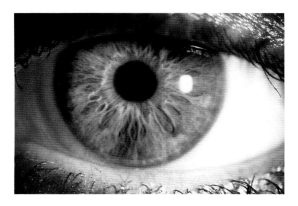

Figure 30.14 Clear pupil lens on eye. (courtesy of R. Payor).

age of light which is absorbed. By comparison, a clear spectacle lens loses 6% transmission by reflection. Transmission curves of tinted hydrogel contact lenses have been reported by different investigators.

Results show that although lenses of similar colour have similar transmission curves, the absorption peaks and corresponding wavelengths of the dyes differ greatly between manufacturers (Hammack & Lowther, 1986). Lenses with a minimum average light transmissibility of 95% have sufficient tint to improve handling without affecting iris colour (Lowther, 1987). Lenses which are intended to enhance eye colour (number 2 or 3 intensity) have 75–85% average transmission. However, the peak absorption can result in much lower transmissions at a specific wavelength (Anonymous, 1985; Lowther, 1987).

UV lenses

Due to differences in the dyes and/or monomers which are used the absorption properties are slightly different from one manufacturer to another. For example, the UV-BLOCK lens (Vistakon/Johnson & Johnson) shows little radiation transmittance below 380 nm while the cut-off for the PERMAFLEX UV lens (Cooper Vision) is slightly more gradual, with 5% transmittance at 360 nm (Bruce & Dain, 1988).

Identifying a UV lens can often be accomplished by viewing the fluorescence of the crystalline lens with a UV lamp while the lens is in place. Relative to no lens or a non-UV-absorbing lens, the UV absorber will decrease the normal crystalline lens fluorescence. Further *in vivo* determination can be accomplished by instilling high molecular weight fluorescein and viewing the lens with a UV lamp with and without a cobalt filter (Benjamin, 1986). When a UV-absorbing lens is illuminated with UV radiation, the fluorescent pattern of the post-lens tear pool is not present. However, when illuminated by light passing through a cobalt filter, the fluorescent pattern under the lens can be viewed. A technique for evaluating lenses *in vitro* has also been described (Bruce & Dain, 1988). A clear control lens and the lens to be identified can be examined in front of a fluorescein solution contained between two glass microscope slides. This method allows for ready evaluation of both rigid and hydrogel lenses.

30.3.5 FITTING PHILOSOPHIES

Tinted contact lenses are most often offered in the same lens parameters and specifications as clear lenses. Most manufacturers add the dye to an already existing and proven clear lens design. The addition of a tint does not affect the fitting performance of the contact lens. Movement, centration, lag and percentage tightness can be predicted using a clear trial lens of identical specifications. As with any soft lens, the fitting goal should be to use the flattest lens that provides good vision, fit, comfort and physiological response. The criteria of a well-fitted tinted

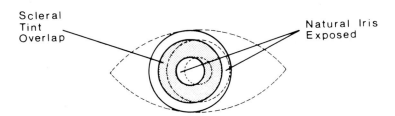

Figure 30.15 Cosmetic result of clear pupil tinted lens decentration (courtesy of A. Hanks).

soft lens are listed below:

1. Full corneal coverage.
2. Good centration (concentric about the visible iris).
3. Centration of the pupillary zone of the lens over the pupil of the eye (for 'clear' pupil lenses).
4. Satisfactory movement in up gaze. Lenses should exhibit 0.2 to 0.5 mm of movement in up gaze.
5. Satisfactory lens lag (in up gaze), a lens lag of 0.5 to 1.0 mm is ideal.
6. Satisfactory comfort response by the patient.
7. Satisfactory vision response by the patient (vision should be at least comparable to best spherical spectacle acuity).

Opaque lenses, by definition, are only available in the clear pupil variety. Therefore, care must be exercised to ensure that the pupillary zone of the lens is centred over the pupil of the eye (Jurkus, 1986b). Special consideration may be needed for the type of lighting conditions that will be most frequently encountered by the patient who wears these lenses, since this could affect visual performance, as well as cosmetic appearance (Kerr, 1987).

30.3.6 VISION

Full iris pattern

As with tinted spectacle lenses, full iris tinted soft contact lenses do not produce a change in visual acuity. Further, contrast sensitivity function (CSF) curves indicate that there is no difference between clear and tinted lenses (Lowther, 1987).

Clear pupil

As previously mentioned, lenses of the clear pupil variety require special fitting considerations relative to lens pupil diameter and centration. A decentred lens can affect visual function, but usually this is a qualitative loss rather than a quantitative one. Patients will describe a vague complaint of a haze or a spider web-type of appearance in a certain field of gaze.

Peripheral 'haziness' of vision is a common finding in opaque lens wearers. One study reported haziness in 72% of MYSTIQUE (Cooper Vision) and 59% of DURASOFT 3 COLORS (Wesley-Jessen) trials (Gauthier *et al.*, 1990). Slight aperture decentration may be acceptable and a 2-week patient adaptation period normally overcomes this effect (Melton, 1987). If a patient experiences chronic hazy vision, the lens should be checked for decentration. Centring the lens, so that the lens pupillary axis coincides with the patient's pupillary axis, will reduce subjective complaints (Daniels & Mariscotti, 1989). This can be accomplished by switching to a different lens type, different pupil size, different base curve/diameter combination (to tighten the fit), and/or to a different manufacturer's product.

In theory, a clear pupil lens could act as an aperture stop and serve to increase depth of focus. Melton (1987) has reported on DURASOFT 3 COLORS (Wesley-Jessen) producing a 'pin-hole' effect on early presbyopic patients. As a result, the add power required is typically 0.50 D less plus than would be predicted. It is stated that this power reduction improves general functioning of the patient.

30.3.7 PERIPHERAL VISION/VISUAL FIELDS

Clinical experience has demonstrated that translucent cosmetically tinted soft contact lenses do not have an effect on visual fields. However, opaque lenses have been shown to cause a disruption of peripheral vision (Anonymous, 1990a).

Recently, several authors have reported on lens induced visual field defects with DURASOFT 3 COLORS (Wesley-Jessen) opaque lenses. The extent and type of defect appear to be dependent on the type of perimeter used and the test conditions employed.

Goldmann visual field testing was performed on ten patients while wearing DURASOFT 3 COLORS (Wesley-Jessen) opaque contact lenses (Insler *et al.*, 1988). Nine out of the ten patients had visual field constriction ranging from 5° to 20°. When the areas inside the three isopters tested (I-4-e, I-3-e, I-2-e) were averaged, the amount of field loss varied from 21% to 47%. Josephson and Caffery (1987) noted a field loss of >10°, as measured with a Dicon autoperimeter. Trick and Egan (1990) found no statistically significant difference between visual field results obtained while wearing a DURASOFT 3 COLORS (Wesley-Jessen) opaque lens versus a clear lens when measured with a Humphrey perimeter. However, subjective evaluation in another study of 68 patients demonstrated that approximately one-quarter of wearers noted a field limitation (Daniels & Mariscotti, 1989). This effect was most noticeable in dusk and evening hours. Therefore, it is recommended to advise opaque lens wearers of potential difficulties in dim illumination conditions.

As previously mentioned, lenses should be fitted in a manner to provide optimal centration of the pupillary zone over the pupil of the eye. Accomplishing this goal will minimize subjective visual complaints and maximize success.

30.3.8   SCOTOPIC VISION

Scotopic vision is unaffected by 'light' tints (intensity number 1). Most 'medium'/number 2 intensity full iris tinted lens wearers function normally while wearing tinted lenses for a variety of night-time activities. However, 'dark'/number 3 intensity lenses may be too dark for dim illumination conditions.

One study examined the effects of tinted contact lenses on the reaction time and recognition probability for red signal lights in normal and color defective observers (Pun *et al.*, 1986). Reaction time was significantly increased when protanopes, protanomal and deuteranopes wore 'dark' (number 3 intensity) tinted contact lenses. Fitters prescribing such lenses should be aware of potential difficulties the lenses may pose for colour-defective individuals, especially under dim illumination conditions (Pun *et al.*, 1986). Alternatively, if a 'dark'/number 3 intensity is chosen, a clear pupil variety may be preferable.

30.3.9   COLOUR VISION

A number of different studies have investigated the effect of full iris tinted soft contact lenses on colour discrimination and colour vision.

The effect of tinted soft contact lenses on colour discrimination was studied using SOFTCOLORS (CIBA Vision) 'dark'/number 3 intensity lenses and the Lanthony New Color Test for 20 subjects with normal colour vision (Tan *et al.*, 1987). No significant difference in test performance was seen for the various tinted lenses and clear control contact lens. 'Medium'/number 2 intensity tinted lens-wearing patients evaluated with the Desaturated Panel D-15 test (Laxer, 1990) and the Farnsworth–Munsell 100 Hue test (Jurkus *et al.*, 1985; Laxer, 1990) also showed insignificant results relative to clear lenses. Results of these studies indicate that there is no effect on colour vision as a result of wearing tinted soft contact lenses.

30.3.10   COLOUR PERCEPTION

While there is no effect on colour vision, some patients do report a transient change in colour perception immediately after inserting full iris tinted contact lenses. This effect is very similar to that which occurs when first putting on a pair of sunglasses, and usually the wearer is unaware that they are viewing the world through a tinted lens.

Reports seem to indicate that these transient changes are noted most often in patients wearing amber, yellow, brown or green colours. One study using a anomaloscope demonstrated an alteration in colour perception occurred with brown and green lenses (Laxer, 1990). In both situations, there was an increase in the luminance of spectral yellow needed to make a match. A complete explanation for these colour perception differences has not been offered. However, it has been suggested that certain shades may affect foveal sensitivity, thereby slowing the adaptation process (Hanks, 1984).

30.3.11   GLARE REDUCTION

Full iris tinted soft contact lenses have been recommended for glare-sensitive subjects, although their effectiveness in reducing glare discomfort is not widely accepted.

One investigation used an Alpascope to study the relief of glare sensitivity with SOFTCOLORS (CIBA Vision) tinted lenses. Results suggested that there was no reduction in glare sensitivity when different intensities of blue or amber lenses were worn (Lutzi *et al.*, 1985a).

Many visual display terminal (VDT) operators complain of glare while working at their VDT units. A number of reports have stated that tinted contact lenses are of benefit to these patients. A clinical trial involving VDT operators showed a majority of the participants felt that amber tinted lenses provided relief from the discomfort glare they experience from fluorescent light while working at a VDT (Mousa, 1987). The investigator felt that the amber lens may decrease discomfort glare by reducing the overall brightness of the office, which is typically over-illuminated for VDT operators, and by eliminating some blue–green light, similar to shooting glasses.

It has been further hypothesized that yellow or amber cosmetic tinted soft lenses may provide clearer vision on a hazy day or under conditions where glare reduction is indicated (Janoff, 1988).

Anecdotal stories exist regarding use of these lenses in patients with corneal opacities, early crystalline lens changes or other media defects which cause debilitating light scatter. A complete physical explanation for these findings has yet to be offered. Additional studies are required to determine if these perceived differences are the result of a simple reduction in the amount of light transmitted through the lens, a placebo effect or some inherent properties of amber tinted lenses (Paramore & King, 1987).

30.3.12   TINT STABILITY

The permanency of colour in a soft tinted lens tends to vary depending upon the manufacturer, as well as the conditions of use (Lutzi *et al.*, 1985b). For the vast majority of lens types, compliance with manufacturers' suggested care systems results in minimal loss of dye from the lenses.

30.3.13   CARE REGIMEN COMPATIBILITY

Testing has been conducted to show that lenses produced by the major manufacturers are compatible with heat disinfection, chemical disinfection, hydrogen peroxide disinfection, surfactant cleaners and enzyme cleaners. While there have been reports that certain lenses are incompatible with certain lens care products, there have been no documented reports which isolate a lens care component apart from the effects of colour matching, weathering and fading.

An *in vitro* evaluation revealed that SOFTCOLORS (CIBA Vision) lenses were stable after 180 cycles when either heat or hydrogen peroxide were employed (Stanek & Yamane, 1985). Another clinical trial clearly demonstrated that 30 cycles of H_2O_2 disinfection had no significant adverse effects upon the transmittance characteristics of the tested lenses (Janoff, 1988). On the other hand,

fellow lens, there may be a noticeable difference when viewed in the storage case. Small differences are generally not apparent on the eye, however, visible *in vivo* discrepancies may necessitate replacing both lenses (Fig. 30.17).

30.4.3 FADING/BLEACHING

Fading or bleaching is defined as a partial or complete loss of color from a tinted lens. This can be caused by exposing lenses to chemical agents which in some way, shape or form, alter the dye and cause a resultant loss of color. Two such agents have been identified and numerous others have the potential for causing a loss of color from tinted lenses.

The first chemical discovered to have an adverse effect on tinted lenses is chlorine. Chlorine is a bleach, and is found in swimming pools, tap water and distilled water. The effect of chlorine on different types of cosmetically tinted contact lenses has been well documented (Hanks, 1984; Liebetreu *et al.*, 1986; Mandell, 1988). Exposure to chlorine, in high enough concentrations, can cause a complete loss of color from the lens, or a loss of color to areas of the lens which are exposed (Fig. 30.18). Most fitters would assume that distilled water, by definition, is

chlorine-free. However, this may not be the case because some bottlers actually add chlorine back into the distilled water in order to ensure sterility of the product at the time of shipment. Distilled water is a common factor with contact lens patients. It is used to mix salt tablet saline, or to dissolve enzymatic cleaners. In light of the controversy over contamination of distilled water and contamination of salt tablet saline, it is recommended that patients use a preserved saline as a rinsing agent, as well as the dilutant for enzymatic cleaners. A recommendation to discontinue the use of distilled water with contact lenses would also be prudent from a medical-legal standpoint.

The second chemical entity found to cause a fading of cosmetically tinted soft contact lenses is benzoyl peroxide. This ingredient is commonly found in dermatological preparations and is utilized for the treatment of mild to moderate acne. It also is responsible for causing a loss of tint from a lens. If benzoyl peroxide is on the fingers of an individual handling a cosmetically tinted lens, patches or areas of tint will be removed from the lens (Fig. 30.19). Table 30.5 lists some of the typical acne medications which contain benzoyl peroxide. Since many teenage patients wearing contact lenses use these acne medications, the practitioner must be aware that

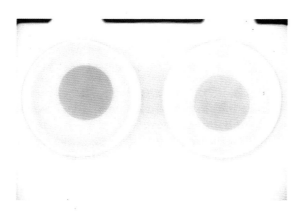

Figure 30.17 Weathering of a tinted soft contact lens: left lens, new; right lens, 12 months old (courtesy of J. Brackbill).

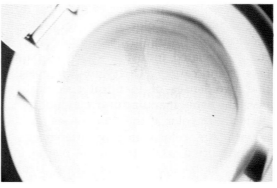

Figure 30.18 Tinted soft contact lens exposed to chlorine (courtesy of R. Payor).

this can be a problem (Lowther, 1987). Thorough hand washing with soap and warm water prior to lens handling will eliminate this situation.

30.4.4 COATINGS

Certain tinted contact lens patients have been noted to experience a coating which builds up on the tinted lens surface (Lowther, 1987). This coating tends to be protein in nature and occurs only on the tinted area of the lens (Figs 30.20 and 30.21). Front surface tinted dispersive/vat dye, covalent bond/reactive dye, and print process lenses have all been involved. If protein is

Table 30.5 Acne medication containing benzoyl peroxide

Medication	% Benzoyl Peroxide
Clearsil	10
Foster Super	10
Noxema Acne-12	10
Topex	10
OXY-10	10
Dry and Clear	10
Propa P.H.Acne	10
Foster Regular	5
OXY-5	5

allowed to build up in large amounts, it can actually cause a distortion of the lens and create an out-of-round shape or rolling up of the lens upon itself (Fig 30.22). The aetiology of this particular phenomenon is unknown. One report suggests that the imprint on DURASOFT 3 COLORS (Wesley-Jessen) acts as a shelf for tear debris, increasing the coating potential in the area of the dot matrix (Daniels & Mariscotti, 1989).

Estimates suggest that this condition occurs in roughly 5–7% of all tinted contact lens wearers, therefore this situation is minimal (Weisbarth, 1986). Clinical experience has shown that once an individual is identified as a 'lens coater', they will continue to coat lenses of the same variety. Often, by

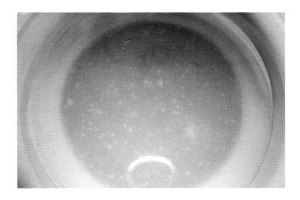

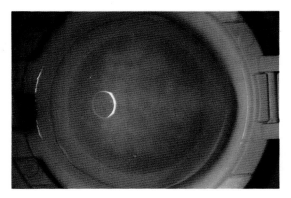

Figure 30.19 Effect of benzoyl peroxide. (a) Tinted soft contact lens exposed to benzoyl peroxide showing patchy fading; (b) tinted soft contact lens exposed to benzoyl peroxide illustrating central fading (courtesy of R. Payor).

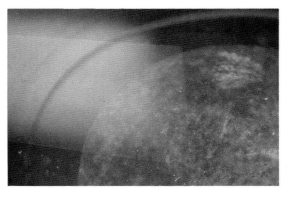

Figure 30.20 Protein coating on surface of tinted soft lens.

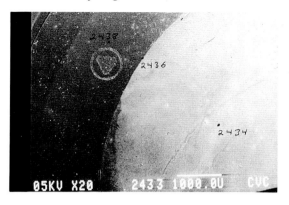

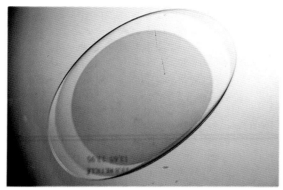

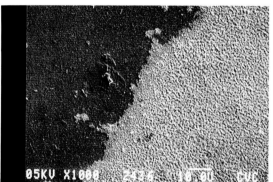

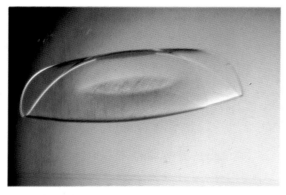

Figure 30.21 Tinted lens coated with protein. (a) SEM photograph depicting junction of clear periphery and tinted portion of lens; (b) enlargement of junction illustrating protein coating on tinted area of lens (courtesy of L. Alvord).

Figure 30.22 Effect of protein coating on a tinted lens. (a) Lens distortion (out of round) caused by coating of tinted area of lens; (b) lens curling secondary to heavy coating on tinted portion of lens (courtesy of J. Brackbill).

switching to another color or another brand of lenses, which uses a different tinting technology, the difficulties can be resolved.

Further, clinical experience has shown that using hydrogen peroxide as the disinfection solution for this type of patient is beneficial. The exact rationale for this proposal has not been offered, however it is felt that since hydrogen peroxide has some cleaning action, it may tend to minimize the build-up of protein on the tinted lens surface.

Patients who exhibit coating tendencies should be instructed to use enzyme on a regular basis, sometimes more frequently than once a week. Subtilisin-containing enzyme tablets, which can dissolved in

hydrogen peroxide, are beneficial since they tend to add to the 'cleaning effect'.

A small percentage of patients who coat lenses do so to such a degree that they create a 'crazing' of the tinted lens surface. This 'crazing' phenomenon corresponds to cracks in the protein coat which parallel the original lathe marks on the surface of the lens (Fig. 30.23). Theoretically, lenses which are manufactured with a molding technology would tend to minimize this condition.

30.4.5 DRYNESS

Some tinted lens wearers complain of a dryness sensation which occurs only with tinted lens wear. When patients are switched to

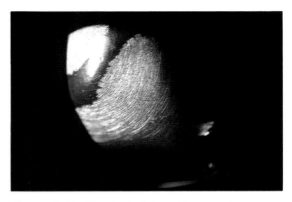

Figure 30.23 'Crazing' of tinted lens surface.

clear lenses of identical parameters, the symptoms are eliminated. Although no firm rationale has been offered, it is most likely that these individuals are marginal dry eye patients and the addition of the lens tint alters the wettability of the lens at a subclinical level, thereby pushing the patient over the 'comfort threshold'. This situation has been noted with all tinted lens types to varying degrees.

In one study evaluating DURASOFT 3 COLORS (Wesley-Jessen), more than one-third of patients had dryness-related symptoms (Daniel & Mariscotti, 1989). It has been suggested that these comfort/dryness problems are secondary to the decrease in pores on the lens surface versus the same lens without the dot matrix (Daniels & Mariscotti, 1989).

Lens lubricants may offer some intermittent relief. Also, as with clear lenses, switching to a higher water content lens or a thicker, lower water content lens may reduce or eliminate the dryness symptoms.

30.4.6 CORNEAL DISTORTION

There have been numerous reports in the literature of tinted contact lenses causing corneal distortion and irregular astigmatism (Lobby, 1987; Lowther, 1987; Smick, 1987; Clements *et al.*, 1988; Mandell, 1988; Schanzer *et al.*, 1989). The majority of these reports are with patients who are wearing cosmetically tinted lenses with a clear pupillary area. The location of corneal distortion is usually in the central portion of the cornea, corre-

Table 30.6 Special applications for tinted soft contact lenses

Lens Type	Application	Reference
Red lens	Color deficiency	Terry, 1988 Wood & Wood, 1991
Reverse piggy-back	Cosmetic eye color change in RGP wearers	Schied, 1989
SUNTACT lens (dark green)	'Sunglass' lens for surfing	Petersen, 1989
JLS lens (aqua)	Color deficiency	Schlanger, 1983, 1984, 1988
Special effect lenses	Motion pictures	Greenspoon, 1987
Custom design lenses	Veterinary applications	Maund, 1989
Experimental lenses	Space programs	Maund, 1989
	Study of visual perception, extraocular movements, color vision, visual deprivation, amblyopia, visual field deprivation, vestibular ocular function	Meshel, 1988
Special design occluder lens	To shield the eyes of animals in captivity whose normal habit is dark ex: deep water sharks	Meshel, 1988
Custom-designed red lenses	Veterinary – pacifying effect on animals, e.g. chickens	Anonymous, 1990b

Narcissus Medical Foundation
1850 Sullivan Avenue, Suite 510
Daly City, CA 94015–1850
USA
(Phone) access + 415 992–9224

Pilkington Barnes-Hind Ltd
1 Botley Road
Hedge End
Southampton SO3 3HB
United Kingdom
(Phone) access + 44 489 785–388

Sola/Barnes-Hind Ltd
8006 Engineer Road
San Diego, CA 92111
USA
(Phone) access + 619 277–9873

Wesley-Jessen
400 W. Superior Street
Chicago, IL 60610
USA
(Phone) access + 312 751–6200

THE SCLERAL RIGID LENS – OPTICAL AND THERAPEUTIC APPLICATIONS

M. Ruben

31.1 DEFINITION

A scleral lens is a lens that obtains its fit and support from the sclera rather than the cornea. This broad definition is true for all scleral rigid lenses even though in part they may have contact with the cornea. The smallest size will be just larger than the limbal–limbal diameter and will be designated '**mini-scleral**'. The largest will be fornix to fornix in size. Therefore there is a range in size from 12.5 mm to 26 mm or more. The soft lenses are mostly scleral in size but, unless they have an unusual thickness that gives rigidity, they mould to the eye and therefore have support and fitting characteristics dependent upon the corneal contact (see Chapter 00).

31.2 EARLY RIGID SCLERAL LENSES

The material used for scleral lenses in the last century and, by some fitters even as late as the 1960s, was glass. Chapter 1 gives details about the development and the individuals involved. In the later half of the nineteenth century the technology for corneal measurement became available, but with glass as the only material the manufacture of a corneal lens, whilst attempted, produced lenses that were intolerable.

To achieve a fit of the eye with glass, the size became larger and this led to the development of the scleral lens. Furthermore, at the same time the early indications for contact lenses were therapeutic and protective, rather than optical, and these conditions were best achieved with a large scleral lens. The philosophy then and even up to the introduction of the ventilated lens in the 1930s, was to produce corneal clearance and scleral contact. Glass is now obsolete as a material for contact lenses and the manufacture of glass scleral lenses will not be described here, as they are no longer fitted. However, the principles learnt from them are now evident in the present generation of rigid scleral lenses, irrespective of the material. Since 1930, although interrupted by the war years, many practitioners have developed the theory and practice of scleral lens fitting, especially since the introduction of plastics. Many fitters did not report or write down their techniques but the reader can refer to Dallos (1937, 1969), Bier (1949), Triesmann (1969, 1970) and Obrig and Salvatori (1957) for further information, and there were many others. Before leaving this aspect it is as well to mention that glass has two good properties not found in all plastics – good

Contact Lens Practice. Edited by Montague Ruben and Michel Guillon.
Published in 1994 by Chapman & Hall, London. ISBN 0 412 35120 X

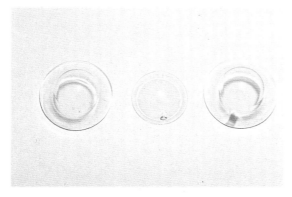

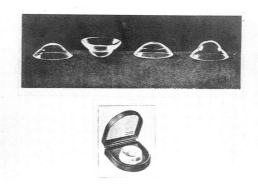

Figure 31.1 (From left to right) A preformed scleral lens with geometric curves surfaces lathe cut. A min-scleral sized lathe cut lens. An impression scleral channelled haptic and lathe cut front optic.

Figure 31.3 Examples of flat and steep fittings from the set shown in Figure 31.2.

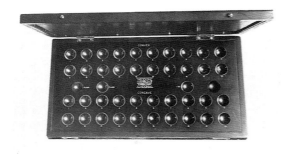

Figure 31.2 A bicurve scleral performed glass trial set (Carl Zeiss circe 1930).

tolerance wettability of the surface, and rigidity of the lens under stress.

31.3 BASIC TERMINOLOGY (FIGS 31.1, 31.2, 31.3 AND 31.4)

The rigid scleral lens can be divided into front and back surfaces and the edge. The edge is less important in the scleral lens than in the corneal, and does not materially alter the function of the lens in the peripheral half millimetre as it can in the corneal lens. Apart from having a smooth, well polished bevel finish, it is not further defined by other terms. Both the front and back surfaces can be subdivided into optic, transition, and haptic portions.

The transition posteriorly is usually further qualified as a limbal transition to denote the eye area it covers. The front transition can also be qualified further by the term optic junction transition zone.

The optic zone, as with the spectacle lens, has an optic centre and a geometric centre. Such terms are necessary because, like the spectacle lens the optic is set into a surround which in the case of the lens is the haptic. The optic zone or portion can be further subdivided into the central and peripheral curvatures.

Since the right and left lenses are of different orientation it is most important that the lenses are marked at 12 o/c on the haptic with either dots or R/L. Other codes can be used.

As almost all rigid scleral lenses have to be modified to obtain a fit it is essential to have a method of identifying any area or point on the lens. The geometric centre may appear the obvious choice for a chief point of refer-

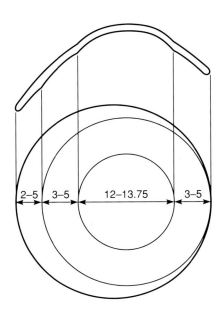

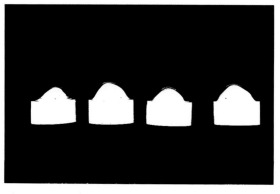

Figure 31.5 The gypsum plaster eye models photographed in profile to show range of shapes seen in clinical practice and how a spherical curve approximated to the corneal cap is eccentric.

Figure 31.4 Construction of a preformed scleral contact lens to show the diameters (chords) of the different zones: back optic chord (diameter) 12 mm to 13.75 mm; haptic chord nasal 3 mm–5 mm; haptic chord temporal 3 mm–5 mm; haptic chord temporal peripheral 2 mm–5 mm.

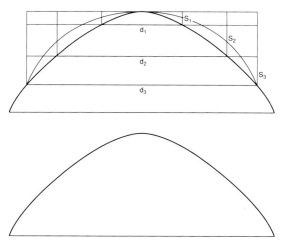

Figure 31.6 Shadowgram of a plaster eye model to show how the lower profile can be analysed to give sagitta measurements over whole scleral lens size optic portion and the corneal apex region. The single curve drawn touches the corneal apex and sclera but nowhere else. This is a section of an eye with moderate cone formation.

ence (Figs 31.3, 31.4, 31.5, 31.6, 31.7, 31.8, 31.9 and 31.10). But most lenses that undergo modifications in parameter of the haptic will suffer a change of the geometric centre. Therefore this text will use the notion of placing, at the earliest phase in manufacture, a back central spherical surface, which can easily have a centre marked when necessary for measurements.

There is an alternative, which will be described in the paragraphs concerned with manufacturing, and that is to identify the limbal ring on the back of the shell, model eye or impression cast of the eye and then find the limbal centre (Fig. 31.11). Having identified the centre as a chief point of reference, any part of the lens can be noted as so many millimetres from the point and in a specified meridian. In a finished lens where the parameter is fixed and will not be altered, millimetres from the edge in a certain specified meridian is an alternative. The measurements on a lens

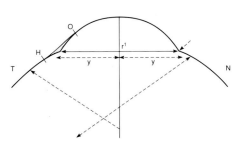

Figure 31.7 The eye model in Figure 31.6, when analysed in another meridian, can give more information as to sagitta of the optic portion. This information has to be averaged in order to manufacture a preformed scleral lens.

are done with a divider and are therefore not along a curvature but are in effect a chord measurement. The other definitions for scleral lenses will be introduced in the text as the manufacturing and fitting procedure is described. It should be noted from Figures 31.2, 31.3 and 31.4 that chord measurements for each part of the lens that are haptic, nasal and temporal plus the optic, do not add up to the total chord for the whole lens, which is the size of the lens, this size measurement being taken from the inside edge of the lens. Furthermore, the optic chord dimension is taken at the junction of the optic with the haptic and, in the finished lens, this has been smoothed away to form the limbal transitions. This is also applicable to the front and back surfaces of the lens. To avoid errors between manufacturer and practitioner it is advised that the lens and/or model be marked with a chinacraft pencil for those areas and points requiring modification. Drawings of the lens are equally valuable for patients' case notes or instructions for the technical work done or ordered.

In summary, the parts of a scleral lens are:

1. Optic (front and back).
2. Haptic (scleral contact portion).
3. Limbal transition (back surface).
4. Optic junction (front and back).
5. Edge bevel.
6. Fenestrations and grooves (channels).

31.4   HAPTIC SHAPE AND SIZE

The haptic parameter is mostly ovoid in shape, the vertical diameter being the smallest. The limiting factors that determine the diameter in any meridian are summarized as follows:

1. **Horizontally**: the eye size and degree of globe protrusion relative to the position of the temporal and nasal check ligaments attached to the orbit. The range of the eye horizontal eye versions.
2. **Vertically**: the extension of the fornices, the superior being much more extensive than the inferior.

Thus the parameter of the haptic will be an irregular oval most extensive superior–temporally and least extensive inferior–nasally (see Figs 31.3, 31.4, 31.12 and 31.13). Secondary factors will modify this basic shape and they are modifications to achieve stability of the lens and centration. There are also modifications to achieve retro – less tear fluid ventilation. These will be dealt with later (see page 707).

31.5   TYPES OF SCLERAL LENSES

The type of lens can be further described by its size or by the mode of manufacture and fitting. The simplest classification is by the process used in manufacture. Thus there are two main types:

1. Preformed:
   i. large scleral;
   ii. mini-scleral.
2. Impression: Cast or moulded scleral.

Irrespective of size or mode of manufacture,

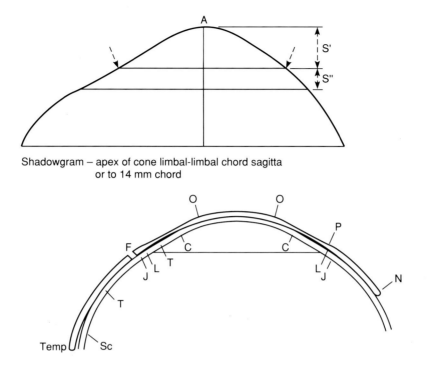

Shadowgram – apex of cone limbal-limbal chord sagitta
or to 14 mm chord

Figure 31.8 The back lens surface design shown gives the blending of the optic/haptic junction to form the clearance over the eye limbus; it should also be noted that the nasal haptic back surface curvature is an offset spherical curve, whereas the temporal is a concentric centred spherical curve. (a) A section of the preformed lens is drawn to show the several points and measurements. This particular form is based upon the data given in Table 31.1 for the small eye fitting with average keratometry 7.2 mm. The front surface is that for a minus lens of haptic thickness 0.6 mm and centre optic thickness 0.3 mm. OO, Front optic diameter; OP, Front peripheral optic; F, Fenestration; CC, Back central optic diameter; CJ, Peripheral back optic; TT, Transition zone; Temp to N, Horizontal size of lens; CC, Corneal apex of eye; L, Limbus of the eye; Sc, Sclera. (b) The back surface design based upon the data given in Table 31.1 for the normal eye size average keratometry 6 mm. In the top diagram the curves are centred and off centred (ipsilateral) to a single central axis.) In the lower diagram the optic portion has been angled 10 to the haptic axis. This is truer in many instances to the eye shape as would be found in keratoconus (see Figure 31.5 for eye profiles).

the finished lens functions the same way and therefore the principles underlying eye tolerance and physiological acceptance of the appliance should be identical. There is the proviso that there are some aspects of fitting best achieved by one process as opposed to another. For example, the impression lens is rarely as thin as a preformed or has as smooth a surface finish and the back optic may be more difficult to centre and work. But on the other hand, the scleral fit of an impression lens, especially in abnormal eyes, can be the only way to achieve a satisfactory lens fitting.

31.6   THE PHILOSOPHY OF SCLERAL LENS FUNCTIONS RELATIVE TO FIT

The scleral lens, from the mini to the full scleral size, can occlude the whole cornea and

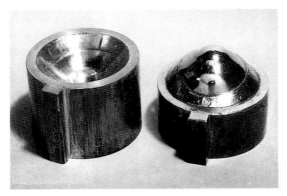

Figure 31.9 The photograph shows a positive and negative dye for the manufacture of scleral lenses. The dyes are made in this instance of printers' metal and several lenses can be made before the dyes lose their form.

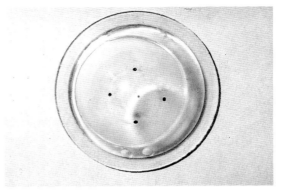

Figure 31.11 A shell cast by the F. Ridley press and before cutting out of the round sheet. Using the inside surface limbal eye markings dividers are used to find the centre that will be used for future orientation of optical surfaces or for later finding the relative vision point which will then become the optical centre.

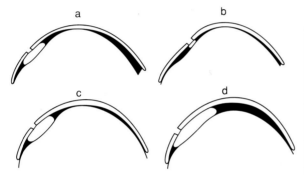

Figure 31.10 The four sections show the eye in different positions and how this affects the relationship of the lens to the eye and therefore the size of the bubble. Note that the fenestration is always open to the bubble and at no time does the bubble cover the cornea centrally.

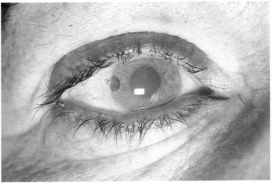

Figure 31.12 A ventilated scleral as worn and the bubble in the primary position is small but enlarged with eye movement. Deepening and widening the transition would have increased the bubble size.

therefore the avoidance of corneal hypoxia and secondary effects on cell metabolism are important aspects to consider. The problems of corneal occlusion have been dealt with from physiological and pathological stand points (see Chapters 42 and 45) with especial reference to the soft and hard corneal lens. But with the rigid scleral they are more important because total occlusion is possible. Furthermore, the scleral lens, because of its size, can transmit by gravity, weight and lid pressure to small zones of eye surface contact and exacerbate, by non-relative eye movements, sheer effects, which can be very traumatic to the cornea or conjunctiva. As this type of appliance is used on diseased eyes and as a basis for shell prosthetics, these effects may not initially have symptoms,

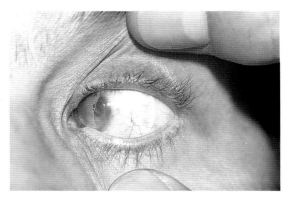

Figure 31.13 A scleral lens at extreme version to show how large the air bubble can become.

2. **Semi-sealed fit**: a lens or shell that has been modified so that the retro-lens tear fluid can escape to the edge (e.g. haptic with posterior grooves, channels or loose fit haptic (sectors)).
3. **Ventilated fit**: a lens that has fenestrations to allow atmospheric air to enter the lens.
4. **Sealed fit**: unless there is some special indication such a fit that totally occludes the eye is not acceptable.

The scleral lens generally fits the sclera slightly flatter than a perfect fit, and this must be especially true at the periphery, so that tear fluid can pass behind the lens. The limbal transition must be wide (2 mm to 3 mm) and deep (0.1 mm to 0.2 mm), the back optic flatter than the average keratometry by at least 1 mm and corneal contact with the lens reduced to a minimum, and then only at the extremes of eye movement. The fenestrations are 1 mm in diameter and placed within the palpebral fissure in the limbal zone. They permit air to enter the lens when the lens moves away from the eye (Bier, 1949; Dallos, 1969). This occurs as the lens edge moves to impinge on the lateral or medial palpebral ligaments (see Figs. 31.8, 31.9, 31.10, 31.14 and 31.15). Alternatively, a degree of misfit which permits the rapid movement of fresh oxygenated tear fluid to behind the lens either from channels or a loose periphery (see Figs. 31.10, 31.12, 31.13, 31.14 and 31.15).

Fluid movement can be tested by the clinician by touching the sclera in the upper fornix just above the lens edge with fluorescein and then timing the filling and the loss of fluorescence from the tear lens space; this should not exceed 1 minute to fill and 5 minutes to empty. The pressure behind a ventilated scleral lens varies with the eye movements from –11 mmHg to +20 mmHg, and this pumping action promotes fluid exchange (Bergman, *et al.*, 1970) (see Fig. 31.2).

since the tissue affected could have lowered sensitivity. Therefore the safe fit is of great importance.

When scleral lenses were used for low refractive errors in the period 1920 to 1960, the investigative techniques for examining the eye tissues response to lens wear were not sophisticated and therefore the literature is not helpful on this aspect. But it was common knowledge that a wearing period of 4 hours produced corneal oedema in the majority of patients. The soft HEMA lens of today would have to be at least 0.3 mm thick to produce the same effect on the normal eye (see Chapters 22 and 42). One can assume from this, and also from the basic research done by Smelzer and Ozaniks (1952) and Smelzer and Chen (1953), that anoxia is a problem with the scleral lens.

31.6.1 THE FIT

It will be of value to define in principle what is the fit of the large rigid scleral lens or shell.

In the first instance, irrespective of whether the lens is manufactured by lathe by impression methods or by a combination of both, there are four acceptable types of fit:

1. **Flush fit**: a shell that follows the shape of the eye surface in parallel.

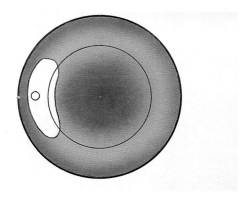

Figure 31.14 This drawing illustrates the size of the bubble with the eye in the primary position and the corneal fit is minimal central clearance which is essential with a ventilated scleral.

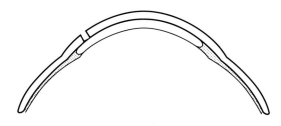

Figure 31.15 If the central clearance is excessive then the bubble can cover the central cornea and prevent clear vision.

31.6.2 FENESTRATION

The following mechanical factors need to be considered in the maintenance of a suitably sized air bubble in the ventilation of the cornea:

1. Position and sizes of fenestrations.
2. Number of fenestrations.
3. Size of air bubble or bubbles.
4. Effect of bubbles on the field of vision.
5. Effect of the tear fluid protein on frothing.
6. Depth of space in the limbal transition.
7. Increase and decrease of bubble on eye movement (Figs. 31.12, 31.13, 31.14 and 31.15.

The fits just described apply to both the preformed and impression scleral lens.

Using PMMA material, and with good fluid and air movement, it has been noted clinically that corneal oedema still ocurrs in many patients after a period of 4 hours. The solution to this problem could be the use of gas permeable materials, preferably thermolabile so that they could be cast manufactured. Because the scleral lens has thicknesses between 0.2 mm and 0.6 mm, the Dk of the material must be high to be of value in the function of gas permeability (see Chapters 3, 32 and 42).

31.7 RETRO-LENS TEAR FLUID FORM AND CONTACT ZONES

The examination of this volume of fluid or its absence is in essence the method of evaluating the fit one has to achieve. The two methods are by use of fluorescein or the use of a fine slit beam of the biomicroscope panned across the lens. Both are combined, but fluorescein alone can be assessed in its geographical distribution and relative density.

1. **Flush fit**: the flush fit should, theoretically, have overall contact. But to achieve function it is flatter than the eye shape and any sealed areas under the lens should either be opened by channels to the periphery or fenestrated.
2. **Semi-sealed fit**: the semi-sealed fit has a fluorescein distribution that shows as minimal clearance over the corneal apex and increasing to the limbus transition. The channel(s) lead from the optic to the haptic periphery. These will be further described later (see page 734).
3. **Fenestrated lens fit**: the fenestrated scleral requires minimal apical clearance and a controlled increase to the limbal transition especially where the fenestration is to be placed (see Figs 31.10, 31.12, 31.13, 31.14 and 31.15). Thus the tear lens has a negative form.

Whilst these appearances are true for the primary eye position, this will change upon eye movement and then care must be taken to see that excessive corneal contact with the lens does not occur. This is often unavoidable in keratoconus and steep grafts.

31.8 PREFORMED SCLERAL LENSES

31.8.1 INDICATIONS FOR PREFORMED SCLERAL LENSES

It is now advisable to consider the commonest uses of rigid scleral contact lenses.

The normal eye fitting for scleral is a rarity and now only takes place for patients using lenses for contact sports, water sports and for actors requiring lenses with special cosmetic effects. More commonly, the scleral is used for the highly myopic or astigmatic eye where the other types of lenses cannot stabilize or obtain satisfactory vision. The keratoconic and grafted corneal eyes are perhaps also in this group. Therefore a preformed fitting set of lenses that do not have lenses for these conditions is of little value.

31.9 MANUFACTURE OF PREFORMED SCLERAL LENSES

Preformed scleral lenses can be manufactured by two methods – cast (or moulded) or lathe generated.

31.9.1 CAST (MOULDED) PREFORMED SCLERAL LENSES

Cast and moulded are synonymous terms, and for scleral lens manufacture are used in two senses – either a sheet of plastic pulled down over a preformed geometric shape or the plastic placed between two shapes that are complementary and are separated by a space. The shapes used for multiple manufacture are called master shapes or dyes.

The masters are made of gypsum or, if many lenses are to be manufactured from the master, then of metal (see Fig. 31.9).

The eye shapes are best called positive dyes. If the dough of plastic in the unpolymerized state is used then the dyes will be of positive and negative design and held in a clamp for polymerization which allows the thickness to be controlled.

If only the positive dye is to be used then the plastic sheet is impressed upon the dye when in a labile state (heated) and then allowed to set. This procedure will be described in greater detail in the section devoted to the fitting of a moulded shell (see page 740).

The preformed trial fitting lenses, irrespective of the type of manufacture, are usually finished with a low optic power unless used specifically for aphakia, when a high plus power is used (e.g. +14 D) with a front optic diameter not larger than 8 mm.

The preformed lens has been used in a range of sizes and shapes as a trial set (Woodward, 1972), mostly for the normal eye.

31.9.2 LATHE GENERATED GEOMETRIC SCLERAL LENSES

The len materials applicable to cutting are: PMMA and gas permeable acrylics.

Geometric lathe cut lenses

The most important features to consider are how to best use the lathe to generate the three back surface portions of the lens (i.e. optic, transition and haptic) and then to control the thicknesses over the whole lens to produce the front surfaces for power requirements and rigidity.

The procedure should also be reproducible within the standards and tolerances required for consistency in fitting. Some of these requirements will be stated:

Optic surfaces ± 0.05 mm radius of curvature
Power ± 0.25 dioptre

the lens in the antero-posterior axis. This can be decreased by altering the vertical to horizontal scleral size ratio. For example, if the lens was 22H/20V then change to 22H/18V or a new lens 23H/20V. New peripheral temporal back curves may then be necessary to avoid increasing the clearance (see Fig. 31.8a).

31.9.16   OPTIC SURFACES

Thus there are several modifications that can be made either by the manufacturer or, preferably, by the practitioner at the chairside. When a good fit has been achieved then the optic centre should be marked on the front surface of the lens. This is easily done by asking the patient to fixate a small spot beam of the slit lamp and using a chinacraft coloured pencil to mark the point on the lens.

The required power is cut on the front surface and the front transition blended to the front haptic. The size of the front optic carrying the power should be at least 5 mm, but for low powers may be as large as 10 mm (negative powered lens). It will occur to the reader that the back and front optic centres may not coincide but since the difference in refraction of tears and lens material is not as great as air to lens, it rarely causes problems. The back optic can be recentred to make both centres coaxial but care must be taken to remove minimal material posteriorly and so alter the clearances to the cornea.

The optics are described in Chapter 7 and particular attention must be paid to the tear lens thickness. If a lens is ordered from spectacle lens power and back vertex distance, only a calculation is required.

31.9.17   DECENTRATION OF OPTIC

It has been stated that the optic visual centre does not coincide with the geometric centre of the optic portion or the geometric centre of the whole lens.

The vision point of the lens is that point

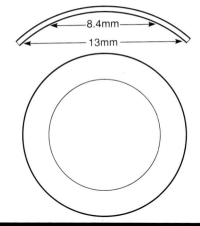

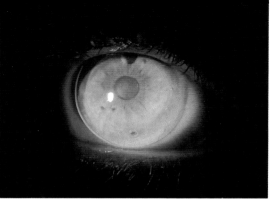

Figure 31.20 (a) Mini-scleral lens – diagrammatic section; (b) mini-scleral lens as fitted to an aphakic eye.

intersected by the vision line of the eye and can only be found by direct observation of the eye and lens when the eye is fixating. This point is usually 1 mm down and in, nasal to the optic geometric centre, and can be placed there for manufacturing purposes unless the fit or a large angle kappa requires another position.

However, optic can be decentred relative to the vision point by a few millimetres (about 5 mm maximum) and, depending upon the lens power, this will induce prismatic deviation. Unlike the spectacle lens the power will be less because of tear fluid

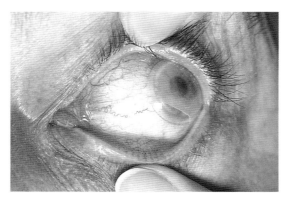

Figure 31.21 Mini-scleral lens on an aphakic eye to show stability even in extreme version and upper lid elevated.

being on the posterior part of the lens (see Chapter 7).

31.10 MINI-SCLERAL (FIGS. 31.20 AND 31.21)

Since these lenses will be preformed they will be dealt with here, and before the moulded scleral lens is described.

There is no standard definition; a mini-scleral lens is stabilized essentially by the sclera, is of rigid form and material, is between the limbal diameter and 16 mm size and is round. This is not a dogmatic definition because change of parameter means that the lens becomes a corneal rigid lens or scleral.

However, because the indications are specific, and the fit likewise, the mini-scleral can be dealt with as an entity.

31.10.1 INDICATIONS FOR MINI-SCLERAL

The indications for scleral lens fitting have already been described in general terms. The mini-scleral is a lens that attempts to give almost the same stability as the larger scleral with the same criteria as to function but with minimal support from the sclera. This is achieved by using a lens that has much less mass than the scleral and a surface that is so much less extensive that the displacement forces are less important.

This type of lens was first used as a sports lens for the normal eye (14 mm size) and subsequently in the 12.5 mm size plus for aphakia (Gordon, 1969; Ruben, 1967). This size of lens was found to be unacceptable to the normal eye except for short periods of wear. But for corneas with lowered sensation, such as aphakia, corneal grafts, refractive keratometry and some keratoconus, even PMMA material was shown to be an all-day wear possibility, sometimes with short periods of rest.

Diseased and physically ugly eyes are also able to fit this type of lens, which can therefore be used as suitable prosthetics. With the use of gas permeable materials this type of lens can be used where there is an indication for scleral lenses and the facility and expertise required for fitting is not available.

31.10.2 DATA FOR PARAMETERS

Because they are likely to be fitted in two types of eye (i.e. aphakia and grafts), two series of trial lenses will be described.

1. **Aphakia:**
    BCOR 8.0 to 9.0 mm (six lenses with 0.2 mm increments)
    BCOD 8.4 mm for all lenses
    PR Add 0.6 mm to BCOR
    Size 13 mm
    Two fenestrations 0.5 mm and 2 mm inset
    Front optic: 8 mm diameter: +14 D power
    Edge thickness 0.2 mm
    Overall sagitta 3.2 to 2.6 mm
2. **General use:**
    BCOR 7.0 to 8.6 mm (nine lenses in 0.2 mm increments)
    BCOD 8.2 mm for all lenses
    PR Add 0.6 mm to all lenses
    Size: two sets of lenses 12 mm and 13 mm

Two fenestrations as above
Front optic: 6 mm diameter: –4 D power
Edge thickness 0.15 mm

Figure 31.20a illustrates the design of such lenses; Figures 31.20b 31.21 give some examples.

31.10.3 FITTING

The aim should be to provide minimal corneal touch and the chief support for the lens should be the sclera and lid superiorly. Thus the fluorescein pattern is, in section, wedge-shaped and open below. The fit must not be so loose that eye movement dislodges the lens from the eye. It is preferable to manufacture the lens in gas permeable materials because of the large size of the lens.

31.11 SUMMARY FOR PREFORMED GEOMETRIC SCLERAL LENSES

This form of lens, and indeed any type of large scleral, is no longer in use for the normal eye with low refractive errors unless there are special indications, as stated previously. Therefore it is not worthwhile designing or having extensive sets of these lenses. The asterisked data in Table 31.1 can be used for normal eye fitting. It is better to use such lenses as a basis and, if necessary, do extensive modifications to obtain a fit. The chief use, therefore, of the preformed lens is to fit the abnormal eye for which there is limited use of soft and corneal lenses. The data and fitting technology can be used to this end. A further extension of the manufacturing technology would be to have optic portions that have an axis at an angle to the haptic axis. This would, in some eyes, give a better fit since the anterior segment is basically a tilted ellipsoid and not shaped around a principal axis. The scleral preformed lenses, with the exception of the mini-scleral, cannot be manufactured to fine tolerances; this applies

to the sizes and optic sagitta in particular. This again could be overcome by advances in technology whenever the scleral form becomes of commercial value and the research and development considered viable. The fitter may therefore find the mini-scleral a useful alternative to the scleral in selected cases.

31.12 THE EYE IMPRESSION (CAST OR MOULDED) OF SCLERAL SIZE

The lens is moulded from an eye model which is based upon the eye impression. For modifications and discussion of the impression problems and technology see Marriot (1966, 1967), Jenkins (1964), Haynes (1968) and Miller *et al.* (1966), who have written extensively on the subject.

Each of the following stages of taking an eye impression can deviate the lens shape from the original eye contours. Fortunately most errors tend to produce a shell that is flatter than the eye shape:

1. Eye impression using ophthalmic alginate or hydrocolloid materials.
2. Model of eye made of gypsum, marking out, modifications, etc.
3. Moulding of a sheet of thermolabile plastic to the eye model.

These procedures results in a plastic shape, which is called the **shell**. The following procedures are then possible:

1. Edging to size parameters.
2. Back central optic by grinding or lathe progression.
3. Blending of transitions, grooves and fenestrations.
4. Fitting to the eye.
5. Refitting and lens copy.
6. Centreing of shell on eye for the front and/or back optic.
7. Front optic.

The technical procedures involved are impression and casting (moulding). It is therefore advantageous to call the scleral lens an impression scleral and confine the terminology of moulding and casting to the manufacturing process.

31.12.1 TERMINOLOGY OF THE IMPRESSION LENS

At this stage it is well to clarify further the lens and shell terminology:

1. A shell is the shape cast from the plaster eye impression model. The fit of the shell without modifications is flush.
2. A scleral contact lens is based upon the shell but in addition has an optic, transition and other modifications. The optic can be front and/or back surface. In the first instance, where the shell fit is flush and the optic power only worked onto the front surface, the lens can be called a flush scleral contact lens (see pages 743–747 for further flush lens definitions).

The indications and function, and indeed the modifications to achieve a fit, are identical to those described for the preformed scleral lens. But because the impression lens requires additional chairside work this will be again described briefly and with reference to the tools used.

31.12.2 TAKING THE EYE IMPRESSION (FIGS 31.21, 31.22, 31.23, 31.24, 31.25 AND 31.26)

The patient is seated comfortably in the chair at a slightly declined angle. The eye is anaesthetized with a local ophthalmic anaesthetic: three drops at 1-minute intervals will suffice, making sure the drop enters the upper fornix. One drop of adrenaline 1/10000 is then instilled; this can be omitted if there is a history of sensitivity but the use of a vasoconstrictor will ensure a better fit. Conjunctival oedema and excessive lacrimation will result not only in a poor impression but in a very flat fit (Miller & Carol, 1967). The excellence of the impression can be judged by the details of the limbal junction and the conjunctival wrinkles impressed into the gel.

The suitably sized tray is then inserted. There are two types of tray:

1. Hollow stem tray for syringe injection of gel.
2. Trays without injection.

The trays should be perforated to allow excess gel to escape (Figs 31.22, 31.23 and 31.24). The tray must be held away from the cornea otherwise an abrasion can occur. The gel material should be mixed according to the manufacturer's instructions and at hand for use immediately the mix is ready. Assistance is necessary for this procedure to avoid mistiming. Once the gel and tray are in position the patient should not alter the eye fixation, which should be in the primary position. An assistant can hold an object for fixation a few metres away from the patient.

Sometimes the patient is impressed under a general anaesthetic, when fixation is not possible. This applies particularly to children.

The manufacturer will state the time for the gel to set but since this is variable, depending upon the temperature of the immediate environment, it is better to test the gel not used and to discover when this is

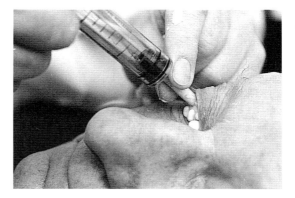

Figure 31.22 Injection of the hydrogel mix into the stem of the tray.

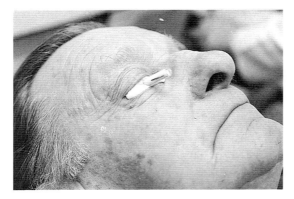

Figure 31.23 Waiting for the gel to set.

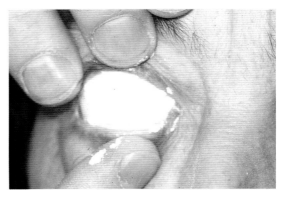

Figure 31.25 A large plastic shell used as a tray. Inserted with the mix.

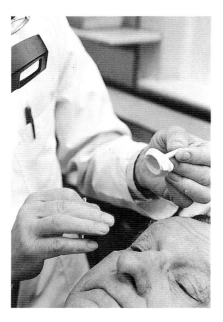

Figure 31.24 The gel and tray removed and impression of the eye obtained.

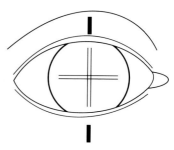

Figure 31.26 Markings on the tray surface to ensure correct orientation.

firmly set. Most gels take only a few minutes to set.

The gel, when set, forms an adhesive bond with the tray and the eye surface. It is important that the tray be removed with the gel intact and not separated in any way. Therefore a blunt-ended muscle hook can be gently inserted beneath the tray and between the conjunctiva and the edge of the gel. The

surface tension will then break and, with a gentle tilt of the tray, holding the stem firmly and with the upper lid retracted, the tray and impression can be slid away from the eye.

This procedure is the basis of a good fitting shell and, without a successful impression, it is not worthwhile proceeding further (Miller *et al.*, 1966).

A worthwhile modification is the placing of a therapeutic soft lens on the eye and the taking of the impression with the lens *in situ*. This ensures a clearance for the shell from the cornea.

31.12.3 THE EYE MODEL (FIGS 31.27, 31.28, 31.29, 31.30 AND 31.31)

The impression, with its tray, is supported in a stand and the mix of dry gypsum powder and water, according to the manufacturer's instructions, is poured into the impression. It is advisable to do this procedure within a few minutes of taking the impression, otherwise the gel will dry and distort its shape.

When the gypsum has set hard the back of the model is marked according to the information drawn on the front of the tray, so denoting the correct orientation, which will eventually be transferred to the shell and then the final lens (see Fig. 31.26).

The front of the gypsum model is examined for detail after it has been removed from the gel impression. If imperfect (usually due to bubble formation) a fresh model can be poured, but the surface of the gel should be wetted.

The front of the gypsum model can now be marked up as to:

1. Edge parameter.
2. Position and extent of transition.

Imperfections of the model can be removed with sandpaper attached to a hand drill (see

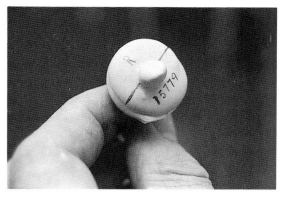

Figure 31.28 The plaster model now set and the markings transferred from the tray to the plaster.

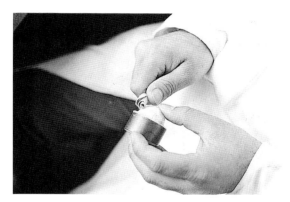

Figure 31.29 The model plaster eye now mounted onto a metal ring for convenience in future handling. The plaster is being smoothed or excess removed to obtain a tighter fitting shell. The sandpaper strip is held in a split pin and rotated in a hand-held spindle.

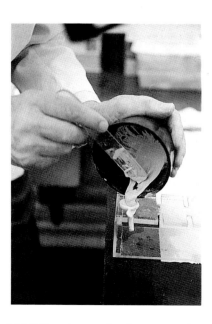

Figure 31.27 Pouring a mix of gypsum plaster and water into the gel impression.

Fig. 31.29). Gross roughness due to conjunctival wrinkling can also be smoothed out, but substantial changes to the model will alter the fit of the shell.

It is as well to note that if substance from the scleral portion of the model is removed then a tighter fitting shell will result, and this can be used when necessary.

The model can also be marked as to the optic zone and the clearance required over this area. Most fitters prefer to fit the shell and mark the shell.

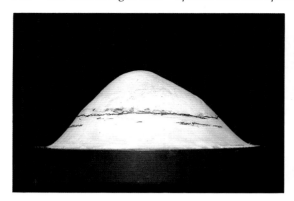

Figure 31.30 An example of an unmounted plaster eye model marked out with the proposed edge parameter (blue) just within the fornix markings (red).

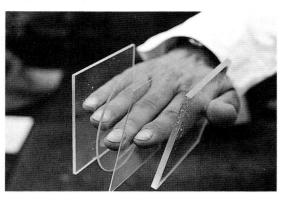

Figure 31.32 A selection of different thickness PMMA plastic sheets for shell production.

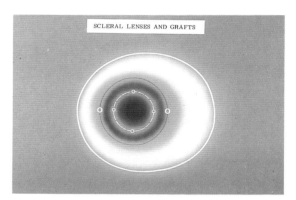

Figure 31.31 The plaster eye model marked out with the suggested limits of the corneal apex (in this case a keratoplasty) as the inner circle with micro fenestrations. The outer circle being the limbus, with two normal fenestrations. The green and black areas simulate proposed zones of contact and clearance. The white is the scleral haptic.

31.12.4   MAKING THE SHELL (SEE FIGS 31.30 TO 31.49)

The PMMA or other thermolabile material to be used is chosen of the thickness desired. These sheets are avaliable from 0.3 mm to 1 mm thick, with 0.6 mm being the most satisfactory. It is possible to make the sheet of variable thickness. Thus for a negative power lens the centre portion can be pre-

pared to be thinner. This will avoid removal of excess material later.

The sheet is heated evenly to between 130 °C and 160 °C, and the exact temperature required to make the whole sheet mouldable but not flowing or burning can only be found by experience, and will depend very much

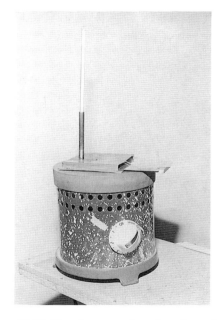

Figure 31.33 Simple oven placed on top of a hot plate. The sheet can reach the temperature required as shown on the thermometer.

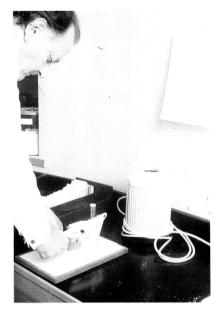

Figure 31.34 An infra-red heater used to heat a plastic sheet which is then placed over the plaster model and the toggle press used to exert even pressure. An asbestos pad or rubber pad can be used to place between the press and the sheet.

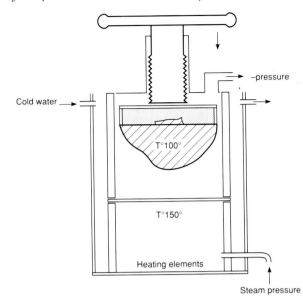

Figure 31.35 A press designed by F. Ridley circa 1955 for applying controlled heat and negative and positive pressures to the casting process.

on the type of heater or oven used and the advice of the plastic manufacturer. After moulding to the plaster cast, the plastic should be allowed to cool slowly (PMMA) and then the required edge parameter marked and the shell cut out.

The shell is now polished and any blemishes removed. The edge is bevelled and polished.

The thickness over the whole shell should be checked and, if at this stage the shell is excessively thick in the haptic, then the front surface should be reduced and the surface polished.

This is now the initial shell ready for fitting. The experienced practitioner will often identify the internal limbal marking and the centre of the optic portion and place a fenestration, if required, at the proposed transition zone at this stage. Depending upon the difficulty of the eye being fitted, and providing it is a scleral lens (and not a flush) that is being fitted, even a back optic

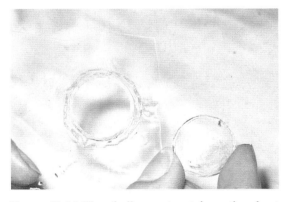

Figure 31.36 The shell as cut out from the sheet after casting.

of a given clearance may also be worked before the first fitting.

31.12.5 THE SHELL FIT OPTIC SURFACES AND THE TRANSITION (FIG 31.32 TO 31.49)

To avoid repetition it will be assumed that the next phase is the shell fitting and the back optic will be worked later. But if the

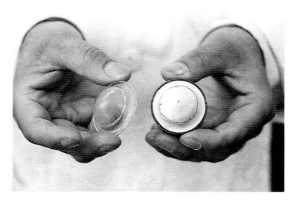

Figure 31.37 The shell approximated to the plaster model to check quality of casting and also to orientate and mark the shell.

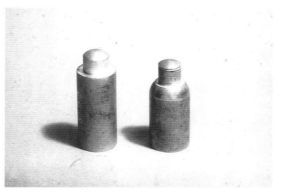

Figure 31.39 Two of the set of spherical surfaced diamond bonded tools for use with the spindle for the process of lapping on curves and grinding out transitions.

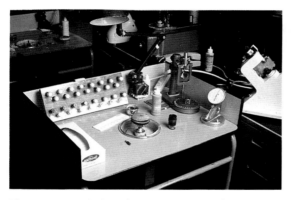

Figure 31.38 A bench set up around an inset vertical spindle with the tools and measuring devices used in the modification of a shell at the chairside.

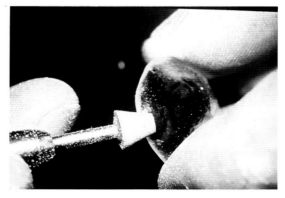

Figure 31.40 A conical tool (carborundum coated) used with a hand-held spindle to edge the lens and which can also be used to flatten the inside haptic at its periphery.

back optic is to be worked at this stage, the transition blended and given clearances, then the shell, after the edge has been cut out and bevelled smoothly, must have the centre of the optic (geometric) marked. This is done by placing four equidistant marks on the limbus, as seen on the inside of the shell. Then, with a divider, the intersecting arcs will place the centre accurately.

This is then marked with a faint burr on the outside. The back optic can now be worked according to the wishes of the practitioner. In most instances this will be done on

a lathe with very careful thickness control so that, at the centre, minimal substance is lost. Alternatively diamond-bonded spherical tools attached to a rotating spindle can be used, again with repetitive thickness measurement to ensure accurate clearance from the model and therefore the cornea. This surface is then polished. Using conoidal carborundum or diamond-coated tools on a hand-driven spindle, the transition is blended and the required clearance achieved. These surfaces are then polished. It is better to use an

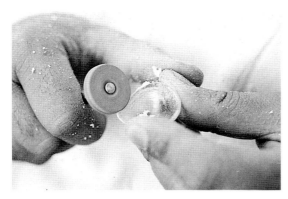

Figure 31.41 A round felt used with polishes to finish the edge.

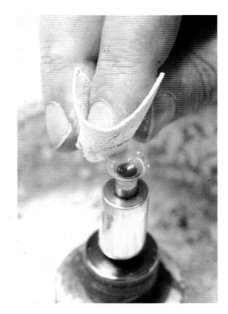

Figure 31.43 The lens is mounted on the spindle with melted wax and the edge is worked on by this alternative way.

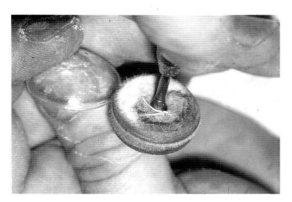

Figure 31.42 A rouged felt used to polish the edge.

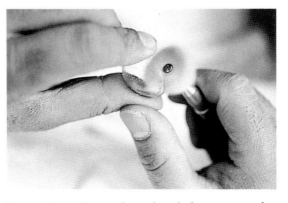

Figure 31.44 Rag and wool ended mops can also be used to polish larger surfaces.

automatic surface polishing machine for all optical surfaces if possible; alternatively the spherical wax or felt coated brass tools can be used.

31.12.6   THE FLUSH FITTING SHELL AND LENS

The definitions of the flush fit lens and shell have been given (see page 739), here the concept and use of such a device will be explained.

Ridley (1958a) introduced the simple shell fit without extensive modifications to provide a protective layer for the several condi-tions of the cornea not then ameneable to treatment, and to provide a splint for the eye and lids after certain surgical procedures – it proved to be most effective in the treatment of bullous keratopathy and alleviated pain. This was followed up by Gould (1970), Girard and Soper (1966) and many others

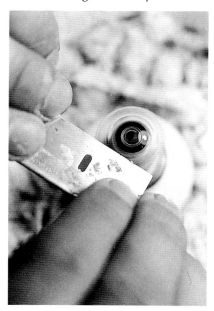

Figure 31.45 The lens is mounted upon the spindle using a spherical tool coated with a thin layer of heated wax (or the surface is gently heated). The photograph shows the razor blade edge being used to remove material and so thin this portion of the haptic.

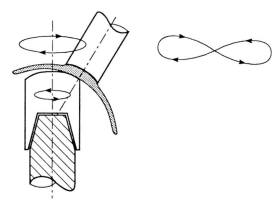

Figure 31.46 The lapping procedure is used in two ways to either steepen a surface when a clockwise rotation is used or to flatten a surface when the peripheral part of the tool is applied in a figure of eight fashion. Much experience is required to impart good optical surfaces and lathe cutting is preferred.

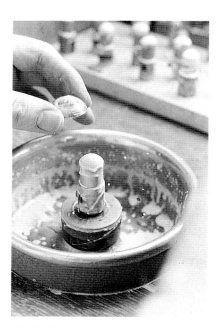

Figure 31.47 The lapping procedure.

involved in treating the complications of surgery of the anterior segment.

If not too large, the shell was a safe device for the cornea that, due to pathology, did not require normal gaseous exchange. The fit would, for the reasons given on page 717, be somewhat flatter than the eye shape and would therefore not seal to the eye.

The hydrophilic soft lens soon superseded the flush fitting shell and advances in cataract surgery technology reduced the incidence of bullous keratopathy. However, there are still a few instances when the flush fit can be of value, for example, in fitting the deformed eye with a prosthesis, or combined with a front optic (Miller, 1968) to correct vision when it has an advantage over the therapeutic soft lens for a diseased cornea. There may be circumstances when a shell used periodically, and not constantly, can be more economic than the soft and more suitable in situations where management is not possible or supplies and facilities are limited.

A hypothesis is that, given a material of sufficiently high gas permeability and given

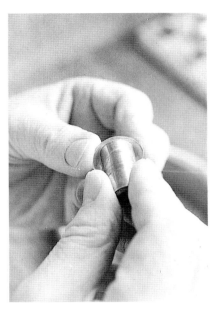

Figure 31.48 The tool is checked against the surface to discover if there is a good result. Carbon paper placed between the lens and tool can reveal areas of contact.

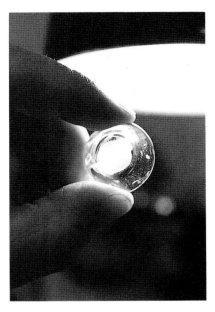

Figure 31.49 The lapped surface before polishing which is best done by machine with spherical wax tools.

a technique for manufacture of individual thin flush fit shells with front optics, then the normal eye can be fitted and tolerate such a lens.

31.12.7   SHELL AND LENS FITTING MODIFICATIONS BY THE CHAIRSIDE

This has in part been described for the preformed lens. The end result must be the same and must achieve a functional and tolerable result (Yorke, 1967).

The shell, when placed on the eye, should touch the sclera, and the optic portion may be seen to be either flush with the cornea or with clearance. In rare instances, the scleral portion will not touch because the whole lens is resting on the cornea. The first modifications will be to achieve scleral touch and minimal central corneal clearance with the eye in the primary position.

The modifications are as follows:

1. Reduce excessive corneal clearance by reducing scleral size.
2. Commence in the sector which appears to be maximal impingement.
3. Minimal decreases in clearance can be achieved by removing material from inside the scleral haptic by grinding and polishing.
4. The back central optic can be recut steeper to increase the optic sagitta and clearance centrally.

If the lens tends, on movement, to slide to one side from the initial insertion position then reduction of the haptic chord of the opposite side may correct this. If the lens rotates about its anterio-posterior axis then reductions of the vertical size can help to stabilize it. If the scleral lens haptic is too flat a fit then the plaster model can be reduced, as explained previously (see page 741), or a new shell made if the manufacturing technique is faulty. Assuming that the shell fit is good and the fenestrations give a small bubble in the primary eye position, which enlarges on the lateral movements of the eye, then the optic can be considered.

31.12.8 OPTIC OF IMPRESSION SCLERAL LENS

At this stage, the shell should have either no back optic but transition and fenestration or, as mentioned (see pages 743–744), a back optic and transition.

In both instances the lens should still have the geometric centre of the optic portion marked on the front surface. With the shell on the eye, the vision point can be marked and its position relative to the geometric centre noted (see page 736).

The practitioner now has to give the manufacturer the ocular refraction (its mean if there is astigmatism) and the new back curve (if desired) for the lens. This can be based upon the keratometry (0.6 mm to 1 mm flatter than average keratometry) or the manufacturer, by use of small-diameter spherical surface gauges, can discover the best approximation to the back 8 mm central portion of the shell and, in the case of keratoconus and grafts, the best over 5 mm chord.

Allowing an approximation for the fluid lens (see Chapter 7) and the lens thickness, the front curve can be calculated and worked onto the lens with the centre at the vision point.

If prism effect or front toric surfaces are required they can be ordered at this time, but some practitioners prefer to keep the initial optics as simple as possible and order modifications to the front optic later.

The front optic junction is blended so as to give a scleral lens haptic of between 0.4 mm and 0.6 mm thickness.

31.13 PATIENT CARE AND MANAGEMENT

This has been dealt with as far as general principles are concerned, in Chapters 25 and 26, but there are a few points that apply specifically to the scleral lens. If the material used absorbs water to any degree then it is advisable to store the lens in a solution with a disinfectant. Since most wearers are not all-day wearers, a solution that gives some protection over a short storage period, and a more effective one for all-night storage, is necessary.

Since this lens as compared with other lens forms has, when on the eye, a semi-sealed retro-lens space, solutions used for insertion must not irritate the cornea. The older procedure used bicarbonate and salt solutions, each 1%, as an insertion solution, but this is no longer commercially available. A good alternative is balanced saline. Ordinary saline is often too acid for comfort. The PMMA lens can be cleaned with detergents and, by the practitioner, with the polishes used in manufacture.

The fenestration can be cleaned with a paint brush (size 0). The methods of insertion and removal follow the general principles. But with the larger lenses the upper lid must be held up and the lens must always be wetted or filled with fluid, then slipped under the upper lid and held there against the eye whilst the lower lid is gently pulled down. Removal is done by a sucker, the lens fitted upwards and then slid down over the lower lid.

31.14 SPECIAL INDICATIONS FOR RIGID SCLERAL LENSES AND THE THERAPEUTIC USES OF SCLERAL LENSES OF RIGID MATERIALS

In Chapter 38 the therapeutic indications and fitting of soft lenses has been dealt with at some length. Historically (see Chapter 1) the rigid scleral preceeded the soft lens (Ridley, 1958a, Gould 1966). Therefore it only remains to decribe those few special cases where rigid scleral is preferable to soft scleral (Ruben, 1989).

They are as follows, but very often the surgeon will, for special reasons, elect to have a scleral rigid lens fitted rather than a soft lens.

1. Burns.
2. Bullous keratopathy.
3. Dry eye.
4. Exposure keratitis.
5. Ocular myopathies and ptosis.
6. Keratoplasty, refractive surgery.
7. Steep, flat cornea and high astigmatism.
8. Division symblepharon.
9. Contact sports and water sports.
10. Services.
11. Prosthetics and occluders.
12. Application of drugs.
13. Electrodiagnostic and experimental lenses.
14. Irregular astigmatism (see Chapter 25).

Non-availability of soft lenses and their correct management is a consideration for using the rigid scleral lens.

31.14.1 BURNS (FIG. 31.50)

Depending upon the extent of the injury to the eye and lid, and the other burn injuries, the team of surgeons, physicians and laboratory scientists will determine, hour-to-hour and then day-to-day, the priorities for the management and initiation of major plastic surgical treatments.

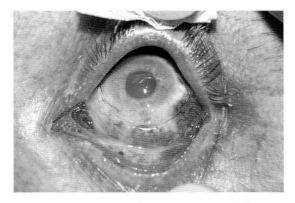

Figure 31.50 Equatorial ring in position following molten metal burn of fornix.

It may, in very extensive injuries, be advised that the eyes or eye affected be covered only with paraffin gauze, and the cornea and conjunctivae protected from drying and infection.

If at some stage the eye is considered in need of a protective shell, this can be combined with a continuous feed of saline or Ringer's solution plus any prophylactic antibiotics. Such shells will prevent undue symblepharon formation. But it must be admitted that the process of symblepharon and conjunctival sclerosis with contraction goes on for several weeks, and therefore the device has to be managed for that time. Later the fluid feed can be discontinued, but in the early stages it acts as an irrigator and keeps the injured eye surface free of debris. Where possible, the shell should be made from a gel impression; when this is not possible the best loose fitting shell should be used. The feed is a capillary tube attached to the face and either fitted to an opening in the shell or to its flattest fitting edge. The other end of the feed is connected to the sterile Ringer's or saline pack that is normally used for intravenous infusions. As the patient progresses, the shell can be altered in shape to give a better fit. Low concentration local steroids are also of value in the early stages.

This treatment can be combined with the plastic lid surgery that may be considered essential. The shell will not be required if the lids or plastic surgery lid replacement provides a tarsorraphy.

31.14.2 BULLOUS KERATOPATHY

Injury of the endothelium, from whatever cause (such as mechanical or chemical burns), are often followed by endothelial degeneration and can result in stromal oedema. The epithelium is lifted by fluid to form bullae, which vary in size from microscopic to large confluent areas; the latter can be exceedingly painful. The soft lens will, in most instances, reduce the pain significantly, and so will the flush fitting shell. In chronic bullous keratopathy not treatable by keratoplasty (and this is true for bullous keratopathy occurring in grafts) the rigid shell may prove to give some vision, whereas the soft lens gives much less.

The shell of rigid material also produces fibrous healing and vascularization of the cornea; close supervision is therefore required. There are some instances when the surgeon

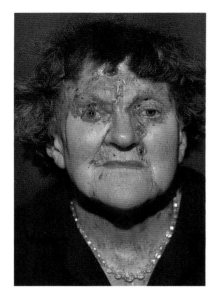

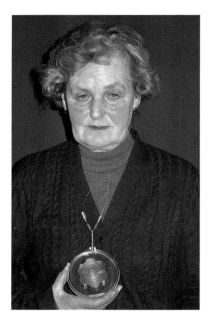

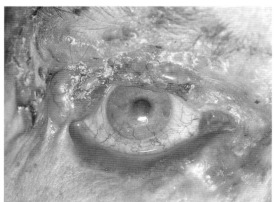

Figures 31.53 and 31.54 Multiple papillomata which caused exposure keratitis treated with scleral contact lenses.

wants this type of healing to occur in the cornea, and then the flush shell is used.

31.14.3 PATHOLOGICAL DRY EYE CONDITIONS (FIG. 31.51 AND 31.52)

These conditions when advanced can cause great distress to the patient. The cornea can become vascularized and sclerosed; the loss of lid movement due to symblepharon for-

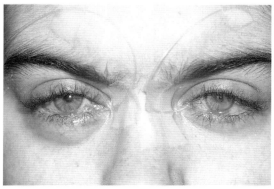

Figures 31.51 and 31.52 Patients with scleral lenses and continuous flow of balanced saline from a pressurized tank and polythene tubing.

mation further exacerbates the disease. Many of these diseases are of collagen tissue and only a few are amenable to systemic treatment. The scleral lens can maintain fluid in contact with the eye surface over long periods of time and provide comfort and vision. Drug treatment can be added to the inside of the lens.

31.14.4 EXPOSURE KERATITIS (FIG. 31.53 AND 31.54)

Once again there are multiple and diverse reasons why the lids may not be able to close and keep the cornea wet. Desiccation of the cornea can lead to scarring and loss of sight, and in some instances perforation and infection. In mild cases of desiccation the soft lens will suffice, providing it is kept wet when worn, but the scleral rigid lens will be of greater value in severe exposure problems.

31.14.5 OCULAR MYOPATHY AND PTOSIS (FIG. 31.55, 31.56 AND 31.57)

Inability to keep the lid open, and in some instances to move the eyes, leads to enforced blindness. There are many ways to give elevation of the lid and sometimes a combination of treatments will give the patient several hours of vision daily. Eyelid operations and the use of spectacles with wire or plastic props can be effective. The danger is that over-elevation leads to corneal desiccation and scarring. The scleral lens fitted with a prop or with a slit above and a thick lip

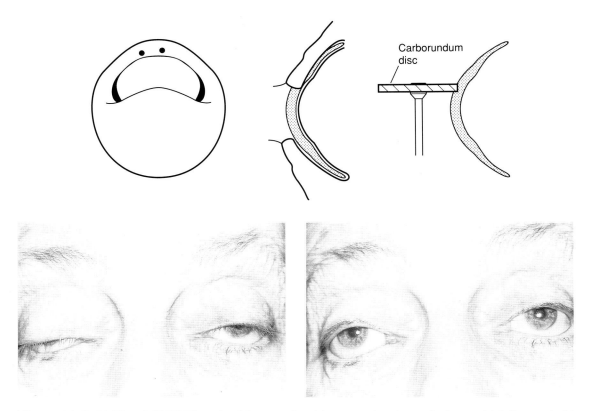

Figures 31.55, 31.56 and 31.57 The scleral lens made with a superior slot and a lower thick lip can hold up the lid as shown in this case of progressive muscular dystrophy.

inferiorly can be a better solution for some patients, and worth trying before surgial intervention.

31.14.6 KERATOPASTY AND OTHER CORNEAL SURGICAL OPERATIONS SUCH AS REFRACTIVE SURGERY

Within this group can be included irregular astigmatism from eye injury or disease (see Chapter 35).

This chapter has described two types of lens that can be effective in optical correction of these conditions. Whenever these conditions cannot be corrected adequately with spectacle lenses, or for reasons of anisometropia and aniseikonia, then the contact lens has to be considered. It is the rigid lens that has to be used to correct the vision since the corneal irregularity will be copied by a soft lens.

Whenever possible the mini-scleral should be tried and, if fitting is still not possible, then the rigid scleral used. This chapter has described lens forms suitable for these problem eye shapes.

31.14.7 STEEP, FLAT CORNEA AND HIGH ASTIGMATISM

Steep and flat corneas are more common in the small and large eye shapes, respectively, and may prove difficult to fit with a conventional small lens or soft lens. The problem is especially worthy of a solution if a high degree of refractive error is present.

Since most of these eyes are otherwise normal and of normal sensitivity, the mini-scleral will not be tolerated and therefore the scleral rigid lens may have to be used.

31.14.8 DIVISION OF SMYBLEPHARON (FIG. 31.58 AND 31.59)

This surgical procedure is done to permit lid and eye mobility and the healing of the conjunctiva or a grafted conjunctiva, and is best achieved with the use of an equatorial ring. If the patient already uses a scleral lens then this can be modified to fit the resected fornix.

The rings can be made in a series of sizes or the peripheral 2 mm of the scleral lens can be cut out for this purpose. They have to be left in place for several weeks.

31.14.9 CONTACT SPORTS AND WATER SPORTS

Soft lenses and even corneal lenses if worn under goggles, are satisfactory for ordinary swimming. But water polo and other water sports require a vision correction that does not under any circumstances become dis-

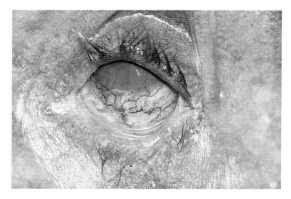

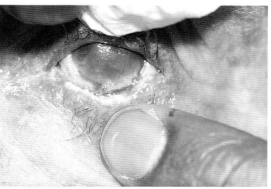

Figures 31.58 and 31.59 The use of equatorial rings to splint the fornix after excision of symblepharon.

lodged, and large rigid sclerals are ideal for this purpose.

The same would apply in certain patients for use in football. All these activities are only of short duration and therefore sensation and physiological tolerance are of secondary consideration.

31.14.10 ARMED SERVICES

The special need for scleral in the armed services is very limited and must only include those tasks of short duration where either the normal eye requires protection or the refractive correction with scleral is required in association with diving or very severe body movements. The conditions for acceptance for service rarely permits scleral rigid lens wear for correction of refractive errors of vision, but their fitting may be advised for personnel who, whilst in the service, develop an eye defect that requires their use (see Chapters 39 and 40).

31.14.11 PROSTHETICS AND OCCLUDERS
(FIGS 31.60, 31.61, 31.62 AND 31.63)

The use of scleral lenses as prosthetic lenses is best dealt with by an ocularist or prosthetics technician. At this time PMMA provides the best material for such devices, surface painting or lamination of colour pigment, and even photographic material, all being possible.

The use of the scleral lens as an occluder is not difficult. It would be of use in those cases where total or partial occlusion is required. Such patients may be sufferers of an extreme degree of photophobia, such as after iridocyclectomy, others may require occlusion for binocular vision problems. The lens can be painted black on the posterior surface and the pigment sealed with polymer. The anterior surface can be painted to the normal eye colouring.

In all these instances the first stage is to obtain a good stable fit that is physiologically functional.

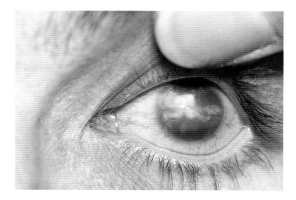

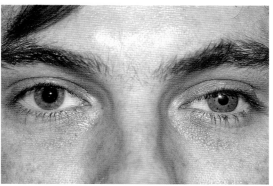

Figures 31.60 and 31.61 The deformed ugly eye can be covered by a flush shell which can then become the basis of a prosthesis.

31.14.12 APPLICATION OF DRUGS

Drug dispensers

At the time of Helmholtz (Circa 1850) it was thought that a glass scleral lens could be filled with a drug containing emollient and placed on the diseased or injured eye to give effective treatment. The absence of antiseptic knowledge would certainly have made such treatments, whilst admirable in theory, less valuable in practice.

It is possible to use the scleral lens in two ways as a drug dispenser:

1. With an irrigator.
2. Direct application.

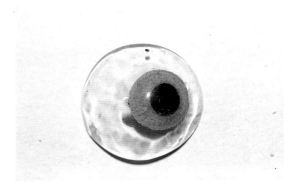

Figure 31.62 An example of a shell prosthesis where the colour was only required over the cornea.

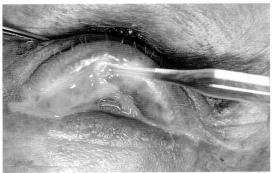

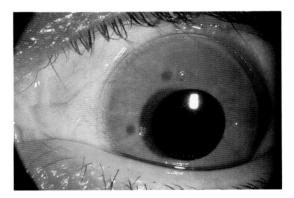

Figure 31.63 The scleral lens used as an optical occluder.

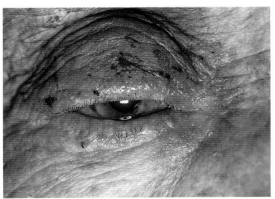

Figure 31.64 and 31.65 The use of imbedded Radon seeds in the treatment of lid tumour which required a protective scleral lens (see text for details).

Radiation therapy (Figs 31.64 and 31.65)

In the treatment of the eye and lids by the various methods of irradiation the scleral lens can be of value. The eye can be protected when only the lid is being treated by the insertion of a lead shell made to the eye shape as a flush fit; the thickness required will be specified by the radiologist. Thin gold laminate covering a PMMA scleral shell and then covered with a thin layer of plastic polymer is another way of achieving the same end. Such protective devices may be required whilst radon seed inserts in the tissue are being treated (Ridley 1958a).

The scleral ventilated or channel lens may be needed to treat the consecutive dry eye that sometimes follows irradiation treatment.

Irrigation drug administration

The scleral lens has to have inlet and outlet tubes of capillary dimensions, and the fluid containing the active ingredients must be fed by gravity (a bag on a stand), by pump or pressure. This treatment is used for burns or after symblepharon excision and allows accurate control of the drug dose.

Direct application

In this treatment the drug is contained in a ointment base, such as paraffin, and applied to the inside of the lens or shell. It could be considered for the treatment of corneal ulceration but it must be noted that the drug concentration or any additives must be less than that used for normal instillation, since if in any way toxic to tissues, the effect can be serious in view of the long period of time the device and drug will be in contact with the tissues.

31.14.13 ELECTRODIAGNOSTIC AND EXPERIMENTAL LENSES

There are now special lenses of soft material made with conductors to pick up potential differences for the measurement of electrooculograms and version electroretinograms. But in those clinics where several tests are to be done each day, the rigid scleral fitted with a conductor of silver may be considered preferable (Byford, 1959; Sundmach 1959). The lenses must be cleaned and disinfected between each application to the eye.

Scleral lenses can be used for a variety of experiments such as controlled flow of fluids and their gaseous estimations across the eye.

31.15 SUMMARY

This chapter has dealt with the fitting of the preformed rigid scleral of large size and also the mini-scleral, mostly made of gas permeable material.

Such lenses, and the data given, are for fitting abnormal eye shapes such as keratoconus and grafted eyes.

The fitting of the impression scleral is also given; this type of lens is preferred if a mini-scleral cannot be fitted. The mini-scleral can be used in a trial set whereas it is unlikely that anyone will have a trial scleral set of sufficient size to be of value in fitting the abnormal eye. Therefore the use of the preformed scleral as described here is by use of data based upon objective and subjective measurements and preferably the eye impression model.

It should be stated that the large scleral lens requires craft and expertise, which are best acquired by serving an apprenticeship to a practitioner who is involved daily in the procedures.

REFERENCES

Bergman, W., Maurice, D.M. and Ruben, M. (1970) The effect of channels of scleral contact lenses on hydrostatic pressures. *Br. J. Ophthalmol.*, **54**, 484.

Bier, N. (1949) The practice of ventilated contact lenses. *Am. J. Optom.*, **26**, 120.

Byford, G.H. (1959) Eye movement recording. *Nature (London)*, **184** (Suppl. 19), 1493–4.

Cooke, G. and Young, G. (1986) Use of computer simulated patterns for fluorescein. *Trans. BCLA.*, 21–6.

Dallos, J. (1937) Fitting of contact glasses. *Trans. Ophth. Soc. UK.*, **57**, 509.

Dallos, J. (1969) Corneal and haptic lenses. *Klin. Mbl. Augenheit.*, **155**, 475.

Forknall, A.J. (1959) Some notes on haptic lenses. *Br. J. Physiol. Optics*, **16**, 96.

Girard, L.J. and Soper, J.W. (1966) Flush fitting scleral contact lenses. *Am. J. Ophthalmol.*, **61**, 1109.

Gordon, S.P. (1969) Perilimbal lenses. *T. Ophth. Soc.*, **89**, 207.

Gould, H. (1966) Treatment of neurotrophic keratitis with scleral contact lenses. Contact lens symposium, Munich.

Gould, H. (1970) Management of dry eye with scleral contact lenses. *Ear, Nose & Throat Monthly*, **49**, 64.

Haynes, P.P. (1968) Eye impression haptic contact lenses. *J. Am. Opt. Assoc.*, **39**, 210.

Jenkins, L. (1964) Fitting of impression scleral contact lenses. *Br. J. Physiol. Optics*, **21**, 163.

Marriott, P.J. (1966) Impression haptic contact lenses. *Cont. J.*, **1**, 8.

Marriott, P.J. (1967) Fitting scleral moulded contact lenses. *Cah. Verres. Cont.* **16**, 2.

Miller, D. (1968) Flush fitting optical scleral contact lenses. *Arch. Ophthamol.*, **79**, 311.

Miller, D. and Carol, J. (1967) Impression techniques and effect on cornea. *Arch. Ophthamol.*, **78**, 331.

Miller, D., Holmberg, A. and Carol, J. (1966) Comparison of two moulding methods. *Arch. Ophthalmol.*, **76**, 422.

Obrig, T.E and Salvatori, P.L. (1957) *Contact Lenses* (3rd edn). Obrig Laboratories, New York.

Ridley, F.T. (1958a) Application of irradiation to Conj Sac *Trans. Ophth. Soc. UK.,* **78**, 171–8.

Ridley, F.T. (1958b) Contact lens in surgical conditions. Barcelona, Barraquer Clinic.

Ruben, M. (1989) *Contact Lenses Colour Atlas* (2nd edn.) Wolfe Medical, London.

Ruben, M. (1967) The apex lens. *Contact Lens,* **1**, 28

Smelzer, G.K. and Ozanics, V. (1952) Oxygen deficiency and contact lenses. *Science (New York),* **115**, 140

Smelzer, G.K. and Chen, D.K. (1953) Physiological changes due to contact lenses. *Arch. Ophthalmol.,* **53**, 676.

Sundmach, E. (1959) Contact lenses for electroretinogram. *Acta. Ophthalmol.,* **37**, (Suppl. 52).

Triesmann, H. (1969, 1970) Personal techniques haptic contact lens fitting. *Contact Lens,* 1; 5; 6; 7; 8: 21; 24; 567

Woodward, E.G. (1972) Preformed scleral lenses. *In Contact Lenses* (eds. A.J. Phillips and A. Stone), Barrie & Jenkins, London

Yorke, H.C. (1967) Shell production and modifications. *Contact Lens,* **1**, 37.

Young, G. (1988) Fluorescein in rigid lens fit evaluation. *Int. Contact Lens Clin.,* **15** (3), 95–100.

GAS PERMEABLE SCLERAL CONTACT LENSES

32

O.D. Schein, P. Rosenthal and C. Ducharme

Although a therapeutic potential has long been recognized for scleral contact lenses, their general acceptance and use have been limited by several factors. First, the skill and time commitment necessary to fit and fabricate such lenses are substantial, restricting their use to only a few dedicated centres. In the United States, this art has essentially disappeared. Second, the application of a polymethyl methacrylate (PMMA) scleral lens, whether molded or preformed, has inevitably been accompanied by physiological limitations (see Chapter 31). These are largely secondary to hypoxia, and are manifested in the short term by corneal epithelial edema, and, chronically, by neovascularization. These predictable complications can be lessened by shortened wearing times or by the use of a variety of gutters and fenestrations that act to increase the exchange of oxygenated tears. In the setting of bilateral severe corneal disease or monocular status, the visual benefits that may be conferred by a scleral lens have frequently justified the risk of these adverse effects. However, these limitations have significantly restricted their use and acceptance.

Ezekiel (1983) in Australia first described the use of rigid gas permeable materials in a preformed scleral lens. He used a low oxygen permeable material (16×10^{-11} cm^2/ml O$_2$/s/ml mmHg at 36 °C) and reported improved com-

fort and wearing time compared with conventional PMMA scleral lenses. Ruben and Benjamin (1985), using the equivalent oxygen percent (EOP) technique, demonstrated the improved physiological performance achieved with preformed RGP materials of low (Boston IV) to medium (Paraperm EW) Dk, even in relatively thick design. Bleshoy and Pullum (1988), monitoring induced corneal swelling by pachometry, confirmed the findings of Ruben and Benjamin (1985). Pullum (1987) described in detail an improved manufacturing technique for RGP scleral lenses, which with other ongoing advances, led to the development of new high Dk RGP scleral lenses.

We are currently evaluating the use of a highly permeable material for use in a scleral design (Schein *et al.* 1990). The Polymer Technology Corporation provides an oversized button of a fluorosilicone/acrylate copolymer (Itafluorofocon B), a highly gas permeable material (110×10^{-11} cm^2/ml O$_2$/ml mmHg at 36 °C). Figure 32.1 shows the lens in profile and Figure 32.2 in schematic form in its relationship to the ocular surface. The lenses are fitted using a specially designed scleral trial diagnostic set. The typical posterior surface can be described as consisting of two primary sections, each having two zones and corresponding radii (Fig. 32.3). The peripheral, or haptic, section encompasses the central haptic radius and the peripheral haptic radius sepa-

Contact Lens Practice. Edited by Montague Ruben and Michel Guillon.
Published in 1994 by Chapman & Hall, London. ISBN 0 412 35120 X

Table 32.1 Clinical characteristics of patients using gas permeable scleral lenses

Patient no., age (years)	Diagnoses and conditioning	Visual acuity		Wearing time (h)	Follow-up (months)
		Spectacle-corrected	Scleral lens		
1,75	Monocular aphakia	*	20/25	12	46
2,72	Aphakia, ruptured globe, scleral buckle, 9 diopters astigmatism, superior limbic staphyloma	*	20/30	12	46
3,19	Marfan's syndrome, bilateral aphakia	20/30 (R.E.) 20/30 (L.E.)	20/25 (R.E.) 20/30 (L.E.)	16	20
4,55	Keratoconus, after penetrating keratoplasty, 10 diopters astigmatism	20/200	20/50	15	36
5,29	After penetrating keratoplasty, after wedge resection, 11 diopters astigmatism	20/200	20/20	12	20
6,24	Keratoconus, apical erosions	20/400	20/40	8	40
7,46	Keratoconus, corneal scar	20/200	20/70	16	33
8,46	Severe myopia, keratoconus, fungal keratitis, after penetrating keratoplasty, 8 diopters astigmatism	20/100	20/30	8	31
9,35	Keratoconus, after superficial keratectomy	20/60	20/25	15	7
10,53	Neurofibromatosis, bilateral cranial nerve V and VII palsies, tarsorrhaphies both eyes	20/200	20/40	16	8
11,22	Corneal anesthesia both eyes, fibrovascular pannus both eyes, tarsorrhaphies both eyes	20/800	20/40	12	4
12,35	Keratoconus, after penetrating keratoplasty, 12 diopters astigmatism	20/200	20/50	8	45
13,45	Keratoconus, after 2 penetrating keratoplasties, 20 diopters astigmatism	20/800	20/20	8	2
14,41	Keratoconus, after thermokeratoplasty, after penetrating keratoplasty, 9 diopters astigmatism	20/80	20/25	12	5
15,43	Keratoconus, after penetrating keratoplasty, after relaxing incision and compression sutures, 8 diopters astigmatism	20/60	20/25	14	7

* Spectacles not feasible because of monocular aphakia.

over-refraction; however, a stable lens fit could not be achieved with corneal PMMA or rigid gas permeable materials. A trial of a rigid lens fit over a soft lens ('piggy-back system') was associated with graft rejection and the development of an elevated scar at the graft–host junction (Fig. 32.4). A gas permeable scleral lens was fitted in a fashion to provide full clearance of the elevated scar, resulting in a comfortable fit, 20/50 acuity and an average daily wearing time of 15 hours over a 2-year follow-up period.

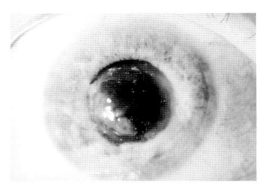

Figure 32.4 Patient with 5 mm corneal graft, irregular astigmatism, and scarring at the graft–host interface.

Case 2

This 48-year-old woman with neurofibromatosis (patient 10) sufferred from bilateral V and VII nerve palsies following surgery for bilateral acoustic neuromas. Multiple, sequential tarsorrhaphies had been performed on both eyes for progressive fibrovascular proliferation of the exposed corneal surface (Fig. 32.5). A diffuse punctate epithelial keratitis was unresponsive to tarsorrhaphy, tear supplements and punctal occlusion. Best corrected visual acuity was 20/200 in each eye. A soft therapeutic

(bandage) lens adhered to the ocular surface, causing epithelial erosions. The tarsorrhaphy was reversed in the right eye and a gas permeable scleral lens was fitted (Fig. 32.4). The lens was fitted to vault the fibrovascular scar. The fluid compartment led to rapid resolution of the punctate keratitis, and her vision returned to 20/40 after incorporation of her myopic correction (– 5.00) into the scleral lens. A reading yields a near acuity of 20/25 allowing her to read for the first time in over ten years. At 1-year follow-up she maintains a wearing time of 16 hours per day.

After initial fitting, the lenses have been remarkably well tolerated. One patient, who had been off topical medications for several years, developed endothelial graft rejection while wearing the lens. This episode responded promptly to topical steroids, and use of the lens has been resumed. No patients have developed ulcerative keratitis or a worsening of the underlying pathology. Several patients with corneal neovascularization have shown partial resolution of corneal vessels. We have experienced one physiological failure. This occurred in a monocular 70-year-old with high myopia, 20 diopters

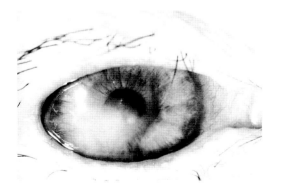 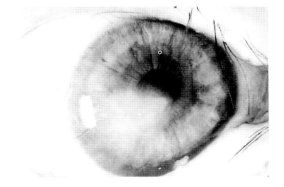

Figure 32.5 (Left) eye of patient with tarsorrhaphy for combined fifth and seventh cranial nerve palsies, corneal scarring, and diffuse punctate keratitis. Visual acuity, 20/200. (Right) Tarsorrhaphy reversed, gas-permeable scleral lens in place. Visual acuity, 20/40.

of astigmatism from a cataract wound inflicted 15 years earlier and aphakic bullous keratopathy affecting the superior 50% of the cornea. Although the gas permeable lens could be comfortably fitted, the region of epithelial edema increased with use of the lens for more than 4 hours, and reversed spontaneously with discontinuation of the lens. This suggests possible limitations in eyes with borderline endothelial function with the current materials.

In addition to refinement in materials and fitting concepts for the gas permeable scleral lens, there is also room for improvement in the composition of the fluid interface. We currently employ non-preserved saline; however, it is quite likely that other preparations, for example a buffered artificial tear solution, might be more healthy for the ocular surface with prolonged use. In addition, if special circumstances dictate the need for still greater oxygen permeability, the use of a liquid perfluorocarbon as an oxygen carrying reservoir has been suggested as a substitute for saline (Refojo *et al.*, 1985).

We are hopeful that evolving strategies employing gas permeable scleral lenses will address the two major therapeutic limitations of conventional corneal lenses in the rehabilitation of patients with significant corneal disease. The first is the setting of abnormal corneal topography where a hard corneal lens over-refraction yields an improvement in visual acuity but cannot be fitted because of positional instability or discomfort (e.g. keratoconus, cornea plana, marginal degenerations, corneoscleral trauma, graft–host interface irregularities). The second major limitation concerns the unsatisfactory performance of therapeutic soft lenses in the presence of corneal exposure or inadequate tear film. These lenses cannot correct visual loss from surface irregularites and frequently adhere in tear-deficient states. The gas permeable scleral lens, with its constant fluid interface may offer significant promise for patients with ocular disorders characterized by dryness or corneal exposure (e.g. keratoconjunctivitis sicca, Stevens–Johnson syndrome, ocular cicatricial pemphigoid, cicatricial trachoma, neurotrophic keratitis, structural lid disease or trauma). Finally, one can imagine potential applications of a gas permeable scleral lens to normal eyes with simple refractive errors in special occupational or sports-related circumstances, in particular aquatic sports or occupations (e.g. deep-sea diving, water polo, etc.).

Pullum *et al.*, (1990, 1991) at Moorfields Eye Hospital in London have also worked with high *Dk* RGP scleral lenses. They have demonstrated that for a *Dk* of approximately 115, the physiological performance achieved is relatively insensitive to thickness differences, 0.15 and 0.30 mm thick lenses producing similar corneal swelling.

REFERENCES

Bleshoy, H. and Pullum, K.W. (1988) Corneal response to gas permeable impression scleral lenses. *J. BCLA.* **11**, 31–4.

Ezekiel, D. (1983) Gas permeable haptic lenses. *J. Br. Contact Lens Assoc.*, **6**, 158–60.

Pullum, K.W., (1987) Feasibility study for the production of gas permeable lenses using ocular impression techniques. *Trans. BCLA Annual Clin. Conf.*, 12, 77–81 (1989).

Pullum, K.W., Hobley, A.J. and Parker, J.H. (1990) Hypoxic corneal changes following sealed gas permeable impression scleral lens wear. *J. Br. Contact Lens Assoc.*, **13**, 83–7.

Pullum K.W., Hobley, A.J., and Davison, C. (1991) 100 + Dk: Does thickness make much difference? *J. Br. Contact Lens Assoc.*, **14**, 17–19.

Refojo, M.F. *et al.*, (1985) Perfluoro-l-methyldecalin as a potential oxygen carrier with fluid scleral lenses. *Curr. Eye Res.*, **4**, 732–3.

Ruben, M. and Benjamin, W. (1985) Gas permeable scleral lenses. *Contact Lens J.*, **13**(2), 5–10.

Schein, O.D., Rosenthal, P. and Ducharme, C. (1990) A gas permeable scleral lens for visual rehabilitation. *Am. J. Ophthalmol.*, **109**, 318–22.

PRESBYOPIA AND THE INFLUENCE OF AGING ON PRESCRIPTION OF CONTACT LENSES

W.J. Benjamin and I.M. Borish

33.1 INTRODUCTION

Deterioration of vision, as a result of aging, is of major concern not only to those directly affected, but to all who wish to continue to age gracefully with the passage of time. In the contact lens arena, the search for an ideal and readily applicable presbyopic correction is a significant factor driving research within the ophthalmic industry.

Presbyopia is but a single ocular change and the purpose of this chapter is to place loss of accommodation in its proper context among the other visual effects associated with aging, so that an optimal influence may be exerted on the materials, design and utilization of contact lenses for individual patients. It is hoped that the reader will realize that 'fitting contact lenses for presbyopia' actually embodies a professional function of a higher order, that of 'prescribing contact lenses for an aging eye' with all of its ramifications included.

33.2 THE AGING EYE AND ITS INFLUENCE ON CONTACT LENS WEAR

33.2.1 EYELIDS AND APPOSITION

As a person ages, changes take place in the ocular adnexia. A reduction occurs in muscle tone, the amount of orbital fat, and elasticity of the skin of the eyelids (Phillips, 1986; Mancil & Owsley, 1988; Soong *et al.*, 1988). The lower lids may vary from their usual setting against the surface of the globe. The lower lids of elderly individuals may not retain sufficient elastic 'memory' to resume their usual place, which may cause the lower lid to loosen from its position normally apposed against the globe of the eye. When contact lenses are worn, the situation may be further aggravated, or even initiated, by insertion and removal procedures which pull the lid away from the globe on a regular basis. The degree of increasing lid laxity ranges from elasticity of the younger eye to eyelids of sufficient retraction to result in ectropion.

Eyelid and punctal appositions are necessary for tear fluid distribution across the ocular surfaces and the contact lens. However, besides its involvement in the wetting of the lenses, inferior eyelid apposition may be important for proper orientation and movement of lenses. The lower lid can be used to help prevent lenses from slipping below the limbus. It is usually assumed that prismatically ballasted lenses are properly oriented before the pupil during reading by

Contact Lens Practice. Edited by Montague Ruben and Michel Guillon.
Published in 1994 by Chapman & Hall, London. ISBN 0 412 35120 X

patient. Several other age-related dystrophies and degenerations of the cornea have been identified (Phillips, 1986; Soong *et al.*, 1988).

A particularly important ocular surface abnormality for contact lens wear, and one that may impact on corneal transmission of light, is the degeneration of subepithelial tissues, including Bowman's membrane, and their replacement by other connective-like tissue resulting in pterygia. These are usually located nasally, but can be temporally, and are often bilateral. While the exact cause is unknown, their origin may be exacerbated by chronic surface dryness, UVR or other radiation. Centration and movement of rigid contact lenses are adversely affected by the presence of pterygia. Fittings of soft contact lenses are influenced not only by pterygia, but by pingueculae that are similarly formed over the nasal and temporal sclera adjacent to the limbus. The wear of rigid and soft lenses may aggravate pingueculae and pterygia by inducing additional mechanical, chemical, allergenic, or wetting-related irritation of these tissues.

33.2.4 AQUEOUS FLUID

Aqueous fluid shows no significant change in transparency with age. It is a clear fluid which helps nourish the posterior cornea and anterior lens and has a half-life of about one hour. While aging does not appear to affect the aqueous itself, it does appear to result in some loss of cells in the outflow pathway and in loss of elastic fibrils in the iris and anterior chamber angle which may result in increased intraocular tension. Because of the growth of the crystalline lens with age, depth of the anterior chamber decreases with age, thus confining the amount of aqueous fluid present.

33.2.5 IRIS AND PUPIL

The entrance pupil of the eye is formed by refraction of the real pupil by the cornea and is just over 3 mm behind the anterior corneal surface. The entrance pupil is very important to contact lens wearers for several reasons. Illumination of the retina is proportional to the square of pupillary diameter. Depths of field and focus for clear vision are inversely proportional to pupil diameter. The lower limit of pupil size for optimum visual acuity is approximately 2 mm, below which effects of reduced retinal illuminance and diffraction outweigh beneficial aspects of an increase in depth of field and reduction of ocular spherical aberration. The entrance pupil also controls blur circle size on the retina for object rays not originating from the far point plane of the eye.

The entrance pupil averages 3.5 mm in diameter in adults under normal illumination and ranges from 1.3 mm to 10 mm. It is usually centered on the optic axis of the eye but is displaced temporally away from the visual axis by 5 degrees, on average. The entrance pupil is decentered approximately 0.15 mm nasally and 0.1 mm inferior to the geometric center of the visible iris circumference (Erickson & Robboy, 1985). In general, the diameter of the pupil gradually becomes smaller during the lifetime of a patient after about the age of 12–18 years. This seems to be a linear relationship in which pupil sizes for light-adapted and dark-adapted eyes at age 20 (means nearly 5 mm and 8 mm, respectively) both diminish to about 2 mm and 2.5 mm, respectively, at age 80 (Loawenfeld, 1979; Pitts, 1982). The progressive change in size is known as senile miosis and is shown in Table 33.1. It is not totally explained by increased iris rigidity or loss of muscle fibers in the iris, but apparently also includes a progressive delayed latency of response time, indicating some neurological involvement (Loewenfeld, 1979).

Pupil size is always changing in the normal eye, due to small slow oscillations, convergence/accommodation (near triad response), and pupillary responses to light. Pupil size can be influenced by drugs and medications and is slightly larger in persons with light irides

Table 33.1 Relation of pupil size to age

Age (years)	Photopic Diameter (mm)	Scotopic Diameter (mm)
20	5	8
40	4	6
50	3.5	5.5
60	3+	4.25
70	2.5	3
80	2+	2.5

(compared to dark irides). Pupils become mydriatic in response to large sensory and psychological stimuli and miotic in response to pain or irritation within the globe (oculopupillary reflex). A recent investigation (Jones, 1990) has shown that pupils are not larger for females (compared to males) and myopes (compared to hyperopes) when accommodation has been accounted for, though these relationships may be present under normal conditions when accommodation is uncontrolled.

It is apparent that the entrance pupil sets the limits of translation and centration of contact lenses on the eye, for the optic zone(s) of a contact lens must be able to sufficiently cover the entrance pupil of the eye to obtain excellent vision. Flare seen by patients wearing rigid contact lenses occurs when the optic zone of the contact lens is smaller than the entrance pupil of the eye, or when the lens is positioned such that its optic zone does not cover the pupil. Optimal diameters of central clear zones of tinted gel lenses are dependent on pupil diameter of each wearer, and can reduce field of view if improperly matched in size or if decentered before the pupil (Josephson & Caffery, 1987). The entrance pupil assumes special importance in the wear of bifocal contact lenses (Erickson & Robboy, 1985; Borish, 1988; Erickson *et al.*, 1988), for its diameter and position relative to the distance and near portions of the contact lens determine effec-

tive visual performance.

A good part of the difficulty of designing and fitting bifocal contact lenses is caused by the fact that entrance pupils vary considerably between individuals and constantly change size in the same individual. Contact lens wear can dramatically enhance vision in a case of an aberrant pupil or iris, such as in aniridia or ocular albinism, for which contact lenses containing apertures can act in lieu of or in addition to, the entrance pupil of the eye to perform its optical function. Cases of anisocoria, polycoria, and distorted pupils can also be managed by placing apertures within contact lenses (Bier, 1981). Positions and sizes of contact lens optical zones relative to size and location of the pupillary reflex can be analyzed with the use of a retinoscope or opththalmoscope, a technique recommended to practitioners (Josephson, 1986).

33.2.6 CRYSTALLINE LENS

The human lens is composed of a single cell type in various stages of cytodifferentiation and retains within it all the cells formed in its lifetime (Marshall *et al.*, 1982). Thus, the lens thickens as one ages and the lens nucleus contains the oldest cells while new cells are added superficially from the anterior epithelium. As cells become older and more embedded they become farther removed from sources of oxygenation and nutrition, therefore, they partially lose structural integrity and become less metabolically active.

The epithelial cell layer of the lens lies only on the anterior surface, posterior to its basement membrane, the anterior lens capsule. It plays a role in the maintenance of the water relationships and resultant transparency of the lens, but its restriction to the anterior surface is not precisely understood, although embryologically, the retina appears to influence the development. Its central zone, roughly equal to the pupil area, is basically static in quantity of cells, although these slowly reduce in number with age. The intermediate area, lying behind the iris, is the major site of cell division in the lens. After division, new cells slowly increase in cytoplasm, extend into the lens equator, and differentiate into lens fibers which extend both anteriorly and posteriorly toward the center of the lens. Ends of these fibers meet at the anterior and posterior 'Y sutures'. As new fibers are formed, older ones are displaced towards the interior, forming the lenticular nucleus.

The lens capsule is the thickest basement membrane in the body. Elasticity of the lens capsule results in accommodation when the zonular tension of the capsule is released at the lens equator by action of the ciliary muscle. Variations of the capsule with age affect transparency very little, but much of the progression of presbyopia is credited to a reduction in elasticity of the lens capsule, thus, its ability to shape the malleable interior matrix of lens fibers is reduced. As the eye ages, the ciliary muscle appears to deteriorate and the interior lens matrix becomes more rigid (less malleable), but the reduced elasticity of the capsule appears to be the major element restraining the accommodative mechanism.

Up to 75% of ultraviolet radiation in the 300–400 nm band is transmitted by the very young lens, but this falls to only 20% by the age of 80. The action of the ultraviolet appears to result in progressive accumulation of fluorescent chromophores which also account for a yellow pigmentation of the lens, most pronounced in the nuclear area (Weale, 1983; Zigman, 1983). Optical density of the lens appears to increase at the rate of 9% per year from age 45 to 63 (Pitts, 1982). When the amount of central yellowing becomes intense, it is visible during biomicroscopy as a brownish color, and the lens nucleus is said to be brunescent. Quite apart from cataract, reduced light transmission especially in the blue wavelengths is a routine age-related phenomenon (Mancil & Owsley, 1988).

33.2.7 VITREOUS

The vitreous is a transparent gel. It contains a few cells generally limited by access to oxygenation and nutrition to positions adjacent to the retina. The vitreous shows little change until the ages of 45–50 when the gel begins to collapse and liquify. In 65% of individuals, by the age of 50, the posterior vitreous detaches from the retinal surface and freed particles of collagen and other particles float across the line of vision (Balazs & Denlinger, 1982).

33.2.8 THE RETINA

The major visual changes which occur with aging are related to: (1) deterioration in the replacement process of photosensitive discs which make up the light-sensitive portions of rods and cones; (2) reduction of the number of cells constituting the retinal pigmentary epithelial layer; and (3) increase in resistance of the sieve-like meshwork of Bruch's layer underlying the epithelium. Photosensitive discs of rods are discrete and, when depleted, are entirely renewable during continued light exposure within approximately two weeks. Those of the cones are not discrete and can only be renewed in the dark over a time period extending from nine months to a year (Marshall, 1977).

Debris of worn-out photosensitive discs is removed by phagocytic action of underlying pigmentary epithelial cells, within which debris undergoes lysitic action. Excess debris known as lipofuscin granules accumulate in the pigmentary cells and are passed by the epithelium through the sieve-like meshwork of Bruch's membrane to the choroid. With aging this replacement action becomes less efficient, as the numbers of the phagocytic pigmentary cells decrease, while at the same time, the sieve of Bruch's membrane becomes resistant to passage of cellular waste particles (Marshall, 1977).

Accumulations of excess debris occur on

the retina when the normal removal system is unable to handle its load. When these accumulations become large enough they are noted during ophthalmoscopy as retinal drusen. Eventually, the accumulation will interfere with retinal attachment and the health of retinal cells most sensitive to supply of oxygen, nutrition, and waste management, i.e. rods, cones and other neural elements. As cones are most susceptible, progressive central macular degeneration is the result. In addition, reduced blood supply through the underlying macular choriocapillaris with aging helps the degenerative process (Bressler *et al.*, 1988; Young, 1988; Friedman *et al.*, 1989). There is a small linear loss of cones up to age 40 after which the loss becomes more rapid, especially in the fovea. Vision of the older eye is directly affected (Marshall, 1977).

Today, we have created artificial lighting which extends the working day of the retina, thus reducing the amount of time available for cones to renew their discs. This imbalance will be continued over our lifetimes, which have also been extended. Therefore, the demands on our retinas have been dramatically increased. We will be able to see in the future if these additional burdens will result in serious visual difficulty.

33.2.9 VISUAL FUNCTION

In addition to the obvious reduction of accommodative amplitude, a number of other changes have been shown to influence the visual capacity of the aging eye. These are manifested essentially in the loss of contrast sensitivity, subsequent inability to cope with reduced illumination, and reduced ability to deal with glare. Visual acuity improves slightly up to the age of 20 years after which it remains normal in the non-pathological eye until about the age of 50, after which it begins to decline. The decline worsens at the age of 65, and visual acuity appears to lose about 7% annually from age 65 to age 85 and

beyond (Pitts, 1982). The loss can be ascribed to the adverse metabolic effects on cones and their decrease in numbers, but also is decidedly influenced by reduced retinal illuminance due to decreased pupil size and reduced transparency of the lens and cornea.

The senotic pupil helps optical imaging by adding to the depth of focus, but, at the same time, impedes it by reducing retinal illuminance. Some authorities state that retinal illumination at age 60 may be only one third of that at age 20. For a subject over 50 years of age, up to twice as much light may be required for the same photopic visual task. Marked increase of background illumination may be required although such an increase may not compensate entirely for visual acuity losses. Some gain is achieved by increasing contrast, but care must be taken to avoid disability glare in doing so. If contrast is reduced by 30% to 40%, target illumination must be increased by 25% to enable equivalent acuity at age 60 to that of age 25 (Pitts, 1982; Weale, 1978). Blackwell & Blackwell (1971) reported that contrast must be increased by a factor of 3.03 in order for 70% of a 60-year-old population to restore visual performance of their eyes at age 20. Table 33.2 shows the contrast alterations necessary at different age levels to achieve equivalent acuity, holding average target illumination constant (Guth, 1957).

Another major deficiency noted in the older eye is the significant decline in the ability to efficiently dark adapt. The miotic

Table 33.2 Age and contrast to achieve equivalent acuity

Age (years)	Relative Contrast Increase
20	1.0
30–40	1.17
40–50	1.2
50–60	1.86
60–70	2.50

pupil is even more pronounced under dark-adapted conditions in comparison to a younger eye, for the pupil fails to dilate as completely. Dark adaptation is slower, diminished in magnitude, and is accompanied by an increase in light scatter by the denser media, particularly of shorter wavelengths. Therefore, illumination utilizing light of longer wavelengths is advantageous. Target illuminance may need to be doubled every 13 years over the age of 20 to achieve equivalent dark-adapted vision.

Uncorrected errors of refraction as well as reduced contrast markedly affect visual acuity of older eyes. Precise correction as well as increased light is needed for best visual acuity by the age of 45 years and upwards. For mesopic vision, one diopter out of focus may require 2–3 times the light, while a two-diopter uncorrected error may call for 5–6 times the light. When prescribing contact lenses, the tendency towards casual refraction, disregard of astigmatic error, use of so-called 'simultaneous vision' bifocals and 'monovision' become much more deleterious to vision when corrections of older eyes are involved. Additionally, the effect of approximate refractions may play a larger role in the presbyopic eye because the eye no longer is capable of adjusting the circle of least confusion to the retina.

33.2.10 THE VISUAL ENVIRONMENT

The influence of factors such as low humidity, high temperature, wind, and dust upon surface wetting, lubrication, and deposition, allergic reactions of the conjunctiva, and visual demands for specific target locations are apparent for contact lenses even before aging and presbyopia are considered. Wetting and lubrication may be more acutely disturbed by the environment when changes in tear flow and quality of the older eye are examined. Awareness of the environmental illumination and task factors which may be part of the patient's individual routine

become important, particularly if the lighting in the practitioner's office and the tests performed in evaluation of vision with contact lenses bear little relation to those conditions actually faced by the patient.

Of vital importance is the realization that mesopic vision and the loss of contrast sensitivity become ever greater handicaps as one ages under the best of conditions, and even when wearing spectacles. For example, matching colors under artificial lighting, detecting low-contrast objects when driving at night or walking into theaters, recovery from oncoming headlights, reading at lower illuminations as with low-contrast menus in dimly lit restaurants, and numerous similar tasks become difficult and exasperating.

As a result, any corrective modality that delivers less than optimal retinal imagery should be of serious concern to practitioners prescribing for the aging eye. The term 'pupil dependency' has been introduced to denote the critical influence of pupil size, position, and contact lens centration on levels of retinal illumination, glare, and contrast when wearing bifocal contact lenses (Borish, 1988). Since many contact lenses designed for presbyopes provide less than optimal optical images to begin with, as will be seen later, their effects on mesopic visual performance must be considered in detail.

33.3 CONSTRUCTS OF BIFOCAL AND RELATED CONTACT LENSES

The older portion of the 'baby boom' generation in the USA has already entered the period of life which necessitates presbyopic correction. Projections of demographic growth indicate that this age group will be the most rapidly increasing proportion of the population in the next decades. Presbyopic correction requires that some form of lens system be used which provides both a focus of the light from distance fixation and a focus of the light from near fixation. In spectacles this is provided by various forms of lens constructions known as multifocals, in which, in a single lens, one or two segments for near and/or intermediate focal points are combined with a major portion of the lens focused for distance, or a progressive channel may connect distance and near focal centers. The eye alternates between desired sections for desired vision. The ideal correction with contact lenses would duplicate or even rise above spectacle performance.

Increased research and development within the contact lens industry has resulted from a general belief that an optically-excellent, comfortable bifocal contact lens would be one outcome of continuing technological advancement. A review of bifocal contact lens patents by the authors has shown an accelerated increase in the number of US patents related to presbyopic correction with contact lenses (Table 33.3). Yet, to date the fitting of bifocal contact lenses has constituted only a small proportion of contact lens practice. Less than 1% of contact lenses prescribed in the USA are bifocal and only 0.5% of persons between the ages of 45 and 64 in Australia wear contact lenses (Back *et al.*, 1989).

Contact lenses are usually divided into two groups of rigid (hard) lenses and soft (flexible) lenses in order to differentiate the properties of each lens group. However, overall optical concepts affecting *bifocal* contact lens designs are similar for both groups. Table 33.4 reveals bifocal designs that are now available to the contact lens practitioner.

Table 33.3 Number of United States patents filed during the last four decades has accelerated from the 1950s to the present

Decade	Number of Patents Related to Bifocal Contact Lenses
1950–1959	2
1960–1969	9
1970–1979	10
1980–1989	24

'Fused segment' bifocals are currently produced only in lenses made of polymethyl methacrylate (PMMA), and represent the only manufacturing method not used in production of today's permeable rigid and soft bifocal lenses. Many of the contact lens bifocal designs have been copied from equivalent spectacle bifocals.

33.3.1 RADIALLY SYMMETRIC CONTACT LENS DESIGNS

'Radially symmetric' bifocal designs are those with multiple refractive zones with outside circular diameters having common geometric centers of curvature at the vertices of each contact lens. With these lenses, refractive power is distributed across optical apertures in concentric iso-power arrangements. Typical subcategories of radially symmetric designs are diagrammatically represented in Figure 33.1. Radially symmetric bifocal lenses, when centered before the pupil, are able to rotate on the eye without causing visual disturbance. They can be made thin and from highly oxygen-permeable materials in order to promote adequate corneal physiology. With the exception of diffractive lenses, radially symmetric bifocals are relatively easy to manufacture and duplicate. As a result they are less costly to the practitioner and patient.

33.3.2 CONCENTRIC BIFOCAL DESIGNS

A concentric bifocal consists of two optical zones of differing refractive powers. The first zone is circular in the center of the lens and is surrounded by a second annular optical zone of different power. Concentric lenses may be distance/center or near/center depending upon whether the central portion of the lens carries the distance or near correction. The refractive power distribution can be placed on the front surface, back surface, or result from a combination of both surfaces (a two-surface design).

Table 33.4 Categories of bifocal and related contact lens designs used in the correction of presbyopia

Radially symmetric presbyopic designs
Concentric bifocal: One-piece or fused (rarely) segment front or back surface
    Distance/center
    Near/center
Progressive (aspheric) multifocal: One-piece design front or back surface
    Distance/center
    Near/center
Diffractive bifocal: One-piece, back surface only
Pinhole contact lenses

Radially asymmetric presbyopic designs
Segmented bifocal: One-piece or fused (rarely) segment front (usually), internal, or back surface
    Atypical bifocals
    Wafer contact lenses

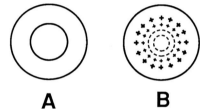 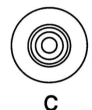 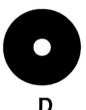

A   **B**   **C**   **D**

Figure 33.1 Radially symmetric presbyopic contact lens designs. (A) Concentric bifocal, (B) progressive multifocal, (C) diffractive bifocal, and (D) pinhole contact lens.

Distance/center and near/center concentrics

Concentric 'distance/center' designs are those in which the central, circular zone contains the eye's distance prescription and the peripheral, annular optical zone contains the eye's near correction. Concentric 'near/center' lenses are those in which the center provides the near power and the annulus the distance power. The difference between these two refractive powers is, of course, the bifocal 'add'. The 'add' power for a conventional concentric bifocal contact lens is created by a difference of surface curvature between the central and peripheral optical zones. The bifocal can be considered to be of 'one-piece' construction. The optical zones are ground into the front surface[P1] or the back surface[P2] of a contact lens in a radially symmetric fashion consistent with ease of manufacture using a lathe.

The relative contribution of the incident light forming each image through a concentric bifocal is proportional to the area of the entrance pupil covered by the respective optical zones contributing to the focus of the distant or the near light. Should the visual requirements merit emphasis of either distance or near vision, the contribution of either optical zone can be increased by enlarging one optical zone in relation to the area of the entrance pupil, while correspondingly reducing the contribution of the other. Concentric bifocal lenses may be employed as either 'simultaneous' or 'alternating' vision lenses, depending on details of dimension and distribution of their key elements. The various types of construction and of manufacturing concentric bifocal lenses are shown in Figure 33.2, and available lenses are listed in Table 33.5.

Front-surface, back-surface, and two-surface concentrics

Distance/center bifocals for which the front surface supplies the add power have front peripheral curves that are steeper than the front central curves in order to supply peripheral adds. The entire back surface of the lens can be appropriately fitted to the cornea, but the near power is gained by producing a lens profile that is drastically thin in the periphery and at the margin of the lens. Because the front surface has a junction between curvatures, these lenses can be less comfortable due to interaction of the junction with the eyelid during blinking. A minus carrier can not be easily added to the design

in order to counteract the deleterious effects of peripheral thinness on vertical centration by interaction of the thinner periphery and edge with the upper lid. The consequent effect on positioning and action of bifocal contact lenses is contingent on the relationship of the shape of the edges to the upper lid and is considered in greater detail later in this chapter.

The peripheral front curvature of a front-surface near/center bifocal is flatter than in the central region, and the surface can be more easily manufactured. In effect, this is a type of minus carrier design in which the minus carrier is enlarged and becomes the annular near correction. Tear fluid tends to fill the anterior curve junction, therefore light scatter and flare at the junction can disturb vision through these lenses. Like any front-surface design having a junction between two different surface curvatures, comfort can be decreased due to eyelid interaction with the surface. For soft lenses, peripheral lens thickness effects of front-surface concentric

Table 33.5 Commonly prescribed concentric bifocals. Many other rigid bifocals are available from your local laboratory on a custom-order basis.

Lens	Manufacturer	Material class	Available parameters, design
Bisoft	CIBA Vision	Soft	4 adds, 3 base curves 1 overall diameter 1 central zone diameter Front surface Distance/center
Spectrum	CIBA Vision	Soft	4 adds, 2 base curves 1 overall diameter 2 central zone diameters Back surface Near/center
Alges	Miami CL Co.	Soft	5 adds, 2 base curves 1 overall diameter 5 central zone diameters Front surface Near/center
Alges Boston bifocal	Miami CL Co.	Rigid	Parameters made to order Front surface Near/center

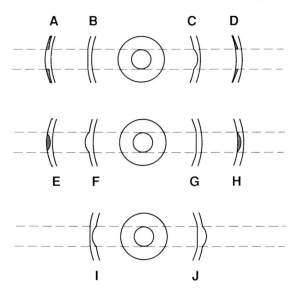

Figure 33.2 Constructs of concentric bifocal contact lenses. Top: Distance/center lenses of front-surface fused (A) and one-piece (B) designs on the left, then back-surface one-piece (C) and fused (D) designs on the right. Middle: Near/center lenses of front-surface fused (E) and one-piece (F) designs on the left, then back-surface one-piece (G) and fused (H) designs on the right. Bottom: Two-surface one-piece concentric designs, near/center on the left (I) and distance/center on the right (J).

designs have less impact on fitting and positioning of the lenses, but junctional tear pooling and superior eyelid interaction may comparatively diminish optical function and comfort of soft lenses even more than for rigid lenses.

Due to the many problems with front-surface concentric designs, most concentric distance/center and near/center bifocals are manufactured using the back surface to produce the add. Manufacture of back-surface distance/center concentric lenses was comparatively easy and these lenses have been available in both soft and rigid forms for many years. The manufacture of near/center back-surface designs became economically feasible relatively recently and several of

these designs are now available even in hydrogel materials. Front surfaces of these lenses can be as smooth and regular as the front surfaces of single-vision contact lenses. Unlike front-surface concentric designs, peripheral lens thickness can be controlled for vertical positioning with a back-surface bifocal by addition of a minus carrier to the front surface, a technique covered later in this chapter.

The transition between distance and near zones on a back-surface bifocal lens is much more abrupt than that on a front-surface lens because the refractive index change at the lens/posterior tear pool interface is much less than the index change at the front surface of the lens in air (in terms of refractive power, the pre-lens tear film is insignificant). The cornea, itself, is insensitive to back-surface junctions under normal circumstances, unlike the eyelid which can be sensitive to lens edges and front-surface junctions. Since the area under the central portion of a concentric bifocal is small (less than the pupil size) in comparison to the peripheral zone, the radius of curvature of the peripheral zone will have a large impact on the lens/cornea fitting relationship.

The add power of a rigid back-surface distance/center bifocal is generally limited to approximately +1.50 D because increased peripheral flattening with higher adds creates an excessively flat-fitting lens with edge lift. If the central back-surface radius is steepened in order to allow for a more appropriate peripheral fit, the central region becomes too steep, creating a large stagnant tear pool adverse to central corneal physiology. Similarly, adds of rigid near/center lenses are also limited to approximately +1.50 D. To achieve a higher add yet maintain an adequate back-surface fit, additional add power may be incorporated into the front surface of these lenses. Concentric distance/center and near/center bifocals can be produced in a 'front- and back-surface', or 'two-surface' design, in which two curvatures are placed on both contact lens surfaces. The total add is a combination of 'adds' derived from the front and back surfaces of each lens. Due to the relative complexity of manufacture when compared to single-surface (front-surface or back-surface) designs, 'two-surface' designs are rarely seen in practice.

Fused versus one-piece concentrics

In PMMA, an annular peripheral segment of higher refractive index can be fused with a distance/center carrier lens of refractive index 1.49, such that the add does not necessitate curvature alterations of either lens surface. Similarly, near/center lenses can be produced with a central fused segment of higher refractive index than the surrounding plastic. Because oxygen-permeable rigid and soft materials are not thermoplastic or thermosetting and, therefore, are not (yet) available fused, this method of producing bifocal lenses with state-of-the-art materials is impractical at this time.

33.3.3 PROGRESSIVE (ASPHERIC) MULTIFOCALS

Progressive bifocal designs are those in which refractive power gradually increases (as compared to the abrupt junction between distance and near portions of the concentric designs described above) into the plus or minus in radial directions peripheral to the geometric center of the contact lens. A progressive bifocal can be made with an aspheric surface on the front or the back of a contact lens. These lenses are, therefore, sometimes called 'aspheric' bifocals and are a type of 'one-piece' design, but without an abrupt junction between curvatures. The authors have classified aspheric bifocals as a separate radially symmetric design, yet they are really 'multifocals' rather than 'bifocals' since they have a progression of powers from center to periphery (Charman & Walsh,

1988). Accepting that progressive lenses are a type of 'bifocal', they could be considered a type of concentric bifocal because their iso-power distributions are concentric around the geometrical center of the lenses.

Distance or near/center, front- or back-surface

Front-surface distance/center aspherics have a front surface which progressively becomes steeper than a spherical surface in the periphery of the lens (oblate), while back-surface aspherics have a back surface which becomes flatter than a spherical surface in the periphery (prolate). In effect, distance/center progressive lenses promote positive spherical aberration and near/center lenses promote negative spherical aberration when compared to lenses made of two spherical surfaces. The aspheric surfaces of progressives are usually elliptical and the degree to which they deviate from a conventional spherical surface in the periphery depends on the surface's eccentricity. As noted in Appendix 33.A, an elliptical surface is specified by its apical radius of curvature, eccentricity and diameter. A list of common aspheric bifocal lenses can be found in Table 33.6.

Back-surface aspheric bifocal contact lenses usually have a 'distance/center' design, in which the posterior surface of the lens is prolate, and, therefore, flattens toward the periphery. The lens/tear pool interface becomes less minus toward the periphery, thus adding plus power in the periphery for a presbyopic correction. To allow for peripheral flattening, the apical radius of a rigid back-surface distance/center progressive lens will be 0.1 to 0.5 mm shorter (steeper) than an equivalent spherical single-vision lens fit, depending on the eccentricity of the aspheric surface. A fluorescein pattern of a rigid progressive distance/center lens is shown in Figure 33.3. Note pooling under the steeper central area of the aspheric lens

Table 33.6 Commonly prescribed progressive (aspheric) multifocal contact lenses. Many additional rigid lenses are also available from your local laboratory on a custom-order basis.

Lens	Manufacturer	Material class	Available parameters, design
PA-1	Bausch & Lomb	Soft	1 add, 1 base curve per distance power, 1 diameter Back surface Distance/center
Unilens	Unilens Corp.	Soft	1 add per distance power 2 base curves, 2 diameters Front surface Near/center
Hydrocurve II	Barnes-Hind	Soft	1 add per distance power 1 base curve, 1 diameter Back surface Distance/center
PS-45	Product Development Corp.	Soft	1 add per distance power 2 base curves, 1 diameter Front surface Near/center
Sof-Touch	N&N Contacts	Soft	1 add per distance power 2 base curves, 1 diameter Back surface Distance/center
VX	GBF Contacts	Rigid	1 add per distance power Parameters made to order Back surface Distance/center
Constavue	Salvatori Ophthalmics	Rigid	1 add per distance power Parameters made to order Front surface Distance/center
VFL-II	Conforma Laboratories	Rigid	1 add per distance power Parameters made to order Back surface Distance/center
Progressive	Miami CL Co.	Rigid	1 add per distance power Parameters made to order Back surface Near center

and under the annular peripheral flatter area.

As with rigid back-surface concentric bifocals, the nominal add power for rigid aspheric back-surface lenses should not be greater than a functional +1.50 diopters or the back surface will not adequately fit the cornea. Nominal add power is the effective add produced by the aspheric surface on the 'typical' patient, considering that refractive power in reality progresses into the plus or minus away from the center of the lens. The add powers of progressive aspheric lenses tend to be low and depend on pupil diameter (Charman & Walsh, 1988; McGill & Erickson, 1988).

Front surface asphericity can also be used

to build more plus refractive power into the periphery of a contact lens. However, the aspheric front surface would need to be steeper in the periphery than in the central portion of the lens (oblate). As this type of surface proves to be difficult to manufacture, most front-surface asperics are near/center lenses made with prolate front surfaces. Should aspheric lenses decenter or translate, unwanted astigmatic error inherent in the periphery will cover the pupil (Charman, 1982; Goldberg & Lowther, 1986).

Progressive 'bifocal' contact lenses are available in rigid or soft materials. In soft lenses, this design has the advantage of fitting nearly like a spherical single-vision gel lens, such that it is easily prescribed if the patient is motivated and can adapt to the simultaneous visual result. While most aspheric bifocal lenses become continuously more plus into the periphery (as in a distance/center design[P3]), the center/near PS-45 hydrogel lens bifocal by Product Development Corporation is said by the manufacturer to have an 'S-shaped' aspheric front-surface curvature that is not elliptical or otherwise conoidal. Beginning at the geo-metric center of the lens, power graduates into the minus in the mid-periphery, but then stabilizes in the mid-periphery at one add power. Vision with this lens should be significantly influenced by pupil size and lens centration.

Modified lens designs

Lenticular contact lens designs are those which limit the effects of refractive power on thickness and shape of lenses by reducing the diameter of the front optic zone. A plus-lenticular lens and a minus-lenticular lens (see Fig. 33.4) both have small front optic zones in comparison to their conventional counterparts. Sagittal depth of the front surface is reduced for the plus-lenticular lens such that center thickness can be reduced. Sagittal depth of the front surface is increased for the minus-lenticular lens so that edge thickness can be reduced. The well-known 'CN bevel' placed on high-minus contact lenses at the practitioner's office to reduce edge thickness is actually a way of creating a minus-lenticular design from a conventional minus lens. Another 'modified' contact lens design uses an aspheric surface (see Appendix 33.1 A).

Ease of manufacture of lenses with 'unconventional' surfaces is greatly enhanced if each surface is of a single construct. Thus, a one-piece spherical or aspheric surface pro-

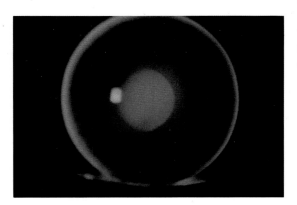

Figure 33.3 Fluorescein pattern of a back-surface distance/center aspheric rigid contact lens. Note the central pooling typical of such designs, due to the steeper apical radius than that normally fitted in a spherical rigid lens design (photo courtesy Mr Mel Sanford of Conforma Labs).

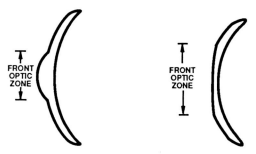

Figure 33.4 (A) Front-surface plus-lenticular; and (B) minus-lenticular contact lenses.

viding the bifocal add can not normally also be lenticular or toric.

33.3.4 HOLOGRAPHIC, OR DIFFRACTIVE BIFOCAL DESIGNS

So-called 'holographic' bifocal contact lenses are of a 'non-translating' variety and function according to a diffractive, or 'zone plate' principle, rather than the usual Fresnel lens principle. The reader can see many concentric optical zones on the rigid diffractive lens shown against a shadowgraph in Figure 33.5A. The authors classify this type of bifocal as a separate radially symmetric design, but it may also be considered a type of concentric design.

Fresnel forms

The well-known Fresnel lens principle, is that in which refractive power is created by a series of annular concentric prisms placed base-to-apex. The annular strips of prism are usually of equal width across the surface of a Fresnel lens. The prismatic power of each strip increases with the diameter of the annulus so that the foci of paraxial and peripheral light rays will coincide. Each annular strip acts independently to the other strips and, therefore, resolution of the lens is diffractively limited by the width of the annuli (Benjamin, 1987). A Fresnel bifocal contact lens could be designed in which alternating annuli contribute to two different refractive powers – one for near and the next for far.

Recent patents have been issued for which a modified form of the Fresnel principle is employed.[P4,P5] The optical surface consists, in one design, of a general base lens for distant vision, into which is interposed a number of smaller circular zones of inner surface curvatures differing from that of the base, designed to coincide in near point foci. In other forms, the shapes of the interposed near sections are varied. The questions raised, of how much diffraction at the numerous interfaces between the two powers, or double imaging of the separate sections will interfere with vision have not been tested since the lenses are not yet available for general use.

Diffractive bifocal designs

The diffractive principle is related to the, Fresnel half-wavelength zone principle, from which flat 'lenses' consisting of annular con-

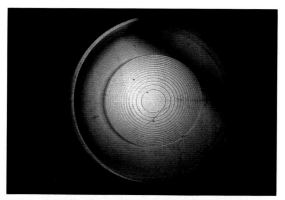

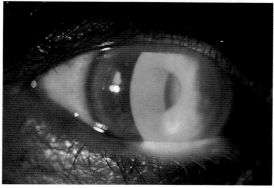

Figure 33.5 Top: A rigid diffractive bifocal lens shown against a shadowgraph. Note that the concentric rings separating one annular zone from another become closer ·together toward the periphery of the optical area. Bottom: When assessed with high-molecular weight fluorescein, a characteristic pattern behind a hydrogel diffractive lens can be seen (fluorescein pattern courtesy Dr N. Rex Ghormley).

centric zones are designed.[P4,P5] Each annular zone represents an optical path length change of one-half wavelength of light, such that light transmitted through the zones undergoes constructive and destructive interference in such a manner as to produce multiple focal points. Because optical path length changes are more easily achieved for peripheral light rays, the half-wavelength annuli become progressively thinner toward the periphery of the lens. However, since the area of the zones holds constant from the center of the lens to the periphery, all of the zones contribute equally to the final image (Benjamin, 1987). A zone plate looks like a square-wave version of a holographic plate, hence application of that term to 'holographic' lenses (Benjamin, 1987; Cohen, 1989; Loshin, 1989).

While the optical system of a 'holographic' bifocal contact lens is more involved than next explained, the optic zone of the lens basically consists of 8 to 20 concentric 'half-wavelength' zones on the back surface of the lens (Fig. 33.5A). The depth of the zones are cut to only a few microns, yet the back-surface annuli result in a unique pattern when the lens/cornea relationship is assessed with high-molecular weight fluorescein (Fig. 33.5B). Front-surface zones are not practical because they provide a rough surface over which the eyelid must blink, the refractive index of the pre-lens medium changes (the front lens surface dries off periodically), and deposition tends to fill in the annular zones. In a typical 'zone plate', either the even- or the odd-numbered zones are blacked out so that light transmitted through the remaining zones can constructively contribute to an image at the focal point of the lens. However, by careful phase shifting, all of the zones of the bifocal contact lens are allowed to transmit light. Half of the strips contribute to the near image (in alternating fashion as in a 'Fresnel lens bifocal') and the other half to the far image. In actuality, about 40% of the light makes up each image, the other 20% is apparently lost to dispersion, neutralization and scatter. In addition, the widths of the annuli have been designed so that the strips act in concert, capitalizing on diffraction so that resolution is not limited by the width of the strips as in a normal Fresnel lens.[P4,P5]

Mention of the word 'holography' usually conjures up an image produced by laser illumination of a hologram film, the image suspended in three dimensions and visible from many perspectives. Such a mental picture is not representative of initial 'holographic' bifocal contact lenses, although the optical principles of the lenses are related to holography in its simplest form. The term 'diffractive' has been adopted to describe these back-surface bifocal lenses in order to differentiate them from other bifocal contact lenses (Benjamin, 1987; Cohen, 1989). Two available diffractive bifocal lenses are the soft Echelon lens (Allergan/Hydron) and the rigid Diffrax lens (Sola/Barnes-Hind).

Several other bifocal designs have been proposed which offer multiple optical zones within the lens aperture. Multiple concentric zones[P6,P7] and multiple non-concentric zones[P8,P9] promise to allow simultaneous vision, but the extent to which these designs might provide excellent vision is yet unknown.

33.3.5 PINHOLE CONTACT LENSES

'Pinhole' contact lenses are not truly bifocals, but increase the depth of field for the patient by creation of an aperture in the center of an otherwise opaque contact lens. The aperture is usually from 1.0 to 2.0 mm in diameter and gives a large field of view (for a pinhole) since it is located only 3 mm in front of the entrance pupil of the eye. To maximize usefulness of the large depth of field, refractive correction prescribed in the contact lens is usually about 0.5 to 1.0 diopter more plus than the distance refraction. The amount of overplus can be adjusted to emphasize a particular working distance most used by the patient. Multiple pinholes or stenopaic slits radiating from a central pinhole, are more complex designs to expand the peripheral field and allow more retinal illumination.

Pinhole contact lenses have several drawbacks. First, retinal illumination is low due to the small aperture diameter and vision in low illumination is thereby severely handicapped. The problems of the older eye, aggravated under mesopic circumstances, are even further compromised. Second, the lens must be fitted tightly to achieve centration and minimal movement. Third, cosmesis is poor unless the aperture is placed in a contact lens made for covering disfigured eyes, for instance, an iris-painted lens or cosmetic scleral shell. For these reasons, pinhole contact lenses are not routinely prescribed and are reserved for special cases (Bier, 1981) in which other bifocal designs are clearly not viable alternatives.

33.3.6 RADIALLY ASYMMETRIC CONTACT LENS DESIGNS

Bifocal lens designs that do not result in concentric iso-power distributions surrounding the geometric center of the lens, are 'radially asymmetric' designs. A bifocal segment contains the near prescription and the carrier portion of the lens contains the distance prescription. The segment's geometrical center does not coincide with the center of the entire contact lens as happens with segments of concentric designs. Each contact lens is expected to translate on the eye so that the entrance pupil is alternately covered by portions of the lens containing distance and near corrections when the patient changes from distance to near vision, and vice versa. Several common radially asymmetric, fused and one-piece segmented bifocal designs are shown in Figure 33.6, though other configurations have been manufactured in the past. A list of common segmented asymmetric bifocals can be found in Table 33.7.

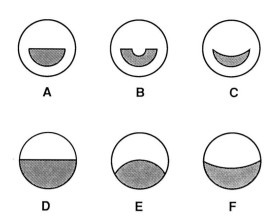

Figure 33.6 Radially asymmetric bifocal segment shapes. Fused: (A) flat top; (B) semi-annular; (C) crescent; and one-piece: (D) flat top; (E) reversed crescent; and (F) crescent.

33.3.7 ACHIEVING ROTATIONAL STABILITY

Radially asymmetric lenses can not be allowed to freely rotate as can radially symmetric bifocals, therefore, some method of maintaining consistent placement of the add below the pupil is required. Several methods of achieving proper rotational stability so that segments stay below the pupil have been attempted (Robboy, 1985):

1. prism ballast or periballast.
2. Inferior metal and other weights.
3. Inferior and/or superior truncation.
4. Inferior and/or superior slab-off.

Prism ballast and periballast

Prism ballast utilizes base-down vertical prism to create a thicker and heavier lower portion of the lens. By gravity, the inferior portion, which contains the bifocal segment, was intended to resist rotation on the eye,[P10] thereby holding the base–apex line vertical. If other parameters of the lens are sufficient, the top of the segment is held below or at the lower margin of the pupil in primary gaze. Segment position is covered later in more

Table 33.7 Commonly prescribed radially asymmetric, segmented bifocal contact lenses. The 'Tangent Streak' is also available as a trifocal with intermediate segment of half the bifocal add. Many other rigid bifocal lenses are available from your local laboratory on a custom-order basis

Lens	Manufacturer	Material class	Available parameters, design
Bi-Tech	Bausch & Lomb	Soft	2 adds, 2 base curves 1 diameter, 2 segment heights Monocentric flat-top segment Periballast Inferior truncation Superior slab-off
True bifocal	Miami CL Co.	Soft	1 add, 3 base curves 3 diameters, 1 segment height Crescent segment Prism ballast Inferior truncation
Synsoft	Salvatori Ophthalmics	Soft	Adds +1.50 to +3.50, 3 base curves 3 diameters, 1 segment height Concentric, annular segment Periballast
Tangent Streak	Fused Kontacts	Rigid	Parameters made to order Segment height +/− 1 mm of center Monocentric flat-top segment Prism ballast Optiioal inferior truncation

detail. A related term is periballast, formed when the distance optical zone on a lens having a minus lenticular flange has been off-set superiorly, so as to expose a large, thick portion of the minus carrier over the inferior portion of the lens. Early in bifocal contact lens history, it was not appreciated that the orientation of a lens was also due to varying eyelid pressures exerted upon the lens surface and not due to gravity alone. The inability of other lens weighting methods, such as metal weights,[P11] to assure correct orientation of a contact lens in the absence of prism ballast was unexplained.

Superior and inferior truncations

Truncations were applied to inferior and superior aspects of bifocal lenses so that contact with the inferior and superior eyelids would help rotationally orient these lenses within the palpebral aperture. Although reasonably effective, the upper truncated edge of a corneal lens proved to be too uncomfortable for most wearers. Inferior truncation proved less irritating and is still used today on several rigid and soft[P12] bifocal lens designs (Robboy, 1985). Thick inferior lens edges created by truncation also tended to keep lenses from sliding under the lower eyelid margin during downgaze at near. Ideally, the edge of the lens at the truncation should be polished flat (Fig. 33.7). If the edge is rolled and tapered such that the edge apex position is too far posterior, the edge will tend to slide underneath the lower eyelid. If the taper produces an edge apex that is anterior, the apex induces discomfort by sharply impinging on the eyelid margin during blinking and inferior gaze.

Even when properly flattened, however, thick truncated edges have proven to reduce

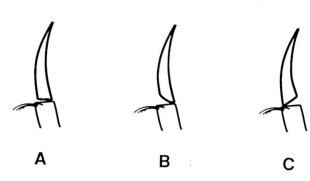

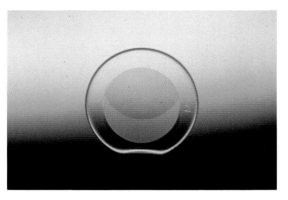

Figure 33.7 Edges of truncation on an asymmetric bifocal should be polished flat (A). Tapered edges can allow lenses to slip below the lower eyelid (B) or cause discomfort (C) (modified from Bier & Lowther, 1977).

Figure 33.9 A soft, prism-ballasted bifocal lens with a crescent segment. Note that the inferior truncation is not appropriately shaped and will cause edge awareness by abutting against the lower lid margin at its lateral pointed ends.

lens comfort. The touch of the lens on the lower lid was often irritating to many wearers, who complained of a constant tickling sensation and whose tear levels were usually reflexly raised. Truncation should leave a curved inferior lens edge that conforms to the curvature of the inferior eyelid margin (Fig. 33.8 and 33.9).

Depending on the sign of the lens refractive power (+ or –), truncation may either lessen or increase the impact of prism ballast. In minus lenses, truncation tends to remove a major amount of the thickest part of the lens. As the apex of a minus lens also thickens toward the edge, the ballasting effect of the lens may be reduced or lost as truncation reduces the thickness difference between the base and the apex (Fig. 33.10A). Because many prism lenses are automatically trun-

cated, it has become customary to increase the amount of prism regularly as the amount of minus increases. In plus lenses, the truncation may assist orientation because it tends to increase the thickness difference between the base and the apex and to lower the center of gravity of the lens (Fig. 33.10B). Since it is desirable to maintain as thin a lens as possible, the least amount of prism which will ballast the lens is recommended. Thus, for minus lenses, inferior truncation has been omitted on many newer translating prism-ballasted bifocal designs.

Superior and inferior slab-off prism

Superior truncation resulted in a thick lens edge over which the superior eyelid had to pass during the blink. Therefore, this design

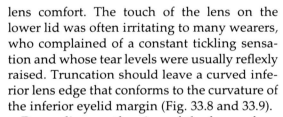

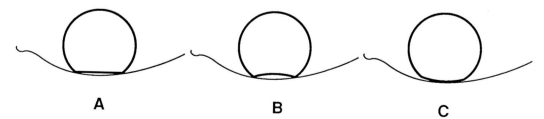

Figure 33.8 The bottom edge of a truncated prism-ballasted lens should conform to the curve of the margin of the lower eyelid, as in (C) (modified from Bier & Lowther, 1977).

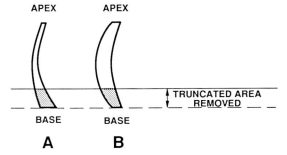

APEX   APEX

TRUNCATED AREA
REMOVED

BASE   BASE

A   B

Figure 33.10 Truncation of a minus lens (A) will reduce the amount of ballast, while truncation of a plus lens (B) will enhance the amount of ballast.

with lens interaction with the inferior eyelid, interactions of prism ballast and superior slab-off are with the superior eyelid. Some of the factors of importance to rotational stability are discussed later in the chapter.

33.4 FUNDAMENTALS AND CONCEPTS

Diverse attempts to correct presbyopia have resulted in the presentation of a large number of hypotheses, many of which are suspect. To adequately understand the premises which underlie appropriate applications of presbyopic correction, it is important that a proper understanding of many of the basic fundamental concepts be understood. Before discussing clinical applications of presbyopic correction, several basic concepts are developed in the following sections.

was dropped in favor of superior slab-off prism, which actually thinned the superior lens edge and helped stabilize axis orientation. Although inferior slab-off was found to help stabilize axis orientation for toric soft lenses (i.e. the CIBA Torisoft lens), the thin inferior edge slipped under the lower eyelid in downgaze. Thus, inferior slab-off was unacceptable for translating bifocal lenses.

Today, axis orientations of most radially asymmetric bifocal contact lenses, whether made of rigid or soft materials, are stabilized by one, two, or all of the design features shown in Figure 33.11: (1) prism ballast in the amount of 0.5 to 3.0 prism diopters; (2) inferior truncation of 1.0 to 2.0 mm; and (3) superior slab-off prism in the amount of 0.5 to 3.0 prism diopters. A method of providing a superiorly located slab-off effect for rigid lenses in the office is by 'CNing' of the apical edge (plus shaping by removing lens material from the front edge of a minus lens). While rotational orientation by inferior truncation is associated

33.4.1 SIMULTANEOUS AND ALTERNATING VISION

Probably no other concept has been more misinterpreted and created more confusion than so-called simultaneous vision. If an individual wears bifocals in the form of spectacles, vision at distance and vision at near is obtained by utilizing that segment of the bifocal focused for the required fixation distance. By this means, all the light passing through the entrance pupil from distance is in focus on the retina when distance vision is desired and all the light from near is in focus when near vision is required. Positioning of

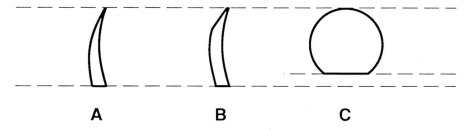

A   B   C

Figure 33.11 Common strategies for obtaining rotational orientation: (A) Prism ballast, (B) superior slab-off prism, and (C) inferior truncation.

the head, and in particular, voluntary movement of the eyes behind the lenses enable vision 'alternation' between distance and near foci to take place.

If an individual is wearing bifocal contact lenses, the lenses ride on the cornea and will move with the eye as it refixates. Movement of the lenses on the cornea is, when attained, beyond voluntary control. If sufficient movement of the lens can be gained so that the segments of different power take a position before the pupil, vision by means of the same 'alternation' as applied to spectacle bifocals may be achieved. This visual process has been titled alternating vision. If the lenses do not move, or move insufficiently, parts of both segments may intersect the pupil. Light from either a distance object or a near one passes through both zones. As fixation is directed to either a distant or a near target, one zone produces a focused image while the other produces a blurred image which overlaps the same retinal elements as does the focused one. An out-of-focus image overlies the focused retinal image of any object of regard, at distance or at near. This process has been called simultaneous vision. The extent of degradation of the resultant retinal image will depend upon the relative amounts of in-focus to out-of-focus light striking the retina. Further degradation is also imposed by light scatter, flare, and diffraction occurring at the junction between the distance and near optical zones. The quality of the image in all instances must be poorer than might have been attained had the pupil been covered by only the portion of the lens providing focused light from the point of fixation.

The simplest method of providing the equivalent of alternating vision is to employ contact lenses for distance vision and to use spectacles over them to provide the necessary power for near vision. However, as noted previously, this has certain disadvantages, possibly completely neutralizing the initial motivation for wearing contact lenses altogether.

Concepts of 'optical' and 'neurological' alternation

The most widely used method to achieve alternating vision is that of 'monovision'. Monovision can be compared to 'simultaneous vision' in that foci from different distances are optically presented to the eyes at the same time. However, whereas in true 'simultaneous vision' each retina receives both focused and unfocused light, in monovision, one eye receives all focused light while the other eye receives all unfocused light depending on the working distance. This actually enables a form of alternating vision to take place, since the patient learns to suppress or ignore vision from the eye which is out of focus. Where 'optical alternation' cannot be achieved by changes in the position of the lenses on the eyes, it is here attempted by 'neurological alternation' of the suppressed eyes. In those individuals in which alternate suppression is not readily achieved, some degradation of vision occurs similar to that described for 'simultaneous vision' in a single eye.

The use of progressive addition lenses in spectacles, in which the power of the lens varies in a continuous channel from the distance towards the near power, has demonstrated that under some distributions of light entering an eye, usable vision can be obtained even though that light results in a mixture of focused and unfocused images. Since many contact lenses, and thus far, all soft lenses, move only slightly on the cornea in an amount insufficient to separately place different optical zones adequately before the pupil, attempts have been and are made to apply this concept to bifocal contact lenses.

If the contact lens does not move or moves only very slightly, usable vision at either far or near fixation requires that sufficient in-focus light strikes the retina from both distances through the same fixed optical system on the cornea. Since a simultaneous vision lens does not change its position on the cornea markedly, it is assumed that at least 50% of the light will be in focus from either distance to provide equally visible images at both near and far. Lenses deliberately designed to achieve this distribution are known as 'simultaneous vision' lenses. Constant repetition of the term 'simultaneous vision' has led to an accepted incorrect assumption that such a process is actually a comparable modality to 'alternating vision', as if both were equivalent alternatives to achieving equal results.

The literature may occasionally state that an alternating lens's visual contribution was augmented by introducing 'simultaneous vision' into the process. It should be apparent from the above, that while 'alternating vision' (in that more of the zone producing a focused image is moved before the pupil) may augment performance of 'simultaneous vision', 'simultaneous vision' (in that more out-of-focus light is introduced into the image) must always degrade 'alternating vision'!

Part of the confusion arises from certain widely presumed misconcepts of retinal imagery. The common premise is that two images lie on the retina, one a focused image and the other an unfocused image, as if two separate films lay at the back of a camera. The brain is assumed to attend to one image while suppressing the other. The physiology of suppressing some parts of monocular stimuli falling on separate retinal receptive fields while concentrating attention upon stimuli falling on other fields, or of suppressing non-identical stimuli in one eye from those in the other on congruent receptors, is accepted (as in monovision, detailed later in this chapter). But here it is postulated that the brain selects one stimulus falling on a receptive field while suppressing an out-of-focus one falling on the same field. Hypothetically, sufficient differences between the two, essentially in intensity and perhaps in color, seem necessary in order that one be suppressed.

Airy's circles and the Rayleigh fraction

It is repeated that, if a simultaneous vision lens is to provide usable vision for both far and near while holding a fixed position on the cornea, at least 50% of the light will have to be in focus from either distance. This will also mean that 50% will be out of focus at either distance. Obviously, the retina is merely a combination of photoreceptors and receptive fields, and the relative stimuli to each are the summation of the amounts of light striking it. In simplified theoretical concept, a point of observation produces an image with a given spread on the retina known as Airy's circle. Two points are discriminated as two points dependant upon the distribution of the light from each of Airy's circles upon the receptive fields they strike. Airy's circle spreads light upon surrounding adjacent receptors, as shown in cross section (Fig. 33.12). The intensity of the sum of the light from both points falling upon the receptor at the midpoint between two other receptors must be sufficiently less than the light falling on each of those two receptors to meet a minimal requirement for detection of contrast.

The ratio of illumination between the light striking the two points and that falling between them to permit detection of two stimuli, is known as the Rayleigh fraction. The actual stimulus on each receptor in the retina consists of the sum of all the light striking each from both the focused and unfocused light passing through the contact lens zones. Westheimer and Campbell (1962) computed the spread of the intensities of two Airy's circles produced by two points on the receptors through a standard sized pupil for light both in-focus and 1.25 D out-of-focus. Borish (1986) showed that the sum of the two equal stimulations (50% in focus and 50% out of focus) falling together upon the same concerned photoreceptors does not produce the necessary Rayleigh fraction. Thus, two closely adjacent points that could be discriminated

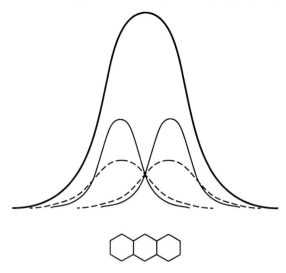

Figure 33.12 Diagrammatic illustration of light distribution centered at three adjacent points on the retina realized as the sum of intensities of Airy's circles produced by 50% light in focus and 50% light out of focus by 1.25 D. Solid lines show cross section of two Airy's circles in focus; dashed lines show two Airy's circles out of focus; heavy solid line equals sum of light of both. Airy's circle proportions traced from Westheimer and Campbell (1962).

under conditions of best correction could not be perceived as two separate points under conditions of simultaneous vision. Therefore, simultaneous viewing of in-focus and out-of-focus images must degrade vision, though in most viewing situations, patients may discriminate between stimuli that are more separated than shown in Figure 33.12. Analysis of modulation transfer functions (Borish & Perrigin; 1985) further lessens the credibility of so-called 'simultaneous vision' in providing clear vision.

Why the 'dirty window' argument doesn't wash

The question arises, then, as to how do so-called 'simultaneous vision' lenses work in those instances in which they have been found effective? One explanation offered is that perceptual processes interpret blurred images sufficiently well to enable such vision to be usable. A visual situation sometimes posed as an example in support of 'simultaneous vision', is the perception of a distant object through a 'dirty' window. It is implied that the visual system attends to the in-focus image while ignoring the blurred image of spots on the window when the eye is focused for distance. When focused at near to view the window surface, the visual system attends to the near image and ignores veiling light from distance. Thus, it is incorrectly assumed, the visual system is capable of providing simultaneous vision that should apply to bifocal contact lens wear.

However, this illustration ignores the basic tenant of the earlier discussion, which is not a question of the qualitative mixture of blurred and clear foci, but of the quantitative relations between the two. Spots on a window block some of the light from distance and present their own retinal images overlying the attenuated distance image on the retina. Because the spots are recognized as entities separate from the distant image, due to their differing binocular disparity as well as other features, the visual system may have a certain capacity to ignore the spots when concentrating on distant objects. If there are a few small spots on the window, the preponderance of light falling on the retina would be from distance, and only a limited amount of pattern recognition would be required to perceive the distance image when the eye is focused for distance vision. Distant targets will be perceived as being 'clear'. When focused for near and viewing spots on the window, illumination from distance provides a lighted background upon which the darker spots are superimposed. As this is a high-contrast situation, views of window spots will also be perceived as being 'clear'. It seems apparent that if window spots became more numerous, perhaps obscuring half of the light from distance, degradation of the distance image would occur and distance vision would be diminished. Even proponents of the 'dirty window' argument must concede, that distance vision through a dirty window is not equivalent to that through a clear window!

Differences in target disparity, color, luminance, shape, size, position and other features, producing high contrast and distinctions between distance and near images, and attenuation of distant light by the opaque nature of the near object are characteristics of the 'dirty window' that may enable the visual system to selectively attend to targets at different distances. But these characteristics are not evident when using a simultaneous bifocal lens, for which the distance and near optical zones produce two overlying retinal images of the same object, significantly differing only in degree of focus. The visual system is not asked, here, to distinguish between two different objects at two different distances and locations, but between similar versions of the same object at an identical retinal position. Comparing vision through a 'dirty window' to that of 'simultaneous vision', is like comparing apples and oranges.

Perhaps a more applicable reason why 'simultaneous vision' bifocals are sometimes satisfying to wearers may be the fact that changes in the size of the pupil (considered below) and centration of the contact lens (considered later in detail) occur despite the inference of 'simultaneous vision'. These optical effects may alter the ratio of focused to unfocused light at specific times and under necessary circumstances so that the focused light exceeds 50% by a sufficient margin to permit the Rayleigh fraction to be achieved. Even when designed and fitted for 'simultaneous vision', bifocal contact lenses move somewhat on the cornea and the pupil changes size, thereby affecting the division of incident light between focused and unfocused retinal images. Thus, interpretation of blur by patients can be augmented by a limited amount of optical alternation.

33.4.2 FACTORS AFFECTING CENTRATION AND ROTATION

Contrary to a once popular assumption, a ballasted contact lens does not appear to react in strict accordance with a simple gravitational effect. If a circular disc which has one side heavier than the other is placed vertically on a wet surface, the disc will rotate so that the heaviest side is down no matter how slight the difference in mass between the two sides. In contradiction, a prism-ballasted bifocal contact lens maintains initial axis orientation even if the wearer stands on his/her head! Similarly, a rigid ballasted lens placed in the eye with the base up does not reorient itself with the head in the normal position, unless forceful blinks by the patient manage to bring the base of the prism out from underneath the upper eyelid. Something prevents gravitational attraction from orienting an inferiorly-weighted bifocal lens of either type of material. One explanation ascribes the effect to capillary attraction of the tear fluid meniscus around rigid lenses and the friction associated with rotation of a soft lens conformed to the cornea. This explanation appears to be partially valid for soft contact lenses. Capillary attraction of a soft lens in which not only a large area conforms to the cornea but a fairly wide band also matches the sclera is a distinct possibility. Obviously these same factors might also apply to frictional resistance.

However, a hard lens usually bears on only a very narrow band of a peripheral curve surrounding the optic zone. The amount of capillary attraction and frictional resistance would appear to be exceedingly slight unless the lens were fitted so tightly that it clamped the cornea or the eye itself were practically dry. In fact, the inevitability of rigid lens movement on the cornea even when undesired for concentric lens designs has consistently been noted. The true cause is easily demonstrated and has probably been observed by many practitioners experienced in the fitting of rigid lenses: If the base of a prism-ballasted rigid lens rides in an eye at an oblique angle (most commonly nasally) it will be observed that usually the upper lid covers the apical area of the lens. If the practitioner lifts the upper lid off the lens, not only does the lens drop somewhat on the cornea, but the base swings back towards the vertical position.

The propensity of the upper lid to pick up a 'minus carrier' peripheral flange, apparently works to attach the nasal side of the lens apex to the upper eyelid and rotates the base towards the nose. This will occur even when the lower eyelid has no contact with the lens. Nasal rotation, therefore, may in part be due to the fact that the muscle force of the upper lid is greater on the nasal side, or that the apical edge of the lens has more minus shape on the nasal side. A ballasted lens which fits intrapalpebrally so that the upper lid does not rest upon it, does not assume a constant oblique angle in a properly lubricated eye unless the 'nasal kick' or 'zipper action' of the lower eyelid during

blinks also acts to nasally rotate the interpalpebral lens. The lens may be similarly rotated without contacting the lower lid, and perhaps for the same reasons, as the upper lid crosses it in the blink, the base tends to reorient after the lid opens. The rigid lens which does not assume proper position when the subject stands on his/her head, or when placed in the eye with the base up, may be merely demonstrating the 'ICLing' concept discussed in the next paragraphs. It is actually impossible for a soft lens to avoid lying under the upper lid, a factor which may make the 'ICLing' concept equally or more important for soft lenses compared to rigid lenses.

The 'ICLing' concept

In the early years of corneal lenses, it was observed that most minus lenses rode relatively high on the cornea while plus lenses often rested at the lower limbus. The initial explanation credited gravity for this effect, on the assumption that the thicker center of

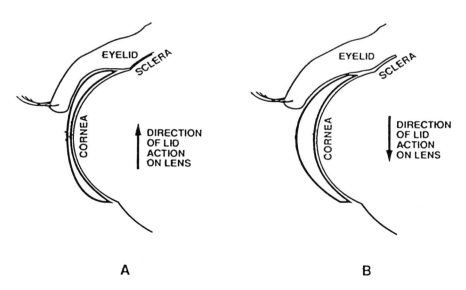

A   B

Figure 33.13 The 'ICLing' concept. The peripheral lens near the edge is pressed between the upper eyelid and globe. Since both sides of the lens are lubricated, eyelid pressure shifts the lens from a thicker to a thinner position between the two. (A) A minus lens will move upward or 'cling' to the superior lid; (B) a plus lens will be 'squeezed' downward.

the plus lens increased the mass of the lens and that the center of gravity of a plus lens rode forward of the cornea while that of a minus lens lay behind it. In 1961, a concept originated that the position of the lens was affected by the shape and thickness of the edge in relation to the pressure or weight of the upper lid. Shick and Borish (1962) experimented with lens designs in which lenses of equal power, thickness, size and other parameters were produced with various edge thicknesses and contours. It was found that plus lenses which rode low when normally constructed, positioned higher on the cornea, if their peripheral zones were reconstructed to resemble the cross-sectional contour of minus lenses. Similarly, minus lenses which tended to ride high, could be repositioned lower on the cornea if their peripheral areas resembled that of normal plus lenses.

The 'ICLing' concept established that the pressure of the upper lid was a major factor in lens positioning (especially vertical centration) and lens rotation. Subsequently, the influence of the superior eyelid on vertical lens translation was also realized (Fig. 33.13). Kessing (1967) later described the space between the conjunctivae lining the upper eyelid, fornix, and globe, his article lending further credence to the concept that edges of minus lenses could be 'squeezed' upwards into an area of lesser pressure between the upper eyelid and the globe. Prescribing contact lenses with the use of the 'ICLing' concept was a technique maintained as a proprietary secret by the Indiana Contact Lens Co. (in which the discoverers had an interest) and information was at first released only in company bulletins to its clients. Using the first three letters of the company name, the technique was called ICLing ('eye cling').

The 'minus carrier' and 'watermelon seed' effects

In the latter part of 1962, a description of the method was published and over the years became universally accepted (Borish, 1962). The proprietary term obviously was not accepted by other manufacturers, who nevertheless utilized the principle. The most widely utilized effect related to the 'ICLing' concept, in which the vertical position of a plus lens was raised with the use of a front-lenticular design having a minus peripheral flange, became known as the 'minus carrier effect'. The technical method of creating peripheral edge thickness varied among different manufacturers from that originally invented (Fig. 33.13A).

Also a result of the 'ICLing' concept, the vertical position of a minus contact lens on the eye could be lowered by providing a progressive thinning of the lens in the periphery toward the margin, such that the upper eyelid did not attach to the lens as readily (Fig. 33.13B). Peripheral thinning can be provided by manufacturing the minus lens in minus-lenticular form, with a front plus peripheral flange. A technique for doing this in the office is by applying a CN bevel, in effect, a plus peripheral flange added by modification of the front surface.

Thinning of the apical margin of a minus lens to resemble the edge of a plus lens lowers the position of the lens on the cornea (Fig. 33.13B). However, this application of the 'ICLing' effect was not widely appreciated until many years after initial publication, after soft lenses were established in the marketplace. Not only could progressive peripheral thinning be achieved with a lenticular design, but the apex of the lens could be designed with: (1) prism ballast or periballast; and (2), superior slab-off prism. For these applications of the 'ICLing' effect, the term 'watermelon seed effect' was coined (Fig. 33.14).

Should a ballasted lens position in the eye so that the segment lies rotated either nasally or temporally, the 'watermelon seed theory' has been interpreted to predict that the upper lid will apply pressure to the thicker edge and cause the lens to then rotate tempo-

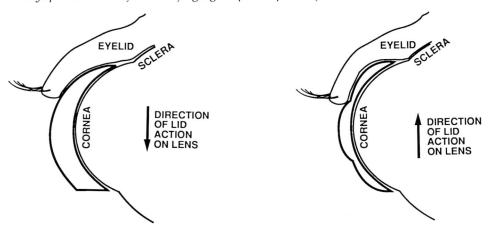

Figure 33.14 'Watermelon seed' effect. The thick inferior aspect of a prism-ballasted lens is 'squeezed' away from the superior eyelid when the apex lies beneath it.

Figure 33.15 'Minus carrier' effect. Thick edge created by minus lenticular flange on a front-surface plus-lenticular lens is drawn superiorly by attachment to the upper eyelid. Vertical lens centration can be elevated or depressed by increasing or decreasing, respectively, the edge thickness of the minus carrier. In other words, the lenticular flange can be made more or less minus.

rally or nasally, respectively, in order to equalize superior eyelid pressure on each horizontal aspect of the lens. Nasal rotation, here, is defined as rotation of the bottom of the lens toward the nose, and temporal rotation is rotation of the bottom of the lens in the opposite direction. For example, nasal rotation of a lens in the right eye would be counter-clockwise as viewed by the practitioner, while of the left eye clockwise. Often, however, the upper lid merely bumps the entire lens into a lower position on the cornea. If the lens is free to move on the cornea, gravity alone tends to rotate the lens so that the base rides down. If the lid passes over the lens or lies upon it, pressure from the upper eyelid will be greatest on the thicker portion of the apical edge of the lens, and the lid will grasp that thicker edge and hold the lens in that position in a 'minus-carrier effect' (Fig. 33.15).

This minus carrier effect will sometimes be manifested if a prism ballasted lens is placed in the eye with the base up. The upper lid may grasp the thickened base and hold the lens in that position (upside down). One reason that patients are often cautioned to be sure that the lens is inserted with the base in an inferior position is to allow a better chance of proper orientation of the segment. During a blink, more powerful pressure or pull seems to be apparent at the nasal portion of the upper lid, while the lower lid appears to exert a 'nasal kick' to rotate the bottom of the lens towards the nose. This tends to produce nasal rotation of the segment during blinking that is especially evident for rigid lenses and less evident for soft lenses. Rigid radially asymmetric segmented bifocal lenses will usually rotate nasally about 5–15 degrees while soft lenses will rotate perhaps 0–10 degrees. Nasal rotation of the segment will probably be even more pronounced during reading. Crescent-shaped segments are deemed better able to provide presbyopic correction, since when such a segment is slightly rotated from the ideal position below the pupil, the pupil will still receive coverage by a portion of the segment during reading.

Segment position and rotation

Segments for rigid asymmetric bifocals are usually custom-ordered so that their vertical axes are off-set nasally from a base-apex line, in order to compensate for nasal lens rotation on the eye (Fig. 33.16). Soft lens bifocals, as they are stocked prescription devices and their segments do not usually rotate far from vertical, are normally available only with segments oriented directly on the base-apex line.

The widest portion of the palpebral aperture may not correspond to the position of the central cornea or the contact lens on the eye. In these situations the 'minus carrier

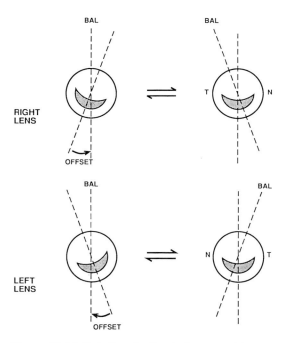

Figure 33.16 Rotational off-set of segment to compensate for nasal rotation of asymmetric bifocal lenses, shown for left and right lenses at the left. Note the segment should be off-set clockwise from the base–apex line (BAL) on a right lens which is rotating nasally, while the segment on the left lens should be rotated counter-clockwise. When the segments rotate into position, shown 'on the eye' to the right, they are positioned below the pupil.

effect' (Fig. 33.15) and the 'watermelon seed effect' (see Fig. 33.14) caused by the superior eyelid can produce seemingly inexplicable rotations of prism-ballasted bifocal lenses. It is not always possible to fit a lens such that the segment is directly inferior to the pupil. However, later, it will be seen that modifications of the upper edges of a rigid lens can help to better orient a lens which tends to ride out of position.

Edge thicknesses of contact lenses depend not only on the amount of slab-off prism and prism ballast but on the other characteristics which make up the structure of a contact lens. The refractive power of a lens, its critical thickness, diameter, and the base curve chosen for the patient will all have their impacts on shape of a conventional contact lens, its mass, and thickness, at any point. For a minus lens, the 'point of critical thickness' is at the center, therefore, center thickness (CT) is the minimum lens thickness. For a plus lens, the 'point of critical thickness' is at the edge of the most plus meridian, therefore, edge thickness (ET) is the minimum lens thickness. Practitioners versed in the art of contact lens design are able to manipulate parameters of the lens in order to achieve an appropriate lens shape, size, thickness, and mass for their patient. The formulae for these purposes are given in Appendix 33.A.

33.4.3 SEGMENT TRANSLATION

The understanding of what is truly responsible for the positioning of a translating bifocal has recently undergone considerable re-evaluation. For many years, the traditional concept noted in the previous paragraphs, has been that the lens should be fitted in a position relative to the lower eyelid, so that upon declination of the eye into a lowered reading position, the lower edge of the lens abuts the lower lid, and as the eye continues to move downward, the movement of the lens is impeded. The lens is moved superiorly relative to the pupil, and the pupil takes up a final position behind the reading segment.

However, it was observed that nearpoint vision could sometimes be attained through a segmented bifocal at the primary plane, without lowering the eyes. Nasal rotation of contact lenses during convergence has been noted for annular designs and also mentioned in relation to the blink in ballasted lenses. Apparently, the act of convergence will rotate the lenses sufficiently, in some cases, so that sufficient proportions of these segments rest before the pupil to permit vision at a nearpoint. Recently, attention has been called to the fact that the lower lid also moves downward with the eye, raising the question of the role the lower lid actually plays in changing the segment position. Measurements were made of 107 subjects of varying ages and both sexes via specially designed photography which enabled the positions of the line of sight and of the lower lid to be measured in both the primary and the reading positions (Borish & Perrigin, 1987). It was discovered that the median difference between the amounts of vertical movement of the line of sight and of the lower lid was less than one millimeter when alternating from a distance target to a reading position. The median differences and standard deviations of these movements are given in Table 33.8, and the range of values is shown in Figure 33.17.

It is immediately apparent that only one

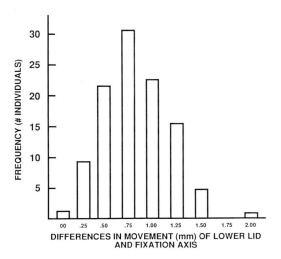

Figure 33.17 Differences in the amount of movement (mm) of the fixation axis and the lower lid when alternating from distance to near (reading) fixation in 107 human subjects (modified from Borish & Perrigin, 1987).

subject of the 107 would have displaced a bifocal lens by as much as 2 mm via interaction with the lower eyelid alone. However, the findings were further refined by comparing each individual's specific projected lens movement against that individual's pupil area to calculate the percentage of the pupil which the bifocal would have covered by lens movement of the amount indicated. The results are shown in Figure 33.18. Again, it is apparent that only two subjects would have had more than 50% of their pupils covered by the segment at the reading position if they depended upon the lower lid alone to superiorly shift the lens from a distance position just below the pupil. Other factors in addition to the lower lid presumably must be involved in the translation of a segmented

Table 33.8 Median and standard deviations of difference in millimeters between lid and fixation movement for 107 subjects

	n	Median	SD
Total	107	0.8314	0.3471
Under Age 40	83	0.7807	0.3362
Over Age 40	24	0.9937	0.3446
Males	52	0.7907	0.3379
Females	55	0.8613	0.3530

bifocal such that optimal alternating vision is achieved.

Normally about 20% of a rigid or soft segmented bifocal is covered by the superior eyelid. As previously noted, the superior eyelid controls rotational stability to a large extent. It also controls vertical positioning of the bifocal lens, therefore, segment position via the 'minus carrier effect' and the 'watermelon seed effect', particularly in cases where the lens edge slips under the lower lid (for instance, a soft lens on anything but a lowly positioned inferior lid margin) or if the lens edge does not contact the inferior lid margin (for instance, a rigid lens with lower eyelid positioned below the limbus). Sometimes, vertical centration of translating bifocals in straight-ahead and near gaze conditions can be achieved by modifying the 'minus carrier effect' or the 'watermelon seed effect' of the upper eyelid (see Figs. 33.13, 33.14 and 33.15).

Clinical experience has shown that plus lens wearers have had greater difficulty in utilizing translating bifocal contact lenses than have minus lens wearers. This cannot be ascribed solely to the difference in thickness of the base of the lens or the weight of the lens, but is due to lack of centration and translation as an effect of a conventional design. Many of these cases can be solved by introducing a minus carrier in the correct amount of peripheral minus power and annular width in order to properly position the plus lenses. For minus lenses which are overly attached to the upper eyelid, the proper amount of plus flange in terms of power and annular width can help these lenses center and translate an appropriate amount. The implication is obvious that the upper lid must play a most significant role in the centration and translation of bifocal contact lenses through the 'minus carrier' and 'watermelon seed' effects.

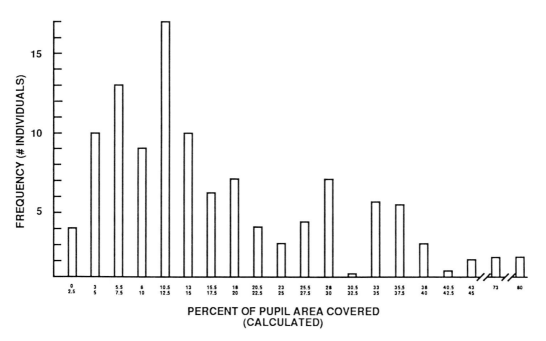

Figure 33.18 Percentage of pupil area that would have been covered by a bifocal segment if dependent solely upon the difference in movement between the fixation axis and lower lid. Values calculated from each subject's pupil diameter and movement difference (modified from Borish & Perrigin, 1987).

33.4.4 BACK SURFACE POWER

Many concentric distance/center and near/center bifocals are manufactured using the back surface to produce the add.[P2] Fannin and Grosvenor in their book, *Clinical Optics*, have developed a unique approach to illustrate how the posterior surface of a back-surface one-piece concentric distance/center bifocal provides the correct add when placed on the eye (Fannin & Grosvenor, 1987). The approach involves the lacrimal lens theory and comparison of the 'exploded' and 'unexploded' views of the lens/cornea optical system shown in Figure 33.19. A question is asked by Fannin and Grosvenor: Should the back surface periphery be made flatter or steeper than the central area in order to provide plus power for near vision?

The answer to this question has been known for many years, However, many clinicians who use the lacrimal lens concept for fitting rigid lenses will reply to this question that the back peripheral curve should be steeper to induce plus power. Their rationale is that the lacrimal lens (viewed 'exploded' as if in air) will be more plus and will, therefore, add plus to the overall lens/cornea optical system. However, the refractive powers of contact lenses must be held the same in order to compare optical effects of back surface curvatures with the lacrimal lens concept. When back surface curvature is steepened and lens power remains the same, more negative power is imparted to the optical system (viewed 'unexploded' at the lens-tear pool interface) which is counteracted by a simultaneous alteration of the front surface power into the plus by approximately three times that magnitude.

Back-surface bifocals have the same front surface for central and peripheral lens areas. Increased front surface curvature to overcome increase in minus by steepening of the back surface is not present, therefore, the lacrimal lens theory has been said not to apply. The correct answer to the question posed by Fannin and Grosvenor is that the peripheral curvature of the posterior distance/center lens surface should be flattened! The contact lens-tear pool interface will then impart less minus (more plus) to the overall optical system, given that the front surface curvature of the periphery remains the same as that at the center of the lens. The peripheral back-surface curvature for a concentric near/center bifocal will, of course, need to be steeper than the central curvature in order to provide the appropriate add power. The situation merely emphasizes the realization that when light passes from a less dense to a denser

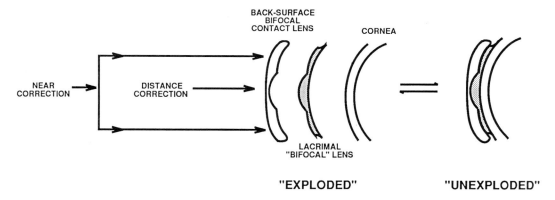

Figure 33.19 A back-surface rigid one-piece bifocal of concentric distance/center design. The posterior peripheral curve must be flatter than the central curve in order to impart plus power to the peripheral add.

medium (as from air to the lens), a steeper curvature at a convex interface results in an increase in plus power, but when light travels from a denser to a less dense medium (as from the lens into tear fluid), a steeper convex surface will produce greater minus power.

The example provided by Fannin and Grosvenor (1987) may also be ameliorated using an 'exploded' view. Calculations are shown in Table 3.9 for a back-surface distance/center rigid lens with a typical +2.00 add when the central back curve radius is 7.50 mm and the lens material has a refractive index of 1.47. The refractive power difference, in air, between the back-surface bifocal lens center and periphery will be 1.4 times the magnitude and of opposite sign than the power difference between the center and periphery of the lacrimal lens in air. Therefore, the 'lacrimal lens concept' gives the correct response when the power change in air between the periphery and center of the contact lens is taken into account! The practitioner need only combine the plus 'add' of the contact lens in air (measured with a lensometer) with the calculated minus 'add' produced by the lacrimal lens (using a keratometric base curve-to-diopter conversion chart) (Benjamin, 1990)!

33.4.5 ACCOMMODATIVE DEMANDS: CORNEAL AND SPECTACLE PLANES

The vertex distance at which a correcting lens is placed influences the magnitude of refractive power required for optimum refractive correction of an eye for distance vision. In a similar manner but in a differing amount, vertex distance also influences the amount of correction required for an object at near. Vertex distance has a lesser impact on optimal refractive correction for near vision (compared to its impact at distance) when considering a plus lens and a larger impact for a minus lens. The difference between distance and near refractive corrections is actually accommodative demand when only the distance correction is worn by a patient, but must be referenced to the vertex plane in which correction was determined. Therefore, accommodative demand at the corneal plane is less for a myopic eye corrected by a spectacle lens than for an emmetropic eye. A spectacle-corrected hyperopic eye has a higher corneal accommodative demand at near than does an emmetropic eye (Neumuller, 1938; Alpern, 1949; Westheimer, 1962; Hermann & Johnson, 1966).

Actual calculations of accommodative demand at the corneal plane are found in the optics chapter of this book. As one might guess, corneal accommodative demand differences between ametropes and emmetropes are further magnified as distance to near objects is reduced (Neumuller, 1938; Alpern, 1949; Westheimer, 1962; Hermann & Johnson, 1966). For the clinician, however, it might be advantageous to refer to Table 33.10 in which hyperopic and myopic spectacle corrections at 15 mm are listed that induce differences in corneal accommodative demand of +/- 0.25, 0.50, 0.75 and 1.00 D from that

Table 33.9 Differences between peripheral (near) and central (distance) refractive powers (the bifocal 'adds') for a concentric back-surface bifocal. The back curve radius is 7.50 mm in the center and 8.42 mm in the periphery. The refractive index of the lens material is 1.47 and of the lacrimal lens 1.3375

'Add' of contact lens in air (Lensometer reading)	'Add' of lacrimal lens in air (Calculated)	'Add' of lens/tear interface (Wet cell reading)
+ 6.85 D	− 4.92 D	+ 2.00 D

tions required to accurately do so (Campbell, 1984) make the wet cell clinically impractical for many refractive power assessments. In addition, magnification of measurement error with the wet cell by a factor of 4 or more results in excessive error when converting from refractive power in water (saline) to refractive power in air. However, an interesting feature of 'diffractive' contact lenses, indeed, nearly all back-surface bifocals (to include one-piece and fused-segment back-surface designs), is that the near 'add' power may be determined directly on the lensometer with the use of a 'wet cell'.

Back-surface bifocals are designed to produce the correct 'add' powers when their posterior surfaces are immersed in tear fluid. The index of refraction ($n = 1.336$) of tears is similar to that of water (saline) bathing the posterior surface of the lens in a wet cell ($n = 1.333$). Therefore, the refractive power of the add of a back-surface bifocal contact lens (the difference between the distance and near powers) is correct when read through a lensometer (focimeter) with the use of a wet cell, although the distance power must be corrected (by a factor of 4 or more).

For instance, let us assume that the refractive index of a soft back-surface bifocal is such that a 4× correction factor should be used to convert power in saline to power in air. If the practitioner reads -0.87 D and $+0.87$ D with a focimeter for the distance and near images through a wet cell, then the add is $+1.75$ D (-0.87 to $+0.87$ D). However, the distance power is -0.87 D multiplied by 4, the correction factor, or -3.50 D. The lens is -3.50 D with $+1.75$ D add on the eye. Had the distance and near powers been obtained in air, the add (in air) would have been $+7.00$ D.

Verification of add power for rigid back-surface bifocals has been practical for many years. Distance and near powers were easily determined in air and other parameters of rigid lenses were easily assessed in order to verify lens design, therefore, refractive power of the bifocal 'add'. Use of a wet cell to verify adds of rigid back-surface bifocal contact lenses was possible but not necessary.

Wet cells have assumed special importance with the introduction of hydrogel back-surface bifocals, such as the diffractive Echelon lens by Allergan-Hydron (Loshin, 1989). Clinically speaking, accurate assessment of gel lens power in air and design parameters necessary for add verification are beyond the capabilities of normal office instrumentation. But with the wet cell, add power can be verified directly and accurately without the need for correction factors notorious for otherwise reducing the wet cell's practical value. In addition, because the back surfaces of rigid diffractive bifocals (Diffrax rigid lens, by Sola/Barnes-Hind) are also not adequately assessed with current office instrumentation, in-office add verification may be efficiently performed with the wet cell when such rigid lenses are prescribed (Benjamin, 1990).

An interesting exception to direct wet cell measurement of add power is the near/center spectrum lens by CIBA Vision. Though technically a back surface design, the back curvatures are thought to conform to the cornea such that add is produced by a front surface curvature change only when on the eye. Thus, the wet cell does not give the equivalent of an 'in eye' add measurement. The lens is a back surface bifocal off the eye, but functions as a front surface bifocal on the eye.

33.5 FITTING AND CORRECTION

Although the majority of individuals who wear spectacle corrections for presbyopia wear some form of multifocal lens, a large number still derive their desired purpose by using lenses for distance in one pair of spectacles and lenses for near in another. Instead of alternating between two portions of a single lens, they alternate between two separate devices. This same alternation between separate devices, each for a specific function, can be applied to contact lenses.

33.5.1 SPECTACLE OVER-CORRECTION

Correction of presbyopia can be achieved by wearing a spectacle correction which provides the near addition before distance vision contact lenses. Many patients who were successful contact lens wearers prior to development of presbyopia have opted to wear spectacles for near vision. This is the least complicated method of achieving presbyopic correction for those currently wearing contact lenses and results in fewer problems for the patient and practitioner.

The approach has several additional advantages: (1) the patient does not discontinue wear of contact lenses; (2) the patient's visual system and ocular physiology are not disrupted by various techniques of using contact lenses for distance *and* near vision which will be covered later in this chapter; (3) there is minimal, if any, change in the way the patient wears contact lenses; (4) several types of spectacle corrections can be obtained, such as single-vision lenses for near, half-eye spectacles, bifocal or trifocal lenses having plano power at distance, and even progressive-addition lenses; bifocal lenses can be prescribed with intermediate near power in the major portion of the lens to be used for vision at intermediate distances; (5) near and reading powers can be easily and cost-effectively interchanged, duplicated, or altered in response to various and changing visual requirements of the patient; (6) a wider range of near vision and binocular requirements can be met.

The categories of over-correction for use in presbyopia are:

1. Spectacle over-corrections.
2. Contact lens over-corrections:
   i. binocular over-plus;
   ii. monocular over-plus or monovision.

Spectacle over-correction for near is perhaps the best presbyopic option for contact lens wearers who have excessive visual demands at near, such that other contact lens alternatives are likely to be less effective. This method of correction is also best for patients who may or may not already have contact lenses and who have little visual demand at near. Other patients may feel that spectacle over-correction defeats the purpose of beginning or continuing wear of contact lenses. A requirement that spectacles had to be worn in addition, might cause the typical presbyope to think twice before even engaging in contact lens wear. Therefore, the search still continues for an acceptable way to correct presbyopes at distance and at near without the use of spectacle lenses.

In the immediate first stages of presbyopia, binocularly over-plussing in the minimal amount of +0.25 to +0.75 diopters may reduce the need for separate distance and near contact lens powers. Binocular over-plus is usually a short-term solution that will not save most patients from making an ultimate decision about presbyopic correction. For patients without clear distant vision needs or visual tasks requiring frequent change in fixation from far to near, this mode of correction may allow them to never require more specialized presbyopic correction. However, for most, minimal over-plus only forestalls the inevitable for a very short duration.

33.5.2 MONOVISION

When minimal over-plus no longer provides acceptable vision to the presbyopic patient, other options for providing alternation from the distance focus to the near focus may be considered. One of these is to provide two single-vision contact lenses, one of which is worn on one of the eyes and has full distance correction; the second lens is worn on the other eye and has full near correction. This method of correcting presbyopia is called the monovision technique. It is likely that the 'monocle' reading lens, which dates back perhaps over 100 years, is the spectacle lens ancestor of monovision contact lens wear (Snyder, 1989).

It has been said by others that monovision is a variant of 'simultaneous vision' assuming that the two eyes are simultaneously focused at different working distances, rather than than each eye simultaneously focused at both distances. It is true that presentation of the two images is optically simultaneous. However, alternation takes place between the 'neural images' of the two eyes during monovision, as it is assumed that the central vision of the eye that is not in focus, will be suppressed. Thus, it is actually a way of forcing a patient's visual system to alternate central suppression between the two eyes when visual attention is alternated between distance and near targets. Therefore, to the extent that it is successful, monovision is a type of 'alternating vision' in which the visual neurological system provides the alternation.

Defining the dominant eye

Since the distance eye is the eye used for sighting and localization of ambulatory field, and since these should be qualities of a 'dominant eye', the lens correcting the distance vision is often recommended for the 'dominant eye'. There are many ways to differentiate between the 'dominant' and 'non-dominant' eyes of a patient. The practitioner will find that results of various methods do not all agree when tested on any particular patient. Many practitioners, however, use a 'distance parallax' test to determine ocular dominance.

The difficulty in truly determining the dominant eye by most tests is that the methods also usually involve 'body' dominance since a hand and arm of the subject is employed in pointing to or holding something as part of the process, plus the fact that the subject is cued or instructed as to what to see. One test which avoids these taints was designed by Ogle *et al.* (1967) for evaluating

fixation disparities. This test ably serves the purpose of designating the dominant eye when the dominant eye is defined as that eye which receives the image on the fovea whereby projection and localization of a perceived object is attained.

In Ogle's eye dominancy test, two vertical lines are presented to each eye. The distance between the two lines is not the same in each target. The right line of each target bears an identifying mark, for one an 'X' is immediately below the line and for the other an 'O' is immediately above the line. When the images are fused as in a stereopsis target, the subject sees two lines, but may see the 'X' directly under one, while the 'O' is above and slightly to one side of the line; or, the subject might perceive the 'O' directly above one line, while the 'X' is below and to the side as seen in Figure 33.20.

The eye whose symbol lies directly above or below the fused line is the dominant eye. Occasionally, neither identifying mark is either directly above or below the line, indicating that neither eye is dominant. Figure

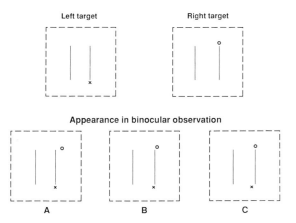

Figure 33.20 Test for ocular dominancy adapted from Ogle (1957). Top: Disparate vertical line targets have a different separation for one eye than for the other. Bottom: Eye dominancy is determined by the binocularly perceived position of the identifying marks (X and O) above and below the right line.

33.21 illustrates the explanation of the test. The dominant eye receives the line on its foveal area of fixation and projects the line straight ahead along its line of sight. The symbol directly above or below the line is in the same vertical plane as the line on the fovea and is therefore also projected straight ahead. The line on the other eye strikes the retina to the side of its foveal fixation point. Falling on Panum's area it is nevertheless fused with the line seen by the dominant eye. However, the symbol aligned with it also strikes the retina to one side of the foveal vertical axis. Having nothing to correspondingly fuse with, it is located as expected by the normal laws of projection to the side of the fused line.

A convincing practical clinical method of determining which eye is to be fitted for distance and which eye for near, is to alternately use monocular plus build-up on each eye under binocular conditions at distance, sometimes called 'plus acceptance to blur' (Ghormley, 1989). The distance eye is the eye that requires the least amount of plus for the patient to detect blur at distance under binocular conditions. The near eye is the eye that requires the most plus in order that the patient detect blur at distance. This method is most suited for monovision, for in actuality, correction will result in a large plus build-up over the non-dominant eye! The test effectively determines which eye is most able to tolerate extra plus power.

Fitting the dominant eye for distance assumes that use of this eye should be superior for spatial-locomotor activities. The practitioner also needs to consider the refractive condition and anticipated use of vision with monovision before assigning the eyes to distance and near vision. Other methods of determining the 'near' and 'distance' eyes are: (1) to have the dominant eye focused at the distance (far or near) most used by the patient (Schor *et al.*, 1987); (2) to correct the most myopic eye for near (Snyder, 1989); and (3) to correct the left eye for distance as it is

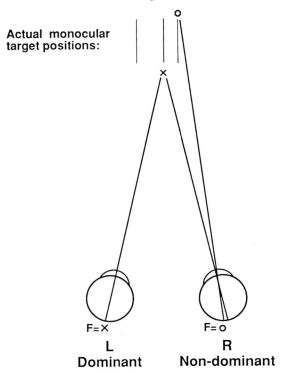

Actual monocular target positions:

F=✕   F=○
L   R
Dominant   Non-dominant

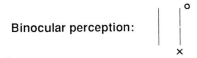

Binocular perception:

Figure 33.21 Diagram explaining the dominancy test. The two right target lines presented to the eyes fall within Panum's area and are thus perceived as one line projecting from the fovea (F) of the dominant eye. The identifying marker of the dominant eye (in this case, ✕) is seen in the same direction as the line. The identifying marker (○) of the non-dominant eye, having no corresponding image on the other eye, is perceived in its original direction.

most important for driving (even though the right eye may be important for the rear-view mirror inside an automobile) (Harris & Classé, 1988). Ghormley (1989) recommends that anisometropic patients be fitted with the least hyperopic, most myopic eye for near vision in order to lessen the difference in refractive power between contact lenses on the two eyes. The 'near eye' might be best situated on the side in which a patient routinely distributes reading material, such as a computer operator who consistently types from material placed on the left (Ghormley, 1989). In this case, use of the right eye for near vision might create confusion between the eye best situated to see the material (O.S.) and the eye from which the patient's visual attention must be directed in order to focus at the near target (O.D.).

To what must the patient adapt?

Occasionally, eye care practitioners will see presbyopic patients who are emmetropic in one eye and myopic in the other eye. These patients have a naturally occurring 'monovision' and can get by without optical correction. The patients have adapted to ametropia over their lifetimes and once they became presbyopic have little visual disturbance or discomfort with the monovisual situation.

On the other hand, patients who are suddenly thrust into monovision have significant visual and adaptative problems to overcome. After all, the patient's visual system is thrown into a situation that most patients would reject if their motivations to be rid of spectacles were not paramount! The practitioner must select patients, educate them, and prescribe monovision contact lenses carefully in order not to overly upset the visual systems of his/her patients. It is best to place diagnostic monovision contact lenses on a patient and have the patient walk around the office and observe effects of the lenses. In this manner, the practitioner can predict how the patient might adjust to monovision before prescribing lenses. Even then, a significant proportion of monovision prescriptions will require that patients endure weeks of adaptation and a few patients will be unable to adapt to the new visual situation. Most pre-selected patients,

however, will be able to pass through an adaptation period within a few days. Success rates with monovision have been quoted at 75% to 80% and greater with pre-selected patients (Ghormley, 1989; Snyder, 1989). Patients should be warned that they may go through a period of disorientation and perhaps hazy or blurry vision.

Monovision contact lens wear reduces the degree of stereopsis elicited by most patients (Lebow & Goldberg, 1975; Beier, 1977; McGill & Erickson, 1988). The amount of decrease is usually small but becomes more significant with increased add power in the non-dominant eye. Monovision compromises binocular visual acuity especially under low-contrast conditions, for as the amount of near add is increased, contrast sensitivity tends to reduce to that of the in-focus eye (Loshin *et al.*, 1982). Monovision patients sometimes complain of episodes in which their vision is momentarily blurred because they are no longer completely binocular. As only one eye can be focused at any particular target, the contralateral (out-of-focus) eye can not cover for minor tear film disturbances or foreign substances in the tear film that move across the central visual field of the in-focus eye and blur the in-focus retinal image. Monovision with toric (astigmatic) soft and rigid contact lenses is difficult for patients because of the variable vision achieved by each toric lens as cylinder axes rotate in and out of position before the eyes. Performance of most near point tasks is slightly reduced in monovision, but the degree of reduction becomes greater for tasks that require excellent visual resolution (Loshin *et al.*, 1982; Sheedy *et al.*, 1988). One would expect performance of tasks requiring excellent depth perception to also be reduced when wearing monovision contact lenses (Lebow & Goldberg, 1975; Beier, 1977).

It has been concluded that the use of monovision does not impair the extent of peripheral monocular or binocular visual fields or peripheral visual acuities of most patients (Collins *et al.*, 1989; Josephson *et al.*, 1989; McGill & Erikson, 1989). The assumption should not be made, however, that peripheral vision is unaffected by the wear of monovision contact lenses. Peripheral detection of targets may, in fact, be impaired by over-plus of the near eye and portions of the distance eye's visual field normally blocked by anatomical features of the patient's face in peripheral gaze (the nose, for instance) will not be adequately covered by the out-of-focus eye. Should a patient detect an object in the binocular field only with the out-of-focus eye, central distance acuity has been reduced in that eye, and eye movement to an extreme temporal gaze may not allow the in-focus eye to compensate. Therefore, monovision contact lens wear becomes a handicap when a patient performs tasks that require excellent peripheral vision (driving, sports activities, etc.).

Two situations that require excellent vision in most respects are driving at night and piloting an airplane at night. Interpretation of visual space is disorganized in normally binocular persons when details about visual space are gained through only one eye. As monovision patients have slight visual decrements in many visual functions, night activities requiring optimum visual function can be problems for monovision wearers. In addition, suppression of blurred, bright high-contrast headlight beams of oncoming vehicles is very difficult. Thus, the out-of-focus image produces glare which psychologically and functionally disturbs many patients. Monovision patients should be advised *not* to drive or be a pilot at night, and if they find themselves doing so, they should be cautious.

Due to the many subclinical binocular problems that can become manifest by creation of visual imbalance between the two eyes, many practitioners do not prescribe their regular distance prescriptions and/or full near adds when using the monovision technique. Typically, full plus refraction or slightly over-plussed correction (by +0.25 or +0.50 D) is prescribed for the distance eye, and the near correction is reduced to the least amount necessary to fulfill the near vision demands of the patient. Recently, however, higher add powers have been recommended on the basis that they stabilize central suppression especially when viewing at near (Heath *et al.*, 1986). Care must be taken when evaluating the results of studies concerning monovision contact lens wear, for the ways in which corrections were determined and prescribed can lead to erroneous correlations of data from different investigations.

For all the detrimental aspects of monovision on the binocular abilities of patients, it is surprising that monovision works so well! In part, this may be due to ability of the visual system to create a limited degree of central suppression of those aspects of the blurred image which may interfere with normal binocular function and to retain those aspects of the blurred image (low spatial frequency elements common to both eyes) which can contribute to overall binocular perception at the cortical level (Heath *et al.*, 1986; Schor & Erickson, 1988). The most successful monovision patients may be those who have *weak* ocular dominance, such that central suppression of the out-of-focus eye is easily alternated between distance and near vision (Schor & Erickson, 1988). In part, also, successful patients have a motivation to overlook the nastier aspects of vision with monovision contact lenses in order to attain freedom from the wear of spectacles and bifocal contact lenses. Simply put, they may only desire vision that is 'good enough' to 'get around'. Thus, presbyopic correction with monovision has been found to be more successful than wearing of bifocal contact lenses which have their own idiosyncrasies and problems (Back *et al.*, 1989).

Some practitioners recommend that patients have either: (1) a distance contact lens for the near eye (a 'third contact lens'); or (2) a spectacle correction for wear with monovision contact lenses, having minus correction over the near eye for distance vision. In theory, these sound like viable options to occasionally compensate for those times when full distance correction in both eyes is required. However, the extent to which a patient might rely on these options is questionable. When a situation arises in which the distance contact lens is desired on the near eye, it is most likely that the circumstance will develop rapidly and/or be fleeting, such that removal of the near lens and replacement with the distance lens is an impractical procedure. Such a 'third contact lens' might be desired when it can be used over longer periods when enhanced distance vision is most required and the ability to see at near is of minimal importance. Spectacle over-correction is more easily used than a 'third contact lens' for moments in which critical distance vision is needed. However, spectacle anisometropia caused by the lenses may disorient the patient due to magnification differences and prismatic effects of the lenses.

Summary

Monovision contact lenses can be recommended to patients who either are not able to wear *or* do not want to wear bifocal contact lenses. Monovision candidates should not have critical visual demands in the areas of visual acuity/resolution, depth perception, and peripheral vision. This would especially be true if critical visual demands occur for long periods of time. Monovision candidates should be willing to experiment with their vision and take the risks, both financial and otherwise, that monovision will prove to be acceptable to them. Presence of pre-existing binocular vision problems will most likely contraindicate monovision contact lens wear, although monovision can be beneficial for patients having constant strabismus (London, 1987). In the absence of effective and comfortable bifocal contact lens correction

for many patients, monovision is a 'stop-gap' measure that affords reasonable vision to those who can overlook its disadvantages in anticipation of receiving spectacle-free presbyopic vision.

Monovision is also the technique preferred by many practitioners who have found successful fitting of bifocals to be not only exceedingly time consuming, but hazardous and unpredictable. Unfortunately, bifocal designs capable of providing excellent distance and near vision thus far fall within the category of 'rigid' lenses which, as a whole, most practitioners are least experienced and skilled in fitting. As most patients are far more effortlessly fitted with 'soft' contact lenses, practitioners lean in the direction which assures readier patient acceptance and tend to resort to monovision as the most likely and easiest to apply within the soft lens modality. Their attitudes may also influence patients to a great extent, and the definition of 'success' with bifocal lenses becomes not the achievement of optimal refractive correction, but the degree to which patients are willing to avoid optimal optical correction in order to wear soft contact lenses.

33.5.3 MODIFIED MONOVISION

Instead of prescribing simple single-vision lenses for each eye, bifocal contact lenses can be biased in an attempt to maximize vision of either eye at the distance most preferred by the patient according to his/her visual requirements. When the powers, lens fit, or parameters of bifocal contact lenses are modified to emphasize distance vision for one eye and/or to emphasize near vision for the other eye, the binocular situation is called 'modified monovision'.

Modified monovision first began with the prescribing of a single-vision lens in the dominant eye for distance vision and an early bifocal lens in the other eye for near vision. Numerous 'modified monovision' patients were fitted with a spherical single-vision soft lens in the dominant eye for distance and the first soft lens bifocal to be widely marketed (the Bausch & Lomb 'PA-1', or 'Progressive Add 1', an aspheric bifocal) in the non-dominant eye. Later, the Ciba Vision 'Bisoft' lens (distance/center concentric bifocal) became the second soft bifocal on the market and also a modified monovision candidate when paired with a spherical single-vision soft lens in the dominant eye. Today, with more soft bifocal designs available, the near eye might be better served with a near/center concentric bifocal lens for which pupil constriction at near helps the process of vision alternation. The distance portion of the bifocal lens can also be powered for an intermediate distance, such that a trifocal range of viewing distances can be provided.

By manipulating various components of a binocular bifocal contact lens prescription, the practitioner may emphasize one eye for distance and the other eye for near, yet maintain a combination of 'alternating' and/or traditional 'simultaneous' bifocal vision for both eyes. This can be brought about either by prescribing lenses of the same type and design (but with different parameters) from the same manufacturer on the two eyes, *or* the eyes can be fitted with lenses of different designs from the same or different manufacturers. It became known that the Bisoft was the better of the two initial soft bifocal lenses for near vision due to availability of more add power and its tendency to translate on the eye. The PA-1 was noted for better distance vision as its nominal add was low and lens movement was minimal. These lenses, then, comprised the first pair of bifocal contact lenses commonly prescribed on alternate eyes for purposes of modified monovision!

A variation of modified monovision, called 'modified trivision', has also been proposed (Pence, 1987). When prescribing 'modified trivision', the dominant eye is given refractive power for full distance correction in the distance portion of the lens and a low add power for an intermediate distance in the near portion, while the non-dominant eye is given a power for the intermediate distance in its distance portion and the required power for near correction in the near portion. The advantage, here, is to provide one power for each eye which corrects for an intermediate distance.

More soft bifocal lenses have come on the market in ever larger supply of various parameters, including distance and add refractive powers, overall diameters, segment heights, segment sizes, and in many different designs. Therefore, opportunities to prescribe modified monovision in a number of different manners has recently come about. Table 33.12 relates many of the methods now available to achieve modified monovision. However, all methods have in common the emphasis of distance vision in one eye and emphasis of near vision in the other eye. Two main themes of pursuing modified monovision are apparent: (1) modification of distance and near refractive powers to achieve the monovision effect; and (2) alteration of fit or segment parameters (segment height, size) in order to achieve the monovision effect.

Summary

Modified monovision is difficult to avoid when fitting bifocal contact lenses and may be much more prevalent that one would ordinarily suspect! Bifocal contact lenses may often fail to provide equal vision at distance and at near for both eyes. Differences between the two eyes in terms of ocular and palpebral anatomical features, normal physiological anisocoria, and variability in stated lens parameters may emphasize one eye for distance and the other for near even when modified monovision is not an intended mode of correction.

Table 33.12 Various forms and examples of 'modified monovision'

Distance eye	Near eye
Single-vision lens	Bifocal lens power(s) biased towards near vision
Bifocal lens power(s) biased towards distance vision	Bifocal lens power(s) biased towards near vision
Large OZ for distance/center	Small OZ for distance/center
Small OZ for near/center	Large OZ for near/center
Low segment height for translation	High segment height for translation
Monofocal lens, concentric progressive, or concentric diffractive lens	Concentric near/center lens with large OZ, or distance/center lens with small OZ

As with any optically simultaneous presentation of images, modified monovision will work better when other alternating qualities of the correction also are apparent. For instance, lens translation and pupil size changes which are in favor of optical alternation may augment the monovisual component of alternation processed by the visual neurological system.

33.5.4 SIMULTANEOUS VISION WITH RADIALLY SYMMETRIC DESIGNS

To achieve 'simultaneous vision', it appears essential that a bifocal contact lens be centered precisely in front of the entrance pupil of the eye at all times, so that the rays from both optical zones may reach the retina. Minimal lens movement should occur upon the blink and during eye rotation. This is generally achieved by fitting the lens more tightly than is optimum for single-vision lenses, and can result in physiological compromise to the cornea. The central optical area should have a diameter somewhat less than that of the pupil, so that light from both distance and near objects can come to a focus at the retina simultaneously through the central zone and the portion of the peripheral zone overlying the pupil. If the area of the peripheral zone overlying the pupil equals the area of the central zone, both distance and near zones will contribute equally and simultaneously to their respective retinal images.

Central optic diameters seem to work best between 2.0 and 3.5 mm, with optimum function generally at 2.5 mm (Erickson & Robboy, 1985). As noted above, some degradation of both clear images results from the overlying blurred image passing through the non-focusing area of the lens. Further degradation is also imposed by light scatter, flare, and diffraction occurring at the junction between the distance and near optical zones. Obviously, variations in pupil size and lens centration will alter the distribution between the two zones and create variable 'simultaneous' vision (Fig. 33.22). The ideal optic diameter is, therefore, individually and continuably variable between patients.

Distance/center lenses

For lenses constructed with the distance portion in the center and the reading power surrounding it (distance/center lenses), the pupil diameter should be large enough (3–5 mm) so that distance and near refractive powers are both adequately represented in the pupil area (Josephson & Caffery, 1986). As the pupil of the aging eye decreases in diameter with the years, maintaining a proportion of light through the annular zone equal to that passing through the central zone will progressively become more difficult. In addition, when fixation is directed at the nearpoint, pupillary constriction as part of the near triad response

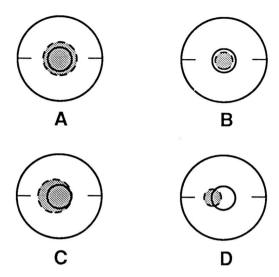

A   **B**

C   **D**

Figure 33.22 Effect of pupil size, pupil size alterations, and lens centration on coverage of central and annular optical zones of a concentric bifocal lens. Darkened circles represent large (A,C) and small (B,D) entrance pupils of the eye, with concentric lenses centered (A,B) and with lenses decentered (C,D).

Near/Center Lenses

For lenses within which the near add is placed at the center, the near triad reflex and bright illumination augment the near image such that a measure of optical alternation is provided. However, bright illumination such as daylight or sunlight may occasionally reduce the acuity for distance as constriction of the pupil reduces the contribution of the distance-powered peripheral zone. In many cases, however, very bright sunlight will produce a pinhole pupil and the resulting distance vision will not be too adversely affected. Of the two concentric designs, center/near lenses have been better accepted by patients requiring better near than distance vision, particularly when used as the near lens for monovision in which the other eye secured the distance vision. Center/near lenses have also been called reversed centrad bifocals (Josephson & Caffery, 1986).

Progressive (aspheric) lenses

As with concentric design bifocal lenses made with spherical surfaces, progressive bifocal contact lenses have been conventionally fitted such that they provide minimal movement and must be centered relative to the entrance pupil of the eye. They, too, are supposed to work on the 'simultaneous vision' principle, in which distance and progressively nearer targets are focused on the retina at the same time. The pupil diameter should be large enough so that distance and near refractive powers are both adequately represented within the pupillary area. Since the add power of the lens is gradually cumulative from the distance center towards the periphery, they provide (or blur?) simultaneous images from many working distances. The maximum amount of add usable is very dependant upon the diameter of the pupil. As many designs are limited in the nominal add power they can provide, the lenses are often usable only for the initial stages of presbyopia. Where the lenses do

tends to reduce the contribution of the outer near segment of the lenses even more and may actually limit vision to the central distance portion alone. Also, presbyopic eyes require an increase in illumination to achieve equivalently efficient vision, but this increased illumination may further constrict the pupils and reduce near vision. One of the few beneficial effects caused by pupil size variation with these lenses, is the sharpening of distance vision under high levels of illumination such as sunlight. Constriction of the pupil provides optical alternation, in the sense that it reduces the contribution of the peripheral near segment's out-of-focus rays. In contrast, however, under dim illumination or at night, when handicapped mesopic vision is involved, dilation of the pupil produces an increase in myopia as the visual contribution of the periphery is increased.

work for higher presbyopic add needs, it is likely that they do so by moving on the cornea to present a more peripheral portion of the lens before the pupil. Various eccentricities of curvatures (see Appendix 33.A) have been introduced into the surfaces of aspheric lenses in an attempt to bring greater peripheral power closer to the distance zone. Because most presbyopic pupils are small, the utility of simultaneous vision with these lenses in medium and higher add powers is limited.

In summary, to obtain simultaneous vision, concentric and progressive bifocal lenses should ideally be immobile on the cornea and centered before a large pupil. However, this is a condition that is incompatible with adequate corneal physiology and tear film dynamics in rigid lens wear. Such minimal lens movement is a condition better met by soft lenses.

Under dim illumination and at night, pupil dilation increases the contribution of the peripheral optic zone. Under bright illumination and when fixating at near, pupil constriction reduces the contribution of the peripheral zone. For lenses exhibiting minimal movement over large pupils, therefore, presbyopic correction with near/center lenses is generally better than with distance/center lenses. Near/center bifocals and diffractive bifocals come the closest to achieving a true simultaneous vision effect when manufactured in soft lens materials.

Diffractive lenses

Freeman (1987) has noted that 'holographic' lenses can be considered 'full aperture' lenses since the resolution is a function of contributions from the entire optic zone such that the entire lens aperture is utilized. Standard simultaneous vision and even alternating vision designs were termed 'reduced aperture' lenses because they limit resolution by the aperture size and are highly dependent upon pupil size and lens centration. The lenses should theoretically function independently of normal pupillary variations and the term 'pupil size independence' has been used in describing them (Benjamin, 1987). In actual usage, although the lenses can be considered 'pupil independent' when centered before the pupil, they do not always seem to perform as expected when displaced on the cornea. Centration appears to be more critical than was anticipated. Young *et al.* (1990) have recently confirmed diffractive lenses to be largely independent, though not entirely independent, of pupil size variations.

Like current simultaneous vision bifocals, 'holographic' bifocals also divide incident light into distance and near images, therefore, vision deteriorates under conditions of reduced illumination. This is of critical importance in presbyopia when more light is required to obtain optimum vision. Diffraction also tends to break white light into its component colors. The computations by which 'diffraction' lenses are designed must make certain assumptions concerning the wavelengths of the rays which will pass through the lens and the orders of diffraction and refraction which will take place. Under certain types of illumination, such as sodium lamps and some types of fluorescent lights, problems of glare and ghost images have been reported.

33.5.5 ALTERNATING VISION BY TRANSLATION OF DISTANCE/CENTER LENSES

Bifocal contact lenses move on the eye away from perfect centration in response to the blink and due to eye movements to various positions of gaze (Fig. 33.23). In fact, the concept of 'centration' is misleading because considerable individual variation of pupil location relative to the center of the cornea exists. The 'average' pupil is slightly nasal and inferior to the center of the visible iris, as has already been noted, such that lenses centered on the cornea will most probably not be centered over the pupil! Scatterplots by Erickson and Robboy (1985) show that bifocal contact lenses rarely center within 0.5 mm of the middle of the pupil.

Patients often complain of distance blur in left and right gaze when wearing distance/center concentric or progressive lenses, due to lens decentration caused by lens lag. This increases the contribution of the near segment covering the pupil. Should distance/center lenses not be perfectly centered even in straight-ahead gaze, additional minus power is often added for distance to lessen the effective amount of add power available at near in an attempt to decrease the distance blur.

In downgaze, contact lenses translate upwards relative to the pupil (Fig. 33.23). During convergence lenses translate slightly temporally relative to the pupil and tend to rotate (bottoms nasally) from their distance vision axis orientation (soft lenses move to a lesser extent than rigid lenses). When wearing concentric distance/center or progressive distance/center lenses, then, each of a patient's lenses will move superotemporally (more superior than temporal) when fixating down and at near on the midline. This will move the

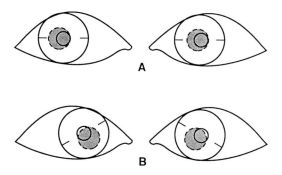

Figure 33.23 Effect of lens lag and rotation on pupil coverage of central and annular optical zones of concentric bifocal lenses with eyes in extreme lateral gaze (A) and in the reading position (B). Note that lens rotation during covergence should not influence vision with symmetric lenses. Darkened circles represent entrance pupils of the eyes.

peripheral refractive areas in most cases to partially or possibly, in a few instances, totally cover the pupil. Therefore, in a distance/center design, so-called 'simultaneous vision' bifocals may often work because of the translation and subsequent vision alternation between distance and near (Borish, 1988).

Translation of radially symmetric lenses

Rigid concentric distance/center lenses can actually be fitted such that they primarily provide presbyopic correction by translation. The degree to which the lenses provide 'alternating vision' is controlled by: (1) the amount and direction of lens translation at near; (2) lens centration over the pupil; (3) pupil size; and (4) lens design and lid contributions, which may abet or hinder such translation. Lenses do not have to translate as much over the cornea to alternate between distance and near zones of correction when an eye has a small pupillary diameter. Because lens translation is at a premium, therefore, patients should be pre-selected to have small pupil diameters when attempting to attain alternating vision. The diameter of the central optical zone should be equal to or only slightly larger than the pupil under average illumination.

The peripheral optical zone of a 'translating' rigid distance/center concentric lens will need to be larger than is optimal for a purely 'simultaneous vision' fitting, for the peripheral zone will be required to cover most of the pupil after translation for near vision. The central optical area may also need to be larger as it should also cover most of the pupil. This may require that a lens of large overall diameter be prescribed, an act that may reduce the amount of translation possible, especially for patients with small palpebral apertures. The lenses may even slide underneath the lower lid during downgaze as they impinge on the superior limbus and bulbar conjunctiva during attempted translation.

An 'image jump' occurs at the junction between distance and near segments of translating concentric lenses due to the fact that the refractive power change occurs at a considerable distance (for a contact lens) from the optic center of the segments. In actual wear, patients rarely report such a jump, since attention is apparently concentrated on securing clear near vision or the junction does not completely translate over the pupil as depicted. The image jump ranges from 0.3 to 1.5 prism diopters according to Prentice's rule:

$$P = hF \qquad \text{(eqn 33.1)}$$

where P, image jump in prism diopters; h, distance of junction from optic center in cm; F, add power in diopters.

The posterior optical zone of a front-surface concentric alternating design will need to be large in order to provide a field of view that will include the front peripheral correction. Correspondingly, the back peripheral curve annulus will be small, or thin, and the base curve will generally need to be slightly flatter than normally prescribed. This necessity reduces a major advantage of front-surface designs, that of providing the practitioner with the ability to optimally fit the lens to the corneal surface. The requirement can not be met with a two-surface bifocal design. Therefore, most concentric bifocal lenses fitted for translation are back surface rigid distance/center lenses.

Near/center 'simultaneous vision' concentric bifocals also translate during downgaze and convergence such that peripheral areas of the lenses cover portions of the pupil. In this case lens translation actually hinders near vision and it is, therefore, important with near/center lenses to minimize lens movement and achieve centration over the pupil. For lenses exhibiting translation especially over pupils with medium to small diameters, distance/center lenses generally provide better presbyopic correction than do near/center lenses. This is one reason why rigid concentric and progressive bifocal lenses are genrally distance/center designs.

Translation of progressives

Progressive lenses are not ordinarily intended for 'alternating vision'. However, as has been noted, the progression of plus power at points increasingly peripheral from the central zone of a distance/center lens and covering the pupil, results in a relatively low nominal add power averaged from a variable pupillary position and size in the reading position. This places any higher add sufficiently peripheral so that the ordinarily miotic pupil of the older eye would tend to prevent most light from entering the pupil through the near periphery of the lens. It would seem that any progressive distance/center lens would have to translate to bring a usable focus to the pupil, unless the eccentricity were so high as to almost place the power circumferentially about the distance. As already noted, this amount of eccentricity would most likely be incompatible with an excellent lens/cornea fitting relationship and would induce larger amounts of unwanted astigmatic error (Charman, 1982; Goldberg & Lowther, 1986) into the periphery of these lenses. Rigid lenses are better able to meet the requirement of lens translation, therefore, most progressive rigid lenses are of a distance/center design.

Progressive near/center lenses would not benefit from lens translation when alternating from distance to near, for this would emphasize the distance peripheral zone at the expense of the near central zone when reading. Therefore, these lenses should be fitted in a manner so as to minimize lens movement, and as with concentric near/center lenses, soft lenses are better able than rigid lenses to meet this requirement.

Summary

As noted just above, radially symmetric distance/center lenses may attain or aid in the attainment of usable far and near vision by translating. An ideal fit would place the junction of the distance and near powers at the bottom of the pupil in distance gaze. The lens should translate so that the portion of the lens which contains the add covers the pupil when viewing at near. Lens movement includes superotemporal translation (for both asymmetric and symmetric distance/center lenses) and rotation (important only for asymmetric lenses). The requirement for translation in response to eye movements is a condition best met by rigid contact lenses and not by soft lenses. In most cases the amount of translation is not enough (even for rigid lenses and certainly not for soft lenses) to entirely cover the pupil with the appropriate aperture for each fixation. However, translation may augment so-called simultaneous vision with these lenses.

33.5.6 RADIALLY ASYMMETRIC BIFOCALS AND ALTERNATING VISION

As with concentric bifocal contact lenses, segments of radially asymmetric designs can be fused in PMMA but are most likely one-piece in permeable materials because of current inability to economically fuse available rigid or flexible (soft) oxygen-permeable contact lens materials. These lenses are more difficult to manufacture than most concentric designs and are, therefore, more costly. Radially asymmetric contact lens bifocals can be produced in front-surface or back-surface forms (Fig. 33.24). As with any front-surface one-piece design, it is difficult to manufacture a minus carrier to be used for control of vertical lens position on the eye. However, back-surface one-piece segments are rarely prescribed because the asymmetric back surface does not allow for an excellent lens/cornea fitting relationship. In comparison to a front-surface one-piece lens, poor fitting of a back-surface lens is exacerbated by the pronounced junction between distance and near zones that is required to achieve the necessary bifocal add when the back surface is immersed in tear fluid on the eye.

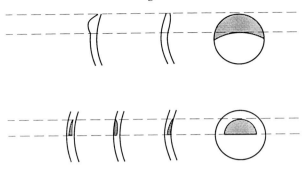

Figure 33.24 Constructs of radially asymmetric, segmented bifocals. Top: fused back-surface, internally segmented, and front-surface lenses. Bottom: one-piece back-surface and front-surface designs.

Surface compatibility

Tear fluid and ocular tissues must be biocompatible with both of the plastic materials used to make a fused bifocal lens. Occasionally, a patient fitted with a normal front-surface fused contact lens may have a tear fluid incompatibility with the segment material, resulting in reduced comfort and increased level of coating or deposition on the segment surface. Of special note is the internal segment fused PMMA contact lens shown in Figure 33.24. This lens design prohibits higher-index plastic used for the segment from contacting the cornea, lids, or tear film of the patient, thereby eliminating exposure of the segment material to the ocular environment. Rigid fused segment bifocals allow placement of a minus carrier on the front surface for vertical positioning of lenses by the superior eyelid and provide an uninterrupted, smooth back surface for optimum fitting on the cornea. Because asymmetric bifocal lenses must maintain stable axis orientations on the eye, a front-surface cylinder may be incorporated into the contact lens prescription.

Now only available in PMMA, fused segment bifocal contact lenses would be welcome additions to the practitioner's bifocal repertoire if they were available in oxygen-permeable rigid materials. Paragon Optical (Mesa, Arizona, USA) has manufactured a fused rigid asymmetric bifocal which shows much promise for the future. The lens is made of an oxygen-impermeable flat-top segment which has been internally fused within a distance carrier of highly oxygen-permeable material. However, this promising lens in only now in the clinical investigatory phase.

Corneal and eyelid physiology

Addition of a superior slab-off prism thins a lens, therefore, corneal physiology in the critical area of the superior cornea is comparatively enhanced. Prism ballast, on the other hand, makes a lens much thicker throughout its vertical dimension, culminating in a very thick inferior aspect. Inadequate corneal oxygenation and mechanical irritation of the inferior limbal area and lower eyelid are two results of soft prism-ballasted bifocal lens wear, with hypoxia

most pronounced at the inferior limbus. Inferior corneal vascularization has been known to occur with soft prism-ballasted lenses especially in extended wear (Westin *et al.*, 1989). It is best, therefore, to limit the daily wearing time of soft prism-ballast lens wearers and to dissuade them from becoming extended wearers of these lenses. Several asymmetric soft bifocal lens designs are shown in Figure 33.25.

Greater corneal swelling has also been shown to occur behind the thicker portions of rigid ballasted lenses as compared to their thinner portions. Although adverse signs are not as great as found with soft lenses, presumably because hypoxia and tear stagnation are not located at the limbal region of the cornea, it appears also advisable that excess thickness be avoided as much as possible. This is especially true for lenses made from oxygen-permeable materials in which thickness directly influences oxygen transmission. Even when manufactured as thin as possible, these lenses require greater thick-

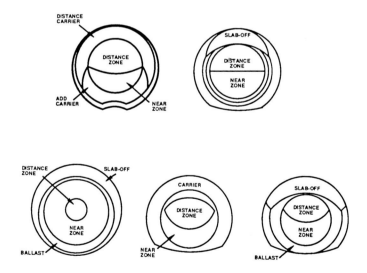

Figure 33.25 Diagrams of several radially asymmetric soft hydrogel bifocal contact lenses, all using various shapes and sizes of optical zones, including several methods for orientation on the eye (modified from Robboy, 1985).

ness, thus, oxygen transmissibility and lens movement on the blink are reduced. As a result, tear exchange is also limited. Corneal physiology suffers and wearing time must be limited to daily wear, or less if the eye is particularly intolerant. The latter adds another argument against the truncation of minus ballasted lenses in which the removal of the thickest part of the base often necessitates increasing the overall amount of prism, thereby increasing the overall thickness of the lens.

Radially asymmetric segmented bifocals are on occasion relatively uncomfortable due to prism thickness and interaction of the thick bottom edges with inferior eyelids, especially when truncated. On the positive side, the distance portion of radially asymmetric segmented bifocals is larger than equivalent symmetric bifocal contact lenses. Therefore, lens lag during various gaze positions and pupil size variations have lesser impact on patient vision (excepting the diffractive bifocal). For the present and future, these translating lenses appear more promising for realistically correcting presbyopia, for when they are fitting appropriately, the patient receives honest-to-goodness alternating vision of high optical quality.

A major disadvantage of radially asymmetric bifocals lies in the fact that they must be made in one-piece, front surface designs in order to optimally fit the cornea and be produced in an oxygen-permeable material. The 'slab off-type' process by which the one-piece reading segment is added, tends to remove most of the prism ballast from the bottom of the lens. To compensate for this, it becomes necessary to introduce a greater amount of prism in the initial single vision blank, which results in much added thickness in the central area of the lens. Since the bottom of the lens is thinned in a one-piece construction, the center of gravity of the lens is left quite high and contributes to the potential for lens rotation on the eye. The fact that the extra thickness works in contradic-

tion to the desired oxygen transmission of the material has already been discussed.

A trifocal form of an asymmetric lens is also available from Fused Kontacts (Chicago, Illinois, USA). Since its need applies essentially to the upper range of add requirements, and the individuals who require such adds also exhibit the smallest pupils, the amount of required translation from one power to another is lessened. This might assist in the fitting, however, the design obviously multiplies the complications associated with the translation of simpler bifocal lenses.

Segment height and position

Near segments of translating bifocals should be placed at the bottom of the pupil in distance gaze and should translate to cover the entire pupil in downgaze when reading (Fig. 33.26). However, near segments of translating contact lenses can cover the inferior 10% to 20% of the pupillary area under normal illumination in straight-ahead gaze if translation is not sufficient in downgaze. The practitioner controls pupil coverage by prescribing the appropriate segment height, which is the distance from the bottom edge of the bifocal lens to the midpoint of the top of the segment (Fig. 33.27). Fitting the segment into the pupil will sometimes disrupt vision of some patients especially if the pupil dilates under dim illumination, so that the segment may need to be lower.

Ideally, translating bifocal lenses should rapidly regain segment position below or toward the bottom of the pupil after the blink. If this is not the case or occurs too slowly, the bifocal height may need to be lowered so that the segment does not intrude as far into the pupil during the blink. Thinning of the apical edge may also be required to reduce the lifting effect of the upper lid via the 'watermelon seed effect'. If the segment does not translate enough or if the pupil is too large, however, the fitting might then

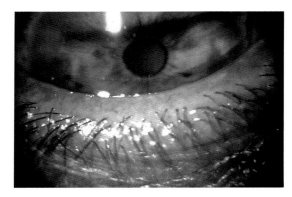

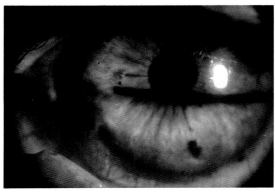

Figure 33.26 The top of a flat-top segment on a soft bifocal contact lens has been marked so that segment position can be seen at the bottom of the pupil in straight-ahead gaze (top) and covering the pupil in the reading position (bottom). This is an ideal case. Oh, what joy there would be if soft lens bifocals translated this much on a significant percentage of presbyopic eyes! (photos courtesy Dr David Westerhout).

introduce more elements of simultaneous vision than would normally be sought and might compromise the vision at either working distance or both.

Image jump and monocentric bifocals

A possible irritation to patients is the small amount of prismatic 'image jump' that occurs when translating from distance to near vision and vice versa. If the optical center of the segment is not at the top of the segment,

image jump will be present and may also increase patient symptoms related to segment coverage of the pupil. Fortunately, radially asymmetric segmented bifocals are available in monocentric one-piece[P13] and fused[P14] designs which eliminate vertical image jump during translation. The distance and segment optical centers of monocentric lenses are at the segment line. These so-called 'No-Jump' designs allow segments to be fitted well into the pupil, perhaps even as much as 25% of the pupil, without adversely affecting distance vision but reducing the amount of translation necessary to cover the pupil during reading. Monocentric segmented bifocal lenses also reduce the visual impact of vertical segment translation during the blink.

Lower lid position

The lower lid acts as a buttress below which the thick edge of a prism-ballasted rigid lens should not travel. Enough space must be allowed between the margin of the lower lid and the pupil so that the segment is not pushed up into the pupillary area in straight-ahead gaze. When fitting rigid (intralimbal) bifocal lenses, this generally means that the lower lid margin should not be more than 1 mm above the inferior limbus. A lower lid margin would be in perfect position if it were at the limbus, while a margin 2 mm or more above the limbus might force the practitioner to consider other bifocal options. If the lower lid lies beneath the limbus, it is assumed that the lower limbal margin of the cornea itself will act as a stop for a rigid lens. Despite proper positioning, an eyelid that is flaccid may permit even a prism-ballasted lens to slip underneath it.

When fitting soft prism-ballasted lenses, slippage below the lower lid margin may be permitted in cases where the margin is above the limbus. The lid margin may approach 1 or 2 mm below the limbus and yet the larger soft lens may still permit adequate segment positioning.

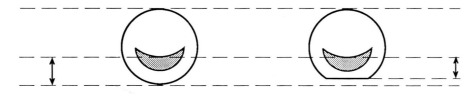

Figure 33.27 Segment height, indicated here by lengths of the arrows, is the distance from the bottom of an untruncated lens to the midpoint of the top of the segment. On a truncated lens, the segment height is measured from the truncated edge.

It is traditionally assumed that a rigid lens fitted interpalpebrally will require the support of the lower lid in order to translate over the pupil for near vision. In this assumption the margin of the lower eyelid should not fall below the limbus and the extent to which it does fall below the limbus should decrease the prospects for successful rigid translating bifocal lens wear. Margins farther than 1 mm below the limbus could require a different bifocal design. It is best to err on the side of having a segment height that is too high when fitting rigid segmented bifocals. A truncation may always be added at the office should the segment height require lowering, however, raising a segment that is too low is not possible. This luxury is not practical for soft lenses which can not be adequately modified in the practitioner's office.

Fitting and evaluation of rigid asymmetric lenses

The authors recommend that the practitioner takes the option of first fitting a patient with single-vision rigid prism-ballasted lenses to determine acceptance of wear and proper physiologic agreement. This also reduces the potential financial gamble. Patients so fitted initially can also be supplied with spectacles to be worn over the contact lenses for close work until a determination has been made. Another result of such a procedure is that many patients will continue to wear single-vision lenses even if a bifocal cannot be found to suit their visual purposes. If a proper and comfortable physiologic fit is achieved, the problem then becomes one of determining whether translation as desired can be attained.

Due to the patient's previous adaptation to rigid lenses, lid tension and reflex tearing, both of which may affect positioning and translation, are at an attenuated and consistent point. As the patient is already wearing lenses with his own distance correction, the add power can be immediately determined by the simple use of trial lenses. Diagnostic bifocal lenses with parameters matching those of the ballasted single-vision lenses can then be tried to test the desired translation. With bifocal diagnostic lenses on, the patient is requested to report the quality of vision in alternate fixations up and back from a distant to a nearpoint chart. The translation of a lens, as a whole, may depend upon the overall diameter of the lens. The lowest position of the lens will likely be either the lower limbus or the lower lid margin. Far from an inexhaustible number of notable problems, several aspects of the fitting of rigid asymmetric bifocals and trouble-shooting tips, are related in the following paragraphs.

1. Problem: Vision is not clear at the distance fixation. The lens rides so that the segment intercepts too much of the pupil. If the lens does not drop far enough on the cornea to enable the segment to clear most of the pupil in the

distance position, and there is room beneath it on the cornea, it may become necessary to attempt to place the lens in the lower position, by: (1) increasing the apical angle by 'CNing' the upper edge, a technique mentioned earlier in this chapter; (2) a new lens can be ordered with a lower segment height; (3) if the upper lid is holding the lens high on the cornea, it may be possible to lessen lid grasp of the lens by reducing the overall diameter of the lens so that less of it fits under the upper lid. This is more likely to prevail if a larger prismatic component is incorporated into the contact lens, thus increasing the apical angle of the front surface. If the upper lid grasp is very tight, however, reducing the size may paradoxically result in raising the lens even more; (4) if the lower lid is too high or otherwise impeding the drop of a truncated lens, applying a slab-off edge to the lower edge of the lens may assist it in slipping under the lid; (5) if the lens is not truncated, it may also be slabbed-off. In some instances, addition of a truncation may also drop the segment lower, though for a minus lens, care should be taken that this does not reduce the ballast too greatly.

2. If vision clears rapidly at each point upon alternation of vision, the translation and segment height are apparently suitable. But problem: If vision is clear at far, then clear at near, but takes too much time to clear when alternating to distance vision, the add is not dropping away quickly enough. The practitioner has several options from which to choose: (1) the segment may be too high and a lower segment height may be tried; (2) a flatter fit may be tried with the lowered segment position; (3) the upper lid may be holding on to the apical edge too much. One technique which has worked effectively for many years in these instances is to CN (polish the front surface to thin the edge) over the entire apical margin. This will reduce the 'minus carrier' effect of minus lenses and cause the upper lid to release its hold on the lens or increase the 'watermelon seed' effect of plus lenses; (4) the prism may be increased to provide both heavier ballast and to present a flatter apical angle to the upper lid at the apical edge.

3. Problem: Vision is clear at far, but not readily attained at near. In this case, the practitioner might: (1) raise the segment height: (2) increase the 'minus carrier' effect of the apical edge by ordering a new lens with a more pronounced minus peripheral flange. Introduction of or increasing the minus carrier is particularly effective with lenses having plus distance corrections; (3) flatten the base curve/cornea relationship; (4) increase the overall diameter to place more of the apical lens area under the upper lid so as to increase lid control over vertical centration. It should be remembered that the actual translation consists of the eye moving downward more than the lens does, not by the lens moving up.

4. Ideally, translating lenses should rapidly regain segment position below the pupil after the blink (Robboy, 1985; Ames *et al.*, 1989). But problem: Vision is unstable when the eyes are redirected at distance and/or particularly after a blink. In this instance: (1) the 'minus carrier' effect of the lid in the blink needs to be reduced by CNing the apical edge, or a new lens may be ordered with less minus apical edge (reduce the minus carrier); (2) increasing the prism ballast may be tried, but this may affect translation at near; (3) a steeper fit may help, or a steeper fit with more prism.

5. Problem: Vision is unstable at near. Here: (1) an increase in 'minus carrier' may help, but care must be taken not to

interfere with distance vision stability. If you order another lens and find that you have increased the minus carrier by too much, the carrier can be trimmed down by CNing; (2) changing the fit by either steepening or flattening will change the translation. Trial lenses with changes in base curve in either direction (flatter and steeper) should be tried; (3) if near vision initially holds fairly well but then is gradually lost as the lens slowly drops, blinking firmly a few times will often restore the position of the segment.

6. Problem: The segment rides at an angle (lens is rotated). As explained earlier, this is most often due to the lifting by the upper lid of a portion of the lens adjoining the nasal side of the apex of the lens. In these instances: (1) an attempt can be made to add weight to the base by increasing the prism, although the disadvantages of extra lens thickness have been mentioned. Caution should be used about increasing the amount of prism. Corneal metabolism may always be disturbed by too much mass; (2) an effective solution used over many years is to reduce the 'minus carrier' lift of the upper lid upon only that portion of the lens involved. In other words, the portion to the side of the apex which is being lifted by the lid is CNed. For example, if the segment is rotated nasally, the nasal side of the apex has been lifted more forcibly by the upper lid, thus rotating the lens. CNing is applied only to the nasal side of the apex. Since a small amount of CNing is performed at a time, the process is repeated and the lens is successively observed in the eye, until a satisfactory rotational position of the segment is achieved.

The same basic technique as has been outlined above, used for years by one of the authors (IMB), may be applied by marking a horizontal line at the desired segment height and filling in the area below this line on the lower front surface of the patient's single-vision prism-ballasted lenses with a red-ink waterproof felt-tipped marking pen. In essence, the practitioner creates an opaque 'executive bifocal segment' on the lens for diagnostic purposes. The ink, when dried, should wet with regular wetting solution. As vision alternates between clear distance vision and a red film obscures the nearpoint, the patient and practitioner can determine the appropriate balance between distance and near vision. The height of the film can be readily changed with this method, until the proper segment height for the patient and with the particular lens design has been achieved. The technique has the advantage of being usable when trial bifocal lenses of the desired parameters are not available, thus saving the expense and delay of ordering a diagnostic bifocal for trial.

33.5.7 TRANSLATION WITH ATYPICAL SOFT LENS BIFOCALS

Many bifocal contact lens designs have come and gone over the last 40 years or so. As mentioned previously, soft lenses are limited in the prospect of achieving 'alternating vision', necessary for producing satisfactory optical results. The authors have selected three atypical bifocals which represent unique attempts to solve the riddle of soft lens translating bifocals.

The first atypical lens is the 'Bayshore bifocal' shown on an eye in Figure 33.28.[P15] This was a radially asymmetric segmented soft lens design which had been made 'triangular' by truncation of superior portions of soft lens material outside of the optic zones of the lens. The idea was to reduce the amount of resistance to upward translation in downgaze through limiting contact of the soft lens with the superior limbus and palpebral conjunctiva. Although reports indicated that alternation did take place, others indicated that drying and reduced wetting of the exposed cornea next to the contact lens resulted in sealing the lens tightly to the corneal surface which eliminated any advantage of translation. Also, the lens required specific material and was exceedingly difficult to manufacture.

Another unique bifocal attempt was the 'laterally translating' soft bifocal lens[P16] depicted in Figure 33.29. The lens consisted of two circular optical zones which were overlapped emphasizing the smaller zone for distance vision and placing the larger zone on the temporal bulbar conjunctiva. In extreme temporal gaze, the lens was to move sufficiently nasally so as to bring the larger near addition over the pupil after which the eye could be brought to fixate a near target. It was hoped that extreme nasal gaze would re-establish the distance zone back before the pupil for distance vision. Translation of this bifocal did not occur as expected.

An interesting idea, horizontal translation was also the object of another patented bifocal design.[P17] In this design, superior and inferior slab-offs were used to rotationally orient a circular lens on the eye. These one-piece lenses were equally divided into left and right halves by a vertical junction having separate distance and near powers, and could be worn with the near powers situated

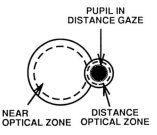
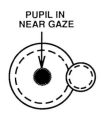

Figure 33.29 Diagram of a 'laterally translating' bifocal[P16]. The patient was to be required to avert gaze horizontally in order to push the near optical zone onto the center of the cornea. Likewise, gaze aversion in the opposite direction might recenter the distance zone before the pupil.

over the nasal halves of the pupils in distance gaze. When converging for near vision, the reader can envision two lenses each translating temporally so that the near optical zones might cover most of the pupils and so augment simultaneous vision at near by translation. Distance vision, on the other hand, would not be augmented.

33.5.8 WAFER CONTACT LENSES

A wafer is a thin crescent, semi-annular, or flat-top lens that can be worn on the front surface of a single-vision contact lens (Taylor, 1962). The wafer is of one refractive power (the presbyopic add) and is by itself not a bifocal, but in combination with a single-vision distance lens is sometimes called a 'piggy-back bifocal'. Center thicknesses of wafers are approximately 0.10 mm, depending on refractive power and diameter. The bottom of a wafer should match the curve of the upper margin of the inferior eyelid and the back curve of the wafer should match the front curve of the single-vision contact lens upon which it rests. A tear film forms by capillary action between the two surfaces and the resultant mucinaceous layer acts as a sort of 'cement' which limits sliding of the wafer across the surface of the single-vision contact lens. In this manner, wafers on

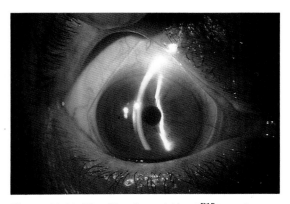

Figure 33.28 The 'Bayshore bifocal[P15]' on the eye of a notable presbyope.

the eye are similar to cemented-segment spectacle lenses, except that the wafer can be moved around on the contact lens surface with forceful manipulation by the practitioner or patient. Prism ballast can be added to a wafer in order to help locate the wafer at the inferior portion of the single-vision distance contact lens.

Theoretically, wafers have several potential advantages. They can be used for diagnostic purposes to cost-effectively ascertain the type of segment, add power, and adaptive ability for patients considering translating bifocals. Wafers can be easily replaced as a patient's add power increases through the years. A patient can be sent home with wafers to assess vision with 'bifocal' contact lenses, before a true bifocal translating lens is ordered. For patients wearing scleral contact lenses, wafers offer one of the few alternatives for presbyopic contact lens correction. In practice, once on the lens, the wafer becomes another asymmetrical design.

It is difficult to position a wafer in the correct inferior position of a distance contact lens on the eye by sliding it around, therefore patients are usually instructed to insert a distance rigid contact lens and wafer together. When used in conjunction with soft lenses or scleral lenses, however, wafers may be inserted after the distance prescription is already on the eye. Wafer lenses have been worn directly on the cornea as presbyopic correction by emmetropes (Taylor, 1965). These lenses are larger than wafers intended to rest on a contact lens surface, but nevertheless tend to slide around and rotate on the cornea due to action of the eyelids especially during blinking.

Wafer lenses are uncomfortable in the eye. Handling of such small and delicate lenses is a problem for patients and practitioners, and manufacture of such minute lenses is exceedingly fine. Extra care and attention to edges of wafers is necessary because they are thin and are easily broken. Because of these drawbacks, wafers are rarely prescribed for presbyopic contact lens correction.

33.5.9 LIQUID CRYSTAL LENSES

A liquid crystal is an optically anisotropic fluid which exhibits birefringence typical of a uniaxial crystal yet also exhibits the fluid properties of an isotropic liquid, hence the term 'liquid crystal'. Liquid crystal materials are made of large, elongated, polar molecules that align with their long axes predominantly oriented in one direction. The direction of alignment may be influenced by physical surroundings of the liquid or by electric fields. Thus, the molecules can be packaged within a display, or as we will see later, a lens, to orient in one direction. This orientation is usually brought about by etched inner surfaces of transparent plates containing a layer of liquid crystal material, the molecules of which align with furrows in the plates caused by etching. An externally applied electric field can swing these polar molecules into other directions by overcoming the normal tendency of the molecules to align with the direction of etching. Because molecules within a liquid crystal material are oriented in one direction, the material exhibits optical anisotropy analogous to that which occurs in stromal lamellae of the cornea.

The attributes of liquid crystals that may be important for use in bifocal contact lenses are: (1) birefringence resulting in ordinary and extraordinary rays of light polarized at right angles to each other; and (2) ability to change orientation of the planes of oscillation of these polarized rays by application of an electric field to the liquid crystal material. The difference of refractive index between birefringent rays of light can be as much as 0.2 or 0.3, which is a large amount relative to birefringence of the cornea (0.0014). A lens made of a birefringent material (liquid crystal or birefringent plastic) would, therefore, have two focal points. Correct design of lens curvatures could result in the appropriate refractive powers for a simultaneous vision bifocal (Hathaway, 1986).

If a polarizer were to be added with its axis

of polarization parallel to the orientation of liquid crystal molecules in a liquid crystal lens ('LC lens'), application of an electric field could determine which polarized rays of light (ordinary or extraordinary rays) were transmitted through the system. Refractive power of the system could be altered from that determined by one refractive index to a power determined by the other. However, only that light oriented to pass through the polarizer would be transmitted. Illumination of the retinal image when wearing such lens systems would be reduced, but two refractive powers would be possible, switchable from one to the other. These lenses could possibly provide alternating vision for patients, but would not be required to translate in order to do so. Lenses of small diameter like this have been constructed to show a possible feasibility of LC lenses for the contact lens field (Hathaway, 1986).

A lens of birefringent material could be sandwiched with an LC lens such that their axes of polarization were parallel (or perpendicular). Polarization of the LC component could be switchable with application of an electric field to be perpendicular (or parallel). If powers of the two components were adjusted carefully, in one orientation the LC lens could counteract the birefringence of the other component (for, say, distance vision), yet strengthen birefringence in the opposite orientation (for near vision).

While many possibilities for LC lenses exist in the ophthalmic field, their optical performance, to date, is limited for several reasons: low resolution, boundary effects of elements containing liquid crystal molecules, reduced effective liquid crystal layer thickness, and inability to apply an electric field evenly across the surface of an LC lens. LC lenses have even been constructed with a Fresnel lens as the substrate upon which the liquid crystal layer lies. While an interesting proposition at this moment, LC lenses need much research and development before they can be ready for the ophthalmic arena (Hathaway, 1987).

33.6 CONCLUSION

From the above it can be seen that few bifocal contact lenses operate adequately and consistently to provide feasible vision by providing purely 'simultaneous' or purely 'alternating' visual effects. It should be pointed out that modified monovision is not always avoided even when bifocal contact lenses are successfully worn. Neither the patient nor the examiner may realize that equal vision at distance and at near for both of the eyes may not be provided through bifocal contact lenses at all times. Differences between the eyes in terms of ocular and palpebral anatomical features, normal physiological anisocoria, wetting or dryness of the tears, and variability in stated lens parameters may tend to vary the extent of translation of the lens in one eye from that in the other or the areas of field of specific segments before the pupils. Vision may be achieved or enhanced unwittingly by only one eye at distance or near even when modified monovision is not an intended mode of correction.

The human binocular visual system operates on the principle of 'alternating vision'. Under optimal binocular conditions, our eyes alter their lines of sight in order to consecutively fixate targets in different directions and at varying distances. Optically, our crystalline lenses are made to alternately focus objects at those distances and our neural systems pay attention to targets at which our eyes are both simultaneously directed and focused. The mode of presbyopic contact lens correction which would most closely simulate that ordinarily obtained would provide as perfect a system of 'alternating vision' as it is possible to attain. The best presbyopic correction would minimize the amount of 'neurological alternation' that must take place to make the optical correction acceptable. However, vision with most current types of bifocal contact lenses is likely to be achieved by variations between all three optical extremes of alternating vision, simultaneous vision, and monovision, according to design, fit, and ocular parameters (Figure 33.30). In other words, any bifocal contact lenses prescription presents a unique combination of optical and neurological alternation for mastery by each patient in order to be successful.

Apparently totally ignored is the fact that the presbyopic patient is not presenting a young eye which just happens to be failing in accommodative ability. The first section of this chapter attempted to indicate that the entire visual operation of the aging eye is involved. Transmission of the media is lessened, retinal sensitivity is diminished, contrast sensitivity is greatly reduced, and mesopic vision is severely affected. Present-day bifocal systems, which tend to present relatively degraded retinal images through imperfect media to already handicapped photoreceptors, may further destabilize an already precarious situation. Unavoidable

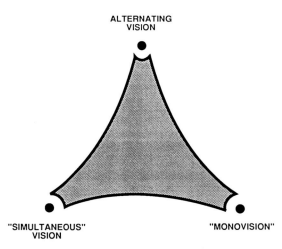

ALTERNATING
VISION

"SIMULTANEOUS"
VISION

"MONOVISION"

Figure 33.30 Most bifocal contact lens prescriptions result in an optical mixture of 'simultaneous vision', 'monovision', and alternating vision. Thus, they provide optical results that lie somewhere in the shaded triangular area depicted here. To the extent that they are successful, simultaneous vision lenses and monovision operate by visual alternation in one form or another.

exigencies of the aging eye demand that augmented rather than diminished images be presented for the correction of presbyopia. Younger presbyopes may initially opt for bifocal contact lens correction, but as the progressive visual effects of aging continue to worsen, most will eventually return to spectacles in order to obtain the optimum optical correction.

A summary of the experiences of practitioners who have attempted to deal with presbyopia via contact lenses indicates that the major methodology used by the majority is monovision in one form or another. The impediment to utilizing bifocal contact lenses arises from several sources. First, patients and professionals have become accustomed to the immediate comfort provided by soft lenses and find them far more preferable as the agent for correction. Most of the contact lenses manufactured in soft lens form provide too little variation in fitting choices, too little option for distinctions in parameters which might make significant differences in individual cases, no practical system of modification, and almost no prognostic certainty to encourage the practitioner to risk his own reputation and the patient's investment. Criteria which might help predict acceptance, guide selection, and reassure practitioner confidence have not been adequately determined.

Secondly, soft lenses are deliberately designed to be fitted and are most comfortable with a relative minimum of movement on the eye. Sufficient translation of lenses on the cornea necessary for 'alternating vision' can be provided only by rigid lenses for most eyes, which unfortunately do not grant immediate comfort. This leaves 'monovision' and 'simultaneous vision' as the only viable presbyopic alternatives, provided, of course, that the patient can learn to 'neurologically alternate' between images.

'Neurological alternation' is most difficult, perhaps even impossible, when images of equal intensity simultaneously overlap on identical monocular retinal fields in the same eye. Most 'simultaneous vision' lenses apparently succeed in modest numbers when pupil dependency and small lens translations are in favor of 'optical alternation', or when used in modified monovision so that a limited 'neurological alternation' can occur, and especially when patients are willing and able to interpret, and/or tolerate, blur. Even diffractive simultaneous vision lenses, which are relatively independent of pupil changes and so can not be yet said to operate by translation, present an imagery which is generally optically suspect. Most practitioners who prefer and chiefly confine themselves to prescription of soft lenses, attain more certain patient satisfaction via 'monovision' than with 'simultaneous vision' or 'translating' soft bifocals. One reason for this is that, in the absence of adequate soft lens translation, neurological alternation between images is better achieved when the images are separately presented to the two eyes. In the presence of alternation, blur interpretation and/or tolerance are not required.

Consequently, only practitioners who have experience or skill in handling initial discomfort challenge themselves to prescribe rigid bifocal designs. Those practitioners who report the greatest success with bifocal contact lenses, indicate that the most predictable modalities available, upon which prognostic indications can genuinely be made, lie within the realm of 'alternating vision' rigid bifocals, with asymmetric designs predominating. 'Success', here, is defined as providing optically excellent distance and near imagery to the eyes and thereby achieving patient satisfaction, but not by inducing the patient to accept optical default in order to achieve comfortable soft lens wear. This may be because many of the practitioners who readily turn to use of rigid lenses are frequently those who dealt with original rigid lenses in the pre-soft lens era and successfully fitted bifocal lenses in the PMMA material. They have had great experience with the fitting of the rigid lens and with the techniques which involve evaluation of and possible changes in lens size, optic zone diameter, base curve fit, width and radius of peripheral curves and a certain amount of hands-on lens modifications performed in the office. Under these situations, the diagnostic and prognostic potentials are greatly enhanced. The optics of 'alternating vision' and rigid lenses are also far more creditable.

Apparently, the potential for widely extending the use of bifocal contact lenses among the great body of practitioners lies in achieving either sufficient translation to attain the required 'alternating vision' in a soft bifocal lens design that maintains soft lens comfort, in achieving initial comfort with a rigid bifocal lens that maintains the level of translation now available, or by matching comfort and translation with some combination of the two materials or their traits. Of course, adequate corneal, eyelid, and tear film physiology must also result from any new contact lens material or design, in order to be successful.

Optically alternating vision could ultimately be achieved other than by translation. In this chapter we have seen that lenses the size of contact lenses can be produced which switch from one refractive power to another. These lenses are not yet suitable in many ways for ophthalmic correction and certainly would not yet be compatible with the ocular and surrounding tissues. Other types of lenses have been proposed which promise to offer the ability to alter refractive power. Future presbyopic corrections may ultimately be found in adaptation of emerging technologies to the contact lens field. In the distant future, pharmacological, surgical, and other optical technologies may so adequately compensate for presbyopia that the bifocal contact lens as we know it today could become obsolete. On the other hand, the search for an immediately comfortable and predictable alternating form of bifocal contact lens may be successful and provide the optimum in presbyopic correction for some time to come.

REFERENCES

Alpern, M. (1949) Accommodation and convergence with contact lenses. *Am. J. Optom.*, **26** (9), 379–87.

Ames, K.S. *et al.* (1989) Factors influencing vision with rigid gas permeable alternating bifocals. *Optom. Vis. Sci.*, **66** (2), 92–7.

Back, A.P., Holden, B.A. and Hine, N.A. (1989) Correction of presbyopia with contact lenses: Comparative success rates with three systems. *Optom. Vis. Sci.*, **66** (8), 518–25.

Balazs, E. and Denlinger, J.L. (1982) Aging changes in the vitreous. In *Aging and Human Visual Function* (eds. R. Sekular, D. Kline and K. Dismukes). Alan R. Liss, New York.

Beier, C.G. (1977) A review of the literature pertaining to monovision contact lens fitting of presbyopic patients. *Int. Contact Lens Clin.*, **4** (2), 49–56.

Benjamin, W.J. (1986) The closed-lid tear pump during rigid extended wear. *Int. Eyecare*, **22**(4), 224–6.

Benjamin, W.J. (1987) 'Full aperture' contact lenses: A 'sneak' preview. *Int. Contact Lens Clin.*, **14** (11), 454–5.

Benjamin, W.J. (1990) Wet cells, back-surface bifocals, and the 'lacrimal lens theory'. *Int. Contact Lens Clin.*, **17** (5&6), 157–8.

Benjamin, W.J. and Rasmussen, M.A. (1985) The closed-lid tear pump: oxygenation? *Int. Eyecare*, **1**(3), 251–7.

Benjamin, W.J. and Simons, M.H. (1984) Extended wear of oxygen-permeable rigid contact lenses in aphakia. *Int. Contact Lens Clin.*, **11**(9), 547–61; Extended wear of rigid lenses in aphakia. A preliminary report. *Int. Contact Lens Clin.*, **11** (1), 44–57.

Bennett, A.G. (1968/69) Aspherical contact lens surfaces, Parts I, II, and III. *The Ophthalmic Optician*, **8** (20), 1037–40; **8** (23), 1297–311; **9** (5), 222–30.

Bier, N. (1981) Albinism. *Int. Contact Lens Clin.*, **8**(5), 10–15.

Blackwell, O.M. and Blackwell, H.R. (1971) Visual performance data for 156 normal observers of various ages. *J. Illumin. Eng. Soc.*, **1**, 3–13.

Borish, I.M. (1962) The ICLing lens. Bulletin #7, Indiana Contact Lens Company, Marion IN; Contact Lens Centering. *Pennsylvania Optometrist*, **22** (5), 9–12.

Borish, I.M. (1986) Presbyopia. In *Rigid Gas-Permeable Contact Lenses* (eds. E.S. Bennett and R.M. Grohe), Professional Press/Fairchild Publications, New York, pp. 381–407.

Borish, I.M. (1988) Pupil dependency of bifocal contact lenses. *Am. J. Optom. Physiol. Optics*, **65**(5), 417–23.

Borish, I.M. and Perrigin, D. (1987) Relative movement of lower lid and line of sight from distant to near fixation. *Am. J. Optom. Physiol. Optics*, **64** (12), 881–7.

Borish, I.M. and Perrigin, D.M. (1985) Observations of bifocal contact lenses. *Int. Eyecare*, **1** (3), 241–8.

Bressler, N.M., Bressler, S.B. and Fine, S.L. (1988) Age-related macular degeneration. *Surv. Ophthalmol.*, **32** (6), 375–413.

Campbell, C.E. (1984) Converting wet cell measured soft lens power to vertex power in air. *Int. Contact Lens Clin.*, **11** (3), 168–71.

Carlson, K.H. *et al.* (1988) Variations in human corneal endothelial cell morphology and permeability to fluorescein with age. *Exp. Eye Res.*, **47**(1), 27–41.

Charman, W.N. (1982) Unwanted astigmatism in lenses with a concentric variation in sagittal power. *Am. J. Optom. Physiol. Optics*, **59** (12), 997–1001.

Charman, W.N. and Walsh, G. (1988) Retinal images with centered, aspheric varifocal contact lenses. *Int. Contact Lens Clin.*, **15** (3), 87–93.

Cohen, A.L., (1989) Bifocal contact lens optics. *Contact Lens Spectrum* **4** (6), 43–52.

Collins, M.J. *et al.* (1989) Peripheral visual acuity with monovision and other contact lens corrections for presbyopia. *Optom. Vis. Sci.*, **66** (6), 370–4.

Creighton, C.P. (1976) *Contact Lens Fabrication Tables*. Alden Laboratories, Inc., Alden, New York.

Ehlers, C.L. and Kupfer, D.J. (1989) Effects of age on delta and REM sleep parameters. *Electroencephalogr. Clin. Neurophysiol.*, **72**(2), 118–25.

Erickson, P. and Robboy, M. (1985) Performance characteristics of a hydrophilic concentric bifocal contact lens. *Am. J. Optom. Physiol. Optics*, **62**(10), 702–8.

Erickson, P. *et al.* (1988) Optical design considerations for contact lens bifocals. *J. Am. Optom. Assoc.*, **59**(3), 198–202.

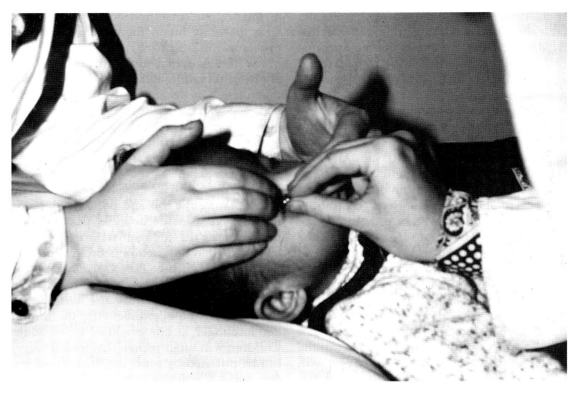

Figure 34.1 A method of soft-lens insertion for a child.

cult on the uncorrected eye, choose a back vertex power on the basis of age and then over-refract; this is much easier than the initial refraction as one is near the end point and the reflex is easier to determine. One wants up to −3.00 dioptres on corrected retinoscopy, to show that the eyes are corrected for within the baby's sphere of interest.

With a high water content soft lens material one's first choice of back optic radius for a baby of 6 weeks of age is 7.00 mm, this increases to 7.20 mm as first choice for a baby of 4 months and 7.30 mm for the 6-month-old. At 1 year the first choice would be 7.60 mm. The criteria are adapted to the individual eyes; for instance the overall size is judged on an assessment of the corneal size. The smallest overall size that is usually fitted to a 6-week-old baby is 12.00 mm, increasing to 13.00 mm with age (Fig. 34.2).

The largest overall size fitted to an aphakic baby is 14.50 mm, and with these larger lenses a bicurve design is needed. When refitting with say a 60% material for daily wear this can be based on the original fitting or the child is refitted as normal.

It is important to have a good stock of lenses for instant fitting and as continual optical correction is essential there should be available a spare set of lenses for each infant at all times. The turnover of lenses tends to be high in the first few months and it can work out at about nine lenses per annum per patient. However, after one year this decreases to less than three lenses per annum (Morris *et al.*, 1979). If there is a particularly large turnover of lenses some infants can be refitted with silicone lenses, these may be more difficult for the infant to displace. The silicone lenses used are usually of around

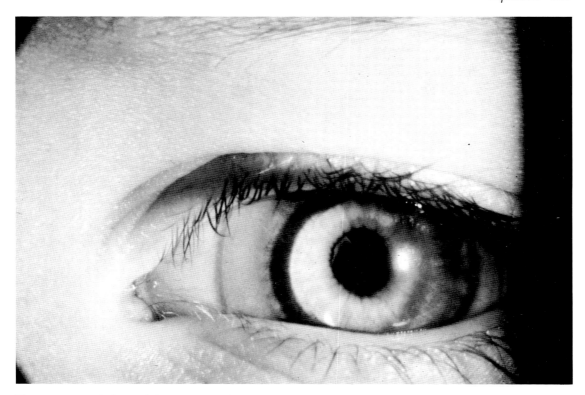

Figure 34.2 Aphakia soft lens on an infant's eye.

11.30 mm in overall size (Wohlk). The steepest back optic radius available is usually around 7.50 mm and this can be used for those patients of 2 years and younger. The 2-to 4-year-olds need a 7.70 mm lens, of 11.70 mm overall size, whilst those older than 4 years usually need a 7.90 mm lens. Danker will also supply aphakic lenses in overall diameter of 10.80 mm. When the lenses are checked the fluorescein minimal apical clearance centrally, minimal bearing in the intermediate zone, peripheral clearance, and moderate edge lift are necessary for a successful fit (Cutler *et al.*, 1985). Silicone lenses do allow an ease of handling compared to a hydrogel lens. The smaller, more rigid silicone lens allows for easier insertion in the small palpebral aperture presented. However, removal due to the greater capillary attraction of the silicone rubber to the eye, can be more difficult until the knack of relieving the suction pressure under the lens with the lids is learnt. The suction effect of silicone rubber can cause red eye problems in some cases.

In the documentation of visual results in a study carried out at Moorfields Eye Hospital the majority, 18%, fell into the 6/36 range of vision. The best vision of those of early onset and little deprivation was 6/12, which is probably adequate to cope with normal education. Even a substantial number of the 6/36 group are coping at a normal school. In the Moorfields study out of 102 patients 69 had a squint; 56 of those were constant and 13 alternating. Patching was carried out in most cases for a few hours a day, but noncompliance was high. Out of 99 patients documented in the same study only 24% did not have nystagmus, 35% had moderate nystagmus which did not reduce with contact lens wear. The major cause of post-offset deprivation in this study was the lenses being out, the majority being lost at some time or other. However, many of the eyes also suffered because of an unattainable retinoscopy reflex due to too small a pupillary gap.

The secondary effects of contact lens wear were also documented. Photophobia was only a problem in 11.65% of those cases documented. Hypoxic ulceration was present in 7.76% of the cases and all had residual effects, i.e. scarring, whilst 9.87% had confirmed infections with 5.59% presumed. It is due to this infection rate that daily wear is suggested as soon as possible or spectacles prescribed. Vascularization was shown to some degree in 25% of cases, this incidence also suggests daily wear is imperative as soon as possible and hard gas permeable lenses may also be indicated as a method of optical correction.

The major cause of abandonment in the study tended to be social problems, continual lens loss from fitting or corneal problems. However, some cases have abandoned after a period of struggle and the child has then come back a few years later and asked him or herself for contact lenses and has been very successful the second time around – motivation is all!

Post-operative and post-corrective problems

Especially in younger children, if the posterior capsule has been left intact as in the aspiration technique, it usually becomes opaque which interferes with refraction and therefore with the prescription of the appropriate contact lens, with the effect that it may cause amblyopia. The contact lens fitter, who frequently sees the patient more often than the surgeon, is very well placed to alert the surgeon to this problem so that appropriate further surgery can be carried out.

Corneal vascularization is frequent with continous wear hydrogel lenses and frequent slit lamp examinations should be undertaken, with the lenses being changed to daily wear, or to high gas permeable hard lenses if necessary. Sometimes contact lens wear has to be abandoned because of vascularization.

Squint occurs frequently and the presence of unilateral fixation, indicating an amblyopic eye, should be noted and the child is preferably managed in conjunction with an orthoptist. Squint surgery may be indicated if the angle is very large which tends to dislodge the lens against the inner canthus, for cosmetic reasons or occasionally in the hope of achieving binocular vision by early surgery.

The ophthalmologist who supervises the child's post-operative management will be keen to learn from the optometrist, the orthoptist and the parents, about the child's vision – if the vision is not up to expected levels, with the child failing to achieve visual milestones, investigations are usually called for into anterior segment, retinal and optic nerve function.

Nystagmus is frequent in congenital cataract and may occur despite optimal management. Whether this is related to amblyopia from early deprivation, or to an associated motor or visual anomaly is not clear. Nystagmus is usually, but not invariably associated with a poor visual prognosis for detailed vision, but is usually compatible with normal vision for navigation. A large amplitide of nystagmus usually correlates with poor acuity.

34.1.3 UNILATERAL APHAKIA

Unilateral cataract is not a very socially significant disease, because it does not affect the child's ability to learn or behave normally, and therefore the justification for treatment of any sort has to be examined carefully. Traumatic cases are usually unilateral, and although they also have a significant effect on the child, it is not all encompassing in the same way as bilateral defects.

The current state of unilateral congenital cataract treatment is still under review due to the generally poor visual prognosis (Burke *et al.*, 1989) but there are increasing numbers of cases in the literature who have good acuities associated with early and vigorous treatment of their aphakia and amblyopia. The fitting of contact lenses is no more difficult than fitting bilateral cases. In unilateral aphakia the absence of accommodation in the aphakic eye results in an optically static eye competing with a dynamic phakic eye. Hence in the congenital cases, although some authors have reported promising results from early detection, surgery, optical correction and occlusion (Beller *et al.*, 1981; Pratt-Johnson & Tillson, 1981; Robb *et al.*, 1987; Birch & Stager, 1988) most would agree that visual results are poor, even with vigorous occlusion therapy, especially if the treatment is started after 6 to 12 weeks of age. The undertaking of occlusion therapy must be carefully monitored to avoid amblyopia in the occluded eye. A contact lens of high power can be used as an occluder in some cases (Ruben & Walker 1967)

34.1.4 TRAUMATIC APHAKIA

Aphakia secondary to trauma may also be treated by soft or rigid contact lenses. Tolerence is, generally speaking, more difficult with these cases so a soft lens is usually the material of first choice if the eye has a reasonably regular surface. In the traumatic cases the later the injury occurs the greater the chance of achieving a reasonable visual result because some vision has already developed, and the effects of the deprivation are less profound. After the injury, the sooner the pupil is cleared and the contact lens fitted following the injury, then the greater the chance of achieving higher levels of acuity and binocular function. The degree of success with contact lens wear in these patients depends on many factors including

the attitude of the child and parent to lens wear. Frequently the patient himself decides that the reward does not justify the effort involved.

34.2 MYOPIA

The correction of high myopia with contact lenses of all types may improve acuity. (Ruben, 1965). However, for the risks to be justifiable, it is essential to demonstrate the superiority of contact lenses over spectacles. Cosmetic indications tend to be important with the parents, however if the child wears spectacles quite happily it is probably best to leave contact lens fitting until a later date, say the teens.

It has been shown that hard contact lenses may have a stabilizing or retarding effect on the progression of myopia (Davis, 1971; Kelly & Butler, 1971; Stone, 1976). Some of these factors may be important in reducing myopia (Davis, 1971):

1. The contact lens has a retaining effect on the curvature or the cornea.
2. Contact lenses do not have the effect of increasing prism or disrupt accommodation–convergence relationships, that may accompany the wearing of spectacles.
3. Contact lenses result in a larger retinal image, as compared with spectacle lenses.
4. Contact lenses seem to exert a gentle massaging effect on the cornea which may have an effect on the corneal metabolism and the curvature.
5. Contact lenses may result in a more natural shift in accommodation–convergence relationship.
6. In progressive myopia, the coats of the eyeball are frequently abnormally soft and distensible. Normally there is no space between eyelid and the cornea; the presence of the contact lens may cause either a pushing back or a holding effect on the stretching.

INTRODUCTION

The term 'abnormal eye' indicates a diseased condition, either active or healed. It can also mean a developmental or congenital anomaly or an eye that has suffered trauma or surgical intervention. The aspect of fitting a contact lens usually requires special consideration. The eye may be abnormal in shape and not able to accept a conventional lens design. It could be that exceptional powers are necessary and outside the normal stocked lens range. But on the other hand the lens may have to be worn on an eye that has pathological tissue and therefore the type of fit, material, and certainly management require special considerations.

In general terms the purpose of the contact lens for this group of conditions is not cosmetic visual. The primary consideration may therefore be to protect the tissues from the lids or environment. In other instances the primary use will be to obtain a vision result. To this end it may be necessary to use supplementary spectacles in addition to the contact lens.

Because the conditions require a contact lens as part of a treatment programme, the motivation on the part of the patient may be at one extreme, antagonistic, because the device may appear unrelated to the disease or, at the other extreme, the patient may become entirely dependent upon the device for useful vision. The motivation in this group of patients often requires special management and is not the same as for the visual cosmetic patient.

It is possible to categorize these patients into a group of indications but the ophthalmologist treating eye disease will often find other examples (see Chapters 35 and 38).

It may appear a paradox that the contact lens is used to treat corneal disease but at the same time it is recognized that the lens can be a cause of disease (Chapters 44 and 45). In some of the eye diseases that the device is used and particularly as a protective the corneal tissue may not be viable and not require oxygen to the same level as required by the normal cornea. For example the soft lens may be used in bullous keratopathy to alleviate pain, and this is the primary function; a visual gain would be a bonus. The corneal epithelium in such an eye could be defunct and separate from the basement membrane due to gross water inhibition of the stroma due to endothelial dysfunction. The function of the lens is then not curative but the alleviation of pain which is important until the final management can be determined. But in all the instances where the corneal epithelium is viable then the considerations regarding hypoxia induced by wear become important and more so if the endothelium is deficient as after graft surgery and aphakia.

Therefore the limitations of lens design and material relative to the possibility of hypoxia occurring must be known and throughout the text this is considered in different contexts (Chapters 3, 22 and 42).

The causes of corneal astigmatism are several (Chapter 35). Most commonly they are from lacerations of the cornea that have healed with surface curvature distortion. Such injuries whilst often accidental could be

Table 35.2 Types of contact lenses used for corneal ectasias (and corrections of irregular astigmatism)

Condition	Lens
Keratoconus – Central cone	Corneal Hard – small size to large depending upon degree of progression – thick spherical soft in early state, toric thick soft, special soft
– Paracentral	Corneal Hard – large size, toric back surface, pseudo-aspherics, to obtain centration
	Scleral large hard (mould to eye fit) when all else fails.
Marginal dystrophy	Corneal hard large size, toric thick Soft.
Keratoglobus	Scleral Hard – mould to eye fit
Melting corneas	Therapeutic soft with local artificial tears and anti-inflammatory drugs
Traumatic ectasia and perforated corneas	Large thick soft to seal cornea
	When cornea healed and if traumatic in origin use hard corneal

loss of vision and that is correctable by contact lenses. Table 35.1 lists the conditions that cause irregular astigmatism and the associated pathology that affects contact lens fitting.

Table 35.2 gives indications of the type of contact lens likely to be used. This chapter will deal in detail with the specific conditions mentioned in Table 35.1 and their management, as outlined in Table 35.3.

Another group of conditions does not have ectatic corneas but does have irregular astigmatism. These are listed in Table 35.4, and will also be covered as to contact lens use.

35.1.1 THE PRIMARY NON-INFLAMMATORY ECTASIAS OF THE CORNEA – KERECTASIAS

Keratoconus

Specialist contact lens practitioners find that this condition affects the majority of patients with an abnormal cornea, and who wear contact lenses, for life. The world contact lens literature contains an overwhelming amount of opinion, some objective but some subjective and of little value to the student of this condition (Fick, 1888; Galt, 1890; Anderson, 1930; Gyorffy 1950, 1951; Ruben 1975, 1979, 1989).

Table 35.3 Irregular astigmatism and no ectasia of cornea

Condition	Type of contact lens
Congenital misplacement of corneal apex	Hard contact lens but of doubtful value
Healed corneal scarring, e.g. wounds, ulceration	Size of contact lens taken will depend upon site and extent of lesion. Hard corneal will give better vision
Surgical sections, e.g. post-cataract and glaucoma operations	Hard corneal of large size even 12 mm
Post-keratoplasty	Depending upon graft size and curvatures from hard corneal to hard scleral
Post-refractive surgery	Large flat back curved corneal
Post-lens implant operation, e.g. tilted implant, anisometropia.	Front toric ballasted hard or soft lens

Table 35.4 Phases in the management with contact lenses of progressive idiopathic keratoconus

Phase	Acuity and motivation	Treatment
Uniocular early	10% loss in one eye	Spectacles if refractive error in other eye
	Pre-puberty one eye	Contact lens pre-puberty to prevent amblyopia or contact lenses in both eyes for cosmesis after puberty
Binocular and early	Up to 20% both eyes loss	Fit contact lenses both eyes
Moderate	Good contact lens acuity, and good tolerance	Continue with contact lens wear and treat hypersensitivity complications
Progression	Good contact lens acuity but poor tolerance poor contact lenses acuity	Consider operation (epikeratoplasty or graft)
Recurrent stromal oedema and hydrops	Severe loss of acuity	Change to soft therapeutic contact lens
		Treat oedema if necessary locally
		Consider operation (penetrating graft)

It must be realized that, as the condition affects young adults and adolescents, who are in great need of normal vision, the motivation for treatment is very high. There is therefore a great deal of frustration in those who fail to obtain sufficient tolerance and anguish from those who overwear or suffer intolerances and complications of wear that make contact lens use impossible. The dependence of the kerataconic individual upon the contact lens must make the practitioner diligent in foreseeing the likely problems that will arise from long-term use of the lens. The practitioner will also see many patients who are already good wearers of lenses fitted by other practitioners. There are many different philosophies as to the correct fit of the keratoconic cornea. Some practitioners assume their methods are correct because the patient achieves good tolerance, but it must be noted that the motivation to wear in this type of patient is high, and therefore many types of lens and material with a great diversity of design and fit are seen to achieve good tolerance.

A teacher has, in honesty, to give students all the current opinions and ideas that appear relevant and must, if evidence is available, indicate preferences for certain lens design and fit for the stages of keratoconic progression. But above all else, a teacher must avoid teaching a dogmatic doctrinal approach, which in my experience is often based upon a mechanical analysis of the diseased cornea.

It is becoming increasingly evident that keratoconus is related to collagen anomaly due to fibroblast dysfunction. The systemic manifestations may, therefore, have to be investigated by a specialist medical physician. Trauma as a cause, including self-inflicted eye rubbing (Ridley, 1961), has been considered seriously; the effect of the contact lens itself has also been considered (Hartstein, 1968).

Fitting the cornea

In the first instance, following the routine examination and where keratoconus is suspected, the corneal shape and thickness must be analysed. It is appreciated that the equipment available to most practitioners, whilst of good quality, may not be designed specifically for some of the investigations to be mentioned. However, this should not be a problem for university centres or specialist

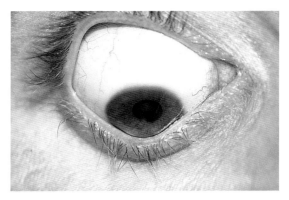

Figure 35.1 The classical sign of the cone is the profile as seen when the lid margin touches the cornea in the depressed position of the eye.

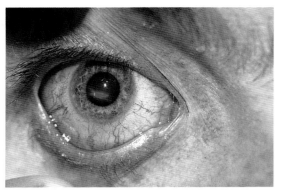

Figure 35.3 An example of advanced cone with stromal and Bowmans membrane scarring. This will severely limit the acuity obtained with a contact lens.

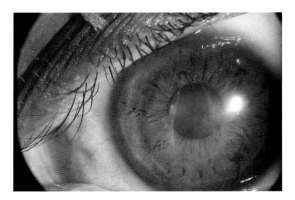

Figure 35.2 Oblique folds in the deeper layers of the stroma and Decscemet's (Vogt lines). The conic cornea was fitted with a contact lens and had periodic episodes of oedema.

5. Sudden change of curvature from cone zone to periphery.
6. Thinning of the cornea at the apex.
7. Evidence of stromal anomaly, such as deep oblique striae (Fig. 35.2).
8. Sub-Bowman's scarring, irregularity of Bowman's membrane (Fig. 35.3).
9. Endothelial cell polymegathy.
10. Fine pigment on the endothelium.

Whilst some of these defects will affect the ability to obtain a fit, others will prevent the attainment of good vision.

The contact lens practitioner should be objective and measure the cornea by methods that can be linked easily to the tolerances of manufacture of a lens on the one hand and to the acceptance of a philosophy of fit that permits a functional result on the other. This combination of objectivity and subjectivity is nowhere better illustrated than in fitting the keratoconic cornea, because the measurement of the keratoconic cornea is often qualitative rather than quantitative.

Retinoscopy

If performed accurately, and providing that corneal transparency permits, retinoscopy will give information about the cone area

tres or specialist practitioners. For a topographical analysis of the cone cornea, see Marechal-Courtois (1969).

The aspects of keratoconus that make the lens fit vary from the routine procedure are:

1. Steeper than normal corneal curvatures (Fig. 35.1).
2. Some displacement of the cone apex from normal centre.
3. Irregular astigmatism.
4. High myopic refraction.

refraction and some ideas about the paracone zone. The degree of astigmatism and its irregularity gives the practitioner a measure of the degree of progression of the disorder. The area over which the abnormal shadow appears also relates to the size of the cone zone and its position. Whilst these interpretations cannot be measured in units, they nevertheless give a great deal of information in a minimal period of examination and do not require sophisticated equipment. Indeed, at one time retinoscopy, together with the examination of the corneal profile, was the only diagnostic sign used by the practitioner.

Keratograms and keratometers

The practitioner should be aware of the two main ways of performing keratometry (see Chapter 00):

1. Measuring corneal curvature over a fixed chord, which is variable in size but usually small compared to the diameter of the cornea.
2. Using a target that varies in size inversely with the degree of steepness of the cornea being measured.

Both principles are used to obtain information over large areas of the cornea. Thus the corneal surface can be made to move around the target, or vice versa, or the target can be increased in size to give information about the central and intermediate areas of the cornea. It is now possible to photograph and record this information, and/or to analyse the results using shape coefficients, so that comparison with the normal or zonal isometers can be recorded. The latter analysis can be programmed into a computer and graphic representation is therefore possible, even with three-dimensional vectors; no doubt the next generation of instrumentation will see storage of corneal curvature shape and representation as halographs, with suitable magnification.

Data that can be visualized and analysed in this way can be matched to a contact lens fitting philosophy relating to a particular lens design, and thus the fit becomes a non-*in-vivo* procedure. However, at present a keratometer used with line of sight fixation gives sufficient information to fit a patient. A reading 5 degrees either side of the central reading can give additional helpful information (see page 000). Most keratometers will not give readings steeper than $r = 5.5$ mm; a supplementary lens in front of the viewing system will give steeper readings. However, in advanced cone, the irregularity and difficulty of the patient to fixate consistently precludes the gathering of useful information.

Topographical techniques (see Chapter 00) will give information that can indicate the area of maximal steepness and degree. Thus these methods are used as follows:

1. Keratometry about the corneal vision point.
2. Siting of the apex.
3. Degree of irregular astigmatism.
4. Recording the progression of the disease.

Trial lens fitting

The use of trial lenses of known design and materials, and the manufacture of the patient's lens to agreed tolerances, will give the best results. It is possible to order lenses from the keratometry or photokeratometry results (providing a consistent and accurate refraction is possible; see Chapters 00 and 00) for each phase of keratoconus.

The trial lenses must consider the following aspects of correction:

1. Steep cornea over small central and paracentral zones.
2. High degrees of astigmatism.

As hard corneal lenses are most useful, they will be considered first, followed by special types of soft and finally by scleral hard lenses. All these lens fits and designs have been dealt with elsewhere for the normal eye and other types of abnormal eye (see Chapters 31 and 35 for additional information).

Keratoconus in most patients is a progressive condition, starting as a uniocular complaint and, in most patients, becoming binocular within a 5-year period. There is therefore a need to reassess the fit and to refit the patient as and when necessary. Furthermore, complications that affect the fit and wear patterns of the lens may, in some instances, be lens-induced and in others result from the basic corneal and lid abnormalities. These will be covered under post-fit management; at present, Table 35.3 – a summarized table of the contact lens treatment – will be of value.

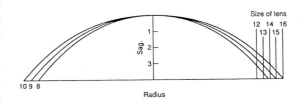

Figure 35.5 The curves and sagitta are those of large corneoscleral lenses and show the choice of back curve and size that could be possible for any given sagitta. Such lenses find use in high irregular astigmatism and abnormal eye shape as to be found after corneal graft surgery, aphakia and traumatic injuries to the eye.

Trial lens designs for hard materials and fitting philosophy

The philosophies, in fact, are related to the degree of cone and the (Figs 35.4 and 35.5) position of the apex. In the first instance, the back curve will be determined largely by the degree of cone progression. On the other hand, the position of the apex will decide how large the lens has to be to obtain stability and acuity. Another factor related to degenerative myopia, if present, or axial myopia due to the cone, is the power the lens has to carry. Thus a high myopic power will be required in such instances if a steep back curve is used, and this will require either a reduced optic or a very thinly designed lens. If not controlled, the lens thickness problem can lead to intolerable non-stable lens fit. The converse of this is to fit a large corneal lens with a back curve flat relative to the keratometry. This will correct a larger portion of the myopia and permit a lens design better tolerated and better centred for acuity correction.

In teaching, two opposing fits have resulted from the above considerations:

1.   The paracone fit, which designs a lens to

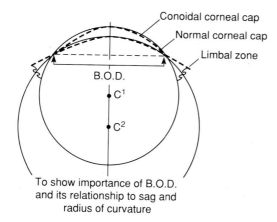

Figure 35.4 The diagram shows two circles with centres on the same axis (C^1 and C^2). The curves correspond respectively to the keratoconic back central optic radius and the normal cornea back central optic radius of corneal fitting lenses. The corneal outlines are shown in dotted outline. The back optic central chord is the same and therefore shows the great increase in sagitta from the normal to the cone fit.

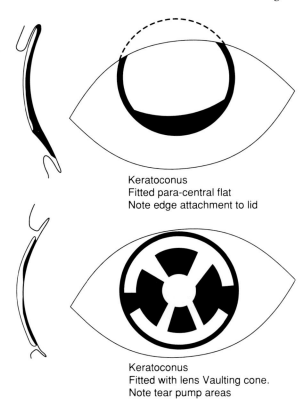

Keratoconus
Fitted para-central flat
Note edge attachment to lid

Keratoconus
Fitted with lens Vaulting cone.
Note tear pump areas

Figure 35.6 The diagram shows the fluorescein retro lens fluid distribution for the two basic fits of the cone eye over the apex and paracone zones. (Top) the paracone fit with its inferior open lens fit and the superior lens to cornea touch and the upper lid to edge stabilising adhesion. (Bottom) the vault type fit with examples of the intermediate clearance and ventilation to the lens periphery.

fit the area of cornea superior and at the sides of the cone, with a large size lens, (Fig. 35.6).

2. The opposing fit, which attempts to vault the apex but at the same time keeping the lens as small as possible in size. The resulting lens often requires reduced front optics and careful thickness control because the power is likely to be high. The fit so obtained is relatively static compared with the paracone fit and therefore a small front optic (even

5 mm) can prove functional. Edge flare and intolerance from the upper lid can be unacceptable.

Trial lenses of both types will make the practitioner's final decision easier, but often this proves too expensive for the practitioner who fits keratoconus infrequently. A compromise lens design that meets both ideas in part is often the end result. A practitioner who has no trial lens can follow the simple rule of fitting the eye with a lens designed from keratometry using the formulation below and then asking for refits based upon modifications judged necessary from the fluorescien patterns (see Chapter 16).

Basic lens design for the vault fit

The lens design is calculated from a knowledge of the overall sagitta and the equivalent central spherical radius and its chord.

In the manufacture of sets of lens for the trial fitting of keratoconus, two series are advised – one set of small size, say 8.7 mm, which will fit corneas with central cones and low powers, and another set of 9.5 mm-sized lenses of high minus power for eccentric cones and high powers.

As an example: vault fit set size 9.5 mm:

$r° = 5.5$ mm sag. $= 2.5$ by equal sagitta increments of 0.05 mm to $r° = 7.5$ mm sag. $= 1.7$

Details of the back surface lens design should be dependent upon a back central optic chord (BCOC) of 5 mm for the steepest lens, increasing to 6.5 mm for the flattest; the axial edge lift being 0.15 mm for all lenses.

The back peripheral curves and centre curves used will be dependent upon the sagitta, and the decision as to whether spherical curves, aspheric or pseudoaspheric curves are used (e.g. tangent periphery or offset spherical). Most specialist practitioners will want to design their own sets of fitting lenses in conjunction with a manufacturer.

Paracone fit

It is not necessary to have a completely new set of lenses designed for this type of fitting.

The conventional 9.5 mm trial fitting set can be extended to include steeper fitting lenses. It is, however, important that the back design is a faithful extension, and therefore the details of the back curve and the edge lift must be known. The steeper lenses should keep the same edge lift as the other lenses, but the central back curve and chord decrease gradually; the steepest lens being one with a back central optic radius (BCOR) = 5.8 and chord 6 mm. These lenses need not have a high minus power.

All corneal trial lenses used solely to access fit can be manufactured in PMMA material.

Peripheral curves

Chapter 5 will give the reader an understanding that the essential features of a back surface are included in the information given of the total diameter, the edge lift and the back optic zone data, either in terms of radius and chord or equivalent aspheric eccentricity. Thus the data for the peripheral curves, whilst variable, are predetermined by the constraints indicated.

There is a choice of peripheral curves – spherical, toroidal, offset spherical, tangential flat or a continuation of the true aspheric. For the small lens, particularly after blending and polishing, it is debatable as to how much difference can be clinically distinguished in fit. However, in the larger sized lens, and especially when the peripheral corneal contact determines the fit, the type of peripheral curve chosen becomes important.

In the vault-type fit, where an apical minimal touch or bare clearance is required, a cone-type periphery is desirable and best found in the aspheric design with an eccentricity of SF = 0.85. The pseudoeccentric curves, such as offset and tangent, are easier to manufacture in the small laboratory and give similar results.

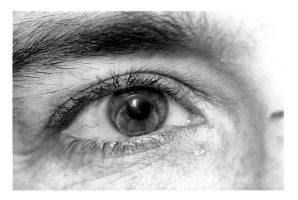

Figure 35.7 A small sized corneal lens sagging downwards from the cone and producing a poorly tolerated lens.

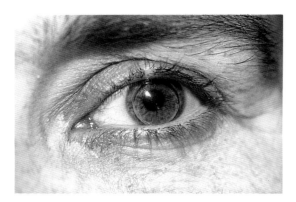

Figure 35.8 A corneal lens of 9.7 mm size fitted to the paracone zone and with peripheral pseudoaspheric curves.

The paracone fit obtains its maximal contact above and around the cone and has a wide zone, which is open below. The conventional aspheric or multicurve surface can give this fit. Very often four curves are required and examples of all these fits are given here, with the back curve formulae.

The practitioner uses the trial lens as a guide to fitting and the modifications asked for of the manufacturer to produce a final lens may require one or more refits. Examples of the type of fit obtained with

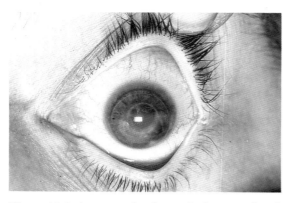

Figure 35.9 An example of a grafted cornea fitted with a corneal lens after suture removal, 10.5 mm size. The graft eye can be fitted with a lens with sutures *in situ* if the knots are buried.

hard corneal lenses are shown in Figures 35.7, 35.8 and 35.9.

Power compensated hard toric corneal lenses

Because the cone surface and remainder of the keratoconic cornea has a toric form in many patients, it is reasonable to use a back toric surface to obtain a fit. This will induce a toric power to correct, and this can be worked onto the front surface. Such lenses do not have to be ballasted because the fit will stabilize the lens. Trial lenses of this type can be made and some basic back curve formulae are given using spherical curves. The difference in meridional radii should either be 1 mm or 2 mm; small differences are not practical:

$$\frac{6.0:7.0}{7.0} / \frac{7.0:8.0}{8.0} / \frac{8.0:9.0}{9.0} / \frac{9.0:9.50}{10.0}$$

by equal increments to:

$$\frac{7.6:7.0}{8.6} / \frac{8.6:8.0}{9.6} / \frac{9.6:9.0}{10.6} / \frac{10.6:9.50}{11.6}$$

Whilst the above formulations are empirical, they at least form a basis for the fitter to determine the final lens best fit.

Silicon rubber lenses

The soft materials available are silicon rubber and the hydrophilic gels. Given an identical lens design, the silicon rubbers are about five times as rigid as the soft gels of low water content (40% approximately). It would therefore be an advantage to try the rubber material lenses before the gels. Unfortunately the rubber lenses are made in few fittings, and then only for the normal eye shape range. Therefore only early keratoconus could be fitted with such lenses. Too flat a fit with a rubber lens is likely to lead to severe epithelial loss over the zone of the contact, which, for the keratoconic eye, will be the apex. On the other hand, the rubber can, if too steep, seal onto the cornea, which could occur with the thin and less rigid than normal cornea. For these reasons, the use of rubber lenses for the fitting of keratoconus is not advised.

Hydrogel lenses

The lens designs used can be of the following:

1. Spherical and aspherical, combined hard and soft.
2. Trapezoid.
3. Toric.
4. Scleral.

Spherical and aspherical

The simplest lens form to ask the manufacturer to make in PHEMA 42% water material is a bicurve back surface with a reduced front optic and centre thickness of 0.25 mm. For the early keratoconic eye a plus power of even higher central thickness can be used with a spectacle lens over-correction to prove the best acuity. It must be noted that for all soft lenses an over-correction in spectacle form is often required.

The following formulae can provide a fitting set:

Thick Soft Lenses

7.50:9.0/8.0:14.0

by equal increments to:

8.30:9.0/8.80:14.50

T_c = 0.25 minutes; P = −15.0 reduced optic to 10 mm; T_e = 0.15 mm.

For more advanced cones as follows:

6.0:7.00/7.50:15.0   Sagitta = 6 mm

to:

8.0:8.7/8.7:15

by equal increments. T_c = 0.30; red optic = 10 mm; P = −8 and −15 D.

Instead of a trial set of such lenses it is possibly better to order one or two lenses about 0.5 mm flatter than av.K. for each eye and refit for the final lens. It must be noted that the rigidity of the lens is related to the thickness and material water content. The rigidity of the lens form when on the eye determines the acuity, and any modifications requested for the final lens or a repeat lens must reproduce the lens thickness to narrow tolerances, or consistent results are not possible. This applies to any equivalent aspheric form.

Combined hard and soft materials

There are several forms of hard centre, soft periphery lens. In its simplest form this could be a thin, high water therapeutic gel lens with a hard gas permeable hard lens fitted onto it. Such a combination will give the acuity of a hard lens and greater comfort than a hard lens by itself. However, there are certain problems with such a combined system. Unless the hard lens is of special design it will have excessive movement and will not stabilize; some patients find that two lenses are impossible to manage.

The hard lens should be at least 10 mm and should not have a flat back edge bevel. It should be fitted steeper than keratometry if

possible, the 'K' reading being taken over the surface of the soft lens. To assist stabilization, the soft lens can be designed with a positive power to provide a more spherical surface onto which to fit the hard lens. Such a reduced optic plus soft lens will have central rigidity compared to thin therapeutic lens.

The only other practical combined lens is one with a hard polymer grafted to a soft, the lens being made out of the combined material; 'Saturn' is the UK tradename of such a lens. The practitioner may find that an insufficient range of fittings may limit the use of what is an excellent solution to the problem of a cone.

Hard gas permeable materials and PMMA

The choice of material for a lens depends upon two factors. First, the material must be least likely to interfere with physiological function of the tissues with which it is in contact, and second, it should give the best fitting and acuity result for the particular lens design used.

In the instance of keratoconus it can be argued that the acuity and fit to produce maximal tolerance are of greater importance than the gas permeability of the material.

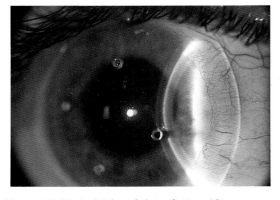

Figure 35.10 A thick soft lens fitting (diameter = 15 mm and C_t = 0.35 mm) PHEMA 42% water. note the fenestrations over the intermediate corneal clearance zones.

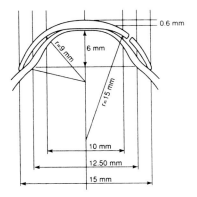

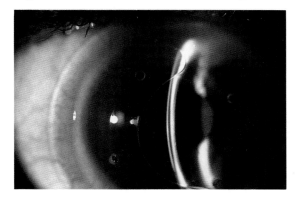

Figure 35.11 A lens design for the thick soft lens material to give central rigidity. The curvatures given are those producing a trapezoid curve and are not those given in the text.

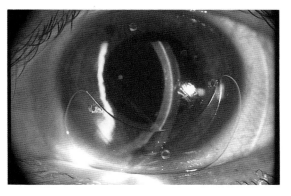

Figures 35.12 and 35.13 The two examples illustrate the large thick soft lens fit which is very similar to that of the hard scleral. Note the bubble formation and the position of the fenestrations.

The two functions are interrelated but decisions often have to be made at the time of refitting. The gas permeable materials, whilst giving greater tolerance, often have the disadvantage of warping when applied to a toric cornea; this is especially true for thin lens design. The use of bitoric lens design can, to a certain degree, avoid this problem. Certainly for small sized thin lenses of low power, PMMA, especially if already well tolerated, should not be changed for larger, thicker gas permeable material, with its wetting and warping problems. It can also be argued that the thin cornea of keratoconus can, under the stress from lens-induced hypoxia, obtain oxygen from the anterior chamber much more easily than the normal cornea. This is a hypothesis, but is nevertheless valid. Thus acuity requirements may have to take precedence over physiological function.

Use of soft materials

Hard materials are first choice for the keratoconic and for that matter all the irregular astigmatic cornea. But because there are tolerance problems softer materials also have to be used. Lenses made of softer materials

softer materials (Figs 35.10, 35.11, 35.12 and 35.13), whilst better tolerated, are unlikely to give good acuity except in the early phases of the disease. The following description of soft lens design and fitting is, in effect, a method to overcome the acuity correction problem. With a few exceptions the lenses described are custom made and are not those in use for the cosmetic correction of refractive errors (Figuccia & Kreis-Gosselin, 1975a,b; Ruben, 1971a, 1975, 1979, 1989).

Soft scleral lenses

Hard scleral lenses will be dealt with in Chapter 31, here soft scleral lenses will be considered (Fig. 35.14).

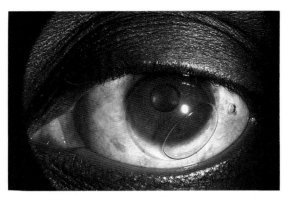

Figure 35.14 The eye with advanced cone has been fitted with a 26 mm size scleral soft PHEMA 42% water lens.

Chapter 31 explains how scleral technology developed. It is therefore apparent that, at one stage, preformed scleral lenses were considered satisfactory for the range of fittings of the normal eye. Dallos developed a fitting set of moulded shapes suitable for the abnormal eye, but even with several hundred shapes it was often impossible to obtain a satisfactory result, hence the use of moulded-to-the-eye fittings of thermoplastic materials such as PMMA.

Given a mouldable material of the conventional thickness of scleral lenses (0.2–1 mm), the need to take impressions of the eye is negated because the soft scleral lens of preformed geometrical shape should itself mould to the eye. Miller *et al.* (1972) reported such a lens made of silica rubber. Ruben made these lenses from gel materials in a large- and mini-scleral form known as the trapezoid-shaped lens.

The formula for a soft scleral of 0.6 mm thick is given below and from this a range of trial lenses can be made. It is suggested that the fitting set have only four lenses and that a final lens is designed from the trial fitting:

9.0/13:23   Sagitta = 6 mm

by equal increments of sagitta to:

9.0:11.0/12.5:23   Sagitta = 10 mm

The lenses must be fenestrated with a 1 mm hole at the optic haptic transition. The fit will appear similar to a hard scleral. There will be an air bubble at the transition and a sufficient looseness of fit is necessary to permit pumping of the retrotear fluid; a front optic of 10 mm diameter will suffice. Reproduction of identical thicknesses in refits is essential.

Soft miniscleral

This lens is based upon scleral lens philosophy but the scleral fit and stability is obtained by using a back peripheral curve steeper than the central back optic.

Formulae for the trapezoid miniscleral lens of hydrogel material

A drawing board or computer can produce a variety of formulae, the following lens forms provide a basis (see Fig. 35.11 for an alternative design):

12.0:8.0/9.0:13.5   Sagitta = 2.8 mm
12.0:8.7/9.0:14.0   Sagitta = 3.0 mm
12.0:8.9/9.0:14.5   Sagitta = 3.4 mm

Thickness = 0.6 mm; PHEMA = 42% water; fenetrated 1 mm at optic junction; power = –4.0 D; red optic = 10 mm; tolerances ± 0.2 mm for size.

The chief problem with the soft scleral is the expense of production and refitting to obtain a result, and the limited life of the lens. If the lens is too thin at the centre, pulsation of vision results with fluctuation of acuity.

Perhaps a hard centre, soft haptic scleral would provide an alternative in the future?

Scleral hard lenses

The manufacture and fitting of scleral lenses has been dealt with in Chapter 31 and therefore this section will only deal with some

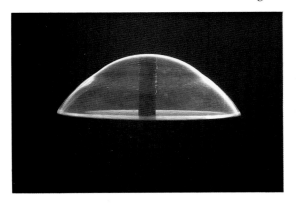

Figure 35.15 The photograph is of a preformed scleral hard gas permeable lens cut from a blank by a lathe. Such lenses have been made from silicon rubber materials by cast methods.

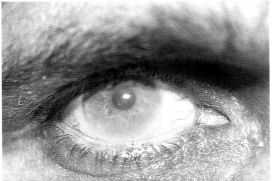

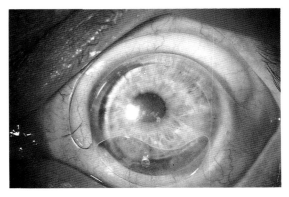

Figure 35.16 A slot ventilated hard PMMA scleral lens made from the eye model by moulding technique.

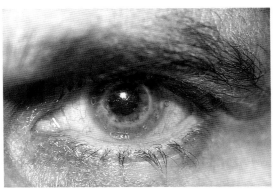

Figures 35.17 and 35.18 Moulded scleral lenses worn by a patient with a keratoconic eye on the left side and grafted cornea on the right. Note that the lens has corneal graft touch which was too excessive whereas the cone eye has satisfactory clearance.

special references to the fitting of keratoconus (Figs 35.15, 35.16, 35.17 and 35.18).

By definition a scleral lens gains stability and support from that portion (haptic) of the lens that is in contact with the sclera. The definition includes all lenses that are larger than the corneal diameter and fulfil that part of the definition that describes stability and support. All soft lenses (except corneal sized lenses) are of scleral size, but in fact are supported by the cornea as well as by the limbal scleral junction. Corneoscleral lenses of 12 to 13 mm could also be described as

scleral, but again they are stabilized by corneal contact. In practice, the true hard scleral is larger than 16 mm in its smallest diameter and the optic portion does not determine the stability of the lens. The moulded-to-eye and preformed fittings have been described. These descriptions are ideal fits, where the apex of the cornea does not contact the back surface of the lens except in exceptional circumstances, or extremes of eye movement. In keratoconus, especially in the advanced cone, the apex of the cornea very often makes contact with the lens and therefore the fit over that zone becomes critical. Methods to achieve this therefore become important.

(even up to 13 mm in diameter) can be considered. In a cornea with a large aphakic section the use of such lenses often gives good results and the full scleral-sized lens is not required. The fitter will find it difficult to obtain centration with high powered hard lenses and should use smaller sized lenses unless toric back surfaces are used.

35.2.7 POST-KERATOPLASTY AND REFRACTIVE SURGERY

The common factor of the astigmatism, whilst in many cases being irregular, can also produce overall an abnormal shaped cornea. For example, in the post-graft keratoconic cornea the centre may still present a very steep curve over a small chord relative to the peripheral cornea. The post-epikeratoplasty and lamellar graft, on the other hand, may present very flat curves over a large zone of the cornea. The thick and even thin soft lens gives bad results as far as the epithelial cell survival is concerned and hard corneal, and even scleral type lens, have to be fitted. Because the cornea can be irregular in limited zones there will be sealed retrolens areas and the fitter should therefore not be afraid to use fenestrations in such lenses, preferably in the intermediate part of the lens and at least 0.5 mm in diameter.

Post-lens implant operation

In all the instances described above, especially when the induced astigmatism due to surgery or trauma affects only one eye, and the other is functional, there is sometimes the additional problem of anisimetropia and anisiekonia, and binocular vision problems if the affected eye gives good acuity with contact lenses. In these rare instances the use of supplementary spectacles and prisms should be considered. In even rarer instances, the use of over-corrections in the contact lens, with neutralization of the over-correction by the spectacle lens to produce a retinal image equalizing effect, will be necessary. These are rare instances, but they do occur in specialist contact lens practice.

In the instance of the pseudolens implant, the astigmatism can be due to tilting of the implant and the correction of this internal astigmatism therefore requires special consideration. Either hard or soft lenses can be used to correct this type of astigmatism and, in both instances, it is necessary to stabilize the lens either by ballast (prisms) or by lens shape and thickness, the astigmatic correction being on the front surface of the lenses. Since, in all these given examples, the restoration of good vision with binocularity is the prime consideration, if it is practical the practitioner can elect to use the spherical powered contact lens combined with a spectacle over-correction for the best results.

REFERENCES

Anderson, J.R. (1930) Contact lenses for conical cornea. *Med. Journal Australia* **1**, 216.

Dolman, C.H. (1969) Contact lens glued to the Bowman's membrane. *Am. Journal Optometry* **46**, 434.

Fick, A.E. (1889) Eine Contactbrille. *Arch. Augenheick* **18**, 279.

Figuccia, R. and Kreis-Gosselin, F. (1975a) Thick soft lenses. ECLSO 5th Am. Gen. Meeting Vienna April 1975.

Figuccia, R. and Kreis-Gosselin, F. (1975b) Essais de correction de keratoconus avec soft contact lenses. *Bul. Soc. Ophthal. de France (Paris)* **5**, 437–443.

Galt (1889) In Fick, A.E. Eine Contactbrille. *Arch. Augenheick* **18**, 279.

Gyorffy, I. (1950) Plastic therapeutic lenses. *Br. J. Ophth.* **32**, 850.

Gyorffy, I. (1951) Role of contact lenses in eye surgery. *Ophthalmologia* **122**, 344.

Hartstein, J. (1968) Keratoconus developing in contact lens wearers. *Arch. Ophth.* **80**, 345.

Marechal-Courtois, C. (1969) A topographical study of the keratoconus cornea. *Amali Oftal Clin Ocul.* **202**, 23.

Miller, D. (1972) Problems with scleral silicon contact lens. *Contact Lens* **3**, 38.

Miller, D., Holmberg, A. and Carol, J. (1966) Comparison of two methods of moulding scleral contact lenses. *Arch. Ophthal.* **76**, 422.

Ridley, F. (1961) Eye rubbing and keratoconus *Br. J. Ophth.* **45**, 631.

Ruben, M.. (1971a) Adhesive keratoprosthesis. *Trans. Ophth. Soc. UK*, **90**, 551.

Ruben, M.. (1971b) Soft lenses. *Trans. Ophth. Soc. UK*, **91**, 59.

Ruben, M.. (1975) Therapeutic uses. In M. Ruben (ed), *Contact Lens Practice*. Baillière Tyndall, London.

Ruben, M.. (1989) Abnormal eye fitting and scleral lenses. In M. Ruben (ed), *Colour Atlas of Contact Lenses*. (2nd ed). Wolfe Medical Publications, London.

CONTACT LENS FITTING POST REFRACTIVE SURGERY

Christine Astin

36.1 INTRODUCTION

Contact lenses represent the best optical method currently available for correcting high degrees of ametropia. When contact lens tolerance is not attainable, refractive surgery offers an alternative to spectacles. Various surgical procedures have been developed, the majority altering the corneal shape or refractive index. Current procedures include: crystalline lens extraction, intraocular and corneal lens implants, corneal wound adjustment, keratoplasty, keratotomy and photoablation using an excimer laser. Considerations when fitting contact lenses to correct residual ametropia following such procedures will be described.

Where possible, contact lens fitting should be avoided on any eye which has undergone refractive surgery because the eye has already suffered trauma and disturbance of its normal physiology. The corneal ability to cope with lens related problems, e.g. infection, neovascularization, corneal distortion, or oedema has been influenced. Lens fitting should be delayed until corneal wounds have stabilized, usually about three months. Early fitting may interfere with stromal healing and epithelial integrity leading to further scarring and an increased risk of infection.

Following refractive surgery the corneal topography stabilizes in a new form. This can facilitate future contact lens fitting, e.g. when corneal transplants are modified surgically to reduce postoperative astigmatism. However, an unusual corneal shape can be produced, e.g. following radial keratotomy. The resultant changes in corneal functioning, strength, sensitivity and response should also be considered when monitoring the lens fit and the ocular condition. A number of these are described below.

36.2 CLEAR LENS EXTRACTION IN HIGH MYOPIA

This method can correct high degrees of myopia but has several complications (Rodriguez *et al.*, 1987). These include loss of accommodation and the refractive change being limited to the crystalline lens power. Lens fitting to correct residual myopia is similar to that for typical low degree myopia (Phillips, 1989). If a limbal incision was performed, there is a greater likelihood of 'against-the-rule' (ATR) astigmatism which encourages the rigid lens to decentre temporally. The fitting could commence once corneal astigmatism has stabilized, e.g. after 4 to 6 weeks postoperatively if the incision is very small as in phacoemulsification (Heslin & Guerriero, 1984; Reading, 1984), after 6 to 8 weeks following limbal incision and after 12 to 16 weeks following corneal incision. After

Contact Lens Practice. Edited by Montague Ruben and Michel Guillon. Published in 1994 by Chapman & Hall, London. ISBN 0 412 35120 X

a large incision, the aphakic eye has a decreased oxygen demand (Guillon & Morris, 1981) and decreased sensitivity following severance of many corneal nerves, which can assist lens adaptation. Preoperatively, contact lens tolerance was influenced by the thick edges and reduced optic zone diameter of the high power lens which are not necessary in the low power lens.

36.3   INTRAOCULAR IMPLANT IN THE PHAKIC EYE

Negative powered anterior chamber intraocular implants to correct high degrees of myopia have been tried more recently by Praeger (1988), Heide *et al.* (1988) and Joly *et al.* (1988) since these implants offer improved predictability of outcome compared to keratomileusis. Baikoff *et al.* (1989) noted that the incision must be wide enough for the entry of the intraocular lens (IOL). The larger the incision, the greater is the likelihood of increased corneal astigmatism, and hence instability of a contact lens at a later date. This technique potentially allows IOL to endothelium contact and prolonged endothelial damage by the support legs of this type of IOL. Any endothelial damage affects the corneal ability to cope with oedema at a later date (Buckley, 1985), so it is important to choose a contact lens of good design and oxygen transmissibility to avoid oedema.

Lens fitting for residual ametropia is affected by the morphology of the wound. Good lens optical quality and surface wettability are advantages. Contrast sensitivity, already reduced by light scatter from the IOL and the crystalline lens, would decrease further if the contact lens surface became very scratched and deposited. Increased risk of limbal pressure would be given by hydrophilic lenses which were tight, thick edged or of poor oxygen transmission, e.g. a thick edged lens would be more liable to cause limbal indentation and peripheral corneal oedema.

36.4   STROMAL LENS IMPLANT

Intralamellar lens implants have been strongly recommended by Choyce (1985) who altered the corneal power by using a rigid polysulphone inlay placed close to Descemet's membrane. There are several problems with this method, e.g. diurnal variation of vision. Climenhaga *et al.* (1988) described polysulphone as impermeable to small molecular weight nutrients such as glucose, water and oxygen passing from the anterior chamber forwards and also to lactic acid from the stroma to the aqueous. Resultant stromal opacities were common. Sometimes these secondary changes gave a significant loss of vision so that penetrating keratoplasty was indicated (Kirkness *et al.* (1985). Amongst the postoperative problems discussed by McCarey *et al.* (1988) and by Shovlin (1989) in a review of the use of these implants, were interfacial scarring, irregular astigmatism and reduced corneal resistance to drying; the latter could be followed by epithelial damage and stromal thinning.

Hydrogel lenticles are also used for intrastromal lens implants in refractive keratoplasty, but reports vary regarding their success in changing corneal power. Werblin *et al.*, (1984) corrected up to 9.0 dioptres of myopia using these implants to flatten the anterior corneal surface. McDonald *et al.* (1983) found minimal refractive change, but Watsky *et al.* (1985) suggested an algorithm to improve predicability. Ohrloff *et al.* (1984) noted opacification, vascularization and chronic inflammation produced by hydrogel lamellar implants. Trials by Beekhuis *et al.* (1986) and McCarey *et al.* (1990) showed minimal interface problems except at the collagen scars at the abruptly cut implant margins, where light scatter increased. As the refractive index was similar to that of the lens, only two-thirds of the desired refractive change was obtained, so residual myopia remained.

If a contact lens must be fitted, a rigid gas

permeable lens is recommended with high transmissibility of oxygen since oxygen transport through the cornea has already been inhibited by the implant. The lens should fit near alignment with the flattest keratometry reading aiming for good tear flow beneath the lens, for further oxygen supply and to assist removal of epithelial debris and lactic acid excreted by the epithelium. A tight lens inhibits the corneal oxygen supply, encouraging the less efficient anaerobic stromal respiration and leading to corneal oedema.

Although not yet adequately investigated, it may be possible for those patients, who even one year postoperatively still suffer from diurnal variations in corneal shape and power, to be fitted with a large diameter (10.0 to 11.0 mm) rigid gas permeable lens. Fitted in alignment to the cornea, this could provide support and help to stabilize the corneal contour. As after most refractive surgery, these implant patients must be particularly cautious during lens insertion and removal. The consequences of daily manipulation of these weakened corneas is unknown. The lens should be easy to remove and undue pressure on the globe avoided. During aftercare the fitter should be extra vigilant for signs of anterior stromal desiccation and thinning which can occur in these cases.

36.5 KERATOMILEUSIS AND KERATOPHAKIA

Barraquer (1981) described keratomileusis as one method of giving a large change in myopia, but it has low predicability. This was demonstrated by Montard and Bosc (1990) and Bosc *et al.* (1990) whose group of 27 cases had a mean preoperative refractive error of −15.5 dioptres yet at one year postoperatively had a mean error of −7.0 dioptres. Most lamellar refractive surgical procedures involve the use of donor tissue (e.g. keratophakia) or host tissue (e.g. keratomileusis) which is frozen so that the curvature

can be adjusted using a cryolathe. Several studies (Schanzlin *et al.* 1983; Baumgartner *et al.* 1984; Baumgartner & Binder, 1985) have noted the adverse effects of these procedures on the corneal structure and transparency. A number of morphological changes were described associated with tissue damage due to freezing, which alters the spacing of the collagen fibrils and damages the stromal keratocytes. Bowman's membrane can also be affected such that re-epithelialization is inhibited. Non-freeze methods which avoid these changes have been used by Hoffmann (1984), Swinger *et al.* (1986) and Zavala *et al.* (1987) but predictability remains poor, so a contact lens may be required to correct residual myopia.

It is advisable to allow 3 to 4 months postoperatively for the host–donor interfaces to heal together. If fitting a hydrophilic lens, pressure on the cornea should be kept to a minimum, e.g. sliding the lens onto the sclera rather than squeezing the lens on the cornea, also by choosing a thin aspheric design lens to give less localized pressure and better oxygen transmission. The first choice lens should be a rigid gas permeable lens of high oxygen transmissibility. There should be adequate edge clearance and well rounded edges so that the lens moves freely over the cornea and allows good tear circulation beneath the lens. A tight or rough edge should be avoided because of the risk of epithelial indentation, of particular concern if disturbing the epithelium over the incision.

The rigid lens should have a back optic zone radius in alignment with the flattest keratometry reading, and show good centration and movement. An elliptical design lens with smooth contours and an adequate back optic zone diameter, e.g. 7.0 to 8.0 mm, would be favourable. After keratomileusis, the corneal curve is flat centrally then steepens near the thicker margin of the keratoplasty, becoming flatter again near the limbus. After keratophakia, the anterior stroma covers a greater volume of tissue, so the cornea is steep centrally then rapidly flattens towards the periphery. These contours should be considered when fitting lenses.

36.6 EPIKERATOPHAKIA

Epikeratophakia ('epi') has been used since 1979 as a simplified alternative to keratophakia and keratomileusis procedures. Kaufman and McDonald (1984) proposed a combination of lenticle implant and epikeratophakia ('epi lens') to give a greater range of correction. It has been described (Werblin & Klyce, 1981, McDonald *et al.* 1987; Durrie *et al.*, 1987) as a suitable alternative to secondary intraocular lenses since epi lens removal is easier. The new corneal power is given by the new anterior contour of the epi lens, produced from donor tissue in a similar manner to contact lens latheing (Kaufman *et al.*, 1990). The recipient area is de-epithelialized thoroughly to avoid risk of epithelial ingrowth and haze later (Morgan & Beuerman, 1986). The epi lens is placed on the recipient cornea, the edge tucked into a shallow peripheral keratectomy groove in a 7.0 to 8.5 mm diameter circle, then sutured in place. The 1.0 mm wide groove acts as the position of scarring links between the donor and the recipient (Fig. 36.1). The epi lens has been lathed from the endothelial surface of the donor cornea so the anterior stroma and Bowman's membrane is intact. Fresh tissue heals quickly, but with lyophilized tissue stabilization of the epi lens epithelium takes four to twelve weeks, so can benefit from the protection of a thin soft therapeutic contact lens in the early stage (Keates & Kelley, 1985).

Visual acuity usually improves to within one or two lines of the final value by the first month after suture removal, performed about 2 months postoperatively, and reaches the final value about 3 months later (Schanzlin, 1986). Anterior surface irregularity and epithelial

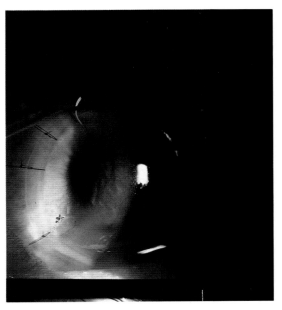

Figure 36.1 Epikeratophakia in groove.

ingrowth often persist so the refractive accuracy and vision quality is disappointing (Werblin *et al.*, 1982; McDonald *et al.*, 1987; McDonnell *et al.*, 1987; Stern, 1988; Halliday, (1990a). Patients with blepharitis and dry eyes, who are more likely to be contact lens intolerant have the greater risk of epithelial instability (Lass *et al.*, 1987). Contact lens options should be thoroughly investigated before embarking on the refractive surgical procedures. However, some patients may need a contact lens to correct residual ametropia and irregular astigmatism.

A minus power epi lens can correct high degrees of myopia, but this is even less stable and predictable (Werblin & Klyce, 1981; McDonald *et al.*, 1985, 1987; Krumeich & Swinger, 1987; Nichols *et al.*, 1988) Astigmatic corrections were very unpredictable (McDonald *et al.*, 1986a; Verity *et al.*, 1986). A sutureless technique may improve accuracy and speed (Rostron, 1988).

For a few keratoconus patients, with minimal corneal scarring yet contact lens intolerance, a plano power epi lens can be used as onlay lamellar transplant (McDonald *et al.*, 1986b; Halliday, 1990b). These aim to support the ectasia and flatten the apical contours to reduce the astigmatism, so spectacle correction or several hours of daily contact lens wear may be re-attempted for optimal visual correction.

36.6.1 CONSIDERATIONS IN FITTING CONTACT LENSES POST-EPIKERATOPHAKIA.

If a plano powered hydrophilic therapeutic lens is fitted, a high water content, good surface quality thin lens should be chosen, suitable for several weeks' extended wear. The lens should be fitted 1.5 to 2.0 mm larger than the visible iris diameter, to give good coverage and centration, usually 0.5 mm movement on blinking and without conjunctival indentation or vessel blanching. The lens fit and condition should be carefully assessed at the postoperative visits, and the lens replaced as required.

When fitting a lens for residual ametropia, several factors should be considered. The corneal topography has been significantly altered so central keratometry is insufficient to guide the first choice of lens. Maguire *et al.*, (1987) analysed the corneal topography of eight eyes following myopic epikeratophakia and found a smaller central optic zone diameter than predicted preoperatively. Beyond this zone, the refractive power of the epi lens surface gradually increased, indicating a progressive steepening and increased power of the corneal curve as the epi lens to host interface margin was approached. Sometimes the epi lens was decentred relative to the visual axis. Their analysis indicated the need to maximize the effective optical zone diameter. Compression of the anterior surface of the epi lens can cause stromal lamellae in the host junction area to compress, resulting in stromal thinning and anterior surface steepening. Compression can be given by a thick contact lens being pushed

onto the cornea by tight lids, especially if the lens is a tight fit or the lens transition rests on the host junction.

At the 6 and 16 month stages, Rao *et al.* (1987) found the epithelial cells were fewer than normal and irregularly arranged with weak interdigitation and poor differentiation of light and dark cells. The epithelial resurfacing and reparative processes were slow. Corneal sensitivity of the epi lenses was reduced, even at 16 months postoperatively. Corneal denervation decreases mitotic activity in the epithelial cells, retards epithelial healing processes and impairs cellular adhesion which may partly cause the abnormal epithelial structure after epikeratophakia. Potential clinical sequelae include increased infection risk, irregular astigmatism, refractory forms of superficial punctate keratopathy, decreased vision, persistant epithelial healing problems and recurrent erosions.

Optical distortion can result from unequal tissue distribution, or tight or unequal suture tension. A thick hydrophilic contact lens could only correct a small amount of the irregular astigmatism. Inadequate oxygen transmission would cause corneal oedema, leading to hazy vision, thickening of the stromal tissue, so increasing stress at the epi lens interface, epithelial disturbance and the risk of neovascularization. Extended contact lens wear should be avoided because it increases corneal oedema and sometimes astigmatism (Kastl, 1986).

A rigid contact lens corrects most of the irregular astigmatism. Oxygen transmissibility and surface wettability are important. Good tear flow beneath the lens is essential for supplying oxygen, flushing debris, removing irritant lens deposits, lubricating lens movement and reducing friction between the epithelial and lens surfaces. A continuous curve or well blended multicurve lens design would encourage smooth lens movement and comfort. A large overall diameter, e.g. 9.0 to 11.0 mm, helps to bridge the operated area and prevent the lens edge eroding the host margin. Following positive power epi lens correction, the cornea is steeply curved centrally and flattens rapidly from the optic towards the host corneal periphery, so the lens contour should follow this to give adequate edge clearance and tear flow beneath the lens. Following myopic correction the corneal topography is flatter centrally and progressively steeper towards the host margin (Maguire *et al.*, 1987). A lens with a flat central curve and decreased edge clearance should give good centration and fit. If bubbles collect under the central optic portion, refitting flatter or fenestrating the lens will assist their escape and so avoid dimpling.

Lembach *et al.* (1989) fitted a number of patients having keratoconic epikeratoplasty. Their ectatic corneas had been flattened from a mean of 6.6 mm ± 0.40 (51.25 dioptres) preoperatively to a mean of 7.1 mm ± 0.40 (47.50 dioptres). Contact lens tolerance was helped by the improved corneal contour and the resultant corneal hypoaesthesia (Koenig *et al.*, 1983). Lembach fitted a lens steeper than the mean keratometry value to show slight apical clearance, good centration and stable visual acuity.

The epi lens may displace as a result of severe trauma before healing. The surgeon may remove it if there are chronic epithelial defects or if the epi lens power *in situ* is markedly inaccurate. Usually the cornea re-epithelializes and within a month returns to spectacle refraction and keratometry readings very similar to preoperative values, although some cases show several dioptres of corneal steepening (Schlichtemeier & Arboegast, 1987). A circular indentation remains at the site of the old groove. A hydrophilic lens easily bridges the groove. A rigid gas permeable lens will need a smooth edge and a diameter larger than that of the circular indentation, so the lens glides over it without eroding the epithelium.

36.7 CORNEAL TRANSPLANT REFRACTIVE SURGERY

Currently, persistent high degrees of astigmatism following penetrating keratoplasty can be reduced by relieving incisions within the transplant margin (Price & Steele, 1987). After 3 months to allow incision healing, contact lens fitting can proceed. The altered corneal contour and physiology can complicate lens fitting (Woodward, 1981; Constad, 1988). A rigid gas permeable lens of good wettability and oxygen transmissibility should be chosen, with a large diameter, e.g. 9.50 to 11.0 mm, so that the lens edge does not disturb the transplant margin. A back optic zone radius on or slightly steeper than the flattest keratometry reading should be selected to ensure good tear flow beneath the lens. When the contours are very irregular, a flexible fitting approach is advisable (Astin, 1985, 1990). Extended wear lenses frequently caused complications including neovascularization, epithelial punctate staining and variable visual acuity (Mannis & Matsumoto 1983).

36.8 RADIAL KERATOTOMY (RK)

Many fitting problems are related to the unusual corneal contour, variable vision and lens instability encountered in the post RK patient (Rowsey & Balyeat, 1982; Astin, 1986, 1989; Rashid & Waring, 1989). Following RK, the corneal rigidity is decreased such that intraocular forces act on the cornea causing mid-peripheral regions to protrude forwards, effectively giving an apical cap of longer radius of curvature than that measured preoperatively. The corneal contour becomes relatively flat centrally and steepens between the mid-region and the corneal periphery. The topography of the central plateau and mid-peripheral 'knee' can be described by central curvature and by eccentricity '*e*', a measure of the curves asphericity or rate of flattening. This is usually described in terms of shape factor 'p', where $p = 1 - e$; so for a sphere $p = 1$, for a prolate (steepening as in RK) ellipse $p > 1$, for an oblate (flattening as in the normal eye) ellipse $0 < p < 1$ (Guillon *et al.*, 1986).

Most contact lens fitting sets have been designed for the oblate elliptical contours of the ametropic eye, so the lens contour flattens accordingly towards the lens edge. Their suitability for RK patients is limited since the lenses often exhibit excess mobility and peripheral fluorescein pooling (Fig. 36.2). The RK contour no longer has a central steeper corneal region to assist correct lens centration, so these lenses often decentre and bridge over the 'knee' region. They may ride low or be held high depending on lid tension and shape. Vision problems with such lenses include: variable vision as the lens rocks, inadequate pupil cover, unstable lens position, tears frothing, dimpling, image flare from the lens periphery, and sometimes greasing as the excess edge standoff stimulates the lid margins.

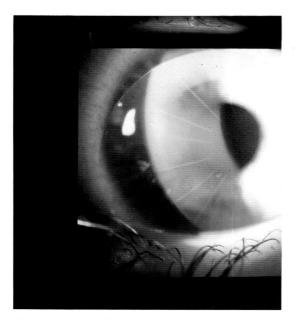

Figure 36.2 Rigid contact lens on cornea, after radial keratotomy.

A minimum edge clearance design, large diameter, rigid, highly oxygen permeable lens, which allows good tear flow beneath the lens and avoids undue pressure on the mid-peripheral region, is recommended (Hoffmann *et al.*, 1986, Astin, 1989; Eggink & Beekhuis, 1989; Rashid & Waring, 1989). Overall diameters are about 9.40 to 11.00 mm (up to 12.80 mm according to Eggink), and back optic zone diameter in the range of 7.50 to 9.00 mm. The initial trial lens has a back optic zone radius (BOZR) of about 0.20 to 0.50 mm steeper than the central keratometry reading. Goldberg (1986) recommended a specially designed lens with a toric or spherical base curve allowing central light corneal bearing and peripheral clearance, to a lesser degree than if an aspheric design lens was fitted. Anderson chose an initial trial lens of BOZR equal to the mid corneal peripheral curve.

Several American practitioners curbed excess lens movement by fitting a lens of BOZR much steeper than the central corneal curvature and often based on the preoperative keratometry readings (Moore, 1988; Rowsey & Rubin, 1988). Shivitz *et al.* (1986, 1987; Shivitz, 1988) advised to wait for 6 months postoperatively then fit a large diameter lens with a BOZR of mean 1.09 mm (5.90 dioptres) steeper than the flattest postoperative keratometry reading. Due to the positive power of the large volume of tears beneath the lens, the contact lens power had to be a higher minus value (range −5.75 to −9.75 dioptres), than the spectacle refraction. Janes and Reichie (1986) aimed for a steep fit using a 9.50 mm diameter lens of BOZR 0.30 mm (1.50 dioptres) flatter than the mean preoperative keratometry reading or based on the peripheral measurement from photokeratoscopy. These steeply fitting lenses inhibited oxygen supply to the cornea via the tears hence causing central corneal steepening, increased myopia, blurred vision and reduced lens tolerance. To mitigate these problems and to allow the escape of bubbles trapped under the lens, fenestration, base curve flattening and increasing the oxygen permeability of the lens were suggested.

Hydrophilic soft lens fitting methods usually followed conventional procedures based on postoperative keratometry (Shivitz *et al.*, 1986; Janes & Reichie, 1986). Vickery (1986) advised using a 15.00 mm diameter, 55% water content soft lens fitting flat so as to align more closely to the flatter than normal curves of the cornea, to minimize limbal pressure and to avoid the disturbed vision given by a steep centrally vaulting lens. Anderson (1988) also advised fitting a soft lens in parallel to the cornea and suggested trying the soft–rigid combination lens, Saturn II. Hydrophilic lenses are more susceptible to spoilation and retention of foreign bodies, and give an increased risk of epithelial erosions, infection, oedema and neovascularization.

Orthokeratology using rigid lenses has been attempted by El Hage and Baker (1986) and Karlin (1986). El Hage and Baker fitted a lens with a flat central curve and a steep periphery of radius of curvature 0.75 mm less than the BOZR. They aimed to apply controllable pressure on the corneal periphery to achieve a new quasi-spherical corneal shape and reduce the hypermetropia of patients over-corrected by the RK. Forced keratoreformation by a tight lens would increase the risk of corneal oedema and irregular astigmatism related to the decreased mechanical stability of the cornea. Astin (1991) showed that, even several years postoperatively, certain patients can experience flattening of the central cornea and reduction of residual myopia, even wearing correctly fitted lenses aimed to cause least corneal stress. Edwards and Schaefer (1987) also noted corneal flattening following soft lens wear.

The structure and function of the cornea is disturbed by radial keratotomy (Bores *et al.*, 1981; Rowsey & Balyeat, 1982) and risks of keratitis, persistant corneal oedema and infections are increased (Waring, 1984). Contact lens wear on the RK eye increases the risk of corneal disturbance and infection, particularly if the lens is tight, overworn, or of poor condition or the lens hygiene is inadequate. A number of complications of lens wear after RK have been described including the increased incidence of neovascularization along the radial scars after soft and extended contact lens wear (Bores *et al.*, 1981; Katz *et al.*, 1982; Anderson, 1988; Ruben & Chu, 1989).

36.9   PHOTOABLATION BY EXCIMER LASER

As yet, this method has only had a short trial so there are few patients fitted with contact lenses for residual ametropia. As the ocular use of lasers developed, several investigations into the effects of excimer laser surgery on the cornea arose (e.g. Trokel *et al.*, 1983; Marshall *et al.*, 1985, 1986; Puliafito *et al.*, 1985; Seiler *et al.*, 1988). The results of two trials by McDonald *et al.* (1990a,b), one on monkeys, the other on blind human eyes, indicated that excimer laser corneal photoablation produced moderate power changes and central flattening, which regressed then stabilized 17 weeks later. Good healing and long-term corneal clarity were shown. Residual myopia was corrected by a repeat procedure. The diameter of the ablated area was 4.0 to 5.0 mm. For a 4.0 mm diameter ablation zone, the tissue depth removed ranged from 11 µm (–2.0 dioptres) to 46 µm (–8.0 dioptres). The greater the refractive change the less predictable the result. Wound healing studies have shown two healing phases, the first being re-epithelialisation followed by stromal remodelling involving epithelial and polymorphonuclear (PMN) cells; the second occuring approximately 33 days postoperatively, which revealed between the epithelium and the stroma the emergence of a combined layer of epithelial cells, keratocytes and PMN (Marshall *et al.*, 1988; Courant *et al.*, 1990; Fantes *et al.*, 1990; Malley *et al.*, 1990).

Little is known of the long-term effects of deprivation of Bowman's membrane and whether this may reduce resistance to infection, therefore it is unwise to subject the eye to contact lens wear, with the accompanying risk of lens related epithelial erosion, oedema and disturbance. Keratometry only measures the central flattened corneal region, so peripheral measurements using the keratoscope would give some guidance. A thin hydrophilic lens would easily drape over the unusual corneal contour. A rigid gas permeable lens would bridge over the central ablated corneal zone, retaining a positive powered tear lens beneath, so the contact lens will need extra negative power. As following other refractive surgery, good lens quality, fit and oxygen transmission are essential.

ACKNOWLEDGEMENTS

Thanks are due to Mr J.K. Dart FRCS, for his valuable advice, and to Miss S. Hickson MBCO for assistance with the literature search.

REFERENCES

Anderson, A.E. (1988) A fundamental approach to post radial keratotomy contact lens fitting. *C.L. Forum*, **December**, 46–8.

Astin, C.L.K. (1985) The use of Saturn II lenses following penetrating keratoplasty. *Trans. Br. C.L. Assoc. Conf.*, 2–5.

Astin, C.L.K. (1986) Considerations in fitting contact lenses to patients who have undergone radial keratotomy. *Trans. Br. C.L. Assoc. Conf.* 2–7.

Astin, C.L.K. (1989) Contact lenses in abnormal conditions – Post radial keratotomy. In *Contact Lenses*. (eds. A.J. Phillips and J. Stone), Butterworths, London, pp.772–82.

Astin, C.L.K. (1990) Fitting corneal grafts-some unusual cases. *J. Br. C.L. Assoc.*, **13** (1), 88–90.

Astin, C.L.K. (1991) Keratoreformation by contact lenses after radial keratotomy. *Ophthal. Physiol. Optic. J.*, **11**, 1.

Baikoff, G., Joly, P., Arne, J.L. *et al.* (1989) *Surgical correction of high myopia with A.C. lenses in phakic eyes (survey of 100 cases in a multicentre study)*. A.R.C.S., Washington.

Barraquer, J.I. (1981) Keratomileusis for myopia and aphakia. *Ophthalmology*, **88**, 701–8.

Baumgartner, S.D. and Binder, P.S. (1985) Refractive keratoplasty. The histopathology of clinical specimens. *Ophthalmology*, **92**, 1606–15.

Baumgartner, S.D., Zavala, E.Y. and Binder, P.S. (1984) Refractive keratoplasty, keratophakia in a nonhuman primate. *Arch. Ophthalmol.*, **102**, 1671–5.

Beekhuis, W.H., McCarey, B.E., Waring, G.O. and Van Rij, G. (1986) Hydrogel keratophakia: a microkeratome dissection in the monkey model. *Br. J. Ophthalmol.*, **70**, 192–8.

Bores, L.D., Myers, W. and Cowden, J. (1981) Radial keratotomy – an analysis of the American experience. *Ann. Ophthalmol.*, **13** (8), 941–8.

Bosc, J.M., Montard, M., Delbosc, B. *et al.* (1990) Keratomileusis myopique non gel. *J. Fr. Ophtalmol.*, **13** (1/2), 10–16.

Buckley, R.J. (1985) Healthy corneal endothelium and the effects of intraocular surgery. *Trans. Ophthalmol. Soc. U.K.*, **104**, 687–92.

Choyce, D.P. (1985) The correction of refractive errors with polysulphone corneal inlays. *Trans. Ophthalmol. Soc. U.K.*, **104**, 332–42.

Climenhaga, H., Macdonald, J.M., McCarey, B.E. and Waring, G.O. (1988) Effect of diameter and depth on the response to solid polysulphone intracorneal lenses in cats. *Arch. Ophthalmol.*, **106**, 818–24.

Constad, W.H. (1988) Fitting post-op keratoplasty patients with RGP contact lenses. *Contact Lens Forum.*, **December**, 40–3.

Courant, D., Fritsch, P., Azema, A. *et al.* (1990) Corneal wound healing after photokeratomileusis treatment on the primate eye. *Laser and Light in Ophthalmology*, **3** (3), 187–99.

Durrie, D.S., Habrich, D.L. and Dietze, T.R. (1987) Secondary intraocular lens implantation vs epikeratophakia for the treatment of aphakia. *Am. J. Ophthalmol.*, **103**, 384–91.

Edwards, G.A. and Schaefer, M.K. (1987) Corneal flattening associated with daily wear soft contact lenses following radial keratotomy. *J. Refract. Surg.*, **3**, 54–8.

Eggink, F.A.G. and Beekhuis, W.H. (1989) Adaptation de lentilles de contact apres keratotomie radiaire. *Contactologia*, **11F**, 164–8.

El Hage, S. and Baker, R.N. (1986) Controlled keratoreformation for postoperative radial kera-

radial keratotomy. *C.L. Forum*, **December**, 38–9.

Shivitz, I.A., Russell, B.M., Arrowsmith, P.N. and Marks, R.G. (1986) Optical correction of postoperative radial keratotomy patients with contact lenses. *C.L.A.O. J.*, **12**, 59–62.

Shivitz, I.A., Arrowsmith, P.N. and Russell, B.M. (1987) Contact lenses in the treatment of patients with overcorrected radial keratotomy. *Ophthalmology*, **94**(8), 899–903.

Shovlin, J.P. (1989) The use of alloplastics: a new realm of refractive surgery? *Int. C.L. Clin.*, **16**(10), 304–6.

Stern, G.A. (1988), Update on the medical management of corneal and external eye diseases, corneal transplantation and keratorefractive surgery. *Ophthalmology*, **95**(6), 842–53.

Swinger, CA., Krumeich, J. and Cassiday, D. (1986) Planar lamellar refractive keratoplasty. *J. Refract. Surg.*, **2**, 17–24.

Trokel, S.L., Srinivasan, R. aand Braren, B. (1983) Excimer laser surgery of the cornea. *Am. J. Ophthalmol.*, **96**, 701–15.

Verity, S.M., Hansen, J. and Kaufman, H.E. (1986) Preliminary results of toric epikeratophakia. *Invest. Ophthalmol. Vis. Sci.*, **27** (Suppl.), 14.

Vickery, J.A. (1986), Post radial keratotomy and the soft lens. *C.L. Forum.*, **October**, 34–5.

Waring, G.O. III. (1984) Evolution of radial keratotomy for myopia. *Trans. Ophthal. Soc. U.K.*, **104**, 28–42.

Watsky, M.A., McCarey, B.E. and Beekhuis, W.H. (1985) Predicting refractive alterations with hydrogel keratophakia. *Invest. Ophthalmol. Vis. Sci.*, **26**, 240–3.

Werblin, T.P. and Klyce, S.D. (1981) Epikeratophakia: the surgical correction of myopia. I. Lathing of corneal tissue. *Current Eye Research*, **1**(10), 591–7.

Werblin, I.P., Kaufman, H.E., Friedlander, M.H. and McDonald, M.B. (1982) Epikeratophakia: The surgical correction of aphakia. III. update 1981. *Ophthalmology*, **89**, 916–20.

Werblin, T.P., Fryczkowski, A.W. and Peiffer, R.L. (1984) Myopic correction using alloplastic implants in nonhuman primates – a preliminary report. *Ann. Ophthalmol.*, **16**(12), 1127–30.

Woodward, E.G. (1981) Contact lens fitting after keratoplasty. *J. Br. C. L. Assoc.*, **4**(2), 42–9.

Zavala, E.Y., Krumeich, J. and Binder, P.S. (1987) Laboratory evaluation of freeze vs nonfreeze lamellar refractive keratoplasty. *Arch. Ophthalmol.*, **105**, 1125–8.

ORTHOKERATOLOGY

L.G. Carney

37.1 HISTORICAL PERSPECTIVES

Techniques to either halt the progression of myopia or to eliminate existing myopia have long been sought after. There are patients who have a strong desire to be able to function effectively without the need for their refractive error correction, and many are prepared to go to extraordinary lengths to achieve this. Techniques such as crystalline lens extraction, scleral reinforcement and the like were in (limited) use long before the current interest in emmetropization became apparent.

The refractive state of the eye is, of course, not dependent on a single factor, but rather it reflects the interaction of a series of optical variables. However, the fact that the anterior corneal surface is by far the most powerful refractive element and is also an easily accessible tissue has made it attractive as a means of manipulating refractive errors (Hirsch, 1965).

It is a well-established fact that the wearing of contact lenses, particularly PMMA lenses, and also rigid gas permeable lenses can induce changes in corneal curvature, refractive error and visual acuity. In routine contact lens fittings, such changes would be considered an undesirable side effect and, indeed, an indication of a misfitting lens, being one of the precursors to spectacle blur. Changes in corneal curvature and refractive error of as much as 2.50 D were commonly reported: occasionally large amounts of corneal astigmatism, up to 6.00 D, were found (Hartstein, 1965). Both the nature of the changes and their causes have been investigated in detail, but are still not completely defined. The original clinical impression that there was often a myopia reduction from normal rigid contact lens wear was investigated but not totally borne out. Nevertheless, the recognition of these changes led ultimately to the notion of purposeful manipulation of corneal shape (Coon, 1982).

It was in 1962 that Jessen formalized the idea with a description of his efforts to induce useful corneal shape changes. Orthokeratology was eventually defined as the 'reduction, modification or elimination of a visual defect by the programmed application of contact lenses'. In response to the critical scrutiny that their claims aroused, most orthokeratology descriptions now tend to emphasize the reduction or modification, rather than elimination, of refractive errors (Paige, 1985).

Since the formation of the Society of Orthokeratology in 1962, an extensive literature has developed, but, as described below, it is often an unsatisfactory literature. A multiplicity of techniques have been described, many evolving as empirical solutions to difficulties as they arise. In recent times, however, several extensive studies of the procedures have been completed.

It has been suggested that orthokeratology, in its use of contact lenses as 'splints', should

Contact Lens Practice. Edited by Montague Ruben and Michel Guillon.
Published in 1994 by Chapman & Hall, London. ISBN 0 412 35120 X

be considered a 'surgical therapy', and hence it is an inappropriate technique for the treatment of a condition that is 'neither a disease nor a deformity' (Safir, 1980). However, this is not a commonly accepted opinion, particularly given the current emphasis on true surgical procedures included in keratorefractive surgery. Stated broadly, orthokeratology is not a therapeutic treatment of myopia, but only an attempt to control corneal shape through a vision correction appliance. In describing the procedures of orthokeratology and then reviewing its successes and limitations, it is worthwhile to bear in mind the alternatives. The efficacy, complications and ethics of the use of this procedure all need to be seen in the light of the desire of some patients to function free of the need for refractive error corrections and the individual practitioner's analysis of the costs and benefits of the alternatives.

37.2   OBJECTIVES

The objectives of orthokeratology, along with the principles of its action, would seem clear enough. However, both have undergone revision throughout the development of the procedures. The early 'orthofocus' techniques of Jessen (1962) and colleagues had the precisely stated objective of producing a long-standing emmetropic state. This was subsequently 'softened' to the perhaps more achievable objective of a reduction or modification of the existing refractive status. More recently, the better recognition of the limits of the refractive changes achieved, both in magnitude and permanence, has been incorporated in the more usual notion of reduction or elimination of the lower errors coupled with the halting of the progression of development of higher errors (Paige, 1985). The role of factors other than central corneal radius of curvature changes has further clouded the specific objectives.

More generally, then, the aim of orthokera-

tology can be considered as the attempt to exert *some control* over refractive error, primarily by encouraging useful corneal shape changes.

37.3   TECHNIQUES

One of the striking facts in the orthokeratology literature is the multiplicity of techniques advocated. This could perhaps be considered a strength of the process, in that it then is presumably not very practitioner dependent. However, in reviewing the principles and achievements of orthokeratology, it must more properly be considered a weakness. The absence of a strong theoretical basis on which to proceed is a heritage of the empirical beginnings of the technique. Whenever a procedure such as this seeks to attain the status of routine clinical practice, there should first be an identification of those variables that influence the success or otherwise of the procedure, and its predictability. This apparently has not been achieved in orthokeratology. This variability of technique also hinders proper analysis of the described achievements.

To demonstrate this variability of technique, some lens fitting features utilized over the years by a series of orthokeratologists are listed in Table 37.1.

It becomes clear from this compilation that a large range of lens parameters could be utilized in an orthokeratology fitting. This variability in lens design, yet still followed by the production of desirable refractive changes, is in keeping with the lack of success in identifying the influential lens parameters. In particular, the large range of base curve/corneal curvature relationships needs to be borne in mind when assessing the mode of action of these lens fittings.

The empirical adoption of adjunct procedures such as the use of a low calcium diet (Nolan, 1971) does little to encourage confi-

Table 37.1 Some relevant characteristics of a series of orthokeratology fitting techniques

Author	Base Curve	Lens Diameter	Lens Changes
Jessen (1962)	Plano lens: tear layer corrects myopia	7.6 to 9.2 mm	None
Nolan (1971)	As for Jessen, if myopia < −2.25 D	7.7 to 9.8 mm	Alter wearing time; retain lens fit
Paige (1981)	(i) As for Nolan (Plus lens increment) (ii) on K to 0.75 D flat	8.6 to 8.8 mm	Alternate these two lenses
Neilson, *et al.* (1964)	0.12 D to 0.37 D flat	Base curve +1.3 mm (8.5 to 10.2 mm)	Flatten 0.50 D
May and Grant (1977)	Alignment fit (base on PEK)	Base curve +1.8 mm (8.5 to 10.2)	When 0.25 D change occurs
Gates (1971)	1.50 D flat	8.7 to 9.6 mm	No lens changes; retainer lenses when error is 0.50 D
Fontana (1972)	One-piece bifocal, central zone 1.00 D flat	9.6 mm	Flatten 1.00 D
Ziff (1976)	On K to 1.00 D flat	8.8 mm	When K changes, or to induce change
Nolan (1972)	1.00 to 1.50 D steep	7.5 to 8.5 mm	Flatten 0.25 D to 0.50 D
Coon (1984)	Alignment	OZD=70% of lens area	Reduce OZD
Carter (1977)	1.00 to 1.50 D flat	8.9 to 9.3 mm	CAB lenses; re-fit when cornea flattens 0.50 D
Harris and Stoyan (1992)	1.00 to 1.50 D flat	9.5 mm	Moderate to high *Dk* material; flatten 0.50 D

dence in the techniques as being theoretically sound.

Attempts have been made to identify the common features among these fittings, but other than the need for relatively thick, dimensionally stable lenses, little is evident (Watkins, 1977).

There are few detailed reports of the use of rigid gas permeable contact lenses for orthokeratology. The information available does suggest that their use has the same effectiveness as for PMMA lenses. The crucial aspect in lens choice for orthokeratology is not oxygen availability, but the use of an appropriate lens design (Buffington & Lilley, 1989; Paige & Mustaler, 1986). Harris and Stoyan (1992) suggested that a myopia reduction of up to 5.00 D or 6.00 D could be achieved with an 'Ortho–K3' design (with an intermediate zone that is 3.00 D steeper than the base curve) in a rigid gas permeable material of moderate to high oxygen permeability, although the average change reported for eight patients was still only 2.00 D. An additional suggested application of rigid gas permeable lenses is the elimination by orthokeratology of any residual refractive errors after radial keratotomy procedures (Buffington, 1988).

Several 'timing' aspects of orthokeratology fittings also reveal marked differences in approach. There is variability, for example, in opinion as to when changes in lens fittings should be made. While some would suggest that a new lens design is to be used only when there has been a desirable refractive and corneal shape change, others would suggest that in the absence of such changes, a thicker or flatter lens is to be used with the express purpose of better inducing these changes (Ziff, 1976). The number and timing of lens re-fittings also vary with the practitioner; suggestions of re-fitting intervals from 6 weeks to 6 months are common. The overall duration of the program could typically be from 1 to 2 years, although other possibilities are given. This last feature is dependent on the practitioner's perception of the stabilization of these changes, and is inter-related to the need for and use of retainer lenses, to be discussed below.

37.4 THE ACHIEVEMENTS

Before looking at the results of the experimental studies, the achievements of an orthokeratology fitting program can first be assessed by a review of the reported desirable changes and their magnitude. The influences of time since lens removal and retainer lens use will be considered separately. The problems associated with much of the literature here, namely the frequent dependence on individual case reports and the use of incomplete and inconsistent data, have been commented upon often (Polse, 1977; Binder *et al.*, 1980). However, numerous reports do

not give sufficient information to gain an understanding of the expectations of those using an orthokeratology program.

Isolated case reports have documented myopia decreases of as much as 4.00 D, resulting in 20/20 unaided vision. However, the average refractive error change to be expected is quite probably considerably less than this. As shown in Table 37.2, the usual decrease in myopia is approximately 1.00 D to 2.00 D. This value is in keeping with an Orthokeratology Position Paper (1981). The absolute limits of the refractive error changes are most often given as 4.00 D myopia, 2.50 D astigmatism (axis direction not always stated) and 2.00 D hyperopia. However, the practical values for astigmatic correction, and certainly hyperopic correction, are difficult to determine because of the scarcity of the data.

The values of the keratometric changes in corneal curvature are given on average as about 1.00 D of flattening in the correction of myopia (Table 37.2). This dioptric value is less than that of the refractive changes, as discussed later. Astigmatism is often diminished as the cornea becomes more spherical in form, although the induction of significant amounts of corneal astigmatism is often an acknowledged difficulty.

Table 37.2 Refractive error, corneal curvature and unaided vision changes through orthokeratology fittings

Author	Refractive Error Decrease (D)	Corneal Curvature Decrease (D)	Unaided Vision Increase* (Snellen Lines)
Neilson *et al* (1964)	0.75	1.12	8
Grant & May (1971)	0.92	1.36	7.1
May & Grant (1977)	2.00	1.25	9
Harris (1978)	2.00	1.25	9
Freeman (1976)	1.63	0.82	–
Kirscher (1976)	1.25	0.81	–
Patterson (1975)	1.15	0.94	–
Coon (1984)	0.73	0.03	5.5
Harris & Stoyan (1992)	2.00	1.12	7.2

* Unspecified often as to test target configuration.

The resulting unaided vision from these orthokeratology procedures is, of course, a function also of the original magnitude of ametropia. As such, it varies in most studies from 20/20 to 20/100. It might have been more useful to always consider these changes in terms of visual improvement, but the lack of standardized testing procedures precludes this having much value. 'Lines of vision' improvement cannot be adequately interpreted. The occasionally used practice of supplying the patient with a letter chart seriously confounds subsequent vision testing (Fontana, 1972).

All of these changes are influenced by an understanding of their permanence and stability, but are considered here without indication of any regression or the need for retainer lenses.

37.5 SOME DIFFICULTIES AND THEIR MANAGEMENT

It is repeatedly stated in the orthokeratology literature that it is a safe procedure, without risk. Contact lenses are, however, well known to have occasional complications associated with their use and can compromise corneal integrity. The question, then, is whether there is any *greater* risk when an orthokeratology fitting procedure is adopted.

There appear to be no reports, by either opponents or proponents, of pathological complications during the orthokeratology procedure. The fact that repeated monitoring and re-fitting of the patient is taking place should influence this. When such examinations are carried out frequently and conscientiously, then the development of any potentially serious changes would be recognized early and appropriate action taken. Perhaps, then, a more appropriate question to consider is whether significant numbers of patients need to discontinue use of their lenses because of a developing loss of corneal integrity. Although general information on this is unavailable, one aspect which has received scrutiny is the appearance of corneal distortion.

The occurrence of corneal warping is an occasional complication of routine contact lens wear, and one that can be difficult to manage. Rigid lenses, particularly if misfitted, are known to be able to induce large amounts of predominantly with-the-rule or irregular astigmatism, which can be semi-permanent (Hartstein, 1965). Such astigmatic changes have been recognized as an undesirable side-effect of orthokeratology fittings, most noticeably with poorly centering lenses. Techniques for its management have included the use of reverse toric lens designs (Fontana, 1978) and the more exotic one of having the patient looking repeatedly from side to side to mimic in the horizontal meridian the vertical action of the lids on the lens (Paige, 1976).

Perhaps the major criticism of orthokeratology has been not the ability to induce refractive changes or their predictability (although these are both of concern), but rather the permanence and stability of any changes. From the work of orthokeratologists, it soon became clear that, in the majority of cases, any desirable refractive changes dissipated in time if contact lens wear ceased totally. This is in agreement with the work of Rengstorff (1967) for more routine contact lens fittings. The technique adopted to counteract such effects was to *not* cease contact lens wear, but rather reduce the lens wearing time. The use of 'retainer' lenses was modified in individual cases so that the least wearing time compatible with the maintenance of maximum refractive changes was sought.

Some practitioners have advocated the use of retainer lenses during sleep. The availability of rigid gas permeable lenses has made the overnight use of rigid contact lenses as retainer lenses, or even as the primary orthokeratology procedure, a more realistic one. This is a more physiologically justified technique than in the case of PMMA lenses.

Various wearing schemes have evolved around the overnight application of contact lenses. For example, Paige and Mustaler (1986) recommend the fitting of rigid gas permeable lenses to both eyes of the patient, with one lens being worn on a daily-wear basis and the second lens worn on an extended wear basis. Alternation of which eye wore the lens overnight was used to produce optimum orthokeratology effects.

There is no consensus on what constitutes the best fitting of a retainer lens. It is acknowledged, however, that the majority of patients need to wear such lenses on a regular basis. Opponents of the orthokeratology process point out that this seems to defeat the objective of freedom from refractive correction; supporters counter that there are still periods of improved unaided vision which may be socially or occupationally of benefit (Paige, 1985).

37.6 UNDERSTANDING THE OBSERVATIONS

The relationship of the observed keratometry changes to those of the refractive errors is a topic that has been debated. The ratio of these changes has been variously determined as 1:1 through 1:5. This has led to the suggestion that there may be other quite potent inputs to the refractive changes besides that of corneal curvature. Corneal thickness, anterior chamber depth, axial length, ciliary tonus and intraocular pressure have all been proposed. Not only does it become difficult to substantiate these changes or establish mechanisms of action, but it is probably not necessary to evoke them. The major influence of contact lens wearing, at least in the mature eye, is a corneal one, particularly acting on anterior corneal topography. Studies finding an imbalance between anterior corneal curvature and refractive error changes are typically dependent on keratometry findings, and fail to consider the irregular topographical

changes likely to result from these mechanical manipulations (Erickson, 1978). Other difficulties inherent in establishing a curvature/refraction relationship include the use of an assumed but constant calibration refractive index for keratometry, spectacle lens effectivity changes, and the sometimes neglected need for meridional analysis of these changes.

There has also from time to time been conflict over the magnitude of vision improvement compared to the refractive changes. These reports often suffer from a lack of standardization of the vision tests, as mentioned above, and also from probable practice effects and possible bias from their unmasked nature.

A difficulty impeding a more general acceptance of orthokeratology has been the lack of predictability of the effects. Routine fitting of corneal contact lenses has shown that any given base curve/corneal curvature relationship can variously produce corneal flattening or steepening and astigmatic increase or decrease (Bailey & Carney, 1977). Since there is then no obligatory response, controlling the appropriate corneal change is not a precise procedure. While the direction of change can be somewhat variable, the magnitude of any changes shows extreme individual variations. And finally, the likelihood and magnitude of regression to the original refractive state is also not yet well-defined. Some of the influences on these changes can be inferred, but there remains a substantial individual effect, leading to unpredictability of results.

Of those influences on the refractive changes that have been investigated, the base curve/corneal curvature relationship is the best established. The variability of successful techniques and the results on predictability just mentioned both indicate, however, its lack of universality. Other influences, both ocular (such as ocular rigidity, blinking behavior) and of the contact lens (such as lens diameter, lens mass), have been investigated, again without conclusive results. The complexity of these influences and the individuality of the corneal response culminate in the unpredictability of the process. While peripheral corneal analysis has indicated a lack of responsiveness if corneal shape is spherical (Freeman, 1976), the fact that subsequent peripheral corneal changes do not correlate well with refractive changes makes interpretation difficult. This means that appropriate guidelines for patient selection are necessarily unavailable or imprecise. One can gauge, from the pre-fitting refractive error and visual acuity, the *average* residual error and unaided vision likely to result. It is only from the practitioner's judgment that the likelihood of any given patient achieving these results can be assessed, and with what combination of fitting and management characteristics it would be achieved.

37.7 SOME INDEPENDENT STUDIES

Most of the orthokeratology literature, as one would expect, has come from those committed to the program as a safe and effective one. The lack of impartial research, with appropriate experimental design, statistical analysis and interpretation of results, has been a source of controversy. This need has been addressed in more recent times by several studies.

When the efficacy of a treatment procedure is in dispute, there are certain basic principles of the experimental design needed to provide a result that is scientifically and clinically valid. Amongst these are the use of control populations, masking procedures to avoid bias, matching of sample populations, randomizing treatments and using adequate sample sizes. In the case of an orthokeratology investigation, the timing and nature of the 'treatment' and the management of attrition from the population are crucial additional considerations. Not all factors have always been appropriately managed.

The first comprehensive study was that of Kerns (1976/78), whose extensive work, while drawing criticisms on some aspects of the experimental design, did give a more substantial basis on which to evaluate the capabilities and limitations of orthokeratology. He used three patient groups: 3 patients wearing spectacles, 13 patients wearing conventional contact lenses and 18 patients undergoing the orthokeratology program. Those in the orthokeratology group at first wore conventional contact lenses, then wore lenses fitted according to the general principles of Neilson *et al.* (1964) for an average of about 1000 days, and finally underwent recovery without contact lens wear. Only the results for the orthokeratology group are summarized here.

The findings for these changes in refractive error (spherical equivalent), horizontal and vertical keratometry, and unaided vision (Snellen lines) at the end of the orthokeratology treatment and following recovery are shown in Table 37.3.

Kerns was able to show that myopia was reduced, the major change being in the first 300 days; unaided vision also was improved,

Table 37.3 Summary of some results from study by Kerns (1976–78)

	At Completion of Orthokeratology Phase	At Completion of Recovery Phase
Change in refractive error (spherical equivalent)	0.98 D (decrease)	0.60 D (decrease)
Change in horizontal keratometry	0.63 D (decrease)	0.39 D (decrease)
Change in vertical keratometry	0.15 D (increase)	0.41 D (increase)
Change in unaided vision (Snellen lines)	4.29 (improvement)	3.09 (improvement)

the major change being in the first 200 days. However, two eyes appeared to show little effect; six eyes developed corneal astigmatism to such an extent that those patients were removed from the program; and following the total cessation of lens wear (not the usual orthokeratology procedure) the refractive error and unaided vision improvements quickly began to dissipate. At 56 days after lens removal, one eye had a plano refraction and two eyes achieved 20/20.

Binder *et al.* (1980) reported a masked study involving 20 patients undergoing orthokeratology and 10 conventional contact lens fittings. When those undergoing orthokeratology reached the retainer lens stage, the lenses were removed for six months. There was a substantial improvement in unaided vision and refractive error. Of these patients, 55% were able to achieve at least 20/25 and 70% were able to achieve at least 20/40 at some time in the program. Although corneal astigmatism was increased, it was not as marked a change as reported by Kerns. These authors found that their population could be divided into three subgroups: five patients failed to respond to the treatment, six showed a partial response, and nine showed a good response. Again, there was a rapid return towards baseline values when lens wear ceased.

The Berkely orthokeratology study (Brand *et al.*, 1983; Polse *et al.*, 1983a, b) again used treatment and control contact lens groups. Those in the orthokeratology program underwent adaptation to lenses for an aver-

age of 2.3 months, orthokeratology treatment for 1 year, gradual lens withdrawal for an average of 26.4 days, and final monitoring for an average of 68.6 days. Thirty patients completed this program, and results for changes in refractive error (spherical equivalent), horizontal and vertical keratometry, and unaided vision (log of the minimum angle of resolution) at the end of the orthokeratology treatment and at recovery are shown in Table 37.4. Polse and colleagues (1983a, b) conclude that myopia is reduced by an average of approximately 1.00 D; this is not permanent, and undergoes recovery; no large shifts in corneal astigmatism were observed.

These studies also contain comments on the quality of vision resulting from the refractive error shifts. The vision changes are reported both as variable and producing visual results subjectively described as of diminished quality.

37.8   MYOPIA CONTROL IN CHILDREN

Orthokeratology attempts to reduce or eliminate refractive error in adults or children. In the case of children, however, little published information is available to assess the suitability of these refractive error reduction techniques, as distinct from the fortuitous halting of the progression of myopia. Roth (1980) found that a controlled refractive error reduction was possible in only a few specific cases.

Another quite distinct application of rigid contact lenses is in the control of myopia

Table 37.4 Summary of some results from Berkeley orthokeratology study

	At Completion of Orthokeratology Phase	At Completion of Recovery Phase
Change in refractive error (spherical equivalent)	0.97 D (decrease)	0.19 D (decrease)
Change in horizontal keratometry	0.52 D (decrease)	0.09 D (decrease)
Change in vertical keratometry	0.38 D (decrease)	0.03 D (decrease)
Change in unaided vision (log minimum angle of resolution)	0.26 (improvement)	0.06 (improvement)

development in children. Here the aim is not necessarily to reduce the myopia, but rather to prevent the progression of myopia. Anecdotal reports of such an effect of contact lens wear were common in the early contact lens literature, although the need for properly controlled studies was soon recognized.

An early detailed study of this effect of contact lens wear was by Kelly *et al.* (1975), who found a positive effect of contact lenses on myopia progression. On the other hand, Baldwin *et al.* (1969) had found only minor differences between contact lens wearers and spectacle wearers.

Perhaps the most detailed and well-controlled study of this possible advantage of contact lens wear was by Stone (1976) who found that rigid contact lenses did indeed have a retarding effect on myopia development, but the effect was small (about 0.22 D per year less increase in myopia in contact lens wearers).

Rigid gas permeable contact lenses were used in a recently reported study on myopia control (Grosvenor *et al.* 1991). This study generally confirmed the findings of Stone (1976), who had used PMMA lenses. After 44 months of contact lens wear, myopia increased by only 0.76 D. Within 2.5 months of ceasing lens wear, a further 0.27 D increase occured. When contact lens wear was resumed, a 0.02 D decrease in myopia occured over the following 8 months. These authors also confirm Stone's contention that the slowing of myopia progression in children is only partially explained by corneal curvature changes as measured by keratometry, but believe it is directly related to apical curvature changes.

A positive effect of rigid contact lenses, both PMMA and gas permeable, on myopia development in children is therefore likely. However, the use of rigid contact lenses in the young brings with it the risk of unwanted side-effects. Careful monitoring both of corneal integrity and of regularity of the corneal shape is essential.

37.9 SURGICAL ALTERNATIVES: A COMPARISON OF EFFICACY

There is a long history of surgical interventions to induce refractive changes. However, over the last few years the field of keratorefractive surgery had expanded dramatically, both in terms of its options and its general acceptance. A comparison of the results achieved by some of these surgical techniques with those from orthokeratology is thus worthwhile, and keeps orthokeratology practice in perspective. Such a comparison, for myopic corrections only and for the more prominent procedures only, is given in Table 37.5.

Efficacy of the procedures is an important issue, but safety aspects should also be addressed. A complete discussion of this is beyond the scope of this chaper, but all procedures have significant complications associated with them. Under- and over-corrections of the refractive error occur as do instabilities of the refractive correction. As well, pathological complications, including vascularization, epithelial damage, perforations and infection, have been reported.

In comparison to orthokeratology, the range of possible refractive corrections is certainly greater with keratorefractive surgery, but inaccuracy and instability of the refractive correction occur, and the scope and incidence of complications must be considered.

37.10 THE BALANCE SHEET

The achievements and limitations of orthokeratology are now becoming more evident. In many cases, it is possible to effect a reduction in the amount of myopia. This appears to be, on average, about a 1.50 D change; larger changes have been reported, up to 4.00 D, but these are isolated cases and may be at the expense of visual quality. Associated with this is an improvement in unaided vision. The possibilities for correc-

Table 37.5 Some comparative results of representative orthokeratology and refractive surgery studies for the correction of myopia

Technique	Condition	Baseline refractive error (D)	Change in keratometry	Change in refractive error (D)	Reference
Orthokeratology	At completion of orthokeratology phase	−2.70 ± 1.13	0.45	0.97	Brand *et al.* (1983)
Orthokeratology	At completion of recovery phase	−2.70 ± 1.13	0.06	0.19	Brand *et al.* (1983)
Radial keratotomy	1 year post-surgery	−2.00 to −3.12	2.54 ± 0.85	2.73 ± 0.84	Waring *et al.* (1985)
Radial keratotomy	1 year post-surgery	−3.25 to −4.37	2.85 ± 1.01	3.41 ± 1.16	Waring *et al.* (1985)
Radial keratotomy	1 year post-surgery	−4.50 to −8.00	3.47 ± 1.17	4.49 ± 1.39	Waring *et al.* (1985)
Radial keratotomy	3 years post-surgery	−2.00 to −3.12	2.81 ± 0.90	2.84 ± 0.97	Waring *et al.* (1987)
Radial keratotomy	3 years post-surgery	−3.25 to −4.37	3.14 ± 1.20	3.66 ± 1.31	Waring *et al.* (1987)
Radial keratotomy	3 years post-surgery	−4.50 to −8.00	3.70 ± 1.27	4.69 ± 1.71	Waring *et al.* (1987)
Radial keratotomy	5 years post-surgery	−2.00 to −3.12	–	2.92 ± 1.10	Waring *et al.* (1991)
Radial keratotomy	5 years post-surgery	−3.25 to −4.37	–	3.84 ± 1.35	Waring *et al.* (1991)
Radial keratotomy	5 years post-surgery	−4.50 to −8.00	–	5.00 ± 1.79	Waring *et al.* (1991)
Myopic epikeratoplasty	3 months post-surgery	−14.00 ± 6.40	3.60	11.20	Lass *et al.* (1987)
Myopic epikeratoplasty	12 months post-surgery	−14.00 ± 6.40	3.20	6.30	Lass *et al.* (1987)
Photorefractive keratotomy	6 months post-surgery	−6.49	–	4.56	Sher *et al.* (1991)
Photorefractive keratotomy	6 months post-surgery	−11.59	6.14	10.69	Sher *et al.* (1991)
Photorefractive keratotomy	6 months post-surgery	−3.00	–	2.28 ±	Gartry *et al.* (1991)
Photorefractive keratotomy	6 months post-surgery	−6.00	–	3.72 ±	Gartry *et al.* (1991)

tion of hyperopic and astigmatic errors are less precisely defined.

There are, however, certain drawbacks evident from the use of these techniques. The sought after visual improvements do not always occur. It is probable that around 50% of patients will show useful changes; unfortunately, identification of those patients likely to show these responses is not easily achieved. Second, the visual improvements, when they occur, tend to be variable so that any given patient's unaided vision can fluctuate from day to day. Third, there is the possibility of corneal damage, particularly corneal warping, from the mechanical stresses placed upon it.

The topic of permanency is also crucial to an evaluation of orthokeratology's worth. The vast majority of patients will require ongoing use of contact lenses for part of most days. If lens wear totally ceases, recovery towards pre-fitting characteristics is usual and quick. Orthokeratologists would, nevertheless, maintain that the periods of non-retainer lens use are worthwhile ones.

The benefits of the treatment are, therefore, very real but very limited. Emmetropia can be achieved, but even for low-magnitude myopia it does not always follow and is rarely lasting. For higher values of refractive error, a limited improvement in unaided vision is the result. Persistence of these changes is not to be expected without continuing use of contact lenses. The means of achieving these changes are tedious, slow and costly. Both the control over the changes and guidelines for selection of patients and lenses are imprecise.

The viewpoint of certain patients that emmetropia, or at least improved unaided vision, as a goal worthy of considerable effort is exemplified by the current interest in the use of refractive surgery procedures. Indeed, orthokeratology has even been proposed as a means of managing under- or over-corrections resulting from such refractive surgery (Buffington, 1988). Orthokeratology will remain for some a useful means of pursuing this goal of improved unaided vision; prospective candidates must be made aware of its effectivess and its limitations.

REFERENCES

Bailey, I.L. and Carney, L.G. (1977) A survey of corneal curvature changes from corneal lens wear. *Contact Lens J.*, **6**(1), 3–13.

Baldwin, W.R., West, D., Jolley, J. and Reid, W. (1969) Effects of contact lenses on refractive, corneal and axial length changes in young myopes. *Am. J. Optom., Arch. Acad. Optom.*, **46**, 903–11.

Binder, P.S., May, C.H. and Grant, S.C. (1980) An evaluation of orthokeratology. *Ophthalmology*, **87**, 729–44.

Brand, R.J., Polse, K.A. and Schwalbe, J.S. (1983) The Berkely orthokeratology study, Part I: General conduct of the study. *Am. J. Optom. Physiol. Opt.*, **60**, 175–86.

Buffington, R.D. (1988) Orthokeratology and the post-RK patient. *Contact Lens Spectrum*, **3**(6), 71–3.

Buffington, R.D. and Lilley, J.Y. (1989) A predictable approach to orthokeratology. *Contact Lens Spectrum*, **4**(5), 67–9.

Carter, T. (1977) Gas-permeable lenses – orthokeratology. *Contacto*, **21**(4), 30–3.

Coon, L.J. (1982) Orthokeratology, Part I. Historical perspective. *J. Am. Optom. Assoc.*, **53**, 187–95.

Coon, L.J. (1984) Orthokeratology, part II. Evaluating the Tabb method. *J. Am. Optom. Assoc.*, **55**, 409–18.

Erickson, P.M. (1978) Accounting for refractive changes in orthokeratology. *Contacto*, **22**(5), 9–12.

Fontana, A. (1972) Orthokeratology using the one-piece bifocal. *Contacto*, **16**(2), 45–7.

Fontana, A. (1978) Using reverse cyclons to control or eliminate corneal astigmatism. *Contacto*, **22**(1), 21–2.

Freeman, R. (1976) Retainer wear in orthokeratology. *Optom. Weekly*, **67** 594–6.

Gartry, D.S., Kerr Muir, M.G., Lohmann, C.P. and Marshall, J. (1992) The effect of topical corticosteroids on refractive outcome and corneal haze after photorefractive keratectomy. *Arch. Ophthamol.*, **110**, 944–52.

Gates, R.C. (1971) Orthokeratology and the Air Force. *Contacto*, **15**(4), 8–16.

Grant, S.C. and May, C.H. (1971) Orthokeratology: Control of refractive errors through contact lenses. *J. Am. Optom. Assoc.*, **42**, 1277–83.

Grosvenor, T., Perrigin, J., Perrigin, D. and Quintero, S. (1981) Rigid gas permeable contact lenses for myopia control: Effects of discontinuation of lens wear. *Optom. Vis. Sci.*, **68**, 385–9.

Harris, D. (1978) Corneal changes in myopia reduction. *Contacto*, **22**(5), 26–33.

Harris, D.H. and Stoyan, N. (1992) A new approach to orthokeratology. *Contact Lens Spectrum*, **7**(4), 37–9.

Hartstein, J. (1965) Corneal warping due to wearing of corneal contact lenses. *Am. J. Ophthalmol.*, **60**, 1103–4.

Hirsch, M.J. (1965) The prevention and/or cure of myopia. *Am. J. Optom.*, **42**, 327–36.

Jessen, G.N. (1962) Orthofocus techniques. *Contacto*, **6**, 200–4.

Kelly, T.S., Chatfield, C. and Tustin, G. (1975) Clinical assessment of the arrest of myopia. *Br. J. Ophthalmol.*, **59**, 529–38.

Kerns, R. (1976/78) Research in orthokeratology, Parts 1 to 8. *J. Am. Optom. Assoc.*, **47**, 1047–51; **47**, 1275–85; **47**, 1505–15; **48**, 227–38; **47**, 345–59; **48**, 1134–47; **48**, 1541–53; **49**, 308–14.

Kirscher, D. (1976) Orthokeratology: Reduction of refractive error with contact lenses. *J. Orthokeratol.*, **2**, 47–60.

Lass, J.H., Stocker, G., Fritz, M.E. and Collie, D.M. (1987) Epikeratoplasty. *Ophthalmology*, **94**, 912–25.

May, C. H. and Grant, S.C. (1977a) A three-eyed view of orthokeratology. *Contact Lens Forum*, **2**(3), 33–40.

Neilson, R.H., Grant, S.C. and May, C.H. (1964) Emmetropization through contact lenses. *Contacto*, **8**(4), 20–1.

Nolan, J. (1971) Orthokeratology. *J. Am. Optom. Assoc.*, **42**, 355–60.

Nolan, J. (1972) Orthokeratology with steep lenses. *Contacto*, **16**(3), 31–7.

Orthokeratology position paper (1981) *Orthokeratology*, **5**, 126.

Paige, N. (1976) The use of transverse axial oscillatory ocular movements to prevent or reduce corneal astigmatism during orthokeratological processing. *Contacto*, **20**(6), 29–30.

Paige, N. (1981) Three-step orthokeratology: a simplified system. *Contacto*, **25**(3), 28–9.

Paige, N. (1985) Why ortho-K? *Contact Lens Forum*, **10**(11), 65–7.

Paige, N. and Mustaler, K.L. (1986) Orthokeratology: A retrospective study. *Contact Lens Spectrum*, **1**(9), 24–8.

Patterson, T.C. (1975) Orthokeratology: Changes to the corneal curvature and the effect on refractive power due to the saggital length change. *J. Am. Optom. Assoc.*, **46**, 719–29.

Polse, K.A. (1977) Orthokeratology as a clinical procedure. *Am. J. Optom. and Physiol. Opt.*, **54**, 345–6.

Polse, K.A., Brand, R.J., Schwalbe, J.S., Vastine, D.W. and Keener, R.J. (1983a) The Berkeley orthokeratology study, Part II: Efficacy and duration. *Am. J. Optom. Physiol. Opt.*, **60**, 187–98.

Polse, K.A., Brand, R.J., Vastine, D.W. and Schwalbe, J.S. (1983b) Corneal change accompanying orthokeratology. *Arch. Ophthalmol.*, **101**, 1873–8.

Rengstorff, R.H. (1967) Variations in myopia measurements: an after-effect observed with habitual wearers of contact lenses. *Am. J. Optom.*, **44**, 149–61.

Roth, H.W. (1980) Orthokeratology on children; experience with myopia progressiva. *Contact Lens J.*, **9**(8), 6–7.

Safir, A. (1980) Orthokeratology. A risky and unpredictable treatment for a benign condition. *Surv. Ophthalmol.*, **24**, 291; 298–302.

Sher, N.A., Barak, M., Daya, S., *et al.*, (1992) Excimer laser photorefractive keratectomy in high myopia. *Arch. Ophthalmol.*, **110**, 935–43.

Sher, N.A., Chan, V., Bowers, R.A., *et al.*; (1991) The use of the 193 nm excimer laser for myopic photorefractive keratectomy in sighted eyes. *Arch. Ophthalmol.*, **109**, 1525–30.

Stone, J. (1976) The possible influence of contact lenses on myopia. *Br. J. Physiol. Opt.*, **31**, 89–114.

Waring, G.O., Lynn, M.J., Gelander, H. *et al.* (1985) Results of the prospective evaluation of radial keratotomy (PERK) study one year after surgery. *Opthalmology*, **92**, 177–98.

Waring, G.O., Lynn, M.J., Culbertson, W. *et al.* (1987) Three-year results of the prospective evaluation of radial keratotomy (PERK) study. *Opthalmology*, **94**, 1339–54.

Waring, G.O., Lynn, M.J., Nizham, A., *et al.*, (1991) Results of the prospective evaluation of radial keratotomy (PERK) study five years after surgery. *Ophthalmology*, **98**, 1164–76.

Watkins, J.R. (1977) The one commonality among the various fitting techniques that make ortho-K work. *Contacto*, **21**(2), 26–31.

Ziff, S. (1976) Ziff orthokeratology procedures. *Optom. Weekly*, **67**, 430–4.

T.John, Eleanor F. Mobilia and K.R. Kenyon

38.1 INTRODUCTION

Therapeutic hydrophilic contact lenses have added a new dimension to the management of certain corneal diseases. Although soft contact lenses were developed primarily for correction of refractive errors, their usefulness as an optical bandage has been well established. These hydrogel lenses are soft and comfortable and are tolerated by most diseased corneas.

More than quarter of a century ago, Wichterle and Lim (1960) introduced the first hydrophilic soft contact lens. Four years later, Rycroft (1964) first commented on the usefulness of soft contact lenses in patients with ocular pemphigoid and Stevens–Johnson syndrome. Ruben, in 1966, used soft contact lenses in patients with pemphigoid. In the 1970s, numerous investigators (Leibowitz & Rosenthal, 1971; Gasset & Kaufman, 1970, 1971, 1973) reported various uses of therapeutic soft contact lenses in corneal diseases. As newer lenses are manufactured, they are studied clinically for their usefulness and advantages over existing lenses. The present-day lenses are far superior to those originally introduced in the 1960s and have greater clinical application in the treatment of ocular surface diseases.

38.2 THERAPEUTIC EFFECTS OF BANDAGE LENSES (FIG. 38.1)

1. Bandage soft contact lenses relieve ocular pain arising from exposure of nerve endings associated with corneal epithelial defects and the rubbing action of eyelids during blinking. Examples of such conditions include bullous keratopathy, recurrent corneal erosion and persistent epithelial defects. In addition, symptoms related to filamentary keratitis are relieved when a bandage lens is used, and the filaments often disappear.

2. Bandage lenses facilitate corneal epithelial healing in corneal ulceration and other epithelial defects by protecting the unstable ocular surface from the eyelids. By the same mechanism, they also prevent epithelial cell detachment from the anterior corneal stroma in cases of recurrent erosion.

3. Therapeutic lenses provide adequate hydration to the corneal surface. This is done by preventing ocular surface drying through evaporation and by providing a water reservoir, especially in lenses of high water content.

4. By replacing an irregular corneal surface with a smooth surface, the lens corrects anterior irregular astigmatism. Although these lenses are not fitted primarily for refractive purposes, they may improve vision under such conditions.

5. Following application of tissue adhesive to the cornea, the surface of the polymerized 'glue' is very irregular. A bandage lens covers this irregular surface, pro-

Contact Lens Practice. Edited by Montague Ruben and Michel Guillon.
Published in 1994 by Chapman & Hall, London. ISBN 0 412 35120 X

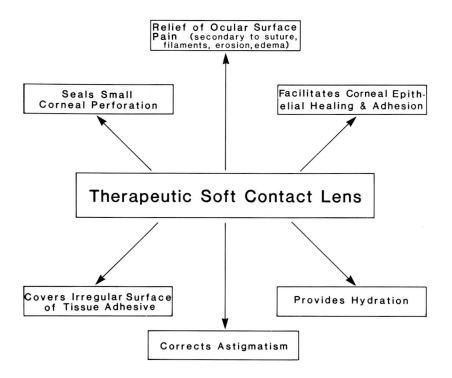

Figure 38.1 Therapeutic effects of bandage lenses.

vides comfort, and prevents the glue from being dislodged by blinking of the lids.

6. A small corneal perforation can be sealed by an appropriate therapeutic soft contact lens.

38.3 CLASSIFICATION OF THERAPEUTIC LENSES

The newer hydrogel materials developed during the last 20 years have resulted in three generations of plastic materials, used in lenses for both therapeutic and refractive purposes.

The first-generation lenses were made of poly (hydroxyethyl methacrylate) (PHEMA), which had a water content of 38% to 40%.

The Bausch & Lomb (B&L) Plano-T lens from this group was the first soft contact lens developed for therapeutic use. The second-generation lenses had a higher water content – 45% to 55% – and were made of a copolymer of HEMA and *N*-vinyl pyrrolidone. An example is the Griffin lens (also known as the Bionite lens or the Natura lens, and presently called Softcon Lens/American Optical Co.). The third-generation lenses have an even higher water content – 70% to 80% – they are made of non-HEMA copolymers. The thin-membrane lenses also belong to this group and have a lower water content of 30% to 40%.

Current therapeutic lenses can be classified into three major groups: low-, medium-, and high-water-content (Table 38.1). The

Table 38.1 Therapeutic hydrophilic soft contact lenses

Product/ Manufacturer	Material	Production Method	Water Content (%)	Central Thickness (mm)	Diameter (mm)	Base curve (mm)
Low water content						
Plano-U/ Bausch & Lomb	Polymacon	Spin-cast	38.6	0.07	12.5	8.6(P.A.R)
Plano-U3/ Bausch & Lomb	Polymacon	Spin-cast	38.6	0.07	13.5	9.2(P.A.R)
Plano-B4/ Bausch & Lomb	Polymacon	Spin-cast	38.6	0.12	14.5	9.9(P.A.R)
Plano-O4/ Bausch & Lomb	Polymacon	Spin-cast	38.6	0.06	14.5	8.4(P.A.R)
Plano-T/ Bausch & Lomb	Polymacon	Spin-cast	38.6	0.15	14.5	8.0(P.A.R)
CSI-T/Syntex	Crofilcon A	Lathe-cut	38.5	0.035	13.8 14.8	8.0, 8.3, 8.6, 8.9 8.6, 8.9, 9.35
Softsite Bandage Lens/ Softsite Contact Lens Laboratory	Hefilcon B	Lathe-cut	45.0	0.06–0.07 15.5	13.5 9.5, 9.8	8.6
Medium water content						
Softcon-EW/ American Optical Corp.	Vifilcon A	Lathe-cut	55.0	0.06–0.12	14.0	8.1, 8.4, 8.7
Hydrocurve-EW/ Barnes Hind Hydrocurve Inc.	Bufilcon A	Lathe-cut	55.0	0.08	14.0 14.5	8.5 8.8, 9.1
High water content						
Sauflon/American Medical Optics	Lidofilcon B	Lathe-cut	79.0	0.16	14.3	8.1, 8.4, 8.7
Permalens/ CooperVision	Perifilcon A	Lathe-cut	71.0	0.24	13.5 14.2 15.0	7.7, 8.0, 8.3 8.6 9.0

EW, extended wear; P.A.R., posterior apical radius.

low-water-content lenses contain 38% to 45% water, the medium-water-content lenses 55%, and the high-water-content lenses 70% to 79%. The low-water-content lenses are thinner than the high-water-content lenses (Table 38.1). All these lenses are manufactured by the lathe-cut method, except the Bausch & Lomb series of therapeutic lenses, which are spin-cast. The smaller-diameter lens is the Plano U (12.5 mm). Various base curves are available for most of these lenses.

38.4 LENS SELECTION

Various parameters, including water content, diameter, and thickness, are considered in selecting a lens to treat a specific corneal disease. For example, a patient with dry eyes often requires a high-water-content lens, whereas a patient with a peripheral corneal ulcer needs a larger diameter for adequate corneal coverage. As an adequate fit must be obtained, a randomly chosen lens will not be optimum. Many of the problems relating to therapeutic lenses are secondary to inadequate lens fitting. It is beyond the scope of this chapter to provide a detailed description of the fitting procedures, but the general principles of lens-fitting apply. For example, to prevent an excessively tight fit, the flattest lens that is stable on the eye should be used. In certain conditions a particular lens fit is desired; for example, in recurrent erosion with surface defect, one would be reluctant to choose a lens with a loose fit, which moves excessively and retards proper healing of the corneal epithelium. In this case a stable lens that moves very slightly with the blink on up gaze would be the preferred fit. In treating a small corneal perforation, a lens that would seal the wound is preferred and not a lens that vaults over the perforation area.

Among the low-water-content lenses, the Plano-T lens is widely used as a therapeutic lens. It is relatively thick (0.15 mm) and has a fairly large diameter (14.5 mm) and a posterior apical radius (PAR) of 8.0 mm. With advancing technology, thinner low-water-content lenses are being manufactured, e.g. Plano U and O series (B&L), the CSI-T lens (Syntex), and the Softsite bandage lens (Softsite Contact Lens Laboratory), which increases oxygen transmission to the cornea. The B&L lenses are comfortable, and the bevel and knife-edge design produces little or no lid sensation. These lenses have a relatively tight fit and minimal movement on the cornea. Of the low-water-content therapeutic lenses, all the B&L lenses are manufactured by the spin-casting method, and the CSI-T and the Softsite bandage lenses are lathe-cut. The Softsite bandage lens is a thin lens with a relatively higher water content of 45%; it is available in two diameters, 13.5 and 15.5 mm. In general, the low-water-content lenses provide better visual acuity, and the CSI lens gives the best acuity, since

there is some PMMA in the polymer which makes it more rigid than the HEMA lenses.

Although an ultrathin lens is best tolerated by the cornea, it can wrinkle and roll on itself when the corneal surface is irregular. The stability of an ultrathin lens can be increased by using a thin lens with a minus power. This increases the lens weight and adds to its stability. Also, a reduction in the central thickness of the lens increases its oxygen permeability. Alternate choices would include a high-water-lens, e.g. Sauflon, Permalens, a thicker B&L lens, or a CSI lens that is thicker in the center.

The medium-water-content lenses include the Softcon and Hydrocurve. The Softcon has a water content of 55% and is now available in an ultrathin series. The Hydrocurve lens used to be available in the larger diameters of 15.5 and 16.0 mm; currently the Hydrocurve-EW plano lens is available only in 14.0 and 14.5 mm diameters. Although this lens is FDA approved for extended wear, it is not currently approved for therapeutic use. The high-water-content lenses contain up to 79% water. Their central thickness ranges from 0.16 to 0.18 mm. The Sauflon lens diameter is 14.3 mm, and the Permalens 13.5, 14.2 and 15.0 mm. In most cases, Permalens provides a good fit. When a high-water-content lens is required, Sauflon is a good choice; it has a 79% water content and is well tolerated.

38.5 INDICATIONS FOR THERAPEUTIC SOFT CONTACT LENSES

1. Bullous keratopathy.
2. Recurrent corneal erosion.
3. Persistent corneal epithelial defect:
   i. trauma;
   ii. infection:
      a. bacterial;
      b. viral (e.g. herpes simplex);
      c. fungal;
   iii. chemical burn;

iv. post-surgery:
   a. penetrating keratoplasty;
   b. vitrectomy;
   c. epikeratophakia;
v. dry eye syndrome;
vi. neuroparalytic keratitis;
vii. anterior segment necrosis;
viii. corneal ulcer.
4. Dry eye syndromes:
   i. keratitis sicca;
   ii. Sjögrens syndrome;
   iii. ocular pemphigoid;
   iv. Stevens–Johnson syndrome.
5. Filamentary keratitis:
   i. idiopathic;
   ii. keratitis sicca;
   iii. superior limbic keratitis;
   iv. corneal edema;
   v. corneal abrasion;
   vi. post-surgery;
   vii. viral infection.
6. Penetrating corneal wounds.
7. Following ocular surgery:
   i. penetrating keratoplasty;
   ii. cataract surgery;
   iii. epikeratophakia;
   iv. stripping of corneal membrane;
   v. postoperative wound leak.
8. Entropion.
9. Vernal catarrh.
10. Topical drug delivery.

38.5.1 CORNEAL EDEMA, BULLOUS KERATOPATHY

The use of hydrophilic contact lenses as bandage lens in patients with bullous keratopathy provides significant ocular comfort and/or visual improvement (Fig. 38.2). Bullous keratopathy results from fluid accumulation and the formation of corneal epithelial bullae, secondary to corneal endothelial decompensation from different causes, such as Fuchs' dystrophy, and aphakic or pseudophakic bullous keratopathy. With corneal endothelial decompensation, both the pump and barrier functions of this monolayer of cells is lost with fluid access into the stroma, resulting in corneal stromal swelling and corneal epithelial edema. Initially, fluid accumulates within the basal epithelial cells, then intercellularly, and finally it collects subcellularly, resulting in lifting up of the epithelium and the formation of corneal epithelial bullae. Corneal epithelial bullae cause marked surface irregularities with irregular corneal astigmatism and a decrease in visual acuity. When a hydrophilic contact lens is used in this condition, it provides a smooth refractive surface, corrects small degrees of irregular astigmatism, and improves vision, especially in the early stages of bullous keratopathy. In Gasset and Kaufman's (1971) series, 43% (21 patients) attained a visual acuity of 20/40 or better after bandage lens therapy. Often the visual acuity is not improved to this extent, unless the edema is very mild with only minimal compromise of existing visual acuity. These bandage lenses are usually well tolerated without causing further corneal epithelial insult or ulceration. With progressive fluid accumulation within the corneal epithelium, these bullae coalesce to form larger bullae that then rupture, resulting in corneal surface defects and exposure of bare nerve endings leading to ocular discomfort and pain. Although the exact mechanism by which a soft contact lens relieves pain is not known, it is most likely by protecting the exposed free nerve endings. Several studies have shown the beneficial effect of a bandage lens in relieving ocular pain associated with bullous keratopathy, (Gasset & Kaufman, 1970, 1971; Leibowitz & Rosenthal, 1971).

A hydrophilic soft contact lens is not indicated in all cases of corneal edema and bullous keratopathy. In the very early stages, with minimal corneal edema, the use of lubricating ointments or hypertonic agents alone may suffice. Blurred vision from corneal edema may be more noticeable in the morning upon arising, due to the decreased surface evaporation at night when the eyelids are closed during sleep. Vision usually clears later in the day due to surface evapora-

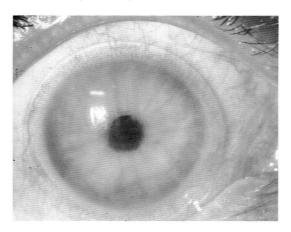

Figure 38.2 A bandage soft contact lens often relieves the pain associated with bullous keratopathy and corrects irregular astigmatism in the early stages.

tion. Five per cent sodium chloride solution may be used as frequently as every 15 minutes on awakening and less often as the day progresses. About two weeks of therapy may be necessary before documenting clinical improvement. In addition, 5% sodium chloride ointment may be used at night before retiring. Increasing the rate of corneal surface evaporation by using a hair dryer to blow warm air over the ocular surface has also been tried. When there is associated anterior uveitis, the use of cycloplegic agents would provide comfort. Although the use of prophylactic antibiotics is controversial, their use is probably advisable in the setting of a decompensated corneal epithelium with a bandage lens.

In advanced stages of bullous keratopathy, when there is increased corneal edema, the cornea swells posteriorly, resulting in folds in Descemet's membrane. The nonstretchable Bowman's layer prevents swelling of the cornea anteriorly. When there are Descemet's membrane folds and/or corneal scarring and opacities from longstanding bullous keratopathy, the use of a bandage lens usually will not improve vision,

although it may provide ocular comfort. If a corneal transplant is planned in the near future, a thin bandage lens should be chosen rather than a thicker lens, since the latter has a greater tendency to cause corneal neovascularization.

38.5.2 RECURRENT CORNEAL EROSION

A hydrophilic soft contact lens as a bandage lens is useful in the management of certain cases of recurrent erosions of the cornea (Fig. 38.3). This syndrome is characterized by recurrent episodes of spontaneous, acute corneal epithelial breakdown, accompanied by sudden onset of pain, photophobia, lacrimation, and blepharospasm. These recurrent epithelial erosions usually occur in the early morning hours upon awakening and opening the eyelids. The eyelid movement may cause the poorly adherent corneal epithelium to peel off from the underlying structures, with the acute onset of symptoms. Recurrent erosion may be associated with a previous history of sudden, sharp, corneal trauma, such as a corneal abrasion from a fingernail, a branch of a tree or plant, or the edge of a piece of paper (Chandler, 1945). Recurrent corneal erosion may also be related to corneal epithelial basement membrane dystrophy or to a combination of previous ocular trauma on pre-existing epithelial basement membrane dystrophy. In such a case, examining the cornea of the fellow eye may be helpful in making the diagnosis. In cases of previous trauma alone, corneal changes would be unilateral, unlike the bilateral corneal changes usually noted in epithelial basement membrane dystrophy. Recurrent erosion has also been described in metaherpetic keratitis (Kaufman, 1964).

Khodadoust *et al.* (1968) showed that, following epithelial scraping in rabbits, the new epithelial layer became firmly adherent within a week in the presence of intact basement membrane. However, when the basement membrane was removed by superfi-

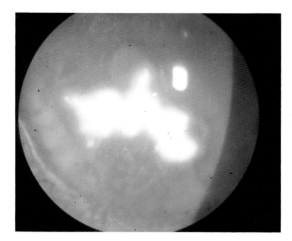

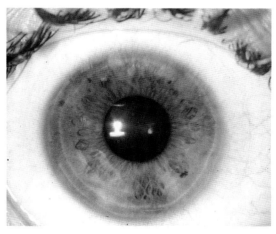

Figure 38.3 (a) Slit-lamp photograph of a patient with recurrent corneal erosion showing fluorescein staining of the epithelial defect. (b) Same cornea 48 hours after start of bandage lens therapy.

cial keratectomy, the regenerating epithelium had to secrete its own new basement membrane, and the epithelial adhesion was subnormal for many weeks to many months (6 weeks in some cases). Basement membrane deficiency has also been detected in human epithelial recurrent erosion syndrome (Goldman *et al.*, 1969; Fogle *et al.*, 1975). Among other corneal dystrophies, mapdot–fingerprint dystrophy, Reis–Bücklers dystrophy and lat-

tice corneal dystrophy may be especially prone to spontaneous recurrent erosions of the corneal epithelium. A common critical factor that plays a role in recurrent erosions is the incompetent or incomplete formation and maintenance of basement membrane complexes (Fig. 38.4), which contribute to the weak epithelial adhesion.

Various therapeutic modalities have been used in the management of recurrent erosions; they include hypertonic ointments, lubrication, patching, mechanical or chemical debridement, cauterization, hydrophilic soft contact lens therapy and lamellar keratoplasty. Small erosions of the cornea can often be managed by applying a pressure-patch with an antibiotic or lubricating ointment. Large areas of nonadherent epithelium should be mechanically debrided under topical anesthesia. A Weck-cel sponge can be used for the gentle debridement, avoiding any additional damage to the critical basement membrane. Epithelial fragments may be removed with a jeweler's forceps. Sharp instruments such as a scalpel blade or Kimura spatula as well as chemical cauterization such as iodine should be avoided. Following the removal of the patch, artificial tears during the day and 5% sodium chloride ointment or lubricating ointment at night may be used. Prophylactic antibiotic drops or ointment may be utilized, especially in the presence of an epithelial defect. A cycloplegic agent should be used in the presence of concomitant anterior uveitis to provide relief to the patient. When the above management fails or there is an increased frequency and/or prolonged duration of attacks, a hydrophilic soft contact lens should be considered. Lubrication (including ointments) and prophylactic antibiotic plus corticosteroids and a cycloplegic agent, when indicated, should be continued. The bandage lens should be used for a mininum of 3 to 4 months to provide adequate time for the elaboration of new basement membrane by regenerating epithelium and hemidesmo-

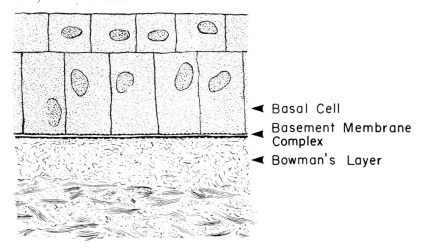

Figure 38.4 Components of a normal corneal attachment complex that play important roles in the pathophysiology of recurrent erosions (courtesy Dr Lawrence Hirst).

somal attachments between basal epithelial cells and the underlying basement membrane and the restoration of tight epithelial–stromal adhesion (Kenyon, 1979). Upon termination of lens wear, lubricating ointment should be used at night for several months.

The use of extended-wear ultrathin therapeutic soft contact lenses of low water content (B&L U or O series, Syntex, CSI, etc.) to provide an optical bandage to shield against the 'windshield-wiper' action of the blinking eyelids over loosely attached or non-adherent regenerating epithelium has significantly reduced morbidity and simplified therapy of many recurrent erosion and persistent epithelial defect problems (Dohlman *et al.*, 1973; Cavanagh *et al.*, 1976; Kenyon, 1982). In contrast to a success rate of 34% of patients with recurrent corneal erosion syndrome using conventional hydrogel lenses (Dohlman, 1974), a success rate of 71% was achieved with ultrathin lenses in recurrent corneal erosions (Mobilia & Foster, 1978). Ultrathin lenses that offer increased oxygen permeability (Mobilia *et al.*, 1977; Holly & Refojo, 1972), substantially decrease corneal edema associated with continuous-wear soft contact lenses in recurrent corneal erosion

syndrome (Mobilia & Foster, 1978). Two relative disadvantages of these ultrathin lenses are the difficulty in handling them and an increased rate of lens loss by patients. Another interesting clinical finding associated with ultrathin soft contact lenses is corneal wrinkling, which is reversible on discontinuation of lens use and has no lasting effect on vision. The handling difficulty when using the ultrathin lenses (0.035–0.04 mm, center thickness) can be overcome by the use of a slightly thicker lens such as Softcon EW with a central thickness of 0.1 mm and a 55% water content. This lens is a good compromise between the extremely thin, low-water-content lenses and the thicker, high-water-content lenses. We reported a 75% success rate in treating corneal epithelial surface disorders with a Softcon EW lens as a bandage lens, and the results are comparable with studies using other thin-design lenses (Mobilia & Kenyon, 1984).

38.5.3 PERSISTENT CORNEAL EPITHELIAL DEFECT

Persistent epithelial defects (PEDs) of the cornea can be a chronic management problem. Additionally, increased vulnerability of the cornea to infection accompanies an epithelial defect. PED has a high incidence of corneal ulceration and perforation, which may be accelerated by the use of topical corticosteroids. Cavanagh *et al.* (1976) reported that 41 of 72 eyes with PED in herpetic keratitis showed melting of the cornea, and 20 eyes perforated. Hence, it is important to understand the pathophysiology of these lesions, in order to manage these difficult cases better.

PED may result from trauma, such as corneal abrasion, or may be associated with recurrent erosion syndrome. It may be a sequel to infections with bacterial, viral (e.g. herpetic corneal disease) (Fig. 38.5), or fungal agents involving the cornea. Other causes include chemical burns (Fig. 38.6), thermal burns (Fig. 38.7), post-surgery (e.g. following corneal transplantation, post-vitrectomy in diabetics (Fig. 38.80, epikeratophakia), dry eye syndromes, neuroparalytic keratitis (e.g. following 5th or 7th cranial nerve injury), and anterior segment necrosis. A leading cause of PED is herpetic keratitis. In

Cavanagh *et al.*'s (1979) series of 202 patients with PED, almost half the cases were associated with herpetic corneal disease.

Epithelial wound healing involves epithelial cell movement, mitosis, resynthesis of basal lamina, formation of hemidesmosomes which bind the basement membrane to Bowman's layer, and anchoring fibrils which play a role in anchoring epithelial basement membrane to the anterior corneal stroma. In PED, cell regrowth may be inhibited by humoral factors such as prostaglandins and catecholamines associated with the inflammatory process seen in PED (Cavanagh *et al.*, 1979). When the epithelial cells regenerate in an attempt to close the surface defect(s), these cells should be protected from the rubbing action of the eyelids during blinking. They should also be in contact with the corneal surface for adequate time to reform the basal attachment complexes. Under these circumstances the use of a therapeutic bandage lens would help in healing the epithelial defect.

A chemical burn to the eye is often associated with chemosis and/or corneal epithelial

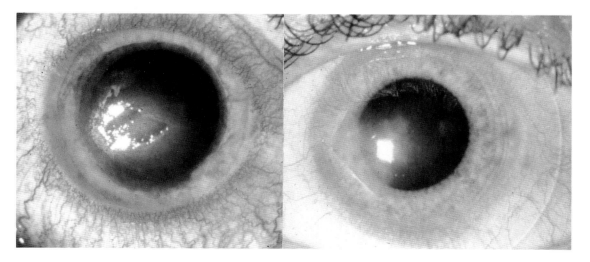

Figure 38.5 (a) An important cause of persistent epithelial defect of the cornea is metaherpetic keratitis following herpes simplex virus infection. (b) The use of a therapeutic lens is often beneficial in the healing of the ocular surface defect.

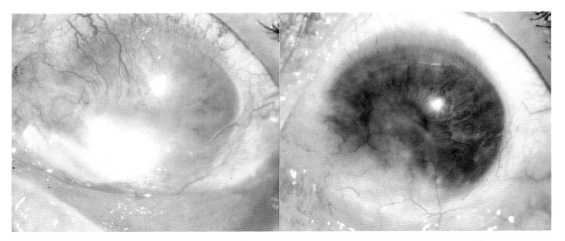

Figure 38.6 (a) Chemical burn with a persistent epithelial defect of the cornea, which has healed following the use of a therapeutic lens (b).

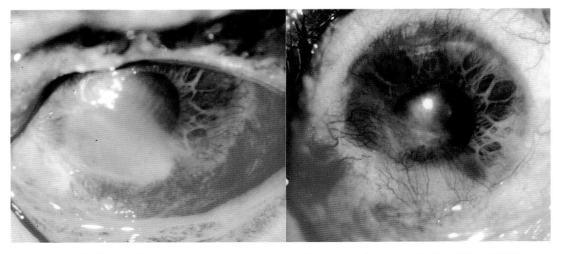

Figure 38.7 (a) Thermal burn of the cornea has resulted in a persistent epithelial defect. (b) Following therapy with a bandage contact lens, the epithelial defect has healed with corneal neovascularization.

damage from the chemical insult. If chemosis is present, a smaller lens that would just cover the limbus should be chosen, the B&L U lens with a diameter of 12.5 mm, for example. If there is a peripheral corneal ulcer with an epithelial defect, it is usually best to choose a low-water-content lens, in order to promote corneal neovascularization. Following the application of a contact lens, the eye

often becomes more inflamed initially, but then usually quietens down. The lens should have an adequate diameter to cover the corneal lesion. A B&L plano B4 or plano T is a good lens to try in these cases; both have a diameter of 14.5 mm.

In diabetes mellitus the corneal epithelium has a poor adhesion to the underlying stroma (Kenyon *et al.*, 1978) and hence is easily

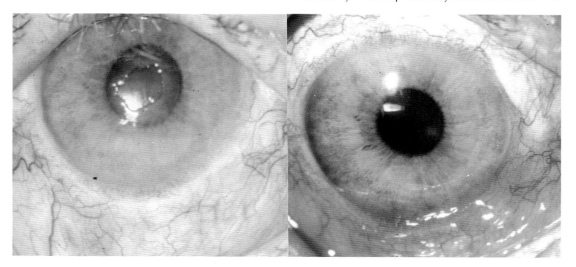

Figure 38.8 (a) Central corneal epithelial defect following vitrectomy in a diabetic patient. (b) Same eye, 2.5 weeks after start of bandage lens therapy. The soft contact lens has contributed to the healing of the epithelial defect.

removed in sheets during operative procedures, which may result in PED during the postoperative period (Brightbill *et al.*, 1978; Foulks *et al.*, 1979). Ultrastructural studies of diabetic corneal epithelial scrapings from patients undergoing vitreoretinal surgery revealed a continuous layer of basement membrane attached to the sheet of epithelium, with basement membrane thickening, multiple laminations, and anchoring fibrils (Fig. 38.9) (Kenyon *et al.*, 1978). It is thus evident that in diabetic cornea there is an inherent weakness in the attachment of the epithelial basement membrane to the underlying Bowman's layer and anterior corneal stroma. It is important to try to avoid removal of the epithelium during surgery, to use Healon, gelfoam, or SCL intraoperatively, and to decrease operative time, in order to minimize the epithelial insult to diabetic patients. If PED develops in these patients, the postoperative use of a therapeutic hydrophilic soft contact lens would be beneficial.

A therapeutic hydrophilic lens may be useful in metaherpetic keratitis with a PED.

If short-term patching fails in healing a small epithelial defect, or if the defect is large, a bandage lens should be tried. Since topical steroids should be avoided in the presence of an epithelial defect, to prevent accelerated stromal melting and ulceration, systemic steroid is preferred for control of uveitis, when present. However, if topical steroids are required at doses in excess of prednisolone acetate 1% or dexamethasone 0.1%, then concomitant use of an antiviral agent is mandatory. Additionally, antibiotics and a cycloplegic agent may be used. Once the epithelial defect has healed and the uveitis has subsided, both topical and systemic steroids are tapered and discontinued. Tapering of topical steroid should be gradual over weeks to months to prevent recurrent inflammation.

In neuroparalytic keratitis from facial nerve palsy, a large-diameter contact lens is preferred, so that at least part of the lens is beneath the palpebral conjunctiva. Since there is exposure of the cornea and surface evaporation of water from the soft contact lens, frequent instillation of artificial tears

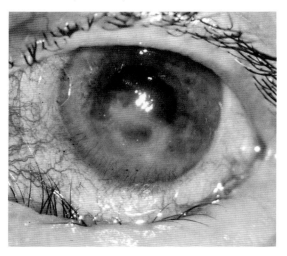

Figure 38.20 In cases of entropion, a bandage lens can protect the corneal surface from the mechanical trauma of the eyelashes. This patient had an epithelial defect and corneal ulceration secondary to the mechanical trauma of the lower lid eyelashes.

(Podos *et al.*, 1972), fluorescein (Waltman & Kaufman, 1970), acetazolamide (Friedman *et al.*, 1985) and tobramycin (Matoba & McCulley, 1985), but the effect is not always predictable. Various factors, including the type of contact lens and the concentration gradient and molecular weight of the drug, influence the rate of uptake and release (Praus & Krejči, 1977). These studies have shown that it is safe to use topical medications in the presence of a soft contact lens, and that it is not necessary to remove the therapeutic soft contact lens. To record intraocular pressure, a Mackay–Marg tonometer can be used over a therapeutic soft contact lens to provide a fairly accurate reading over a range of 10–50 mmHg (Meyer *et al.*, 1978).

38.6 COMPLICATIONS OF THERAPEUTIC LENSES

Complications of therapeutic soft contact lenses include lens intolerance, corneal vascularization, lens deposits, and corneal infec-

tions. For detailed discussions, refer to Chapter 00. Some of the complications, such as neovascularization and corneal edema secondary to a therapeutic lens, may not be distinguishable from the primary corneal disorder with similar changes. Whenever necessary, the therapeutic lens should be discontinued. A close follow-up of these patients is important, especially since contact lenses fitted on a compromised or diseased cornea can predispose to major infectious complications.

REFERENCES

Binder, P.S., Abel, R.A. Jr. and Kaufman, H.E. (1975) The effect of chronic administration of a topical antibiotic on the conjunctival flora. *Ann. Ophthalmol.*, **7**, 1429–35.

Bloomfield, S.E., Gasset, A.R., Forstot, S.L. and Brown, S.I. (1973) Treatment of filamentary keratitis with the soft contact lens. *Am. J. Ophthalmol.*, **76**, 978–80.

Bodner, B.I. (1984) Selection and fitting of therapeutic lenses. In *Contact Lenses: The CLAO Guide to Basic Science and Clinical Practice*, Vol. 2 (eds O.H. Dabezies, Jr., H.D., Cavanagh, R.L. Farris and M.A. Lemp), Grune & Stratton, Orlando, FL.

Brightbill, F.S., Myers, F.L. and Bresnick, G.H. (1978) Postvitrectomy keratopathy. *Am. J. Ophthalmol.*, **85**, 651–5.

Brown, S.I., Bloomfield, S., Pearce, D.B. and Tragakis, M. (1974) Infections with the therapeutic soft lens. *Arch. Ophthalmol.*, **91**, 275–7.

Cavanagh, H.D. (1978) Therapeutic hydrogel lenses. In *Clinical Ophthalmology, Vol. 4: External Diseases; The Uvea.* (ed. T.D. Duane), Harper and Row, Hagerstown, MD.

Cavanagh, H.D., Pihlaja, D., Thoft, R.A. and Dohlman, C.H. (1976) The pathogenesis and treatment of persistent epithelial defects. *Trans. Am. Acad. Ophthalmol. Otolaryngol.*, **81**, 754–69.

Cavanagh, H.D., Colley, A. and Pihlaja, D.J. (1979) Persistent corneal epithelial defects. *Int. Ophthalmol. Clin.*, **19**(2), 197–206.

Chandler, P.A. (1945) Recurrent erosions of the cornea. *Am. J. Ophthalmol.*, **28**, 355–61.

Dohlman, C.H. (1974) Complications in therapeutic soft lens wear. *Trans. Am. Acad. Ophthalmol. Otolaryngol.*, **78**, 399–405.

Dohlman, C.H., Boruchoff, S.A. and Mobilia, E.E.

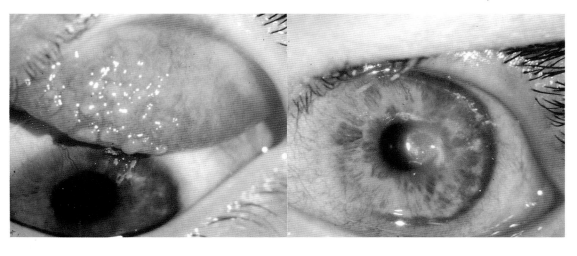

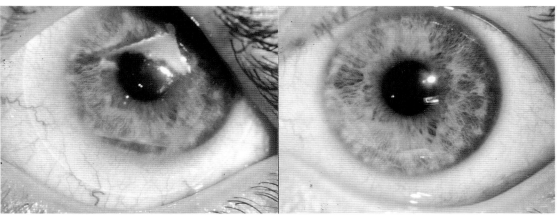

Figure 38.21 (a) Large conjunctival papillae in a patient with vernal keratoconjunctivitis. (b) Same patient with shield ulcer of the cornea. (c) The corneal surface has healed after treatment with a bandage soft contact lens. Also seen is a good corneal light reflex (d).

(1973) Complications in use of soft contact lenses in corneal disease. *Arch. Ophthalmol.*, **90**, 367–71.

Dohlman, C.H. (1978) Punctal occlusion in keratoconjunctivitis sicca. *Trans. Am. Acad. Ophthalmol. Otolaryngol.*, **85**, 1277–81

Fogle, J.A., Kenyon, K.R., Stark, W.J. and Green, W.R. (1975) Defective epithelial adhesion in anterior corneal dystrophies. *Am. J. Ophthalmol.*, **79**, 925–40.

Fogle, J.A., Kenyon, K.R. and Foster, C.S. (1980) Tissue adhesive arrests stromal melting in the human cornea. *Am. J. Ophthalmol.*, **89**, 795–802.

Foulks, G.N., Thoft, R.A., Perry, H.D. and Tolentino, F.I. (1979) Factors related to corneal epithelial complications after closed vitrectomy in diabetics. *Arch. Ophthalmol.*, **97**, 1076–8.

Freeman, J.M. (1975) The punctum plug: Evaluation of a new treatment for the dry eye. *Trans. Am. Acad. Ophthalmol. Otolaryngol.*, **79**, OP874–9.

Friedman, Z., Allen, R.C. and Ralph, S.M. (1985) Topical acetazolamide and methazolamide delivered by contact lenses. *Arch. Ophthalmol.*, **103**, 963–6.

Gasset, A.R. and Kaufman, H.E. (1970) Therapeutic uses of hydrophilic contact lenses. *Am. J. Ophthalmol.*, **69**, 252–9.

Gasset, A.R. and Kaufman, H.E. (1971) Bandage lenses in the treatment of bullous keratopathy. *Am. J. Ophthalmol.*, **72**, 376–80.

Gasset, A.R. and Kaufman, H.E. (1973) Hydrophilic lens therapy of superficial sterile corneal ulcers. *Ann. Ophthamol.*, **5**, 139–42.

Goldman, J.N. Dohlman, C.H. and Kravitt, B.A. (1969) The basement membrane on the human cornea in recurrent erosion syndrome. *Trans. Am. Acad. Ophthamol. Otolaryngol.*, **73**, 471–81.

Holly, F.J. and Refojo, M.E. (1972) Oxygen permeability of hydrogel lenses. *J. Am. Optom. Assoc.*, **43**, 1173–80.

Kaufman, H.E. (1964) Epithelial erosion syndrome: Metaherpetic keratitis. *Am. J. Ophthalmol.*, **57**, 983–7.

Kenyon, K.R. (1979) Recurrent corneal erosion. Pathogenesis and therapy. *Int. Ophthalmol. Clin.*, **19** (2), 169–95.

Kenyon, K.R. (1982) Decision-making in the therapy of external eye disease: Noninfected corneal ulcers. *Ophthalmology*, **89**, 44–51.

Kenyon, K.R., Wafai, Z., Michels, R., Conway, B. and Tolentino, E. (1978) Corneal basement membrane abnormality in diabetes mellitus. *Invest. Ophthalmol. Vis. Sci.*, **17 (ARVO Suppl.)**, 245.

Khodadoust, A.A., Silverstein, M., Kenyon, K.R. and Dowling, J.E. (1968) Adhesion of regenerating corneal epithelium: The role of basement membrane. *Am. J. Ophthalmol.*, **65**, 339–48.

Leibowitz, H.M. (1972) Hydrophilic contact lenses in corneal disease. IV. Penetrating corneal wounds. *Arch. Ophthalmol.*, **88**, 602–6.

Leibowitz, H.M. and Rosenthal, P.R. (1971a) Hydrophilic contact lenses in corneal disease: I. Superficial, sterile, indolent ulcers. *Arch. Ophthalmol.*, **85**, 163–6.

Leibowitz, H.M. and Rosenthal, P. (1971b) Hydrophilic contact lenses in corneal disease: II. Bullous keratopathy. *Arch. Ophthalmol.*, **85**, 283–5.

Lemp, M.A. (1978) Bandage lenses and the use of topical solutions containing preservatives. *Ann. Ophthalmol.*, **10**, 1319–21.

Matoba, A.Y. and McCulley, J.P. (1985) The effect of therapeutic soft contact lenses on antibiotic delivery to the cornea. *Ophthalmology*, **92**, 97–9.

Messner, K. and Leibowitz, H.M. (1971) Acetylcysteine treatment of keratitis sicca. *Arch. Ophthalmol.*, **86**, 357–9.

Meyer, R.F., Stanifer, R.M. and Bobb, K.C. (1978) Mackay-Marg tonometry over therapeutic soft contact lenses. *Am. J. Ophthalmol.*, **86**, 19–23.

Mobilia, E.F. and Foster, C.S. (1978) The management of recurrent corneal erosions with ultrathin lenses. *Contact & Intraocular Lens Med. J.* **4** (1), 25–9.

Mobilia, E.F. and Kenyon, K.R. (1984) A new bandage lens for treatment of corneal disease: Softcon®. XT. *CLAO J.*, **10**, 353–5.

Mobilia, E.F., Dohlman, C.H. and Holly, F.J. (1977) A comparison of various soft contact lenses for therapeutic purposes. *Contact & Intraocular Lens Med. J.*, **3**(1), 9–15.

Pfister, R.R. and Burnstein, N. (1976) The effect of ophthalmic drugs, vehicles, and preservatives on corneal epithelium: A scanning electron microscope study. *Invest. Ophthalmol.*, **15**, 246–59.

Podos, S.M., Becker, B., Asseff, C. and Hartstein, J. (1972) Pilocarpine therapy with soft contact lenses. *Am. J. Ophthalmol.*, **73**, 336–41.

Praus, R. and Krejči, L. (1977) Elution and intraocular penetration of the ophthalmic drugs of different molecular weights from the hydrophilic contact lenses through the intact and injured cornea. *Acta Univ. Carol. [Med. Monogr.] (Praha)*, **23**, 3–10.

Rao, G.N., John, T., Ishida, N. and Aguavella, J.V. (1985) Recovery of corneal sensitivity in grafts following penetrating keratoplasty. *Ophthalmology*, **92**, 1408–11.

Refojo, M.F., Dohlman, C.H. and Koliopoulos, J. (1971) Adhesives in ophthalmology: A review. *Surv. Ophthalmol.*, **15**, 217–36.

Roberts, C. and Kenyon, K.R. (1964) Applications of tissue adhesive in anterior segment surgery. In *Advanced Techniques in Ocular Surgery* (eds. F.A. Jakobiec and J. Sigelman), W.B. Saunders, Philadelphia, pp. 39–52.

Ruben, M. (1966) Preliminary observations of soft (hydrophilic) contact lenses. *Proc. Roy. Soc. Med.*, **59**, 530–1.

Rycroft, B.W. (1964) Anterior chamber lenses. *Highlights Ophthalmol.*, **7**, 253–4.

Tseng, S.C.G. (1985) Staging of conjunctival squamous metaplasia by impression cytology. *Ophthalmology*, **92**, 728–33.

Waltman, S.R. and Kaufman, H.E. (1970) Use of hydrophilic contact lenses to increase ocular penetration of topical drugs. *Invest. Ophthalmol.*, **9**, 250–5.

Wichterle, O. and Lim, D. (1960) Hydrophilic gels for biological use. *Nature*, **185**, 117–18.

PART NINE

Special Applications

INTRODUCTION

Two chapters comprise this section. Chapter 39 deals with the use of contact lenses in the work environment, more specifically in industry where they, at times, afford some protection but more commonly where they have to be used under adverse circumstances such as a dry atmosphere or in the presence of fumes. Chapter 40 deals with the use of contact lenses in the armed forces, where special requirements are made, such as long periods of wear in the combat and training field for the infantry, or when very special environmental conditions are encountered, such as in the air force when the oxygen level may be low and/or the lens exposed to very high gravitational forces.

S.-E.G. Nilsson

The widespread use of contact lenses has prompted studies concerning the risks and advantages of contact lens wear at work. Are the risks associated with contact lens wear greater at work than at home? If so, are there certain situations that are clearly dangerous? On the other hand, are there other situations when a contact lens may protect the eye? A number of experimental and clinical studies were performed in our laboratory to answer these and other questions. The results are reviewed in this chapter.

39.1 CONTACT LENSES IN RELATION TO MECHANICAL TRAUMA TO THE EYE

39.1.1 SPLINTERS

Does a contact lens increase or decrease the risk of corneal perforation by metal splinters? Highgate (1974) considered hard lenses to be protective in certain cases, whereas soft lenses were not. We studied this experimentally (Nilsson et al., 1981). A moderately pointed metal projectile, 20 mm in length and 1 mm in diameter, was accelerated axially and at right angles against the eyes of anaesthetized rabbits by using a specially designed air-pistol. The projectile could be given increasing energies from 3 to 44 mJ by varying the pressure of the compressed air. Either the cornea was naked, or fitted with a low water content soft lens, a high water content soft lens or a hard (PMMA) lens.

Figure 39.1 shows the energies needed to give rise to corneal perforation. There was no significant difference in energies required to cause perforation of the naked cornea, the cornea fitted with a high water content lens, or with a hard lens. However, when the cornea was fitted with a low water content lens significantly ($P < 0.05$) more energy was needed for perforation. It may be noted that significantly ($P < 0.001$) less energy was required to splinter a hard lens than to give rise to corneal perforation. This is important, since splinters from the hard lens generally penetrated the corneal tissue and, at higher energies, often followed the metal projectile into the eye, complicating the damage.

It may be concluded that a low water content lens offered certain, significant protection against corneal perforation, that a high water content lens did not make any difference, and that a hard lens was often associated with more complicated damage because of splinters.

39.1.2 BURNING GRIT PARTICLES, ETC.

The eyes of anaesthetized rabbits, fitted with contact lenses, were exposed to massive bursts of particles, produced by grinding and cutting discs (Nilsson et al., 1981). All par-

Contact Lens Practice. Edited by Montague Ruben and Michel Guillon.
Published in 1994 by Chapman & Hall, London. ISBN 0 412 35120 X

the NSPB announced its stand on contact lens use in industry:

> Because of increased risk to eyes, the NSPB strongly advises that the use of contact lenses of any type by industrial employees while at work should be prohibited, except in rare cases. The NSPB recommends that any exceptions be verified in writing to the employer by the physician or optimetrist who sanctions the use in a specific industrial environment. Contact lenses do not provide eye protection in the industrial sense; their use without eye and/or face protective devices of industrial quality should not be permitted. . . . To be of industrial quality, safety eyewear devices must meet or exceed *all* requirements of the American National Standard Practice for Occupational and Educational Eye and Face Protection, Z87.1–1979, or later revisions thereof, as published by the American National Standards Institute, Inc.

As examples of risks involved, NSPB lists trapping of particles beneath lenses, irritation by chemical fumes that may cause excessive tearing and dislodge lenses, delay in removing lenses after splashes of chemicals and spectacle blur.

Furthermore, NSPB states, that 'All individuals who are permitted to wear contact lenses while working in an industrial setting should be identified'.

In the NIOSH/OSHA Pocket Guide to Chemical Hazards (DHEW (NIOSH) Pub. No. 78–210), as referred to in the US National Society to Prevent Blindness News Release, February 1980, the following statement applies to almost all of the 380 chemicals listed, 'Contact lenses should not be worn when working with this chemical'. In addition, OSHA prohibits wear of contact lenses when a respirator is being used in a contaminated atmosphere.

In 1985 the Swedish National Board of Occupational Safety and Health issued recommendations for the use of contact lenses in the working environment. These recommendations are somewhat more liberal than the American ones and more in accordance with the results of my own as well as of other studies referred to in this presentation.

39.10 GENERAL CONCLUSIONS

Table 39.1 summarizes in a fairly general way what has been put forward in more detail in the text. Based upon recent scientific studies it seems justifiable to state that contact lenses, mainly soft ones, may be used more widely in the work environment than was thought before. In certain cases, they even offer some protection. Furthermore, contact lenses generally allow a closer fitting of protective eyewear than glasses, which is advantageous.

REFERENCES

(1974) Contact lenses and electrical arcs. *Welding Inst. Res. Bull.*, **15**, 43–4.
(1974a) Contact lens hazard. *Qual. Eng.*, **38**, 95.
(1974b) Contact lens hazard. *Qual. Eng.*, **38**, 150.
(1975) Flash and contact lenses. *Occup. Safety Health*, **5**, 11.
(1977) An industrial atrocity story! *Occup. Safety Health*, **7**, 85.
Andrasko, G. and Schoessler, J.P. (1980) The effect of humidity on the dehydration of soft contact lenses on the eye. *Int. Contact Lens Clin.*, **7**, 210–12.
Bennett, Q. (1985) Contact lenses for diving. *Aust. J. Optom.*, **68**, 25.
Bennett, Q.M. (1988) The use of contact lenses for diving (sport and commercial). *Contact Lens J.*, **16**, 171–2.
Brennan, N.A., Efron, N., Bruce, A.S., Duldig, A.I. and Russo, N.J. (1988) Dehydration of hydrogel lenses: environmental influences during normal wear. *Am. J. Optom. Physiol. Optics*, **65**, 277–81.
Castren, J. (1984) The significance of low atmospheric pressure on the eyes with reference to soft contact lenses. *Acta Ophthalmol.*, **Suppl. 161**, 123–7.
Cedarstaff, T.H. and Tomlinson, A. (1983) A comparative study of tear evaporation rates and

water content of soft contact lenses. *Am. J. Optom. Physiol. Optics*, **60**, 167–74.

Coe, J.E. and Douglas, R.B. (1982) The effect of contact lenses on ocular responses to sulphur dioxide. *J. Soc. Occup. Med.*, **32**, 92–4.

Contact Lens Association of Ophthalmologists (1983) Policy statement on arc welding and contact lens wear. *CLAO J.*, **9**, 343.

Cordrey, P. (1977) Arc flash and the contact lens wearer – a modern myth. *Eye-1*, **4**, 3–4.

DeDonato, L.M. (1982) Changes in the hydration of hydrogel contact lenses with wear. *Am. J. Optom. Physiol. Optics*, **59**, 213–14.

Diefenbach, C.B., Soni, P.S., Gillespie, J. and Pence, N. (1988) Extended wear contact lens movement under swimming pool conditions. *Am. J. Optom. Physiol. Optics*, **65**, 710–16.

Efron, N., Brennan, N.A., Lowe, R., Truong, V.T., O'Brien, K., Murphy, P. and Carney, L.G. (1986) Clinical significance of hydrogel lens dehydration. *Am. J. Optom. Physiol. Optics*, **63**, 58P.

Eng, W.G., Harada, L.K. and Jagerman, L.S. (1982) The wearing of hydrophilic contact lenses aboard a commercial jet aircraft: I. Humidity effects on fit. *Aviat. Space Environ. Med.*, **53**, 235–8.

Fatt, I. and Forester, J.F. (1972) Errors in eye tissue temperature measurements when using a metallic probe. *Exp. Eye Res.*, **14**, 270–6.

Fox, S.L. (1973) *Industrial and occupational ophthalmology*. C C Thomas, Springfield, IL.

Galkin, R.A. and Semes, L. (1983), Risk of loss of Soflens® during water skiing. *J. Am. Optom. Assoc.*, **3**, 267–9.

Guthrie, J.W. and Seitz, G.H. (1975) An investigation of the chemical contact lens problem. *J. Occup. Med.*, **17**, 163–6.

Hapnes, R. (1980) Soft contact lenses worn at a simulated altitude of 18,000 feet. *Acta Ophthalmol.*, **58**, 90–5.

Highgate, D.J. (1974) Contact lenses at work. *Occup. Health Safety*, **3**, 8–11.

Hill, R.M. (1983) Dehydration deficits. *Int. Contact Lens Clin.*, **10**, 364–5.

Hill, F.M. and Leighton, A.J. (1965) Temperature changes of human cornea and tears under a contact lens. I. The relaxed open eye, and the natural and forced closed eye conditions. *Am. J. Optom.*, **42**, 9–16.

Johnsson, H. (1977) Hur farlig är en ljusbåge? *Elteknik Med Aktuell Elektronik*, **11**, 28–9.

Kok-van Alphen, C.C., van der Linden, J.W., Visser, R. and Bol, A.H. (1985) Protection of the police against tear gas with soft lenses. *Military Med.*, **150**, 451–4.

Lövsund, P., Nilsson, S.E.G., Lindh, H. and Öberg, P.Å. (1979a) Temperature changes in contact lenses in connection with radiation from welding arcs. *Scand. J. Work Environ. Health*, **5**, 271–9.

Lövsund, P., Nilsson, S.E.G. and Öberg, P.Å. (1979b) Temperature changes in contact lenses in connection with radiation from infrared heaters. *Scand. J. Work Environ. Health*, **5**, 280–5.

Lövsund, P., Nilsson, S.E.G. and Öberg, P.Å. (1980) The use of contact lenses in wet or damp environments. *Acta Ophthalmol.*, **58**, 794–804.

Mandell, R.B. (1975) Sticking of gel contact lenses. *Int. Contact Lens Clin.*, **2**, 28–9.

Martin, D.K. and Holden, B.A. (1983) Variations in tear fluid osmolality, chord diameter and movements during wear of high water content hydrogel contact lenses. *Int. Contact Lens Clin.*, **10**, 332–42.

National Society to Prevent Blindness (USA) (1972) Position statement – contact lenses in industry. *Ind. Med.*, **41**, 38–9.

National Society to Prevent Blindness (USA) (1980) *NSPB announces stand on contact lens use in industry*. News Release, February.

Nilsson, K. and Rengstorff, R.H. (1979) Continuous wearing of Duragel contact lenses by Swedish air force pilots. *Am. J. Optom. Physiol. Optics*, **56**, 356–8.

Nilsson, S.E.G. and Andersson, L. (1982) The use of contact lenses in environments with organic solvents, acids or alkalis. *Acta Ophthalmol.*, **60**, 599–608.

Nilsson, S.E.G. and Andersson, L. (1986) Contact lens wear in dry environments. *Acta Ophthalmol.*, **64**, 221–5.

Nilsson, S.E.G., Lövsund, P. and Öberg, P.Å. and Flordahl, L.-E. (1979) The transmittance and absorption properties of contact lenses. *Scand. J. Work Environ. Health*, **5**, 262–70.

Nilsson, S.E.G., Lövsund, P. and Öberg, P.Å. (1981) Contact lenses and mechanical trauma to the eye. An experimental study. *Acta Ophthalmol.*, **59**, 402–8.

Nilsson, S.E.G., Lindh, H. and Andersson, L. (1983) Contact lens wear in an environment contaminated with metal particles. *Acta Ophthalmol.*, **61**, 882–8.

Novak, J.F. and Saul, R.W. (1971) Contact lenses in industry. *J. Occup. Med.*, **13**, 175–8.

Orsborn, G.N. and Zantos, S.G. (1986) The relationship between lens movement and tear exchange under hydrogel contact lenses. *Am. J. Optom. Physiol. Optics*, **63**, 56P.

Orsborn, G.N. and Zantos, S.G. (1988) Corneal desiccation staining with thin high water content contact lenses. *CLAO J.*, **14**, 81–5.

Peterson, W. (1989) Contact lenses and surfing. *Contact Lens Spectrum*, **4**, 59.

Sander, H. and Brewitt, H. (1984) Thermographische Untersuchungen zum Verhalten von Kontaktlinsen am Auge. *Contactologia*, **6**, 60–4.

Socks, J.F. (1982) Contact lenses in extreme cold environments: response of rabbit corneas. *Am. J. Optom. Physiol. Optics*, **59**, 297–300.

Socks, J.F. (1983) Use of contact lenses for cold weather activities: results of a survey. *Int. Contact Lens Clin.*, **10**, 82–90.

Solomon, J. (1977) Swimming with soft lenses. *South J. Optom.*, **19**, 13–18.

Soni, P.S., Pence, N.A., DaLeon, C. and Lawrence, S. (1986) Feasibility of extended wear lens use in chlorinated swimming pools. *Am. J. Optom. Physiol. Optics*, **63**, 171–6.

Terry, J.E. and Hill, R.M. (1978) Human tear osmotic pressure. Diurnal variations and the closed eye. *Arch. Ophthalmol.*, **96**, 120–2.

Wesley, N.K. (1966) Chemical injury and contact lenses. *Contacto*, **10**, 15–20.

T.J.P. Rouwen

40.1 INTRODUCTION

40.1.1 SPECTACLES

In modern combat situations visual performance of the individual soldiers becomes increasingly important. More sophisticated weapons with directional devices demand good visual functions from the operator. The use of spectacles in the Military Service is accompanied with a number of disadvantages. Spectacles are often incompatible with eye pieces of telescopic sights for target acquisition or night vision. In tracked vehicles, helicopters and modern jet-fighter aircraft the vibration makes the wearing of spectacles an annoyance.

The protection of the eye becomes more important as more and more laser range-finder beams are used in the battle-field and flashes of exploding grenades and missiles become more intense. Protective ocular devices, gas-protection face-masks, head-gear, oxygen delivery masks as well as diving goggles do not integrate very well with most spectacles. This is also true during heavy weather conditions, afloat and during parachute-jumping. Bifocals are not suitable for use in cockpits with overhead instrument panels.

The US Army mentioned 79 items of equipment incompatible with spectacle wear, while in 13 military occupations spectacle wear was contra-indicated (Reinke, 1970).

Spectacles often induce annoying reflections from the rear or the front of the lens. These reflections cannot be completely banished by the use of anti-reflecting coatings. Spectacles can be lost or broken, while pieces of a broken spectacle lens can damage the eye. Restrictions of the visual field due to the spectacle frame or temples, radial and oblique astigmatism, occurring through the periphery of the spectacle lens, constitute significant disadvantages during certain tasks, requiring optimal visual performance. Changes in temperature, especially in arctic conditions, being part of the work terrain of the marine corps, fogs up spectacle lenses. Also in moist or rainy weather conditions, visual performance with spectacles is greatly reduced.

Combat spectacles must always be compatible with the standard type of gas-protection mask. Not only the gas-protection mask alone, but also the combination with combat spectacles, should be leak-proof. Combat spectacles also need an extra provision to prevent their loss, e.g. during heavy weather conditions on board ship or during parachute-jumping. In helicopters the protection of the helmet against acoustic ear damage is reduced by the introduction of spectacle temples.

40.1.2 CONTACT LENSES

All these factors stimulated the interest of servicemen for contact lens wear as an alter-

Contact Lens Practice. Edited by Montague Ruben and Michel Guillon.
Published in 1994 by Chapman & Hall, London. ISBN 0 412 35120 X

native to spectacles. As a result, contact lens wear in the Services is rapidly increasing. However, adverse environmental conditions also affect the wearing of contact lenses, although in some circumstances contact lenses definitely perform better than spectacles. For example, the use of soft contact lenses whenever tear-gas (CN or CS gas) is present in the environment, offers the wearer a real protection against irritation, also when protective masks are used. (Kok Van Alphen *et al.*, 1985). Gas-protection masks are never totally leak-proof and an increase in ocular irritation is the result. Also these masks limit the physical performance of the wearer. Thus they have to be removed as soon as possible. Tear-gas concentrations, which can be tolerated when inhaled, continue to produce corneal oedema and conjunctival irritation leading to blurred vision. This can be effectively prevented by wearing soft hydrogel lenses. Contact lenses are also capable of protection of the cornea against small foreign body injuries, compared with the naked eye (Nilsson *et al.* 1981).

However, with respect to ocular protection, spectacles (preferably polycarbonate) are of course superior. On the other hand, eye protection is often offered by special helmet-visors and other devices, making protective spectacles superfluous. According to Nilsson, even soft lenses protect the eye against small high velocity foreign bodies. (Nilsson *et al.*, 1983)

Many iron slivers, which have to be dug out of the cornea, could have been captured by a contact lens. Explosives going off in the proximity of the eye scatter small fragments and gunpowder globules to various depths in the ocular tissues (Fig. 40.1).

Any substance being present between the source and the eye tends to absorb kinetic energy, thus reducing the energy needed to penetrate the cornea. Of course a hard lens absorbs more of this energy, while pieces of the broken lens in the eye are not as harmful as one might expect.

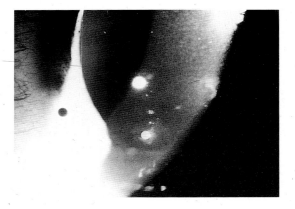

Figure 40.1 Fragments and gunpowder globules, from an exploding bomb, in the ocular tissues.

40.2   THE SITUATION IN THE ARMY

In most armies, contact lens wearers continue to wear their lenses, in spite of the fact that they have been provided with combat spectacles. In the Dutch army the Canadian type of combat spectacles are used (Fig. 40.2). The design of this frame is cosmetically not very attractive. Spectacle-wearing military personnel also tend to wear their civilian spectacles during active duty.

40.2.1   FIELD MANOEUVRES

During military manoeuvres an entirely different situation exists. The lack of sanitary facilities and running water during military manoeuvres constitutes a complicating factor for contact-lens-wearing military personnel. Soldiers are also afraid of losing lenses when they have to be removed at night in poorly-lit shelters, and many leave their lenses at home or in their barracks for the above mentioned reasons. Rengstorff (1965b) found that 44% of all contact-lens-wearing soldiers did not wear their lenses during military exercises, while about 7% lost their lenses during the basic training (Rengstorff 1965a,b, 1972). At that time all lenses were made of polymethyl methacrylate.

In 1982, van Norren held a mail survey of

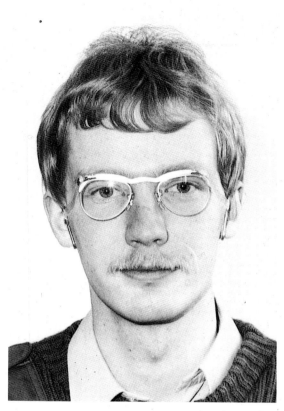

Figure 40.2 Canadian type of combat spectacles.

just under 1000 servicemen and a small inquiry under soldiers, who had just finished a large field exercise that lasted 10 days (van Norren, 1984). He found that soldiers favoured soft contact lenses and were also afraid of losing lenses (especially hard lenses) during field exercises.

In 1983 we collected data from 476 contact lens wearers entering the Military Service during two months, as well as from 168 recruits wearing spectacles (Rouwen *et al.* 1983).

In 1984 we followed a group of contact lens wearing Dutch soldiers ($n = 69$) during a 3-week field manoeuvre in Germany (Rouwen *et al.*, 1986). They were examined in advance in the Netherlands as well as during the manoeuvre in Germany. Most of the

numbers in the text are from the above mentioned surveys and observations.

Van Norren found that 20% of the contact-lens-wearing servicemen did not plan to wear their lenses during military manoeuvres (hard contact lens wearers 19%, soft contact lens wearers 20%). Additionally 23% terminated lens wear during the manoeuvre or wore spectacles now and then! (hard contact lens wearers 28%, soft contact lens wearers 17%). This was affirmed in our own investigation (Rouwen *et al.*, 1986), in which 21% of the contact lens wearing soldiers had no intention of wearing their lenses during manoeuvres (soft contact lens wearers 26%, hard gas permeable (HGP) contact lens wearers 30%, but none of the PMMA wearing group). The reasons are obvious: many experienced cleaning difficulties (11% of the soldiers in the field; almost all were soft lens wearers). Others lost their lenses, about 9% during a 3-month period, without manoeuvre (during which 15% of all spectacle wearing subjects broke one or more glasses!), but as much as 10% during a large scale NATO manoeuvre lasting 10 days, according to van Norren (15% of all hard lens wearers and 3% of all soft lens wearers).

During the 3-week shooting series in Germany, 6% of all subjects wearing contact lenses lost one or more lenses. In our series, only hard lenses were lost. This indicates that the chance of losing a lens increases considerably during a manoeuvre.

We also found more complaints about foreign bodies behind lenses: 11% before the manoeuvre and 26% during the manoeuvre. On the other hand, complaints about decreased vision and burning/irritation actually decreased during the manoeuvre. Complaints were more common in the group wearing soft lenses more than 1 year old. This could have something to do with the fact that contact lens wearers often report more comfortable wear during out-door activities, possibly due to stimulation of tearing because of the wind, higher levels of air humidity and increased blinking rate. The group wearing PMMA lenses always wore their lenses; in most instances for a long time. In addition, they often did not possess civilian spectacles and, because of the considerable amount of spectacle blur, they could not adapt to their combat spectacles.

We found spectacle blur in both eyes in 13.6% of all PMMA contact lens wearing subjects (compared to 5.5% for HGP lenses and 1.2% for soft lenses). In our first study the recruits were refracted after exactly three days without their contact lenses, which has been an arbitrary period in the Dutch Army. From this viewpoint it is obvious that PMMA lenses should not be fitted in Army personnel.

40.2.2   OCULAR COMPLICATIONS

Another question which had to be answered was whether there was a possibility of an increase in ocular complications of contact lens wear during military manoeuvres (or during war-time with comparable circumstances, but of course outlasting these manoeuvres).

This was not investigated earlier, so we undertook our second study (Rouwen *et al.*, 1986). In our first study we found that recruits entering the Dutch Army already show ocular complications of contact lens wear:

Corneal neovascularization: 4.8% (PMMA: 0.8%, HGP: 0%, soft hydrogel lenses: 10.6%)
Conjunctival injection: 5.9% (PMMA: 0.9%, HGP: 0.6%, soft hydrogel lenses: 4.4%)
Giant papillary changes of the superior tarsal conjunctiva: 18.1% (PMMA: 5.7%, HGP: 2.4%, soft hydrogel lenses: 9.9%)
All corneal opacifications: 3.9% (PMMA: 0.9%, HGP: 0% and soft hydrogel lenses: 3.0%)

In general the differences between the hard lenses on the one hand and the soft lenses on the other hand are statistically significant.

Corneal staining was present in 38% of all PMMA-wearing subjects and in 14% of all HGP-lens-wearing subjects, the difference being statistically significant ($P = 0.02$, Chi-square test for contingency tables).

Corneal staining constitutes an extra risk of corneal infection, especially during field manoeuvres under less sanitary conditions.

In the second study we focused on ocular complaints, visual acuity changes, corneal curvature changes and changes in fluorescein staining and neovascularization during the shooting series. We were able to show a significant increase in corneal staining for all types of contact lenses during the field manoeuvre. Also, during this study, PMMA wearers showed more epithelial staining in comparison to HGP contact lenses. Epithelial staining was even less in subjects wearing soft contact lenses.

Again, corneal neovascularization was found almost exclusively in soft contact lens wearers. The degree of neovascularization did not alter in most subjects, who already showed some neovascularization before the manoeuvre. Clinically significant neovascularization (grade II in our study) occurs in 2% of all cases during the pre-examination and in 5% of all cases during the field manoeuvre. This difference was not statistically significant. Keratometry measurements were taken immediately after removal of the lenses before and during the field manoeuvre. These measurements were made in two groups: one wearing lenses in the field, and one who left their lenses at home. Surprisingly, curvature changes were seen more often in the soft lens wearers than in the hard lens wearers (both in the first and the second group). For all lens types, curvature changes were more pronounced in the group who ceased lens wear during the manoeuvre.

Because of the overall wearing comfort, insensibility for environmental dust and less epithelial staining, both before and during the field manoeuvre, we prefer soft lenses for use during military exercises. Two significant problems remain: first, visual acuity with soft lenses is often less than with hard lenses, especially with soft lenses older than one year. Visual acuity also tends to deteriorate during the field manoeuvre. Second, handling of soft lenses in poorly lit shelters, without running water for cleaning the hands, is very difficult.

40.2.3 EXTENDED WEAR

Both problems could be solved by the fitting of extended wear soft contact lenses for selected subjects with careful follow-up.

We looked for lenses suitable for a flexible wearing regimen: daily wear during barrack residence and extended wear during military exercises. For this experiment we used methyl methacrylate-*N*-vinylpyrrolidone (MMA-NVP), 70% water content lenses (Rouwen & Rosenbrand, 1986). They appeared to be strong enough for daily wear during barrack residence and featured a *Dk*-value high enough to make extended wear possible. As an alternative, extra-thin 38% water content lenses could also be used, but, in practice, the superior handling characteristics of the thicker 70% water content lenses proved to be an important factor. Twenty-eight soft-contact-lens-wearing soldiers were refitted with the high water content lens. Many subjects (93% of all eyes) already showed ocular pathology as a result of the wearing of old, coated or misfitted soft lenses. Nevertheless, the subjects were very enthusiastic about the lenses, especially when worn during exercises on an extended wear basis. In fact many subjects also wore their lenses continuously during barrack residence or off-duty leisure activities.

The lenses provided superior wearing comfort, especially after longer wearing periods. Mechanical damage of the lenses during the 3-month study period did not occur. Given the state of the corneal health at the beginning of the study, the success rate of 71% was considered good.

Maintenance of the best possible visual acuity was a difficult matter. Actually, on average, the decrease in visual acuity during the 3-month follow-up was significant. On the first day, 84% scored visual acuity 20/20 or better, while on the last day 64% scored 20/20 or better (Chi-square test for contingency tables, $P < 0.05$.)

In most cases a decrease in visual acuity could be linked to lens spoilage, which constitutes another problem with these lenses: the formation of jelly bumps contributed significantly to the reduction of the success rate. Twenty-three per cent of all lenses showed jelly bumps, also 23% of all lenses were coated with protein and 7% had rust particles incorporated in the lens matrix. This is somewhat more than reported by other investigators in other studies with MMA-NVP lenses (Barner *et al.*, 1980; Nilsson & Persson, 1986). The predominance of the male sex, dirty environment and the absence of the use of a daily cleaner or weekly protein cleaner in our study may serve as an explanation for this observation.

Surprisingly, we observed no clinically evident oedema during the study; pachymetry even showed a decrease of corneal thickness after 1 and 3 months.

Corneal curvature changes also occurred, but there was no significant trend in either steep or flat direction. Two slit lamp findings – epithelial microcysts and punctate corneal staining – showed a significant increase during the study.

40.2.4 HGP CONTACT LENSES

As these lenses are not suited for every candidate (because of corneal astigmatism, pre-existent lens-related abnormalities, such as giant papillary conjunctivitis and tear film abnormalities) we also tried HGP lenses for the use in the military service. We followed a group of soldiers, who had been provided with gas-permeable lenses by our own department. They were compared with a group of PMMA-lens-wearing soldiers.

The lenses used were lathe-cut from a siloxanyl–acrylate material: Sil-O$_2$-Flex, Dk-value:12.2 (10^{11} ml O$_2$/cm^2/s/ml mmHg), wetting angle 25 degrees and water content 0.2%. These lenses were cut with a full aspheric base curve with eccentricity values ranging from 0.4 to 0.6. These lenses cannot be worn while asleep, but they permit extended wear periods of more than 24 hours while awake, which is a prerequisite for military servants.

It turned out that 96% wore their lenses all waking hours. Visual acuity with these lenses was very good (Table 40.1) and only 11% judged visual acuity with their spectacles as being insufficient (compared to 22% of the group of PMMA-wearing subjects). This was very important because 11% had to remove the lenses once in a while during military manoeuvres, another 11% experienced severe eye trouble and often replaced the lenses by their (combat) spectacles and 7% stated that lens wear was impossible and used spectacles instead. Only 19% never experienced any foreign bodies behind the lens. So it was obvious that, with this particular hard-lens-related problem, despite the aspheric design with minimal edge stand-off, we made little progress since the Fort Dix report of Rengstorff in 1965a. Rengstorff stated that 99% of the PMMA-wearing military personnel admitted irritation due to dust and sand.

In our study epithelial staining was less in the group soldiers wearing HGP lenses (15% compared to 38% of the PMMA-wearing soldiers, $P < 0.005$, Chi-square test for contingency tables). However, GPC was more prevalent in this HGP lens wear group (13% compared to 1%, $P < 0.05$). Others have shown that HGP contact lenses are more sensitive to protein coating, which could account for this finding (Caroline, 1984).

Within the framework of an FDA approval study to establish the safety and efficacy of a Boston IV HGP contact lens with an aspheric design, we also fitted about 20 active soldiers with this lens and followed them for 6 months. The first 3 months the lenses were worn exclusively on a daily wear regimen, while the last 3 months were on a mixed daily wear/extended wear basis. Most subjects had never worn contact lenses before and we had the impression that the initial tolerance of these lenses was nearly as good as with soft lenses.

Visual acuity was again superior to visual acuity with the 70% water content MMA-NVP soft contact lenses (Table 40.1). In the entire group under investigation (including the civilians, $n = 46$), visual acuity with lenses was as good as with spectacle Rx, actually increasing during the 3-month daily wear study period. Visual acuity with spectacle Rx immediately after lens removal during and at the end of the study was as good as before fitting lenses, suggesting the complete absence of spectacle blur.

Table 40.1 Visual acuity after (at least) 3 months' wear

	Boston IV aspheric HGP(%)	Sil-O$_2$-Flex aspheric HGP(%)	PMMA spheric (%)	BL70 soft E.W.(%)
V.A.> = 6/6	82.9	94	70	63
V.A.< 6/6 but > = 6/8	15.3	2	20	33
V.A.< 6/8	1.8	4	10	4
Total	100	100	100	100
Number of eyes		136	52	56

E.W., extended wear; V.A., visual activity.

Subjects with a considerable amount of corneal astigmatism experienced good visual acuity with their lenses. This is important, because in previous studies we calculated that 20% of 456 contact-lens-wearing recruits showed a refractive astigmatism equal or in excess of half their spherical value. Based on other calculations, we concluded that one out of five contact lens candidates could *not* satisfy the visual demands in the Military Service when fitted with spherical soft lenses. In Figure 40.3 the fluorescein pattern is shown of a soldier with more than 4 dioptres of corneal astigmatism. Despite the fact that the aspheric Boston IV lenses lifted off inferiorly, actually allowing an air bubble under the lens, the lenses could be worn all waking hours without adverse effects and also improved his vision from 12/20 with spectacle *Rx* to 20/20 with contact lenses. During the first 3 months (daily wear) the success rate was 93%. The reasons for failure being wearing discomfort, insufficient motivation or uncorrected residual astigmatism. Neither of these subjects exhibited moderate or severe adverse slit lamp findings. After 3 months' daily wear we found no corneal vascularization and in 17.5% of all eyes some epithelial staining and in 2.6% of all eyes minimal papillary changes, none of these findings leading to a decrease in wearing comfort or reduction of the wearing time.

After 3 months of daily wear, extended wear candidates were selected in the sense that they had to be successful daily wear patients. They were instructed to return for an examination the next day, and they slept in their lenses. They were allowed to clean their lenses as often as needed. An abrasive type of contact lens cleaner was chosen for its superior cleaning activity. Considering the subjective experience of the individuals, the results of the extended wear HGP experiment were very encouraging. Slight discomfort, experienced during daily wear, actually disappeared during extended wear. The possibility of extended wear during military

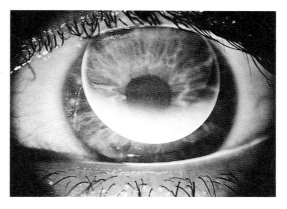

Figure 40.3 Aspheric Boston IV HGP lens on toric cornea.

manoeuvres came in very handy, while the lenses needed only minimal amounts of care-solutions whenever they had to be removed. During follow-up examinations the same complications were seen as with daily-wear, but were slightly more common, and a few new complications were seen, such as lens sticking with corneal compression, corneal oedema with vertical striae, the visibility of the anterior epithelial mosaic pattern (Fischer–Schweitzer pattern), crystalline deposits on the corneal epithelium and rather large microcysts of the epithelium.

Other investigators found similar complications with extended wear HGP contact lenses (Levy, 1985). These findings warned us to be very careful with HGP extended wear in areas where the patient cannot easily seek professional attention. Irrespective of the above mentioned precautions, we are still on the look out for better HGP materials with higher *Dk* values and lower wetting-angles in order to make HGP extended wear safe enough for the military environment.

40.2.5 COLD ENVIRONMENTS

In the extreme cold environment, important for units of the Marine Corps, HGP contact lenses and soft lenses can be used without any problem (Socks, 1982). By increasing the temperature of the precorneal tear-film, contact lens wearing soldiers are also somewhat protected against freezing of the cornea.

40.2.6   WARM ENVIRONMENTS

In hot climates, the contact-lens-wearing soldier meets more problems with his lenses. Under these conditions, low water content (38%) soft lenses are more suited than high water content lenses, because of the increased rate of evaporation. HGP contact lenses might be tolerated under these conditions, but dust and sand often cause real problems.

40.2.7   LENS CARE REGIMEN

When fitting active military personnel with contact lenses, the lens care regimen is also important. One cannot expect the soldier to carry extra large amounts of rinsing solutions, nor will he be able to use an electrically operated disinfection unit. Care regimens based on hydrogen-peroxide (H_2O_2) are also less suited in the military environment. When the soldier constantly moves about, with an irregular mapping out of the day, it is difficult to organize the daily care regimen properly. At times there will be no time for the neutralization procedure. Care regimens should be simple, reliable, safe and flexible. The fact that HGP lenses can be stored and inserted with tap-water in case of emergency is an important asset.

In Holland, according to our advice, the Directorate of Military Health Services recently officially allowed the wearing of contact lenses during military duty. In West Germany ophthalmologists of the Military Hospitals only accept the extended wear soft contact lens for military purposes (Marquardt, 1976; Roth, 1982). In general, the NATO members, France and the Warsaw Pact members all tolerate contact lens wear in the Army.

40.2.8   RECOMMENDATIONS

1. All recruits entering the Army and wearing contact lenses, should be examined biomicroscopically. Visual acuity with and without lenses and with optimal refractive correction should be determined and keratometry measurements should be taken after lens removal.
2. Based on the above mentioned data, all contact-lens-wearing soldiers should be provided with adequate (spare) combat spectacles.
3. At the present time, only high water content MMA-NVP soft lenses and HGP lenses with *Dk* values exceeding 12 (10^{-11} ml O_2/cm^2/s/ml mmHg) are recommended for use during military manoeuvres. This means that all Army personnel wearing other lenses have to be refitted with these lenses or have to return to (combat) spectacle wear, if they wish so. To reduce the possibility of lens loss HGP contact lenses with a large diameter (9.2 mm or more), preferentially with an aspherical base curve, are to be favoured. Personnel working under special conditions receive an individual permission for wearing lenses.

40.3   THE SITUATION IN THE AIR FORCE

40.3.1   SPECTACLES

Most of the statements in the previous paragraph are also valid for Air Force personnel. Although stringent ophthalmic criteria exist for the candidate pilot, it is very well possible that a minor myopia will develop after some years of active duty. The use of correction spectacles for air-crew members does possess some specific disadvantages:

1. The spectacle frame may interfere with personal safety equipment, such as light weight visor, oxygen mask, NBC protec-

tive mask, nuclear flash goggles or night vision equipment.

2. Some spectacle frames displace during high +Gz loads. (+ Gz = gravitational forces directed caudally.) Observations during centrifuge training show frames to slip up or down at +Gz loads over +5Gz.

3. During night and instrument flying the reflection of the many optic systems in a modern fighter-aircraft may create a disorientation hazard when the pilot is wearing glasses, even when these glasses are provided with an anti-glare coating.

4. Changing temperatures and air-flow directions in the cockpit may blur the glasses due to condensation of water vapour.

40.3.2   CONTACT LENSES

Most of the above mentioned disadvantages could be overcome by the use of contact lenses. Research conducted on the use of hard contact lenses in jet-aircraft was already started in the 1940s. Initially, this research was focused on scleral lenses. The limited wearing time was considered as an important contraindication for use in the Air Force (Duguet, 1952). Corneal PMMA contact lenses were tested for use in the jet-fighter cockpit by Draeger *et al.* in 1980.

Although the corneal PMMA lenses realized much more wearing comfort and permitted a longer wearing period, they are not generally accepted as useful for pilots (Chevaleraud & Perdriel, 1976). This attitude is based mainly on the properties of small PMMA lenses such as spectacle blur, irritation of foreign bodies behind the contact lens and the chance of corneal abrasion and the possible loss of the lens during flight.

Indeed ground-staff and helicopter pilots cannot tolerate hard lenses, whether gaspermeable or not: dust in the vicinity of aircraft take-off almost certainly gets under the lens.

With the advent of soft lenses, most researchers focused on these lenses for use in the Air Force. Crosley *et al.* (1974) proved that soft lenses can be used by helicopter air-crew without difficulty, except for the maximum wearing time. He stated that this should be 72 hours without lens removal, but this was impossible with the standard low-water content soft lenses he used. Furthermore, he mentioned the possibility of lens dehydration under the influence of a reduced blink rate and a tendency to stare during a flight under stress. Nilsson and Rengstorff reported successful continuous wearing of 74% water content soft lenses by a Swedish Air Force pilot (Nilsson & Rengstorff, 1979). Brennan and Girvin subjected pilots wearing soft lenses to several adverse conditions to be encountered in military aviation (Brennan & Girvin, 1985). They used high water content lenses (both 50% and 75%) in order to make continuous wear for periods of at least 48 hours possible. The subjects were subjected to ambient corneal hypoxia in the hypobaric chamber, simulating heights of 12 000 feet and 27 000 feet, to rapid decompression (from 8000 feet to 38 000 feet), to pressure breathing, to extreme hot (50 °C) and cold (–26 °C) environments, to vibration and +Gz acceleration forces. Rapid decompression is done in order to discover possible gas-bubble formation under the lenses. They subjected the test pilots to +4Gz and +6Gz for 20-s periods. Maximum displacement was 1.5 mm at +4Gz and 1.75 mm at +6Gz. Rapid decompression induced no bubble formation under the lens and visual acuity remained stationary. They concluded that soft lenses performed very well under these circumstances.

Polishuk and Raz also demonstrated the efficacy of standard soft lenses in military aviation and argued that contact lenses also offer an advantage over spectacles in the case of a crash (Polishuk & Raz, 1975). They, however, also found that 17% of their pilots rejected the lenses, because vision was unsatisfactory. Spherical soft lenses do not give sufficient optical correction for pilots with a refractive astigmatism of 0.5 dioptre or more. Toric soft lenses are often impractical for small amounts of astigmatism or show visual instability, especially during aerobatics with rotation of gravitational forces (Hart, 1984).

40.3.3   TRIAL IN THE ROYAL DUTCH AIR FORCE

This was one of the reasons for us to repeat the examinations of Draeger *et al.* (1980) and Brennan and Girvan (1985), but with the use of aspheric HGP lenses. Our test pilot was a 36-year old myopic Royal Netherlands Air Force fighter pilot. He had worn PMMA

lenses during flight in the past, but was now trained for flying the F-16, a 'high sustained gravity' aircraft (Punt *et al.*, 1985). He was refitted with rather large (9.8 mm) aspheric HGP lenses and both the old and the new pairs of lenses were marked, for enhanced visibility (Fig. 40.4).

Acceleration forces

For evaluation, the human centrifuge of the Dutch National Aerospace Medical Center was used (Fig. 40.5). The fully computer-controlled equipment allows +Gz acceleration forces of more than +10Gz with high onset rates of +3.5Gz per second. A video camera with a zoom lens recorded the behaviour of the contact lenses on the eye. Our

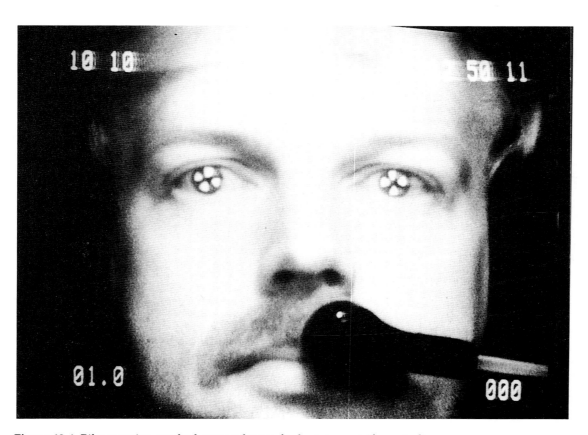

Figure 40.4 Pilot wearing marked contact lenses for human centrifuge studies.

pilot was able to reach +8.6Gz peak-levels and +6Gz levels for 30 s, during which he performed horizontal gaze movements. Before and after each test session, visual acuity, refraction and keratometry were repeated and lenses and eyes examined biomicroscopically.

We found that the vertical displacement of the PMMA lenses (diameter 9.2 mm) was significant (4.5 mm at peak-value of +8.6Gz), while extreme horizontal gaze movements almost caused the lenses to slip from the cornea. Through blinking action the lenses returned to the cornea. In general, the movements were unstable, jerky and strongly influenced by blinking action and facial tension. There was no apparent decentration of the aspheric HGP lenses, neither during peak levels of +8.6Gz, nor during horizontal gaze movements (movement was not more than 1.5 mm from the central position). Even if a conventional small PMMA lens is not totally lost from the cornea during +Gz acceleration forces, the large aspherical contact lens, with its large optical zone diameter, will reduce the risk of glare from the edge of the lens, especially during night flights. The lens was fitted subpalpebrally and with little edge lift, reducing the chance of lens loss.

Rapid decompression

During rapid decompression, gas bubbles temporarily appeared under the lens, disappearing very rapidly, while they did not influence the visual acuity (Fig. 40.6).

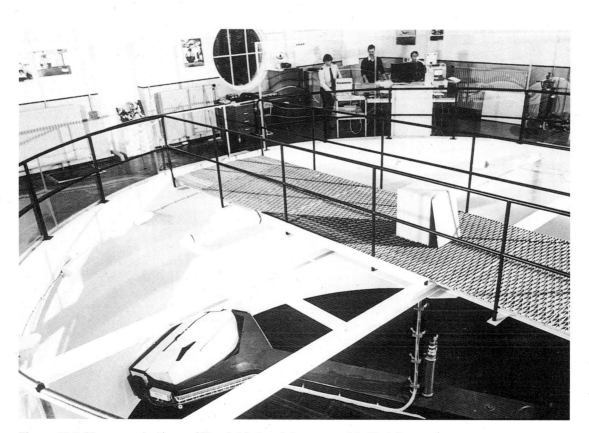

Figure 40.5 Human centrifuge of Dutch National Aerospace Medical Center.

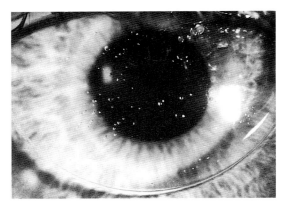

Figure 40.6 Gas bubbles beneath aspheric HGP contact lens during rapid decompression.

40.3.4   EFFECTS OF HIGH ALTITUDE FLYING

Another problem for the fighter pilot wearing contact lenses, is the danger of corneal hypoxia, due to the hypobaric effects of high altitude flying. In military aircraft the cockpit pressure varies with the altitude because the cockpit is only partially pressurized. This often means that the pressure continuously drops, until a certain altitude is reached; the system then keeps the pressure on a constant level with increasing altitude. Climbing beyond another fixed altitude means that the cockpit pressure further decreases. Above 10 000 feet (3048 m, 522 mmHg air pressure, 110 mmHg PO_2) pure oxygen breathing is necessary to avoid the effects of hypoxia. However, the eyes are exposed to the hypobaric atmospheric pressure in the cockpit. Eng *et al.* demonstrated that soft lens (38% water content) wearability was not affected by simulated altitudes of 20 000 feet and 30 000 feet. (Eng *et al.*, 1978; Flynn *et al.*, 1988) This corresponds to aircraft altitudes of 35 000 feet and 50 000 feet, respectively (10 668 m and 15 240 m). Only a moderate increase in scleral injection was seen, but visual acuity, refraction, keratometry and biomicroscopy were unaffected. Hapnes kept his five subjects somewhat longer (4 h instead of the 3 h) in the hypobaric chamber and found that all ten eyes showed objective changes behind the standard soft HEMA lenses (Hapnes, 1980). The simulated altitude was 18 000 feet. The hypoxia problem was further complicated by reduction of water-vapour levels in the cockpit, with resultant evaporation of the tear film. This was only investigated in the cabins of commercial jet-aircrafts, but humidity levels in military aircrafts are also very low. Low humidity has a negative effect on the fit of soft lenses and wearing comfort of both soft and hard lenses.

40.3.5   PARACHUTE JUMPING

Rippel reported about parachute jumping and the wearing of contact lenses (Rippel, 1979). He concluded that hard contact lenses are very well tolerated during parachute jumping.

The wearing of contact lenses for military aviation is not officially allowed in most countries. In the UK contact lenses are allowed for Army Air crew, and Braithwaite (1983) gives some recommendations based on flying experience of seven contact-lens-wearing Army pilots since 1974.

40.3.6   RECOMMENDATIONS

1. All recruits entering the Air Force and wearing contact lenses, should be examined as detailed on page 938.
2. Based on the above mentioned data, all contact lens wearing Air Force personnel should be provided with adequate (spare) combat-spectacles.
3. At the present time, only high water content MMA-NVP soft lenses and large aspheric HGP lenses with Dk values exceeding 12 (10^{-11} ml O_2/cm^2/s/ml mmHg) are recommended for use during active duty. This means that all Air Force personnel wearing other lenses have to be refitted with these lenses or have to return to (combat)

spectacle wear, if they wish so. Pilots may need special spectacles to fit under their helmets. Personnel working under special conditions receive an individual permission for wearing lenses.

40.4 THE SITUATION IN THE NAVY

More than in the Army and Air Force, naval personnel are short of professional care for longer periods. On the other hand, all naval units have their own medical service, manned by a physician and trained male nurses. The general practitioner will be able to treat simple daily wear contact-lens-related complications, such as overwear, traumatic erosions because of faulty insertion, allergic reactions, lens removal problems, etc. Although the circumstances are ideal for extended wear, except in warm climates, the lack of professional care, attainable in a matter of hours, precludes the use of the different types of extended wear lenses on board of a ship. Whenever adequate spare spectacles are at hand and the individuals are very carefully instructed not to wear their extended wear soft lenses in a red or painful eye, high water content lenses are probably safe for extended wear in healthy eyes of naval personnel. The frequency of the follow-up visits constitutes a problem for naval personnel, especially in the first few months after the initial fitting.

The chance of lens loss in the wet environment is clearly present for all types of hard lenses. This was investigated for both hard and soft lenses and with the use of water with various salt concentrations by Lövsund *et al.*, (1980). In practice, none of the soft lenses and all hard lenses were lost from the eye in 15 min test periods with the eyes blinking and moving under water. Others reported soft contact lens wear during scuba (self-contained underwater breathing apparatus) diving, both in sea-

water and in chlorinated swimming pools (Williamson, 1971). There were no problems, with or without the use of a facemask. It seems that soft contact lens wear can even prevent discomfort due to splashes of sea water in the eye. The resulting tearing of the eye diminishes the visual acuity. This was important enough to fit competition catamaran sailors and windsurfers in Holland with (plano-) soft lenses as protective devices. Divers using contact lenses also experience decompression phenomena when they return to the surface, much like pilots, who suddenly lose their cockpit pressure. These effects were studied in hyperbaric chambers by Simon and Bradley (1978, 1980). Soft lenses, PMMA lenses and PMMA lenses with central fenestration were used. They observed fine (nitrogen) bubbles beneath the hard lenses during standard decompression procedures. The bubbles cleared after 30 min at sea level, but slit lamp examination at this time showed nummular patches of epithelialoedema in the areas overlain by the bubbles and persisting up to 2 hours after diving. Subjects experienced ocular discomfort, halos, specular highlights and decreased visual acuity. Bubbles were not seen under soft lenses or fenestrated (a single central 0.4 mm hole) PMMA lenses. Data, concerning the fit of these PMMA lenses are lacking, but the authors themselves already suggested that the insufficient precorneal tear exchange with these particular lenses probably caused the bubble formation and retention.

40.4.1 RECOMMENDATIONS

See page 938.

ACKNOWLEDGMENTS

I am grateful to Dr H. Punt, ophthalmologist, for his continuous stimulation to examine contact lens wear in the Services; Professor Dr A.Th.M. v. Balen and Dr P.C. Maudgal, ophthalmologists, for critically reading this chapter and their suggestions. Rob M. Rosenbrand, Ron J.P. Beerten and Alfred W. v/d Hulst, optometrists and contact lens specialists helped during the trials. The Inspectorate of the Military Health Services of the Royal Dutch Army and personnel of the Dr A Mathijsen Military Hospital in Utrecht contributed to the organization of the trials.

REFERENCES

Barner, S., Marner, K. and Fahmy, J.A. (1980) Clinical experience with continuous wear hydrophilic contact lenses in aphakia. *Acta Ophthalmol.*, **58**, 83–9.

Braithwaite, M.G. (1983) The use of contact lenses by Army Air crew. *J.R. Army Med. Corps.*, **129**, 43–5.

Brennan, D.H. and Girvin, J.K. (1985) The flight acceptability of soft contact lenses. An environmental trial. *Aviat. Space Environ. Med.*, **56**, 43–8.

Caroline, P.J. (1984) Focus on rigid gas-permeable CLs and surface deposits. *The Dispensing Optician*, **X**, 20–4.

Chevaleraud, J.P. and Perdriel, G. (1976) Aptitude au vol et lentilles de contact souples. *AGARD Conf. Proc.*, **191**, C6-1–C6-3.

Crosley, J.K., Braun, E.G. and Bailey, R.W. (1974) Soft (hydrophilic) contact lenses in U.S. Army Aviation: An investigative study of the Bausch and Lomb Soflens. *Am. J. Opt. Physiol. Opt.*, **51**, 470–7.

Draeger, J., Schroeder, U. and Vogt, L. (1980) Untersuchungen ueber die Vertraeglichkeit von Kontaktlinsen in der Luft und Raumfahrt. *Klin. Mbl. Augenheikd.*, **176**, 421–6.

Duguet, J. (1952) Practicability of contact lenses for pilots. *J. Aviat. Med.*, **23**, 477.

Eng, W.G., Rasco, J.L. and Marano, J.A. (1978) Low atmospheric pressure effects on wearing soft contact lenses. *Aviat. Space Environ. Med.*, **V**, 73–75.

Flynn, W.J., Miller, R.E., Tredici, T.J. and Block, M.G. (1988) Soft contact lens wear at altitude: effects of hypoxia. *Aviat. Space Environ. Med.*, **59**(1), 44–8.

Hapnes, R. (1980) Soft contact lenses worn at simulated altitude of 18,000 feet. *Acta Ophthalmol.*, **58**, 90–5.

Hart, L.G. (1984) Contact lenses and other ophthalmic innovations and their relationship to the flight environment. *Can. Aero. Space J.*, **30**, 120–7.

Kok van Alphen, C.C., Linden, J.W., Visser, R. and Bol, A.H. (1985) Protection of the police against tear gas with soft lenses. *Military Med.*, **150**, 451–4.

Levy, B. (1985) Rigid gas-permeable lenses for extended-wear: a 1 year clinical evaluation. *Am. J. Opt. Physiol. Opt.*, **62**, 880–94.

Lövsund, P. Nilsson, S.E.G. and Öberg, P.A. (1980) The use of contact lenses in wet or damp environments. *Acta Ophthalmol.*, **58**, 794–804.

Marquardt, R. (1976) Kontaktlinsen- Ihr Fuer und Wider. *Wehrmed Mschr.*, **6**, 170–4.

Nilsson, S.E.G., and Persson, G. (1986) Low complication rate in extended wear of contact lenses. *Acta Ophthalmol.*, **64**, 88–92.

Nilsson, K. and Rengstorff, R.H. (1979) Continuous wearing of duragel contact lenses by Swedish Air Force pilots. *Am. J. Optom. Physiol. Opt.*, **56**, 356–8.

Nilsson, S.E.G., Lövsund, P. and Öberg, P.A. (1981) Contact lenses and mechanical trauma to the eye. *Acta Ophthalmol.*, **59**, 402–9.

Nilsson, S.E.G., Lindh, H. and Anderson, L. (1983) Contact lens wear in an environment contaminated with metal particles. *Acta Ophthalmol.*, **61**, 882–8.

Polishuk, A. and Raz, D. (1975) Soft contact-hydrophilic lenses in civil and military aviation. *Aviat. Space Environ. Med.*, **46**, 1188–98.

Punt, H., Heuvel, A.C.H., Biggelaar, H.H., Hoekstra, G.J. and Rouwen, A.J.P. (1985) Dynamic behaviour of spherical and aspherical contact lenses exposed to +Gz acceleration forces. *AGARD Conference Proceedings*, **379**, 16-1–16-5.

Reinke, A.R. (1970) Contact lens for military environment: requirement survey and study of feasibility (ACN 17167). United States Army Combat Developments Command, Medical Service Agency, Fort Sam, Houston, Texas, September, 1970.

Rengstorff, R.H. (1965a) The Fort Dix report – a longitudinal study of the effects of contact lenses. *Am. J. Optom.*, **42**, 153–63.

Rengstorff, R.H. (1965b) Contact lenses and basic training in the US army. *Mil. Med.*, **130**, 419–21.

Rengstorff, R.H. (1972) Spectacles and contact lenses: a survey of military trainees. *Mil. Med.*, **137**, 13–14.

Rippel, W. (1979) Kontaktlinsen und Fallschirmspringen. *Klin. Monatsbl. Augenheilkunde*, **174**, 284–6.

Roth, H.W. (1982) Kontaklinsen fur Soldaten – Neue wehrmedizinische aspekte. *Wehrmed. Mschr.*, **13**(3), 95–7.

Rouwen, A.J.P. and Rosenbrand, R.M. (1986) High water content soft lenses used for flexible daily/ extended wear for military personnel. *Int. Eyecare*, **2**, 435–40.

Rouwen, A.J.P., Pinckers, A.J.L.G., Pad Bosch, A.A.I., Punt, H., Doesburg, W.H. and Lemmens, W.A.J.G. (1983) Visual acuity, spectacle blur and slit-lamp biomicroscopy on asymptomatic contact-lens wearing recruits. *Graefe's Arch. Clin. Exp. Ophthalmol.*, **221**, 73–7.

Rouwen, A.J.P., Punt, H., Pinckers, A.J.L.G., Doesburg, W.H. and Lemmens, W.A.J.G. (1986) Contact lens wear during military field manoeuvres. *Contactologica*, **8**, 136–41.

Simon, D.R. and Bradley, M.E. (1978) Corneal edema in divers wearing contact lenses. *Am. J. Ophthalmol.*, **85**, 462–4.

Simon, D.R. and Bradley, M.E. (1980) Adverse effects of contact lens wear during decompression. *JAMA*, **244**(11), 1213–14.

Socks, J.F. (1982) Contact lenses in extreme cold environments: Response of rabbit corneas. *Am. J. Optom. Physiol. Opt.*, **59**(4), 297–300.

van Norren, D. (1984) Contact lenses in the military service *Am. J. Optom. Physiol. Opt.*, **61**, 441–7.

Williamson, D.E. (1971) Soft contact lenses and scuba diving. *The Eye, Ear, Nose and Throat Monthly*, **50**, 64–8.

PART TEN

Performance, Adverse Effects and their Management

INTRODUCTION

This part of the text considers the adverse effects that the contact lens can have upon vision and the eye tissues. It is not difficult to measure the more obvious aspects such as acuity, field of vision, contrast sensitivity, mesopic vision, and halation in different contrast illumination situations of the target (Chapter 41). It is even possible to measure the relative magnifications of the contact lens as compared with spectacle vision. But the everyday situation of performing highly critical tasks at work and at home all demand different degrees of visual function, and cannot be measured statistically. The problems of changes in binocular vision have already been alluded to in Part Eight. There are also the difficulties that may be experienced when changing from contact lens vision to spectacle vision due to alteration of the corneal curvature (Chapter 44) or induced stromal oedema (Chapter 45). On the other hand, the patient may adapt rapidly to contact lens vision, with all its advantages of field, free ocular motility and acuity. In particular, patients may find it impossible to return to spectacle vision, even if advised by the practitioner.

The aetiology of contact-lens-induced pathology and lens spoilation is fully discussed in Chapters 45, 46 and 47. The clinician has to determine whether the cause is inherent in the tissue and not related primarily to the contact lens wear, or is the device and its manner of use as the primary initiator of the eye pathology.

The upset of the normal protective mechanisms of the eye can lay the eye and adnexa open to infection with serious consequences (Chapter 46). Therefore great emphasis is laid upon the hygiene routines and standards. This is evident at all stages of manufacture, practitioner procedures and patient lens care. There are some special instances when extra precautions become necessary. They are in all instances of overwear such as continuous (extended) night and day (Chapter 43), where eye disease is already a factor, and in those systemic disorders that have a history of infection hazards, such as debility of any aetiology and metabolic disorders such as diabetes mellitus. The above considerations may be obvious to most practitioners. There are other hazards that are inherent such as allergic and also toxic reaction to preparations or atmospheric pollution (Chapter 39).

As a protection against the hazards inherent in the lens material, lens design and the preparations to be used there has arisen regulatory conditions imposed upon the manufacturer and even the practitioner. Such problems are sometimes issued as standards for quality but at other times as licensing regulations. To meet the requirements of the latter, it is often necessary for the manufacturer to test the product extensively by laboratory, animal and human controlled trials. But even so, the products require ongoing reportage by a licensing authority to ensure that late or missed adverse effects can be assessed.

In spite of all the controls that attempt to ensure safety and efficiency of a product there are patients who ignore or misunderstand directions by the practitioner, and eye pathology can result. The incidence of severe and irreversible eye disease is rare, but the practitioner has to be ever-vigilant to prevent its occurrence.

It does appear that the major causes of adverse reactions that produce eye pathology are hypoxia and trauma of a mechanical type followed by infection. These causes can to a large degree be overcome by materials that are gas permeable and by a good lens design and fit. Yet, even so, there will remain the periodic episodes of eye dryness and lower than normal oxygen tension, systemic metabolic anomalies, drugs and many other factors that will turn the balance and produce tissue pathological changes. There therefore always remains a small element of risk with contact lens wear.

M. Guillon

41.1 INTRODUCTION

Over the years the evaluation of the visual performance of contact lenses has been given a relatively low priority compared to other aspects of contact lens performance such as comfort and adverse corneal effects. Vision-related problems, however, are not unexceptional. In clinical practice it is not unusual to find patients with general symptoms of visual decrement or with symptoms for specific environmental conditions (e.g. night driving) who also have an acuity of 6/6 or better when tested with a conventional visual acuity chart (Ruben, 1979). At times patients also report much better vision quality and satisfaction with contact lenses than with their previous spectacle correction, when again, the visual acuity tested on a conventional chart is often equivalent. Finally, at times refitting with a different lens design and/or material is attempted because of vision problems, but the improvement in conventional visual acuity is only marginal and the decision to proceed with the refit becomes a difficult one.

In clinical research, when the efficacy of contact lenses is evaluated as part of large clinical trials, in particular when the research is for licensing purposes (Food and Drug Administration, 1984) conventional visual acuity is the only visual criteria used despite the shortcomings mentioned previously. It is only during investigations dealing specifically with contact lens visual performance that more sophisticated clinical techniques (Guillon *et al.*, 1988) have been used to critically assess that aspect of lens performance. However, many of the past clinical investigations have lead to contradicting conclusions, due in part to non-standardized testing conditions, and also in many cases to the small sample size used and/or the poor statistical treatment of the results.

The above situation has lead to practitioners talking about qualitative loss of vision (Kreis-Gosselin, 1978; Ruben, 1979) without a quantifiable decrease of performance. This has been particularly prevalent with soft contact lenses and therefore we sometimes hear that soft lenses produce poor visual quality. In this chapter we will therefore:

1. Review the factors that influence contact lens visual performance.
2. Describe the different techniques used to assess contact lens visual performance and the results obtained to date.
3. Propose a protocol applicable to routine clinical practice.

The scope of our discussion will be limited to central visual performance of single vision lenses. The peripheral visual performance, measured in terms of field of vision, is

Contact Lens Practice. Edited by Montague Ruben and Michel Guillon.
Published in 1994 by Chapman & Hall, London. ISBN 0 412 35120 X

already better with contact lenses than with glasses (Ruben, 1979) due to the absence of the limiting spectacle frame even for those cosmetic lenses with an opaque periphery (Josephson & Caffery, 1987). The correction of presbyopia with contact lenses is the subject of Chapter 33.

41.2 FACTORS AFFECTING CONTACT LENS VISUAL PERFORMANCE

The factors that affect contact lens visual performance fall into two broad categories: environmental and contact-lens- and/or eye-related factors. The environmental factors are imposed by the various conditions under which contact lenses are used. These latter factors must be taken into consideration by any comprehensive testing routine. The contact lens and/or eye related factors are those that need to be identified and their effects quantified by any useful testing routine.

41.2.1   ENVIRONMENTAL FACTORS

Introduction

There are four main environmental factors to consider: (1) the overall luminance; (2) the contrast of the visual scene or task; (3) the presence or absence of glare: and (4) the time allowed to carry out the visual task of interest. The first two factors are the most influential.

Luminance

Luminance is the one single factor that has the largest changes and the greatest influence on contact lens visual performance. Contact lenses are required to perform at high mesopic level of 0.4 to 3 cd/m² during night driving (Commission Internationale de l'Eclairage, 1977), at low photopic level for visual display work (Illuminating Engineering Society, 1981), at average photopic level of up to 150 cd/m² during more general

indoor tasks (Illuminating Engineering Society, 1981), and at high or even very high photopic levels outdoor, 1100 to 32,000 cd/m² under the midday sun (Commission Internationale de l'Eclairage, 1977). Changes in luminance affect visual performance by creating different levels of retinal illuminance and by altering the pupil diameter.

The variation in pupil diameter is particularly important. The aberrations of both the ocular system (Ivanoff, 1956; Jenkins, 1963; Campbell & Green, 1965; Howland & Howland, 1977; Millodot & Sivak, 1979; Walsh and Charman, 1985) and the contact lens (Westheimer, 1961; Woo & Sivak, 1974; Bauer, 1979; Campbell, 1981; El Nashar & Larke, 1986; Cox, 1990; Charman, 1991) are brought into effect when the pupil is dilated under low luminance conditions. The ocular system that was thought to mainly suffer from positive spherical aberration at distance (Ivanoff, 1956; Millodot & Sivak, 1979) has been shown in recent studies, using sophisticated techniques, to exhibit different types of aberrations including oblique astigmatism, spherical aberration and coma (Howland & Howland, 1977; Walsh & Charman, 1985; Charman, 1991). Such aberrations in general are detrimental to the visual performance when the pupil diameter is greater than 4 mm (Riggs, 1965). Similarly contact lenses exhibit complex aberrations (El Nashar & Larke, 1986). The spherical component of such aberrations for conventional hard and soft lenses creates significant visual performance losses for pupils of 6mm or more (Cox, 1990).

The variation in retinal illuminance also significantly affects performance in the absence of significant changes in pupil diameter. The visual acuity varies with luminance for average photopic levels before reaching a near plateau. That plateau differs depending upon the contrast of the optotype. Low contrast optotypes on average reach a plateau at a higher luminance (200 cd/m²) than high contrast optotypes (160 cd/m²)

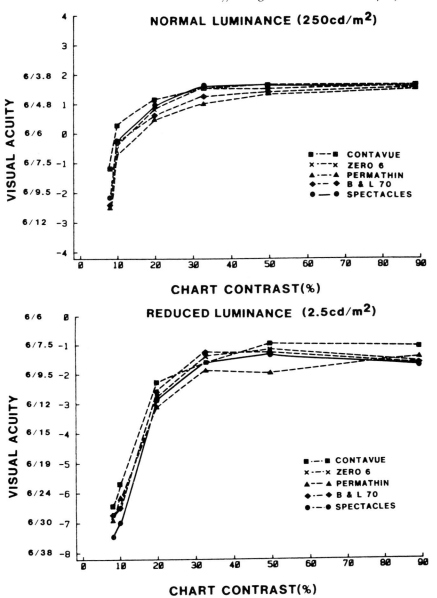

Figure 41.1 Visual acuity results recorded in VA units (– 10 logarithm of the minimal angle of resolution) spectacles and various soft contact lenses. (a) At high luminance (250 cd/m²); (b) at low luminance (2.5 cd/m²) (by courtesy of Guillon *et al.*, 1988).

(Richards, 1977). The subject's age, is also a factor (Chapter 33); older people who have lower ocular media light transmittance need a higher optotype luminance before reaching

a plateau, all other conditions being equal (Richards, 1977).

A study comparing the contrast sensitivity obtained with spectacles, soft and rigid gas permeable contact lenses (Guillon *et al.*, 1983) has demonstrated the important effect of luminance on contact lens performance, revealing significant differences in performance for distance vision at low luminance but not at high luminance. Similarly the magnitude of the differences in visual acuity achieved with various soft lenses was shown to be greater at low luminance (2.5 cd/m^2) than at high luminance (250 cd/m^2) (Figs 41.1 and 41.2) (Guillon *et al.*, 1988; Guillon & Sayer, 1988).

Contrast

Visual tasks vary significantly in contrast from a value as high as 90% for high quality print down to 60% for a newspaper

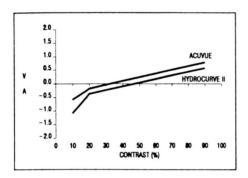

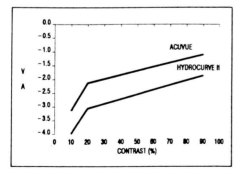

Figure 41.2 Visual acuity results recorded in VA units (– 10 logarithm of the minimal angle of resolution) for Acuvue™ and Hydrocurve II™ soft contact lenses. (a) At high luminance (250 cd/m^2); (b) at low luminance (2.5 cd/m^2) (by courtesy of Guillon & Sayer, 1988).

print and as low as 5% for a dull object in fog. Most tasks have a contrast between 90% and 10%. A recent study has shown that, for conventional soft contact lenses, the VA achieved both under high luminance (250 cd/m^2) and low luminance (2.5 cd/m^2) was practically constant for optotypes varying in contrast from approximately 30% to 90% (Guillon *et al.*, 1988) but that below 30% the visual acuity (VA) decreased rapidly (Fig. 41.1). A greater difference in VA was recorded for the low contrast charts than the high contrast charts indicating that such differences in VA between contact lenses are due to diffusive blur and not to uncorrected refractive errors. The validity of this differential diagnosis was demonstrated by Ho and Bilton (1986), who compared the relative loss in visual acuity produced by spherical defocus (refractive blur) and by an evenly diffusing media on Logmar VA charts for three different contrasts (high, medium and low) (Fig. 41.3). This finding suggests that conventional soft contact lenses of different types produce retinal images of different qualities. This helps to explain the increase in symptoms experienced by some patients while wearing contact lenses and carrying out tasks under low contrast conditions.

The threshold of contrast detection has been directly tested for different types of contact lenses by contrast sensitivity (CS) evaluation. Such evaluation without doubt is more sensitive than conventional visual acuity measurement, in particular for testing taking place at spatial frequencies between 3 and 6 cycles per degree (Applegate & Massof, 1975; Mitra & Lamberts, 1975; Woo & Hess, 1979; Bernstein & Brodrick, 1981; Guillon *et al.*, 1983; Kirkpatrick & Roggenkamp, 1985; Tomlinson & Mann, 1985; Gundel *et al.*, 1988; Nowozyckyj *et al.*, 1988). However, in the author's experience CS testing is more difficult to carry out in clinical pratice but not more sensitive than

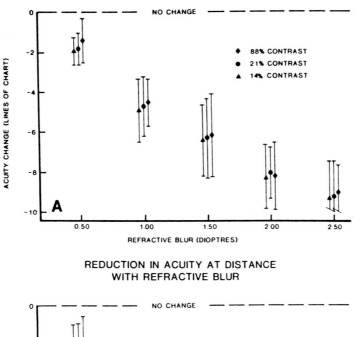

REDUCTION IN ACUITY AT DISTANCE
WITH REFRACTIVE BLUR

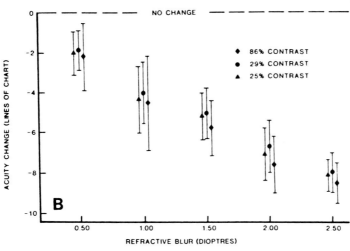

REDUCTION IN ACUITY AT NEAR
WITH REFRACTIVE BLUR

Figure 41.3 Visual acuity loss recorded in line of visual acuity for Logmar charts of different contrasts. Loss produced: (a) by increasing refractive blur (spherical defocus) and (b) by increasing diffusive blur (diffusing media) (by courtesy of Ho & Bilton, 1986).

an extensive routine based upon VA measurements under different contrasts. Also the clinical implications of any difference recorded by contrast sensitivity testing are more difficult to interpret than those recorded by visual acuity measurements. Further contrast sensitivity tests visual performance at contrast thresholds which are well below the contrasts normally encountered in every-day life.

Glare

Glare complaints, in particular those due to oncoming headlights during night driving with rigid contact lenses, are common complaints reported in clinical practice.

The presence of glare creates disability by light scattering within the ocular media and/or the contact lens. Hence the greater the glare problem the worse the light transmission of the eye/contact lens system. The disability produced increases when the eccentricity of the glare source decreases (Applegate & Wolf, 1987) or when the intensity of the glare source increases (Miller *et al.*, 1967) with reference to the visual task. The important characteristic concerning glare is that the disability is not due to the intrinsic intensity of the source itself but to the relative intensity of that source compared to the luminance of the visual task. The phenomenon has been clearly demonstrated for contact lenses by Applegate (Applegate & Wolf, 1987; Applegate & Jones, 1989), who reported that a fixed luminance light source only created glare for low luminance background conditions. These results explain in turn why the most commonly reported symptom is glare at night, when it is easy to create a relatively high glare source.

Presentation time

A visual task near the patient threshold for that task will be more difficult to perform when presented for a short period of time than when a longer exposure period is allowed. This difficulty in performing a task with reduced exposure time is compounded by any fluctuation in vision that occurs in time with lenses exhibiting poor mechanical performance. Such cases include rigid gas permeable (RGP) lenses, with an unstable flat fit or excessive lens flexure, and RGP or soft lenses with uncorrected astigmatism. But even for well fitting lenses, RGP lenses, because of their large blink-induced move-

ments, have been shown to perform worse than spectacles and/or soft lenses (Ridder & Tomlinson, 1991). This aspect of clinical performance is particularly relevant for situations where the visual task is presented for a short time period only, such as drivers that attempt to read a road sign or airline pilots.

41.2.2   CONTACT LENS AND CORNEA RELATED FACTORS

Causative factor classification

Visual performance achieved with any corrective lens and in particular with contact lenses is dependent upon the quality of the retinal image. Any contact lens or cornea related factor that contributes to a degradation of that retinal image creates a subjective impression of blur. Such factors are numerous but fall into two broad categories: (1) refractive; and (2) diffusive (non-refractive).

The two testing routines most commonly used to quantify losses in visual performance have been visual acuity and contrast sensitivity, and both differentiate between these two types of blur. The VA evaluation routine that involves testing with charts of different contrasts permits that differentiation and quantifies each type of blur (Ho & Bilton, 1986). Refractive blur creates a VA loss of similar magnitude for all contrasts whereas diffusive blur creates a loss of VA that increases in magnitude as the chart contrast decreases. Hence the loss of high contrast VA with a contact lens compared to the VA obtained with the best sphero-cylindrical refraction is an indication of refractive blur. The differential loss of VA between high and low contrast for the same two corrections is due to diffusive blur (Fig. 41.4). Contrast sensitivity also leads to a differential diagnosis between the two types of blur. Refractive blur creates a CS loss that increases when the target spatial frequency increases (Campbell

& Green, 1965). Non-refractive blur, such as that produced by ocular aberrations present with a dilated pupil, exhibit similar losses for mid and high spatial frequencies (Green & Campbell, 1965).

For each type of blur the causative factors are numerous. Refractive blur may be due to uncorrected spherical or astigmatic refractive errors, whereas non-refractive blur may be due to the contact lens directly or to the adverse effects induced by contact lens wear. Several contact lens factors responsible for non-refractive blur have been identified, they include: poor material homogeneity, poor surface quality (poorly finished or distorted lenses, poorly wettable and/or heavily deposited lenses) and aberrations. The adverse effects produced by the action of the contact lens on the cornea and which are responsible for non-refractive blur are also numerous. They include the osmotic changes that create vision loss in patients with epithelial oedema, and the gross mechanical changes produced by the adverse mechanical effects of RGP lenses with low or no clinically useful oxygen permeability such as CAB or PMMA.

VA HCSP = High Contrast Spectacle VA
VA LCSP = Low Contrast Spectacle VA
VA HCCL = High Contrast Contact Lens VA
VA LCCL = Low Contrast Contact Lens VA
Refractive Blur = VA HCCL − VA HCSP
Diffusive Blur = (VA LCCL − VA LCSP) − (VA HCCL − VA HCSP)
eg:
VA HCSP = +1.2
VA HCCL = +1.0
VA LCSP = −4.0
VA LCSP = −5.0
Refractive Blur = (+1.0) − (+1.2) = −0.2
Diffusive Blur = [(−5.0) − (−4.0)] − [(+1.0) − (+1.2)] = − 0.8

Figure 41.4 Differentiation between types of blur induced by contact lenses using VA measurement routine. VA recorded in VA units (− 10 the logarithm of the minimum angle of resolution).

Refractive Blur

Refractive blur with contact lenses concerns in the majority of cases residual astigmatism and/or induced astigmatism.

The problem of residual astigmatism is very well known with soft contact lenses which conform closely to the cornea (Tomlinson, 1976; Garner, 1977) and transfer the near totality of the corneal astigmatism to their front surface, hence do not correct astigmatism even with the relatively thick early soft lens designs (Grosvenor, 1972; Harris *et al.*, 1979). A point of interest however, is that the refractive cylinder determined by subjective refraction is always smaller than the cylinder determined by over-keratometry. For a corneal astigmatism of 1.50 DC the front contact lens surface keratometric cylinder is identical but the over-refraction cylinder is only one dioptre (Grosvenor, 1972). In the early days practitioners attempted to mask astigmatism by using thick lens designs with some success. The approach was to increase the lens thickness from a normal value of 0.17 mm to approximately 0.30 mm to correct an astigmatism of 2.00 DC to 2.50 DC (Boyd, 1974; Kreis-Gosselin, 1978). That modality of correction, however, was not universally accepted. Morrison (1973) suggested that patients subjectively accept less than an optimal correction, in particular, they accept some degree of uncorrected astigmatism which is not detected with conventional VA charts.

Both Morrison (1973) and Grosvenor (1972) concluded that conventional VA measurements lead to an underestimation of any astigmatism present.

Induced and/or residual astigmatism are optical problems which are rare with rigid lenses but not absent (Chapter 28). There are three main instances in which such problems are encountered. First, for those patients with a spherical or near spherical spectacle refraction and significant corneal astigmatism, a spherical rigid lens is contraindicated. In such a case the lenticular astigmatism is equal or near equal in magnitude to the corneal astigmatism. A conventional rigid lens corrects the corneal astigmatism and induces an astigmatism equal to the lenticular astigmatism. The lens of choice is in that case a spherical soft contact lens. Second, patients with an astigmatic spectacle correction and a spherical or near spherical cornea will have some residual astigmatism with conventional rigid lenses. The refractive astigmatism being in that case of lenticular origin will mean that a spherical rigid lens will have no alleviating effect on that astigmatism. The easiest alternative is a front toric soft contact lens or if a rigid lens is selected a more complex correction with a stabilized, most likely truncated and/or prism ballasted front surface toric lens will be required. The third case, which also involves patients with lenticular astigmatism, is when the spectacle and corneal cylinders are significantly different. The refractive astigmatism will not be fully corrected by a spherical rigid contact lens and will require the same approach as the previous case.

Diffusive blur

Direct effects

Poor material homogeneity The problems associated with poor material homogeneity are always possible with complex polymers such as those used in contact lens manufacturing. Non-homogeneity creates irregular power variations and internal light scatter that can produce diffusive blur. However with modern manufacturing technology and good process control the problems that concerned clinicians involved with early hydrogel lens fitting are now mostly just points of an historic interest. One particular contribution has been the understanding (Sammons, 1981, 1988) of the non-isotropicity of soft lens hydration. Anisotropicity is usually corrected by using different radial and axial

swell factors for calculating the parameters of lathe cut lenses or the parameters of the moulds for lenses to be cast moulded as xerogel. Recently the problem has been bypassed by producing lenses in their final hydrated form, in a process known as soft moulding (Sammons, 1989).

Poor lens *in vivo* wettability Good *in vivo* wettability of contact lenses is an essential factor to achieve good visual performance. Micro-irregularities are present both at the surface of the cornea and contact lenses, and only their coverage by a continuous tear film gives to those surfaces their good optical properties. Any disruption in the continuity of the tear film will produce a diffusive blur by either creating an irregular highly refractive surface that produces significant distortions and/or high amount of light scattering (Holly, 1981). Such disruptions are usually associated with a decrease in the stability of the pre contact lens tear film (PLTF) and are of real concern. With contact lenses, the stability of the tear film is intrinsically significantly poorer than that of the cornea. This is well illustrated by the much shorter pre-lens tear film break-up time than the pre-ocular tear film break-up time for both RGP (Guillon, 1986) and soft (Guillon & Guillon, 1989) contact lenses (see Chapter 21).

The problem of poor surface characteristics as a cause for a decreased visual performance has been reported from the early days of soft contact lens fitting (Gasson, 1974). But a formal association between vision quality and keratometric image quality was demonstrated only much later (Knoll, 1984). However, one must avoid a simplistic approach as to the factors responsible for contact lens surface anomalies that produce a decrease in visual performance. If we accept the premise that for any contact lens material the smoother the surface the better the wettability, several variables may play a part. Lens manufacturing process may be a factor with cast moulding and spin casting achieving better surface quality than latheing and polishing (Sammons, 1985). Normal lens usage, via repeated lens manipulation, produces both scratches and deposits for RGP (Allary *et al.*, 1989; Guillon *et al.*, 1989a) and soft (Guillon *et al.*, 1989b) lenses. This in turn has been shown to destabilize the PLTF and to affect visual performance (Doane *et al.*, 1990). Lens mobility if excessive, particularly for RGP lenses where the near permanent lens movement does not allow, as for hydrogel lenses, enough time for the PLTF to form evenly and continuously, also contributes to a reduced visual performance.

Aberrations The exact role of contact-lens-induced aberrations is presently difficult to quantify from the limited information available in the literature. That area of investigation more than any other has led to contradictory findings. Several points can be made regarding the information to date. First, a number of investigations have measured contact lens aberrations in air, which does not correspond to their condition of use (Westheimer, 1961; Bauer, 1979). Second, when *in situ* conditions of use have been considered, wrong assumptions have been made in the calculations, such as spherical corneal and/or non representative lens parameters (Campbell, 1981). Finally, a too simplistic analysis has often been proposed, with only one aberration, usually a spherical aberration, being analysed (Westheimer, 1961; Woo & Sivak, 1976; Bauer, 1979; Campbell, 1981; Cox, 1990). One exception has been the work of El Nashar (El Nashar & Larke, 1986) who calculated the wavefront aberration of a cornea and a soft contact lens from photokeratoscopic measurements. The analysis of the wavefront aberration is to be commended, as it permits to quantify all the aberrations that affect an optical system and is not restricted to one or two which may be assumed to play a primordial role (Charman, 1991). Unfortunately in the El Nashar study the corneal and contact lens front surface were considered in isolation and not as part of the whole ocular image forming system.

The literature also includes claims from various workers that for both rigid (Kerns, 1974) and soft (Evans, 1983; Evans & Morrison, 1984, Lydon 1990) lenses an aspheric front surface improves visual results for patients with residual astigmatism with conventional spherical lenses.

The question of aberrations with contact lenses needs to be totally re-evaluated using a global approach involving the measurement of the overall contact lens and ocular aberrations *in situ*. Presently we can only indirectly extrapolate the relative effect of the image quality produced by the different lens types by reviewing the available information concerning the visual performance achieved with those different lenses. From our current information we can, however, state that as expected, contact lens aberrations are mainly a problem with dilated pupils under low luminance. However the results of some visual performance investigations using low contrast targets suggest that even at normal luminance aberrations may play a part (Guillon & Schock, 1991)

Indirect contact lens effects on the cornea

The indirect adverse effects of contact lenses on visual performance have been known to clinicians from the early days of contact lens practice, their exact mechanism however has taken much longer to identify. The two major adverse effects have been coloured haloes around lights during wear and spectacle blur at contact lens removal. Coloured haloes have been reported with conventional hard contact lenses, both scleral and corneal (Dallos, 1946; Obrig', 1947) and early design soft lenses of low oxygen transmissibility (Jenkins & Mulcahy, 1979).

Coloured haloes are usually reported around oncoming headlights or street lights at night. In the clinic they are best detected in a dimly lit room while the patient looks at a small bright light source.

The first important diagnostic sign is the

presence of coloured rings. That sign is the differentiating sign from colourless rings around lights at times reported by rigid lens wearers under similar conditions. The latter rings are due to flare produced at the edge of the optic zone when the zone is too small and/or when the lens is decentred. The second differential diagnostic sign for rigid lenses is the associated abnormal biomicroscopic signs referred to as central corneal clouding (CCC) (Mandell & Polse, 1971; Mandell, 1974). The appearance of CCC is a haze in the central cornea when the cornea is observed in sclerotic scatter against the background of the black pupil (Chapter 18). Several erroneous theories to explain those haloes have been put forward in the past. It is only recently that diffraction taking place at the level of the basal epithelial cells was put forward as the most likely cause (Miller & Benedek, 1973); this theoretical prediction was later proven indirectly with rabbit corneas (Lambert & Klyce, 1981) and more recently with human (Cox & Holden, 1990). In fact the discussion regarding the causative factors and the corneal layers responsible for visual losses was ongoing for many years using various investigational techniques, in particular glare sensitivity (Miller *et al.*, 1967; Lancon & Miller, 1973) contrast sensitivity (Hess & Garner, 1977; Hess & Carney, 1979; Carney & Jacobs, 1984) and light scattering measurement (Elliott *et al.*, 1991). The overall evidence indicates that both osmotic and hypoxic oedemas are responsible for vision losses but that the former produces the greater effects, the layer mainly responsible for such losses being the epithelial layer.

Spectacle blur at contact lens removal (Rengstorff, 1968, 1969a, 1971) is due to the distorted and changing corneal surface that does not allow the formation of a sharp retinal image with conventional spherocylindrical spectacle lenses and/or a stable refraction. Spectacle blur has only been reported with contact lenses of low or no oxygen transmissibility. The distortion is due to the mechanical effect of the lens on an oedematous cornea, that seems to be less resistant to mechanical trauma. This explains its absence with high *Dk* RGP lenses, that supply enough oxygen to the cornea for the maintenance of a normal metabolism, and with soft lenses that do not produce a noticeable mechanical effect.

41.3 INVESTIGATIONAL TECHNIQUES AND LENS PERFORMANCE

At least five different clinical techniques have been used to assess contact lens visual performance: (1) conventional visual acuity; (2) contrast sensitivity; (3) low contrast visual acuity; (4) border enhancement detection and (5) glare sensitivity.

41.3.1 CONVENTIONAL VISUAL ACUITY

Conventional visual acuity measurements using high contrast optotypes ($> 90\%$) viewed under high luminance conditions (> 160 cd/m^2) constitutes the most common evaluation of contact lens visual performance. However, those optotypes are very insensitive at detecting any anomaly other than those due to the refractive blur produced by uncorrected spherical or astigmatic refractive errors or very gross vision loss due to diffusive blur. For those reasons conventional VA testing in contact lens practice is only useful to detect refractive blur, or wherever conventional VA is affected after all refractive errors have been fully corrected it is indicative of a major diffusive blur problem.

These limitations of the technique outlined above has curtailed its usefulness to only the early investigations of the visual performance with soft contact lenses. Those conventional VA measurements demonstrated the detrimental effects of uncorrected astigmatism (Grosvenor, 1972; Morrison, 1973; Boyd, 1974; Kreis-Gosselin, 1978) and diffusive blur losses associated with early spun cast (Knoll *et al.*, 1970) and lathe cut (Sarver, 1972; Wechsler, 1978) lenses. Such losses have not been confirmed with modern designs both spun cast, lathe cut and cast moulded (Hill, 1980; Watson *et al.*, 1981).

41.3.2 CONTRAST SENSITIVITY

Contrast sensitivity (CS) has been used extensively to critically assess the visual performance achievable with contact lenses and at times has been considered the panacea. There are a number of remarks to make with regard to that technique in the context of contact lens visual performance. First, it has been commented that CS is superior to visual acuity when testing contact lens visual performance. We agree, with that expected finding, where the time consuming CS measurements bring more information than the rapid technique of conventional single visual acuity measurement. It must be remembered also that CS tests performance at contrasts corresponding to the threshold of detection and not at contrasts commonly encountered during normal contact lens use. A further comment concerns the CS routine employed to test contact lens visual performance. CS was shown very early on to be affected by optical blur such as that due to contact lens or associated effect only in the mid

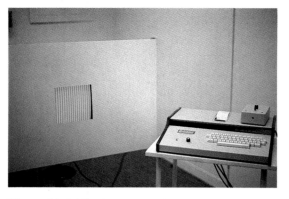

Figure 41.6 Nicolet system for computer generation of contrast sensitivity testing patterns.

to high frequencies (Green & Campbell, 1965; Campbell & Gumbish, 1966), the low frequency being insensitive to optical blur. Despite those findings, current investigation routines still involve low frequency testing, whereas measurements should really begin at spatial frequencies at least 2 cycles per degree.

The early contact lens investigations were based upon very few patients and lacked rigorous statistical treatment. However they revealed trends suggesting that:

1. Interpalpebral fit PMMA lenses and early design spun cast soft lenses produced lower CS responses in particular for mid-frequencies in the absence of any difference in VA (Applegate & Massof, 1975), specially under low luminance for spun cast soft lenses (Rosenblum & Leach, 1975).

2. Soft contact lens symptomatic patients had a greater loss in CS compared to spectacles than asymptomatic patients (Woo & Hess, 1979).

More rigorous studies have permitted us to conclude that:

1. The loss of performance with rigid contact lenses, compared to spectacles, is greater under low than high luminance (Millodot, 1969; Guillon *et al.*, 1983).

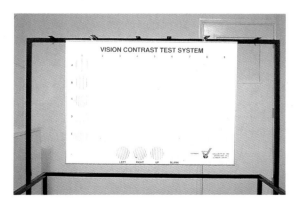

Figure 41.5 VistechTM, printed contrast sensitivity chart.

Conversely, for lathe cut soft lenses either no difference in performance was recorded compared to spectacles (Guillon *et al.*, 1983) or contact lenses gave a better performance than spectacles under low luminance (Millodot, 1975; Guillon, *et al.*, 1988).

2. The visual performance of spherical contact lenses is similar to spectacles and remains unchanged for lathe cut lenses of different thickness and water content (Tomlinson & Mann, 1985). That performance is predictable long term from early measurements (Nowozckyj *et al.*, 1988). Some studies, however, still lead to controversial findings. For example Grey (1986a,b) testing a group of unadapted patients concludes that the visual performance over the first hour of wear was correlated to the corneal swelling produced (Grey, 1986c). This would suggest that stromal oedema is responsible for such visual loss and that the lenses used produced severe swelling in one hour (7%–10%). Epithelial oedema induced by tear osmotic changes, which is well known during adaptation, would seem a far more probable explanation than the 2% to 4% stromal oedema measured.

3. Gundel *et al.*, (1988) showed that both modern lathe cut and cast moulded lenses performed equally to spectacles at all spatial frequencies.

The suggestion for a relevant routine to test critically new designs is therefore to test only mid to high spacial frequencies at high and low luminances. The most useful clinical approach is to use printed CS (Fig. 41.5) tests rather computer produced VDU-based tests which are more amenable to research practice (Fig. 41.6).

41.3.3 LOW CONTRAST VISUAL ACUITY

The evaluation of contact lens visual performance with low contrast VA charts is

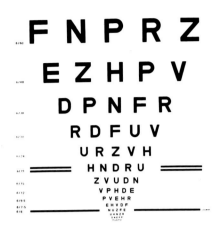

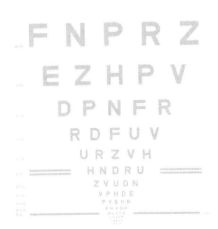

Figure 41.7 Bailey–Lovie type logarithmic progression visual acuity charts (a) high contrast (90%) and (b) low contrast (10%).

favoured by the author for the routine clinical situation. It has several advantages over CS: (1) patients are familiar with the proce-

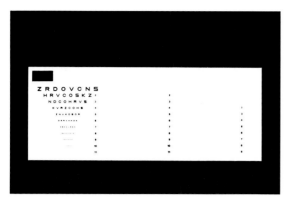

Figure 41.8 Regan logarithmic high (90%), low (6% and 4%) contrast visual acuity charts.

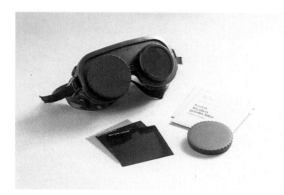

Figure 41.9 Modified welding goggles and neutral density filters used for low luminance measurements.

dure; (2) the procedure is relatively rapid; and (3) patients are tested at contrast levels comparable to every day activities. Further low contrast VA charts are as sensitive as CS charts at detecting differences in performance (Guillon, unpublished data) and also differentiate between the different types of blur (Ho & Bilton, 1986).

A number of studies to date have shown different aspects of the effects of diffusive blur:

1. Among leading daily wear soft lenses, some lathe cut lenses outperform spun cast lenses when tested on the same patients. Similarly Acuvue disposable lenses produced by cast moulding directly in their final form outperforms spun cast lenses (Guillon & Schock, 1991) and lathe cut (Guillon *et al.*, 1993a,b). We believe the cause for those differences to be peripheral aberration.

2. Extended wear RGP lenses give as good a visual performance as spectacles and produce a recovery in visual performance when long-term PMMA wearers are refitted (Guillon & Allary, 1990; Guillon *et al.*, 1993c). Recovery from corneal distortion induced by PMMA lenses is felt to be the cause of the difference in performance.

3. Worsening lens wettability with wear has been shown to be associated with visual losses (Doane *et al.*, 1990; Guillon *et al.*, 1992).

The VA technique used by the author is highly specific and identifies under which environmental condition (luminance/contrast combination) the performance of any lens may be defective. The routine proposed is to use a conventional high contrast chart (90%) and a low contrast chart ($\leq$ 10%), testing being carried over at two luminance levels, 250 and 2.5 cd/m^2. The methodology to follow involves the use of VA charts with logarithmic progression that create equal steps between the various lines each containing the same number of letters, either five (Bailey & Lovie, 1976) (Fig. 41.7) or eight (Regan & Neima, 1988) (Fig. 41.8). A number of those charts are now available commercially. The lighting system should be set for the high luminance measurements and altered by using neutral density filters (Guillon & Sayer, 1988) (Fig. 41.9). The methodology adopted requires the measurement VA to the nearest letter to achieve maximum test sensitivity (Guillon & Schock, 1991). In that way, the method has been shown to be highly reliable at detecting differences in performance (Guillon & Schock, 1991; Guillon *et al.*, 1993a). Some authors have added a glare source to test performance but we have not found that necessary.

REFERENCES

Allary, J.C., Mapstone, V., Guillon, J.P. and Guillon, M. (1989) Rigid gas permeable lens surface evaluation. *Trans. Br. Contact Lens Assoc. Ann. Clin. Conf.* **6**, 18–19.

Applegate, R.A. and Jones, D.H. (1989) Disability glare and hydrogel lens wear revisited. *Optom. Vis. Sci.*, **66**, 756–9.

Applegate, R.A. and Massof, R.W. (1975) Changes in the contrast sensitivity function induced by contact lens wear. *Am. J. Optom. Physiol. Opt.*, **52**, 840–46.

Applegate, R.A. and Wolf, M. (1987) Disability glare increased by hydrogel lens wear. *Am. J. Optom. Physiol. Opt.*, **64**, 309–12.

Bailey, I.L. and Lovie, J.E. (1976) New design principles for visual acuity charts. *Am. J. Optom. Physiol. Opt.*, **53**, 740–5.

Bauer, G.T. (1979) Longitudinal spherical aberration of spherical soft contact lenses. *Int. Contact Lens Clin.*, **6**, 143–150.

Bernstein, I.R. and Brodrick, J. (1981) Contact sensitivities through spectacles and soft contact lenses. *Am. J Optom. Physiol. Opt.*, **58**, 309–13.

Boyd, M.M. (1974) Optical quality of lathe cut compared with molded soft contact lenses. *Trans. Am. Acad. Ophthalmol. Otol. Laryngol.*, **78**, 412–18.

Campbell, C.E. (1981) The effect of spherical aberration of contact lens to the wearer. *Am. J. Optom. Physiol. Opt.*, **58**, 212–17.

Campbell, F.W. and Green, D.G. (1965) Optical and retinal factors affecting visual resolution. *J. Physiol. Lond.*, **181**, 576–93.

Campbell, F.W. and Gumbish, R.W. (1966) Optical quality of the human eye. *J. Physiol. Lond.*, **186**, 558–73.

Carney, L.G. and Jacobs, R.J. (1984) Mechanisms of visual loss in corneal oedema. *Arch. Ophthalmol.*, **102**, 1068–73.

Charman, W.N. (1991) Wavefront aberration of the eye: a review. *Optom. Vis. Sci.*, **68**, 574–83.

Commission Internationale de l'Eclairage (1977) *Recommendations for the lighting of roads for motorized traffic. CIE publications, no. 12* (2 edn), TC 46, Commission Internationale de l'Eclairage, Paris.

Cox, I. (1990) Theoretical calculation of the longitudinal spherical aberration of rigid and soft contact lenses. *Optom. Vis. Sci.*, **67**, 277–82.

Cox, I. and Holden B.A. (1990) Can vision loss be used as a quantitative assessment of variable oedema? *Int. Contact Lens Clin.*, **17**(4), 176–9.

Dallos, J. (1946) Sattler's veil. *Br. J. Ophthalmol.*, **30**, 607–12.

Doane, M.G., Timberlake, G.T. and Bertera, J.M. (1990) Low contrast visual acuity loss associated with in-vivo contact lens drying. *Inv. Ophthal. Vis. Sci.*, **31**, 407.

El Nashar, N.F. and Larke, J.P. (1986). Wavefront aberration in hydrogel lens wearing eye. *Am. J. Optom. Physiol. Opt.*, **63**, 409–12.

Elliot, D.B., Mitchell S. and Whitaker D. (1991) Factors affecting light scatter in contact lens wearers. *Optom. Vis. Sci.*, **68**, 629–33.

Evans. T.C. (1983). The CALS lens: Optical and perceptual considerations in aspheric topography. *Can. J. Optom.*, **45**, 21–7.

Evans, T.C. and Morrisson, I. (1984) Sensitivity to retinal defocus with aspheric soft lenses – predictions and clinical validation. *Am. J. Optom. Physiol. Opt.*, **61**, 729–36.

Food and Drug Administration (1984) *Testing guidelines for Class III contact lenses.* Food and Drug Administration, Rockville, MD.

Garner, L.F. (1977) Front surface topography of spherical flexible contact lenses on the eye. *Aust. J. Optom.*, **60**(2), 40–5.

Gasson, A. (1974) A comparative appraisal of Hydron, Sauflon and 'Soflens' soft lenses. *Ophthal. Opt.*, **15** (August 10), 738–54.

Green, D.G. and Campbell, F.W. (1965) Effects of focus on visual performance to a sinusoidal modulated spatial stimulus. *J. Opt. Soc. Am.*, **55**, 1154–7.

Grey, C.P. (1986a) Changes in contrast sensitivity during the first hour of soft lens wear. *Am. J. Optom. Physiol. Opt.*, **63**, 702–7.

Grey, C.P. (1986b) Changes in contrast sensitivity when wearing low, medium and high water content soft lenses. *J. Br. Contact Lens Assoc.*, **9**, 21–5.

Grey, C.P. (1986c) The effects of soft lens parameters on the contrast sensitivity function. *Trans. Br. Contact Lens Assoc. Conf.*, 48–54.

Grosvenor, T. (1972) Visual acuity astigmatism and soft contact lenses. *Am. J. Optom. Arch. Am. Acad. Optom. Opt.*, **49**, 407–12.

Guillon, J.P. (1986) Tear film structure and contact lenses. In *The Preocular Tear Film, in Health,*

Disease and Contact Lens Wear (ed. F.J. Holly), Dry Eye Institute, Lubbock, TX.

Guillon, M. and Allary, J.C. (1990) Refitting PMMA wearers with extended wear RGP lenses. *Optom. Vis. Sci.*, **67**, 142.

Guillon, M. and Guillon, J.P. (1989) Hydrogel lens wettability during overnight wear. *Opthal. Physiol. Opt.*, **9**, 355–9.

Guillon, M. and Sayer, G.S. (1988) Critical assessment of visual performance in contact lens practice. *Contax*, **May**, 9–13.

Guillon, M. and Schock, S.E. (1991) Soft contact lens visual performance: a multicentre study. *Optom. Vis. Sci.*, **68**, 96–103.

Guillon, M., Lydon, D.P.M. and Wilson, C. (1983) Variations in contrast sensitivity function with spectacles and contact lenses. *J. Br. Contact Lens Assoc.* **60**(3), 120–4.

Guillon, M, Lydon, D.P.M. and Solman RT (1988) Effect of target contrast and luminance on soft contact lens and spectacle visual performance. *Cur. Eye Res.*, **7**, 635–48.

Guillon, M., Guillon, J.P., Mapstone, V. and Dwyer, S. (1989a) Rigid gas permeable lenses in vivo wettability. *Trans. Br. Contact Lens Assoc. Ann. Clin. Conf.*, **6**, 24–6.

Guillon, J.P., Guillon, M., Dwyer, S. and Mapstone, V. (1989b) Hydrogel lens in vivo wettability. *Trans. Br. Contact Lens Assoc. Ann. Clin. Conf.*, **6**, 44–5.

Guillon, M., Allary, J.C., Guillon, J.-P. and Osborn, G. (1992) Clinical management of regular replacement. Part 1. Selection of replacement frequency. *Int. Contact Lens Clin.*, **19**(5/6), 104–20.

Guillon, M., Guillon, J.-P. and Shah, D. (1993a) Visual performance stability of disposable contact lenses. *Int. Contact Lens Clin.*, **20**, 7–17.

Guillon, M., Guillon J.-P. and Shah, D. (1993b) Visual performance stability of planned replacement daily wear contact lenses. *Int. Contact Lens Clin.*, in press.

Guillon, M., Allary, J.C., Guillon, J.-P. and Kreis-Gosselin, F. (1993c) Extended wear with rigid gas permeable contact lenses. *Pract. Optom.*, **4**(1), 40–6.

Gundel, R.E., Kirshen, S.A. and Diverglio, D. (1988) Changes in contrast sensitivity induced by spherical hydrogel lenses on low astigmats. *J. Am. Optom. Assoc.*, **59**, 636–40.

Harris, M.G., Goldberg, T., McBride, D. and Thromburg, L. (1979) Residual astigmatism and visual acuity with hydrogel contact lenses: a comparative study. *J. Am. Optom. Assoc.*, **50**, 303–6.

Hess, R.F. and Carney, L.G. (1979). Vision through an abnormal cornea: a pilot study of the relationship between visual loss from corneal distortion, corneal oedema, keratoconus and some allied corneal pathology. *Inv. Ophthalmol. Vis. Sci.*, **18**, 476–83.

Hess, R.F. and Garner, L.F. (1977) The effect of corneal oedema on visual function. *Inv. Opthalmol. Vis. Sci.*, **16**, 5–13.

Hill, J.F. (1980) Clinical comparison of the (Polymacon) spincast hydrogel contact lenses to the (Polymacon) lathe cut hydrogel lenses. *Am. J. Optom. Physiol. Opt.*, **57**, 523–6.

Ho, A. and Bilton, S.M. (1986) Low contrast charts effectively differentiate between types of blur. *Am. J. Optom. Physiol. Opt.*, **63**, 202–8.

Holly, F.J. (1981) Tear film physiology and contact lens wear II: Contact lens tear film physiology. *Am. J. Optom. Physiol. Opt.*, **58**, 324–30.

Howland, H.C. and Howland, B. (1977) A subjective method for the measurement of the monochromatic aberration of the eye. *J. Opt. Soc. Am.*, **67**, 1508–18.

Illuminating Engineering Society (1981) *IES Lighting Handbook*. Illuminating Engineering Society, New York.

Ivanoff, A. (1956) About the spherical aberration of the eye. *J. Opt. Soc. Am.*, **46**, 901–3.

Jenkins, T.C.A. (1963) Aberrations of the eye and their effects on vision. *Br. J. Physiol. Opt.*, **20**, 59–91.

Jenkins, L. and Mulcahy, B.L. (1979) Practical observations of fitting low plus soft lenses. *J. Br. Contact Lens Assoc.*, **2**, 35–6.

Josephson J.E. and Caffery B.E. (1987) Visual field loss with colored hydrogel lenses. *Am. J. Optom. Physiol. Opt.*, **64**, 38–40.

Kerns, R.L. (1974) Clinical evaluation of the merits of an aspheric front surface contact lens for patients manifesting residual astigmatism. *Am. J. Optom. Physiol. Opt.*, **51**, 750–7.

Kirkpatrick, D.L. and Roggenkamp, J.R. (1985) Effects of soft contact lenses on contrast sensitivity. *Am. J. Optom. Physiol. Opt.*, **62**, 407–12.

Knoll, H.A. (1984) Relation between qualitative vision and qualitative over keratometry in hydrogel contact lens wearers. *Am. J. Optom. Physiol. Opt.*, **61**, 448–52.

Knoll, H.A., Harrington, B. and William III Jr (1970) Two years experience with hydrophilic contact lenses. *Am. J. Optom. Physio. Arch. Am.*

Acad. Optom., **47**, 1000–4.

Kreis-Gosselin, F. (1978) *Visual acuity and soft lenses in soft contact lenses* (ed. M. Ruben), Bailliere Tyndall, London.

Lambert, S.R. and Klyce, S.D. (1981) The origins of Sattler's veil. *Am. J. Ophthalmol.*, **91**, 51–6.

Lancon, M.R. and Miller, D. (1973) Corneal hydration, visual acuity and glare sensitivity. *Arch. Ophthalmol.*, **90**, 227–30.

Lydon, D. (1990) Improved optics and control of astigmatism without cylinders. *Trans. Br. Contact Lens Assoc. Ann. Clin. Conf.*, 41–3.

Mandell, R.B. (1974) *Symptomatology and Post-fitting Care in Contact Lens Practice. Hard and Flexible lenses.* (ed. R.B. Mandell) Charles C Thomas, Springfield, II.

Mandell, R.B. and Polse, K.A. (1971) Corneal thickness changes accompanying central corneal clouding. *Am. J. Optom. Arch. Am. Acad. Optom.* **48**, 129–32.

Miller, D. and Benedek, G. (1973) *Intraocular Light Scattering*. C.C. Thomas, Springfield, IL.

Miller, D., Wolf, E., Geer, S. and Vansallo, V. (1967) Glare sensitivity related to use of contact lenses. *Arch. Ophthalmol.* **78**, 448–50.

Millodot, M. (1969) Variation of visual acuity with contact lenses: a function of luminance. *Arch. Ophthalmol.*, **82**, 461–5.

Millodot, M. (1975) Variation of visual acuity with soft contact lenses: a function of luminance. *Am. J. Optom. Physio. Opt.*, **52**, 541–4.

Millodot, M. and Sivak, J. (1979) Contribution of the cornea and lens to the spherical aberration of the eye. *Vis. Res.*, **19**, 685–7.

Mitra, S. and Lamberts, D.W. (1975) Contrast sensitivity in soft lens wearers. *Contact Intraocular Lens Med. J.*, **27**, 315–22.

Morrisson, R.J. (1973) Comparative studies: visual acuity with spectacles and flexible lenses, ophthalmometer reading with and without flexible lens. *Am. J. Optom. Arch. Am. Acad. Optom.*, **50**, 807–9.

Nowozyckyj, A., Carney, L.G. and Efron, N. (1988) Effect of hydrogel lens wear on contrast sensitivity. *Am. J. Optom. Physiol. Opt.*, **65**, 263–71.

Obrig, T.E. (1947) Solutions used with contact lenses. *Arch. Ophthalmol.*, **38**, 668–74.

Regan, D. and Neima, D. (1983) Low contrast acuity charts as a test of visual function. *Ophthalmology*, **90**, 1192–200.

Rengstorff, R.M. (1968) Contact lenses and after effects – some temporal factors which influence myopia and astigmatic variations. *Am. J.*

Optom. Arch. Am. Acad. Optom.*, **45**, 364–73.

Rengstorff, R.M. (1969a) Variations in corneal curvature measurements: an after effect observed with habitual wearers of contact lenses. *Am. J. Optom. Arch. Am. Acad. Optom.*, **46**, 45–51.

Rengstorff, R.M. (1969b) Relationship between myopia and corneal curvature changes after wearing contact lenses. *Am. J. Optom. Arch. Am. Acad. Optom.*, **46**, 357–62.

Rengstorff, R.M. (1971) Variations in astigmatism overnight and during the day after wearing contact lenses. *Am. J. Optom. Arch. Am. Acad. Optom.*, **48**, 810–13.

Richards, O.W. (1977) Effects of luminance and contrast on visual acuity, ages 16 to 90 years. *Am. J. Optom. Physiol. Opt.*, **54**, 178–85.

Ridder, W.H. III and Tomlinson, A. (991) Blink induced temporal variations in contrast sensitivity. *Int. Contact Lens Clin.*, **18**, 231–7.

Riggs, L.A. (1965) Visual acuity. In *Vision and Visual Perception* (ed. C.H. Graham), Wiley, New York, pp. 321–49.

Rosenblum, W.M. and Leach, N.E. (1975) The subjective quality (SQF) of B&L Softlens. *Am. J. Optom. Physiol. Opt.*, **52**, 658–62.

Ruben, M. (1979) Visual disturbances from contact lenses. Turnville Memorial Lecture. *Ophthal. Opt.*, **19**(6), 186–94.

Sammons, W.A. (1981) A mathematical description of soft lens hydration (Part 1). *Am. J. Optom. Physiol. Opt.*, **58**, 718–24.

Sammons, W.A. (1985) Contact lens surface texture. *J. Br. Contact Lens Assoc.*, **8**, 31–9.

Sammons, W.A. (1988) The Nissel Memorial Lecture. Manufacturing materials, methods and measurements. *Trans. Br. Contact Lens Assoc. Sci. Meeting.* **12**, 12–19.

Sammons, W.A. (1989) Soft lens expansion . . . twenty years on. *Trans. Br. Contact Lens Assoc. Ann. Clin. Conf.*, **6**, 39–43.

Sarver, M.D. (1972). Vision with hydrophilic contact lenses. *J. Am. Optom. Assoc.*, **43**, 316–21.

Tomlinson, A. (1976) The flexure and toricity of best, flat and steep fitting hydrogel lenses on the eye. *Br. J. Physiol. Opt.*, **30**, 101–7.

Tomlinson, A. (1991) Vision with contact lenses. *Trans. Br. Contact Lens Assoc. Ann. Clin. Conf.*, In press.

Tomlinson, A. and Mann, G. (1985) An analysis of visual performance with soft contact lenses and spectacles correction. *Ophthal. Physiol. Opt.*, **5**, 53–7.

Walsh, G. and Charman, W.M. (1985) Measurements of the axial wavefront aberration of the human eye. *Ophthal. Physiol. Opt.,* **5**, 23–31.

Watson, E., Ruben, M. and Guillon, M. (1981) Lens flexure effects with lathe cut and spin cast lenses. *Int. Contact Lens Clin.,* **8**(5), 24–33.

Wechsler, S. (1978). Visual acuity in hard and soft contact lens wearers: a comparison. *J. Am. Optom. Assoc.,* **49**, 251–5.

Westheimer, G. (1961) Abberrations of contact lenses. *Am. J. Optom. Arch. Am. Acad. Optom.,* **38**, 445–8.

Woo, G. and Hess, R. (1979) Contrast sensitivity function and soft contact lenses. *Int. Contact Lens Clin.,* **6**, 171–6.

Woo, G.C.S. and Sivak, J.G. (1976) The effect of hard and soft contact lenses (Soflens™) on the spherical aberration of the human eye. *Am. J. Optom. Physiol. Opt.,* **53**, 459–63.

EFFECTS OF CONTACT LENSES ON CORNEAL PHYSIOLOGY

M.R. O'Neal and J.A. Bonanno

42.1 INTRODUCTION

The cornea has high metabolic activity and needs both nutrients and oxygen to stay healthy and transparent (Maurice, 1984). The cornea gets most of its nutrients from the eye's anterior chamber, located directly behind the cornea, while oxygen gets into the cornea mostly by diffusion across its front surface. Many of the corneal changes from contact lens wear appear to be due to hypoxia (i.e. decreased oxygen) under the lens at the anterior corneal surface (Holden, 1989). Since oxygen plays such a primary role in corneal health, this discussion on corneal physiological changes with lens wear will begin with hypoxia and corneal edema before addressing the corneal layers.

42.2 CORNEAL SWELLING

42.2.1 EARLY STUDIES

The most studied and measured aspect of corneal response to contact lens wear has been changes in corneal thickness. Early corneal physiological research found that normal corneal hydration is necessary for the maintenance of optical transparency (Maurice, 1957), and that corneal hydration is linearly related to corneal thickness (Hedbys & Mishima, 1966). A number of apparatus and techniques for corneal thickness measurement were developed and have been described in detail by Mishima (1968). The development of the electronic optical pachometer (based on the Haag–Streit pachometer, Mishima–Hedby's method) by Mandell and Polse (1969) allowed a practical method of measuring corneal thickness, and thus monitoring the physiological change in corneal hydration with contact lens wear.

One of the earliest corneal slit lamp observations noted with the wear of PMMA lenses was a whitish haze, appearing in the apical area of the cornea. Known as central corneal clouding (CCC), this hazy area usually disappeared within several hours after the lenses were removed. Mandell and Polse (1971) found that PMMA lens daily wear resulted in about 6% corneal edema and accompanied the observation of central corneal clouding with these lenses. Much earlier, Smelser and Ozanics (1952) had been the first to relate the central corneal clouding to oxygen insufficiency (i.e. hypoxia) at the epithelial surface. Polse and Mandell (1971) established further that corneal hypoxia was the cause of the corneal swelling with PMMA lens wear. They found less corneal edema when a PMMA lens wearing eye was exposed to a high oxygen level during lens wear.

Contact Lens Practice. Edited by Montague Ruben and Michel Guillon.
Published in 1994 by Chapman & Hall, London. ISBN 0 412 35120 X

42.2.2   MINIMUM CORNEAL OXYGEN REQUIREMENT

Goggle hypoxia studies

When the amount of oxygen at the anterior corneal surface is below a critical level, fluid moves into the cornea and it begins to swell. The rate and amount of corneal swelling is dependent upon the degree of hypoxia, with the maximum swelling generally occurring by 3 hours (Fig. 42.1), (except longer for very low oxygen) when a goggle is used to expose the eye to lower oxygen levels (Holden *et al.*, 1984). In addition, there is a wide range between individuals in the corneal swelling response to the same oxygen level (Fig. 42.2); as first demonstrated by Mandell and Farrell (1980) and confirmed by others (Sarver *et al.*, 1983; Holden *et al.*, 1984). This large inter-subject variability in corneal swelling response also occurs with the same contact lens, particularly during closed eye wear (O'Neal *et al.*, 1984).

This swelling response variability may be one reason why it has been so difficult to determine the minimum oxygen level to prevent corneal edema; along with goggle experiment variables such as subject tearing, length of exposure, and the humidity, temperature, and flow rate of the gas at the cornea. Mandell (1988) has plotted the data of a number of researchers (Fig. 42.3), which shows the interstudy range of corneal swelling measured for the percent oxygen concentrations used and the different zero swelling oxygen levels found. The goggle hypoxia studies have suggested the critical oxygen level to be from about 3–4% (Mandell & Farrell, 1980) to a group mean of 10% and as high as 21% for some subjects (Holden *et al.*, 1984), and more recently even 18% oxygen (Brennan *et al.*, 1988).

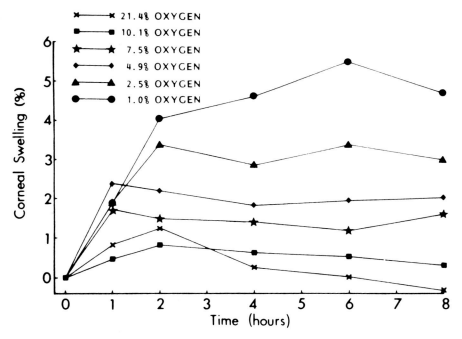

Figure 42.1 Corneal swelling over time for exposure to reduced oxygen pressure using goggles. Maximum corneal swelling occurs by 3 hours, except for lower oxygen levels (from Holden *et al.*, 1984).

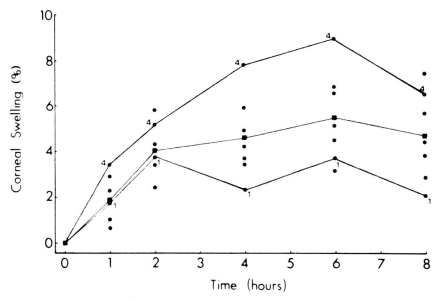

Figure 42.2 Intersubject variability in corneal swelling response for subjects exposed to 1.0% oxygen for 8 hours using goggles (from Holden *et al.*, 1984).

Other hypoxic criteria

Other studies have used different methodologies and criteria for corneal hypoxic compromise, including reduced epithelial mitotic rate (Hamano *et al.*, 1983), epithelial glycogen reduction (Uniacke *et al.*, 1972), and reduced epithelial metabolic rate (Masters *et al.*, 1982). These studies generally show that almost any level of hypoxia produces a change, however small, in corneal physiology; and it may be argued that the amount of oxygen normally available from the atmosphere, 21% or 155 mmHg PO_2, is the true minimal oxygen requirement (Efron & Brennan, 1987). However, many people living at high altitudes, where the oxygen pressure is reduced, do not appear to suffer undue corneal distress and complications; and the minimal oxygen tension to prevent any cornea change may bear little relation to the 'critical' oxygen tension to prevent corneal damage.

42.2.3   OXYGEN AVAILABILITY AND EDEMA WITH CONTACT LENSES

Open eye lens wear

The primary source of oxygen to the cornea is from the ambient air, and with contact lenses the oxygen gets behind the lens to the cornea either by diffusion through the lens or along with fresh tears during blinking. During open eye contact lens wear, the oxygen under the PMMA lens is due to tear exchange with blinking, as PMMA lenses are impermeable to oxygen. On the other hand, the oxygen under hydrogel lenses is virtually only from diffusion through the lens, since soft lenses have only a negligible (1%) tear exchange (Polse, 1979). Both tear exchange and diffusion occur during open eye wear of rigid gas permeable (RGP) lenses, allowing for higher levels of oxygen under RGP lenses and less swelling. For example, corneal edema of about 6% was found with daily wear of

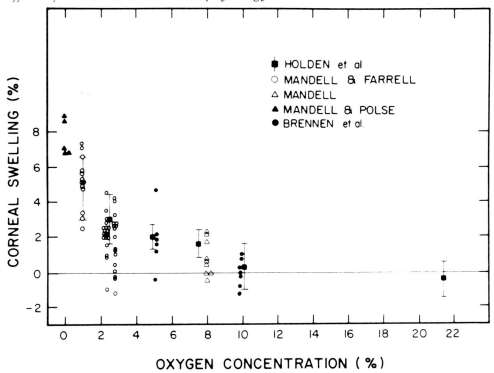

Figure 42.3 Relationship between corneal swelling after 3 hours and oxygen pressure at the corneal surface (from Mandell, 1988).

thicker, low water content single vision hydrogel lenses (Carney & Bailey, 1972), while in general little if any edema occurs with daily wear of RGP lenses (Vreugdenhil *et al.*, 1990).

Closed eye lens wear

The oxygen tension in air is about 155 mmHg, and is also called the 'driving force' of oxygen. However, during closed eye lens wear (i.e. sleep), the oxygen comes from the lid conjunctiva; and the oxygen tension at the corneal surface drops to only about one-third as much, 40–55 mmHg (Efron & Carney, 1979). This decrease in oxygen driving force greatly reduces the oxygen under the lens while the eye is closed (O'Neal *et al.*, 1983). The relationship between lens oxygen transmissibility (i.e.

oxygen availability) and corneal swelling during eye closure has been determined by O'Neal *et al.* (1984) (Fig. 42.4). They measured rather high (up to 15%) levels of corneal swelling with the lower oxygen transmission lenses worn with the eye closed. It should be noted that this 15% corneal swelling with closed eye wear is much higher than the 8% corneal edema found at even the zero oxygen level in the goggle experiments. On the other hand, they also found that wear of a high oxygen transmission lens resulted in corneal edema similar to that found during normal sleep without lenses. These findings suggest that other factors, which are related to lens oxygen (and other gas) transmission, besides direct hypoxia must be affecting the cornea during closed eye contact lens wear.

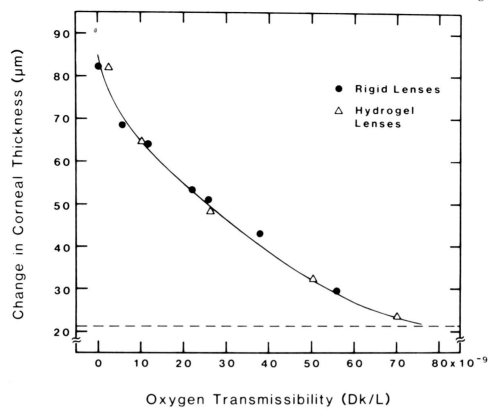

Figure 42.4 Corneal swelling versus lens oxygen transmissibility following 3 hours of eye closure while wearing rigid or hydrogel contact lenses (adapted from O'Neal *et al.*, 1984).

42.2.4 TOPOGRAPHICAL CORNEAL SWELLING

Central corneal clouding is often observed in patients wearing standard PMMA contact lenses. The clouding is easily observed to be confined to the area of the epithelium directly beneath the contact lens. Mandell and Polse (1971) had shown that the concommitant stromal swelling was also confined to the area of clouding without any significant spread of edema to the corneal periphery. In contrast, measurements of central and peripheral swelling in patients wearing daily-wear soft lenses showed a relatively uniform amount of swelling (Sanders *et al.*, 1975). These differences in epithelial and stromal edema between hard and soft lenses

helped to explain why refractive and keratometric changes were more prevalent following PMMA lens wear than hydrogel lens wear.

With the advent of extended wear and its associated peripheral neovascularization and infiltrates, attention was again drawn to peripheral corneal edema. The question arose as to whether patients fitted with high minus extended wear lenses developed relatively more peripheral edema and were thus at greater risk for developing complications. Studies by Bonanno and Polse (1985), Bonanno *et al.* (1986) and Holden *et al.* (1985a) showed consistently less edema peripherally than centrally even with −9.00 D lenses (Fig. 42.5). Peripheral and central swelling increased directly with lens power, however central swelling increased more rapidly. This was true even for lens designs where central oxygen transmissibility (*Dk/L*) was constant across all lens powers, e.g. Bausch and Lomb 'O' lens. Thus central swelling is best predicted by an average *Dk/L* rather than the local *Dk/L* at each lens position. These studies concluded that the peripheral cornea was restrained from swelling relative to the center due to an edge 'clamping' effect, presumably derived from the tight interweaving of collagen fibers at the limbus. Any increased complication rate shown with high minus hydrogel lenses thus could not be easily

ascribed to peripheral edema *per se*, but more likely to the overall deficit of oxygen supply.

42.3 CORNEAL HYDRATION CONTROL

42.3.1 NORMAL FUNCTION

Although there has been a substantial amount of research, the exact basis for all aspects (i.e. normal function, edema, and recovery) of corneal hydration control remains elusive and not fully understood. Both passive and active mechanisms function in control of corneal hydration. The active ion fluid pump sites for removal of

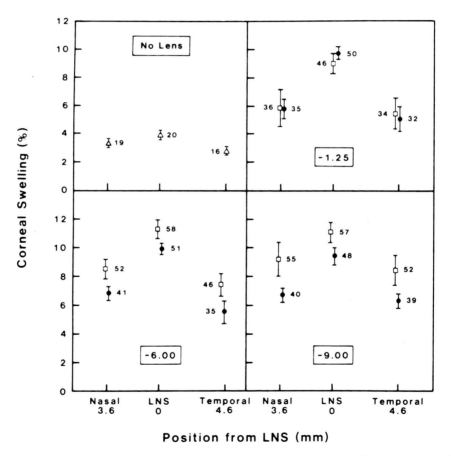

Figure 42.5 Comparison between central versus nasal and temporal corneal swelling after 3 hours of closed eye without (upper left) and with soft lenses (upper right and lower two panels) (from Bonanno & Polse, 1985).

water from the cornea are located in the endothelium (Maurice, 1962), while both the epithelium and endothelium offer a passive resistance to the flow of water into the cornea (Mishima & Hedbys, 1967). The polysaccharides in the corneal stroma create a natural tendency for the stroma to imbibe water, called the swelling pressure (Hedbys & Dohlman, 1963) or imbibition pressure (Hedbys *et al.*, 1963), that results in a 75–80% normal water content. There is also a passive fluid evaporation from the anterior corneal surface that can have a considerable effect on corneal thickness (Mishima & Maurice, 1961). These active and passive mechanisms were combined by Maurice (1962) into the 'pump-leak' theory of corneal hydration control, in which there is a constant leak of fluid into the cornea that is balanced by the endothelial pump. The primary passive (hydraulic) leak of fluid into the cornea appears to occur through the endothelial intercellular spaces, while the active (localized osmotic) flow of fluid out is thought to be across the cell membranes (Fischbarg *et al.*, 1977, Fischbarg & Lim, 1984).

When the eye is closed (i.e. during sleep) the cornea normally swells about 3% (Mertz, 1980). The cause of this swelling is generally thought to be a return of the cornea to normal hydration (Maurice, 1984) due to a decrease in tear tonicity (Chan & Mandell, 1975). This reverses the normal corneal thinning that occurs after eye opening (Mandell & Fatt, 1965), from the slightly hypertonic tears caused by tear evaporation (Mishima & Maurice, 1961). The cornea appeared to receive sufficient oxygen from the palpebral conjunctiva to prevent hypoxia (Efron & Carney, 1979); however, the recent research on minimum critical oxygen tension suggests the oxygen level needed may be above the amount supplied by the palpebrae. Sweeney and Holden (1991) recently re-examined the factors involved in normal closed eye edema; with the results suggesting approximately one-half of the edema is due to hypoxia plus about equal contributions from lower tear osmolality, increased humidity and higher temperature.

42.3.2 MECHANISMS OF CORNEAL SWELLING

Classic hypoxic swelling mechanism

The generally accepted mechanism for corneal swelling from hypoxia, as proposed by Klyce (1981), is that an osmotic imbalance is created in the cornea due to an increase in lactate from cell anaerobic metabolism. The metabolism of glucose, which diffuses into the cornea from the anterior chamber, supplies the energy necessary for healthy cellular activity. The cornea has a high rate of aerobic glycolosis that is almost entirely located in the epithelial layers, with little occurring in the stroma (Langham, 1952). With decreased oxygen levels, glucose metabolism shifts to anaerobic glycolosis, resulting in more of the pyruvic acid being formed into lactic acid. Since the epithelium is relatively impermeable to lactic acid, it moves by diffusion across the stroma and through the endothelium into the aqueous humor. Presumably, it is at the endothelial/aqueous interface that the lactate generated osmotic imbalance results in a net inflow of fluid into the cornea.

Contact lens swelling mechanisms

A number of studies using an *in vitro* rabbit cornea model with gas-impermeable lenses have investigated possible mechanisms for contact lens induced corneal edema. The amelioration of the edema by lactate dehydrogenase inhibitors, which retards lactate production (Rohde & Huff, 1986), and the temperature dependency (i.e. cold reduces edema) of the swelling (Huff, 1990) support the idea that the lens-induced edema is due to the osmotic load from stromal lactate accumulation. Further, Huff (1991a) recently evaluated a host of possible pharmacological mechanisms for lens-induced edema; eliminating any role for cytotoxic mechanisms and again concluding the edema appears to involve hypoxic lactate accumulation. Also, since little swelling was found when the endothelium was replaced with silicone oil, the fluid uptake was confirmed to occur across the endothelium (Huff, 1990).

Early models of oxygen tension distribution across the cornea by Fatt and co-workers (1974) indicated the oxygen level at the corneal endothelium would remain normal during anterior corneal hypoxia. However, some measurements have shown a decrease in oxygen tension in the anterior chamber with contact lens wear (Barr & Silver, 1973; Stefansson *et al.*, 1983). It is possible then that hypoxia at the posterior corneal endothelium due to front surface hypoxia might affect the endothelial ion-based fluid pump that actively moves fluid out of the cornea. Indeed, rabbit corneas exposed to hypoxia with contact lens wear showed a reduction in endothelial pump site density (MacDonald & McCarey, 1988). However, Huff's (1990) study also found that acute, short-term lens-induced edema does not require inhibition of endothelial (nor epithelial) ion transport.

The corneal endothelial fluid pump mechanism is known to be affected by pH changes; with both the transendothelial potential and fluid transport being pH sensitive (Fischbarg & Lim, 1974). Bonanno and Polse (1987a,b) found an acidic shift in stromal pH with both hypoxia and contact lens wear (see page 980). Thus, one possiblity is that epithelial surface hypoxia leads to acidification of the stroma which then affects the endothelial fluid pump. However, Huff (1991b) has reported that contact lens-induced stromal edema and acidosis are dissociable *in vitro*, as the same level of rabbit corneal edema occurred even when the acidic shift was prevented by buffering. In addition, Bonnano's laboratory (Giasson & Bonnano, 1991) measured an acidic shift in

rabbit corneal epithelial pH with gas-impermeable contact lenses but found little if any change in the aqueous humor pH, suggesting anterior corneal pH changes may have little effect on pH at the posterior cornea (i.e. endothelium). On the other hand, Cohen *et al.* (1991) found a slower recovery from corneal swelling with 7% CO_2 (i.e. lower stromal pH obtained) versus normal oxygen perfused human cornea *in vivo* with goggles, suggesting stromal acidosis may affect corneal hydration control.

Interestingly, Huff (1990) also reported a high level of corneal swelling with lens wear even without the presense of the corneal epithelium (i.e. replaced by silicone oil), suggesting there may be a significant role for the stroma in lens-induced corneal edema. He argues that the origin of the accumulated lactate may be the stroma rather than the epithelium, citing a number of factors, including that the normoxic epithelial and stromal lactate production are similar, the stroma has lower PO_2 during hyoxia, and the effect of lactate dehydrogenase to produce lactate is greater in the stroma than the epithelium. Indeed, much earlier, Langham (1965) had suggested the high metabolic activity of the stromal keratocytes should be considered as a factor in corneal hydration.

42.3.3 RECOVERY FROM CORNEAL SWELLING (DESWELLING)

Swelling recovery time course

After the edema inducing stimulus is removed, human *in vivo* corneal recovery (i.e. deswelling) follows a nonlinear time course with the rate of recovery decreasing as the cornea thins back to normal thickness (Fig. 42.6) (O'Neal & Polse, 1985). There have been a wide range of recovery times reported, even from similar levels of edema, and the cornea in some studies was found to become thinner than baseline (O'Neal *et al.*, 1984). Mandell *et al.* (1989) have refined recovery analysis using a coupled exponential model, which includes a more exact determination of the corneal open-eye steady state thickness (OESS) and the percent recovery per hour (PRPH) of corneal thickness that can be used from any level of induced edema. Their research group found a PRPH of about 50–60%/h in young adults (Cohen *et al.*, 1990), and suggest the interstudy variability in recovery rates and reported overshoot in recovery is primarily due to differences in baseline thickness measurement procedures.

Swelling recovery mechanisms

In one of the first studies on the mechanisms involved in human corneal recovery and hydration control, O'Neal and Polse (1985) used a comparison between open and closed eye recovery (Fig. 42.6) supplemented with a calculational approach based on published values for membrane permeability and swelling pressures, including animal data. Simplistically, since stromal swelling pressure decreases as hydration increases (Hedbys & Dohlman, 1963), the 'leak' into the cornea is less with edema and becomes

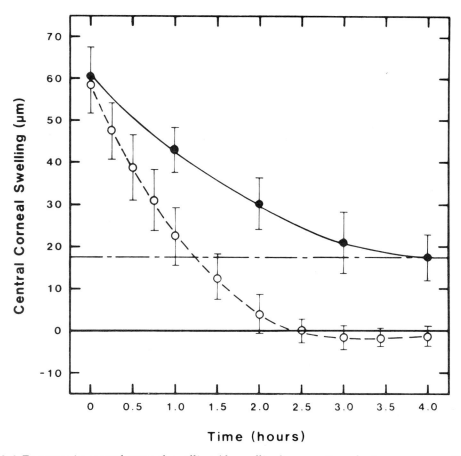

Figure 42.6 Decrease in central corneal swelling (deswelling) versus time during recovery with the eyes open (open circles) and closed (filled circles) following corneal swelling induced with hydrogel lenses worn with the eyes closed (from O'Neal *et al.*, 1985).

greater as the cornea thins; and a 'steady state' endothelial pump rate would thus move the excess water out at an ever decreasing rate. In addition, their calculations suggest evaporation plays a major role in open eye corneal recovery.

In the O'Neal and Polse (1985) study, they found a similar time course of recovery for closed eye versus humidified open eye environments, indicating the slower closed eye recovery was not caused by the reduction in oxygen that occurs with eye closure. Further, there was good agreement between the calculated fluid flow out of the cornea that would occur with a steady state pump and the measured outflow with corneal thinning during recovery with the eyes closed. They conclude this finding suggests that the human endothelial pump functions at one speed regardless of the level of corneal hydration, which is in agreement with the results of Baum *et al.* (1984) for the rabbit cornea. Open eye corneal swelling recovery was much faster than closed eye recovery (Fig 42.6), and they hypothesized the difference was due to evaporation. Again, the corneal thinning calculated due to evaporation was in close agreement with that reported by Mishima and Maurice (1961) for the rabbit. From these findings, O'Neal and Polse (1985) lastly determined that the endothelial pump provided only about one-fifth the recovery from 60 μm of edema, with the bulk of recovery due to evaporation.

However, others have not been able to replicate the finding that humidified open eye recovery follows the same time course as closed eye recovery; but instead followed normal humidity open eye recovery (Cohen *et al.*, 1990). This difference may be due to the procedure in the O'Neal and Polse (1985) study of the subject's eyes being closed between the high-humidity room and thickness measurement room, resulting in slight hypoxia and/or tear hypotonicity changes that have been found to occur rapidly on eye closure (Benjamin, 1990). Regardless, the small degree of hypoxia suggested by Sweeney and Holden (1991) may not severely affect corneal recovery with the eyes closed, but suggests some of the O'Neal and Polse (1985) conclusions may need further evaluation on other factors (e.g. stromal pump rate change, etc.), in addition to steady state pump rate and evaporation; although, the good agreement between their calculations and published data cannot be ignored.

42.4 EPITHELIUM

42.4.1 EPITHELIAL EDEMA

PMMA lens wearers have often observed increased glare or halos surrounding bright lights especially following long periods of lens wear. Observations with the clinical slit lamp using sclerotic scatter showed a grey epithelial haze in these patients. The haze is limited to the area of lens coverage and has therefore been termed central or circular corneal clouding. The cause of the haze was recognized early on by Smelser (Smelser & Ozanics, 1952; Smelzer & Chen, 1955) as being due to epithelial hypoxia. Finkelstein (1952) shortly afterward made subjective measurements of the half angle subtended by the halos and concluded that they arose from a cellular layer with individual scatterers of 10 microns in diameter.

Definitive demonstration of the basal epithelium as the site of the scattering was later given by Lambert and Klyce (1981). Using a laboratory specular microscope they photographed the change in light scatter at the basal epithelium of an isolated rabbit cornea before and after hypoxia. Treating the photographs as interference gratings, they determined that the grating would give rise to halos corresponding in size to that seen subjectively. Presumably, the increased production of lactate by the hypoxic epithelium induces an accumulation of fluid between the epithelial cells as the lactate is transported out of the cells. The difference in

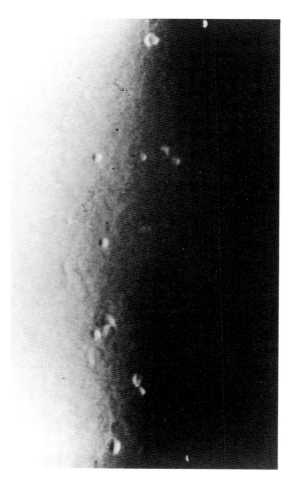

Figure 42.7 Epithelial microcysts (courtesy of Doctor Brien Holden).

refractive index between intra- and extracellular space then leads to increased scatter between the cells. The net result is a meshwork of polygonal light scatterers acting as an interference grating.

42.4.2 EPITHELIAL MICROCYSTS

Epithelial microcysts are commonly observed in extended wear patients (Zantos and Holden, 1978) (Fig. 42.7). Discontinuation of lens wear reduces the number of cysts slowly over a number of months (Kenyon *et al.*, 1986). The

mechanism by which cysts form and the persistance of the cysts well past the normal epithelial turnover time remains a mystery. These observations may be related to a reduction in epithelial mitotic activity by hypoxia (Hamano *et al.*, 1983) and the prolonged cell residence time (i.e. increased cell turnover time), observed in contact lens wearers (Lemp & Gold, 1986). The reduction in mitotic activity and prolonged residence time seems to imply also a reduction in healing time during lens wear (Zimny & Salisbury, 1982), which then leaves the cornea more susceptible to infection.

42.4.3 CORNEAL SENSITIVITY

Contact lens wear can produce other morphological and functional changes in the corneal epithelium for which the etiology is less certain. Reduction in corneal sensitivity is common among contact lens wearers. Millodot and O'Leary (1980) attribute these observations to corneal hypoxia. Bergenske and Polse (1987) later concurred, showing that PMMA lens wearers refitted with gaspermeable lenses regained normal touch thresholds, indicating the mechanical rubbing of the lens on the cornea did not alone decrease sensitivity. In an earlier experiment, however, Polse (1978) had found little or no reduction in sensitivity in subjects with their epithelium made hypoxic by exposure to nitrogen gas. The explanation for these apparently different effects on sensitivity may be due to gas exchange. Higher amounts of carbon dioxide accumulate at the cornea under lenses than in goggles hypoxia and leads to lower pH (see later this page), which may alter corneal sensitivity.

42.5 STROMA

42.5.1 STROMAL STRUCTURE

The stroma comprises the bulk (90%) of the cornea and is composed of 100 to 200 parallel collagen fibrils, lamellae. These are surrounded by matrix of glycosaminoglycans (GAG) having keratocytes dispersed throughout the matrix. The stromal polysaccharides attract water to give rise to the corneal swelling pressure. The stroma has classically received little interest in contact lens wear. However, recent studies suggest the stroma may play a greater role in the corneal response to contact lenses than previously thought. The stroma has been reported to have a high level of glucose consumption (Zurawski *et al.*, 1988), suggesting metabolic activity that could be affected during hypoxia. Indeed, Holden *et al.* (1985c) reported a thinning of the stroma with long term soft lens extended-wear. A possible etiology for such stromal thinning is a loss of stromal matrix GAGs, which was found with corneal edema (Kangas *et al.*, 1988) and with extended wear of contact lenses (Cejkova *et al.*, 1988).

42.5.2   STROMAL pH

Recently, Bonnano and Polse (1987a) used a non-invasive fluorometric slit lamp based technique to measure *in vivo* human corneal pH. They found that corneal hypoxia created with 100% nitrogen gas exposure in goggles produced a small drop in stromal pH from the normal 7.5 to 7.35 (Fig. 42.8a). The pH returned to normal 20 minutes after goggle removal. This acidic shift could be due to the production of lactic acid that builds up in the stroma. With thick soft contact lens wear and the eyes open the pH is reduced even further, to about 7.15 (Fig. 42.8b) (Bonnano & Polse, 1987b). They determined this increase in acidic pH change with lens wear is due to carbon dioxide accumulation under the contact lens.

42.6   ENDOTHELIUM

42.6.1   ENDOTHELIAL ASSESSMENT

The corneal endothelium is composed of a monolayer of primarily hexagonal cells that functions as both a passive barrier to fluid entering the cornea and as an active metabolic fluid pump to maintain normal corneal hydration (Maurice, 1984). Because of this primary fluid control function, any alteration of the corneal endothelium due to contact lens wear is of particular interest.

With the advent of the specular microscope, assessment of the endothelium has attempted to determine clinically relevant measurements that would differentiate between a normal and compromised endothelium. To this end, endothelial photomicrographs (Fig. 42.9a,b) have been used to make measurements of endothelial cell density and changes in cell morphometry, including cell shape (pleomorphism) and size (polymegathism). The typical area photographed is about 200 microns wide by 800 microns, and a tracing of about 100 cells is made from a magnified image of the photomicrograph. Contact lens wear appears to alter some morphological characteristics of the endothelium and not others (as described by these endothelial parameters), and thus may affect endothelial function. Both general morphological changes and highly localized endothelial changes have been documented with contact lens wear.

42.6.2   ENDOTHELIAL BLEBS

Zantos and Holden (1977) first reported the localized appearance of small black spots or breaks in the endothelial mosaic of soft lens wearers, which they termed endothelial 'blebs', (Fig. 42.10). The blebs appeared within 30–60 minutes of lens wear, and were gone in a similar time period. The appearance of transient endothelial blebs were also seen in hard lens wearers (Barr & Schoessler, 1980). Holden *et al.* (1985d) later showed that three separate conditions: (1) lens wear; (2) hypoxia produced by nitrogen gas; or (3) exposure to 10% CO_2 in the presence of excess oxygen, all produced blebs. They concluded that the most likely common effect of the three treatments was a decrease in cor-

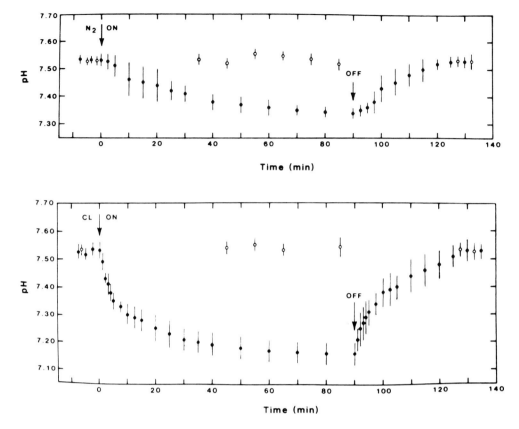

Figure 42.8 Human *in vivo* stromal pH changes with (a) 100% nitrogen gas across test cornea (filled circles) and normal air across control cornea (open circles) with goggles, and (b) thick soft lens on lens wearing eye (filled circles) and no-lens control eye (open circles) (from Bonanno & Polse, 1987).

neal pH (i.e. blebs were caused by a decrease in corneal pH rather than hypoxia *per se*).

Bonanno and Polse (1987b) showed shortly thereafter that the stromal pH does indeed drop during lens wear and that the effects of hypoxia and CO_2 accumulation were additive. How might the increased corneal acidity lead to bleb formation? One possibility is that the endothelial intracellular pH is also dropping in response to the drop in extracellular pH. This may directly interfere with cellular volume regulation causing the cells to swell. Another possibility is that the cells try to regulate intracellular pH by mechanisms such as Na^+/H^+ exchange which bring Na^+ into the cells and thus induce

swelling osmotically. Whatever the actual cause, it is clear that acute or chronic changes in corneal pH could have deleterious effects on endothelial function.

42.6.3 ENDOTHELIAL MORPHOLOGICAL RESPONSE

Endothelial cell density

The cell density is about 3000 cells/mm^2 in the normal endothelium and decreases with age (Yee *et al.*, 1985). Within the general morphological response to contact lens wear, corneal endothelial cell density does not appear to decrease with either PMMA

cell size with the discontinuance of lens wear. This non-recovery of polymegathism has been found regardless of lens type, length of lens wear, or time since stopping lens wear Holden *et al.*, 1985b; MaRae *et al.*, 1986). Indeed, following long term PMMA lens wear, the increased endothelial polymegathism was still present 7 years after stopping wear (Yamauchi *et al.*, 1987). Thus, at least some of the polymegathistic changes in the corneal endothelium due to contact lens wear appear to be permanent.

42.6.4   ETIOLOGY OF ENDOTHELIAL MORPHOLOGICAL RESPONSE

Endothelial polymegathism is known to occur in a variety of conditions, in addition to those already noted (contact lens wear, aging, cataract surgery, intraocular lens implant), including diabetes mellitus (Schultz *et al.*, 1984), glaucoma (Markowitz & Morin, 1984), and keratoconus (Spring, 1982), among others. For contact lenses, the evidence strongly suggests that the corneal endothelial changes are induced by the corneal hypoxia that occurs with contact lens wear. Kamiya (1982) has related the endothelial changes with contact lens oxygen transmissibility and found less endothelial changes with RGP lenses than with PMMA lens wear. The role of contact lens hypoxia in increased polymegathism is further supported by the finding of Schoessler *et al.* (1984) that no polymegathistic change occurred with silicone elastomer contact lenses, which have very high oxygen transmissibility. The mechanism of these hypoxic changes is open to conjecture, and may be due to any of a number of processes including cell metabolism interference related to the buildup of carbon dioxide and acidic pH change (Bonanno & Polse, 1987a,b).

42.6.5   CLINICAL SIGNIFICANCE OF ENDOTHELIAL MORPHOLOGICAL CHANGE

Studies suggest that endothelial function is affected by contact lens wear. Although the actual cellular changes remain unknown, endothelial function appears to be related to particular morphological changes and not others. Fluorophotometric studies to assess endothelial permeability have given conflicting results. Carlson *et al.* (1988) did not find a difference in fluorescein permeability for a group of PMMA, soft, or RGP lens wearers, while one group of researchers report an increase in the endothelial permeability to fluorescein for PMMA and soft lens daily wear (Lass *et al.*, 1988) and soft lens extended-wear (Dutt *et al.*, 1989). Shaw *et al.* (1978) did not find a relationship between preoperative endothelial cell density and postsurgical corneal edema, suggesting cell density may not be of primary importance in maintaining normal corneal hydration.

A number of studies have, however, indicated that endothelial polymegathism is correlated with corneal swelling recovery. Rao *et al.* (1979) found greater corneal swelling following cataract surgery and intraocular lens implantation in patients having more preoperative endothelial polymegathism, suggesting that the 'functional reserve' of the endothelium is compromised with polymegathism. O'Neal and Polse (1986) found slower corneal deswelling in a group of normal older subjects compared to young normals during both open eye and closed eye recovery following hypoxic stress with a thick soft lens. This apparent decrease in endothelial pump rate in the normal older subjects was also accompanied by more polymegathism than the young normals. In addition, Sweeney *et al.* (1985) also induced corneal edema with a thick lens in normals and found both the amount of corneal swelling and deswelling rate to correlate inversely with the degree of polymegathism. For long term contact lens wear, Polse *et al.* (1990) found that PMMA and extended lens wear years of hypoxia corresponded to increases in endothelial polymegathism and PRPH deswelling stress test (see corneal deswelling section). These findings suggest that contact lens wear alters the endothelial cell mosaic and affects corneal function, and may compromise the ability of the cornea to recover from edema if future corneal surgery is required.

42.7 CONCLUSION

Corneal hypoxia with contact lens wear has been found to cause significant and wide ranging changes in corneal physiology. Not discussed, but of current interest in corneal research is the role of hypoxia stimulated corneal epithelium biologically active cytochrome P450 arachidonic acid metabolites, 12(R)HETE and 12(R)DiHETE, in corneal hypoxic complications and their alleviation (Davis *et al.*, 1990, 1991). And the possible relationship of long-term corneal hypoxia and endothelial polymegatism with the corneal exhaustion syndrome (Holden & Sweeney, 1988) that occurs after 10–15 years of PMMA and low oxygen transmission soft lens wear (Pence, 1988). It is possible that the much faster and more complete recovery from overnight corneal swelling with RGP versus soft lens extended wear (O'Neal, 1988) will help to reduce the hypoxic sequelae. As Holden (1989) suggests, in light of the evidence it would seem prudent for the contact lens practitioner to prescribe lens and wearing regimen combinations that avoid unnecessarily compromising corneas with long-term hypoxia.

Dr O'Neal is a Lt Colonel in the USAF. The views expressed in this article are those of the author and do not reflect the official policy or position of the Department of Defense of the United States Government.

REFERENCES

Barr, J.T. and Schoessler, J.P. (1980) Corneal endothelial response to rigid contact lenses. *Am. J. Optom. Physiol. Opt.*, **57**, 267–74.

Barr, R.E. and Silver, I.A. (1973) Effects of corneal environment on oxygen tension in the anterior chambers of rabbits. *Invest. Ophthalmol.*, **12**, 140–4.

Baum, J.P., Maurice, D.M. and McCarey, B.E. (1984) The active and passive transport of water across the corneal endothelium. *Exp. Eye Res.*, **39**, 335–42.

Benjamin, W.J. (1990) Influence of eyelid closure on tear prism fluid osmolality. *ARVO Abstracts, Invest. Ophthalmol. Vis. Sci.*, **31**(Suppl.), 408.

Bergenske, P.D. and Polse, K.A. (1987) The effect of rigid gas permeable lenses on corneal sensitivity. *J. Am. Optom. Assoc.*, **58**, 212–15.

Bonanno, J.A. and Polse, K.A. (1985) Central and peripheral corneal swelling accompanying soft lens extended wear. *Am. J. Opt. Physiol. Opt.*, **62**, 74–81.

Bonanno, J.A. and Polse, K.A. (1987a) Effect of rigid contact lens oxygen transmissibility on stromal pH in the living human eye. *Ophthalmology*, **94**, 1305–9.

Bonanno, J.A. and Polse, K.A. (1987b) Corneal acidosis during contact lens wear: effects of hypoxia and CO_2. *Inv. Ophthalmol. Vis. Sci.*, **28**, 1514–20.

Bonanno, J.A., Polse, K.A. and Goldman, M.M. (1986) Effect of soft lens power on peripheral corneal edema. *Am. J. Opt. Physiol. Opt.*, **63**, 520–6.

Brennan, N.A., Efron, N. and Carney, L.G. (1988) Corneal oxygen availability during contact lens wear: A comparison of methodologies. *Am. J. Optom. Physiol. Opt.*, **65**, 19–24.

Carlson, K.H., Bourne, W.M. and Brubaker, R.F. (1988) Effect of long-term contact lens wear on corneal endothelial cell morphology and function. *Invest. Ophthalmol. Vis. Sci.*, **29**, 185–93.

Carney, L.G. and Bailey, I.L. (1972) Hydrophilic contact lenses – their effect on the cornea. *Aust. J. Optom.*, **55**, 161–3.

Cejkova, J., Lojda, Z., Brunova, B., Vacik, J. and Michalek, J. (1988) Disturbances in the rabbit cornea after short-term and long-term wear of hydrogel contact lenses. Usefulness of histochemical methods. *Histochemistry*, **89**, 91–7.

Chan, R.S. and Mandell, R.B. (1975) Corneal thickness changes from bathing solutions. *Am. J. Optom. Physiol. Opt.*, **52**, 465–9.

Cohen, S.R., Polse, K.A., Brand, R.J. and Mandell, R.B. (1990) Humidity effects on corneal hydration. *Invest. Ophthalmol. Vis. Sci.*, **31**, 1282–7.

Cohen, S.R., Polse, K.A., Janic, G., Brand, R.J. and Bonanno, J.A. (1991) Stromal acidosis reduces corneal hydration control. *ARVO Abstracts,*

EXTENDED OR CONTINUOUS WEAR LENSES 43

M. Guillon and M. Ruben

43.1 INTRODUCTION

43.1.1 DEFINITION AND GENERAL REMARKS

The criteria and problems concerning the daily wear of contact lenses are dealt with throughout the text of this book, daily wear being considered the conventional type of wear. This chapter addresses extended wear, which is the continuation of daily wear into sleep. An alternative to the use of the term extended wear is continuous wear, which was originally used to describe this manner of wearing contact lenses (Ruben, 1975, 1978). This latter term has now been abandoned, or at least relegated to those lenses used for therapeutic purposes, not generally removed by the patient but by the practitioner during routine after-care visits.

The 24-hour cycle varies in every human according to their individual needs and tasks. In addition, physiological functions of the human vary widely according to the degree of activity and periods of rest. The metabolism of the body is able to cope with such extremes in demand by supplying nourishment and gases for energy and cell survival and reproduction. Variations in these supplies will affect the body's ability to cope with changes to its environment. Accordingly, in part because of the limitation of current lenses and also because of the

environmental condition of wear, if one has compensated to the daily wear of contact lens, it does not infer that the same success will be achieved during extended wear. In addition to the differences between the daily and extended wear modalities, it is important to also consider the variability which exists within each of these modalities, as well as between individuals. For example, sleeping habits can differ with regard to the number of hours of sleep as well as the environment of the bedroom. Furthermore, the quality of sleep can also vary, i.e. deep, undisturbed as compared to light and disturbed (Ruben, 1975, 1978). Some people regularly take medicines before retiring, which can affect tear flow and lens tolerance (Fraunfelder, 1982). Furthermore, the daily period may, for some people, end with a contact lens that is at the limits of tolerance while others have no problems with the lens or the eye tissues. It is sufficient to say that a patient who may be an ideal daily wearer, with the night period being a rest period before recommencing lens wear, can tip the balance to the onset of pathology of the superficial eye tissues due to physiological stress when proceeding to extended wear.

It is obvious that the influence of many of these factors on the individual's response to both daily and extended wear is still unknown. Consideration of these factors

Contact Lens Practice. Edited by Montague Ruben and Michel Guillon.
Published in 1994 by Chapman & Hall, London. ISBN 0 412 35120 X

becomes most important when there is evidence of lens intolerance and tissue damage. Because individual behaviour is so variable, investigative methods using small sample sizes without objectivity can often be considered of little value when determining population responses to lens wear.

This chapter will deal with extended wear, where the closed eye condition is of primary concern. The use of the extended wear lenses as therapeusis in certain eye diseases is described in Chapter 38; because the tissues for these eyes are very different to those of normal eyes the discussion in this chapter is limited to the normal eye. Extended wear lenses have been used in the special instances of abnormal eyes such as infantile and senile aphakia; those aspects are treated in Chapter 34.

This chapter will state those aspects that are particularly germane to extended wear; the general information for daily wear does, in the main, remain valid for extended wear.

A century ago, at the commencement of glass scleral lens history, only a few hours' wear at a time was possible. Some 50 years later, with better technology and an understanding of tear fluid exchange, wearing times for a few patients could be extended to all day wear. There were even instances of extended wear periods with scleral lenses (Ridley, 1963) and most practitioners of that era could report such experiences by patients but they were rarely recorded. One of us (M.R.) knew a patient who was shipwrecked in the 1939–1945 war and, for 14 days, wore the scleral lenses continuously, albeit in an exhausted and abnormal physical state, with no long-term deleterious effects on the eye or vision. There have been many instances of extended wear with the PMMA corneal lens, especially in aphakia (Cassidy, 1969). In most cases the patient ignored instructions but at times extended wear occurred because of unusual circumstances, such as arm injury or travel. In some instances this was achieved by periodic dislodgement of the lens from the cornea into the fornix and then relocation at wakening. Such periods of extended wear sometimes lasted for several years without undue injury to the eye tissues. On the other hand there are instances of tragic consequences (Ruben *et al.*, 1976; Cooper & Constable, 1977; Zantos & Holden, 1978; Weismann *et al.*, 1984; Chalupa *et al.*, 1987), which will be discussed later in this chapter.

In 1968, a health minister asked what state contact lens knowledge had reached, the answer given then was 'for the patient with a normal refractive error satisfactory daily wear is achieved in 75% of patients motivated to contact lenses'. The minister then said 'Is this the ultimate state of the art and science of contact lens practice?' The answer was 'No, we are at the penultimate state, the ultimate state will be when a lens is inserted and left indefinitely'. We have yet to reach that ideal state.

43.1.2 THE EFFECTS OF CLOSED EYE WEAR

To understand the underlying problem of the closed eye state and contact lens wear the reader is referred to Chapters 3, 4, 14, 15, 22 and 42.

To examine the problems of the closed eye state and its effect on the eye, techniques to both quantitatively and qualitatively measure the eyes' responses are employed. These techniques are both well defined and standardized in order that the objectivity of studies and their conclusions are truly valid. Investigators have used, for example, oxygen uptake of the cornea (Efron & Carney, 1981; Efron & Ang, 1990), biomicroscopic appearance of the corneal layers (Holden & Zantos, 1979; Holden *et al.*, 1985b,d), cell morphology and cell counts (Schoessler, 1983; Carlson & Bourne, 1988; Carlson *et al.*, 1988; MacRae, *et al.*, 1989), corneal thickness measurements (Hirji & Larke, 1978; Sorensen & Corydon, 1979; Schoessler & Barr, 1980; Holden *et al.*, 1983, 1985a,c; O'Neal *et al.*, 1984), corneal sensitivity measurements (Millodot, 1984), corneal stromal acidosis measurements (Bonanno & Polse, 1987), tear film measurements (Guillon & Guillon, 1989, 1991) and visual performance assessment by variable contrast visual acuity and contrast sensitivity, in order to understand the response of the living human eye which has been subjected to extended wear. Various investigators have also attempted to evaluate the different states of wear patterns and conditions. Thus using one type of lens as a standard some investigators have compared open eye wearing times with closed eye and others have differentiated the closed eye state from the closed eye in the sleep cycle. It is easy to extrapolate numerous experimental variants such as lens material, degrees of lens gas occlusion, fits of the lens, age and sex differences. There emerge some obvious conclusions from this vast amount of research. The 'single' most important factor is the oxygen deprivation caused by lens wear. This results in stromal water imbibition which, in most normal corneas, resolves but at least creates temporarily corneal thinning (Hirji, 1979, Sorenson & Corydon 1979, Schoessler & Barr, 1980; Holden *et al.*, 1985a;) that disappears (Holden *et al.*, 1985a) over a period of several months, when the contact lens wear is discontinued. The thinning is estimated at 0.4% per year of wear (Holden *et al.*, 1985a). The long-term effects of closed eye wear also result in changes to the endothelial cell morphology (Schoessler, 1983; Holden *et al.*, 1985a,b; Carlson & Bourne, 1988; Carlson *et al.*, 1988; McRae *et al.*, 1989), epithelial cell loss (Holden *et al.*, 1985a,b), abnormal epithelial microcytic formations (Zantos & Holden, 1978) and decreased epithelial adherence to the basement membrane (Madigan *et al.*, 1987)) and other disturbances such as decreased endothelial function estimated at 1.1% per year of extended wear (Polse *et al.*, 1990). All the previous effects are described in detail in this chapter. In some instances, an anterior ocular inflammatory reaction can result (Benjamin, 1991).

The principal forms of contact lens inflammatory reactions are contact lens induced papillary conjunctivitis (CLPC) (Mackie & Wright, 1978; Kotow *et al.*, 1987) chronic red eyes (Grant *et al.*, 1987; Graham *et al.*, 1988) and even corneal infiltration (Litvin, 1978; Josephson & Caffery, 1979; Zantos, 1983, 1984; Gordon & Kracher, 1985; Nilsson & Persson, 1988; Stapleton *et al.*, 1989) and infection (Ruben, 1976; Cooper & Constable, 1977; Zantos & Holden, 1978; Weismann *et al.*, 1984; Chalupa *et al.*, 1987; Ruben, 1989; Schein *et al.*, 1989; Benjamin, 1991; Dart *et al.*, 1991; Guillon & Benjamin, 1991).

Information concerning the 'sealed' eye may be of help in understanding the process of extended wear. The diseased cornea has often been protected by the surgical procedure of tarsorrhaphy. This technique rarely produces complete sealing and therefore an abnormal hypoxic state does not occur. Experimentally, however, animals' eyes can be completely sealed and even so it must not be assumed that hypoxia alone produces the pathological inflammatory reaction that often results, since complete sealing permits little evaporation of water and an accumulation of debris and toxic metabolites all of which can produce an inflammatory reaction of the cornea. It is perhaps a clue as to what can happen when the cornea is completely sealed by a contact lens over a long period of time.

43.2 THE LIDS' MECHANICAL ACTIONS AND EXTENDED WEAR

43.2.1 INTRODUCTORY REMARKS

The lid mechanical action plays an important part in successful extended wear and two aspects must be considered to fully understand its clinical implications. It is firstly the role of the normal blink action in creating contact lens movement which is essential to ensure the elimination of debris post closed eye wear, but also the effect of the closed eyelid for long periods of time at night.

43.2.2 OPEN EYE BLINK ACTION

Reflex blinking

The normal blink which occurs in most humans during the open eye cycle is a rapid downwards movement of the lids followed by an upward phase (Doane, 1980). The closure is however usually only partial, the upper lid not contacting the lower lid before starting its upward motion. Normal blinking is also associated with a retro movement of the globe of 1.5 to 2.0 mm on average. This backward movement of the globe is produced by the contraction of the extraocular muscles (Riggs *et al.*, 1987) rather than the action of the eye lids pressing on the globe. It is an unconscious reflex stimulated by tear drying, and the environmental atmosphere such as irritants and air movement. The reflex is easily over-ridden by nervous system status such as anxiety or fatigue. The evaluation of the true blink rate is very difficult (Carney & Hill, 1982; Greene, 1986). In fact a specific blink rate does not exist. Even under controlled conditions, the blink rate shows very variable interblink intervals and even sometimes erratic rates exist. Such variations are even greater when all the factors listed above are left uncontrolled as in the normal situation.

The implications for extended wear of those findings are that a predictable post eye sleep blink rate cannot be relied upon to eliminate metabolic by-products that may have built up between the contact lens and the cornea. Also, the blink rate cannot be measured in order to predict its efficiency in a normal clinical situation. This leaves the clinician with the sole tool of observing the presence or absence of trapped debris early in the morning to assess the efficiency of the tear induced flushing system.

Forced blinking

The forced eyelid closure is never (Carney & Hill, 1982), or possibly only rarely, present during normal eye closure (Abelson & Holly, 1977). The forced eyelid closure creates forces much higher than normal eyelid closure, the ratio varying between 2.5 and 4 times, according to the authors Moller (1954) and Miller (1967). Often this results in the eyelid margin impinging against the tear film creating its subsequent disruption. Also the eyelids can remain closed at the will of the individual and in hysterical states this closure may last for several minutes.

From an extended wear viewpoint, the role of the forced blink is clinically important. For rigid gas permeable (RGP) lenses, patients should be instructed to force blink at waking to identify whether or not lens binding has taken place and to ensure that the lens dislodges rapidly, otherwise manual lens removal becomes necessary. Obviously, if lens binding occurs repeatedly, refitting or abandonment of extended wear is required. However, in our experience lens binding, which affects a minority of patients, occurs infrequently and cannot be predicted, hence the importance of the forced blink. For soft contact lenses, those patients that show a slow elimination of back surface debris, if maintained on extended wear with the same lens type, should be instructed to force blink on several occasions upon waking and during the early morning period of wear; repeated debris build up behind the lens is a case for refitting or abandoning extended wear (Mertz & Holden, 1981).

43.2.3 OVERNIGHT LID ACTION

As the individual enters the unconscious state of sleep the lids close lightly and the eyes rotate upwards. The lids are never completely closed. In fact in some individuals the lids remain opened to variable degrees and the inferior cornea is exposed. This can result in chronic, minute, inferior corneal epithelial erosions.

Therefore the criteria found from investigations of the closed eye state wearing contact lenses when awake cannot be directly applied to the asleep state, in particular when the eyes are tightly or even lightly patched.

43.3   EFFECTS OF SLEEP ON THE CLOSED EYE ENVIRONMENT

The closed eye state in sleep is different to the closed eye state when awake because the state of unconsciousness associated with sleeping corresponds to an overall alteration of the body metabolism that varies throughout the sleeping period. During the sleeping period the subjects go through two general states of sleep based upon eye movement (Hartmann, 1965). Initially the eye moves upwards as per the Bell phenomenon and the subject goes through a period with no or very few eye movements. This period, known as the non-rapid eye movement (NREM) period is divided into four stages of variable duration corresponding, it is believed, to increasing depths of sleep. After that, a period of conjugate rapid eye movements (REM) that, on average, corresponds to about 20% of the sleeping period among adults (Aserinky & Kleitmann, 1955) takes place. During that latter period, the amplitude and variation of the eye movements are highly variable and unpredictable with the majority of movements in an oblique direction, versus 25% to 35% in the vertical plane and 5% to 15% in the horizontal one (Jacobs *et al.*, 1971). An important point however to remember is that, within the normal population, there are very large variations between individuals in both the usual lengths of sleep and in the sleeping patterns (Hartmann *et al.*, 1971). In general, short sleepers and very long sleepers, spend the same absolute amount of time in deep sleep (NREM Stage 4), hence the percentage of NREM Stage 4 is

markedly decreased for the long sleeper. For REM however, a similar percentage of time is spent in that phase by both types of sleepers, leading to a much shorter absolute REM period for short sleepers (Hartmann *et al.*, 1971). Daytime or, in particular, evening activity also affects the sleep response in particular with regards to drug usage. Barbiturates and alcohol both increase total sleep, whereas marijuana seems to decrease REM sleep.

The sleep cycle is accompanied by a general slowing of bodily activity and metabolism, the respiratory rhythm can periodically go into apnoea resulting in increased PCO_2 and decreased PO_2, and the body tissues and organs are well able to adapt to these changes in the sleep state. Certainly the respiration is regular and deep, heart rate regular and slow (Snyder *et al.*, 1964) and the blood pressure below waking level (Williams & Cartwright, 1969) during the NREM period. Those activities become more variable and a shadow respiration takes place during REM (Snyder *et al.*, 1964; Williams & Cartwright, 1969).

But even overnight studies with patients asleep in the laboratory, which are the best type of studies to consider the effects of sleep on extended wear, have their limitations. Because of the fixed sleeping period, usually eight hours, most often imposed in those studies, to control the experimental conditions, the information obtained is that of the effect of a given lens type for a period of eight hours wear overnight and not the effect of that lens type during normal closed eye wear for a given patient or population. To achieve this, one should monitor the patient's response at their natural waking as some patients normally sleep for less than six hours, others more than nine. Even under those conditions to avoid inaccuracies, it is necessary to pre adapt the subjects to sleep in the clinic as it has been shown during sleep study that the first night data is unreliable (Agnew *et al.*, 1966; Mendels & Hawkins 1967; Schmidt & Kaelbling 1971). During the first night in the clinic there is a reduction in deep (Phase 4) NREM, hence a reduction in the period with the lowest metabolic demand. This could lead to the production of more oedema than during normal closed eye wear. These problems are best considered under the headings of the corneal hypoxia and water evaporation problems.

43.4   CORNEAL OXYGENATION AND EXTENDED WEAR

43.4.1   INTRODUCTORY REMARKS

Clinical experience shows categorically that there is a wide range of responses to the same lens worn by different patients on an extended wear basis. All involved in the field agree that the level of adverse tissue response, including possible acute eye infections, is associated with the hypoxic corneal stress, that is the relative lack of oxygen necessary to fulfil the corneal metabolic requirements and the individual capacity to deal with this stress. In this section we will review the information available concerning corneal oxygen demand that must be fulfilled, corneal oxygen supply and the contact lens oxygen transmissibility criteria to fulfil this demand. However, rather than being principally interested in average responses which are the driving criteria in contact lens design, we will consider the information available from the viewpoint of the overall population. Whereas we are aware of the failings of the current materials available at present and support the push towards contact lenses with higher gas transmissibility, we would like to avoid a dogmatic approach and suggest reasons for the limited adverse effects of current clinically successful extended wear patients on the one hand and the need, for some other patients, of contact lenses with even higher gas transmissibility than presently suggested. Those aspects will be reviewed from the standpoint of the possible effects on clinical performance.

43.4.2   OXYGEN CONSUMPTION

The first factor to consider when aiming to assess the adequacy of oxygen transfer by a contact lens is the oxygen consumption of the cornea. More specifically, the oxygen consumption by the epithelium and anterior two-thirds of the stroma (Fatt *et al.*, 1974) which have been shown to receive their oxygen from the atmosphere, hence to be directly interfered by the presence of a contact lens. Many studies using similar methodologies have addressed this question. Basically an oxygen sensor measures the rate of use of oxygen from a reservoir, either a sealed scleral contact lens (Hill & Fatt, 1963a) or, most commonly, a thin plastic membrane (Hill & Fatt, 1963b). The results from some of those studies are summarized in Table 43.1 (Hill, 1966; Larke *et al.*, 1981, Quinn & Schoessler, 1984; Fitzgerald & Efron, 1986). These show that, because of the inherent inaccuracy of the method, no absolute value can be given as a criteria for corneal oxygen requirement hence for contact lens oxygen transmissibility. Of great interest here is that in the absence of contact lenses, even amongst a highly homogeneous population of young males (Larke *et al.*, 1981) there is already a very large intersubject variability with approximately a three-fold difference in oxygen consumption (Figure 43.1). This difference in oxygen consumption seems linked to the subject and remains fairly constant during waking hours or from day to day (Larke *et al.*, 1981). Contrary to general opinion, oxygen consumption seems fairly age independent (Quinn & Schoessler, 1984) and similar for the central and peripheral cornea (Fitzgerald & Efron, 1986).

How can such data be interpreted for closed eye wear and what are its implications?

If we assume that oxygen consumption under closed eye conditions is related to the oxygen consumption under open eye conditions then we can understand that:

Table 43.1 Human corneal atmospheric oxygen consumption in the absence of contact lenses in μl/cm²/h. (95% range calculated from standard deviation values.)

Reference	Population	Mean	Standard deviation	Range
Hill & Fatt, 1963a		4.8		3.7–7.8
Hill, 1966		1.5		1.4–2.0
Larke, *et al.*, 1981	*n* = 68 males Age 18–25 years	6.3		3.0–9.0
Quinn & Schoessler, 1984	*n* = 50 Age 11–52 years	1.7		1.3–2.1
Fitzgerald & Efron, 1986	*n* = 10 Age 17–24 years	6.2	± 0.79	4.4–8.0

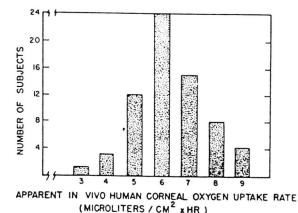

Figure 43.1 Oxygen uptake rate distribution for young male non contact lens wearing population (*n* = 68) (by courtesy of Larke *et al.*, 1981).

1. Some patients with low oxygen consumption tolerate well current extended wear contact lenses with minimal adverse effects contrary to the research predictions.
2. Consumption seems stable for a given individual, hence the evaluation of contact lens performance by the clinician at the start of extended wear should be a good indicator of long term performance.
3. Corneal consumption is similar for the central and peripheral cornea, hence transmissibility requirements should

apply to the whole cornea and not only to the central 6 mm.

The limitation of the extrapolation of the current data to the quantification of the corneal oxygen consumption under normal closed eye conditions without contact lenses are in two opposite directions. Several factors indicate that oxygen consumption under closed eye situations decreases. Hill and Fatt, for example, have shown that when the oxygen tension at the anterior corneal surface decreases from 155 mmHg to 50 mmHg the oxygen consumption decreases from 4.8 to 1.5 μl/cm²/h (Hill & Fatt, 1963a). Does that mean that under closed eye situations the oxygen consumption is one-third of the consumption under open eye? Also, as indicated earlier, respiration and general metabolism (Snyder *et al.*, 1964) decrease during sleep, hence one would assume that the corneal metabolism and corneal oxygen consumption also decrease under the same conditions. The sole information suggesting a reverse effect is the effect of temperature. Under open eye conditions the normal temperature varies from 33 °C to 36 °C whereas under closed eye the corneal temperature should be higher as it is equal to the palpebral conjunctiva that it contacts (Freeman & Fatt, 1973). This only creates a 0.5 °C difference but if we consider that a 2 °C increase in temperature results in a 20% increase in corneal metabolic activity (Freeman & Fatt, 1973) this difference is not negligible.

43.4.3 SOURCES AND LEVELS OF OXYGEN SUPPLY IN THE ABSENCE OF CONTACT LENSES

The oxygen supply of interest in contact lens practice, as indicated earlier, is the oxygen supplied at the corneal front surface and utilized by the epithelium and anterior two-thirds of the stroma. The source of that oxygen is the atmospheric oxygen during open eye wear (Smelser, 1952) and the capillary blood vessels of the palpebral conjunctiva (Langham, 1952) during closed eye wear. Because of the different sources of oxygen and their uncontrolled nature, the amount of oxygen available to the cornea varies according to environmental conditions, and also mainly diurnally during the repeated daytime and night-time wear cycle, during which the oxygen available when the eyes are closed at night, is estimated to be one-third of the oxygen available, when the eyes are opened. There resides the main challenge to successful extended contact lens wear.

The oxygen available to the exterior corneal surface has been expressed in various forms. Most commonly in equivalent oxygen percentage (EOP) (21% for the normal atmosphere) or as partial pressure of oxygen (PO_2) in millimetres of mercury (mmHg) (155 mmHg for the normal atmosphere) or in kilo Pascals (kPa) (21 kPa for the normal atmosphere). In this chapter we will use partial pressure values in mmHg, the unit used in most of the publications quoted.

During daytime wear, the oxygen available to the cornea will vary according to differences in atmospheric pressure. Hence, the value usually given for the PO_2 of 155 mmHg is for sea level under normal atmospheric pressure. So even at sea level, the PO_2 may vary by up to 10%, purely due to variation in atmospheric pressure. The greatest variation for atmospheric differences takes place however with altitude because of the decrease in the concentration of oxygen; this can lead to a significant decrease in the oxygen available as pointed out by Hill (1978) (Table 43.2). An activity becoming increasingly common that involves a decrease in the oxygen available to the cornea is long haul commercial flying where the cabin is equivalent to an altitude of 8000 feet (2450 m) equivalent to more than 25% reduction in oxygen available to the cornea. So, during long flights or during travel to altitude such as during skiing holidays, the recovery from overnight corneal swelling may be slowed down resulting in clinical complications for bordercase wearers.

The critical situation with regard to the oxygen available to the cornea is during sleep. Tests on rabbits (Fatt *et al.*, 1974) which suggested that the PO_2 at the anterior corneal surface during sleep was 55 mmHg were confirmed for humans in several studies (Fatt, 1968; Efron & Carney, 1979; Holden & Sweeney, 1985; Holden *et al.*, 1985b; Isenberg & Green, 1985; Mader *et al.*, 1987; Efron

Table 43.2 Atmospheric oxygen available during open eye wear at various altitudes (from Hill, 1978)

Altitude ft (m)	Location	Oxygen available(%)	Oxygen available compared to sea level(%)
0 (0)	Sea level	21	100
5 000 (1 550)	Denver, Colorado, USA	18	86
7 500 (2 300)	Mexico City, Mexico	16	76
11 000 (3 350)	Cuzco (Peru)	14	67
29 000 (8 650)	Mt Everest	7	33

& Ang, 1990) (Table 43.3). With the exception of one study (Efron & Ang, 1990), those studies are in good agreement with regard to the average palpebral oxygen tension of 55–60 mmHg. We believe that the different mean value obtained by Efron and Ang is probably, or at least partially, due to the small sample size tested ($n = 10$) and the very large standard deviation achieved.

From a clinical viewpoint, however, the most important data is that of Isenberg & Green (1985) because of the large sample size involved. This data (Fig. 43.2) shows that the palpebral PO_2 decreases from an average of approximately 65 mmHg at 20 years of age down to approximately 40 mmHg at 70 years of age, confirming the suggestion made by one of us (MR) as to the possible effect of arteriosclerosis on the availability of palpebral conjunctival oxygen (Ruben, 1978). Potentially, therefore, a greater percentage of presbyopic patients wearing contact lenses on an extended wear basis will run the risk of hypoxic problems that young patients. This problem is compounded by the fact that most presbyopics will use a monovision correction for which positive contact lenses with lower overall gas transmissibility are often needed. The second aspect of Isenberg and Green's data, confirmed by Efron and Ang, is the very large inter-patient variation that exists even within the same age group – at least a two-fold range for a normal young contact-lens-wearing population. The supply of oxygen by the palpebral capillaries hence is a very important factor in the difference between extended wear success and failure. The last very important clinical implication of the data on oxygen supply during closed eye wear concerns the effect of changes in altitude (Mader *et al.*, 1987). For example, going from sea level to altitudes encountered during a skiing vacation such as 1800 to 3000 m decreases the PO_2 palpebral oxygen from 60 mmHg to approximately 48 mmHg and 40 mmHg respectively (Fig. 43.3). It would be interesting to know whether patients who have adapted to high altitude show the same decrease or if they have developed a compensating mechanism. Certainly one should make extended wear patients that intend to go to high altitudes aware of the possible risks of hypoxic problems due to the combined open and closed eye effects of the reduction in PO_2 at the corneal front surface. However, what still remains unknown are the effects of sleeping on the oxygen supplied, in terms of the partial pressure of oxygen of the palpebral capillaries during sleep, and oxygen demands and whether those changes are connected.

Table 43.3 Human palpebral partial pressure of oxygen in mmHg

Reference	Population	Mean	Standard deviation	Range
Fatt & Beiber, 1968	$n=1$	55.5		
Efron & Carney, 1979	$n=1$	56.7		
Holden & Sweeney, 1985	$n=16$ Age 18–21 years	61.4	±6.9	47.6 – 75.2
Isenberg & Green, 1985	$n=101$ Age 10–84 years	58 (Torr)	± 14 (Torr)	30.0 – 86.0* (Torr)
Mader *et al.*, 1987	$n=12$ Age 18–36 years	60 (Torr)		45.0 – 85.0*
Efron & Ang, 1990	$n=10$ Age 18-25 years	37.4	± 20.9	00.0 – 84.6**

* Observed range from original graph.
** 95% range calculated from standard deviation values.

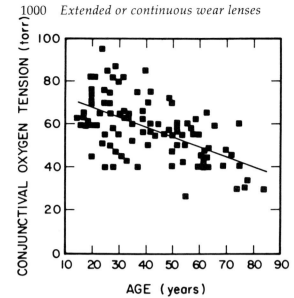

Figure 43.2 Palpebral conjunctival partial pressure of oxygen usage for normal population ($n = 101$) (by courtesy of Isenberg & Green, 1985).

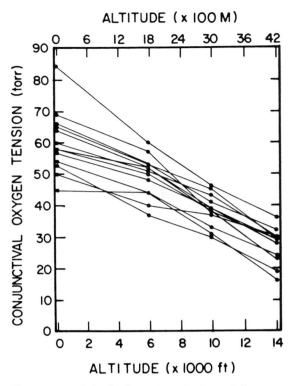

Figure 43.3 Palpebral conjunctival partial pressure of oxygen versus altitude for two young adults (by courtesy of Mader *et al.*, 1987).

43.4.4   EFFECTS OF CONTACT LENS WEAR ON GAS TRANSMISSION

Any contact lens acts as a relative barrier to the free movement of gas, principally oxygen and carbon dioxide, to and from the cornea. Such a relative barrier affects the cornea most critically during closed eye wear. In that situation the driving force for the movement of these gases, due to the relative pressure differential of these gases over the corneal surface, is greatly reduced. For oxygen, the external pressure decreases from approximately 155 mmHg to less than 55 mmHg (Fatt, 1968; Fatt, 1989a) and for carbon dioxide the external pressure increases from less than 0.5 mmHg to approximately 33 mmHg (Efron & Ang, 1990) in the closed eye. The net result of the decrease in relative pressure of oxygen and carbon dioxide during closed eye is a compromised metabolism for which the most obvious clinical manifestation is corneal swelling.

The relative barrier effect of any contact lens is therefore measured by its transmissi-

bility for any gas of interest. Such a transmissibility is expressed in terms of Dk/L (Fatt, 1978) in cm $\times$ ml O_2/s/ml/mmHg where D is the diffusion coefficient of the gas in question, k its solubility and L the thickness of the contact lens. The higher the transmissibility the lower the barrier effect. Several criteria have been given as to a safe minimum for extended wear (O'Neal & Polse, 1985; Holden & Mertz, 1984) and are a help as to predicting the potential performance of any lens type under consideration. This topic has been discussed in detail in Chapters 3 and 5, but as a guideline for clinicians (Holden & Mertz, 1984; O'Neal & Polse, 1985). One could summarize that:

1.   An oxygen transmissibility $> 100 \times 10^{-9}$ cm/ml O_2/s/ml/mmHg should be

the target *Dk/L* for extended wear contact lenses. Such lenses would allow a metabolism similar to that without contact lenses for the whole population.

2. An oxygen transmissibility of approximately 85×10^{-9} cm $\times$ ml O_2/s/ml/ mmHg is sufficient to maintain a normal corneal metabolism for the average wearer.

3. An oxygen transmissibility of at least 70×10^{-9} cm $\times$ ml O_2/s/ml/mmHg is necessary to maintain a normal corneal metabolism for those wearers with the lowest oxygen requirements.

4. An oxygen transmissibility of approximately 35×10^{-9} cm $\times$ ml O_2/s/ml/ mmHg creates a closed eye corneal metabolic compromise that is reversible during open eye wear for the average wearer.

5. The carbon dioxide transmissibility is approximately 21 times that of oxygen for hydrogel contact lenses (Fatt, 1968; Fatt *et al.*, 1969; Ang & Efron, 1989; Fatt & Fink, 1989) whereas their relative movement across the cornea is approximately 7. For hydrogel lenses the limiting physiological factor is therefore the oxygen transmissibility.

6. The carbon dioxide transmissibility for RGP lenses is of the order of 7 times that of oxygen. Both should therefore be considered when testing new RGP materials to determine the critical lens parameters.

In the end the clinician must therefore determine how much corneal swelling is permissible for any given patient over the short and long term to prevent irreversible pathology. This will then be the criteria for safe extended wear. A concept that could be useful to the practitioner would be that of the 'occlusion factor'. A lens that would allow normal metabolism similar to no lens wear, let's say a lens with a *Dk/L* 100×10^{-9}, would have an occlusion factor of 0%, whereas a lens creating 15% overnight swelling such as PMMA would have an occlusion factor of 100%.

43.5 LENS DESIGN AND MATERIALS IN EXTENDED WEAR

43.5.1 INTRODUCTION

The lens design and material criteria for extended wear have been dealt with in Chapter 5. The pertinent issues discussed here will concern specific lens design potentials and an historical view of the progress made to date. However, before embarking upon the discussion of specific designs and materials, it is important to remember the three key contact lens design principles for extended wear:

1. Optimize oxygen transmissibility to permit a normal corneal metabolism.

2. Ensure adequate lens movement to eliminate the metabolic by-products that may be trapped between the contact lens and the cornea (Mertz & Holden, 1981).

3. Avoid any adverse mechanical tissue reaction that could be produced by excessive evaporation with hydrogel contact lenses (Zantos *et al.*, 1986; Holden *et al.*, 1986; McNally *et al.*, 1987; Orsborn & Zantos, 1988; Guillon & Guillon, 1990) or adherent RGP contact lenses (Swarbrick & Holden, 1987; Swarbrick, 1988; Kenyon *et al.*, 1989).

43.5.2 RIGID SCLERAL LENSES

Corneal metabolic considerations

Few authors have attempted to fit patients with gas permeable scleral lenses (Ezekiel, 1983; Pullum *et al.*, 1989; Schein *et al.*, 1990); their application is not patient elective but mainly due to the diseased or distorted eye. Recent material (Pullum *et al.*, 1990) and manufacturing technique (Pullum *et al.*, 1991) developments have lead to lenses with high oxygen transmissibility that should make their use in extended wear, which may be clinically useful in some cases, feasible.

In the most recent investigation, (Pullum *et*

al., 1991) the lenses tested had respective central Dk/L of 38.3×10^{-9} and 76.7×10^{-9} cm $\times$ ml O_2/s/ml/mmHg. Such values are well above Holden and Mertz (1984) criteria for no open eye corneal swelling (24.1 ± 2.7 cm $\times$ ml O_2/s/ml/mmHg or 8% closed eye corneal swelling (34.3 ± 5.2 cm $\times$ ml O_2/s/ml/mmHg, the latter even approaching the target DkL for 0% closed eye swelling (85.0 ± 3.3 cm $\times$ ml O_2/s/ml/ mmHg. The limited data available suggests that, at least for the open eye situation, no significant corneal swelling takes place with such lenses ($\approx$ 1%) and that such swelling could well be due to osmotic tear changes that took place because the subjects tested were non habitual wearers. However one should keep in mind that with such totally occlusive sealed scleral contact lenses a significant tear reservoir exists between the contact lens and the cornea. This reservoir may well be initially beneficial and act as a secondary source of oxygen, helping to achieve a low corneal swelling, but once this source is depleted the reservoir, with a thickness of 0.10 to 0.5 mm, may act as a secondary barrier to oxygen flow with a Dk/L of 15 to 79 $\times$ 10^{-9} cm $\times$ ml O_2/s/ml/mmHg due to the limited permeability of tears (Fatt & St Helen, 1971). Recent results confirm the limitations of scleral lenses to transmit oxygen, demonstrated earlier with moderate Dk materials. Such lenses manufactured with limbal and apical thin zones of 0.1 mm did not permit one of us (MR) to achieve even a few hours' wear without marked oxygen deprivation.

Mechanical considerations

In Chapter 31, dealing with daily wear, the acceptable fit for a rigid lens is described as one that permits a flow of retro-lens tear fluid to the periphery. This is obtained by the lens rocking about either a fulcrum or an axis, thus a 'donkey pump' action occurs with eye movement but not with eye fixation or normal lid blinking unless slits or holes are made in the lens. During sleep, eye movements are mini-

mal for most of the time, as indicated earlier. In such a situation, the relatively large post lens tear reservoir may also result in a build up of large amounts of acid leading to further corneal swelling (Bonanno & Polse, 1987a). Furthermore, the cell debris and degenerate mucous may eventually form an accumulation of metabolic by-products of a 'turbid' nature, in particular with sealed lenses.

Channelled or ventilated scleral lenses may be preferable for extended wear as they would favour tear exchange at eye opening that would avoid the long term accumulation of metabolic by-products. In addition to these unwelcome complications mentioned, when the lids are closed with a scleral lens *in situ*, the lid pressure on the contact lens front surface would tend to squeeze out retrolens fluid without permitting re-entry and a retro-lens negative pressure would result producing unacceptable adverse corneal mechanical effects. In part, some of these effects can be seen in the scleral 'prop' lens fitted to cases of myotonic dystrophia.

Even if the above problems can be overcome, scleral lens fitting for extended wear will remain limited to a small number of clinical cases. The complexity of preformed or moulded lens fitting makes this modality of correction commercially non-viable in the main but worthwhile for some cases.

Silicon rubber material, which would avoid all the problems associated with oxygen supply (Miller, 1972), was once experimentally made in large scleral lens design. This study was, however, limited and fitting problems encountered prevented the achievement of conclusive results; no oxygen estimations were made.

43.5.3 RIGID HIGH GAS PERMEABLE CORNEAL LENSES

Historical review and general material classification

From the early 1970s, a range of hard lens

copolymers has become available with gas permeable properties. Whereas early materials such as cellulose acetate butyrate (CAB) had negligible oxygen transmissibility compared to PMMA, recent developments have lead to lenses with a transmissibility well above those achieved with current hydrogel lenses. Current rigid gas permeable (RGP) lenses, in the main, fall into two categories, silicone/acrylate (S/A) and fluorosilicone/acrylate (F/S/A).

Following the use of PMMA lenses in some cases of extended wear (Dickinson, 1955; Dick 1958; Magatami, 1960), the pioneering work on the use of RGP lenses for cosmetic extended wear originates from Canada. Two optometrists, Levy and Fonn, reported early success in the first half of the 1980s (Fonn & Holden, 1986) using silicone acrylate materials (Levy, 1983, 1985). Fluoropolymers (Keates *et al.*, 1984), because of their high oxygen permeability, were thought at one time to be the family of materials with the best potential for RGP extended wear. However, due to other problems, those lenses were available commercially only for a short period of time but are not currently used; they will therefore not be discussed in detail here.

Corneal metabolic considerations

The first criterion to consider when selecting a RGP material for extended wear, as for hydrogel lenses, is its oxygen permeability. Only the materials with the highest Dk should be used as current clinical evidence suggests the criteria set by Holden and Mertz (1984) of a $Dk/L > 85 \times 10^{-9}$ cm $\times$ ml O_2/s/ml/mmHg for hydrogel lenses is also applicable to RGP lenses. It has been shown that RGP and hydrogel lenses of similar Dk/L give similar overnight swelling (O'Neal *et al.*, 1983, (1984); Sweeney & Holden, 1983; Tomlinson & Armitage, 1985). RGP lenses have, however, two characteristics that may suggest that a lower Dk/L could be acceptable.

The typical lens design for extended wear has a diameter of 9.5 to 10 mm, resulting in only 60% corneal coverage leading to a lower overall hypoxic load than hydrogel lenses of similar Dk/L that cover the whole cornea. The large blink induced lens movement present on eye opening produces an efficient pump that helps to resolve any closed eye induced overnight swelling faster than for hydrogel lenses (Andrasko, 1986; Holden *et al.*, 1988). Conversely there are several negative factors to keep in mind for RGP materials. The key factor concerning performance is the lens transmissibility (Dk/L) and not the lens permeability (Dk). Because typical RGP lenses are much thicker (typical centre thickness for negative lenses 0.15–0.20 mm) than hydrogel lenses (typical centre thickness for negative lenses 0.04–0.12 mm) the Dk of RGP lenses will need to be commensurably higher that the permeability of hydrogel lenses to achieve similar transmissibility. Further, there has been some controversy (Guillon & Holden, 1985) and significant disparities in the determination of the Dk of RGP materials over the years (Holden *et al.*, 1990). Often nominal values and certainly early measurements (Fatt, 1984) that did not take into consideration all the relevant measurement factors lead to an overestimation of the 'effective' Dk (Holden, *et al.*, 1985c) of RGP materials. For Dk values that have been obtained using the polarographic method first described for contact lenses by Fatt (Fatt & St Helen, 1971) one must ensure that the data given has been corrected for 'boundary effect' and 'edge effect'. Even when those correction factors have been applied for the high Dk material, the polarographic method has been considered to be of low repeatability. This has led the International Standards Organisation (ISO) (1991) and the Committee Européen de Normalisation (CEN) on contact lenses to put forward an alternative method for high Dk RGP materials based on coulometric measurements, first introduced to the contact lens industry by Winterton (Winter-

requiring a more precise fitting than hydrogel lenses. The combination of these two mechanical properties creates lens adherence in a slightly too steep fitting lens or a slightly too flat fitting lens that decentres. A wide range of lens designs with diameters which vary from smaller than the cornea with the initial Mueller Welt lenses (Black, 1972; Long, 1974), to full size scleral lens diameter (Miller, 1972) including semi-scleral diameters from 11.7 mm to 14.2 mm have been used without alleviating the lens binding problem. The fitting increment was always positive, the larger the diameter the greater the step. For example, an increment of + 0.10 to + 0.20 mm was chosen for a corneal diameter design ($\approx$ 11.7 mm) and +0.70 mm for a semi scleral contact lens ($\approx$ 14.2 mm). Lens adherence usually involved very high forces, the lens becoming totally immobile and almost impossible to remove compared to a tight hydrogel contact lens. This adherence created an occlusive effect producing discomfort, corneal distortion, corneal abrasion and, in extreme cases, acute red eyes. In fact, most of the clinical successes with silicone rubber lenses have been achieved with aphakic patients using corneal lenses. Because of the lens thickness, these lenses have a rigidity close to RGP lenses and behave in a similar mechanical fashion, demonstrating less lens adherence.

The second problem that affects silicone rubber lenses is the hydrophobic nature of the material. Various processes, including oxidation by ionic treatment and grafting of hydrophilic surfaces (Ruben & Guillon, 1979b), have been tried to compensate for the material hydrophobicity but without total success. Usually the treatment was initially efficient, producing a good hydrophilicity that deteriorated rather rapidly. The deterioration lead to the appearance of hydrophobic zones and to the accumulation of principally a lipidic film, some mucus deposits on the front surface of the lens and discrete debris on the back surface. The latter is thought to be necrotic epithelial cells or other by-products of the corneal metabolism (Ruben & Guillon, 1979b; Blackhurst, 1985). The appearance of deposits was particularly problematic with some lens types where the surface quality observed under magnification was debatable (Hamano et al., 1979; Ruben & Guillon, 1979b).

The material being more rigid than hydrogel materials and the lens thickness varying between 0.12 and 0.30 mm for a negative contact lens, one could anticipate more astigmatism correction than hydrogel contact lenses, but certainly far less than RGP lenses. Finally, at least initially the increased rigidity resulted into slightly less comfortable contact lenses than hydrogel lenses.

43.5.5 SOFT HYDROPHILIC LENSES

Historical review

The concept of extended wear is closely associated with the development of hydrogel lenses. Wichterle and Lim, who introduced the first hydrophilic contact lens (1960), already thought of that lens as a 'fit and forget' lens without quite achieving it. In fact, some 30 years later, this goal still eludes us, despite the tremendous efforts made to achieve it and numerous steps in progress accomplished. It was a British optometrist, John De Carle, who was the first to develop a material (De Carle, 1972a, b) for wearing during sleep. The material was Permalens, a 74% water content material which due to its higher water content achieved a higher oxygen transmissibility than the other lenses of that time. In that range of water content, most of the early progress was due to the UK with the development of even higher water content materials, Sauflon 85 by Cordrey (Cordrey & Mikucki, 1975) later modified by Highgate and Franklin (Highgate, 1978) and marketed as Duragel 75 or Scanlens. It was only later that the very thin lenses made from the original HEMA material by Wichterle and Lim by the spin casting process were introduced for extended wear use. This type of lens was often referred to as hyperthin. At about the same time mid-water content materials, also in a relatively thin design, were introduced for extended wear. It is this group of materials and lens designs that is currently most commonly used for extended wear and with which the concept of disposable lenses worn for a single 7-day period and discarded was introduced with the Acuvue Lens. We will review, by water content groups, the advantages and disadvantages and describe the geometry employed with the different groups of hydrophilic materials available for extended wear (Coon *et al.*, 1979).

The distinction between the various groups is arbitrary. From a clinical and design viewpoint we will consider lenses with > 60% water content to fall in the high water content category, those with > 45% water content and < 60% to constitute the mid water content category and those with < 45% to be in the low water content category.

High water content materials

A common characteristic of all high water content lenses is their relatively thick design. For negative lenses the centre thicknesses encountered are commonly between 0.14 and 0.18 mm. Usually, the higher the water content, the greater the thickness. Such a feature partially offsets the advantages due to the high water content with regard to oxygen transmissibility; so, more recently, slightly thinner lenses such as the Igel Prima lens designed by one of us (MG) with a centre thickness of 0.12 mm and a thin mid-peripheral design due to a tricurve front surface high water content of 67% have become available. The initial reason for using a relatively thick design was the high fragility of the materials such as Permalens or Sauflon 85 or the natural collagen materials (Hill & Brezinski, 1986). That initial problem was, however, rapidly solved even for the

same families of materials with Permaflex or Sauflon 70. The current limits on how thin a lens can be are the evaporative properties of those materials (see Chapters 5 and 21) that create corneal staining if the design chosen is too thin (< 0.1 mm). The advantages of such relatively thick designs are the rigidity of the lens, giving the lens good handling characteristics, and on-eye lens movement if properly fitted. The latter ($\approx$ 0.50 mm at blink) permits the elimination of metabolic by-products between the contact lens and the cornea following closed eye wear. The relative disadvantages of these designs, in addition to the reduced Dk/L of the lens, are the increased lens awareness reported when compared to thin low water content lenses, and the necessity to achieve an accurate fitting. With the exception of the initial Permalens design proposed by De Carle (De Carle, 1975) who used tightly fitting corneal diameter lenses (total diameter 11.50 to 12.50 mm) to minimize trauma, all the other designs share an alternative common concept (De Carle, 1978). The lenses are semiscleral diameter lenses (total diameter 13.50 to 14.50 mm) and are fitted as loosely as possible. This requires the use of more than one back optic radius (BOR) for each lens design; these are most commonly between 8.40 and 9.20 mm. The more rigid the lens, the greater the number of alternate BORs required.

The high water content materials for extended wear fall into two broad categories with regard to their surface characteristics: materials that are surface charged (ionic) such as Permalens, and those that are not (non-ionic) such as Bausch and Lomb 70. The nature of the surface is the basis of the most commonly used classification to date (see Chapter 47 Part 3) and impart specific properties. Ionic materials are those that attract the most proteins and consequently are required to be changed most frequently; they also permit the most rapid formation of a biofilm and therefore should be favoured for

disposable or frequent replacement programmes where lenses are replaced regularly
(i.e. once a week). Finally, all the high water
content materials have a tendency to be heat
sensitive, decreasing in size from the vial to
the eye, hence requiring to be made in a
greater nominal diameter than low water
content lenses to achieve the same on eye
diameter.

Low water content materials

The low water content materials are usually
HEMA based materials and therefore non-
ionic. For extended wear all the low water
content lenses have an identical hyperthin
design with a centre thicknesses of 0.035–
0.045 mm for negative lenses. Because of the
difficulties in manufacturing associated with
the exact thickness control required, most
lenses of that type are either manufactured
by spincasting (e.g. Bausch and Lomb O_3
and O_4) or cast moulding (e.g. Allergan Zero
4). As indicated elsewhere (see Chapter 5),
such a feature leads to an over-estimation of
the oxygen available to the cornea as the
relative increase in thickness at the lens
periphery greatly reduces the overall lens
oxygen transmissibility. The other problem
associated with hyperthin low water content lenses is that they wrap around the
cornea and conjunctiva and make lens
movement very limited to non-existent.
This phenomenon may lead to a greater
difficulty in eliminating debris after overnight wear.

The advantages of the low water content
lenses are the ease of fitting, usually a single
BOR is available (and suitable to fit the great
majority of eyes as the lens wraps to the eye),
and also the very good degree of comfort
achieved due to the minimal lens movement
and extremely thin lens edge.

Mid-water content materials

The mid-water content contact lenses are
now the most commonly used lenses for

extended wear. These lenses that appear as a
compromise between the two groups
described above are in fact an optimization
of the relative material properties of each.
The lenses can be made thin enough (0.055 to
0.07 mm centre thickness) to allow optimal
comfort with minimal lens edge awareness
and good corneal wrapping leading to an
easy lens fit, hence incorporating the many
benefits of low water content lenses. At the
same time the oxygen transmissibility in
particular in the low negative power range
(up to − 4.00 DS) is similar and sometimes
superior to that achieved by the high water
content lenses.

The material gas permeability increases
exponentially with water content. Hence an
increase of 20% in water content, which
corresponds to the materials with the highest
H_2O content currently available (75–80%)
would increase the permeability by 100%.
However such extreme water content materials (Stein & Slatt, 1984) are usually fragile and
very sensitive to on eye water losses forcing
them to be made in a thickness of approximately 0.20 mm. The oxygen transmissibility
is inversely proportional to thickness. Hence
by reducing the thickness from 0.20 mm to
0.07 mm one increases oxygen transmissibility by 285%, offsetting the advantage of the
high water content contact lenses. Obviously
this concerns only the lens transmissibility at
its centre, but even if due consideration is
given to the lens average thickness (≈ 0.10
mm for a 55% water content versus ≈ 0.24
mm for a 75% water content) the overall
balance is still in favour of the mid-water
content lenses.

The mid water content lenses available
are most commonly ionic lenses such as the
disposable lenses (Acuvue 58%; New Vues
55%) and made by cast moulding the
former in its final form (soft moulding), the
latter by conventional technique. However
non-ionic materials with lenses made by
lathing are also available (Hydrocurve II
55%).

43.6   LONG TERM EFFECTS OF EXTENDED WEAR

43.6.1   INTRODUCTORY REMARKS

The effects of extended wear contact lenses fall into two broad categories of chronic and acute effects and will be discussed in that way in this chapter. The chronic effects are principally morphological and functional changes affecting ocular tissues and associated with the hypoxia produced by current extended wear lenses, but also include the palpebral changes that are thought to be partly related to the nature of the contact lens surface that contacts the lids for extended periods of time. The acute effects are possibly of greatest concern as they are of various degrees of severity including potentially sight threatening infective keratitis. The various effects mentioned above are described elsewhere in the book. Ocular tissue changes are being dealt with in Chapters 19 and 42, and lid changes and acute reactions in Chapter 46. They will therefore be discussed here only with regard to the specific case of extended wear.

The clinical implications of this section for the management of extended wear patients are numerous. The key to management of extended wear is to establish the relative risk of extended wear compared to other modalities of ametropic correction. Without doubt, the relative risk of complication is greater for extended than for daily contact lens wear, but the information reported as to the safety of extended wear must be put into its true context. The studies dealing with acute effects are mostly referral studies and, in many cases, may give a biased view of the true safety of extended wear. The studies on the chronic effects of extended wear often relate to subtle changes that, although not desirable, in the main do not warrant the discontinuation of contact lens wear. Unfortunately there are very few long term extended wear studies involving large num-

bers of patients but those tend to report good long term clinical acceptance. In the USA one such study (Koetting *et al.*, 1988) reported on 500 extended wear patients (418 hydrogel wearers and 82 RGP wearers) with an average extended wear use of 2½ years. Successful criteria was taken from continued overnight wear by patients reporting satisfactory comfort and vision and the absence of clinically unacceptable changes when the cornea was observed by the practitioner. The success achieved according to the clinical criteria outlined above may appear high at 79.6% but it is in fact quite representative of large clinical studies with extended wear. Two European studies (Nilsson & Persson, 1986; Rengstorff *et al.*, 1987) published at the same time for extended wear for a high water content hydrophilic material (Scanlens 75) confirms these findings. The first study (Nilsson & Persson, 1986), which was a prospective study of 100 patients over 2 years of extended wear, reported an 88.4% success according to similar criteria. The second study (Rengstorff *et al.*, 1987), which was a retrospective study of 2000 extended wear patients with an average of 4.5 years of extended wear, achieved a success rate of 87% when taking an habitual 14 days uninterrupted wear as minimal criteria for long term wear.

43.6.2   CHRONIC EFFECTS

Cornea

Epithelium

The long term use of hydrogel extended wear contact lenses reduces the oxygen uptake rate that is considered the key indicator of the epithelial metabolic rate (Holden *et al.*, 1985b) by approximately 15%. Such a decrease in metabolic rate would seem to lead to a thinning of the epithelium by 6% after 5 years of extended wear (Holden *et al.*, 1985a). However, such findings require confirmation in humans as the mean loss recorded (3 μm) is within the experimental uncertainty of the measuring technique used in that study.

An undisputed side effect of the abnormal metabolism is the appearance of abnormal microcytic formations (Zantos & Holden, 1978) that develop at the level of the deep epithelial layers and tend to migrate towards the epithelial surface. The exact nature of the microcysts is not known, but they are thought to be an accumulation of metabolic by-products that are trapped within the epithelium (Zantos, 1983). Microcysts, which can be seen by retro-illumination (Chapter 18), are reported to be present with all hydrogel extended wear contact lenses (Zantos, 1983; Kenyon *et al.*, 1986). They are usually thought to appear after three months of extended wear, but recent studies have reported their appearance after as little as one week of extended wear (Epstein & Donnenfeld, 1989; Veys, 1991; Efron & Veys, 1992). The clinical implications of microcysts depend upon their severity. Less than 50 microcysts per cornea is considered normal in extended wear (Zantos, 1983). Above that number proactive action is recommended, the objective being to increase the oxygen available to the cornea. Such effect can be achieved in several ways: (1) refitting with an extended wear lens with a higher oxygen transmissibility, which usually involves an RGP lens; (2) increasing the frequency of lens removal to every two or three days out of every seven; (3) reverting to flexible wear (occasional overnight wear) or daily wear; (4) discontinuing lens wear for a while. The choice of action will depend upon the severity of the microcytic reaction. With the exception of increasing the frequency of lens removal, where conflicting results have been achieved (one study showing improvement (Holden *et al.*, 1989) and the other no improvement (Kenyon *et al.*, 1986), all approaches have categorically shown some remedial effect. Whenever effective remedial

action takes place microcysts take approximately six months to totally disappear (Humphreys *et al.*, 1980; Zantos, 1983; Holden *et al.*, 1985a). When contact lens wear is first discontinued microcysts initially increase significantly in number before disappearing. When the remedial action is the discontinuation of contact lens wear the peak increase in microcysts is between one and two weeks post-contact-lens wear. No convincing explanation has been given for that phenomenon. Microcysts are usually not associated with significant corneal staining.

Another indication of the level of the epithelial metabolic rate is the sensitivity of the cornea. Corneal touch threshold measurements show that hydrogel extended wear decreases corneal sensitivity (Larke & Hirji, 1979). However, this loss of sensitivity, in the case of extended wear, may well be due to a morphological tissue change with a decrease in the density of the epithelial nerve endings (Hamano, 1984). No data is available for extended wear RGP but if we extrapolate the data obtained for daily wear (Millodot, 1974; Millodot *et al.*, 1979), we expect greater losses with RGP than with hydrogel lenses of similar oxygen transmissibility.

For both RGP and soft lens types, the clinical implication of the decrease in innervation and resulting loss of sensitivity is a possible delay before the patient becomes aware of any discomfort associated with an acute corneal adverse effect. This obviously would contribute to the greater severity of acute adverse effects with extended wear.

All the above effects which are associated with corneal hypoxia have been identified with hydrogel soft lenses, similar effects can be expected with the first generation of RGP lenses that have similar transmissibility. Accordingly, one would anticipate lesser problems with the new generation of RGP materials that produced none or a very low hypoxia.

Another structural modification in extended wear that has been demonstrated in the animal model has been a decrease in hemidesmose junctions that hold cells together (Madigan, 1989). This decrease is associated with a decreased adherence of the epithelium to the underlying structures; such loss of adherence is related exponentially to the transmissibility of the lenses used (Sweeney, *et al.*, 1987). It is thought that, if also true in humans, this decrease in epithelial adherence due to hypoxia could be a significant contributing factor to the increased incidence of corneal ulceration in extended wear. For corneal sterile ulcers an epithelial anomaly will make deeper tissue defects more likely. For infective ulcers, the epithelial anomaly will provide a portal of entry for any infective agent that may be present.

The other main epithelial change associated with extended wear, epithelial staining, has, in addition to a hypoxic cause, a supplementary element and therefore must be discussed separately. Whereas the aetiology of corneal staining is common to hydrogel and RGP extended wear, being in both cases an inadequate maintenance of a continuous stable tear film over the contact lens and the cornea between blink, the morphological appearance and lens factors involved are totally different (Chapter 21). With hydrogel contact lenses that fully cover the cornea, staining is most frequently encountered in the upper and lower quadrant of the cornea, often in an arcuate fashion following the upper and lower lid tear prism edge. Such staining, sometimes called superior epithelial arcuate limbal staining (SEALS) (Hine *et al.*, 1987), is due to the instability of the tear which is greatest in that region of the eye (Guillon *et al.*, 1990). Induced corneal staining for hydrogel lenses is not mechanical in nature as suggested by some but is the result of an unstable hydration gradient that reaches the lens back surface (Fatt, 1989b) and creates the resulting staining. Past studies (Orsborn & Zantos, 1988) have shown that such staining is highly patient depen-

dent and for lenses of equal thickness more marked with high water content lenses and for a given material more marked for thinner lenses. For hydrogel extended wear when such staining is unacceptable in severity, usually the only suitable solution is to refit the patient with a different lens material and/or design. The changes necessary to correct that problem result in a decrease in oxygen transmissibility and therefore, even when successful may still compromise successful extended wear.

With RGP lenses, staining is most often encountered in the horizontal meridian just outside the edge of the contact lens. This staining, usually called '3 and 9 o'clock staining', always begins as a punctate staining and in problematic cases develops into a coalescent staining, even triggering corneal neovascularization that becomes clinically unacceptable. The staining initially develops because the tear film cannot produce a continuous film in that area during the inter-blink period and is compounded by the blink action that covers that area last (Guillon & Guillon, 1988). Three and 9 o'clock staining, which was a significant problem with PMMA, and had greatly reduced with daily wear RGP lenses, has again become a significant problem with extended wear RGP lenses (Zantos & Zantos, 1985; Seger & Mutti, 1986; Zabkiewig, *et al.*, 1986; Schnider, 1987). In addition to the patient poor tear characteristics the main cause for the variations in staining incidence is the difference in peripheral design for daily and extended wear RGP lenses (Chapter 5). The greater the edge clearance of the lens the higher the incidence of peripheral desiccation. Both PMMA and RGP lenses for extended wear have greater edge clearances, produced by flatter peripheral curves and/or wider peripheral zones, than daily wear RGP lenses. In the case of RGP lenses for extended wear the reason for such a change in design is to avoid lens binding during overnight wear. Two other contributing factors are a

Table 43.5 Relative risk of ulcerative keratitis for different lens types reported in the literature

Relative risks	Authors		
	Schein *et al.*, 1989	Benjamin, 1991	Dart *et al.*, 1991
Daily wear RGP			1.0
Daily wear soft		1.0	
Used for daily wear:	1.0		3.6
Used overnight:	9.3		
Extended wear RGP			
Extended wear Soft		4.2	20.8
Used for daily wear:	2.7		
Used overnight in general:	12.6		
Used overnight for consecutive nights:			
1	3.0		
2–7	8.4		
8–14	24.9		
> 15	29.8		

authors feel that extended wear of hydrogel lenses, because of the hypoxic conditions and associated chronic effects they produce and the increased risks of acute adverse effects, should not be the first modality of choice. The relative risks of the various modalities of wear should be explained to these patients and in an attempt to convince them to opt for daily wear and/or flexible wear where lenses are only occasionally worn overnight. Usually novice contact lens wearers are concerned with the notion of extended wear with RGP lenses, hence this option is not usually considered by them.

For current daily wearers the physiological limitations of hydrogel lenses still apply but it has been shown that if the patient is already a successful asymptomatic daily wearer, the chances of successful extended wear are greater (Guillon *et al.*, 1992). The authors are therefore more inclined towards extended wear in particular if, for professional reasons (e.g. on call for more than 24 hours), or specific hobbies (e.g. sailing), the management of daily wear lenses is not practical. For current symptomatic daily lens wearers, extended wear is not recommended. Overall these patients achieve a lower suc-

cess rate than previous asymptomatic patients and regularly contaminate their lenses, requiring careful and thorough lens care and frequent replacement (Guillon *et al.*, 1991).

For current RGP wearers our experience over the last three years led us to a far more positive approach to RGP extended wear. Because of the very good physiological performance achieved with lenses of the latest generation and the very low incidence of acute adverse effects, any successful daily RGP patient with the correct ocular characteristics that attends for a routine aftercare visit and requires a change of lenses for fitting reasons or because of damage, is explained the relative advantages and disadvantages of RGP extended wear and given the opportunity to opt for RGP extended wear lenses.

Ideally the patients selected for extended wear should satisfy all the criteria as to normality of the tissues that will be in contact with the lens. The tear formation and tear film should be normal and ocular allergies well controlled if present. There should not be any evidence of vernal conjunctivitis or untreated papillitis. The daily environment should not expose the eyes to prolonged drying spells, chemical or dust pollution. The patient should not be on heavy medication that produces decreased lacrimation such as beta-blockers that regulate cardiovascular disease or tranquillizers.

43.8.2 LENS DESIGN AND MATERIAL SELECTION

Lens design and materials used for extended wear have been described earlier. From the lenses currently available the choice of lens will depend, amongst other considerations, on the patient's prescription. For patients with astigmatism greater that 0.75 D, RGP lenses are the first and possibly the only choice. Current toric hydrogel lens designs seem too thick to achieve an acceptable physiological response for the average patient. For patients with 0.75 D or less astigmatism both hydrogel and RGP lenses are fitted. One important factor is the patient's previous wearing modality; patients tending to be fitted with lenses of a similar type to those they currently wear. For new wearers the relative advantages and disadvantages are stressed and the decision is made during consultation with the patient. Whenever a hydrogel lens is selected, the authors prefer to opt for a thin mid-water content or a high water content lens rather than a hyperthin low water content lens that produces a higher corneal swelling. Further, as the regular replacement of conventional contact lenses or the use of disposable contact lenses has been shown to reduce the incidence of all extended wear chronic and/or acute adverse effects associated with the status of the contact lens surface (Kotow, *et al.*, (1987a) the authors only fit patients with extended wear, if they agree to follow that process. For RGP the choice of material is determined by its Dk, that should be greater than 75, and mechanical properties. As for hydrogel lens wearers, RGP lens wearers would benefit from frequent replace-

ments, at least every 6 months, as the performance of these lenses has been shown to decrease after 3 to 4 months of wear (Guillon & Guillon, 1991). The discussion on the recommendations and management of regular replacement is described later.

43.8.3 LENS FITTING AND DISPENSING

Lens fitting has already been described in detail in Chapter 27 and further comments have been made in this chapter in the section on lens design (see pages 1002–8). With regard to the criteria to fulfil for an optimal fit with extended wear lenses, the key to success, in addition to the requirements of daily wear, is to ensure that, both for hydrogel and RGP, the lens fit is mobile soon after waking in order to eliminate any trapped debris that could create a toxic adverse reaction. Because the critical aspect of extended wear performance is the ocular and lens response to overnight wear, we include the first night of wear and the ensuing visit in the fitting process. Potential extended wear patients are told that the decision to fit them with extended wear can only be made after evaluating the first night's performance both for hydrogel and RGP lenses. With the advent of disposable lenses, potential hydrogel wearers are issued with a first pair of lenses that can be discarded at low cost if the trial is not successful. For RGP lenses, failure to achieve overnight wear due to lens binding does not preclude the same lens to be perfectly suited to daily wear use, hence avoiding excessive trial cost to the patient. The last phase of the fitting process after the first night's wear takes place as early as possible after waking to assess the signs of overnight wear. Particular attention is paid to detect any sign of residual gross oedema. If striae are present after two hours of open eye wear, that particular lens fitting is unacceptable. The other aspects reviewed are the lens mobility and any sign of lens adherence with RGP lenses or possible tight lens syndrome with hydrogels.

Lens dispensing modalities have been described in detail in Chapter 25 and apply here. All instructions must be given verbally and in writing, particularly for extended wear patients, who have a greater risk of developing adverse reactions. Also, because lens removal with extended wear is infrequent, it is even more important than for daily wear, for which repeated use increases the handling ability, to ensure total proficiency in lens handling before the patient leaves the office.

The information for extended wearers includes some relevant to daily wearers. The following information is required:

1. Lens handling and care instructions, including the names of the specific products to use. Also when the fitting is completed a full prescription must be issued to the patient to enable any practitioner that may have to deal with the patient, in particular in an emergency, to have all the relevant details available. Some practitioners, especially when using new products or undertaking trials, insist on the patient signing a waiver form to protect them from legal implications such as claims of lack of professional care or mismanagement. In those instances where patients suffered eye lesions, legal claims have been made against the practitioner and the manufacturer and even in few instances against the Government Licensing Authority.

    In this area, two steps specific to extended wear have been added for both hydrogel and RGP to the usual daily wear instructions. The care instructions include the use of an unpreserved, single aqueous eyedrop, usually normal saline, to be used nightly before retiring and soon after waking. Also, for RGP, the patients are instructed to check for lens binding on waking.

2. Information on the relative risk of daily and extended wear for various chronic and acute adverse effects, in particular, microbial ulceration with emphasis being put on the importance of compliance for problems with use and long term success. Advice on the steps to take in case of emergency is also given.

3. Information on the initial maximum length of wear without removal. In all cases the maximum allowed wearing period without removal is 6 nights and 7 days for both hydrogel and RGP lenses. Hydrogel wearers and new contact lens wearers progress immediately to their first night of wear with no previous adaptation to daily wear. RGP wearers must initially adapt to daily wear. Despite the good physiological response achieved with RGP lenses, physical tolerance of the lenses does not allow immediate extended wear.

    Whereas the signing of an informal statement of the risks does not remove any rights of the patients and therefore does not unduly protect the practitioner we favour that approach for extended wear. Our reasons for that approach is to reinforce to the patients the importance of following instructions and to restate the increased risks associated with extended wear.

4. Advice as to the likely replacement frequency. Our research work over the last few years (Guillon *et al.*, 1992) has shown that the frequency of replacement is highly patient dependent. Our concept is not based upon a fixed replacement for all patients for a given lens type, but on an individualized replacement programme for each patient. Our aftercare routine involves the monitoring of the lens surface characteristics and on-eye wettability (Chapter 21), and the patient subjective response. The patients are initially issued with no replacement instructions and the fre-

quency of replacement will be the longest period without any change in performance from that achieved with the new contact lens. The performance is considered to be worse that optimal if any of the following take place:

i. The subjective comfort and/or subjective vision ratings, which are rated on a five-point scale (excellent, very good, good, fair and poor), decrease by two or more grades (i.e. very good to fair);

ii. The best correctable visual acuity shows a loss of at least one visual acuity line,

iii. The lens surface deposits observable with the slit lamp biomicroscope which are classified on a six-point scale (none, very slight, slight, moderate, severe and very severe) and show an increase of at least two grades (e.g. very slight to moderate).

iv. The wettability, defined by the prelens tear film break up time, is less than 10 seconds and shows a decrease of more than 25% from the value achieved with the new lens (Chapter 21).

For a given lens type (04 series Bausch & Lomb lenses) used on an extended wear basis, depending on the patient, the optimal replacement period varied between 3 days and 3 months (Guillon *et al.*, 1992).

43.8.4 AFTERCARE VISITS

Regular aftercare visits are essential for long term successful extended wear. In the initial period the visits are necessary to decide upon the optimal replacement period. After this the visits are to ensure that no clinically unacceptable adverse effects develop. Our routine includes aftercare visits after 1 day, 1 week, 1, 3 and 6 months, and at least 6-monthly afterwards. All these visits should take place as early in the morning as possible. They should also be performed

towards the end of the wearing cycle of a regularly replaced lens rather than at the beginning in an attempt to check on the continued absence of lens spoilation.

The conclusion is that for the cosmetic visual patient, great care must be observed in the use of extended wear and the patient must be encouraged to seek professional advice whenever any unusual symptoms become manifest.

REFERENCES

Abelson, M.B. and Holly, F.J. (1977) A tentative mechanism for inferior punctate keratopathy. *Am. J. Ophthalmol.*, **83**, 866–75.

Agnew, H.W., Webb, E.R. and Williams, R.L. (1966) The first night effect and EEG study of sleep. *Psychophysical*, **2**, 263–6.

Allansmith, M.R., Korb, D.R., Greiner, J.U., Henriquez, A.S., Simon, M.A. and Finnemore, V.M. (1977) Giant papillary conjunctivitis in contact lens wearers. *Am. J. Ophthalmol.*, **83**, 697–708.

Ames, K.S., and Cameron, M.H. (1989). The efficiency of regular lens replacement in extended wear. *Int. Contact Lens Clin.*, **16**(4), 104–11.

Andrasko, G.J. (1986) Corneal deswelling response to hard and hydrogel extended wear lenses. *Invest. Ophthalmol. Vis. Sci.*, **27**, 21–3.

Andrasko, G.J. (1990) Peripheral corneal staining: edge lift and extended wear. *Spectrum* **5**(8), 33–5.

Ang, J.H.B. and Efron, N. (1989) Carbon dioxide permeability of contact lens materials. *Int. Contact Lens Clin.*, **16** (2), 48–58.

Aserinsky, E. and Kleitmann, N. (1955) Two types of ocular mobility occurring in sleep. *J. Appl. Physiol.*, **8**, 1–10.

Barishak, Y., Zavaro, A., Samra, Z. and Sompolinsky, D. (1984) An immunologic study of papillary conjunctivitis due to contact lenses. *Curr. Eye Res.*, **3**, 1161–8.

Barr, and Schoessler, J.P. (1980) Corneal endothelial response to rigid contact lenses. *Am. J. Optom. Physiol. Opt.*, **57**, 267–74.

Becker, W.E. (1959) *Silicone Contact Lens.* US Patent No. 834752.

Benjamin, W.J. (1991) Assessing the risks of extended wear. *Optom. Clin.*, **1**(3), 13–31.

Bennett, E.S. and Ghormley, N.R. (1987) Rigid

extended wear. An overview. *Int. Contact Lens Clin.*, **14**, 319–32.

Black, C.J. (1972) *Silicone Lenses in Soft Contact Lenses* (eds. A.R. Gassett, and H.E. Kaufman), C.V. Mosby, Saint Louis.

Blackhurst, R.T. (1985) Personal experience with hydrogel and silicone extended wear lenses. *Contact Lens Assoc. Ophthalmol. J.*, **11**, 136–7.

Bonanno, J.A. and Polse, K.A. (1987a) Effect of contact lens transmissibility on stromal pH. *Invest. Ophthalmol. Vis. Sci.*, **28**, 163.

Bonanno, J.A. and Polse, K.A. (1987b) Corneal acidosis during contact lens wear. Effect of hypoxia and CO_2. *Invest. Ophthalmol. Vis. Sci.*, **28**, 1514–20.

Bonanno, J.A. and Polse, K.A. (1987c). Measurement of in vivo human corneal stromal pH: open and closed eye. *Invest. Ophthalmol. Vis. Sci.*, **28**, 522–30.

Brennan, N.A., Lowe, R., Efron, N., Ungerer, J.L. and Carney, L.G. (1987). Dehydration of hydrogel lenses during overnight wear. *Am. J. Optom. Physiol. Opt.*, **64**, 534–9.

Campbell, R.C. (1987) Corneal ulcers in contact lens wearers. *Contact Lens Spectrum*, **2**(11), 28–31.

Carlson, K.H. and Bourne, W.M. (1988) Endothelial morphologic features and function after long term extended wear of contact lenses. *Arch. Ophthalmol.*, **106**, 1677–9.

Carlson, K.H. Bourne, W.M. and Brubaker, R.F. (1988) Effect of long term contact lens wear on corneal endothelial cell morphology and function. *Invest. Ophthalmol. Vis. Sci.*, **29**, 185–93.

Carney, L.G. and Hill, R.M. (1982) The nature of normal blinking patterns. *Acta Ophthalmologica*, **60**, 427–30.

Cassidy, J.R. (1969) Correction of a phobia with corneal contact lenses. *Am. J. Ophthalmol.*, **68**, 319–23.

Chalupa, E., Swarbrick, H.A. Holden, B.A. and Sjostrand, J. (1987) Severe corneal infections associated with contact lens wear. *Ophthalmology*, **94**, 17–22.

Cho, M.H. Norden, L.C. and Chang, F.W. (1988) Disposable extended wear soft contact lenses for the treatment of giant papillary conjunctivitis. *Southern J. Optom.*, **6**(1), 9–12.

Cohen, E.J., Gonzales, C., Leavitt, K.G., Arentsen, J.J. and Laibson, P.R. (1991) Corneal ulcers associated with contact lenses including experience with disposable lenses. *Contact Lens Assoc. Ophthalmol. J.*, **17**, 173–6.

Comité Européen de Normalisation (1991) *Contact lens determination of oxygen permeability and transmissibility by coulometric method.* CEN TC 170 SC7/WG4 N40.

Coon, L.J, Miller, J.P. and Meier, R.F. (1979) Overview of extended wear contact lenses. *J. Am. Optom. Assoc.* **50**, 745–9.

Cooper, R.L. and Constable, I.J. (1977) Infective keratitis in soft contact lens wearers. *Br. J. Ophthalmol.*, **61**, 250–4.

Cordrey, P.W. and Mikucki, W. (1975) *Hydrophilic co-polymers and articles formed therefrom.* British Patent 2,391,438.

Cox, I. and Ames, K. (1989) Effect of eye patching on the overnight corneal swelling response with rigid contact lenses. *Optom. Vis. Sci.*, **66**, 207–8.

Croin, F., Guillon, M., Polse, K. and Brand, R. (1990) Transient effect of extended wear on corneal function. *Optom. Vis. Sci.*, **67**, 198P.

Dart, J.K.G. (1986). Complications of extended wear hydrogel contact lenses. *Contax*, **March/April**, 11–19.

Dart, J.K.G., Stapleton, F. and Minassian, D. (1991) Contact lenses and other risk factors in microbial keratitis. *Lancet*, **338**, 650–4.

Davies, I. (1990) The limbus revisited. *J. Br. Contact Lens Assoc.*, **13**, 32–5.

De Carle, J. (1972a) Developing hydrophilic lenses for continuous wear. *Contacto*, **16**(1), 39–42.

De Carle, J. (1972b) *Improvements in or relating to hydrophilic polymers and contact lenses manufactured therefrom.* British Patent 1,385,677.

De Carle, J. (1975) Oxygen permeability and physical fitting considerations in hydrophilic contact lens wear. *Contacto*, **19**(6), 55–8.

De Carle, J. (1978) Hydrophilic lenses for constant wear. In *Soft Contact Lenses: clinical and applied technology*, Bailliere Tyndall, London.

Dick, R.B. (1958) Contact lenses in constant use for a three month period. A case report. *Am. J. Optom. Arch. Am. Acad. Optom.*, **35**, 240–50.

Dickinson, F. (1955) Experiences with the microlens. *Br. J. Physiol. Opt.*, **12**, 62–75.

Doane, M.G. (1980) Interaction of eyelids and tears and the dynamics of the normal human eyeblink. *Am. J. Ophthalmol.*, **89**, 507–11.

Dunn, J.P., Mondino, B.J. Weissman, B.A., Donzis, P.B. and Kikkawa, D.O. (1989) Corneal ulcers associated with disposable hydrogel contact lenses. *Am. J. Ophthalmol.*, **108**, 113–17.

Dutt, R.M., Stocker, E.G., Wolff, C.H., Glavan, I. and Lass, J.M. (1989) A morphologic and fluophotometric analysis of the corneal endothelium in long term extended wear soft contact lens wearers. *Contact Lens Assoc. Opthalmol. J.,* **15** (2), 121–3.

Efron, N. and Ang, J.H.B. (1990). Corneal hypoxia and hypercapnia during contact lens wear. *Optom. Vis. Sci.,* **67**, 512–21.

Efron, N. and Carney, L.G. (1979) Oxygen tension measurements under soft contact lenses with blinking. *Int. Contact Lens Clin.,* **6** (6), 25–9.

Efron, N. and Carney, L.G. (1981) Models of oxygen performance for the static, dynamic and closed lid wear of hydrogel contact lenses. *Aust. J. Optom.,* **64**, 223–33.

Efron, N. and Veys, J. (1992) Defects in disposable contact lenses can compromise ocular integrity. *Int. Contact Lens Clin.,* **19**(1), 8–18.

Epstein, A.B. and Donnenfeld, E.D. (1989) Epithelial microcysts associated with Acuvue disposable contact lenses. *Contact Lens Forum,* **3**, 33–6.

Ezekiel, D. (1983) Gas permeable haptic lenses. *J. Br. Contact Lens Assoc.,* **4**, 158–61.

Fatt, I. (1968) Steady state distribution of oxygen and carbon dioxide in the in vivo cornea II. The open eye in nitrogen and the covered eye. *Exp. Eye Res.,* **7**, 413–30.

Fatt, I. (1978) Gas transmission properties of soft contact lenses. In *Soft contact lenses.* (ed. M, Ruben), Bailliere Tindall, London, pp.225–43.

Fatt, I. (1979) Negative pressure under silicone rubber contact lenses. *Contacto,* **23**, 6–9.

Fatt, I. (1984) Oxygen transmissibility and permeability of gas permeable hard contact lenses and materials. *Int. Contact Lens Clin.,* **11**, 175–83.

Fatt, I. (1989a) Successful fit of an extended wear contact lens depends on physiological conditions of the eye. *Contact Lens J.,* **17** (7), 230–5.

Fatt, I. (1989b). A predictive model for dehydration of an hydrogel contact lens in the eye. *J. Br. Contact Lens Assoc.* **12** (2), 15–31.

Fatt, I. and Fink, S.E. (1989) The ratio of carbon dioxide to oxygen permeability of RGP contact lens materials. *Int. Contact Lens Clin.,* **6**(11), 347–52.

Fatt, I. and St Helen, R. (1971) Oxygen tension under an oxygen permeable contact lens. *Am. J. Optom. Physiol. Opt.,* **48**, 545–55.

Fatt, I., Bieber, T.M. and Pye, S.D. (1969) Steady state distribution of oxygen and carbon dioxide in the in-vivo cornea of an eye covered by a gas permeable contact lens. *Am. J. Optom. Physiol. Opt.,* **46**, 3–14.

Fatt, I. Freeman, R.D. and Lin, D. (1974) Oxygen tension distribution in the cornea. A re-examination. *Exp. Eye Res.,* **18**, 357–65.

Fish, B. (1990) Corneal ulcers and contact lens wear. *Contact Lens Spectrum,* **5** (5), 49–57.

Fitzgerald, J.P. and Efron, N. (1986) Oxygen uptake profile of the human cornea. *Clin. Exp. Optom.,* **69**, 149–52.

Fitzgerald, J.K. and Jones, D.P. (1978) Oxygen flow data can be misleading. *Int. Contact Lens Clin.,* **5**, 134–8.

Fonn, D. and Holden, B.A. (1986) Extended wear of hard gas permeable contact lenses can induce ptosis. *Contact Lens Assoc. Ophthalmol. J.,* **12**, 93–4.

Fraunfelder, F.T. (1982) *Drug induced ocular side effects and drug interaction* (2nd edn), Lea and Febiger, Philadelphia.

Freeman, R.D. and Fatt, I. (1973) Environmental influences on ocular temperature. *Invest. Ophthalmol. Vis. Sci.,* **12**, 596–602.

Fromer, C.H. and Klintworth, G.K. (1976) An evaluation of the role of leucocysts in the pathogenesis of experimentally induced corneal vascularisation. III Studies related to the vaso proliferative capability of polymorphonuclear leucocysts. *Am. J. Pathol.,* **82**, 157.

Ghormley, N.R. (1988) The fluoroperm family: Part One. *Int. Contact Lens Clin.,* **15**, 239–40.

Ghormley, N.R. (1989) The Advent™ contact lens. Clinical viewpoints. *Int. Contact Lens Clin.,* **16**, 194–6.

Gonnering, R., Edelhausser, H.F., Van Horn, D.L. and Durant, W. (1979) The pH tolerance of rabbit and human corneal endothelium. *Invest. Ophthalmol. Vis. Sci.,* **18**, 373–90.

Gordon, A. and Kracher, G.P. (1985) Corneal infiltrates and extended wear contact lenses. *J. Am. Optom. Assoc.* **56**, 198–201.

Graham, C.M., Dart, J.K.G., Buckley, R.G., Franks, W., Adams, C.G.W., Wilsonholt, N. and Minassian, D. (1988) Estimating the risks of contact lens wear. *J. Br. Contact Lens Assoc. Trans. Int. Contact Lens Conf.,* **11**, 102–5.

Grant, T., Kotow, M. and Holden, B.A. (1987) Hydrogel extended wear, current performance and future options. *Contax,* **May**, 5–8.

Greene, P.R. (1986) Gaussion and Poisson blink statistics; a preliminary study. *IEEE Trans. Biomed. Eng. BME.,* **33**, 359–66.

Guillon, M. (1991) Acuvue clinical research update. *Optician,* **202** (5317), 13–15.

Guillon, M. and Allary, J.C. (1991) Refitting daily (RGP and PMMA) wearers with high Dk RGP extended wear lenses. *J. Br. Contact Lens Assoc.*, in press.

Guillon, M. and Benjamin, W.J. (1991) Contact lenses and keratitis. Letter to the editor. *Lancet*, **338**, 1146.

Guillon, M. and Guillon, J.P. (1988) Pre-lens tear film characteristics of high Dk rigid gas permeable lens. *Am. J. Optom. Physiol. Opt.*, **65**, 73.

Guillon, M. and Guillon, J.P. (1989) Hydrogel lens wettability during overnight wear. *Ophth. Physiol. Opt.*, **9**, 355–9.

Guillin, J.P. and Guillon, M. (1990) Corneal desiecation staining with hydrogel lenses. Tear film and contact lens factors. *Ophthal. Physiol. Opt.*, **10**, 343–50.

Guillon, M. and Guillon, J.P. (1991) Disposable contact lenses. Contact lenses and tear film interactions. *Invest. Ophthalmol. Vis. Sci.*, **32** Suppl., 1114.

Guillon, M. and Holden, B.A. (1985) The HGP Dk Controversy. *Int. Eye Care*, **1**, 505.

Guillon, M. and Lydon, D.P.M. (1986) Tear layer characteristics of rigid gas permeable lenses. *Am. J. Optom. Physiol. Opt.*, **63**, 527–35.

Guillon, J.P., Guillon, M. and Malgouyres, S. (1990) Corneal desiccation staining with hydrogel lenses, tear film and contact lens factors. *Ophthal. Physiol. Opt.*, **10**, 343–50.

Guillon, M., Allary, J.C., Guillon, J.P. and Orsborn, G. (1992) Clinical management of regular replacement, Part I, Selection of replacement frequency. *Int. Contact Lens Clin.*, **19**(5/6), 104–20.

Hamano, T. (1984) Effects of contact lens wear on the corneal nerves. *Folia Ophthalmol. Jap.*, **35**, 1951–5.

Hamano, H., Heri, M., Hirayama, K. and Itsumaga, S. (1979) Scanning electron microscope observation of corneal surface after wearing hard, soft and silicone rubber lenses. *Contacto*, **21**, 16–21.

Hartmann, E. (1965) The D state; a review and discussion of studies on the physiologic state consistent with dreaming. *New Engl. J. Med.*, **273**, 30–5; 87–92.

Hartman, E.H., Baekeland, F., Zwilling, G. and Hoy, P. (1971) Sleep need: how much and what kind? *Am. J. Psychiatr.*, **127**, 1001–8.

Henry, V.A., Bennett, E.S. and Forrest, J.F. (1987) Clinical investigation of the Paraperm extended wear rigid gas permeable contact lens. *Am. J. Optom. Physiol. Opt.*, **64**, 313–20.

Henry, V.A., Bennett, E.S. and Sevigny, J. (1989) Rigid extended wear problem solving. *Int. Contact Lens Clin.*, **17**, 121–33.

Henry, V.A., Bennett, E.S. and Sevigny, J. (1990) Rigid extended wear problem solving. *Int. Contact Lens Clin.*, **17**(3), 121–33.

Highgate, D.J. (1978) Contact lens materials. Potential for future developments. *J. Br. Contact Lens Assoc.*, **1**(3), 27–32.

Hill, R.M. (1966) Respiratory profiles of the corneal epithelium. *Am. J. Optom. Arch. Acad. Optom.*, **43**, 233–7.

Hill, R.M. (1978) 'Life style' as a contact lens fitting variable. *Aust. J. Optom.*, **61**, 242–3.

Hill, R.M. and Brezinski, S.D. (1986) The great water race. *Contact Lens Spectrum*, **1**(9), 21–2.

Hill, R.M. and Fatt, I. (1963a) Oxygen uptake from a reservoir of limited volume by the human cornea *in vivo*. *Science*, **142**, 1295–7.

Hill, R.M. and Fatt, I. (1963b) How dependent is the cornea on the atmosphere? *J. Am. Optom. Assoc.*, **34**, 873–5.

Hine, N., Back, A. and Holden, B. (1987) Aetiology of arcuate epithelial lesions induced by hydrogels. *J. Br. Contact Lens Assoc. Transac. Br. Contact Lens Assoc. Conf.*, **12**(4), 48–50.

Hirji, N.K. (1979) *Some aspects of the design and the ocular response to synthetic hydrogel contact lenses intended for continuous usage*. PhD Dissertation, University of Aston, Birmingham.

Hirji, N.K. and Larke, J.R. (1978) Thickness of human cornea measured by topographic pachometry. *Am. J. Optom. Physiol. Opt.*, **55**, 97–100.

Holden, B.A. (1983) Ocular changes associated with the extended wear of contact lenses. *Ophthalmic Optician*, **23**, 140–2.

Holden, B.A. (1989) The Glenn A Fry Award Lecture 1988: Ocular response to contact lens wear. *Optom. Vis. Sci.*, **66**, 717–23.

Holden, B.A. and Mertz, G.W. (1984) Critical oxygen levels to avoid corneal oedema for daily and extended wear contact lenses. *Invest Ophthalmol Vis. Sci.*, **25**, 1161–7.

Holden, B.A. and Swarbrick, H.A. (1987) 'Rigid gas permeable lens binding: significance and contributing factors. *Am. J. Optom. Physiol. Opt.*, **64**, 815–23.

Holden, B.A. and Swarbrick, H.A. (1989) Extended wear lenses. In *Contact Lenses. 'A textbook for practitioner and student* (3rd edn) (eds. A.J. Phillips and J. Stone), Butterworths, London, 555–94.

Holden, B.A. and Sweeney, D.F. (1985) The oxygen tension and temperature of the superior palpebral conjunctiva. *Acta Ophthalmologica*, **63**, 100–3.

Holden, B.A. and Zantos, S.G. (1979) The ocular response to continuous wear of contact lenses. *The Optician* **177** (4581), 50; 52–3; 56–7.

Holden, B.A., Mettz, G.W. and McNally, J.J. (1983) Corneal swelling response to contact lenses worn under extended wear conditions. *Invest. Opthalmol. Vis. Sci.*, **24**, 218–26.

Holden, B.A., Sweeney, D.F., Vannas, A., Nilsson, K.T. and Efron, N. (1985a) Effects of long term extended contact lens wear on the human cornea. *Invest. Opthalmol. Vis. Sci.*, **26**, 1489–501.

Holden, B.A., Vannas, A., Nilsson, K. Efron, N. Sweeney, D., Kotow, M., Lahood, D. and Guillon, M. (1985b) Epithelial and endothelial effects from extended wear of contact lenses. *Curr. Eye Res.*, **4**, 739–42.

Holden, B.A., Lahood, D. and Sweeney, D. (1985c) Does Dk/L measurement accurately predict overnight edema response? *Am. J. Optom.*, **62**, 95P.

Holden, B.A., Williams, L. and Zantos, S.G. (1985d). The etiology of transient endothelial changes in the human cornea. *Invest. Ophthalmol. Vis. Sci.*, **26** 1354–9.

Holden, B.A., Sweeney, D.F. and Seger, R.G. (1986) Epithelial erosions caused by thin high water contact lenses. *Clin. Exp. Optom.*, **69**, 103–7.

Holden, B.A., Sweeney, D.F., Lahood, D. and Kenyon, E. (1988) Corneal deswelling following overnight wear of rigid and hydrogel contact lenses. *Curr. Eye Res.*, **7**, 49–53.

Holden, B.A., Grant, T., Kotow, M., Schneider, C. and Sweeney, D. (1989) Epithelial microcysts with daily and extended wear of hydrogel and rigid gas permeable contact lenses. *Invest. Ophthalmol. Vis. Sci.*, **30**, 372.

Holden, B.A., Newton-Howes, J., Winterton, I., Fatt, I., Hamano, H., Lahood, D., Brennan, N.A. and Efron, N. (1990) The Dk project. An interlaboratory comparison of Dk/L measurements. *Optom. Vis. Sci.*, **67**, 476–81.

Humphreys, J.A., Larke, J.R. and Parrish, S.T. (1980) Microepithelial cysts observed with extended contact lens wearing subjects. *Br. J. Ophthalmol.*, **64**, 888–9.

International Standards Organization (1991) *Contact lens determination of oxygen permeability and transmissibility by coulometric method*. CEN TC 172/SC7 WG4 N57.

Isaacson, W.B. and Rodriquez, O. (1989) Flexible fluoropolymer. A new category of contact lens. *Contact Lens Spectrum*, **4**, 60–4.

Isenberg, S.J. and Green, B.F. (1985) Changes in conjunctival oxygen tension and temperature with advancing age. *Crit. Care Med.*, **13**, 383–5.

Jacobs, L., Feldmann, M. and Bender, M.B. (1971) Eye movements during sleep. The pattern in the normal human. *Arch. Neurol.*, **25**, 151–9.

Josephson, J.E. and Caffery, B.E. (1979) Infiltrative keratitis in hydrogel lens wearers. *Int. Contact Lens Clin.*, **6**, 223–42.

Josephson, J.E., Zantoss, S., Caffery, B. and Herman, J.P. (1988) Differentiation of corneal complications observed in contact lens wearers. *J. Am. Optom. Assoc.*, **59**, 679–85.

Kamiya, C. (1982) A study of corneal endothelial response to contact lenses. *Contact Lens J.*, **8**(2), 92–5.

Keates, R.H., Ihlenfeld, J.V. and Issacson, W.B. (1984) An introduction to fluoropolymer contact lenses; a new class of material. *Contact Lens Assoc. Ophthalmol. J.*, **10**, 332–4.

Kenyon E., Polse, K.A. and Seger, R.G. (1986) Influence of wearing schedule on extended wear complications. *Ophthalmology*, **93**, 231–6.

Kenyon, E., Polse, K.A. and Mandell, R.B. (1988) Rigid contact lens adherence: incidence, severity and recovery. *J. Am. Optom. Assoc.*, **59**, 163–74.

Kenyon, E., Mandell, R.B. and Polse, K.A. (1989) Lens design effects on rigid lens adherence. *J. Br. Contact Lens Assoc.*, **12**(2), 32–6.

Klyce, S. (1981) Stromal lactate accumulation can account for corneal oedema osmotically following epithelial hypoxia in the rabbit. *J. Physiol.*, **321**, 49–64.

Koetting, R.A., Metz, G. and Seibel, D.B. (1988) Clinical impressions of extended wear success relative to patient age. *J. Am. Optom. Assoc.*, **59**, 164–5.

Kotow, M., Holden, B.A. and Grant, T. (1987a). The value of regular replacement of low water content contact lenses for extended wear. *J. Am. Optom. Assoc.*, **58**, 461–4.

Kotow, M., Grant, T. and Holden, B.A. (1987b). Avoiding ocular complications during hydrogel extended wear. *Int. Contact Lens Clin.*, **14**, 95–9.

Laing, R.A., Sandstrom, M.M., Berrospi, A.R. and Leibowitz, J.M. (1976) Changes in the corneal endothelium as a function of age. *Exp. Eye Res.*, **22**, 587–94.

Langham, M.E. (1952) Utilization of oxygen by the

component layers of the living cornea. *J. Physiol.*, **117**, 461–70.

Larke, J.R. (1985a) Corneal swelling and its clinical sequence. In *The Eye in Contact Lens Wear*. Butterworths, London.

Larke, R.J. (1985b) Anterior limbus. In *The Eye in Contact Lens Wear*. Butterworths, London.

Larke, J.R. and Hirji, N.K. (1979) Some clinically observed phenomena in extended contact lens wear. *Br. J. Ophthalmol.*, **63**, 475–7.

Larke, J.R. Parrish, S.T. and Wigham, C.G. (1981) Apparent human corneal oxygen uptake rate. *Am. J. Optom. Physiol. Opt.*, **58**, 803–5.

Lass, J.H., Dutt, R.M., Spurney, R.V., Stocker, E.G. Wolfe, C.H. and Glavan, I. (1988) Morphologic and Fluorometric analysis of corneal endothelium in long term hard and soft contact lens wearers. *Contact Lens Assoc. Ophthalmol. J.*, **14**(2), 104–9.

Levy, B. (1983) The use of a gas permeable hard lens for extended wear. *Am. J. Optom. Physiol. Opt.*, **60**, 408–9.

Levy, B. (1985) Rigid gas permeable lenses for extended wear. A 1 year clinical evaluation. *Am. J. Optom. Physiol. Opt.*, **62**, 889–94.

Litvin, M. (1978) Subepithelial infiltrates and soft lenses. *J. Br. Contact Lens Assoc.*, **1**, 31–4.

Long, W.E. (1974) An update of the silicone lens status. *Contacto*, **18**(3), 35–7.

Mackie, I.A. and Wright, P. (1978) Giant papillary conjunctivitis (secondary vernal) in association with contact lens wear. *Trans. Ophthalmol. Soc. UK*, **98**, 3–9.

Marcrae, S.M. Matsuda, M. and Shellans, S. (1989) Corneal endothelial changes associated with contact lens wear. *Contact Lens Assoc. Ophthalmol. J.*, **15**, 82–7.

Macrae, S. Herman, C., Doyle, R. Lippman, R., Whipple, D., Cohen, E., Egan, D., Wilkinson, C.P., Scott, C., Smith, R. and Phillips, D. (1991) Corneal ulcer and adverse reaction rates in premarket contact lens studies. *Am. J. Ophthalmol.* **111**, 457–65.

Mader, T.H., Friedl, K.E., Mohr, L.C. and Bernard, W.M. (1987) Conjunctival oxygen tension at high altitude. *Aviation, Space and Environmental Med.*, **58**, 76–9.

Madigan, M. and Holden, B.A. (1988) Factors involved in loss of epithelial adhesion with long term continuous hydrogel lens wear. **29**, 253.

Madigan, M.C. Holden, B.A. and Kwok, L.S. (1987) Extended wear of contact lenses compro-

mises corneal epithelial adhesion. *Curr. Eye Res.*, **6**, 1257–60.

Magatani, H. (1960) Limitless wearing of contact lenses without interruption. *Contacto*, **4**(31), 81–7.

Mandell, R.B., Polse, K.A., Brand, R.J., Vastine, D., Demartini, D. and Flom., R. (1989) Corneal hydration control in Fuch's dystrophy. *Invest. Ophthalmol. Vis. Sci.*, **30**, 845–2.

McMonnies, C.W. (1983) Contact lens induced corneal vascularisation. *Int. Contact Lens Clin.*, **10**, 12–21.

McMonnies, C.W., Chapman-Davies, A. and HOLDEN, B.A. (1982) The vascular response to contact lens wear. *Am. J. Optom. Physiol. Opt.*, **59**, 795–9.

McNally, J.J., Chalmers, R. and Payor, R. (1987) Corneal dessication staining with thin high water contact lenses. *Clin. Exp. Optom.*, **70**, 106–11.

Mendels, J. and Hawkins, D.R. (1967) Sleep laboratory adaption in normal subjects and depressed patients ('The first night effect'). *Electroenceph. Clin. Neurophysical.*, **22**, 556–8.

Mertz, G.W. and HOLDEN, B.A. (1981) Clinical implications of extended wear research. *Can. J. Optom.*, **43**, 203–5.

Miller, D. (1967) Pressure of the lid on the eye. *Arch. Ophthalmol.*, **78**, 328–32.

Miller, D. (1972) Problems with silicone lenses. *Contact Lens J.*, **3**, 38–42.

Millodot, M. (1974) Effect of soft contact lenses on corneal sensitivity. *Acta Ophthalmologia*, **52**, 603–8.

Millodot, M. (1984) Clinical evaluation of an extended wear lens. *Int. Contact Lens Clin.*, **11**,. 16–23.

Millodot, M., Henson, D. and O'Leary, D.J. (1979) Measurements of corneal sensitivity and thickness with PMMA and gas permeable contact lenses. *Am. J. Optom. Physiol. Opt.*, **56**, 628–32.

Moller, P.M. (1954) Tissue pressure in the orbit. *Acta Ophthalmologica*, **32**, 597–602.

Nilsson, S.E.G. and Persson, G. (1988) Low complication rate in extended wear of contact lenses. *Acta Ophthalmologica*, **64**, 88–92.

O'Neal, M.R. and Polse, K.A. (1985) In-vivo assessment of mechanisms controlling corneal hydration. *Invest. Ophthalmol. Vis. Sci.*, **26**, 849–56.

O'Neal, M.R., Polse, K.A. and Fatt, I. (1983) Oxygen permeability of selected GPH polymers and prediction of tear layers oxygen tension. *Int. Contact Lens Clin.*, **10**, 256–66.

O'Neal, M.R., Polse, K.A. and Sarver, M.D. (1984) Corneal response to rigid and hydrogel lenses during eye closure. *Invest. Ophthalmol. Vis. Sci.*, **25**, 837–42.

Orsborn, G.N. and Zantos, S.G. (1988). Corneal desiccation staining with thin high water content lenses. *Contact Lens Assoc. Ophthalmol. J.*, **14**, 81–4.

Perryman, F. (1988) The management of GPC with disposable lenses. *Optician*, **196** (5177), 21–2.

Poggio, E.C., Glynn, R.J., Schein, O.D., Seddon, J.M., Shannon, M.J., Scandinno, V.A., Kennyon, K.R. (1989) The incidence of ulcerative keratitis among users of daily wear and extended wear soft contact lenses. *New Engl. J. Med.*, **321**, 779–83.

Pole, J. and Lowther, G.E. (1989) One week vs two-week hydrogel extended wear schedules. *J. Am. Optom. Assoc.*, **89**, 515–19.

Polse, K.A. and Mandell, R.R. (1976) Etiology of corneal strain accompanying hydrogel lens wear. *Invest. Ophthalmol. Vis. Sci.*, **15**, 553–6.

Polse, K.A., Sarver, M.D., Kenyon, E. and Bonanno, J. (1987) Gas permeable hard contact lens extended wear: ocular and visual responses to a 6-month period of wear. *Contact Lens Assoc. Ophthalmol. J.*, **13**, 31–8.

Polse, K.A., Brand, R., Cohen, S. and Guillon, M. (1990). Hypoxic effects on corneal morphology and function. *Invest. Ophthalmol. Vis. Sci.*, **31**, 1544.

Pullum, K.W., Parker, J.H. and Hobley, A.J. (1989) Development of gas permeable impression scleral lenses. The Josef Dallas Award Lecture, Part One. *Trans. Br. Contact Lens Assoc. Ann. Clin. Conf.*, **12**, 77–81.

Pullum, K.W., Hobley, A.J. and Parker, J.H. (1990) Hypoxic corneal changes following sealed gas permeable impression scleral lens wear. *J. Br. Contact Lens Assoc.*, **13**, 83–7.

Pullum, K.W., Hobley, A.J. and Davison, C. (1991) 100 + Dk. Does thickness make much difference? *J. Br. Contact Lens Assoc.*, **14**, 17–19.

Quinn, T.G. and Schoessler, J.P. (1984) Human corneal epithelial oxygen demand population characteristics. *Am. J. Optom. Physiol. Opt.*, **61**, 386–8.

Rao, G., Shaw, E., Arthur, E. and Aquavella, J. (1979) Endothelial cell morphology and corneal deturgescence. *Am. J. Opthalmol.*, 885–99.

Rengstorff, R.M., Nilsson, K.T. and Sylvander, A.E. (1987) 2000 extended wear cases: A retrospective survey of contact lens complications. *J.

Br. Contact Lens Assoc.*, **10**(1), 13–15.

Ridley, F. (1963) Scleral contact lenses. *Arch. Ophthalmol.*, **70**, 740–5.

Riggs, L.A., Kelly, J.P., Manning, K.A. and Moore, R.K. (1987) Blink related eye movements. *Invest. Ophthalmol. Vis. Sci.*, **28**, 334–40.

Rivera, R.K. and Polse, K.A. (1989) Effects of hypoxic dose levels on corneal response in RGP extended wear. *Optom. Vis. Sci.*, **66**, 165.

Roth, H.W. (1990) The aetiology and pathogenesis of corneal ulcers in contact lens wearers. *Contactologia*, **12**, 110–14.

Ruben, M. (1975) The factors necessary for constant wearing contact lenses. *Aust. J. Optom.*, **58**, 436–42.

Ruben, M. (1978) Some criteria for continuous wear of contact lenses. *Aust. J. Optom.*, **61**, 308–12.

Ruben, M. (1989) Adverse reactions to contact lens wear. In *Colour Atlas of Contact Lenses and Prosthetics* (2nd edn), Wolfe Medical, London, 150–81.

Ruben, M. and Guillon, M. (1979a) 'Silicone rubber' lenses in aphakia. *Br. J. Ophthalmol.*, **63**, 471–4.

Ruben, M. and Guillon, M. (1979b) Silicone rubber lenses – a review. *Aust. J. Ophthalmol.*, **7**, 215–20.

Ruben, M., Brown, N., Lobascher, D., Chaston, J. and Morris, J. (1976) Clinical manifestations secondary to soft contact lens wear. *Br. J. Ophthalmol.*, **60**, 529–31.

Sakamoto, R., Miyanaga, Y. and Hamano, H. (1990) Corneal swelling and deswelling with overnight wear: a soft and rigid lens comparison. *Optom. Vis. Sci.* **67**, 99P.

Sarver, M.D. (1971) Striate corneal lines among patients wearing hydrophilic contact lenses. *Am. J. Optom and Physiol. Opt.*, **48**, 762–3.

Schein, O.D., Glynn, R.J., Poggio, E.C., Seddon, J.M. and Kenyon, K.R. (1989) The relative risk of ulcerative keratitis among users of daily wear and extended wear soft contact lenses. A case control study. *New Engl. J. Med.*, **321**, 773–8.

Schein, O.D., Rosenthal, P. and Ducharme, C. (1990) A gas permeable scleral contact lens for visual rehabilitation. *Am. J. Ophthalmol.*, **109**, 318–22.

Schmidt, H.S. and Kaelbling, R. (1971) The differential laboratory adaption of sleep parameters. *Biol. Psychiat.*, **3**, 33–5.

Schnider, C.M. (1987) An overview of RGP extended wear. *Contax*, **May**, 10–12.

Schoessler, J.P. (1983) Corneal endothelial polymegathism associated with extended wear. *Int

Contact Lens Clin., **10** (3), 7–15.

Schoessler, J.P. and Barr, J.T. (1980) Corneal thickness changes with extended contact lens wear. *Am. J. Optom. Physiol. Opt.,* **57**, 729–33.

Schoessler, J.P. and Woloschak, M.J. (1981) Corneal endothelium in veteran PMMA contact lens wearers. *Int. Contact Lens Clin.,* **8**(6), 19–25.

Schoessler, J.P. Woloschak, M.J. and Mauger, T.F. (1982) Transient endothelial changes produced by hydrophilic contact lenses. *Am. J. Optom. Physiol. Opt.,* **59**, 764–5.

Seger, R.G. and Mutti, D.O. (1986) Corneal swelling and epithelial compromise with hard gas permeable contact lenses. *J. Br. Contact Lens Assoc. Transac. Br. Contact Lens Assoc. Conf.,* **9**, 92–4.

Simons, R., Thomas, A.R.S. and Holden, B.A. (1977) A preliminary study of ion exchange capacities of some soft contact lens materials. *Am. J. Optom Vis. Sci.,* **60**, 263–6.

Smelser, G.R. (1952) Relation of factors involved in the maintenance of optical properties of cornea to contact lens wear. *Arch. Ophthalmol.,* **47**, 328–43.

Snyder, F., Hobson, J.A., Morrison, D.F. and Goldfrank, F. (1964) Changes in respiration, heart rate and systolic blood pressure in human sleep. *J. Appl. Physiol.,* **19**, 417–22.

Sorensen, T. and Corydon, L. (1979) Corneal changes in central thickness during permanent lens wear. *Contacto,* **23**(6), 28–30.

Spoor, T.C., Hartel, W.C., Wynn, D. and Spoor, D.K. (1984) Complications of continuous wear soft contact lenses in non-referral population. *Arch. Ophthalmol.,* **102**, 1312–13.

Staarman, M.T. and Schoessler, J.P. (1991) Contact lenses and eye closure: comparative analysis using three different methods to induce corneal swelling. *Optom. Vis. Sci.,* **68**, 374–9.

Stapleton, F., Dart, J. and Minassian, D. (1989) Contact lens related infiltrates. Risk figures for different lens types and association with lens hygiene and solution contamination. *J. Br. Contact Lens Assoc. Trans Br. Contact Lens Assoc. Trans Br. Contact Lens Conf.,* **12**, 52–5.

Stein, H.A. and Slatt, B.J. (1984) Soft lenses. In *Fitting Guide for Rigid and Soft Contact Lenses. A practical approach.* CV Mosby, London.

Swarbrick, H.A. (1988) A possible etiology for RGP lens binding (adherence). *Int. Contact Lens Clin.,* **15**(1), 13–19.

Swarbrick, H.A. and Holden, B.A. (1987) Rigid gas permeable lens binding significance and contributing factors. *Am. J. Optom. Physiol. Opt.,* **64**, 815–23.

Sweeney, D.F. and Holden, B.A. (1983) The closed-eye swelling response of the cornea to Polycon and Menicon O_2 gas permeable hard lenses. *Aust. J. Optom.,* **66**, 186–9.

Sweeney, D.F., Holden, B.A. Vannas, A., Efron, N., Swarbrick, H., Kotow, M. and Chan, T. (1985) The clinical significance of corneal endothelial polymegathism. *Invest. Ophthalmol. Vis. Sci.,* **26**, 53.

Sweeney, D.F., Holden, B.A. and Madigan, M. (1987) The effect of oxygen transmissibility on epithelial adhesion with continuous contact lens wear. *Invest. Ophthalmol. Vis. Sci.,* **28** Suppl., 258.

Tomlinson, A. and Armitage, B. (1985) Closed eye response to a tertiary butyl styrene gas permeable lens. *Int. Eye Care,* **1**(4), 320–3.

Vannas, A., Holden, B. and Makitie, J. (1984) The ultrastructure of contact lens induced changes. *Acta Ophthalmologica,* **62**, 320–33.

Veys, J. (1991) *Ocular response to defective disposable contact lenses.* Paper given at the European Symposium on contact lenses, Geneva, Switzerland, October, 1991.

Weismann, B.A., Mondino, B.J., Petit, T.H. and Hofbauer, J.D. (1984) Corneal ulcers associated with extended wear soft contact lenses. *Am. J. Ophthalmol.,* **97**, 476–81.

Wichterle, O. and Lim, D. (1960) Hydrophilic gels for biological use. *Nature,* **185**, 117–18.

Williams, D.H. and Cartwright, R.D. (1969) Blood pressure changes during EEG monitored sleep. *Arch. Gen. Physiol.,* **20**, 307–14.

Williams, L. and Holden, B.A. (1986) The bleb response of the endothelium decreases with extended wear of contact lenses. *Clin. Exp. Optom.,* **63** (3), 90–2.

Winterton, L.C., White, J.C. and Su, K.C. (1987) Coulometric method for measuring oxygen flux and Dk of contact lenses and lens materials. *Int. Contact Lens Clin.,* **14**, 441–52.

Winterton, L.C., White, J.C. and Su, K.C. (1988) Coulometrically determined oxygen flux and resultant Dk of commercially available contact lenses. *Int. Contact Lens Clin.,* **15**, 117–23.

Yee, R.W., Matsuda, M., Schultz, R.O. and Edelhauser, H.R. (1985) Changes in the normal corneal endothelial cellular pattern as a function of age. *Curr. Eye Res.,* **4**, 671–8.

Zabkiewicz, K., Swarbrick, H. and Holden, B.A. (1986) Clinical experience with low to moderate Dk hard gas permeable lenses for extended wear. *J. Br. Contact Lens Assoc. Transac Br.*

Contact Lens Assoc. Conf., **9**, 101–2.

Zantos, S. (1983) Cystic formations in the corneal epithelium during extended wear of contact lens. *Int. Contact Lens Clin.*, **10**, 128–46.

Zantos, S. (1984) Management of corneal infiltrates in extended wear contact lens patients. *Int. Contact Lens Clin.*, **11**, 604.

Zantos, S.G. and Holden, B.A. (1978) Ocular changes associated with continuous wear of contact lenses. *Aust. J. Optom.*, **61**, 418–26.

Zantos, S.G. and Zantos, P.O. (1985) Extended wear feasibility of gas permeable hard lenses for myopes. *Int. Eyecare*, **1**, 66–75.

Zantos, S., Orsborn, G., and Walter, M. (1986) Studies on corneal staining with thin hydrogel contact lenses. *J. Br. Contact Lens Assoc.*, **9**, 61–4.

in corneal shape beyond the limited central area measured by the keratometer. With orthokeratology the limit of induced refractive seems to be limited to that which occurs when changing the cornea from its normal aspheric shape to a spherical shape (Freeman, 1978). This is likely to be true with inadvertent changes with rigid lens wear.

44.2 REFRACTIVE AND CORNEAL CURVATURE CHANGES WITH PMMA LENS WEAR

Long-term wear of PMMA corneal contact lenses cause greater refractive changes than RGP or hydrogel lenses. Immediately on lens removal the change in refractive error from baseline varies with individuals. Some will show an increase in myopia and others a decrease. A number of studies have shown an average decrease (Amano *et al.*, 1968; Goldberg, 1968; Pennington, 1969) while others an average increase (Rengstorff, 1965a,b; Naito, 1970; Grant & May, 1972) in myopia. With most studies, the average change on immediate removal is less than 1.00 D. The average change can be misleading as when some patients have an increase in myopia and others a decrease, the average may indicate no change. It is not unusual to have individuals change by 2.00 to 3.00 diopters in spherical power as well as have significant cylindrical changes over time. The cylindrical changes are usually with-the-rule changes and can be several diopters (Pratt-Johnson & Warner, 1965; Rengstorff, 1965b; Hartstein, 1965, 1967). The magnitude of the increase in cylinder appears to be related to number of years of lens wear (Rengstorff, 1965b, Ing, 1976). These with-the-rule astigmatic changes are often associated with high riding, flat fitted lenses and are usually more permanent changes than the spherical changes.

The corneal asphericity, the rate of change of the corneal radius from the center towards the periphery, can be altered by contact lens

wear. Carney (1975a) found an average decrease in corneal asphericity (a steepening of the peripheral cornea). In comparing the asphericity change for lenses fitted steeper, with alignment or flatter than the cornea, he found the least change in asphericity for the flatly fitted lens with both the alignment and steep lenses showing greater changes. Hovding (1983) found a significant decrease in the corneal asphericity with PMMA lens wear. In studying corneal changes during orthokeratology, a reduction in the asphericity is also found (Freeman, 1978; Kerns, 1977; Binder *et al.*, 1980; Grant, 1980).

There have not been many studies looking at the time course for the development of refractive change with lens wear. Carney (1975b) found an average increase in myopia of 0.50 D within a few days of wear in a group of newly fitted patients. He did not find any significant additional change over the three months of the study. With respect to cylindrical change, there was an increase in cylinder for the first 4–5 weeks of lens wear. Rengstorff (1967) in studying the recovery of refractive changes found a difference between the group that had worn lenses a year or less and those wearing lenses for longer periods. However, he did not find differences between those wearing lenses from a year to 2.5 years and those wearing lenses from 3 to 6 years. The orthokeratology studies (Kerns, 1978; Polse *et al.*, 1983) show that with efforts to change corneal curvature with progressive lens changes, there is little change after the first several months of wear. Polse *et al.* (1983) found that the changes in refractive error occurred during the first 132 days of therapy with little or none during the next 241 days of therapy. Therefore, it appears that the majority of changes occur quickly, less than a year, after initiating lens wear. Obviously there are large individual differences in the time course.

The way in which the lens is fitted can have an effect on the refractive error change induced. Carney (1975a) found that lenses fitted flatter than the cornea caused a decrease in myopia while those fitted to match the corneal curvature (on K) or steeper caused an increase in myopia. For the patients on which the lenses were fitted steeper than K, there was a slight decrease in cylindrical correction while the alignment and flat fitting lenses caused an increase in cylindrical correction.

The centration of rigid lenses appears to have an effect on the type and amount of corneal and refractive change. It is often seen where flat, high riding PMMA lenses cause large amounts of with-the-rule corneal toricity. This was indicated by Kerns (1978) in his study of orthokeratology. Wilson *et al.* (1990a, b) using the sophisticated Corneal Modeling System to analyze the corneal topography, found that with distorted corneas due to lens wear there was a correlation between the corneal shape and the resting position of the rigid lens. They also suggest that lens decentration is a risk factor for development of cornea distortion.

The corneas of patients wearing PMMA contact lenses appear to be in a state of flux. There is a diurnal variation in the refractive state (Rengstorff, 1970, 1978; McLean & Rengstorff, 1978). On average there is less myopia on awakening in the morning, prior to lens placement. The amount of myopia increases during the day with lens wear reaching maximum, on average 1.00 D increase, in the mid afternoon and then decreasing slightly until lens removal prior to retiring. During sleep the amount of myopia further reduces to the morning level (Fig. 44.1). Such diurnal changes do not occur with patients not wearing contact lenses.

An important clinical concern is the rate of recovery of the refractive error after discontinuing lens wear. Rengstorff studied this

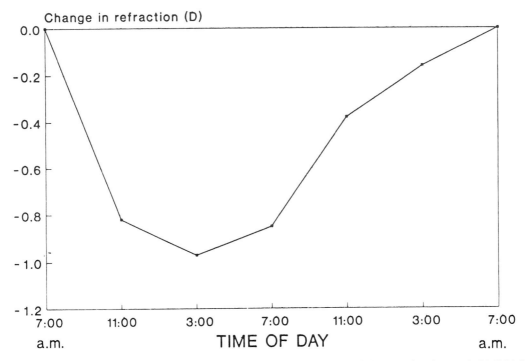

Figure 44.1 Average change in refractive finding (increase in myopia) during the day with PMMA lens wear (after Rengstorff, 1970).

extensively. He found in a study of 100 subjects that following discontinuance of lens wear there was a decrease in the myopia over a three-day period with an average decrease of 0.62 D with some patients changing four diopters or more (Rengstorff, 1965a, 1967, 1969). The amount of myopia then increased over the next 3 weeks reaching an equilibrium at a level relatively close to that found on immediate lens removal (Fig. 44.2). Polse *et al.* (1983) found that the majority of the induced refractive change regressed following 90 days of no contact lens wear. These changes indicate the importance of not prescribing spectacle corrections after 2 or 3 days of no lens wear and that the changes may take weeks to months to stabilize.

It is suggested that cylindrical changes increase and are more permanent when contact lens wear is abruptly discontinued than if lens wear is gradually discontinued (Rengstorff, 1975, 1977; Arner, 1977).

For long term PMMA wearers the best correctable spectacle visual acuity will often be reduced due to distortion of the cornea. Rengstorff (1965a) found that on immediate lens removal a significant number of patients had distorted corneas (Fig. 44.3). He also found 39% of the eyes had only 20/25 or worse acuity with the number decreasing to only 4% after 14 days of no lens wear (Fig. 44.4) (Rengstorff, 1965a, 1966). Therefore, in addition to the refractive fluctuations there may be reduced acuity with the best correction.

44.3 REFRACTIVE CHANGES WITH RIGID GAS PERMEABLE LENSES

Rigid gas permeable (RGP) lenses have greatly reduced the clinical problems of refractive changes and spectacle blur with contact lens wear. Sevigny (1983) found an increase in minus correction over a three-

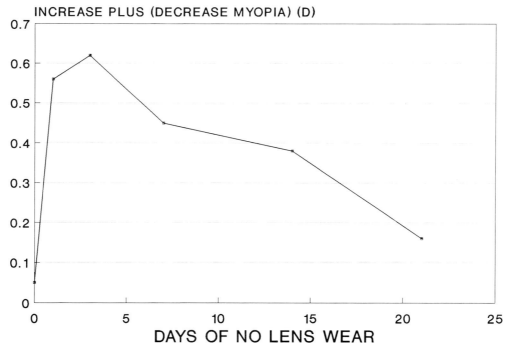

Figure 44.2 Decrease in myopia after the discontinuation of PMMA lens wear (after Rengstorff, 1965a).

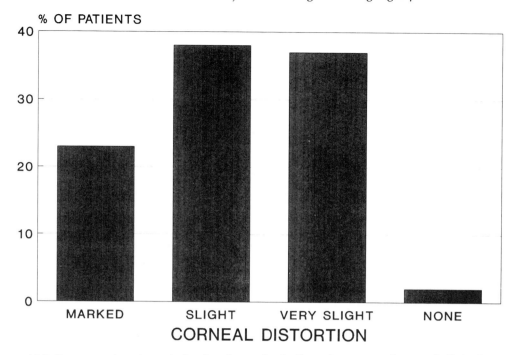

Figure 44.3 Per cent of patients judged to have the indicated amount of corneal distortion on lens removal following long term PMMA lens wear (after Rengstorff, 1965a).

month period with 50 patients wearing daily wear Boston lenses (*Dk* 12) of 0.15 D. The lenses were fitted on K. In another study with Boston II lenses on daily wear on one eye and Boston IV lenses on extended wear on the opposite eye, Sevigny found a decrease in myopia of 0.22 D with the Boston II lenses and only slightly more, 0.30 D, with the Boston IV lenses (Sevigny, 1986). In the same study he found a slight increase in with-the-rule refractive cylinder, 0.18 D, with both lens types and wearing schedules. The corneal curvature showed only a 0.07 D average flattening with daily wear. This shows, as with PMMA lenses, that the corneal curvature change is only about one-half of the refractive change (Williams, 1976; Kroll, 1978; DeRubeis & Shily, 1985). A 0.13 D increase in corneal toricity was found with the Boston II lenses.

DeRubeis and Shily (1985) found that patients fitted with Boston II lenses did not show any change in the radius of curvature of the horizontal meridian and the vertical meridian flattened by 0.31 D.

In a study comparing silcon resin rigid lenses with PMMA, CAB and Polycon I lenses, there was generally less than 0.25 D increase in minus with all the gas permeable lenses over the six months of the study (Lowther & Paramore, 1982). The change in cylindrical refraction was less than 0.30 D with all the gas permeable lenses. Obviously these lenses are low *Dk* materials compared to many being used today and they still caused little refractive change. The clinical impression is that the higher *Dk* materials cause even less refractive change.

Comparison of Polycon II lenses with Boston IV, Paraperm EW and Equalens over a three-month period indicated that there were no average sphere power changes at

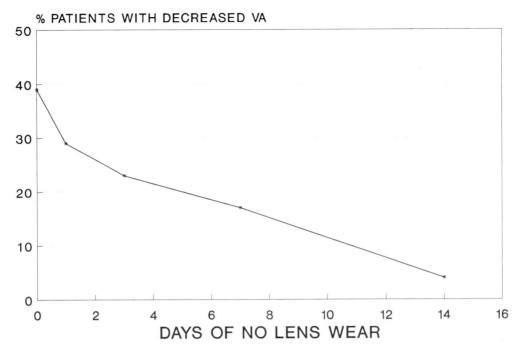

Figure 44.4 Per cent of long term PMMA wearing patients with visual acuity reduced to 20/25 or worse after the given days of no contact lens wear (after Rengstorff, 1965a).

any visit with any lens type over 0.25 D (Pole & Lowther, 1987). In addition, there was little change in the refractive cylindrical power, the greatest change being 0.344 D with most lens types and different wearing times showing less than 0.25 D increase in cylinder. There was little change in the central K readings with lens wear. Some corneas flattened slightly while others steepened slightly in the horizontal meridian, however, it was less than 0.25 D. The vertical meridians generally flatten, often up to about 0.30 D.

In a study of myopia control in children with Paraperm O$_2$+ RGP lenses, Perrigin *et al.* (1990) found an average corneal flattening of 0.37 D over a 3-year period. They also found that the contact lenses decreased the rate of myopia progression as compared to spectacle wearing children.

44.4   REFRACTIVE CHANGES WITH DAILY WEAR HYDROGEL CONTACT LENSES

Hydrogel contact lenses have little effect on corneal curvature and refractive findings as compared to PMMA lenses, however, they may cause small changes. Small decreases in myopia (on average up to 0.50 D) and flattening of the corneal curvature have been shown with standard thickness hydrogel lenses (0.10 mm or greater center thickness) during the initial wearing period, up to as long as 6 weeks wear (Grosvenor, 1975; Hill, 1975; Hovding, 1983). This initial decrease in myopia is attributed to the overall corneal swelling that develops with these lenses. Following this initial decrease in myopia a long term increase in myopia with corneal steepening occurred (Grosvenor, 1975; Harris *et al.*, 1975; Hill, 1975; Miller *et al.*, 1980).

This increase in myopia averages about 0.50 D. A study by Barnett and Rengstorff (1977) discovered the initial flattening of the corneal curvature but found a gradual increase in myopia over three months without the initial decrease. They did not find a good correlation between corneal curvature changes and refractive changes. Hovding (1983) did not find any change in corneal asphericity with hydrogel lens wear, however, Miller *et al.* (1980) found an increase in asphericity after 7 months of extended wear.

In studying five hydrogel lens wearers who had developed corneal distortion, Wilson *et al.*, (1990a) using the Corneal Modeling System, found that the corneas of these patients took an average of 5.2 weeks to return to normal. In comparison, corneal distortion due to PMMA lens wear required an average of 14.7 weeks to return to normal while three corneas warped with CAB lens wear required an average of 10.1 weeks. This more sensitive method of measuring corneal shape showed that minor changes last longer than are detected by normal refraction or keratometer readings. These corneas were apparently fairly severely distorted, more than is normally found.

The above reported increases in myopia occurred with relatively thick hydrogel lenses. Hill (1976) found that patients fitted with ultrathin hydrogel lenses, center thickness 0.06 mm, did not demonstrate either corneal curvature or refractive changes. He also found that patients previously fitted with thicker hydrogel lenses with the resultant increase in myopia would show a resolution of the change when refitted with thin lenses. These results point to the requirement of corneal edema which occurs with the thicker lenses, as well as with PMMA lenses, in the initiation of refractive changes. Since a majority of hydrogel lenses fitted today are thin, and/or high water content, we seldom see significant refractive changes with daily wear hydrogel lenses.

Hydrogel lenses can cause corneal distortion as well as regular changes. Tinted lenses with clear pupils have caused an imprinting of the cornea with resultant distortion and often mild visual acuity loss of about one line (Lowther, 1987; Clements *et al.*, 1988). These changes were due to the stiffer tinted portion indenting the cornea via the lid pressure. Significant corneal wrinkling has also been reported with thin, clear lenses (Lowe & Brennan, 1987) that reduced the acuity to 6/120 (20/400). This indicates that in susceptible subjects corneal distortion can occur with hydrogel lenses.

44.5 REFRACTIVE CHANGES WITH EXTENDED WEAR RIGID LENSES

Extended wear appears to cause somewhat greater changes in corneal curvature and refractive error than daily wear. Zantos and Zantos (1985) found that the central corneal curvature flattened by an average of 0.28 D over a 5-week period for patients on extended wear but only 0.03 D for daily wear. In the same patients the refractive error showed an average decrease of 0.54 D with extended wear but only 0.25 D with the daily wear patients. In a similar study by Orsborn *et al.* (1986) using several different materials, it was found that there was slightly greater corneal flattening with extended wear than daily wear. They did not find a significant difference in the refractive finding, however, there was a trend towards more myopia. Henry *et al.* (1987) using Paraperm EW lenses found an average flattening of the horizontal meridian of 0.33 D and 0.43 D in the vertical meridian after 12 months' wear with a resultant decrease in corneal toricity of 0.19 D. The equivalent sphere refraction decreased by 0.30 D (less myopia) and the refractive astigmatism decreased by 0.37 D. Polse *et al.* (1988) found a slight flattening in the flat meridian of the cornea (0.24 D) and slight steepening in the vertical meridian (0.13 D) over a 5-month period. They found slightly less change in refractive error than corneal curvature change. In another study (Levy, 1985) no significant change in corneal curvature or refractive change occurred over a 1-year period.

44.6 REFRACTIVE CHANGES WITH EXTENDED WEAR HYDROGEL LENSES

Miller *et al.* (1980) found an average increase in myopia of 0.26 D in a group of patients wearing hydrogel lenses on an extended wear schedule for 7 months. A similar steepening of the corneal curvature was also found. It is often found that extended wear patients will need more minus power over months or years of wear. Often clinicians will change lens power when lenses need replacement and over time not realize the full extent of change. This gradual increase in myopia has been termed 'myopic creep'.

Rengstorff and Nilsson (1985) found little change in refraction and corneal curvature following discontinuance of hydrogel extended wear over a 7-day period. The trend was towards decreasing myopia and increasing with-the-rule astigmatism.

REFERENCES

Amano, J. and Tankaka, K. (1968) Examination of patient after long wear of contact lenses. *Contacto*, **12**(3), 3–8.

Arner, R.S. (1977) Corneal deadaptation – the case against abrupt cessation of contact lens wear. *J. Am. Optom. Assoc.*, **48**(3), 339–41.

Barnett, W.A. and Rengstorff, R.H. (1977) Adaptation to hydrogel contact lenses: Variation in myopia and corneal curvature measurements. *J. Am. Optom. Assoc.*, **48**(3), 363–6.

Binder, P.S., May, C.H. and Grant S.C. (1980) An evaluation of orthokeratology. *Am. Acad. Ophth.*, **87**, 729–44.

Carney, L.G. (1975a) Corneal topography changes during contact lens wear. *The CL J.*, **5**, 5–16.

Carney, L.G. (1975b) Refractive error and visual acuity changes during contact lens wear. *The CL J.*, **5**, 28–34.

Clements, D., Augsburger, A., Barr, J.T. and Marshall, D. (1988) Corneal imprinting associated with wearing a tinted hydrogel lens. *CL Spectrum*, **3**(6), 65–7.

DeRubeis, M.J. and Shily, B.G. (1985) The effects of wearing the Boston II gas permeable contact lens on central corneal curvature. *Am. J. Optom. Physiol. Optics*, **62**(8), 497–500.

Freeman, R. (1978) Predicting stable changes in orthokeratology. *Contact Lens Forum*, 321–31.

Goldberg, J.B. (1968) Corneal curvature and refractive state changes induced by contact lenses observed immediately after removal and related to time. *Optom. Weekly*, **59**(15), 31–5.

Grant, S.C. (1980) A safe and effective treatment for a disabling problem. *Survey Ophth.*, **24**, 291–7.

Grant, S.C. and May, C.H. (1972) Orthokeratology – control of refractive errors through contact lenses. *Optician*, **163**(4214), 8–11.

Grosvenor, T. (1975) Changes in corneal curvature and subjective refraction of soft contact lens wearers. *Am. J. Optom. Physiol. Optics*, **52**(6), 405–13.

Harris, M.G., Sarver, M.D. and Polse, K.A. (1975) Corneal curvature and refractive error changes associated with wearing hydrogel contact lenses. *Am. J. Optom. Physiol. Optics*, **52**(5), 313–19.

Hartstein, J. (1965) Corneal warping due to contact lenses. *Am. J. Ophth.*, **60**(6), 1103–4.

Hartstein, J. (1967) Astigmatism induced by corneal contact lenses. In *Current Concepts in Ophthalmology* (eds B. Becker and R.C. Drews), C.V. Mosby, St Louis, pp 207–9.

Henry, V.A., Bennett, E.S. and Forrest, J.F. (1987) Clinical investigation of the paraperm EW rigid gas permeable contact lens. *Am. J. Optom. Physiol. Optics*, **64**(5), 313–20.

Hill, J.F. (1975) A comparison of refractive and keratometric changes during adaptation to flexible and non-flexible contact lenses. *J. Am. Optom. Assoc.*, **46**(3), 290–4.

Hill, J.F. (1976) Variation in refractive error and corneal curvature after wearing ultra-thin hydrophilic contact lenses. *ICLC*, **3**(6), 23–9.

Hosaka, A. and Chuang, C. (1971) Changes of ocular refraction in long-term lens wearers. *J. Jap. Contact Lens Soc.*, **13**, 116.

Hovding, G. (1983) Variation of central corneal

curvature during the first year of contact lens wear. *Acta Ophth.*, **61**, 117–28.

Ing, M.R. (1976) The development of corneal astigmatism in contact lens wearers. *Ann. Ophth.* **8**(3), 309–14.

Kerns, R.L. (1976) Research in orthokeratology-Part III: Results and observations. *J. Am. Optom. Assoc.*, **47**(12), 1505–15.

Kerns, R.L. (1977) Research in orthokeratology, Part V: Results and observations – Recovery aspects. *J. Am. Optom. Assoc.*, **48**(3), 345–59.

Kerns, R.L. (1978) Research in orthokeratology – Part VIII: Results, conclusions and discussion of techniques. *J. Am. Optom. Assoc.*, **49**(3), 308–14.

Kroll, J.R. (1978) Preliminary report on refractive changes in orthokeratology patients using automated refractors. *Ophth. Optician*, **18**(1), 39.

Levy, B. (1985) Rigid gas-permeable lenses for extended wear – A 1-year clinical evaluation. *Am. J. Optom. Physiol. Optics*, **62**(12), 889–94.

Lowe, R. and Brennan, N.A. (1987) Corneal wrinkling caused by a thin medium water content lens. *ICLC*, **14**(10), 403–6.

Lowther, G.E. (1987) A review of transparent hydrogel tinted lenses. *Contax*, **March**, 6–9.

Lowther, G.E. and Paramore, J.E. (1982) Clinical comparison of silcon resin lenses to P.M.M.A., C.A.B. and Polycon lenses. *ICLC*, **9**(2), 106–20.

McLean, W.E. and Rengstorff, R.H. (1978) Evaluating the effects of wearing contact lenses: Morning and afternoon testing. *J. Am. Optom. Assoc.*, **49**(3), 305–6.

Miller, J.P., Coon, L.J. and Meier, R.F. (1980) Extended wear of hydrocurve II_{55} soft contact lenses. *J. Am. Optom. Assoc.*, **51**(3), 225–32.

Naito, Y. (1970) Cases changed from myopia to hyperopia or mixed astigmatism due to a long wearing of contact lenses. *J. Jap. Contact Lens Soc.*, **12**, 135.

Orsborn, G.N., Andrasko, G.J. and Barr, J.T. (1986) RGP lenses: Daily wear vs. extended wear. *CL Spectrum*, **1**(4), 32–49.

Pennington, N.R. (1969) A comparison of three corneal lens forms. *Aust. J. Optom.*, **52**(8), 229–37.

Perrigin, J., Perrigin, D., Quinter, S. and Grosvenor, T. (1990) Silicone-acrylate contact lenses for myopia control: 3 year results. *Optom. Vis. Sci.*, **67**(10), 764–9.

Pole, J.J. and Lowther, G.E. (1987) Clinical comparison of low, moderate and high rigid gas permeable lenses. *CL Forum.*, **12**(7), 47–51.

Polse, K.A., Brand, R.J. Schwalbe, J.S. *et al.* (1983)

The Berkeley orthokeratology study, Part II: Efficacy and duration. *Am. J. Optom. Physiol. Optics*, **60**(3), 187–98.

Polse, K.A., Rivera, R.K. and Bonanno, J. (1988) Ocular effects of hard gas-permeable-lens extended wear. *Am. J. Optom. Physiol. Optics*, **65**(5), 358–64.

Pratt-Johnson, J.A. and Warner, D.M. (1965) Contact lenses and corneal curvature changes. *Am. J. Ophth.*, **60**(5), 852–5.

Rengstorff, R.H. (1965a) The Fort Dix Report – a longitudinal study of the effects of contact lens wear. *Am. J. Optom.*, **42** 153–63.

Rengstorff, R.H. (1965b) Corneal curvature and astigmatic changes subsequent to contact lens wear. *J. Am. Optom. Assoc.*, **36**(11), 996–1000.

Rengstorff, R.H. (1966) A study of visual acuity loss after contact lens wear. *Am. J. Optom. Arch. Am. Acad. Optom.*, **43**(7), 431–40.

Rengstorff, R.H. (1967) Variation in myopia measurements: An after effect observed with habitual wearers of contact lenses. *Am. J. Optom.*, **44**(3), 149–61, 1967.

Rengstorff, R.H. (1969) Relationship between myopia and corneal curvature changes after wearing contact lenses. *Am. J. Optom. Arch. Am. Acad. Optom.*, **46**(5), 357–62.

Rengstorff, R.H. (1970) Diurnal variation in myopia after the wearing of contact lenses. *Am. J. Optom. Arch. Am. Acad. Optom.*, **47**, 812–15.

Rengstorff, R.H. (1975) Prevention and treatment of corneal damage after wearing contact lenses. *J. Am. Optom. Assoc.*, **46**(3), 277–8.

Rengstorff, R.H. (1977) Astigmatism after contact lens wear. *Am. J. Optom. Physiol. Optics*, **54**(11), 787–91.

Rengstorff, R.H. (1978) Circadian rhythm: Corneal curvature and refractive changes after wearing contact lenses. *J. Am. Optom. Assoc.*, **49**(4), 443–4.

Rengstorff, R.H. and Nilsson, K.T. (1985) Long-term effects of extended wear lenses: Changes in refraction, corneal curvature, and visual acuity. *Am. J. Optom. Physiol. Optics*, **62**(1), 66–8.

Sevigny, J. (1983) The Boston lens clinical performance. *ICLC*, **10**(2), 73–81.

Sevigny, J. (1986) Clinical comparison of the Boston IV contact lens under extended wear vs. the Boston II lens under daily wear. *Int. Eyecare*, **2**(5), 260–4.

Williams, B. (1976) Orthokeratology update. *Contacto*, **20** (11), 34–8.

Wilson, S.E., Lin, D.T.C. Klyce, S.D. *et al.* (1990a)

Topographic changes in contact lens induced corneal warpage. *Ophthlmology*, 97, 734–44.

Wilson, S.E., Lin, D.T.C. Klyce, S.D. *et al.* (1990b) Rigid contact lens decentration: A risk factor for corneal warpage. *The CLAO J.*, 16(3), 177–82.

Zantos, S.G. and Zantos, P.O. (1985) Extended wear feasibility of gas permeable hard lenses for myopes. *Int. Eyecare*, 1(1), 66–76.

R.C. Tripathi, Brenda J. Tripathi and Sharon Fekrat

In the past 20 years, great strides have been made in contact lens technology, but this progress has been overshadowed by a multitude of lens-related ocular sequelae. Contact lenses are foreign bodies on the eye, and the success of their wear depends on the ocular tolerance to a given contact lens. Contact lenses can induce significant changes in the eye, and in vision, that may range from reversible abnormalities to chronic and insidious pathologic tissue damage. However, the ocular pathology differs depending on the type of lens, the duration of wear, host defenses, and the lens-care regimen used.

The various contact lens induced ocular abnormalities may be broadly categorized according to the pathogenetic mechanisms that produce them, e.g. mechanical, inflammatory, infectious, and metabolic.

45.1 MECHANICAL DAMAGE

Mechanically induced consequences of contact lens wear may be patient-related or lens-related.

45.1.1 PATIENT-RELATED

Irrespective of the type of lens worn, the patient may damage the ocular tissues when the lenses are inserted or removed. Traumatic subconjunctival hemorrhages occur more often with scleral lenses than they do with corneal lenses, and especially if the lens is lodged in the conjunctival fornices (Ruben, 1975). Partial-thickness corneal abrasions involve the surface and polygonal layers of the corneal epithelium (Fig. 45.1). The loss of anterior corneal squamous epithelium is manifested as secondary corneal edema and may lead to infectious lesions. Full-thickness abrasions are manifested as loss of the entire corneal epithelium with or without involvement of the basal lamina and/or Bowman's zone of the stroma. Such lesions heal by migration of neighboring cells, and their bundles of cytoskeletal filaments extend along the base and out into the leading edges of the cells (Zimny & Salisbury, 1982). In all lens fittings and lens handling, the epithelial barrier must be respected (Tripathi, 1974). Long fingernails, cosmetic contaminants, impatience, poor lighting and vision, as well as an individual's intolerance or abusive wear may all contribute to patient-related ocular damage.

45.1.2 LENS-RELATED DAMAGE

Mechanical pressure of the lens on the cornea reduces the sensitivity of the cornea and its tolerance of contact lens wear. The danger of this corneal adaptation is that surface lesions may remain unrecognized by the patient

Contact Lens Practice. Edited by Montague Ruben and Michel Guillon.
Published in 1994 by Chapman & Hall, London. ISBN 0 412 35120 X

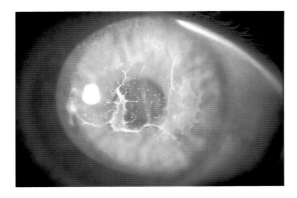

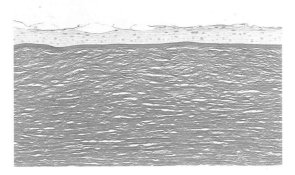

Figure 45.1 (a) Clinical appearance of epithelial lesion secondary to contact lens wear. Fluorescein staining shows a pseudodendritic pattern of epithelial loss and focal defects (courtesy Jeffrey Harris). (b) Superficial epithelial defect manifesting as loss of surface cells and cystic swelling of individual cells (original magnification × 50).

until the deeper ocular tissues become involved. However, a reduction in sensitivity may not be due solely to adaptation, but may occur because the nerve endings undergo trophic changes that are caused by repeated trauma, pressure, or chronic epithelial edema.

Dry eye

Tears act as a lubricant for contact lenses, and the mechanical tolerance of wear depends on the integrity of the tear film. The precorneal tear film also protects the epithelium from

osmotic damage that may occur because of evaporation.

The disruption of the normal contour of the tear film is the earliest complication of contact lens wear. Recent studies of tear composition in contact lens wearers indicate that the precorneal film is altered, and that this may be a significant cause of dry eye (Farris, 1986). Patients who use daily-wear hard or extended-wear soft contact lenses develop elevated mean tear osmolalities that disrupt the tear film. The resulting dry eye and the movement of the lens over the dry cornea can result in suppression of surface cell desquamation and can reduce the number of microvilli; this causes the cell surface to become smooth (Francois *et al.*, 1974). Ocular surface-drying effects combined with inadequate flushing result in trapping of debris beneath the lens and lead to additional corneal trauma. Moreover, an inadequate tear film can lead to keratinization and ulceration.

In the presence, or even in the absence, of dry eye, small lenses and thick edges of the lenses contribute to localized tear film dysfunction and surface desiccation. Local areas of the epithelium adjacent to corneal lenses and areas under fenestrations in haptic lenses may become desiccated. In these 'dry spots' (Ruben, 1989), abnormal surface cells with substantially reduced numbers of microvilli are observed (Bergmanson *et al.*, 1984), (Fig. 45.2). The loss of lipid film in such areas further prevents the serous and mucoid tear layers from adhering to the epithelium and contributes to the development of punctate epithelial necrosis and erosions (Ruben, 1975). Histologically, basal cell edema of the epithelium is present, and the cells have a tendency to become separated from the basement membrane, with loosening of their hemidesmosomes (Fig. 45.3).

With prolonged wear of hard contact lenses, pterygium may form as a result of a chronic conjunctival inflammatory reaction and growth of vessels into an adjacent desic-

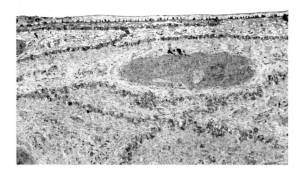

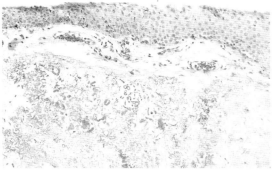

Figure 45.2 Corneal epithelium showing loss of microvilli from its most anterior layer of cells. Transmission electron micrograph (original magnification × 4000).

Figure 45.4 Section of a pterygium-like growth on the cornea. The epithelium is irregularly hyperplastic and Bowman's zone below is destroyed. Blood vessels are present in the subepithelial fibrous tissue beneath which extensive elastotic degeneration is evident as abundant curvilinear structures (original magnification × 50).

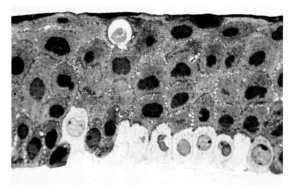

Figure 45.3 Light micrograph of corneal epithelium showing an intraepithelial microcyst (top). Extracellular edema is represented by dilated intercellular spaces, and intracellular edema (hydropic degeneration) is manifest as swollen, pale basal cells. Note that the basement membrane of the basal cells is partly detached (below) in the region of the degenerating basal cells (original magnification × 1425).

Alterations in the blink reflex

The blink reflex, a major means of good tear distribution and flow, is as important as is good tear formation. An increase in the blink frequency may be due to the mere presence of a foreign-body feeling when a new contact lens is in the eye. In some patients, this can give rise to prolonged blepharospasm just before or after the initial insertion (Ruben, 1975; Tripathi, 1975). After the adaptation period, however, a persistent increase in blinking frequency may be due to a lens which is too mobile or too tightly fitting. Contact lens wear can alter the normal blink reflexes as a result of the associated decrease in sensitivity of the cornea, conjunctiva, and lid. Because the contact lens may replace the protective function of the blink reflex, the incidence of corneal injury may be increased.

With every blink, imperfections in the lens material (caused by defects or distortion in the plastic, or by lens deposits) can abrade the protective epithelium of the cornea. Moreover, foreign bodies trapped under the lens, such as dust particles, cosmetics, dried secretions, and dead cells from the kerato-

cated area at the limbus. Histologically, the subepithelial substantia propria shows elastotic changes (basophilic degeneration) and breakdown of collagen. The invasion of the superficial cornea is preceded by dissolution of Bowman's membrane, which leads to permanent scarring (Fig. 45.4).

conjunctiva, can contribute to similar lesions. The subsequent corneal cell damage is evident as a localized epithelial defect or as superficial punctate or linear keratitis. These lesions usually resolve after removal of the offending agent (Ruben, 1975).

Changes in the corneal stroma

The maintenance of the thickness of the cornea depends partly on blinking. In wearers of hard corneal contact lenses, and sometimes even in soft-lens wearers, if the blink rate is decreased, the 3 and 9 o'clock limbal zones are often not wetted by the quick, inadequate blinks. The epithelium in these areas exhibits punctate irregularities that overlie a thinned area of dehydrated stroma resulting in depression of the surface, termed 'dellen'. Histologically, the dellen consists of a partial or full-thickness epithelial defect with shrinkage of the underlying stromal tissues or even collapse of fibrils from dehydration with or without marginal ulceration (Ruben, 1975). Depending on the degree of inadequacy of corneal wetting, similar stromal thinning and degeneration may also occur more centrally.

Deep corneal stromal opacities in long term contact lens wearers have been documented. The whitish opacities are located in the central cornea, directly adjacent to Descemet's membrane. On replacement of HEMA and PMMA lenses with gas-permeable rigid lenses, the lesion gradually diminishes or resolves. The possible etiologic factors include thimerosal toxicity and endothelial hypoxia (Remeijer *et al.*, 1990).

Superficial corneal mosaic

In normal eyes, the superficial corneal mosaic results from massaging of the cornea with the lid closed and disappears soon after discontinuation of the external pressure. In the presence of keratoconus this is observed without massaging or external pressure. In contact lens wear, however, the superficial corneal mosaic manifests itself because of the mechanical pressure exerted by the lens on the underlying corneal surface (Tripathi, 1975). The structural basis for this mosaic pattern lies in the particular arrangement of collagen lamellae that continue obliquely from the anterior stroma into Bowman's zone (Bron & Tripathi, 1969) (see also Chapter 12).

Spectacle blur

The mechanical pressure of the contact lens on the corneal epithelium is responsible for spectacle blur. Immediately after removal of the lenses, the patient may experience transient blurred vision with spectacles that may persist for several minutes or a few hours. Spectacle blur over this time span is considered normal in clinical practice and must not be confused with the more permanent epithelial edema of contact lens wear, known as Sattler's veil (see page 1057).

Changes in corneal curvature

There has been increased awareness of the potential for significant distortion of the cornea with the use of contact lenses. The corneal changes involved should be differentiated from the edema and molding that are responsible for the rapidly reversible spectacle blur (Tripathi, 1975; Levenson, 1983).

Significant irregular astigmatism may develop with long-term wear of PMMA contact lenses because of alterations in the corneal contour that may reduce the best-corrected vision with spectacles and prompts permanent dependence on contact lenses. The mechanism is based on the interplay of individual corneal characteristics with the contact lens-induced disruption of corneal metabolism and the mechanical pressure of the lens on the cornea. The contact lens decreases the corneal oxygen supply and thus causes depletion of glycogen stores, which leads to secondary disruption of the corneal water regulation (Levenson, 1983; Ruben, 1989) and thus to epithelial and stromal edema. The swollen stromal tissue is distorted as a result of the mechanical forces exerted by the contact lens. In a susceptible cornea, this interaction may initiate a decompensation of certain contour maintaining factors and may even culminate in keratoconus (Hartstein, 1968; Macsai *et al.*, 1990).

Reversible changes in the corneal curvature, however, have been observed in patients who wear soft, hydrophilic contact lenses (Levenson, 1983). Also, gas-permeable hard lenses produce less corneal edema than do PMMA lenses (Mandell, 1979; Ruben, 1989); therefore, with gas-permeable lenses, the cornea becomes less malleable and more capable of resisting structural alterations induced by the contact lens. The material of gas-permeable hard lenses is treated chemically to give them a hydrophilic surface which conforms to the contour of the cornea better than does a standard hard lens (Refojo, 1972).

Wrinkling

'Wrinkles' are seen on the corneas of most contact lens wearers because the edge of the lens disrupts loose epithelium. These wrinkles disappear upon removal of the lens (Ruben, 1975).

Lens deposits, mechanical erosion, and corneal scarring

Deposition of protein, mucin, calcium, lipid, or other constituents of the tear film on contact lenses is a common complication of soft contact lens wear (Tripathi *et al.*, 1980, 1988, 1991; Tripathi & Tripathi, 1984). These superficial deposits can cause mechanical erosion and inflammation, resulting in a corneal scar that may interfere with vision.

'Mulberry' deposits are commonly found on soft contact lenses, especially when the lenses are worn over an extended period (see Chapter 47 Part 2). These deposits are composed primarily of lipids and mucoproteins which originate from the tear film, possibly combined with some calcium (Tripathi *et al.*, 1980, 1988; Tripathi & Tripathi, 1984; Weissman *et al.*, 1986). They may induce corneal erosion with consequent scar formation.

Ptosis

Ptosis in association with contact lens wear (Fonn & Holden, 1986) has been observed secondary to entrapment of the contact lens under the upper lid (Sebag & Albert, 1982) and to the disinsertion of the aponeurosis of the levator palpebrae superioris muscle as a result of excessive eyelid manipulation during lens insertion (Epstein & Putterman, 1981). The extended wear of a rigid gas-permeable (RGP) contact lens can also induce ptosis in a patient who has lid edema that may be associated with chronic eyelid irritation by the lens edge.

Overwear

Patients who overwear PMMA hard contact lenses are more likely to sustain mechanical injury to the cornea than are those who overwear hydrogel soft lenses (Hamano *et al.*, 1985). The resulting corneal epithelial trauma may be caused by overnight wear of a lens, by any sudden increase in wearing time, or by mechanical rubbing of a poorly fitted contact lens.

Histologic examination of the corneal epithelium in rabbits subjected to contact lens wear shows hyperkeratinization of the corneal epithelium, disappearance of the intercellular glycoproteins, and rupture of desmosomes and alpha-keratin filaments after 8 hours of hard-lens wear or 10 hours of soft-lens wear; new silicone lenses produce the fewest alterations (Francois, 1983). Scanning electron microscopy documented increased numbers of intermediate (Type III) and dark (Type II) cells with increased wearing time and preceding desquamation (Francois, 1983).

Disturbances of the normal structure of the epithelium interfere with the capacity of the cells to withstand further trauma. Because the epithelium normally acts as a barrier to the entry of fluid, such denuded areas cause localized stromal edema and swelling. However, soon after the epithelium regenerates, the edema disappears.

In the early stages of regeneration, the epithelium may be dislodged easily by hasty insertion of the contact lens, which causes corneal erosions. The regenerated epithelium may not achieve normal adherence to Bowman's layer and may form subepithelial vesicles which coalesce. This phenomenon is probably related to a decrease in the blink reflex and a change in the dynamics of tear flow, both of which are seen with contact lens wear.

Tight lens syndrome and tight upper eyelids

The tight lens syndrome, which also can result in corneal abrasions, is found in association with both hard and soft hydrophilic contact lenses. The pressure of the lens over a zone of contact will, if the force is strong enough, eventually cause epithelial desquamation and necrosis, loss of water from the stroma, and sometimes even stromal scarring. This syndrome is seen most frequently in aphakic or bandage extended-wear patients (Lohman, 1986), and it usually occurs after the lens has been worn for one or two days. With removal of the lens, some additional epithelium may be torn away from Bowman's layer.

In soft-lens wearers, an abrasion resembling a discrete arc near the superior corneo-scleral limbus has been documented as the effect of a tight upper eyelid, which presses the contact lens mechanically against the cornea and produces an opacity in the 11 o'clock and 1 o'clock meridians (Horowitz *et al.*, 1985).

Perilimbal hyperemia

Trauma to the limbal zone from corneal or scleral contact lenses may result in hyperemia and discomfort. A rapidly moving edge of a large corneal lens, for example, may impinge upon the perilimbal blood vessels and cause pericorneal hyperemia with stromal ingrowth of limbal vessels. An intracorneal hemorrhage may be induced by superficial corneal vascularization in the superior limbic area from the prolonged use of extended wear soft contact lenses (Laroche & Campbell, 1987).

Corneal microcysts, vacuoles, and bullae

Formation of cysts in the corneal epithelium has been documented in long-term wearers of contact lenses (Zantos, 1983). On slit-lamp examination, intraepithelial microcysts appear as translucent dots dispersed across the central and mid-peripheral areas of the cornea. These microcysts differ from vacuoles and bullae in that they are of varying optical densities. Microcysts originate in the deep epithelial layers and migrate anteriorly with the evolution of the epithelial cells to the surface layer (see Fig. 45.3). It has not yet been clearly delineated whether the microcysts are the result of chronic epithelial trauma or whether they occur because of an abnormality in epithelial cell growth. However, the formation of microcysts is presumed to be a consequence of disruption and necrosis of the epithelium from physical trauma and prolonged hypoxia (Zantos, 1983; Tripathi, 1975). Pseudoepitheliomatous hyperplasia, metaplasia, and dysplasia can occur with prolonged wear of contact lenses (Tripathi *et al.*, 1988). No evidence exists presently to support the notion that chronic trauma to the epithelium by contact lenses can induce erratic cell growth characteristic of carcinoma.

Intraepithelial cysts, with or without cellular debris, have been documented in monkeys after 12 hours of wearing RGP contact lenses (Bergmanson *et al.*, 1984) Microscopic examination of these cysts demonstrated their formation within surface epithelial cells. The investigators postulated that, because RGP lenses allow for the corneal oxygen requirement, the cause of the cysts is the traumatic effect of the rigid lens itself (Bergmanson *et al.*, 1984).

Epithelial vacuoles have distinct edges and are demonstrable by unreversed illumination, which indicates that their refractive index is lower than that of the surrounding corneal tissue. The incidence in patients using extended wear contact lens has been reported as 32%. An association with concavities in the corneal surface due to air bubbles beneath the lens has been described (Zantos, 1983).

Epithelial bullae of unknown etiology are oval with indistinct edges, and they frequently coalesce into clusters. They have flattened profile and are located in the epithelial or subepithelial space. The incidence in contact lens wearers is very low unless they are associated with other causes, such as chronic hypoxia and bullous keratopathy.

Eyelid edema

Lid edema is commonly associated with wear of haptic hard lenses. The pathogenesis is due to mechanical irritation of the palpebral and fornix conjunctivae. The conjunctiva usually exhibits a follicular reaction with excess mucoid production.

45.2 INFLAMMATORY REACTIONS

Contact lens wear can induce inflammatory reactions of various types (e.g. allergic, mechanical) in the absence of microorganisms.

45.2.1 PYOGENIC GRANULOMA

A pyogenic granuloma may develop in association with extended wear of a soft contact lens (Hamburger, 1986). Because the granuloma is usually attached to the upper tarsus, the mechanical effect of this lesion produces further ocular irritation and corneal compression. The lesion may develop concurrently with giant papillary conjunctivitis (GPC); therefore, a causal relationship may exist. Often the granuloma is the consequence of an idiosyncratic, overwhelming inflammatory response (Hamburger, 1986). Pyogenic granuloma may also be associated with ruptured chalazions.

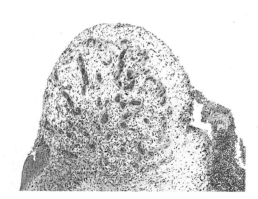

Figure 45.5 Histologic section of pyogenic granuloma protruding through a gap in the epithelial layer of the conjunctiva (present on either side of the lesion). The surface of the granuloma is devoid of the epithelial covering. In the stroma, numerous dilated capillaries are seen together with inflammatory cells and loose fibrous tissue (original magnification × 25).

Histologically, the granuloma consists of small caliber, dilated, endothelium-lined vascular channels that contain red blood cells (Fig. 45.5). The surrounding stroma of loose connective tissue shows an inflammatory infiltrate, consisting predominantly of polymorphonuclear leukocytes, lymphocytes, and plasma cells. The growing surface of the granuloma lacks an epithelial covering. The absence of contact inhibition by epithelial cells, along with chronic irritation, is probably responsible for the progression of pyogenic granuloma.

45.2.2 GIANT PAPILLARY CONJUNCTIVITIS

This disorder, which may eventually induce intolerance of the contact lens, is an external ocular inflammatory response probably due to increased amounts of coating on the surface of worn contact lenses. It is associated with the development of large papillary excrescences in the upper palpebral conjunctiva (Fig. 45.6). The giant papillae (more than 0.3 mm in diameter) are similar clinically and histologically to the cobblestone papillae observed in vernal conjunctivitis. GPC occurs in approximately 10% of persons who wear soft contact lenses and in 1% to 5% of those who wear hard lenses (Grutzmacher, 1989); it has also been reported recently in association with the wear of rigid gas-permeable contact lenses (Douglas *et al.*, 1988).

Histologically, the conjunctival epithelium overlying the giant papillae is thickened and irregular with an occasional tendency toward epidermalization and a decrease in the number of goblet cells (Fig. 45.7). Mast cells are regularly present in the epithelium, and the papillae harbor eosinophils, basophils, polymorphonuclear leukocytes, lymphocytes, and plasma cells both in the epithelium and stroma (Allansmith *et al.*, 1977). In the early stages of GPC, hyperemia of the upper tarsal conjunctiva appears, with small strands of mucus across the smooth conjunctiva. As the disorder progresses to the middle stage, opacification of conjunctival tissue occurs because of the infiltration of inflammatory cells. The collagen structures or papillae then emerge from the tarsal plate and push aside the normal micropapillae. In the advanced stage, proliferation of fibroblasts and increased mucus production are observed (Allansmith & Ross, 1988).

GPC is thought to be a delayed hypersensitivity reaction characterized by an abundance of basophils and a possible IgE humoral component (Allansmith & Ross, 1988), which are triggered in response to the methyl methacrylate-related antigens or to immunogenic accretions on the lens surface (Srinivasen *et al.*, 1979). The mechanical irritation of the lenses and the contact lens solutions used are probably also implicated in this process.

45.2.3 ALLERGIC CONTACT CONJUNCTIVITIS

The preservative chlorhexidine gluconate may be responsible for many cases of allergic contact conjunctivitis. This preservative

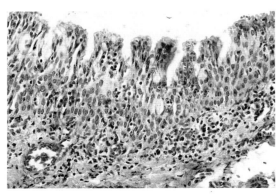

Figure 45.7 Conjunctival papillae seen in histologic section. The papillary projections are supplied by capillaries, the epithelium is hyperplastic, and the subepithelial stroma is infiltrated with inflammatory cells and also contains large caliber vessels (original magnification × 100).

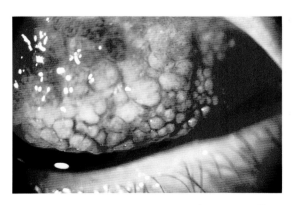

Figure 45.6 Clinical appearance of giant papillary conjunctivitis.

binds to soft contact lenses and is slowly released during lens wear. Small amounts of chlorhexidine then bind to the corneal epithelium. In some patients, this allergy is manifested as a follicular conjunctivitis with punctate keratitis and subepithelial infiltrates (Binder *et al.*, 1981).

45.2.4 UVEITIS

No proven cases of uveitis as a consequence of contact lens wear have been described (Ruben, 1975). However, it may occur secondary to contact lens-induced keratitis or corneal ulcer.

45.3 INFECTIONS

The contact lens wearer is prone to infection from pathogenic as well as opportunistic microbes (bacteria, viruses, fungi, or parasites) because the eye and lids are in a compromised state (Tripathi & Tripathi, 1984; Tripathi *et al.*, 1989). Infection of the eye may be the result of contact lens wear or may be due to the use of contaminated solutions.

45.3.1 CONTACT LENS WEAR

Irrespective of contact lens wear, conjunctivitis, keratitis, and blepharitis are common eye complaints which may lead to severe complications. The wearing of contact lenses, however, can only exacerbate these signs and symptoms, and it may lead to further complications with severe consequences.

In all contact lens wearers, the corneal epithelium has an increased susceptibility to infectious processes. When worn for several hours, the contact lens increases the temperature of the surface epithelium and decreases the oxygen tension, thus promoting the growth of various infectious agents. As discussed previously, the corneal microtrauma and resulting epithelial defects predispose the eye to microbial invasion. In eyes with lenses, tear lysozyme and immunoglobulins are prevented from covering the whole cornea; this is especially true for large soft lenses, under which little or no tear flow can be demonstrated. This situation fosters an ideal medium for corneal infection and delays the healing process even when the infection is controlled. The composition of tear immunoglobulins in contact lens wearers, however, is not significantly different from that in normal individuals (Mannucci *et al.*, 1984).

Bacterial blepharoconjunctivitis

Bacterial blepharoconjunctivitis may be caused, for example, by the introduction of virulent bacteria on a lens, which are capable of initiating the breakdown of the integrity of the conjunctival epithelium or attaching to focal epithelial defects caused by lens trauma. The dry eye and the decrease in blink frequency seen in lens wearers also predispose the conjunctiva to infection.

Most bacteria cause nonspecific histopathologic changes of varying severity, characterized by fibrinopurulent exudate, edema, epithelial and stromal necrosis, and reactive hyperemia.

Infectious corneal ulcers

Ulcerative keratitis is an ulceration of the corneal epithelium with concomitant involvement of the stroma, which, if not treated immediately, may progress to permanent loss of vision. The cause is thought to be microbial (Schein *et al.*, 1989). These infectious corneal ulcers are associated more frequently with the use of soft than with that of hard contact lenses. Because repeated overnight hypoxic stress leads to epithelial breakdown, extended wear patients are particularly at risk, with *Pseudomonas aeruginosa* being the pathogen most frequently isolated (76%) (Donnenfeld *et al.*, 1986). *Serratia marcescens* (Lass *et al.*, 1981), *Bacillus coli, Candida, Aspergillus, Streptococcus* and *Staphylococcus epidermidis* also have been documented frequently as etiologic agents (Tripathi *et al.*, 1990). The annual incidence of ulcerative keratitis is estimated at 20.9 per 10 000 persons using extended-wear soft contact lenses and 4.1 per 10 000 persons using daily-wear soft lenses (Poggio *et al.*, 1989).

Slit-lamp examination of the cornea reveals dense focal infiltrates with a loss of corneal luster. Depending on the stage of the process, hypopyon may be observed (Fig. 45.8). These lens-related ulcers will progress rapidly to panophthalmitis, culminating in corneal perforation and loss of the globe if they are not treated promptly (Ruben, 1975; Grutzmacher, 1989; Tripathi & Tripathi, 1984). Ulceration (Fig. 45.9) may leave a scar, which adversely affects vision.

The contact lens provides a site for adherence of bacteria. Contact lens coatings, especially mucin, facilitate the adherence of *Pseudomonas* to soft contact lenses (Ramphal *et al.*, 1981; Tripathi & Tripathi, 1984; Stern & Zam, 1986; Tripathi *et al.*, 1990). Experimental evidence suggests that corneal epithelial trauma is a necessary prerequisite for *Pseudomonas* corneal ulceration, because the infection begins with bacteria adhering to injured epithelial cells (Donnenfeld *et al.*,

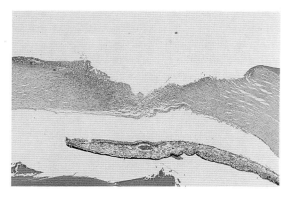

Figure 45.9 Histologic section of an eye passing through a central corneal ulcer. The crater-like lesion resulted from necrosis and destruction of the stroma, and provided a weak point for perforation of the globe (original magnification × 10).

1986). Scanning electron microscopy has demonstrated poor adherence of *Pseudomonas* to a stroma denuded of the corneal epithelium, but large numbers of organisms were seen adhering to the edge of the injured epithelium in the mouse cornea (Stern *et al.*, 1982).

A *Pseudomonas* corneal ulcer has also been reported after the use of an extended-wear RGP contact lens (Ehrlich *et al.*, 1989). Insertion and removal of a contaminated lens may cause epithelial injury and set the stage for development of the infected corneal ulcer. It has been recommended that, for a decrease in the incidence of these bacterial ulcers, pressure patching be avoided in contact lens patients who have corneal abrasions (Clemons *et al.*, 1987).

45.3.2 CONTACT LENS AND ITS SOLUTIONS

The contact lens itself or the storage case and solutions can become contaminated with microorganisms and instigate an infectious process.

Hydrophilic soft contact lenses facilitate the growth of bacteria, fungi, and spores on their surfaces. Those hydrophilic materials that contain water-soluble additives produce

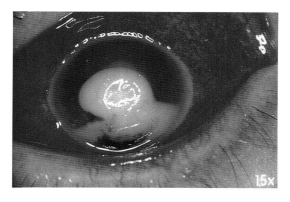

Figure 45.8 Clinical appearance of a corneal ulcer with central necrosis and hypopyon.

vacuoles in which organisms may thrive. Some soft hydrophilic contact lenses, either daily or extended wear, contain low concentrations of PVP which can act as a nutrient broth for many bacteria (Ruben, 1975; Tripathi *et al.*, 1980, 1988; Tripathi & Tripathi, 1984). Even with the use of disinfection techniques, long-term infections caused by spores resistant to these methods are possible. The invasion of a soft contact lens by uncommon invaders, such as the fungus *Exophiala jeanselmei*, has been documented (Hurtado & Magran, 1989). This is a reminder than any organism may cause ocular damage in contact lens wearers.

Many solutions that do not contain preservatives can grow pathogens once their container has been opened (Ruben, 1975). The use of distilled water for storage is a potential source of infection. Moreover, this and other homemade saline solutions, as well as the contact lens case, may become contaminated with various organisms (Tripathi & Tripathi, 1984; Grutzmacher, 1989) which, in the presence of an epithelial defect, will initiate a microbial infection.

Acanthamoeba keratitis

Inoculation of the cornea with *Acanthamoeba*, a free-living ameba found in water and soil, will result in a recalcitrant keratitis that may be misdiagnosed clinically as viral (especially *Herpes simplex*), fungal, or bacterial (especially *Mycobacterium*) keratitis. Another causative agent is *Paecilomyces lilacinus* (Starr, 1987). Although daily-wear soft contact lenses are associated most commonly with *Acanthamoeba*, this condition is also known to occur in patients who use extended-wear soft lenses, hard lenses, RGP lenses, and hybrid (Saturn II) lenses (Tripathi *et al.*, 1989). The highest incidence has been reported with use of extended-wear soft contact lenses and the lowest incidence was observed with hard contact lens wear (Chalupa *et al.*, 1987).

Infection with this organism is of particular concern because the ameba is able to change from a chemotherapeutically susceptible trophozoite to a resistant cyst form (Moore *et al.*, 1985). The trophozoites found in corneal epithelial cells are polygonal, measure 15 to 45 µm in length, and have a single nucleus with one or more prominent nucleoli. The cytoplasm contains numerous mitochondria, endoplasmic reticulum, food vacuoles with phagocytosed material in different stages of digestion, and other organelles (Tripathi *et al.*, 1989). The wall of the *Acanthamoeba* cysts (which measure up to 7 µm wide and 16 µm long) consists of an outer layer (ectocyst) and a stellate, polygonal inner layer (endocyst). Often the cyst wall is wrinkled and folded irregularly, and some organisms show remnants of organelles, such as a nucleus, mitochondria, membrane-bound vacuoles, and ribosomes (Fig. 45.10).

On biomicroscopic examination, a chronic keratoconjunctivitis may be evident (Fig. 45.10a). The affected cornea demonstrates patchy, irregular, focal, multifocal, or dendritiform ulceration, or it may be intact. Stromal haze develops slowly, and there may be a mild nonsuppurative keratitis, with single or multiple superficial stromal infiltrates comprised mostly of polymorphonuclear leukocytes. Subsequently, a corneal ring infiltrate and a low-grade anterior uveitis develop (Tripathi *et al.*, 1989). In advanced cases, severe iritis, hypopyon, and necrotizing stromal perforation may occur. As the infection progresses through the stroma, infiltration of polymorphonuclear leukocytes with stromal necrosis develops (Tripathi *et al.*, 1989).

Because *Acanthamoeba* keratitis may be confused with the clinical manifestations of other forms of bacterial, fungal, or viral keratitis, a definitive diagnosis is essential. The diagnosis is based on the clinical findings, the smear and culture, and special stains used on tissue sections examined by

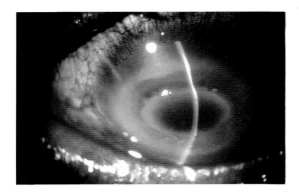

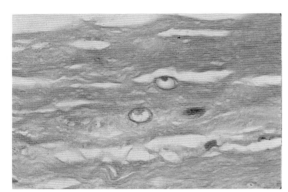

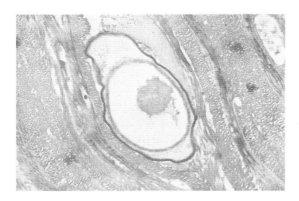

light and electron microscopy (Fig. 45.11). Indirect immunofluorescence staining provides a reliable diagnosis (Tripathi *et al.*, 1989).

45.4 METABOLIC DAMAGE

Many biochemical alterations in the corneal epithelium and in the aqueous humor as a result of contact lens wear have been documented. These changes may be caused by the contact lens itself or by the toxicity of the components of the cleaning solution.

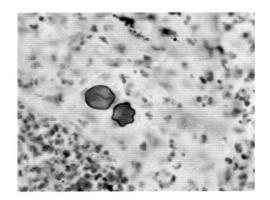

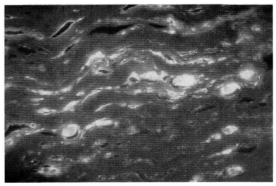

Figure 45.10 (a) Biomicroscopic appearance of corneal ulcer caused by *Acanthamoeba*. Note the characteristic ring-shaped ulcer. (b) Histologic section of corneal stroma from a case of *Acanthamoeba* keratitis. Two *Acanthamoeba* cysts (center) are seen (original magnification × 250). (c) Transmission electron micrograph of an intrastromal, double-walled cyst of *Acanthamoeba* (original magnification × 9000).

Figure 45.11 (a) Epithelial scraping from a patient with *Acanthamoeba* keratitis. Two cysts are seen (center) in this stained preparation (original magnification × 250). (b) Immunofluorescent staining of *Acanthamoeba* in the corneal stroma (original magnification × 160).

45.4.1 CONTACT LENS-INDUCED METABOLIC DAMAGE

The corneal epithelium requires a high oxygen tension to support the aerobic metabolism that is indispensable for the cornea to maintain its transparency (Zimny & Salisbury, 1982). If this requirement is not met adequately, corneal edema, neovascularization, mitotic arrest, morphologic and functional alterations in the endothelium, and bullous keratopathy may result.

Corneal epithelial edema

The cornea becomes edematous during sleep because of the relative hypoxia during lid closure, but gradually resumes its normal thickness upon awakening (Tripathi, 1975). Epithelial edema of contact lens wear, known as Sattler's veil, is also a response of the corneal epithelium to anterior hypoxia. Its occurrence depends on the degree of transmission of oxygen through the lens and the duration of wear (Tripathi, 1975). Whereas PMMA lenses transmit very little oxygen, and RGP and hydrophilic soft lenses facilitate somewhat more oxygenation, silicone lenses allow oxygen to pass freely through the lens material. Extended wear and tight fitting of the contact lens interfere with the uptake of atmospheric oxygen by the epithelium, which leads to depletion of glycogen, an increase in the amount of lactic acid, and accumulation of fluid within the corneal epithelial cells (Ruben, 1975; Tripathi, 1975).

In its early stages, intracellular edema results in a reversible disorganization of corneal structure, with vertical striae in Descemet's membrane, that temporarily compromises transparency (Smith, 1969). As the edema progresses to hydropic degeneration, disruption of cell membranes occurs and eventually gives rise to liquefaction, degeneration, and cystic changes in the epithelium (Tripathi, 1975). Such changes in the basal cells lead to loosening of their cohesion

with the basement membrane and may contribute to the formation of epithelial erosions. In chronic edema, intraepithelially proliferating fibrous tissue and degenerative pannus (Fig. 45.12) may become thick enough to increase light scatter substantially and thus interfere with the optical function of the cornea.

Neovascularization

New-vessel formation associated with contact lens-induced hypoxia may occur as a vascularized pannus along the limbus or may be in a deeper location (Fig. 45.13). In daily contact lens wear, chronic dilatation of the limbic capillary network may be a precursor to new-vessel growth, with subsequent chronic vascularization (McMonnies *et al.*, 1982). Intracorneal hemorrhages may be a consequence, as seen in 'gas keratitis' resulting from the wear of haptic lenses and, in normal corneas, from contact lens trauma of these perilimbal vessels (Laroche & Campbell, 1987).

The presence of a contact lens on the eye results in some degree of corneal anoxia (Levenson, 1983; Hamano *et al.*, 1985). Increasing oxygen deprivation by extended

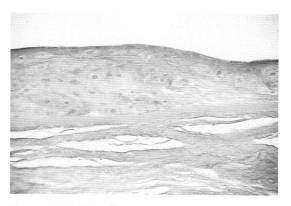

Figure 45.12 Histologic section of a fibrous pannus (below) associated with finger-like projections of basement membrane and fibrous tissue into the epithelium (above) (magnification × 100).

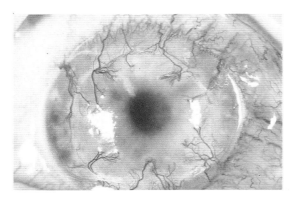

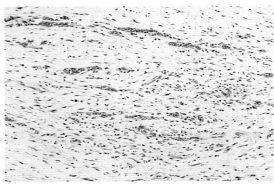

Figure 45.13 (a) Clinical appearance of stromal vascularization (courtesy of G.N. Rao). (b) Histologic section of corneal stroma showing neovascularization together with chronic inflammatory cell infiltrate (original magnification × 50).

lens wear leads to conjunctival injection and, in some cases, corneal neovascularization. With the reduction in the oxygen supply to the cornea, anaerobic metabolism becomes favored by the cell, with concomitant suppression of aerobic metabolism (Connor & Zagrod, 1986). A considerable amount of lactic acid is thus formed in the cornea, especially when scleral lenses are worn (Ruben, 1989). As a consequence, the cornea may be invaded by blood vessels superficially in the perilimbal area; alternatively, deeper in the stroma, looping of stromal vessels, or formation of collaterals, or isolated branching from a single feed may occur. The aftermath of corneal vascularization may be the presence of ghost vessels and a perivascular fibrotic sheathing.

Corneal epithelial mitoses

Extended wear of soft contact lenses has been shown to suppress epithelial mitoses in the rabbit cornea (Hamano & Hori, 1983). The basal layer of the epithelium uses the greatest amount of oxygen; its high consumption is necessary for viability and for the mitotic process of epithelial regeneration.

Morphologic and functional alterations in corneal endothelium

Contact lens wear induces transient as well as permanent morphologic changes in the corneal endothelium (Carlson *et al.*, 1988; Matsuda *et al.*, 1988.) With daily-lens wear, PMMA and soft contact lens wearers have manifested reversible morphologic changes in the corneal endothelium, known as the endothelial bleb response, which do not affect the barrier or pump function of the endothelium (Lass *et al.*, 1988). Such changes are not observed to any significant extent, however, with highly gas permeable silicone lenses. The cause is thought to be the relative endothelial hypoxia associated with changes in the pH and with the accumulation of lactic acid and/or carbon dioxide within the endothelium (Holden *et al.*, 1985). Clinically, the 'blebs' appear as small, nonreflective areas scattered throughout the endothelial mosaic. With continued lens wear, they increase in both size and number. Electron microscopy reveals edema within the rabbit endothelium; this alters the posterior endothelial cell border and separates it from Descemet's membrane (Vannas *et al.*, 1984).

Alterations in endothelial cell morphology (Fig. 45.14) observed after extended wear of PMMA, RGP, and soft lenses include increased polymegethism (variation in cell size, which is presumed to compromise the cellular functional reserve) and pleomor-

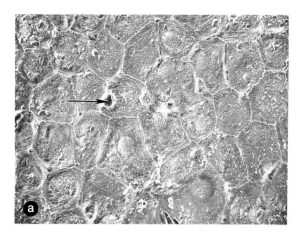

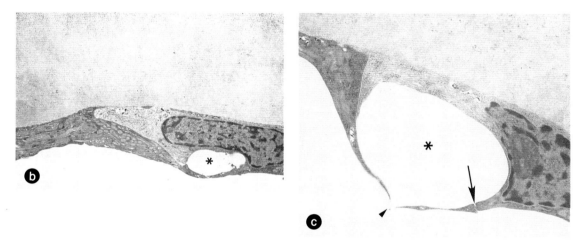

Figure 45.14 The corneal endothelium in an elderly aphakic soft contact lens daily wearer (courtesy Bergmanson, 1992). (a) Scanning electron microscopy reveals variability in cell size, shape, and marked polygonality. The rupture of an intercellular cyst (arrow) has left a small crater (original magnification ✕ 800). (b) Transmission electron micrograph showing intercellular edema (asterisk). The cellular overlapping is due to oblique the section of adjacent cell surfaces (original magnification ✕ 18 000). (c) High magnification extracellular edematous space (asterisk) between two neighboring endothelial cells. A tight junction (arrow) and a localized thinning (arrowhead) of the cyst wall suggest that this is the point where the vacuolar space is likely to burst. Transmission electron micrograph (original magnification ✕ 30 000).

phism (variation in cell shape), with no apparent difference in endothelial cell density (Holden *et al.*, 1986; Schoessler, 1987). The cause of these morphometric abnormalities is uncertain, but may be related to chronic hypoxic stress (MacRae *et al.*, 1985).

When a contact lens is placed on the eye, the level of oxygen dissolved in the aqueous humor is decreased (probably the result of greater utilization by the stroma). Because the aqueous humor bathes the posterior surface of the endothelium, a reduction in the oxygen tension in the aqueous humor places the endothelium in a hypoxic environment (Connor & Zagrod, 1986). It may be noted that corneal endothelial pleomorphism also develops with age.

Significant aberrations in the endothelial barrier and pump functions have also been documented with long-term contact lens wear (Lass *et al.*, 1988). Corneal thickness and hydration are maintained within a narrow range by an energy-dependent metabolic pump in the endothelium (Mishima & Kudo, 1967; Maurice, 1984). If the pump fails, fluid enters the stroma and disrupts the organization of collagen fibrils (Fig. 45.15); this results in loss of the endothelial barrier function and in corneal opacification.

Bullous keratopathy

Endothelial pleomorphism has been implicated in apparently spontaneous bullous keratopathy that sets in after long-term contact lens wear (Roth, 1986).

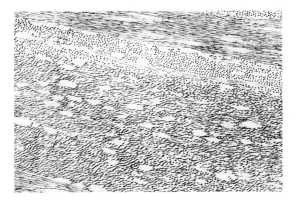

Figure 45.15 Stromal edema as seen by transmission electron microscopy. Note numerous electronoptically empty areas (lakes) and irregularity in the arrangement of the stromal collagen fibers. The swollen corneal stroma, together with the mini-lakes, accounts for stromal haze seen in corneal edema. (original magnification ×39 000).

45.4.2 TOXICITY OF CONTACT LENS SOLUTIONS

The various chemicals, antibacterial preservatives, buffers, emulsifiers, and chelators in contact lens solutions may induce toxic or allergic ocular reactions in susceptible patients.

Hydrogen peroxide

Exposure of the eyes to a 3% hydrogen peroxide solution used as a disinfectant for daily- and extended-wear hydrogel contact lenses may result in permanent corneal damage. In cell cultures of human corneal epithelium, a single dose of hydrogen peroxide at concentrations as low as 30 ppm caused cell retraction as well as cessation of cell movement and of mitotic activity (Tripathi & Tripathi, 1989a) (Fig. 45.16). Cell death occurred by 4 to 5 hours. This sequence of events was more rapid with higher concentrations of hydrogen peroxide (Fig. 45.16). Because hydrogen peroxide can also directly damage DNA, this agent may be capable of causing a number of corneal disorders. Contact lens wearers should be aware of the deleterious effects of residual peroxide, because concentrations as high as 400 ppm have been purported not to elicit an appreciable discomfort response (see Tripathi & Tripathi, 1989a).

Benzalkonium chloride and chlorobutanol

Both of these preservatives are commonly contained in the artificial tear solutions used by contact lens patients for dry eyes. Primary cultures of human corneal epithelial cells treated with 0.01% benzalkonium chloride (BAK) and 0.5% chlorobutanol demonstrate immediate cessation of normal cytokinesis and mitotic activity, followed by epithelial degeneration by 2 hours and 8 hours, respectively (Tripathi & Tripathi, 1989b). This correlates clinically with potentiation of existing

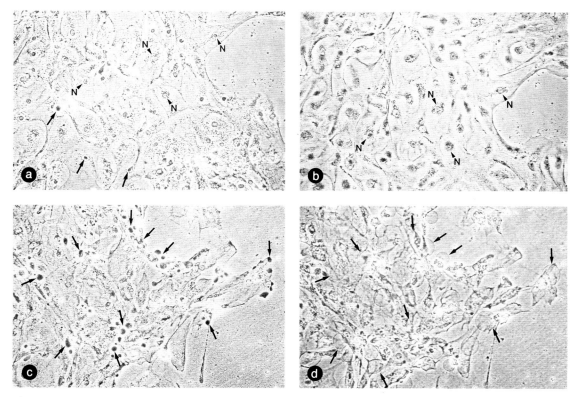

Figure 45.16 (a) Primary confluent culture of human corneal epithelium. The cells are epithelioid in shape, have a wide cytoplasmic span, and contain a relatively small, centrally located nucleus (N). (b) After 5 hours exposure to 30 ppm hydrogen peroxide, the cells show indistinct borders, retraction, granularity of the cytoplasm, shrinkage and pyknosis of nuclei (N), and a few dense refractile spots on the cell surface (arrows). Same field of view as seen in (a). (c) Human corneal epithelial cells *in vitro* after 1.5 hours exposure to 50 ppm hydrogen peroxide showing numerous optically dense, refractile spots (arrows) on the cell surface. (d) After 5 hours exposure to 50 ppm hydrogen peroxide,the cells show degenerative changes that include indistinct cell outline, granularity of cytoplasm, as well as nuclear pyknosis. The optically dense spots seen in (c) have developed into large, optically lucent vesicles (arrows). Phase-contrast micrographs (original magnification × 140) (from Tripathi & Tripathi, 1989a).

epithelial defects and delay in wound healing.

Benzalkonium chloride disrupts the lipid layer of the tear film, which results in rapid break-up of the tear film with free evaporation of water (Tripathi & Tripathi, 1989b). This process hastens drying of the cornea. If BAK is used by patients who already have a defective epithelium, more serious complications may result. The detergent effect of BAK (Pfister & Burstein, 1976) accounts for much

of its epithelial toxicity, the effects of which include severe loss of epithelial microvilli, disruption of cell membranes, and death and desquamation of surface epithelial cells. Cultured human corneal epithelial cells exposed to a single dose of 0.01% BAK for 2 hours showed marked retraction, a rounded or elongated profile, as well as vacuolation and pyknosis of the nuclei. The extracellular spaces were enlarged and were traversed by elongated intercellular bridges (Tripathi &

Tripathi, 1989b) (Fig. 45.17).

Chlorobutanol promotes disorganization of the lipid structure of cell membranes which leads to increased cell permeability (Tripathi & Tripathi, 1989b). Moreover, chlorobutanol inhibits utilization of oxygen by the cornea. Cultures of human corneal epithelial cells exposed to a single dose of 0.5% chlorobutanol for 24 hours showed some cell retraction. The cells also developed small, refractile vacuoles, and the nuclei appeared relatively normal. Another feature of chlorobutanol cytotoxicity is the conspicuous membranous blebs that appear after 3 to 5 hours of exposure (Fig. 45.18). The mechanism of bleb formation remains unknown.

Thimerosal

Thimerosal, an organic mercurial preservative commonly found in many ophthalmic solutions at concentrations of 0.001% and 0.004%, is known to be responsible for some

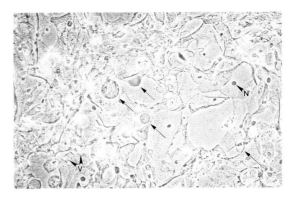

Figure 45.18 Two-week-old confluent culture of human corneal epithelial cells exposed to a single dose of 0.5% chlorobutanol for 24 hours. The cells show some retraction and contain small, refractile vacuoles (V) and nuclei (N) that are relatively intact. Conspicuous membranous blebs (arrow), which first appear after 3 to 5 hours of exposure, are an additional feature of chlorobutanol cytotoxicity. Phase-contrast micrograph (original magnification × 190) (from Tripathi & Tripathi, 1989).

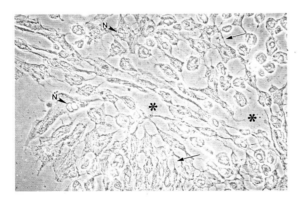

Figure 45.17 Two-week-old confluent culture of human corneal epithelial cells exposed to a single dose of 0.01% benzalkonium chloride for two hours. The cells show marked retraction, a rounded or elongated profile, and vacuolation and pyknosis of the nuclei (n). The intercellular spaces are enlarged (asterisk) and are bridged by elongated intercellular junctional complexes (arrow). Phase-contrast micrograph (original magnification × 225) (from Tripathi & Tripathi, 1989).

of the toxic and many of the hypersensitivity reactions of the ocular surface (Mondino & Groden, 1982). Cell cultures of rabbit corneal epithelium demonstrated a toxic effect after exposure to a 0.004% thimerosal solution for 90 minutes (Burnstein & Klyce, 1977). Long-term animal and human studies on such exposure *in vivo*, however, are lacking.

In some vulnerable wearers of daily soft contact lenses, pseudodendrites develop after exposure to thimerosal (Udell *et al.,* 1985). These transient lesions, which are thought to be related to the toxicity of the preservative, resolve after discontinuation of lens wear. Extended-wear contact lens patients may be less susceptible to these dendriform lesions because they have minimal exposure to this preservative and because the extended-wear lens exerts a bandage healing effect.

Hypersensitivity reactions may also result from exposure to thimerosal. In some patients, a follicular conjunctivitis results (Tosti & Tosti, 1988); in others, conjunctival hyperemia and corneal infiltrates have been observed (Mondino & Groden, 1980). A superior limbic keratoconjunctivitis (SLK) syndrome, which should not be confused with the classical form of SLK (Theodore, 1963), has also been documented in some soft contact lens wearers (Miller *et al.*, 1982; Bloomfield *et al.*, 1984). The clinical manifestations include superior conjunctival inflammation as well as punctate staining of the conjunctiva and superior cornea, which may progress to formation of superior pannus that involves the central cornea (Stenson, 1983). As the keratitis extends toward the

central cornea, it brings with it vascularization, scarring, and, occasionally, surface breakdown. Light and transmission electron-microscopic examination reveals keratinization of the corneal epithelium with intracellular edema in some patients, and acanthosis, pseudoepitheliomatous hyperplasia, and acute inflammation in others (Fig. 45.19). The superior limbal and bulbar conjunctival changes may mimic the classic form of SLK; however, the latter usually exhibits a diffuse inflammation and a papillary reaction of the superior tarsal conjunctiva, and it is also often seen in association with contact lens wear (Sendele *et al.*, 1983).

45.5 CONCLUSION

Contact lens wear constitutes the introduction of a foreign body in the keratoconjunctival sac that creates uncommon pathophysiologic alterations which may be associated with a variety of complications. Epithelial trauma contributes to the metabolic and morphologic changes due to hypoxia that have been documented with contact lens wear. The microtrauma and the altered metabolism related to the lens design and methods of insertion set the stage for further injury, infection, and inflammation of a stressed epithelium in the contact lens wearer. The deeper stroma and other associated ocular injuries, and their sequelae, are often consequential.

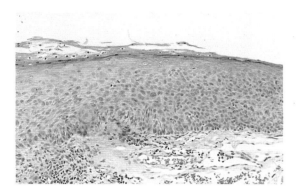

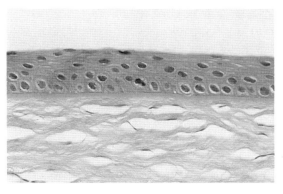

Figure 45.19 (a) A hyperplastic epithelium showing increased number of cells and a mitotic figure (center) in the basal layer (original magnification × 160). (b) An epithelial dysplasia with surface keratinization of the cells and subepithelial infiltration by inflammatory cells are seen in this histologic section (original magnification × 50).

REFERENCES

Allansmith, M.R. and Ross, R. N. (1988) Giant papillary conjunctivitis. *Int. Ophthalmol. Clin.*, **28**, 309–15.

Allansmith, M.R. *et al.* (1977) Giant papillary conjunctivitis in contact lens wearers. *Am. J. Ophthalmol.*, **83**, 697–708.

Bergmanson, J.P.G. *et al.* (1984) Corneal epithelial response of the primate eye to gas permeable corneal contact lenses: a preliminary report. *Cornea.*, **3**, 109–13.

Binder, P.S. *et al.* (1981) Keratoconjunctivitis and

soft contact lens solutions. *Arch. Ophthalmol.*, **99**, 87–90.

Bloomfield, S. *et al.* (1984) Contact lens induced keratopathy: a severe complication extending the spectrum of keratoconjunctivitis in contact lens wearers. *Ophthalmology*, **91**, 290–4.

Bron, A.J. and Tripathi, R.C. (1969) Anterior corneal mosaic. Further observations. *Br. Ophthalmol.*, **53**, 760–4.

Burnstein, N.L. and Klyce, S.D. (1977) Electrophysiologic and morphologic effects of ophthalmic preservatives on rabbit cornea epithelium. *Invest. Ophthalmol. Vis. Sci.*, **16**, 899–911.

Carlson, K.H. *et al.* (1988) Effect of long term contact lens wear on corneal endothelial cell morphology and function. *Invest. Ophthalmol. Vis. Sci.*, **29**, 185–93.

Chalupa, E. et al. (1987) Severe corneal infections associated with contact lens wear. *Ophthalmology*, **94**, 17–22.

Clemons, C.S. *et al.* (1987), *Pseudomonas* ulcers following patching of corneal abrasions associated with contact lens wear. *CLAO J.*, **13**, 161–2.

Connor, C.G. and Zagrod, M.E. (1986) Contact lens-induced corneal endothelial polymegathism: functional significance and possible mechanisms. *Am. J. Optom. Physiol. Opt.*, **63**, 539–44.

Donnenfeld, E.D. *et al.* (1986) Changing trends in contact lens associated corneal ulcers: an overview of 116 cases. *CLAO J.*, **12**, 145–9.

Douglas, J.P. *et al.* (1988) Giant papillary conjunctivitis associated with rigid gas permeable contact lenses. *CLAO J.*, **14**, 143–7.

Ehrlich, M. *et al.* (1989) *Pseudomonas* corneal ulcer after use of extended-wear rigid gas-permeable contact lens. *Cornea*, **8**, 225–6.

Epstein, G. and Putterman, A.M. (1981) Acquired blepharoptosis secondary to contact-lens wear. *Am. J. Ophthalmol.*, **91**, 634–9.

Farris, R.L. (1986) The dry eye: its mechanisms and therapy, with evidence that contact lens is a cause. *CLAO J.*, **12**, 234–45.

Fonn, D. and Holden, B.A. (1986) Extended wear of hard gas permeable contact lenses can induce ptosis. *CLAO J.*, **12**, 93–4.

Francois, J. (1983) The rabbit corneal epithelium after wearing hard and soft contact lenses. *CLAO J.*, **9**, 267–74.

Francois, J. *et al.* (1974) Keratoconjonctivite seche experimentale (étude microscopique et histochimique). *Ann. Oculistique*, **207**, 185–200.

Grutzmacher, R.D. (1989) Ocular disease from wearing contact lenses. *Contact Lenses*, **86**, 90–100.

Hamano, H. *et al.* (1985) Adverse effects of contact lens wear in a large Japanese population. *CLAO J.*, **11**, 141–7.

Hamano, H. and Hori, M. (1983) Effect of contact lens wear on the mitoses of corneal epithelial cells: preliminary report. *CLAO J.*, **9**, 133–6.

Hamburger, H.A. (1986) Pyogenic granuloma associated with extended wear contact lenses. *CLAO J.*, **12**, 99–100.

Hartstein, J. (1968) Keratoconus that developed in patients wearing corneal contact lenses. *Arch. Ophthalmol.* **80**, 728–9.

Holden, B.A. *et al.* (1985) The etiology of transient endothelial changes in the human cornea. *Invest. Ophthalmol. Vis. Sci.*, **26**, 1354.

Holden, B.A. *et al.* (1986), The endothelial response to contact lens wear. *CLAO J.*, **12**, 150–2.

Horowitz, G.S. *et al.* (1985) An unusual corneal complication of soft contact lens. *Am. J. Ophthalmol.*, **100**, 794–7.

Hurtado, I. and Magran, B.L. (1988) Invasion of a soft contact lens by *Exophiala jeanselmei*. *Mycopathologia*, **105**, 171–3.

Laroche, R.R. and Campbell, R.C. (1987) Intracorneal hemorrhage induced by chronic extended wear of a soft contact lens. *CLAO J.*, **13**, 39–40.

Lass, J.H. *et al.* (1981), Visual outcome in eight cases of *Serratia marcescens* keratitis. *Am. J. Ophthalmol.*, **92**, 384–90.

Lass, J.H. *et al.* (1988) Morphologic and fluorophotometric analysis of the corneal endothelium in long-term hard and soft contact lens wearers. *CLAO J.*, **14**, 105–9.

Levenson, D.S. (1983) Changes in corneal curvature with long-term PMMA contact lens wear. *CLAO J.*, **9**, 121–5.

MacRae, S. *et al.* (1985) The effect of contact lenses on the corneal endothelium. *Invest. Ophthalmol. Vis Sci.*, **26** (Suppl.), 275.

Macsai, M.S. *et al.* (1990) Development of keratoconus after contact lens wear. *Arch. Ophthalmol.*, **108**, 534–8.

Mandell, R.B. (1979) Oxygen-transmitting hard contact lenses. *J. Am. Optom. Assoc.*, **50**, 323–4.

Mannucci, L.L. *et al.* (1984) The effect of extended wear contact lenses on tear immunoglobulins. *CLAO J.*, **10**, 163–5.

Matsuda, M. *et al.* (1988) Corneal endothelial changes associated with aphakic endothelial cell morphology and function. *Arch. Ophthalmol.*, **106**, 70–2.

Maurice, D. (1984) The cornea and sclera. In *The Eye*, vol. 1B (ed. H. Davson), Academic Press, London, pp. 1–158.

McMonnies, C.W. *et al.* (1982) The vascular response to contact lens wear. *Am. J. Optom. Physiol. Opt.*, **59**, 795–9.

Miller, R.A. *et al.* (1982) Superior limbic kerato-conjunctivitis in soft contact lens wearers. *Cornea*, **1**, 293–9.

Mishima, S. and Kudo, T. (1967) In vivo incubation of rabbit cornea. *Invest. Ophthalmol.*, **6**, 329.

Mondino, B.J. and Groden, L.R. (1980) Conjunctival hyperemia and corneal infiltrates with chemically disinfected soft contact lenses. *Arch. Ophthalmol.* **98**, 1767–70.

Mondino, B.J. and Salamon, S.M. (1982) Allergic and toxic reactions in soft contact lens wearers. *Surv. Ophthalmol.*, **26**, 337.

Moore, M.B. *et al.* (1985) *Acanthamoeba* keratitis associated with soft contact lenses. *Am. J. Ophthalmol.*, **100**, 396–403.

Pfister, R.R. and Burstein, N. (1976) The effects of ophthalmic drugs, vehicles, and preservatives on corneal epithelium: A scanning electron microscope study. *Invest. Ophthalmol.*, **15**, 246–58.

Poggio, E.C. *et al.* (1989) The incidence of ulcerative keratitis among users of daily-wear and extended-wear soft contact lenses. *N. Engl. J. Med.*, **321**, 779–83.

Ramphal, R. *et al.* (1981) Adherence of *Pseudomonas aeruginosa* to the injured cornea: a step in the pathogenesis of corneal infections. *Ann. Ophthalmol.*, **13**, 421–5.

Refojo, M. (1972) Physiochemical properties of hydrophilic soft contact lenses and their physiological implications. *J. Am. Optom. Assoc.*, **43**, 262–5.

Remeijer, L. *et al.* (1990) Deep corneal stromal opacities in long-term contact lens wear. *Ophthalmology*, **97**, 281–5.

Roth, H. (1986) Pseudobullous keratopathy: a rare complication of contact lens wear. *Contactologia*, **8**, 116–17.

Ruben, M. (1975) Intolerance and eye disease due to contact lens wear. In *Contact Lens Practice. Visual Therapeutic and Prosthetic*, (ed. M. Ruben), Bailliere Tindall, London, pp. 257–77.

Ruben, M. (1989), Adverse reactions to contact lens wear. In *Color Atlas of Contact Lenses and Prosthetics*, (ed. M. Ruben), C. V. Mosby, St Louis, pp. 150–82.

Schein, O.D. *et al.* (1989) The relative risk of ulcerative keratitis among users of daily-wear and extended-wear soft contact lenses: a case-control study. *N. Engl. J. Med.*, **321**, 773–8.

Schoessler, J.P. (1987) The corneal endothelium following 20 years of PMMA contact lens wear. *CLAO J.*, **13**, 157–60.

Sebag, J. and Albert, D.M. (1982) Pseudochalazion of the upper lid due to hard contact lens embedding. Case reports and literature review. *Ophthalmic Surg.*, **13**, 634–6.

Sendele, D.D. *et al.* (1983) Superior limbic kerato-conjunctivitis in contact lens wearers. *Ophthalmology*, **90**, 616–22.

Smith, J.W. (1969) The transparency of the human cornea. *Vision Res.*, **9**, 393.

Srinivasan, B.D. *et al.* (1979) Giant papillary conjunctivitis with ocular prostheses. *Arch. Ophthalmol.*, **97**, 892–5.

Starr, M.B. (1987) *Paecilomyces lilacinus* keratitis: two case reports in extended wear contact lens wearers. *CLAO J.*, **13**, 95–101.

Stenson, S. (1983) Superior limbic keratoconjunctivitis associated with soft contact lens wear. *Arch. Ophthalmol.*, **101**, 402–4.

Stern, G.S. and Zam, Z.S. (1986) The pathogenesis of contact lens-associated *Pseudomonas aeruginosa* corneal ulceration 1. *Cornea*, **5**, 41–5.

Stern, G.S. *et al.* (1982) Adherence of *Pseudomonas aeruginosa* to the mouse cornea. *Arch. Ophthalmol.*, **100**, 1956–8.

Theodore, F.H. (1963) Superior limbic keratoconjunctivitis. *Eye, Ear, Nose, Throat Monthly*, **42**, 25–8.

Tosti, A. and Tosti, G. (1988) Thimerosal: a hidden allergen in ophthalmology. *Contact-Dermatitis*, **18**, 268–73.

Tripathi, B.J. and Tripathi, R. C. (1989a) Hydrogen peroxide damage to human corneal epithelial cells in vitro. *Arch. Ophthalmol.*, **107**, 1516–19.

Tripathi, B.J. and Tripathi, R. C. (1989b) Cytotoxic effects of benzalkonium chloride and chlorobutanol on human corneal epithelial cells in vitro. *Lens and Eye Toxicity Res.*, **6**, 395–403.

Tripathi, B.J. *et al.* (1990) Adhesion of bacteria to contact lenses. In *Contact Lenses: Basic Science and Clinical Practice*, (ed. O. H. Dabezies), Little, Brown, and Co., Boston.

Tripathi, B.J. *et al.* (1993) Cytotoxicity of ophthalmic preservatives on human corneal epithelium. *Lens. Eye Tox. Res.*, **9**, 361.

Tripathi, R.C. (1975) Applied physiology and anatomy. In *Contact Lens Practice. Visual Thera-*

peutic and Prosthetic, (ed. M. Ruben), Bailliere Tindall, London, pp. 24–55.

Tripathi, R.C. and Tripathi, B. J. (1984) Lens spoilage. In *Contact Lenses, A Clinical Handbook of The Contact Lens Association of Ophthalmologists of America*, (ed. O. H. Dabezies), Grune and Stratton, New York, pp. 1–36.

Tripathi, R.C. *et al.* (1980) The pathology of soft contact lens spoilage. *Ophthalmology*, **87**, 365–80.

Tripathi, R.C. *et al.* (1988) Physiochemical changes in contact lenses and their interaction with the cornea and tears. A review and personal observations. *CLAO J.*, **14**, 23–32.

Tripathi, R.C. *et al.* (1989) Contact lens-associated *Acanthamoeba* keratitis: a report from the USA. *Fortschr. Ophthalmol.*, **86**, 67–71.

Tripathi, R.C. *et al.* (1991) Contact lens deposits and spoilage: identification and management. *Int. Ophthalmol. Clin.*, **31**, 91.

Udell, I.J. *et al.* (1985) Pseudodendrites in soft contact lens wearers. *CLAO J.*, **11**, 51–3.

Vannas, A. *et al.* (1984) The ultrastructure of contact lens induced changes. *Acta Ophthalmol.*, **62**, 320.

Weissman, B.A. *et al.* (1986) Corneal scar caused by a 'mulberry' contact lens deposit. *Cornea*, **6**, 69–74.

Zantos, S.G. (1983) Cystic formations in the corneal epithelium during extended wear of contact lenses. *Int. Contact Lens. Clin.*, **10**, 128–46.

Zimmy, M.L. and Salisbury, C. (1982) Effects of soft contacts on corneal wound healing in rabbits. *Cornea*, **1**, 301–7.

COMPLICATIONS OF SOFT CONTACT LENSES 46

K.R. Kenyon and T. John

46.1 INTRODUCTION

Following the development of hydrophilic soft contact lenses for cosmetic daily wear in the 1960s, improvements in lens materials and design have extended the utility of soft lenses to include therapeutic extended wear for a variety of corneal and external ocular abnormalities and cosmetic extended wear for myopes and aphakes. With the ever-broadening benefits of soft lens wear comes an inevitably increasing litany of lens-related complications (Dohlman, 1974; Ruben *et al.*, 1976). Many of these disorders are, enhance, or mimic inflammatory or infectious problems of the cornea and conjunctiva, and it is important for contact lens practitioners to recognize such problems, as prompt treatment can often avoid sight-threatening sequelae. Adopting Stenson's (1984) approach, we classify the complications as patient-, lens-, or care-related:

1. Patient-related:
   i. compromised cornea – pre-existing disease;
   ii. frequent medications – antivirals, antibiotics, corticosteroids;
   iii. bacterial superinfection;
   iv. chronic blepharitis;
   v. keratitis sicca;
   vi. poor compliance with lense care regimen;
   vii. poor hygiene.

2. Lens related:
   i. Lens:
      a. manufacturing imperfection;
      b. improper fit;
      c. deterioration;
      d. microbial and fungal colonization;
      e. deposits;
   ii. cornea:
      a. epithelial defect;
      b. edema (epithelial, stromal);
      c. endothelial blebs;
      d. endothelial pleomorphism;
      e. neovascularization;
      f. EKC-like syndrome;
      g. decreased sensation;
      h. subepithelial opacification.

3. Care-related:
   i. Hypersensitivity:
      a. thimerosal, chlorhexidine;
   ii. Infectious keratitis:
      a. bacterial infection;
      b. fungal infection;
      c. parasitic infection (including *Acanthamoeba*).

46.2 PATIENT-RELATED COMPLICATIONS

Just as the most effective treatment of complications is their avoidance, it is important to exercise clinical judgment in patient selection for soft lens wear. Thus, corneas in patients requiring *therapeutic bandage lenses* are at high risk to develop complications, as

Contact Lens Practice. Edited by Montague Ruben and Michel Guillon.
Published in 1994 by Chapman & Hall, London. ISBN 0 412 35120 X

they are compromised by pre-existing disease and there is often concomitant use of antibiotics, antivirals, or corticosteroids. For example, we might expect that a patient with a persistent corneal epithelial defect secondary to recurrent herpes simplex keratitis and chronically requiring multiple topical medications is at greatly increased risk to develop a major lens-related complication such as bacterial superinfection (Boisjoly *et al.*, 1983). These patients clearly demand extraordinarily close surveillance. Similarly, in the *extended-wear aphakic population*, age-related disorders of chronic blepharitis and keratitis sicca in an elderly or incapacitated patient, who is often unable to comply with lens care regimens and who may have poor personal hygiene, are increased risks. *Cosmetic daily wearers* of soft lenses may manifest chronic staphylococcal or seborrheic blepharitis and mild dry-eye conditions that can compromise lens wear capability. However, proper attention to these pre-existing ocular surface disorders may allow satisfactory lens wear.

46.3　LENS-RELATED COMPLICATIONS

This class of problems includes manufacturing imperfections, lens-fitting difficulty, lens deterioration secondary to age or sterilization, microbial and fungal spoilage, and deposits. With both spin-cast and lathe-cut lenses, *manufacturing imperfections* can include surface scratches and edge defects that produce irritative signs and symptoms in the cornea and conjunctiva.

46.3.1　LENS FITTING

Lens fitting is of obvious importance as an improper fit can limit tolerance and predispose to anterior segment complications. Even with appropriate fitting, many patients complain of irritation and discomfort during the first night or two of adaptation to extended wear. This problem seems somewhat more prevalent with normal than with damaged corneas. Recurrent erosions in particular are most difficult to deal with, as frequently the patients do well until the middle of the first night of lens wear when they awaken with severe pain. Rather than remove the lens, however, it is advisable to consider cycloplegia, lubrication, and perhaps steroids, because the lens will become more comfortable during the ensuing two days. This phenomenon is probably due to a process of adaptation by the cornea to an inadequate oxygen supply. After Sarver's description of corneal edema with soft lenses, studies have demonstrated that there is very little exchange of tears to enhance oxygen underneath hydrophilic lenses, perhaps only 1% tear replacement per blink. The initial effect of such oxygen deprivation is epithelial edema, and prolonged oxygen deprivation or a level of available oxygen significantly below the minimal threshold will cause full-thickness stromal edema. Since the tear pump mechanism is less effective with hydrophilic lenses, lens manufacturers have resorted to reducing lens thickness or increasing lens hydration to increase the amount of oxygen passing through a lens. Thus, we contrast the thin (central thickness <0.04 mm), relatively low-water-content lens, such as the CSI Syntex or the B&L 03/04, and the relatively thick, high-water-content (70%–85% hydrated) lens, such as the Cooper Permalens. This initial adaptive response to relative hypoxia presumably also accounts for the finding of corneal endothelial blebs, which Zantos and Holden (1978) described as occurring immediately after soft contact lenses were placed on the eye. These blebs seem to represent focal endothelial cell edema, and they subside within approximately 30 minutes and apparently have no sequelae, as long-term specular microscopy of both hard and soft contact lens wearers fails to demonstrate any reduction in endothelial cell population density (although some endothelial pleomorphism may be observed).

46.3.2 TIGHT LENS SYNDROME

Another fitting problem is the so-called *tight lens syndrome* (Fig. 46.1). After initial application of a lens that appears to be an adequate fit, and especially with higher water-content lenses, if the water content drops, the lens can tighten. This in turn can cause the conjunctiva to swell and further tighten the lens. In addition, high-water-content lenses are very sensitive to pH, such that as anaerobic metabolic products accumulate, the lens may steepen and tighten. An accumulation of these toxic metabolic waste products beneath the lens can be observed. In addition to discomfort, the eye becomes inflamed. When examined by slit lamp, the lens itself appears in good condition but does not move with the blink. Treatment is simply lens removal without medication, as the condition will subside and the eye can be refitted, perhaps with a very thin lens. In the chronic state, the tight lens syndrome can also stimulate stromal *neovascularization* (Fig. 46.2). Although this is seldom clinically significant, a progressive ingrowth of vessels extending more than 2 mm from the limbus may require discontinuation or reduction of lens wear if fit cannot be improved.

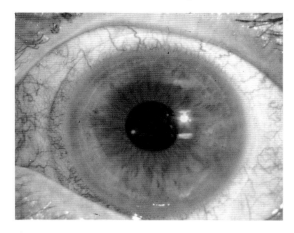

Figure 46.2 Corneal neovascularization involving the superficial and deep corneal stroma, associated with soft contact lens wear (courtesy of Dr G.N. Rao).

46.3.3 CORNEAL NEOVASCULARIZATION

Corneal neovascularization associated with soft contact lens (SCL) wear can involve the superficial or deep corneal stroma, or both. Although corneal neovascularization is usually minimal in aphakic patients fitted with extended wear-lenses (Stark *et al.*, 1979), it may be of greater concern in corneas fitted with a soft contact lens following penetrating keratoplasty where deep stromal neovascularization may increase the risk of graft rejection. Lemp (1980) reported an 89% incidence of graft vascularization in corneal transplant patients fitted with extended-wear soft contact lenses. With the use of corneal fluorescein angiography in SCL-induced graft vascularization following penetrating keratoplasty, the vascularization was found to be more extensive than was clinically apparent and the 'new vessels' were incompetent and leaky (Mackman *et al.*, 1985). Rarely, lipids (especially cholesterol) can leak from the incontinent new vessels and become permanently deposited within the stroma. Thus, in patients with significant graft vascularization secondary to SCL wear, alternative methods of visual correction such as spec-

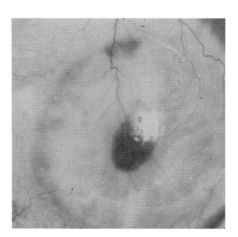

Figure 46.1 Clinical appearance of a 'tight lens syndrome' with prominent conjunctival injection.

tacles or gas-permeable contact lenses should be considered. ·

46.3.4 SUBEPITHELIAL INFILTRATES

A variant of the acute red eye, occurring for the most part in extended-wear patients, is unilateral conjunctival inflammation, frequently associated with *subepithelial infiltrates* of inflammatory cells in the corneal stroma that usually presents upon morning awakening. The contact lens itself is usually in good condition but appears to fit tightly on the eye with limited motion. Corneal epithelial edema may be present. The small stromal infiltrates are usually peripheral but may localize centrally and often have a granular quality that can be difficult to differentiate from adenoviral keratoconjunctivitis (Fig. 46.3) (Mondino & Groden, 1980). As Binder and associates (1981) pointed out, this epidemic keratoconjunctivitis (EKC)-like syndrome most often develops in patients using preserved solutions for soft lens disinfection, and if thermal disinfection was substituted the syndrome did not recur when the lenses were replaced. Corneal hypoxia, as well as other alterations marked by stromal infiltrates, also appears to be involved in this condition. Such hypoxia-related reactions seem to occur less often with very thin lenses because their relatively improved oxygen permeability can satisfy the respiratory needs of the cornea. Thus, discontinuation of the lenses for a brief time and avoidance of potentially toxic or allergic preservatives are usually adequate therapy. It is, of course, always vital to rule out an infectious etiology, especially in the presence of stromal infiltrates with overlying epithelial defects.

Changes in the corneal epithelium occur following SCL wear. In owl monkeys (*Aotus tivergatus*) fitted with hydrogel contact lenses, thinning of corneal epithelium from epithelial cell flattening and loss of superficial cells were demonstrated using transmission electron microscopy (Bergmanson *et al.*,

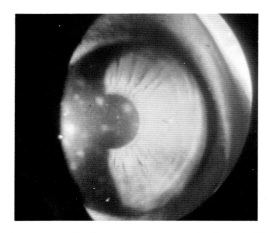

Figure 46.3 Slit lamp appearance of subepithelial infiltrates associated with SCL which can be confused with epidemic keratoconjunctivitis (EKC).

1985). Factors involved in corneal epithelial thinning without edema may include anoxia, lid pressure, lens weight, negative suction, abrasion from lens movement, and abnormal metabolism. Other epithelial changes include punctate epithelial keratitis (Fig. 46.4), corneal microcysts (Fig. 46.5), filamentary keratitis (Fig. 46.6), epithelial hypertrophy, decreased corneal sensation, and subepithelial opacification. (Binder, 1979).

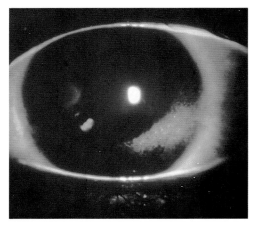

Figure 46.4 Corneal epithelium shows punctate epithelial keratitis (SPK) secondary to SCL wear.

Figure 46.5 SCL usage can result in microcyst formation of the corneal epithelium (courtesy of Dr S. Zantos).

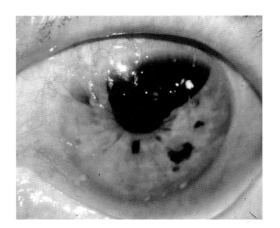

Figure 46.6 Filamentary keratitis.

46.3.5 LENS AGING

With *lens aging*, deterioration of the polymer structure can affect fit, power, and surface characteristics. The lens polymer structure tends to break down with time, and this deterioration is accelerated by thermal (in comparison with chemical) disinfection. Among the clinical clues of deterioration are yellowish discoloration, increased lens movement, surface cracks (Fig. 46.7), edge nicks, and increased surface coating and

deposit formation (Fig. 46.8). The breakdown of polymer structure also provides crevices that become excellent growth sites for the proliferation of microorganisms, especially fungi (Fig. 46.9). Such *microbial spoilage* seems more prevalent in extended-wear cases and represents a potential hazard for infectious keratitis.

Certainly the most prevalent cause of lens spoilage is the formation of debris and insoluble *deposits* on the lens surface. Patients with dry eyes and incomplete blink seem more predisposed to deposit formation. There is some evidence that HEMA materials form deposits more quickly than the CSI polymer, so that the CSI lens may be appropriate for trial in individuals who have a chronic recurrent deposit problem. Although most deposits occur on the front lens surface, back surface deposits also appear and are more troublesome as they can be abrasive or perhaps toxic to the corneal epithelium. Several morphologic varieties of surface deposits have been described. Diffuse proteinaceous products can usually be removed or prevented with the use of enzyme cleaners. Combinations of lipid and mucoprotein deposits occur in various forms ranging from a greasy film to discrete globu-

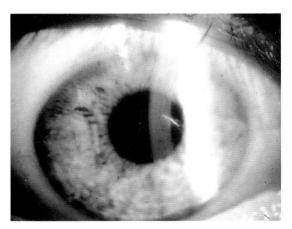

Figure 46.7 Slit lamp photograph showing surface crack in a soft contact lens.

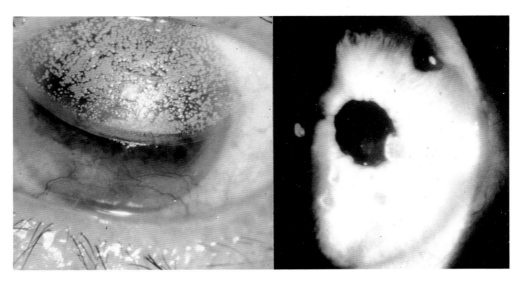

Figure 46.8 Deposits on the surface of a soft contact lens may be small and diffuse (a), or larger and segmental (b).

lar spots (Fig. 46.8). These are removable with detergents, but are difficult to eliminate as they may be related to an excessively oily component of the tear film in predisposed patients. Finally, calcium phosphate or carbonate deposits may result in discrete surface elevations that cannot be removed effectively.

46.3.6 MICROBIAL SPOILAGE

Research in our laboratory (John *et al.*, 1989a) has shown that both Gram-positive and Gram-negative bacteria, including *Pseudomonas aeruginosa* and *Staphylococcus aureus*, adhere to the surface of new and used contact lenses when exposed to bacteria *in vitro* (Fig. 46.10). The bacteria adhered to the uneven contact lens surface in aggregates. Some bacteria had filamentous processes by which they attached to the SCL surface (Fig. 46.10). These lenses also had scattered small deposits. Bacterial adherence has been noted on the granular surface coating of SCLs from asymptomatic contact lens wearers and SCL-associated giant papillary conjunctivitis

(Fowler *et al.*, 1979). Experimental bacterial adherence to corneal epithelium has also been demonstrated. *In vivo* studies in mice have shown that *P. aeruginosa* adheres to injured corneal epithelium (Ramphal *et al.*, 1981; Stern *et al.*, 1982). Among Gram-positive bacteria, *S. aureus* has been shown to adhere to rabbit corneal epithelial cells in an *in vitro* system (Johnson *et al.*, 1984). *In vitro* adherence of *Moraxella bovis* to intact bovine corneal epithelium has also been reported (Jackman & Rosenbusch, 1984), as well as adherence of both Gram-positive and Gram-negative bacteria to human corneal epithelial cells (Reichert & Stern, 1984). Contact lenses with bacteria attached to them may prove to be a significant factor in vision-threatening corneal ulceration in the presence of corneal epithelial surface injury, irregularity, or epithelial defect.

Unlike bacteria, fungal invasion of contact lenses is uncommon (Berger & Streeten, 1981; Churner & Cunningham, 1983) and corneal involvement by the fungus is even less common (Yamamoto *et al.*,

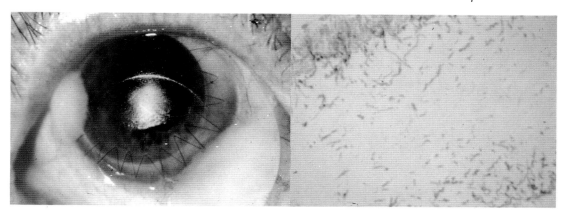

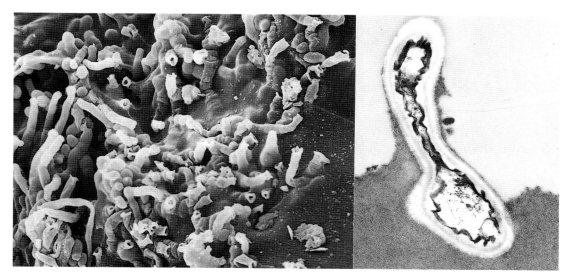

Figure 46.9 (a) Clinical photograph of a fungally invaded soft contact lens over a clear corneal transplant. (b) Cross-section of an extended-wear SCL showing fungal invasion into the lens matrix (Gomori methamine silver stain, × 300). (c) Scanning electron micrograph of the surface of a SCL showing numerous fungal elements encrusting the lens surface (× 1500). (d) Transmission electron micrograph showing penetration of the lens surface by a fungal hypha (× 15 200).

1979). Rarely, actinomycetes can invade a contact lens. However, when corneal involvement occurs, management becomes difficult and may even require a penetrating keratoplasty to salvage the eye. *Acanthamoeba castellanii* cysts and trophozoites can also adhere firmly to soft contact lenses when exposed to these lenses *in vitro* (John *et al.*, 1989b). To minimize or prevent potential corneal complications associated with SCLs, therefore, it is essential to stress to the patient the importance of a strict lens-care regimen and early medical attention when symptoms develop. Sterilization procedures for soft contact lenses should have adequate anti-fungal capability. The use of a hydrogen peroxide disinfection system for at least 45 minutes has been recommended against fungi (Penley *et al.*, 1985).

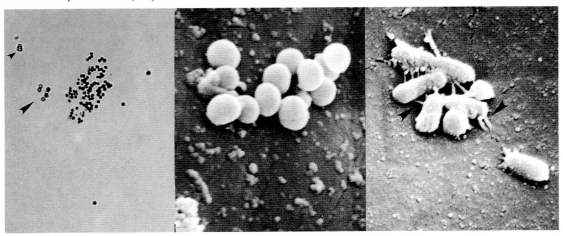

Figure 46.10 (a,b) *Staphylococcus aureus* adherent to the surface of a used SCL following exposure of the CL to the organism. Also seen by light microscopy (a) are surface deposits (arrowheads). These small surface deposits are better seen under SEM (b). (a: Gram stain, × 2000; b: × 10 400). (c) *Psudomonas aeruginosa* adherent to the surface of a used CL exposed to this organism *in vitro*. The Gram-negative rods are seen to adhere to the lens surface with filamentous processes (arrowheads) (SEM, × 12 000).

46.4   CARE-RELATED COMPLICATIONS

The third major area of complication concerns the care and maintenance of the hydrogel. Specifically, we can consider two broad areas, *hypersensitivity or toxic reactions* to lens materials or to the chemicals involved in lens-care solutions, and *infectious keratitis*, which may or may not be related to improper sterilization technique. Certainly the most widely recognized care-related problem currently involves hypersensitivity reactions to thimerosal-containing lens-care solutions (Fig. 46.11) (Abelson *et al.*, 1983). Chlorhexidine has also been implicated to a lesser extent. The incidence of thimerosal hypersensitivity, well documented in the dermatologic literature, ranges from about 7% in the United States to as high as 15%–25% in a Scandinavian study. Although metallic mercury is moderately allergenic, it is generally accepted that sensitivity to the thiosalicylate moiety of thimerosal is greater than sensitivity to elemental mercury. Although the precise immunologic mechanism is still

speculative, it is likely that type 3 hypersensitivity (antigen–antibody complex) and type 4 hypersensitivity (cell-mediated immunity or delayed hypersensitivity) may play an important role in ocular allergic responses to preservatives commonly found in ophthalmic preparations. Thus, after microbial infection, poorly fitting lenses, and other causes of inflammation have been ruled out, thimerosal hypersensitivity should be suspected in any soft lens wearer who uses care solutions containing preservatives and who develops red eyes. The patient may experience a sudden onset of ocular itching and irritation. Alternatively, subacute or chronic conjunctival hyperemia, limbal follicles, or superficial punctate keratopathy may develop. There is no clinical evidence of infection, and there is neither giant papillary conjunctivitis nor superior limbic keratoconjunctivitis. Prolonged exposure intensifies the reaction, leading to bulbar conjunctival follicles and corneal infiltrates with the long-term potential for corneal neovascularization. Thimerosal sensitivity can be differentiated from toxic reactions by the absence in the latter of itching and bulbar follicles and by the immediacy of the toxic reaction which occurs as soon as the lenses are inserted. Allergic reactions typically develop 36–48 hours after lens insertion. In diagnostically difficult cases, allergic reactions can sometimes be confirmed by conjunctival inoculation of the incriminated lens-care solution (Wilson *et al.*, 1981). Management of such cases involves discontinuation of lenses until the clinical signs and symptoms subside and the use of preservative-free solutions in the lens-care regimen. Non-preserved saline solutions (e.g. Unisol®) and solutions containing preservatives other than thimerosal (e.g. Clerz® and Pliagel®, both sorbate-preserved) should be used in conjunction with heat sterilization. The lenses themselves should be purged by boiling in preservative-free saline or in a weak solution of hydrogen peroxide. Some patients may need new lenses. Finally, although sorbate and polyquat are promising with respect to their decreased allergenicity, the possible development of hypersensitivity to these and other preservatives must always be borne in mind.

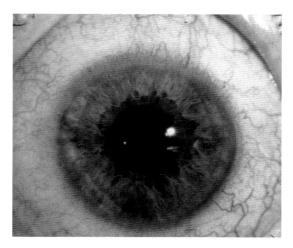

Figure 46.11 Clinical appearance of thimerosal sensitivity.

Another clinical entity that is seemingly allergic in nature is *superior limbic keratitis* (SLK) in contact lens wearers (Fig. 46.12). Our own experience now numbers more than 50 patients who presented with symptoms of irritation and decreased lens tolerance (Sendele *et al.*, 1983). Inflammation of the bulbar conjunctiva was limited to the superior sector, which was hyperemic and minimally keratinized. The corresponding superior limbal area was elevated by gelatinous epithelium and micropannus. The pannus may extend several millimeters onto the superior cornea, and there is diffuse superficial punctate keratitis, usually limited to the superior one-third to one-half of the cornea. A subepithelial, V-shaped releucency is sometimes apparent. Corneal filaments are unusual. The tarsal conjunctiva may exhibit a fine, velvety, papillary pattern, but giant papillae or follicles are not characteristic. In several respects these clinical findings are identical to those seen in the idiopathic SLK of Theodore. This SLK variant typically occurs both in cosmetic hard lens wearers who change to soft lenses and use either preserved saline or other chemical-containing care solutions, and in successful soft lens patients who switch from unpreserved saline to preserved care solutions. Indeed, we have never observed this problem in patients using unpreserved saline and heat sterilization. Ocular and skin testing disclosed approximately one-third of patients to be sensitive to thimerosal, and none was reactive to other common contact lens preservatives. The only effective treatment is total abstinence from lens wear for several weeks to months. Adjunctive therapy with topical antibiotics or steroids is of no benefit. The overall prognosis is good with complete resolution of signs and symptoms often requiring several months to occur but with excellent visual recovery. Many of these patients are eventually able to return to successful soft lens wear using non-preserved maintenance systems, or they can use gas-permeable or hard lenses. Recognition of this problem is important, as diagnostic confusion with other forms of chronic keratoconjunctivitis may result in inappropriate management and continued exposure has been reported in rare cases to stimulate corneal scarring with permanent visual reduction.

Giant papillary conjunctivitis (GPC) is undoubtedly the most common complication of soft lens use (Fig. 46.13) (Allansmith *et al.*, 1977). Fortunately, most of these patients are asymptomatic. GPC can occur with all soft lenses and even, rarely, with hard or gas-permeable lenses, although among soft lenses the frequency appears less with high-water-content polymers. As the condition requires months to years to develop, it is not surprising that the condition is most common in cosmetic wearers and exceedingly rare in therapeutic lens patients. GPC-like reactions have also been observed in response to other foreign materials, including nylon sutures and ocular prostheses. Clinically, these patients complain of varying degrees of itching, upper lid swelling, red-

ness, mucoid discharge, decreased vision due to lens coating, and decreased lens tolerance. The bulbar conjunctiva and cornea are usually only minimally inflamed. However, with eversion of the upper lid, papillae greater than 1 mm in diameter are evident. These giant papillae appear identical to those seen in vernal conjunctivitis, and in many respects the pathophysiology of this condition resembles a delayed cutaneous basophilic hypersensitivity. Deposits on the contact lens surface are a constant feature of GPC, and it is thought that the combination of protein build-up on the lens and the mechanical factor of lens edge design can abrade the tarsal conjunctival epithelium, creating a portal of entry for the protein antigens coating the lens. This induces an immune response in the lymphoid tissue of the upper tarsal conjunctiva, in turn causing antibody production which makes the giant papillae grow. The immune response may then release chemotactic factors that draw inflammatory cells into the tissue and mast cells to migrate to abnormal positions. The mast cells degranulate, releasing vasoactive

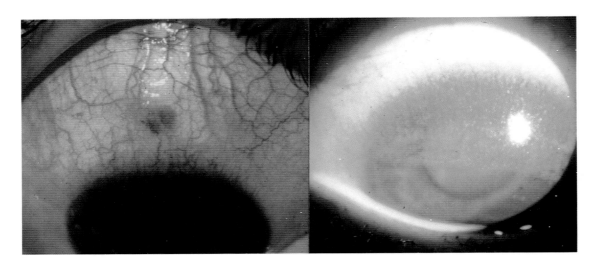

Figure 46.12 (a) Contact lens related superior limbic keratitis (SLK) showing prominent injection of superior bulbar conjunctiva and superior limbal micropannus formation. (b) SPK localized to the superior portion of the cornea, seen with fluorescein staining.

substances and inflammatory mediators, predominantly histamine. This mediator alone can account for the itching, erythema and edema. In addition, mediators released by degranulating mast cells result in eosinophilic infiltration of the tissue. Eosinophil-derived factors, such as major basic protein, neurotoxic factors, and myeloperoxidase-superoxide anion, may cause ocular tissue damage (Udell *et al.*, 1981) and contribute to the tissue changes seen in giant papillary conjunctivitis.

In regard to therapy, cleaning of lens deposits may help to remove protein build-up, and hence more frequent enzyme treatment or new lenses may be useful. Larger-diameter lenses with thicker edges may predispose to GPC, and thus therapy can also include changes to a higher-water-content, smaller-diameter, and thinner-edge lens. Some patients will benefit by switching to gas-permeable lenses. As preservative sensitivity has also been implicated in GPC, other patients may be helped by discontinuing preservative-containing solutions. Finally, some practitioners have recommended sodium cromoglycate (Cromolyn), a mast cell stabilizer that is useful in vernal conjunctivitis. In summary, we can consider both mechanical and allergic factors as being responsible for the immunologic response in the upper tarsal conjunctiva. Particular attention to the removal of these antigens and less mechanical stress on the involved tissue are the principles of therapy.

Corneal infection is undoubtedly the most serious complication of contact lens use. Most commonly caused by bacterial microorganisms (with special predisposition for *Pseudomonas*), fungi and parasites (including *Acanthamoeba*) (Schein *et al.*, 1989a), have also been reported. As discussed previously, several associated risk factors may predispose patients to infectious keratitis. In patients with therapeutic lenses, the anatomically and immunologically compromised cornea is at increased risk for superinfection. In these patients, the adjunctive use of prophylactic broad-spectrum antibiotics (such as chloramphenicol or gentamicin) does not appear to change conjunctival culture results; however, most practitioners recommend the appropriate use of prophylactic antibiotics in these high-risk patients. On the other hand, indiscriminate administration of antibiotics for mild conjunctivitis should be avoided since the excessive use of antimicrobial drugs can result in drug toxicity or allergy, or in the emergence of drug-resistant bacterial strains. A second

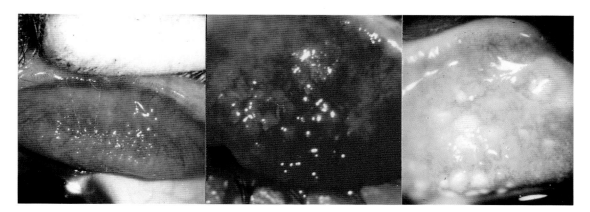

Figure 46.13 (a,b) Giant papillary changes of the tarsal conjunctiva in a SCL wearer, (c) with fluorescein staining.

high-risk group, as noted previously, is the extended-wear aphake. Third, with increasing attention on the toxic and hypersensitivity reactions to lens-care products, there is a tendency to shift toward non-preserved saline solution, with the result that many cases of bacterial keratitis have been reported in patients using non-preserved saline, improperly stored or sterilized, or failing to use accessory thermal disinfection.

Equally important is the recognition that infectious keratitis can occur in healthy patients with healthy eyes who have seemingly not abused either lens wear or lens care (Adams *et al.*, 1983) Holden (1984) estimated the incidence of infectious keratitis in Australia to be one case per 1 million hard or gas-permeable lens wearers, in comparison to 1 per 100 000 daily-wear SCL wearers and 1 per 3 000 extended-wear subjects. Poggio *et al.*, (1989), in a large prospective study carried out in the United States on cosmetic wearers, established the annualized rate of ulcerative keratitis to be 4.1 (95% confidence range 2.9 to 5.2) per 10 000 for daily wear soft contact lenses and 20.9 (95% confidence range 15.1 to 26.7) per 10 000 for extended wear soft contact lenses. Even more ominous is the recognition that the microbial species involved are those most capable of serious sight-threatening sequelae. A number of reviews of infectious keratitis note that the ratio of Gram-positive to Gram-negative infections in the United States is usually about two to one, but a Miami study (Alfonso *et al.*, 1986) of 98 soft lens-wearing patients with microbial keratitis found that 78% involved Gram-negative organisms versus 18% Gram-positive, implying a possibly five-fold increase in Gram-negative organisms. Worse, 93% of the Gram-negatives were *Pseudomonas* with potentially devastating consequences. Similarly, Hassman and Sugar (1983) have reported three cosmetic extended-wear lens patients who developed *Pseudomonas* keratitis. Krachmer and Purcell (1978) recovered *Pseudomonas* from three of

five such CL-related bacterial ulcers. Wilson *et al.*, (1981) observed seven SCL wearers with *Pseudomonas* corneal ulcers associated with the use of saline solutions prepared from distilled water and sodium chloride tablets. Finally, Weissman *et al.*, (1984) reported that 18 bacterial corneal ulcers in extended-wear patients equally divided between myopes and aphakes showed 70% infected with *Pseudomonas*. These authors also raised the question of a potentially increased incidence of this problem with extended wear and related that during the interval they treated these 18 patients, they encountered only 11 daily-wear patients with infectious keratitis. Extrapolating that there are many more daily-wear than extended-wear patients in their population, we have additional 'soft' evidence that bacterial keratitis is an increased risk in extended-wear patients. The increased relative risk, associated with extended wear, suggested by Weissman *et al.*, (1984), has been recently confirmed both in the United States and Europe. Schein *et al.*, (1989b), in a large case control study involving cosmetic wearers, report a relative risk for extended wear contact lenses, compared to daily wear contact lenses, of 3.90 (95% confidence interval 2.35 to 6.48). Interestingly they show in the same study that the problem is not associated with the type of soft contact lens used, but the wearing modality. For example, the relative risk of ulcerative keratitis with extended wear lenses used overnight is 10 to 15 times greater than daily wear lenses used strictly during the day. The relative risk is however not significantly different when extended wear and daily wear contact lenses were both used only during the day. Dart *et al.*, (1991), in the United Kingdom, confirms the increased relative risk of overnight wear. Taking daily wear rigid gas permeable contact lenses as referend, they report a relative risk of 20.8 (95% confidence interval 7.3 to 59.6) for overnight wear soft contact lenses and 3.6 (95% confidence interval 0.9 to 13.9) for daily wear soft contact lenses.

In a recent study, out of 422 patients fitted with extended-wear SCL for aphakia or myopia, 23 patients (5%) developed bacterial corneal ulceration (Aquavella *et al.*, 1985). Forty-three percent of the corneal ulcers were secondary to *P. aeruginosa*. In 43% of the patients with corneal ulcers, a penetrating keratoplasty was required for visual rehabilitation. However, not all corneal ulcers secondary to *P. aeruginosa* have a poor prognosis. If *Pseudomonas* corneal ulcer is detected early and treated appropriately, the condition can resolve without significant visual impairment (Fig. 46.14a). However, delay in initial presentation and commencement of antibiotic therapy can result in severe corneal ulceration and scarring that would require a subsequent penetrating keratoplasty to improve vision (Fig. 14b).

How do we reconcile this conclusion with other large series involving several hundred patients during the initial studies of aphakic Permalenses for whom the incidence of infectious keratitis was very low? (Martin *et al.*, 1983; Lembach & Keates, 1984)? We interpret this as being the result of very close

surveillance and follow-up in these controlled study situations. For example, in Keates' and Lembach's (1984) series of 293 eyes of 137 patients, a total of 2 646 follow-up visits were involved over a 5-year period. In patients followed so intensively, minor complications were probably noted and treated before major problems occurred. In contrast, the studies carried out by Schein *et al.* (1989b) and Dart *et al.* (1991) demonstrated poor compliance and abuse of the lens care system. Adherence to the recommended care regime was variable and a poor adherence was shown to increase the risk of keratitis (Schein *et al.* 1989b). Non-adherence to the wearing schedule was present in both Schein *et al.* (1989b) and Dart *et al.* (1991) studies. In the latter case, 22% of patients used their daily wear lenses overnight.

Thus, as the use of extended-wear lenses proliferates, we must stress caution. In the United States, many patients are wholly unaware of the relatively increased risks with extended-wear contact lenses. The typical American 'one-stop shopping', 'set it and forget it' mentality lures us to overlook the fact that daily care and concern are implicit

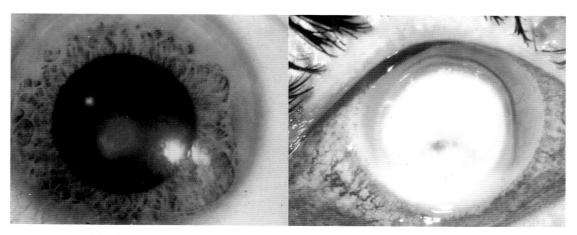

Figure 46.14 (a) Early treatment of extended-wear SCL-related *Pseudomonas* corneal ulcer has resulted in a small scar with no significant visual impairment. (b) Delay in presentation and treatment of *Pseudomonas* corneal ulcer following SCL wear with contaminated home-made saline solution has caused massive stromal necrosis with hypopyon.

even in extended-wear lenses and may lead to carelessness about lens maintenance. The studies of Poggio *et al.* (1989) and Schein *et al.* (1989b) have lead the FDA to change their approval for extended wear contact lenses from 30 days without removal, to 7 days without removal. We note, for example, that many wearers retain their lenses without resterilization for longer than the one week for which they are now approved by the FDA. In our own practice, we limit the duration of extended wear to no more than one week, to over-emphasize the possibility of major complications, and to under-score this with color photographic enlargements of eyes lost to bacterial keratitis. Patients should be admonished not only to return for routine follow-up, but also to 'run, not walk' to your office when even minor irritative problems occur.

In terms of specific therapeutic recommendations, we continue to stress the need for careful patient selection in dispensing extended-wear lenses for myopia or aphakia. Proper lens care and hygiene are important to avoid infection. Careful follow-up to ensure continuing good fit and corneal integrity is vital. Patients must be instructed to remove their lenses at the first sign of redness or discomfort and to see their contact lens practitioner if symptoms do not abate with lens removal. All corneal infiltrates with overlying epithelial defects should be suspected of having bacterial origin and should be scraped for smears and cultures. A high index of suspicion is warranted, since Gram-negative microbes, especially *Pseudomonas*, are frequently isolated. Because of the potential for rapid progression, intensive fortified topical antibiotics (but only rarely subconjunctival antibiotics) and hospitalization are indicated. To ensure broad spectrum coverage, initial treatment should include both an aminoglycoside (tobramycin or gentamicin) and cefazolin, and/or fluoroquinolone with treatment modified pending the clinical course and the results of cultures and sensitivities. Carbenicillin and ticarcillin are synergistic with aminoglycosides, and either may be added when a Gram-negative organism is suspected or proven.

In summary, with the continuing advance of hydrophilic contact lens technology, an ever-increasing number of individuals are turning to soft lenses for therapeutic and cosmetic purposes, as both daily- and extended-wear options make hydrogel lenses a far more attractive alternative to either spectacles or hard lenses. On the downside, however, we continue to appreciate the numerous and sometimes serious complications of soft lenses. Although many problems such as corneal edema and superficial neovascularization are transient and may subside by simple lens abstinence or replacement, others, particularly ulcerative keratitis, pose a real threat to vision. Hence, both patient and practitioner must be aware of these potential complications so that intelligent management decisions can be made regarding contact lens wear.

REFERENCES

Abelson, M.B., Butrus, S.I. and Weston, J.H. (1983) *Thimerosal Update: Thimerosal Hypersensitivity in Wearers of Soft Contact Lenses.* Excerpta Medica, Princeton, NJ.

Adams, C.P. Jr, Cohen, E.J., Laibson, P.R., Galentine, P. and Arentsen, J.J., (1983) Corneal ulcers in patients with cosmetic extended-wear contact lenses. *Am. J. Ophthalmol.*, **96**, 705.

Alfonso, E., Fox, M.J., Mandelbaum, S. and Forster, R.K. (1986) Ulcerative keratitis associated with contact lens wear. *Am. J. Ophthalmol.*, **101**, 423.

Allansmith, M.R., Korb, D.R., Greiner, J.V., Henriquez, A.S., Simon, M.A. and Finnemore, V.M. (1977) Giant papillary conjunctivitis in contact lens wearers. *Am. J. Ophthalmol.*, **83**, 697.

Aquavella, J.V., Rao, G.N. and John, T. (1985) Corneal ulceration associated with extended-wear soft contact lenses. *Geriatric Ophthalmol.*, **1**, 9.

Berger, R.O. and Streeten, B.W. (1981) Fungal growth in aphakic soft contact lenses. *Am. J. Ophthalmol.*, **91**, 630.

Bergmanson, J.P.G., Ruben, C.M. and Chu, L.W.-F. (1985) Epithelial morphological response to soft hydrogel contact lenses. *Br. J. Ophthalmol.*, **69**, 373.

Binder, P.S. (1979) Complications associated with extended wear of soft contact lenses. *Ophthalmology*, **86**, 1093.

Binder, P.S., Rasmussen, D.M. and Gordon, (1981) Keratoconjunctivitis and soft contact lens solutions. *Arch. Ophthalmol.*, **99**, 87.

Boisjoly, H.M., Pavan-Langston, D., Kenyon, K.R. and Baker, A.S. (1983) Super-infections in herpes simplex keratitis. *Am. J. Ophthalmol.*, **96**, 354.

Churner, R. and Cunningham, R.D. (1983) Fungal-contaminated soft contact lenses. *Ann. Ophthalmol.*, **15**, 724.

Dart, J.K.G, Stapleton, F. and Minassian, D. (1991) Contact lenses and other risk factors in microbial keratitis. *Lancet*, **338**, 650–3.

Dohlman, C.H. (1974) Complications in therapeutic soft lens wear. (Symposium: Soft contact lenses). *Trans. Am. Acad. Ophthalmol. Otolaryngol.*, **78**, OP339.

Fowler, S.A., Greiner, J.V. and Allansmith, M.R. (1979) Attachment of bacteria to soft contact lenses. *Arch. Ophthalmol.*, **97**, 659.

Hassman, G. and Sugar, J. (1983) *Pseudomonas* corneal ulcer with extended-wear soft contact lenses for myopia. *Arch. Ophthalmol.*, **101**, 1549.

Holden, B. (1984) *The incidence of corneal infection in contact lens wear*. Fifth International Contact Lens Congress, Surfers Paradise, Australia.

Jackman, S.H. and Rosenbusch, R.F. (1984) *In vitro* adherence of *Moraxella bovis* to intact corneal epithelium. *Curr. Eye Res.*, **3**, 1107.

John, T. Refojo, M.F., Hanninen, L., Leong, F.L., Medina, A. and Kenyon, K.R. (1989a) Adherence of viable and nonviable bacteria to soft contact lenses. *Cornea*, **8**, 21.

John, T., Desai, D. and Sahm, D. (1989b) Adherence of *Acanthamoeba castellanii* cysts and trophozoites to hydrogel contact lenses. *Invest. Ophthalmol. Vis. Sci.*, **30 (Suppl.)**, 480.

Johnson, A.P, Wool, B.M., and Johnson, M.K. (1984) Adherence of *Staphylococcus aureus* to rabbit corneal epithelial cells. *Arch. Ophthalmol.*, **102**, 1229.

Krachmer, J.H. and Purcell, J.J. Jr (1978) Bacterial corneal ulcers in cosmetic soft contact lens wearers. *Arch. Ophthalmol.*, **96**, 57.

Lembach, R.G. and Keates, R.H. (1984) Long-term follow-up of extended wear aphakic Permalenses. *CLAO J.*, **10**, 83.

Lemp, M.A. (1980) The effect of extended-wear aphakic hydrophilic contact lenses after penetrating keratoplasty. *Am. J. Ophthalmol.*, **90**, 331.

Mackman, G., Polack, F.M. and Sidrys, L. (1985) Fluorescein angiography of soft contact lens induced vascularization in penetrating keratoplasty. *Ophthalmic Surg.*, **16**, 157.

Martin, N.F., Kracher., G.P., Stark, W.J. and Maumenee, E. (1983) Extended-wear soft contact lenses for aphakic correction. *Arch. Ophthalmol.*, **101**, 39.

Mondino, B.J. and Groden, L.R. (1980) Conjunctival hyperemia and corneal infiltrates with chemically disinfected soft contact lenses. *Arch. Ophthalmol.*, **98**, 1767.

Penley, C.A., Llabrés, C., Wilson, L.A. and Ahearn, D.G. (1985) Efficacy of hydrogen peroxide disinfection systems for soft contact lenses contaminated with fungi. *CLAO J.*, **11**, 5.

Poggio, E.C., Glynn, R.J., Schein, O.D. *et al.* (1989) The incidence of ulcerative keratitis among users of daily wear and extended wear soft contact lenses. *N. Engl. J. Med.*, **321**, 779–83.

Ramphal, R., McNiece, M.T. and Polack, F.M. (1981) Adherence of *Pseudomonas aeruginosa* to the injured cornea: A step in the pathogenesis of corneal infections. *Ann. Ophthalmol.*, **13**, 421.

Reichert, R. and Stern, G. (1984) Quantitative adherence of bacteria to human corneal epithelial cells. *Arch. Ophthalmol.*, **102**, 394.

Schein, O.D., Ormerod, L.D., Barraquer, E. *et al.* (1989a) Microbiology of contact lens-related keratitis. *Cornea*, **8**(4), 281–5.

Schein, O.D., Glynn, R.J., Poggio, E.C. *et al.* (1989b) The relative risk of ulcerative keratitis among users of daily wear and extended wear soft contact lenses. *N. Engl. J. Med.*, **321**, 773–8.

Ruben, M., Brown, N., Lobascher, D., Chaston, and Morris, (1976) Clinical manifestations secondary to soft contact lens wear. *Br. J. Ophthalmol.*, **60**, 529.

Sendele, D.D, Kenyon, K.R., Mobilia, E.F., Rosenthal, P., Steinert, R. and Hanninen, L.A. (1983) Superior limbic keratoconjunctivitis in contact lens wearers. *Ophthalmology*, **90**, 616.

Stark, W.J., Kracher, G.P., Cowan, C.L., Taylor, H.R., Hirst, L.W., Oyakawa, R.T. and Maumenee, A.E. (1979) Extended-wear contact lenses and intraocular lenses for aphakic correction. *Am. J. Ophthalmol.*, **88**, 535.

Stenson, S (1984) Complications of soft contact lenses. *Ophthalmic Forum*, **2**(2), 74.

et al., 1987). Similarly, silicone contact lenses, rigid gas-permeable (RGP) polymer lenses and hydrogel materials also accumulate lipids (Tripathi & Tripathi, 1984; Hartstein, 1985; Hart *et al.*, 1986, 1987). The mechanism for lipid inter-action with hydrogels might be associated with protein adsorption to the hydrogel lenses (i.e. the adherent proteins could introduce hydrophobic and complexation sites in or on the lenses). Also, the lipids can form three-dimensional aggregates within the lenses. These aggregates probably assemble in the presence of protein and calcium ions. 'Jelly bumps' on contact lenses are thought to be largely lipids and calcium (Hart *et al.*, 1986; Corkhill *et al.*, 1990). Thus lipids have potential mechanisms whereby they can interact with all important lens types, and, indeed, lipid-like deposits are seen on all types of lenses. How-ever, the problem is especially important for silicone and RGP lenses.

47.4   CALCIFICATION AND MINERALIZATION OF BIOMEDICAL DEVICES

Lens deposits containing calcium, magnesium, or sodium have been reported to occur as a result of mineral accumulation from tears. Other compounds containing such substances as iron, mercury, silica, chromium, and copper have been reported in lens deposits, but are attributed to extrinsic factors (Tripathi & Tripathi, 1984). Deposits containing calcium salts are the most common mineralized lens deposits.

Calcification of a biomedical device usually involves the deposition of hydroxyapatite, the form of calcium phosphate commonly encountered in the body, onto the surface of the device (Schoen *et al.*, 1988). This process occurs in a variety of biomaterial devices: bioprosthetic heart valves (Schoen, 1987), mechanical blood pumps (Coleman, 1981; Coleman *et al.*, 1981) intrauterine contraceptive devices (Khan & Wilkinson, 1985), and contact lenses (Ruben *et al.*, 1975).

Heavy, calcified films on hydrogel contact lenses can cause damage to the lens surface because the mineralization may penetrate into the lens matrix (Bowers & Tighe, 1987a). These deposits are commonly composed of calcium phosphate with coprecipitated pro-tein. The main cause of these deposits appears to be the precipitation and growth of calcium phosphate from tears while the lens is in the eye. Some studies suggest that protein films could predispose the lens to a build-up of inorganic material (Bowers & Tighe, 1987a), and other studies report that lipids and lipid–mineral complexes are involved in the nucleation of apatite crystals on medical devices (Owen & Zone, 1981; Schoen *et al.*, 1988).

Bowers and Tighe (1987a) have suggested that the mechanism that leads to corneal calcification might contribute to lens calcifi-cation. In this process, the release of calcium and phosphorus from injured cells increases the local calcium phosphate concentration. This increase, along with the release of cellular enzymes such as adenosine triphos-phatase and alkaline phosphatase, could trigger calcification. These enzymes cause the hydrolysis of pyrophosphates (physiological inhibitors of calcification in soft tissues) to inorganic phosphate. Once it is precipitated, hydroxyapatite grows from slightly supersaturated solutions such as tears.

47.5   MEASUREMENT OF LENS DEPOSITION

In 1891, Lord Kelvin stated, 'When you can measure what you are speaking about, and express it in numbers, you know something about it; but when you cannot measure it, when you cannot express it in numbers, your knowledge is of a meagre and unsatisfactory kind.' Unfortunately, most of the papers reporting on contact lens deposition are qualitative. This lack of quantitative literature exists, in part, because the problems of measuring lens deposition are formidable. For clinical practitioners, nondestructive, qualitative techniques such as slit lamp biomicroscopy, specular microscopy, and light microscopy are easily accessible and simple to perform. However, for a fuller understanding of the composition and cause of deposits, a combination of several quantitative techniques is necessary.

In this section, we present a few comments on how measurements and observations have been made on lens deposits, and the concerns with these measurements. This will help the reader appreciate the literature on this subject. In addition, we suggest specific spectroscopic and biochemical methods that can be used to quantitatively study lenses and lens deposits.

47.5.1 MICROSCOPIC METHODS

A wide variety of microscopic methods have been used to examine gross and fine morphological aspects of the deposits on contact lenses (Tripathi & Tripathi, 1984; Hart *et al.*, 1986; Bilbaut *et al.*, 1986; Klotz *et al.*, 1987). These methods include hand magnifying lenses, slit lamp microscopy, specular microscopy (to 300×), conventional light microscopy (including stereomicroscopy, phase contrast microscopy, polarization microscopy, and staining and immunocytological methods coupled with these microscopies), confocal scanning microscopy, scanning electron microscopy (SEM), and transmission electron microscopy (TEM). The latter two methods can be performed only outside the eye on specially prepared (fixed) lenses. Although these methods have primarily been used in a qualitative fashion, they do provide an overview of the morphologic nature of the deposit and a rough assessment of its magnitude.

Computer image analysis, particularly in conjunction with confocal microscopy, SEM,

and TEM, can provide some level of quantitative information. Although these methods do not work well for analyzing thin, uniform coating deposits (e.g. monolayer films of proteins) on lenses, they can be used to examine granular, electron-dense deposits. Several investigators have used electron microprobe X-ray analysis to examine inorganic deposits on soft lenses (Tripathi *et al.*, 1978; Bilbaut *et al.*, 1986; Tripathi & Tripathi, 1984). By using this technique, Tripathi et al. determined that the principal component of a deposit had a Ca:P ratio of 3:1, consistent with calcium triphosphate (Tripathi *et al.*, 1978). Bilbaut *et al.* used this method to perform semiquantitative elemental analyses on several types of deposits (Bilbaut *et al.*, 1986) Hart *et al.* (1986) studied the calcium composition of jelly bumps with analytical SEM.

47.5.2 SPECTROSCOPIC METHODS

Spectroscopic methods typically measure the energy absorbed or emitted by the deposit on the lens surface. Some of these methods are schematically illustrated in Figure 47.4.

Infrared absorption (IR) has been used in some studies to observe lens deposits (Castillo *et al.*, 1984, 1985, 1986). Specific absorption bands indicative of protein, carbohydrate, lipid, or mineralized materials can be monitored. Studies are complicated by the presence of water and by geometric requirements imposed by the need for extremely thin samples. Most contact lens IR studies are performed using the attenuated total reflectance (ATR) technique (Fig. 47.4a). ATR permits analysis by IR of deposits on only the outermost 1–5 μm of the lens surface. This simplifies sample preparation and examines a relevant region of the lens.

Other spectroscopic methods that can be applied to contact lens studies include electron spectroscopy for chemical analysis (ESCA, a method that measures the outermost 50 Å of a lens) (Ratner & McElroy, 1986),

47.6.1 CLINICAL OBSERVATIONS OF CONTACT LENS DEPOSITS

Systematic descriptions of deposits on contact lenses have been appearing in the literature since at least the early 1970s. Good overviews of the literature that describe clinical observations of contact lens deposits have been published (Wedler & Riedhammer, 1982; Tripathi & Tripathi, 1984; Bowers & Tighe, 1987a, b; Hart & Shih, 1987).

One of the earliest attempts to classify lens coatings and depositions was developed by Rudko and Proby in a 1974 Allergan report. This *in vitro* classification scheme divided lenses into four categories: I = no deposit visible on wet or dry lenses with 15× magnification, II = deposits visible on wet lenses with 15× magnification, III = deposits visible on dry lenses without magnification, and IV = deposits visible on wet lenses without magnification. Contact lens deposits were classified by Tripathi and Tripathi (1984) into categories by type of deposit (similar to Table 47.1). Josephson and Caffery (1989), based upon the slit lamp biomicroscopy examination of lenses in the eye, proposed that lenses be graded as follows: 0 = a smooth, uniformly reflecting surface; 1 = a coarse, hazy surface that is temporarily resolved with each blink; 2 = a stable, nonwetting area of some magnitude; and 3 = gross crystalline or amorphous deposits. Hart recently proposed a biomicroscopy classification method, as presented in Table 47.3.

Papers in the clinical literature on lens deposits fall into a few distinct categories: descriptions of types of deposits, biochemical analyses of deposits, comparisons of various lenses in their tendency to deposit, and management of deposits. Interesting examples in each category are briefly discussed in the following paragraphs.

Studies that describe specific types of deposits on one or many lenses are common. For example, Bowers and Tighe (1987b) examined white spot deposits by means of SEM. They found these elevated deposits to be 40 to 160 µm in diameter and to exhibit a complex three-layer morphology. Other reports consider the discoloration of lenses, related to the material of the lens itself, preservatives, or protein (Stone *et al.*, 1984; Wardlow & Sarver, 1986). Hart *et al.* describe jelly bump deposits (1986) and relate these to patient diet (1987). Use of certain drugs, and high intake levels of cholesterol, protein, and alcohol, all correlated significantly with jelly bump formation.

Papers on the biochemical analysis of deposits provide more specific, but still nonquantitative information. One of the earliest papers presenting a systematic study of lens deposits using biochemical methods was published by Wedler in 1977. By using fluorescein-labeled antibodies, he found albumin, lysozyme, γ-globulin, and γ_1-lipoprotein in all deposits on worn polymacon lenses. He found SDS and dithiothreitol to be effective in removing lens protein, which he subsequently analyzed by using

Table 47.3 Table of lens coating classifications (Hart *in situ* biomicroscopy method)

Grade/type	
I	No tear film break-up ≥ 10 seconds of withheld blinking
II	Tear film break-up on lens between 5 and 9 seconds
III	Tear film break-up on lens between 2 and 4 seconds
IV	Protruding deposit; unwettable; instantaneous tear film break-up

electrophoretic methods. Klotz *et al.* (1987), analyzed the nature of carbohydrate material (probably associated with glycoprotein) by using fluorescein-labeled lectins. Bilbaut *et al.* (1986) studied lens deposits with electron microprobe methods and electrophoresis of SDS-extracted protein. Different deposit morphologies had different compositions, but all deposits contained lysozyme. Although these studies provide specific biochemical descriptions of deposits, none of them allow a quantitative assessment of the various components present.

Comparison papers attempt to reach conclusions as to which type of lens will lead to the lowest level of deposition. For example, Tomlinson and Caroline (1989) compared the contamination resistance of poly(2-hydroxyethyl methacrylate) (PHEMA) (phemfilcon A, actually a HEMA/2-ethoxyethyl methacrylate copolymer), modified HEMA (bufilcon A, a HEMA/diacetone/acrylamide copolymer) and non-HEMA (crofilcon A, a methyl methacrylate/glyceryl methacrylate copolymer) contact lenses. By using a digitizer to count deposits in SEM photographs of several worn lenses (10 patients), the authors concluded that the modified HEMA, and non-HEMA lenses exhibit considerably better deposit resistance than the HEMA lens. Without quantitative analysis of deposit chemistry and larger sample sizes, comparison papers do not provide definitive answers.

A number of papers are available on the management of deposits. Nolan and Nolan (1985) reported that persistent deposits on silicone acrylate lenses and consequent patient discomfort can be controlled only by teaching the wearer to recognize the deposit formation and to use an abrasive cleaning-agent polish to bring the lens back to a 'crystal-like' shine. Another study compared, for 66 wearers, the typical peroxide cleaning method to a procedure using the peroxide cleaning plus a once-per-week enzyme cleaning (Nilsson & Lindh, 1988). The lenses that received the peroxide and enzyme cleaning exhibited lower levels of deposits at six months.

47.6.2 FUNDAMENTAL STUDIES ON CONTACT LENS DEPOSITIONS

Fundamental studies permit lens interactions to be studied in a systematic fashion with appropriate controls and experimental design. However, the relevance of these studies can always be questioned because of the limited availability of pure tear proteins and the inability to properly simulate the ocular environment. Still, these studies can provide important insights that can be tested first in animal models and then in the clinic.

One of the earliest basic studies of protein adsorption to hydrogels of the types used in contact lenses was by Refojo and Holly (1977). They studied the adsorption of albumin, γ-globulins and lysozome to PHEMA and poly(glyceryl methacrylate-co-methyl methacrylate) lens buttons. Based upon contact angle measurements they concluded that protein adsorption readily occurs and that adsorbed proteins can be resistant to removal.

Early studies on protein adsorption to contact lens materials were performed by Royce *et al.* (1982); later, these studies were followed up in a series of more detailed experiments by Bohnert *et al.* (1988). By using ^{125}I-labeled proteins, Royce *et al.* (1982) measured the extent of protein adsorption and noted the following results: during exposure to an artificial tear solution (lysozyme, albumin and IgG in buffer) containing a radiolabeled tag protein, each composition of polymers and copolymers of HEMA and methyl methacrylate (MMA) adsorbed a different total amount of protein, and each adsorbed a different composition of surface protein from the artificial tear mixture.

By using a similar technique, Bohnert *et al.* (1988) found that the majority of adsorbed protein on all MMA-HEMA polymers was

interaction chromatography and stationary phases comparison. *J. Chromatogr.*, **458**, 93–104.

Benedek, K., Dong, S. and Karger, B.L. (1984) Kinetics of unfolding of proteins on hydrophobic surfaces in reversed-phase liquid chromatography. *J. Chromatogr.*, **317**, 227–43.

Benedek, K., Lu, S.M. and Karger, B.L. (1986) Conformational effects in the high-performance liquid chromatography of proteins. *J. Chromatogr.*, **359**, 19–29.

Bilbaut, T., Gachon, A.M. and Dastugue, B. (1986) Deposits on soft contact lenses. Electrophoresis and scanning electron microscopic examinations. *Exp. Eye Res.*, **43**, 153–65.

Binder, P.S. and Worthen, D.M. (1977) Clinical evaluation of continuous-wear hydrophilic lenses. *Am. J. Ophthal.*, **83**, 549–53.

Bohnert, J.L. and Horbett T.A. (1986) Changes in adsorbed fibrinogen and albumin interactions with polymers indicated by decreases in detergent elutability. *J. Coll. Interf. Sci.*, **111**, 363–77.

Bohnert, J.L., Horbett, T.A., Ratner, B.D. and Royce, F.H. (1988) Adsorption of proteins from artificial tear solutions to contact lens materials. *Invest. Ophthalmol. Vis. Sci.*, **29**, 362–73.

Bowers, R.W.J. and Tighe, B.J. (1987a) Studies of the ocular compatibility of hydrogels. A review of the clinical manifestations of spoilation. *Biomaterials*, **8**, 83–8.

Bowers, R.W.J. and Tighe, B.J. (1987b) Studies of the ocular compatibility of hydrogels. White spot deposits – incidence of occurrence, location and gross morphology. *Biomaterials*, **8**, 89–93.

Brash, J.L. (1981) Protein interactions with artificial surfaces. In *Interaction of the Blood with Natural and Artificial Surfaces*, (ed. E.W. Salzman), Marcel Dekker, New York, pp. 37–60.

Briggs, D. (1989) Recent advances in secondary ion mass spectrometry (SIMS) for polymer surface analysis. *Br. Polym. J.*, **21**, 3–15.

Bull, H.B. and Neurath, H. (1937) The denaturation and hydration of proteins. II. Surface denaturation of egg albumin. *J. Biol. Chem.*, **118**, 163–75.

Castillo, E.J., Koenig, J.L., Anderson, J.M. and Lo, J. (1984) Characterization of protein adsorption on soft contact lenses. I. Conformational changes of adsorbed human serum albumin. *Biomaterials*, **5**, 319–25.

Castillo, E.J., Koenig,, J.L. Anderson, J.M. and Lo, J. (1985) Protein adsorption on hydrogels. II. Reversible and irreversible interactions

between lysozyme and soft contact lens surfaces. *Biomaterials*, **6**, 338–45.

Castillo, E.J., Koenig, J.L., Anderson, J.M. and Jentoft, N. (1986) Protein adsorption on soft contact lenses III. Mucin. *Biomaterials*, **7**, 9–16.

Castner, D.G. and Ratner, B.D. (1988) Static secondary ion mass spectroscopy: a new technique for the characterization of biomedical polymer surfaces. In *Surface Characterization of Biomaterials* (ed. B.D. Ratner), Elsevier Press, Amsterdam, pp. 65–81.

Cohen, S.A., Dong, S., Benedek, K. and Karger, B.L. (1983) Multiple peak formation in the reversed phase liquid chromatographic separation of soybean trypsin inhibitor. *Affinity Chromatography and Biological Recognition*, 479–87.

Cohen S.A., Benedek, K.P., Dong, S. Tapuhi, Y. and Karger, B.L. (1984) Multiple peak formation in reversed-phase liquid chromatography of papain. *Anal. Chem.*, **56**, 217–21.

Cohen, S.A., Benedek, K., Tapuhi, Y., Ford, J.C. and Karger, B.L. (1985) Conformational effects in the reversed-phase liquid chromatography of ribonuclease A. *Anal. Biochem.*, **144**, 275–84.

Coleman, D.L. (1981) Mineralization of blood pump bladders. *Trans. Am. Soc. Artif. Int. Organs*, **27**, 708–13.

Coleman, D.L., Lim, D., Kessler, T. and Andrade, J.D. (1981) Calcification of nontextured implantable blood pumps' *Trans. Am. Soc. Artif. Int. Organs*, 27, 97–104.

Corkhill, P.H., Hamilton, C.J. and Tighe, B.J. (1990) The design of hydrogels for medical applications. *CRC Crit. Rev. Biocompat.*, **5**, 363–436.

Davies M.C. and Lynn, R.A.P. (1990) Static secondary ion mass spectrometry of polymeric biomaterials. *CRC Crit. Rev. Biocompat.*, **5**, 297–341.

Deng, X.M., Castillo, E.J. and Anderson, J.M. (1986) Surface modification of soft contact lenses: silanization, wettability and lysozyme adsorption studies. *Biomaterials*, **7**, 247–51.

Desai, N.P. and Hubbell, J.A. (1991) Biological responses to polyethylene oxide modified polyethylene terephthalate surfaces. *J. Biomed. Mater. Res.*, **25**, 829–43.

Dong, D.E., Andrade, J.D. and Coleman, D.L. (1987) Adsorption of low density lipoproteins onto selected biomedical polymers. *J. Biomed. Mater. Res.*, **21**, 683–700.

Galle, P., Berry, J.P. and Escaig, F. (1983) Secondary ion mass microanalysis: applications in biology. *SEM*, **II**, 827–39.

Gombotz, W.R., Guanghui, W. and Hoffman, A.S. (1988) Immobilization of poly(ethylene oxide) on poly(ethylene terephthalate) using a plasma polymerization process. *J. Appl. Polym. Sci.*, **35**, 1–17.

Hart, D.E. and Shih, K.L. (1987) Surface interactions on hydrogel extended wear contact lenses: microflora and microfauna. *Am. J. Optom. Physiol. Optics*, **64**, 739–48.

Hart, D.E., Tidsale, R.R. and Sack, R.A. (1986) Origin and composition of lipid deposits on soft contact lenses. *Ophthalmology*, **93**, 495–503.

Hart, D.E., Lane, B.C., Josephson, J.E., Tidsale, R.R., Gzik, M., Leahy, M.R. and Dennis, R. (1987) Spoilage of hydrogel contact lenses by lipid deposits. *Ophthalmology*, **94**, 1315–21.

Hartstein, J. (1985) Hydrophilic lens deposits. *Ocular Surg. News*, **3**, 38–41.

Horbett, T.A. (1982) Protein adsorption on biomaterials. In *Biomaterials: Interfacial Phenomena and Applications, ACS Advances in Chemistry Series*, Vol. 199 (eds. S.L. Cooper and N.A. Peppas), American Chemical Society, Washington, D. C., pp. 233–44.

Horbett, T.A. and J.L. Brash, (1987) Proteins at interfaces: current issues and future prospects. In *Proteins at Interfaces: Physicochemical and Biochemical Studies, ACS Symposium Series*, Vol. 343 (eds. T.A. Horbett and J.L. Brash), American Chemical Society, Washington, D.C., pp.1–33.

James, L.K. and Augenstein, L.G. (1966) Adsorption of enzymes at interfaces: Film formation and the effect on activity. *Adv. Enzymol.*, **28**, 1–40.

Josephson, J.E. and Caffery, B.E. (1989) Classification of the surface appearance characteristics of contact lenses in vivo. *Optom. Vis. Sci.*, **66**, 130–2.

Khan, S.R. and Wilkinson, E.J. (1985) Scanning electron microscopy, x-ray diffraction, and electron microprobe analysis of calcific deposits on intrauterine contraceptive devices. *Human Pathology*, **16**, 732–8.

Klotz, S.A., Misra, R.P. and Butrus, S.I. (1987) Carbohydrate deposits on the surfaces of worn extended-wear soft contact lenses. *Arch. Ophthal.*, **105**, 974–7.

Lenk, T.J., Horbett, T.A., Ratner, B.D. and Chittur, K.K. (1991) Infrared studies of time-dependent changes in fibrinogen adsorbed to polyurethanes. *Langmuir* **7**, 1755–64.

Lopez, G.P., Ratner, B.D., Tidwell, C.D., Haycox, C.L., Rapoza, R.J. and Horbett, T.A. (1991) Plasma deposition of tetraethylene glycol dimethyl ether for nonfouling biomaterial surfaces *J. Biomed. Mater. Res.*, **26**, 415–39.

Macritchie, F. (1978) Proteins at interfaces. *Adv. Protein*, **32**, 283–326.

Mayhan, K.G., Hahn, A.W., Dortch, S.W., Wu, S.H., Peace, B.W., Biolsi, M.E. and Bertrand, G.L. (1977) The effect of catalyst concentration on the cured properties of a medical grade RTV silicone elastomer. *Int. J. Polym. Mater.*, **5**, 231–49.

Merrill, E.W., Pekala, R.W. and Mahmud, N.A. (1987) Hydrogels for blood contact. In *Hydrogels in Medicine and Pharmacy. Properties and Applications*, Vol. 3 (ed. N.A. Peppas), CRC Press, Inc., Boca Raton, FL, pp. 1–16.

Miller, I.R. (1971) Interactions of adsorbed proteins and polypeptides at interfaces In *Progress in Surface and Membrane Science*, Vol. 4, (ed. J.F. Danielli, M.D. Rosenberg, and D.A. Cadenhead), Weizmann Inst. Sci., Rehovot, Israel, pp. 299–350.

Nilsson, S.E.G. and Lindh, H. (1988) Hydrogel contact lens cleaning with or without multienzymes: a prospective study. *Acta Ophthalmol.*, **66**, 15–18.

Nolan, J.J. and Nolan, J.A. (1985) Managing persistant deposits on silicone/acrylates. *Contact Lens Forum*, **10**, 55–8.

Norde, W. (1986) Adsorption of proteins from solution at the solid-liquid interface. *Adv. Coll. Interf. Sci.*, **25**, 267–340.

Owen, D.R. and Zone, R.M. (1981) Analysis of a possible mechanism of surface calcification on a biomedical elastomer. *Trans. Am. Soc. Artif. Int. Organs*, **27**, 528–31.

Ratner, B.D. and McElroy, B.J. (1986) Electron spectroscopy for chemical analysis: applications in the biomedical sciences. In *Spectroscopy in the Biomedical Sciences*, (ed. R.M. Gendreau), CRC Press, Boca Raton, Fl, pp. 107–40.

Refojo, M.F. and Holly, F.J. (1977) Tear protein adsorption on hydrogels: a possible cause of contact lens allergy *Contact Intraocul. Lens Med. J.*, **3**, 23–35.

Royce Jr., F.H., Ratner, B.D. and Horbett, T.A. (1982) Adsorption of proteins from artificial tear solutions to poly(methyl methacrylate-2-hydroxyethyl methacrylate) copolymers. *ACS Adv. Chem. Ser.*, **199**, 453–62.

Ruben, M., Tripathi, R.C. and Winder, A.F. (1975) Calcium deposition as a cause of spoilation of

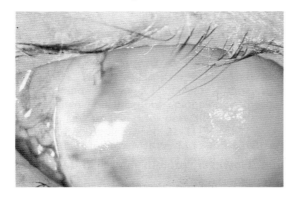

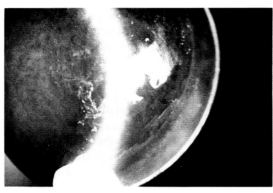

Figure 47.5 (a) An extended-wear hydrogel contact lens worn by the patient. Note the heavy coating by protein film. (b) A protein film deposited on a soft contact lens and examined by slit lamp microscopy. Note also focal opaque calcareous deposits on the lens surface.

more readily than do non-ionic ones (Lowther, 1986).

Other factors that favor protein build-up include the use of thermal disinfection, incomplete blinking, tear deficiency, altered tear composition, chronic allergic conjunctivitis, and giant papillary conjunctivitis. Protein deposits are also a factor in the etiology of giant papillary conjunctivitis (Spring, 1974; Allansmith *et al.*, 1977; Refojo & Holly, 1977; Mondino *et al.*, 1982). Proteins combine with chlorhexidine to form an antigenic complex that may cause protein conjunctivitis (Tripathi *et al.*, 1988). Proteins can also provide a substrate for the colonization

and growth of microorganisms.

The incidence of protein deposits varies from 14% to 80% within three months to one year of wear (Tripathi & Tripathi, 1984). Such protein build-up impairs the transparency of the lens. In addition to optical aberrations such as reduction of visual acuity, proteinaceous deposits cause the lens to feel sticky and produce ocular irritation, as well as other keratoconjunctival symptoms and signs. Furthermore, the deposition of protein can damage the lens material.

Lipid film

Lipid appears as a greasy, smooth, and glistening film, frequently with fingerprint impressions (Fig. 47.6). By polarized light microscopy, these deposits show a 'Maltese cross' birefringence pattern. Lipids may be removed with lipolytic enzymes. However, the breakdown of triglycerides releases free fatty acids which contribute to ocular irritation (Tripathi & Tripathi, 1984). The various lipids which have been identified include phospholipids, triglycerides, cholesterol and its esters, as well as both saturated and unsaturated fatty acids (Tripathi & Tripathi, 1981; Hart, 1984).

Much of the lipid material originates from extraneous sources such as fingers and cosmetics (mascara, eyeliner, pencils, or creams) which contain waxy substances such as phospholipids, lecithin, cholesterol, beeswax, lanolin, spermaceticetyl alcohol, petroleum, cocoa butter, paraffin, diethylene glycol stearate, triethinomine, and stearic acid. The lipids of ocular origin most often are derived from the glands of the lids, i.e. the meibomian glands and the glands of Zeis. These ocular lipids are especially problematic when they are secreted in increased amounts, as occurs in the presence of bacterial conjunctivitis, chronic blepharoconjunctivitis, and meibomianitis (Tripathi & Tripathi, 1984). A lipid-rich tear film favors further deposition of lipids (Josephson &

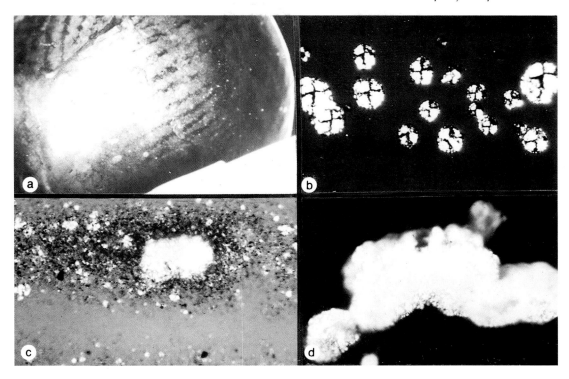

Figure 47.6 Various profiles of lipid deposits on hydrophilic contact lenses. Top left: greasy fingerprint impression (gross view). Top right: characteristic Maltese-cross pattern of lipid deposits on a lens surface as revealed by polarization microscopy (original magnification × 135). Bottom left: surface of a soft lens contaminated with mascara as seen by polarization microscopy which also highlights the lipoidal component of the cosmetic (original magnification × 295). Bottom right: cryosection of contact lens stained with oil red O and viewed with polarized light microscope. The birefringent deposit consists predominantly of lipid that has partly infiltrated the anterior lens matrix (original magnification × 700).

Caffery, 1981). Dry-eye syndrome predisposes to lipid deposition (Doughman *et al.*, 1975), as does a dry atmosphere. Lipids render the lens surface hydrophobic, with resulting dryness and poor wettability. Thus a positive-feedback cycle ensues. Incomplete blinking is another factor associated with lipid deposits (Hart, 1984, Tripathi & Tripathi, 1984). Patients who suffer from nocturnal lagophthalmos and those who use extended-wear lenses are prone to deposition of lipid when the tears dry on the lens surface, for example, during sleep (Wagner *et al.*, 1980; Tripathi & Tripathi, 1981).

Chlorhexidine renders the lens surface hydrophobic and thus lipophilic. Silicone lenses are ordinarily more lipophilic than are other lens materials, especially when their surface coating has become degraded (Tripathi *et al.*, 1980). There seems to be a relationship between lipid deposits and wearers' blood levels of lipoproteins, triglycerides, cholesterol, and alkaline phosphatase. The deposition of lipid is also associated with the use of contraceptive pills (de Vries, 1985) and diuretics (Masterson, 1982).

Bacterial film

Bacteria contaminating soft contact lenses form a translucent film. Gram stain can narrow the differential diagnosis (Fig. 47.7), but culture provides a more definitive identification. Bacteria that contaminate contact lenses include *Staphylococcus aureus, Staphylococcus epidermidis, Streptococcus pyogenes, Streptococcus pneumoniae, Escherichia coli, Corynebacterium xerosis, Neisseria gonorrhoeae, Pseudomonas aeruginosa, Haemophilus* sp. *Proteus* sp., and *Serratia* sp. (Tripathi *et al.*, 1980, Tripathi & Tripathi, 1984). The source of contamination can be normal or abnormal ocular flora as well as extraneous microbes. The wide variation in the normal and contaminating microbial flora, and in the amounts of meibomian and lacrimal gland secretions, may partly explain why lens contamination develops more rapidly in some patients than in others (Tripathi & Tripathi, 1984; Tripathi *et al.*, 1991a,b).

In vivo, the contact lens is an immersed object, and therefore it draws suspended particles, including microbes, to its surfaces. In a new lens, however, the forces of attraction such as gravitation, chemotaxis, London–van der Waals forces, electrostatic interaction, and surface tension are coun-tered by repulsive forces such as negative surface charges of the polymer and steric hindrance (Costerton *et al.*, 1978; Christensen *et al.*, 1985; Tripathi *et al.*, 1991a). Thus, the bacteria will remain at a minimum distance from the lens surface. With time, however, the surface properties of the lens change. The forces of repulsion diminish, and microbes begin to adhere readily. The organisms are often trapped by surface irregularities that result from polymer breakdown or from lens spoilage due to previous deposits (Fig. 47.8).

It is uncertain whether all bacteria can directly digest the lens material. However, *Staphylococcus aureus, Streptococcus pneumoniae, Escherichia coli*, and *Corynebacterium xerosis* produce lipolytic enzymes which can convert triglycerides in the tears into fatty acids. Such fatty acids are not only ocular irritants, but they also interact with the lens material (Tripathi & Tripathi, 1984).

For bacteria to proliferate on a soft contact lens, they must first adhere to the lens surface. Ordinarily, the negatively charged ions of the polymer hydroxyl groups repel the negatively charged bacteria (Tripathi *et al.*, 1991a). This situation is analogous to the mechanisms of adherence of bacteria to cell membranes, which also bear negative charges. In the cell membrane, adherence is effected through ligand–receptor interaction (an interaction exactly comparable to the well-known antigen–antibody reaction). Several ligands which serve as the binding molecules on the bacterial cell wall have been identified. They include proteins (e.g. for some strains of *Escherichia coli* and *Neisseria gonorrhoeae*), the lipid portion of glycolipids (e.g. for group A streptococci and *Staphylococcus aureus*), as well as sugars and other carbohydrates (e.g. for *Streptococcus pneumoniae*) (Tripathi & Tripathi, 1984; Tripathi *et al.*, 1991a). The ligands may or may not be associated with fine surface structures, known as fimbriae or fibrillae, in gram-negative and gram-positive bacteria, respec-

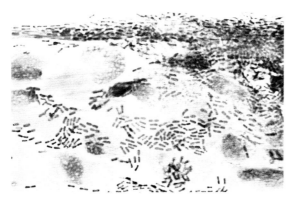

Figure 47.7 Smear prepared from the surface of a soft contact lens. Note numerous Gram-negative bacilliform organisms (*E. coli*) (original magnification × 1850).

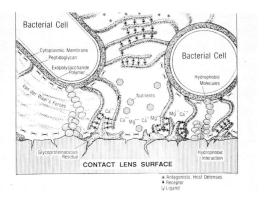

Figure 47.8 Schematic illustration of the mechanism of bacterial adherence. At specific distances the initial repelling forces between like charges on the surfaces of bacteria and the contact lens are overcome by attracting van der Waal's forces and hydrophobic interactions between molecules. Under appropriate conditions, exopolysaccharide polymers develop that further allow ligand-receptor interaction and pertinacious bonding of the bacteria to the contact lens surface. Divalent cations such as Ca^{2+} and Mg^{2+} in the tear film also help to stabilize the bacteria through ion bridging that is operational in the initial adherence process. Various deposits on the lens surface may enhance the adherence by providing receptors for bacterial adhesions, by increasing surface hydrophobicity and by masking the negative charges on the lens surface. F, fimbriae and fibrillae on bacterial cell wall (adapted from Gristina *et al.*, 1985).

tively (Fig. 47.8). The only receptors identified in cells thus far are the sugar residues that are present in the glycolipids or glycoproteins of the cell plasma membrane (Tripathi & Tripathi, 1984; Tripathi *et al.*, 1991a,b). It is possible that, in the case of the soft lens, a coating of glycoprotein or glycolipid is required before bacteria can adhere. However, because it is known that proteins and lipids from ocular secretions are deposited on soft lenses, it is perhaps more likely that the bacterial ligands are attracted directly to the lens surface. Hydrophobic molecules on the bacterial surface also help the organism to approach the negatively charged lens surface (Fig. 47.4).

Another factor which favors bacterial adhesion is the decxreased negative charge in the polymer lattice when the pH falls (Tripathi & Tripathi, 1984). The metabolisc activity of many bacteria produces an acidic environment, and this, in turn, creates a favorable condition for adhesion. Extended-wear lenses are especially likely to be contaminated by bacteria because they are cleaned less frequently than are daily-wear lenses, and they are more prone to organic deposits which favor growth and adherence of microorganisms (Tripathi & Tripathi, 1984). Prophylactic cleaning is important because, once organisms are lodged in crevices and voids, they are not removed by disinfection (Tripathi *et al.*, 1980). Following disinfection, microbial debris and denatured protein on the lens produce irritation or act as an antigenic stimulus. There is no effective means of sterilizing contaminated soft lenses or of rectifying surface and matrix defects; therefore, the only safe remedy is to discard an infected lens (Tripathi & Ruben, 1972; Tripathi *et al.*, 1978, 1980; Tripathi & Tripathi, 1984; Tripathi *et al.*, 1991a).

Calcium film

Calcium forms a white, translucent film with a fine granular surface and appears similar to a protein film (Fig. 47.9). The two often appear concurrently, because protein facilitates the deposition of inorganic minerals by creating a hydrophobic surface. Usually, the calcium film is on the anterior surface of the lens, often in a central location. The calcium in these deposits is mainly of ocular origin. Calcium is normally present in tears; keratoconjunctival tissue is another possible source (Uotila *et al.*, 1972; Ruben *et al.*, 1975; Klintworth *et al.*, 1977; Huth *et al.*, 1980).

A number of factors, such as dry-eye syndrome and elevated tear calcium concentration, may predispose to the formation of calcareous films (which are usually in the form of calcium phosphate). Other factors

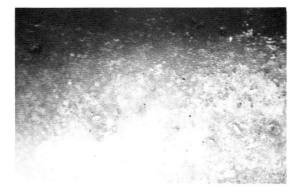

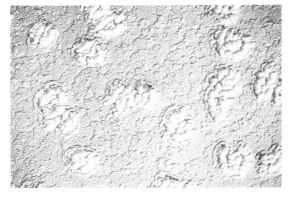

Figure 47.9 (a) Granular calcareous film on a soft contact lens seen *in vivo* by specular microscopy. (b) Mixed deposit of protein film and focal encrusted, calcareous material on the anterior surface of an intact soft contact lens is revealed by Nomarski optics of a light microscope (original magnification × 865).

include a pre-existing protein film, a short tear break-up time, dry atmosphere, incomplete blinking, decreased rate of blinking, inflammation, decreased blood PCO_2, which raises the tear pH, poor oxygen circulation, tight-fitting lenses, the high-plus lenses of aphakics, increased blood calcium and phosphate levels, and decreased blood potassium levels. In the presence of tissue necrosis, enzymes are released which convert pyrophosphates to phosphates, thus favoring calcium phosphate deposition (this mechanism is probably similar to that of dystrophic calcification and band keratopathy). A break-

down of the lens polymer exposes negatively charged hydroxyl sites which attract positively charged calcium ions (Tripathi & Tripathi, 1984). Decrease in temperature also favors calcium deposition. Because the posterior surface of the lens is in contact with the eye, it is warmer than is the anterior surface. The lids, which are warmer than air, cover the lens periphery more often than they cover the center of the lens. The above two factors help to explain the tendency for an anterior/central localization of these deposits. Finally, calcium is deposited with higher frequency in extended-wear than in daily-wear lenses.

The calcium deposits are soluble in dilute hydrochloric acid; however, their removal by this means weakens the lens structure and changes its physical parameters. Sodium edetate (EDTA) and other chelating agents can help remove these deposits, and this is probably one of the reasons for the addition of these agents to commercial cleaning and disinfecting solutions. However, removal of calcium salts leaves pits, voids, and other irregularities in the lens which favor secondary deposition of inorganic and organic substances and microbial infestation (Ruben *et al.*, 1975; Tripathi & Tripathi, 1984; Tripathi *et al.*, 1980, 1988). Calcium deposits (especially calcium carbonate) are partly soluble in hot water; therefore, thermal disinfection is sometimes recommended. However, care must be taken because this process may facilitate the formation of a protein film which can then predispose to further deposition of calcium (Tripathi & Tripathi, 1984).

47.8.2 BARNACLE-LIKE DEPOSITS AND CONCRETIONS

In addition to producing a film, calcium can form glistening, chalky-white granules which look like barnacles with concentric layers or lamellae. The concentric ring pattern is visualized *in vivo* by specular microscopy (Fig. 47.10). With polarized light, these

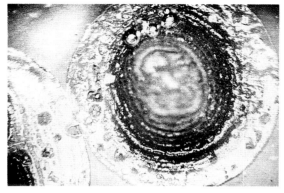

Figure 47.10 Barnacle-like calcareous deposits on the anterior surface of a soft contact lens. A concentric ring arrangement of the calcium carbonate deposit is revealed by specular microscopy (courtesy L. Lohman MD).

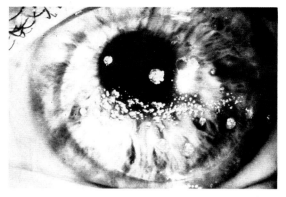

Figure 47.12 Mixed deposits of mucoprotein lipid with and without calcium as seen clinically on the anterior surface of a soft contact lens *in vivo*.

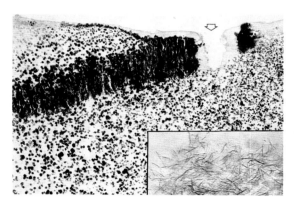

Figure 47.11 Transmission electron micrograph of calcium granules deposited in the anterior lens matrix of a soft contact lens. Arrow denotes a crack in the lens surface (original magnification × 13 250). Inset: needle-shaped crystals of calcium phosphate are resolved by electron microscopy (original magnification × 152 850).

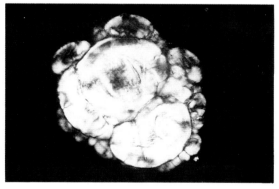

Figure 47.13 A mixed deposit of mucoprotein lipid on the anterior surface of a soft contact lens. A confluent birefringency is revealed by polarized light microscopy (original magnification × 60).

deposits exhibit birefringence. Barnacle-like deposits, which are made up of calcium carbonate, may project exteriorly from the lens surface to become a source of lid irritation and lens intolerance. In addition, when these deposits are present in the central region of the lens, they cause visual aberrations and a reduction in acuity.

Calcium can also be deposited as concretions, made up of calcium phosphate, which are recognizable by stereomicroscopy and by slit lamp biomicroscopy especially with retro-illumination. Deposits of calcium phosphate, whether in the form of concretions or as a film, can extend from just beneath the external surface into the deeper lens matrix as spherules (Fig. 47.11). The formation of such deposits is aided by surface drying and surface degradation of the lens (Tripathi & Tripathi, 1984; Tripathi *et al.*, 1988).

47.8.3 MULBERRY OR JELLY BUMPS

Mulberry deposits (jelly bumps) appear as circular or oval, multilobulated mounds (Fig. 47.12) which range in diameter from 15 μm to 1 mm (average = 0.25 mm). They probably are the most frequent type of lens deposit (Tripathi *et al.*, 1980). Mulberry deposits consist of mixed elements (mucin, protein, and lipid, with or without calcium) (Tripathi *et al.*, 1980; Hart *et al.*, 1986). They are, therefore, referred to as mucoprotein-lipid (MPL) deposits. The proportions of the components determine the appearance of the deposit by polarized-light microscopy. If lipid is the main component, a Maltese cross birefringence pattern will predominate, but more often a confluent pattern is observed (Fig. 47.13). Because these deposits have mixed constituents and because they may penetrate the lens matrix (Fig. 47.14), they are difficult to remove. The use of multiple enzyme systems has been advocated. However, failure to remove the enzymes after cleaning may result in sensitization of the eye. Pancreatin that contains amylase, trypsin, and lipase can dissolve many of these deposits.

High-water-content lenses (daily and extended-wear) are particularly prone to MPL deposits. This is a problem, especially

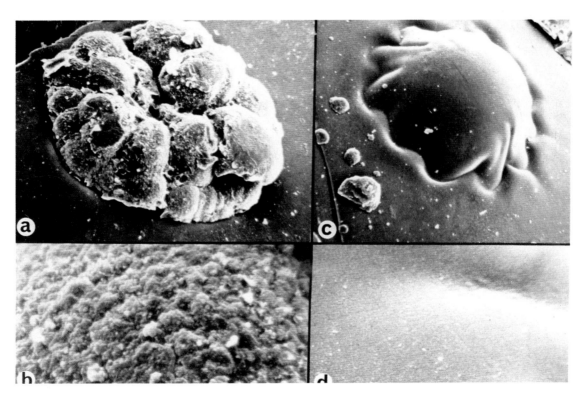

Figure 47.14 Scanning electron microscopy of mucoprotein lipid deposits. (a) Multiobulated configuration (original magnification × 110). (b) higher magnification from (a) showing irregular surface of inspissated mucoprotein (original magnification × 950). (c) Dome-shaped deposit partly embedded in outer lens matrix (original magnification × 110). (d) Higher magnification from (c) showing smooth surface of the deposit indicative of its high lipoidal content (original magnification × 950).

with extended-wear lenses because, in addition to having a high water content, they are cleaned less frequently than are daily-wear lenses. The factors which have been associated with the formation of jelly bumps (when lipid is the predominant component) include decreased tear flow, diminished potassium concentration in tears, diabetes, increased intake of protein, alcohol, or cholesterol, and use of diuretics, anticholinergics, and sympathomimetics, the last probably enhancing depletion of potassium from the tear film (Hart *et al.*, 1987).

47.8.4   STRINGS AND PLAQUES

Mucin deposits appear as yellowish-white strings and plaques (Fig. 47.15). Mucin deposition can be cleaned with mucolytic agents. Derived from the goblet cells of the conjunctiva, the mucoid material is spread or rubbed onto the lens surface by the lids. Excessive production of mucus is a common response of the conjunctiva in most contact lens wearers. Mucin deposits are seen frequently in patients with altered tear function or even minor conjunctival irritation. The deposition of mucin is especially severe in the presence of giant papillary conjuctivitits and vernal conjunctivitis (Tripathi & Tripathi, 1984). Inspissated mucin can form encrusted deposits which erode the lens surface. In addition, mucin deposits are notorious for entrapping foreign bodies, tissue debris, and microorganisms (Fig. 47.16). Such entrapped material induces a foreign-body reaction as well as secondary changes in the cornea, such as epithelial edema and erosion.

47.8.5   MICROFILAMENTOUS DEPOSITS

Fungal contamination appears as fine filaments (mycelia) which can be of various colors, including white, yellow, pink, orange, blue, brown, gray, or black (Fig. 47.17). Fungal culture will provide identification of the specific organism involved. Fungi reported to

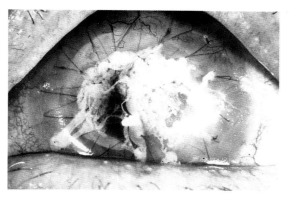

Figure 47.15 Mucin deposits in the form of strings and plaques on the anterior surface of a soft lens worn after penetrating keratoplasty.

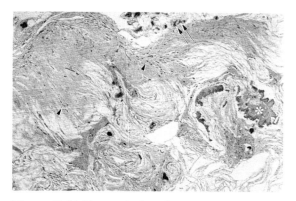

Figure 47.16 Transmission electron micrograph of a mucin deposit on a contact lens showing predominantly a filamentous and granular arrangement of elements. The deposit has entrapped necrotic cells (asterisk), calcareous granules (arrow heads), and microbes (double arrow) (original magnification × 14 800).

have contaminated contact lenses include *Aspergillus niger, Aspergillus fumigatus, Candida albicans, Fusarium verticilloides, Cladosporium cladosporoides, Curvularia lunata, Cephalosporium acremonium, Dermatophilus congolensis, Aureobasidium pullulans, Penicillium* sp., *Rodotorula* sp., and *Ascomycetes* sp. (Bernstein, 1973; Brown *et al.*, 1974; Shapiro, 1974; Palmer *et al.*, 1975; Sagan, 1976; Gasset *et al.*, 1979; Morgan, 1979; Yamamoto *et al.*, 1979; Tripathi *et al.*,

1980; Tripathi & Tripathi, 1984; Berger & Streeten, 1981; Wilson & Ahearn, 1986).

In contrast to bacteria, fungi can adhere to the surface of a relatively clean contact lens and then penetrate into the lens matrix. The pore size of the hydrogel polymer is estimated to be 5 to 7 nm (Gachon *et al.*, 1986). Normally, the intact polymer of lens materials will not permit entry of substances of molecular weight greater than 10 000 (Tripathi *et al.*, 1980). However, fungi can penetrate the lens pores even though the diameters of their mycelia are greater than 5 to 7 nm (Fig. 47.18). These facts support the existence of an active mechanism of adherence and penetration. The fungi initially use mycelial strands and polysaccharide adhesions, as well as ionic bridges, to gain purchase upon the lens surface (Tripathi *et al.*, 1988). Flattened branches or areas on hyphae which resemble appressoria appear to cement the hyphal elements or germ tubes to the soft-lens surface (Simmons *et al.*, 1986). The fungi begin to excrete digestive enzymes which degrade the polymer structure of the lens and allow deeper penetration (Williams, 1981; Tripathi *et al.*, 1988). The fungi which become attached are capable of developing a thickened fibrillar surface layer that confers resistance to cleaning agents and enhances

their adherence to the lens (Tripathi *et al.*, 1988). Such modifications of the surface of the fungi may occur because of the availability of nutrients on the lens. Consequently, lens deposits with surface moieties such as albumin, lysozyme, lactoferrin, and fibronectin, and with increased surface area, promote the adherence of fungi (Butrus & Klotz, 1986).

High-water-content lenses are most susceptible to fungal infection, probably because of their open network of molecules which allows easy passage of nutrients into the lens

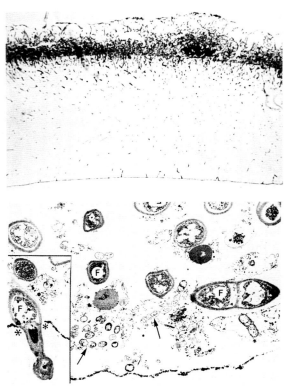

Figure 47.18 Section of soft lens showing fungal filaments proliferating on the anterior lens surface (top) and invading the entire thickness of the lens matrix (original magnification × 112). (b) Transmission electron micrograph of a soft lens showing proliferation of both fungi (F) and bacteria (arrows) on the lens surface. Inset shows infiltration (asterisk) of a fungal hypha into lens matrix (original magnification × 5200).

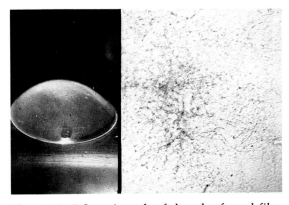

Figure 47.17 Invasion of soft lens by fungal filaments. Left: gross appearance; right: phase-contrast microscopy of the intact lens.

(Yamaguchi *et al.*, 1984; Gachon *et al.*, 1986; Tripathi *et al.*, 1988). The high-water medium may also aid the enzymes excreted by the fungi in their polymer degradation and thus promote colonization with fungi. High-water-content, extended-wear soft lenses are more likely to be contaminated because they are cleaned less frequently than are daily-wear lenses, and are more prone to organic deposits which further favor growth and adherence of the fungi (Tripathi & Tripathi, 1984). Once a lens is contaminated with fungi, it must be discarded because their complete removal is often impossible.

The source of contamination can be abnormal ocular flora or extraneous microbes. Extraneous sources include cosmetics (Wilson *et al.*, 1969, 1971; Gasset *et al.*, 1979; Tripathi *et al.*, 1988) and contaminated areas in the environment, such as the bathroom (Simmons *et al.*, 1986). In contrast to bacteria, fungi are not a part of the normal flora of the eye (Wilson *et al.*, 1969; Ando & Takatori, 1982). The use of lenses infected with fungi only rarely results in fungal infection of the eye, but when it occurs it can be disastrous. Patients should not allow cosmetics to smear the keratoconjunctival surface. Extreme care should be taken to avoid fungal contamination of therapeutic lenses prescribed for patients with corneal disorders. In one case report, a patient with metaherpetic corneal epithelial erosion was using a therapeutic lens contaminated with *Cephalosporium acremonium*, and later required a penetrating keratoplasty because the cornea was invaded by the fungus (Yamamoto *et al.*, 1979).

47.8.6 FOREIGN BODIES

Foreign bodies include silica, iron, and other extraneous substances.

Silica deposits

Silica deposits appear sand-like and are best seen with the stereomicroscope and retro-illumination. Silica deposits are especially common in sand, brick, and masonry workers (Tripathi *et al.*, 1980; Tripathi & Tripathi, 1984). These workers should use protective goggles.

Iron deposits

Iron deposits appear as small rust-colored or red/orange spots or rings, which usually form when iron-containing foreign bodies from the environment become embedded in the lens and then oxidize to form ferrous salts (Tripathi & Tripathi, 1984). Iron has been found in new lenses, having been introduced during the manufacturing process. Rarely, iron salts may accumulate in the lens when an iron foreign body has entered the eye. Small deposits away from the visual axis may cause few problems, but eventually the lens should be replaced. Treatment with reducing agents and with some lens cleaners may temporarily change the color of the iron salts from orange to black. Chemical removal with EDTA is possible, but this will leave a defect in the lens.

Other deposits

Manganese, chromium, cadmium, zinc, silver, and copper have also been detected in soft contact lenses. These elements can induce a foreign-body reaction (Tripathi *et al.*, 1988).

47.8.7 DISCOLORATIONS

Substances which cause discoloration of soft contact lenses include melanin and tyrosine-like pigments, nicotine, adrenochrome, tetrahydrazaline, chlorhexidine, mercury, and diagnostic dyes such as fluorescein and rose bengal.

Melanin and tyrosine-like pigments

Melanin and tyrosine-like pigments appear as a yellow/brown discoloration just below the lens surface, often beginning at the edge of the lens. A blue haze is seen by stereomicroscopy when a dark backround is used. Under ultraviolet light, the lens shows some fluorescence. These pigments are derived from the oxidative polymerization of aromatic compounds in the tears and are exacerbated in lenses that are disinfected thermally. Melanin-like pigmentation of contact lenses is also common among cigarette smokers, with melanin production in the lens probably being stimulated by nicotine and other polycyclic aromatic compounds that are present in tobacco smoke (Tripathi & Tripathi, 1984).

Nicotine

Deposits of nicotine often appear on the lenses of patients who are cigarette smokers (especially those with nicotine-stained fingers), or of those exposed to large amounts of cigarette smoke (Broich *et al.*, 1980; Tripathi & Tripathi, 1984). Nicotine usually appears as a uniform brown discoloration.

Adrenochrome:

A uniform or spotty brown/black discoloration may be seen on the contact lenses of patients who have glaucoma and use epinephrine drops. This discoloration most probably is caused by adrenochrome deposition (Sugar, 1974; Miller *et al.*, 1976; Tripathi & Tripathi, 1984). Epinephrine can undergo oxidation to form melanin pigments, and it is likely that these pigments are responsible for the discoloration. A switch to dipivalyl epinephrine, an epinephrine analog, should be considered because this drug does not result in discoloration of contact lenses (Newton & Nesburn, 1979; Tripathi *et al.*, 1980, 1988). A lens that has already been discolored can be made transparent by immersion in 3% hydrogen peroxide for 5 hours (Miller *et al.*, 1976). However, there have been no studies to determine whether lens defects remain after this process.

Tetrahydrazaline

A brown discoloration can sometimes be seen on the soft contact lenses of patients who use tetrahydrazaline drops (Tripathi & Tripathi, 1984). These drops should not be used during wearing of contact lenses.

Chlorhexidine

A yellow/green discoloration may be seen on the soft contact lenses of patients who use solutions for disinfection, or topical ophthalmic preparations, that contain chlorhexidine. Under ultraviolet light, the lenses display bright fluorescence (Tripathi & Tripathi, 1984). Solutions whose shelf-life has expired or solutions that are discolored green should be discarded because this indicates decomposition of chlorhexidine. Deposition of chlorhexidine on clean lenses causes ocular sensitivity in less than 1 percent of patients (Tripathi & Tripathi, 1984). In lenses with a proteinaceous coating, however, the combination of chlorhexidine with denatured protein may form an active substance with antigenic properties which induces so-called protein conjunctivitis. The presence of chlorhexidine in a hydrogel lens renders the lens hydrophobic and lipophilic. This encourages lipid deposition.

Mercury

Mercury appears as a grey/black discoloration. Most commonly, mercury is derived from solutions containing thimerosal, a mercury-containing preservative. This is especially troublesome when thimerosal-preserved saline is used with thermal disinfection, because thimerosal is decomposed by heat. Free mercury is released and can then precipitate as a mercuric salt – usually water-insoluble black mercuric sulfide. Decomposition can also occur in old or reused solutions. Sulfur-containing rubber, which is sometimes used in vial caps and seals, creates conditions that favor the precipitation of mercuric sulfide. The deposits have a tendency to accumulate gradually in used lenses. Compared with new lenses, used lenses can have a 15-fold increase in thimerosal concentration (Tripathi & Tripathi, 1984).

Deposits of mercury may impair lens transparency, thus causing decreased vision. The most serious side effect of mercury deposits is an often unrealized delayed allergic reaction that compels many otherwise successful soft lens wearers to abandon their lenses. Thimerosal has also been implicated in the etiology of contact lens-associated superior limbic keratoconjunctivitis, epithelial edema, pseudoepitheliomatous hyperplasia, and acute and chronic inflammation, as well as in a decrease in the number of goblet cells (Sendele *et al.*, 1983; Tripathi & Tripathi, 1984). Ocular sensitivity to thimerosal has been demonstrated in several studies (Suzuki, 1972; Mondino & Groden, 1980; Wilson *et al.*, 1981; Sendele *et al.*, 1983; Bloomfield *et al.*, 1984; Tripathi & Tripathi, 1984).

Diagnostic dyes

A yellow/green, red, or blue discoloration may be seen after use of fluorescein, rose bengal, or alcian blue dyes, respectively (Tripathi & Tripathi, 1984). Soft contact lenses should not be worn immediately after examination of the eye with these dyes unless the keratoconjunctival surface has been rinsed thoroughly. Residual dye present in the conjunctival sac, or liberated from devitalized keratoconjunctival tissue, can stain the lenses.

47.8.8 FERN-LIKE DEPOSITS

Sodium deposits, which can be visualized by phase-contrast light microscopy, appear as a fern-like pattern (Fig. 47.19). These deposits arise when sodium salts from tears or from

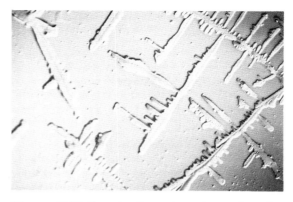

Figure 47.19 Examination of an intact lens by light microscopy using Nomarski optics. Deposits of sodium chloride form a fern-like pattern on the lens surface.

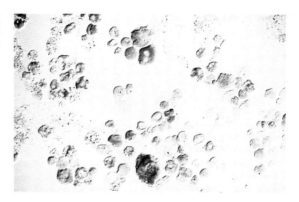

Figure 47.20 Adherence of *Acanthamoeba* to the surface of a soft contact lens as seen by Nomarski optics microscopy. Both the cystic and trophozoite forms are adherent to the lens surface (original magnification × 525).

instilled solutions precipitate on the lens. Dry eye predisposes to this type of deposition (Tripathi & Tripathi, 1984).

47.9 INVISIBLE SPOILAGE

47.9.1 MAGNESIUM

Magnesium tends to accumulate in lenses pre-coated with other deposits or in lenses that contain denatured polymer. Magnesium is detected only by chemical assay. Thermal disinfection with tap water rich in this mineral, such as water in mountainous regions, can be the source of this contamination (Tripathi & Tripathi, 1984).

47.9.2   ACANTHAMOEBA

Many of the contaminants that have been discussed in this chapter are difficult to detect when present in low concentration. An important contaminant is *Acanthamoeba*. This protozoan can be detected by high magnification light microscopy, as well as by scanning and transmission electron microscopy. It occurs in both cyst and trophozoite forms. Many cases of *Acanthamoeba*-induced keratitis have been documented, and more

careful clinical diagnosis may reveal a greater number of lenses which are contaminated with amoebae (Moore *et al.*, 1985; Tripathi *et al.*, 1989).

The cornea may be infected as the result of the interaction between the lens surface and the cornea. In the surface of the corneal epithelium, microscopic breaks and trauma occur because of friction with the lens surface (Tripathi & Tripathi, 1981; Moore *et al.*, 1985). These breaches in the epithelial barrier provide entry points through which amebae can readily pass. The main sources of *Acanthamoeba* are contaminated ophthalmic solutions (e.g. home made saline), tap water, pond water, hot tub water, environmental pollutants, and the nasal and oral cavities. We have shown experimentally that acan-

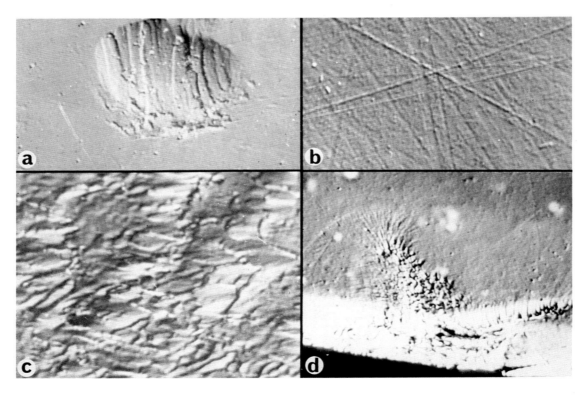

Figure 47.21 Phase-contrast microscopy showing various forms of surface defects on soft lenses. (a) Bubble defect, (b) polishing marks, (c) surface irregularity, (d) crack defect at the edge of the lens (original magnification × 250).

thamoebae adhere to the contact lens surface (Tripathi *et al.*, 1989). The contact lens, therefore, can act as a carrier for the introduction of *Acanthamoeba* into the eye (Fig. 47.20).

47.10 MANUFACTURING AND PHYSICAL DEFECTS, POLYMER IMPURITY, AGING, AND DECAY

Manufacturing defects in lenses include material impurity, texture inhomogeneity, bubble defects, tool marks, nicks, scratches, abrasions, chips, cuts, punctures, cracks, and unfinished lens surfaces (Fig. 47.21). Such defects are very common, and their presence varies widely from one manufacturer to another, depending upon their quality control system and on the type of manufacturing process used (spincasting, lathe-cutting, molding, etc.). During polymerization of the soft-lens material, a monomer impurity can leave potential chemical-binding sites, especially hydroxyl groups, which readily attract positively charged ions, such as calcium, and proteins. The reactive ester groups present in soft lenses may further hydrolyze during the cleaning and disinfection process under acidic or alkaline conditions to liberate ethanol, which diffuses out of the lens material, thus altering the chemical, physical, and optical characteristics of the lens and contributing to its premature aging and decay (Fig. 47.22). With wear and due to the disinfection process, the surface of the lens may become hydrophobic, thus attracting various organic and inorganic deposits.

A soft lens is not indestructible. Although it is convenient to clean lenses by rubbing them between the fingers, physical defects (scratches, abrasions, nicks, crush damage, chips, cuts, and punctures) can result, depending on the condition of the fingers and the amount of pressure applied. Such physical defects account for spoilage in one of every three or four lenses (Tripathi & Tripathi, 1984).

Quality control of the lenses during the

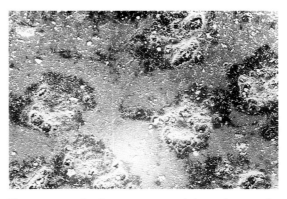

Figure 47.22 Surface erosion and degradation of a worn soft contact lens as revealed by scanning electron microscopy (original magnification × 320).

manufacturing process is the only way to ensure against manufacturing defects. There is no way to manage the aging and decay of lenses. All forms of physical damage to the lenses are irreversible; such damaged lenses should be discarded.

47.11 CRAZING

Rigid gas-permeable lenses have enabled some patients who could not tolerate soft contact lenses, or who were not candidates for such lenses, to become contact lens wearers. However, the rigid gas-permeable lens has not provided the solution for all of the problems that are associated with contact lenses. Although rigid gas-permeable lenses do not become spoiled as often as do soft contact lenses, with age and wear they develop spider-like, interconnecting surface cracks that may extend into the anterior surface of the lens. This phenomenon is known as crazing (McLaughlin & Schoessler, 1987; Lembach *et al.* 1988). The cracks predispose the lens to secondary deposits, and these cause further spoilage. (Fig. 47.23). The exact etiology of crazing is unknown. Some investigators have suggested that crazing stems from the manufacturing process

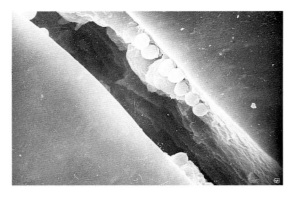

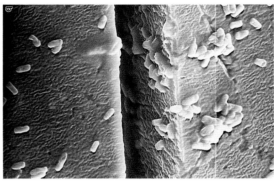

Figure 47.23 Scanning electron microscopy of surface crazing of rigid gas permeable lenses. (a) The crevice contains cocci and a build-up of encrusted material. (b) Both the surface and the crevice is infected by bacilli and a focal encrusted material (courtesy Patrick J. Caroline) (original magnification × 10 000).

(McLaughling & Schoessler, 1987), whereas others believe that it is related to lens wear (Lembach *et al.*, 1988).

47.12 GENERAL CONCEPTS

47.12.1 FDA CLASSIFICATION OF HYDROGEL LENSES

In 1985, the FDA classified hydrogel lenses in the following four groups:

Group 1 – low-water-content,   non-ionic
          polymers

Group 2 – high-water-content,   non-ionic
          polymers
Group 3 – low-water-content,   ionic poly-
          mers
Group 4 – high-water-content,   ionic poly-
          mers

This classification provides a basis for an organized approach to the correlation of lens spoilage with polymer type. Unfortunately, this classification has not been used widely in scientific publications. With regard to lens spoilage, it has been shown that ionic polymers bind lysozyme more readily than do non-ionic polymers; thus lenses in groups 3 and 4 are more susceptible to spoilage from protein films (Lowther, 1986).

47.12.2 SOURCES OF SPOILAGE

In most cases, lens spoilage originates from substances produced by the eye itself. However, a significant part of the lens spoilage material originates from the patient's own hands (this includes especially lipids and microbial contaminants). Therefore, the state of cleanliness of the patient's hands is an important factor in the etiology of contact lens spoilage, so much so that the use of talc-free sterile gloves during lens handling has been suggested (Nesburn, 1979). However, this precaution has rarely been applied because of the additional cost and inconvenience, and because of the requirement of too high a level of manual dexterity for most patients. This practice could also significantly increase the incidence of lens loss. However, in patients who are particularly prone to extraneous lens spoilage, the use of talc-free sterile gloves could potentially eliminate a significant cause of lens spoilage.

47.12.3 FREQUENCY OF LENS REPLACEMENT AND SPOILAGE

Perhaps the most important etiologic factor in the occurrence of lens spoilage is the frequency of lens replacement. There is simply not sufficient time for lenses to become spoiled significantly if they are replaced frequently (e.g. weekly or bi-weekly). Thus the concept of the disposable lens arose (Tripathi *et al.*, 1978, 1980, 1988; Tripathi & Tripathi, 1984). This concept should not be restricted to the soft contact lens, because rigid gaspermeable lenses become spoiled as well. The most common criticism of the disposable-lens concept is that patients will not replace their lenses at the prescribed intervals thereby saving money. Ideally, disposable lenses should be of a quality equal to that of non-disposable lenses. However, this makes it even more tempting to forego lens replacement. There are two prerequisites for the elimination of non-

compliance of lens replacement. First, ocular clinicians must emphasize the hazards of foregoing lens replacement while stressing the benefits of proper use. Second, the lenses must be so inexpensive that it would be virtually unthinkable to risk the health of one's eyes to save such a small amount of money.

Another criticism of disposable lenses is that, when they are used for extended wear, they do not eliminate the potential problems of covering the cornea for long periods of time. It is clear that a large number of patients have tolerated extended-wear lenses well. However, it remains to be seen whether corneal problems are minimized or eliminated by using disposable lenses on a daily-

Table 47.6 Classification of contact lens deposits

Appearance	Cause
Films	
white/translucent	Protein (yellow/white)
	Bacteria (heavy deposit)
	Calcium (chalky or granular)
greasy/smooth/glistening	Lipid
Barnacle-like deposits	Calcium
Concretions	Calcium
Mulberry or jelly bumps	Mucoprotein lipid (with or without calcium)
Strings and plaques	Mucin
Fine filaments	Fungus
Foreign bodies	
red/orange spots or rings	Iron
sand-like	Silica
Uniform discolorations	
gray/black	Mercury
brown hues	Melanin and tyrosine-like pigments (yellow/brown)
	Nicotine (brown)
	Adrenochrome (brown/black)
	Tetrahydrazaline (brown)
yellow/green	Chlorhexidine
	Fluorescein (fluorescent)
red	Rose bengal
blue	Alcian blue
Fern-like deposits	Sodium
Invisible deposits	Magnesium (detected by chemical assay)
	Acanthamoeba (seen under high-magnification light microscopy; appears in cyst and trophozoite forms)
Crazing	Unknown (phenomenon seen on rigid gas permeable lenses)

wear, timed-replacement basis. Although, following this regimen, these patients would continue to purchase lens solutions and, therefore, not realize the savings comparable to those patients who use their lenses on an extended-wear regimen, they would reap the benefits of wearing lenses with minimal deposits.

Table 47.6 is a summary of the appearance and causes of the deposits.

REFERENCES

Allansmith, M.D. *et al.* (1977) Giant papillary conjunctivitis in contact lens wearers. *Am. J. Ophthalmol.*, **83**, 697–708.

Ando, N. and Takatori, K. (1982) Fungal flora of the conjunctival sac. *Am. J. Ophthalmol.*, **94**, 67–74.

Bernstein, H.N. (1973) Fungal growth into a Bionite hydrophilic contact lens. *Ann. Ophthalmol.*, **5**, 317–22.

Berger, R.O. and Streeten, B.W. (1981) Fungal growth in aphakic soft contact lenses. *Am. J. Ophthalmol.*, **91**, 630–3.

Bloomfield, S.E., Jakobiec, F.A., and Theodore, F.H. (1984) Contact lens induced keratopathy: A severe complication extending the spectrum of keratoconjunctivitis in contact lens wearers. *Ophthalmology*, **91**, 290–4.

Broich, J.R., Weiss, L. and Rapp, J. (1980) Isolation and identification of biologically active contaminants from soft contact lenses. *Invest. Ophthalmol. Vis. Sci.*, **19**, 1328–35.

Brown, S.I. *et al.* (1974) Infections with the therapeutic soft lens. *Arch. Ophthalmol.*, **91**, 275–7.

Doughman, D.J. *et al.* (1975) The nature of 'spots' on soft lenses. *Ann. Ophthalmol.*, **7**, 345–53.

de Vries, K.A. (1985) Contact lenses and 'the pill'. *Contact Lens Forum*, **10**, 21–3.

Fowler, S.A., Greiner, J.V. and Allansmith, M.R. (1979) Attachment of bacteria to soft contact lenses. *Arch. Ophthalmol.* **97**, 659–60.

Gasset, A.R., Mattingly, T.P. and Hood, I. (1979) Source of fungus contamination of hydrophilic soft contact lenses. *Ann. Ophthalmol.*, **11**, 1295–8.

Hart, D.E. (1984), Lipid deposits which form on extended wear contact lenses. *Int. Contact Lens Clin.*, **11**, 348–62.

Hart, D.E., Tisdale, R.R. and Sack, R.A. (1986)

Origin and composition of lipid deposits on soft contact lenses. *Ophthalmology*, **93**, 495–503.

Hart, D.E. *et al.* (1987) Spoilage of hydrogel contact lenses by lipid deposits. *Ophthalmology*, **94**, 1315–21.

Huth, S.W., Hirano, P. and Leopold, I.H. (1980) Calcium in tears and contact lens wear. *Arch. Ophthalmol.*, **98**, 122–5.

Josephson, J.E. and Caffery, B.B. (1981) Observation of the lipid layer of the tear film. *Am. J. Optom. Physiol. Opt.*, **58**, 1033.

Klintworth, G.K. *et al.* (1977) Calcification of soft contact lenses in patient with dry eye and elevated calcium concentration in tears. *Invest. Ophthalmol. Vis. Sci.*, **16**, 158–61.

Lembach, R.G., McLaughlin, R. and Barr, J.T. (1988) Crazing in a rigid gas permeable contact lens. *CLAO J.*, **14**, 38–41.

Lowther, G.E. (1986) Hydrogel lens classification. *Int. Contact Lens Clin.*, **2**, 298.

McLaughlin, W. and Schoessler, J. (1987) Manufacturing defect in a rigid gas-permeable lens. *Int. Eye Care*, **14**, 167.

Masterson, C. (1982) Diuretics. *Eye Contact*, **September**, 2.

Miller, D., Brooks, S.M. and Mobilia, E. (1976) Adrenochrome staining of soft contact lenses. *Ann. Ophthalmol.*, **8**, 65–7.

Mondino, B.J. and Groden, L.R. (1980) Conjunctival hyperemia and corneal infiltrates with chemically disinfected soft contact lenses. *Arch. Ophthalmol.*, **98**, 1767–70.

Mondino, B.J., Salamon, S.M. and Zaidman, G.W. (1982) Allergic and toxic reactions in soft contact lens wearers. *Surv. Ophthalmol.*, **26**, 337–44.

Morgan, J.F. (1979) Complications associated with contact lens solutions. *Ophthalmology*, **86**, 1107–19.

Nesburn, A.B. (1979) Complications associated with therapeutic soft contact lenses. *Ophthalmology*, **86**, 1130–7.

Newton, M.J. and Nesburn, A.B. (1979) Lack of hydrophilic lens discoloration in patients using dipivalyl epinephrine for glaucoma. *Am. J. Ophthalmol.*, **87**, 193–5.

Palmer, E., Ferry, A.P. and Safir, A. (1975) Fungal invasion of a soft (Griffin Bionite) contact lens. *Arch. Ophthalmol.*, **93**, 278–80.

Refojo, M.F. and Holly, F.J. (1977) Tear protein adsorption on hydrogels: a possible cause of contact lens allergy. *Contact IOL Med. J.*, **3**, 23–35.

Ruben, M., Tripathi, R.C. and Winder, A.F. (1975)

Calcium deposition as a cause of spoilation of hydrophilic soft contact lenses. *Br. J. Ophthalmol.*, **59**, 141–8.

Sagan, W. (1976), Fungal invasion of a soft contact lens. *Arch. Ophthalmol.*, **94**, 168.

Sendele, D.D. *et al.* (1983) Superior limbic keratoconjunctivitis in contact lens wearers. *Ophthalmology*, **90**, 616–22.

Shapiro, I. (1974) Penicillium species fungus growth on a Bionite hydrophilic contact lens. *Minn. Med.*, 943.

Simmons, R.B. *et al.* (1986) Morphology and ultrastructure of fungi in extended-wear soft contact lenses. *J. Clin. Microbiol.*, **24**, 21–5.

Spring, T.F. (1974) Reaction to hydrophilic lenses. *Med. J. Aust.*, **1**, 449–50.

Sugar, J. (1974) Adrenochrome pigmentation of hydrophilic lenses. *Arch. Ophthalmol.*, **91**, 11–12.

Suzuki, H. (1972) Allergic conjunctivitis and blepharoconjunctivitis caused by thimerosal used as preservant. *Jpn. J. Clin. Ophthalmol.*, **26**, 783–8.

Tripathi, R.C. and Ruben, M. (1972) Degenerative changes in a soft hydrophilic contact lens. *Ophthalmic Res.*, **4**, 185–92.

Tripathi, R.C. and Tripathi, B.J. (1981) The role of lids in soft contact lens spoilage. *Contact and Intraocular Lens Med. J.*, **7**, 234–40.

Tripathi, R.C. and Tripathi, B.J. (1984) Soft contact lens spoilage. In: *Contact Lenses: The CLAO Guide to Basic Science and Clinical Practice*, Vol. 2, (ed. O.H. Dabezies), Grune and Stratton, Orlando, FL, pp.45.1–45.36.

Tripathi, R.C., Ruben, M. and Tripathi, B.J. (1978) Soft lens spoilation. In: *Soft Contact Lenses: Clinical and Applied Technology*, (ed. M. Ruben), John Wiley and Sons, New York, pp.299–334.

Tripathi, R.C., Tripathi, B.J. and Ruben, M. (1980) The pathology of soft contact lens spoilage. *Ophthalmology*, **87**, 365–80.

Tripathi, R.C., Tripathi, B.J. and Millard, C.B. (1988) Physicochemical changes in contact lenses and their interaction with the cornea and tears. *CLAO J.*, **14**, 23–32.

Tripathi, R.C., Monninger, R.H.G. and Tripathi, B.J. (1989) Contact lens-associated *Acanthamoeba* keratitis: a report from the USA. *Fortscr. Ophthalmol.*, **86**, 67–71.

Tripathi, B.J., Tripathi, R.C. Rhee, J.M. (1991a) Adhesion of bacteria to contact lenses. In: *Contact Lenses: The CLAO Guide to Basic Science and Clinical Practice*, (ed. O. Dabezies), Grune and Stratton, Orlando, FL, pp.42.1–42.17.

Tripathi, R.C., Tripathi, B.J., Silverman, R.A. and Rao, G.N. (1991b) Contact lens deposits and spoilage: Identification and management. *Int. Ophthalmol. Clinics*, **31**, 91–120.

Uotila, M.H., Soble, R.E. and Savory, J. (1972) Measurement of tear calcium levels. *Invest. Ophthalmol. Vis. Sci.*, **11**, 258–9.

Welder, F.C. (1977) Analysis of biomaterials deposited on soft contact lenses. *J. Biomed. Mater. Res.*, **11**, 525–35.

Wilson, L.A. and Ahearn, D.G. (1986) Association of fungi with extended-wear soft contact lenses. *Am. J. Ophthalmol.*, **101**, 434–6.

Wilson, L.A. *et al.* (1969) Fungi from the normal outer eye. *Am. J. Ophthalmol.*, **67**, 52–6.

Wilson, L.A. *et al.* (1971) Microbial contamination in ocular cosmetics. *Am. J. Ophthalmol.*, **71**, 1298–302.

Wilson, L.A., McNatt, J. and Reitschel, R. (1981) Delayed hypersensitivity to thimerosal in soft contact lens wearers. *Ophthalmology*, **88**, 804–8.

Yamamoto, G.K. *et al.* (1979) Fungal invasion of a therapeutic soft contact lens and cornea. *Ann. Ophthalmol.*, **11**, 1731–5.

PART 3   CLINICAL ASPECTS OF LENS SPOILATION

G.E. Lowther

Lens deposits, discoloration and aging have been a major clinical problem with hydrogel and rigid gas permeable lenses. To clinically manage this problem one must be able to inspect and identify the deposit. Deposits may be due to poor tear film quality, improper cleaning, use of incorrect care systems and solutions, foreign material from the hands or environment, or medications. Likewise, different materials and wearing schedules can affect the type and amount of deposit. In this chapter the different deposits and discolorations and their causes will be explained.

By being able to identify deposits and knowing the cause, one can give the patient advice on how to prevent or minimize the problem and what cleaner and care system to use to prolong lens life or prevent the recurrence.

47.13   LENS INSPECTION TECHNIQUES

A number of methods can be used to inspect lenses for deposits. The most common clinical method, and often the first method, is to view the lens on the patient's eye with the biomicroscope. If the patient presents for an examination wearing the lenses, it is easy to inspect the lens on the patient. Using low magnification ($\times$10–15) and a relatively wide parallelopiped, the lens can be scanned for deposits and defects. If a deposit is located or if no deposits are visible, higher magnification with a narrow parallelopiped can be

used to look at the surface in more detail. The use of specular reflection from the lens surface allows visualization of small detail that might otherwise be missed.

A clinical method of inspecting the lens off the eye is to hold the lens up with a pair of tweezers and illuminate it from the side with a penlight. It should be viewed against a dark background. When the lens is wet, only a heavy coating can be detected. If one blots the lens with a lint free tissue to remove surface water any significant deposit will be visible. The appearance of the deposit and the area of the lens covered by the deposit can be noted. A hand magnifier of $\times$7–10 magnification, i.e. the type used to measure optical zone diameters, can be used to inspect the deposit in greater detail. The biomicroscope can also be used to examine the lens off the eye.

To study deposits in even greater detail they can be studied under a microscope. A standard light microscope is not satisfactory since most of the deposits are not colored and, therefore, will not show up. The best method to visualize the deposits with a light microscope is to use phase contrast microscopy. With phase contrast any type of deposit is visible. Hydrogel lenses can be placed on a microscope slide and flattened with a cover slip. This does not damage the lens and allows the whole surface of the lens to be scanned without major refocusing of the microscope. If the lens surface is clean and has no scratches, the lens will appear a

Contact Lens Practice. Edited by Montague Ruben and Michel Guillon.
Published in 1994 by Chapman & Hall, London. ISBN 0 412 35120 X

uniform bluish-gray color. Any detail such as scratches or deposits will be visible against this background. Dark field microscopy can also be used but is usually not as satisfactory as phase contrast.

It is useful for clinical recording to use a standard classification of the deposits. One useful method is the modified Rudko system (Table 47.7) (Rudko & Gregg, 1975; Hathway & Lowther, 1976). With this system the heaviness or degree of coating is specified on a scale of I through IV with I being a clean lens, II a coating visible with magnification only when the lens is wet, III a coating visible when the lens surface is blotted and IV a heavy coating visible on a wet lens without magnification. With this system the type of deposit is also indicated as well as the extent of the surface that the deposit covers.

For research purposes scanning and/or transmission electron microscopy can be used to view the lens surfaces or matrix under very high magnifications. With these techniques the detail, and, depending on the microscope, the chemical nature of the deposits can be studied. The use of these instruments requires that the lens be processed in such a way that they can no longer be used by the patient.

47.14 PROTEIN DEPOSITS

Very early in the clinical use of hydrogel lenses it was recognized that proteins from the tear film could deposit on hydrogel lenses (Krezanoski, 1972; Trager, 1972; Uotila & Gasset, 1972; Filippi *et al.*, 1973). The uniform surface coating that is routinely referred to as protein is mostly protein but probably also contains mucopolysaccrides,

Table 47.7 Lens deposit classification system (modification of Rudko classification system)

Code	Heaviness of deposit
I	Clean
II	Visible under oblique light when wet using ×7 magnification
III	Visible when dry with unaided eye
IV	Visible when wet or dry with unaided eye

Code	Type of deposit
C	Crystalline
G	Granular
F	Filmy
P	Plaque
Co	Coating
D	Debris

Code	Extent of deposit
a	0–25% of lens surface
b	25–50% of lens surface
c	50–75% of lens surface
d	75–100% of lens surface

C, crystalline deposits comprised of crystal groups which may be scattered or layered; G, granular deposits consisting of fine granulation; F, film and hazes consisting of coatings that are not granular or crystalline; P, plaques are deposits which cover large portions of the lens and appear as islands or cracks in uniform coatings. Co, Coating is the term applied when a film is dense and uniform covering the entire lens surface D, Debris appears as scattered areas of deposits having no specific symmetry or geometry and occurs at any place on the lens surface.

ions and other tear film components as well.

These protein deposits are the most common deposits seen on hydrogel lenses. On the eye it appears as a fairly uniform coating that results in a rapid break up of the tear film (Fig. 47.24). Viewed off the eye, after blotting the surface, the deposit appears as a whitish coating, usually over a major portion of the lens (Fig. 47.25). When viewed under higher magnification using a phase contrast microscope (Fig. 47.26), the deposit can be seen developing as small spots that coalesce to form the more uniform coating seen clinically. Under higher magnification using a scanning electron microscope, the surface of the deposit appears rough with many small elevations.

When the lens is sectioned and the deposit stained for protein, it can be seen that the coating is limited to the lens surface (Fig. 47.27). It may penetrate the surface slightly but not to a great extent. The fact that the deposit is mainly surface in nature indicates that cleaning is at least feasible.

Numerous studies have investigated the different proteins that make up these uniform surface coatings. Lysozyme, albumin, glycoproteins and globulins have been shown to deposit on hydrogel lenses (Krezanoski, 1972; Lowther, 1975; Refojo & Holly, 1977; Wedler, 1977; Gudmundsson *et al.*,

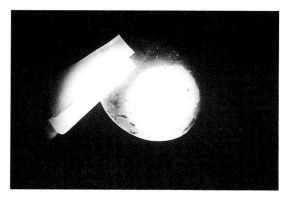

Figure 47.25 Heavily coated hydrogel lens off the eye and held before the biomicroscope after the surface water is blotted off.

1985). Other studies have indicated that lysozyme is the major protein depositing on hydrogel lenses (Karageozian, 1974a, b).

There are several mechanisms by which proteins may interact and attach to lens surfaces. Initial binding may occur due to polar lipid head groups or ionic amino acid side chain groups. Adjacent denatured proteins may form disulfide bonds between peptide chains causing cross-linking of the denatured proteins (Wedler, 1977; Wedler & Riedhammer, 1982). Ionic components (i.e. calcium and magnesium) of the tear film also

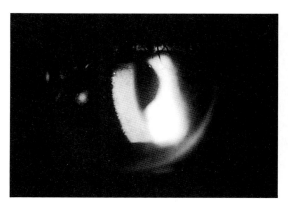

Figure 47.24 Protein coating of a hydrogel lens as seen on the eye with the biomicroscope.

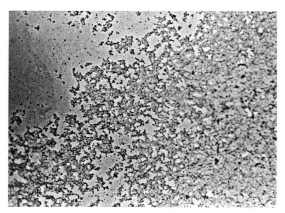

Figure 47.26 Surface coated hydrogel lens surface seen under magnification with a phase contrast microscope at the edge of a coated area.

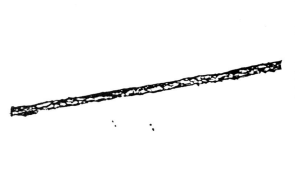

Figure 47.27 A cross section of a coated hydrogel lens with the surface coating stained with a protein stain. The coating is seen limited to the lens surface.

appear to be involved. The ionic components may become concentrated in the lens providing nucleation sites for the binding of the proteins (Wedler, 1977). Calcium has been shown to crystallize on and within hydrogel lenses (Lowther *et al.*, 1975; Lowther & Hilbert, 1975; Hilbert *et al.*, 1976). Lenses coated with known proteins without ionic components do not have the same appearance and apparently do not adhere as tightly to the lens as protein solutions containing calcium salts (Hathaway & Lowther, 1976). The ions may tend to crystallize on the lens surface to help bind the protein.

Other theories are that the presence of enzyme bearing microorganisms are necessary for organic deposits (Liolet *et al.*, 1983) and that blood constituents are involved in the deposits (Morgan *et al.*, 1976). Neither of these theories have been proven or accepted.

Clinically we want to know the factors that increase the rate of the deposit and the materials depositing on the lens in order to properly advise patients on preventing the build-up and what cleaning method is best.

Different polymers tend to attract and hold proteins differently. High water content, ionic lenses bind more protein, especially lysozyme, than do low water content lenses (Stone *et al.*, 1984; Antignani *et al.*, 1985; Fowler *et al.*, 1985). Ionic lens materials, for example those containing methylacrylic acid or other compounds that give a charge to the lens surface, bind more protein than those lens materials that have a neutral surface charge. Therefore, high water content, ionic lenses would be expected to coat more rapidly with a heavier coating. The ionic lenses apparently bind mainly basic proteins, i.e. lysozyme, whereas the neutral lenses bind all of the proteins about equally (Sack, 1985). On the ionic lenses 90% of the lysozyme present is active whereas on the neutral lenses essentially none of the protein is active (Sack, 1985). The fact that lysozyme is selectively bound on ionic lenses and remains active has interesting possibilities with respect to differential antimicrobial effects with different materials, especially with extended wear. Of course, if lenses with protein on the surface are heat disinfected the protein will be denatured and deactivated. Just because a lens material attracts certain proteins or coats to a greater degree while worn does not mean that it is a worse lens. A lens surface must coat to some degree to wet properly and be comfortable. The problem is when it coats to such a degree that the coating interferes with ocular physiology or vision or when the coating becomes denatured on the surface and can not be cleaned off. The full clinical implications of this differential coating is not presently known, but clinicians should be aware of the effect of material on the coating and if a patient has a problem with one type of material to change to a material in a different category. Table 47.8 indicates some of the materials in the different groups.

A clinical factor that will accelerate the rate of protein deposit formation on the lens surface is surface drying. It has been shown that patients with short tear film break-up times (BUT) will develop coatings faster than those with long BUTs. (Dohlman *et al.*, 1973; Lowther, 1975; Doughman *et al.*, 1976; Keot-

Table 47.8 Hydrogel lens groupings

Group I	Group II	Group III	Group IV
Low water, non-ionic	High water, non-ionic	Low water, ionic	High water, ionic
tefilcon (38%)	lidofilcon B (79%)	etafilcon (43%)	bufilcon A (55%)
–CibaSoft	–CW 79	–Hydromarc	–Hydrocurve II 55
–Cibathin	–Sauflon PW	–Visimarc	
–Softcolors			
tetrafilcon A	surfilcon (74%)	bufilcon A (45%)	perfilcon (71%)
–AO Soft	–Permaflex	–Hydrocurve II 45	–Permalens
–Aquaflex		–Softmate	–Permalens XL
crofilcon (39%)	lidofilcon A (74%)	deltafilcon A (43%)	etafilcon A (58%)
–CSI 38	–B&L 70	–Amsoft	–Vistamarc
	–Sauflon 70	–Aquasoft	
hefilcon A&B (43%)	vifilcon A (55%)	droxifilcon A (47%)	ocufilcon C (55%)
–Flexlens	–Softcon	–Accugel	-Ocu–Flex
–Sofsite	–Softcon EW		
–Naturvue			
phemfilcon A (30%)		phemfilcon A (38%)	phemfilcon A (55%)
–Durasoft		–Durasoft 2	–Durasoft 3
–Durasoft TT		–Durasoft 2 toric	–Durasoft 3 Toric
isofilcon (36%)		ocufilcon (44%)	tetrafilcon B (58%)
–AL–47		–Tresoft	–Aquaflex 58
polymacon (38%)		mafilcon (33%)	methafilcon (55%)
–Soflens		–N&N Menicon	–Hydracon
–Hydron			–Metro 55

ting, 1976; Hathway & Lowther, 1978; Holly, 1978; Refojo, 1984). The proteins apparently are concentrated on the lens surface by the evaporation of the water from the tears and the drying denatures the protein on the surface. Ions, such as calcium, may also be crystallized on and in the material by the drying. Once the denatured protein starts to build up on the lens surface, the surface dries more rapidly because the denatured protein is hydrophobic. This accelerates the deposition of more protein. Therefore, patients with short BUTs will most likely deposit protein more rapidly and must be more diligent in their routine lens cleaning.

Another factor that can affect the rate of protein deposits is the type of care system the patient uses. In general, heat disinfection systems will result in more rapid protein deposit. This is because the heat denatures

protein and precipitates ions on the lens surface creating multiple layers of coating and making the coating more difficult to remove. If all of the tear film constituents could be removed prior to heat disinfecting the lenses each day this would not be a problem. The removal of all material from the lens surface prior to disinfection is not possible but routine cleaning prior to heating will certainly prolong lens life.

47.14.1 REMOVING PROTEIN DEPOSITS

One of the most effective means of removing a protein coating is by the use of an enzymatic cleaner. The enzyme breaks down the protein molecule and allows easy removal. If a patient presents a lens with a heavy protein coating one can repeatedly use an enzymatic cleaner to remove it. By allowing the lens to

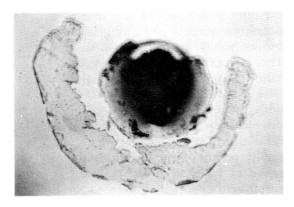

Figure 47.38 A rust spot on the surface of a hydrogel lens with some protein deposit around it.

would get on the patient's hands when handling the bottle and then be transferred to the lenses. The lenses would have a light pink tinge but would fluoresce when placed under an ultraviolet light due to the fluorescent nature of the ink. Therefore, in many cases one must question the patient carefully about chemicals, etc. that they may come into contact with and be a good detective to determine what is discoloring the lenses.

47.19   DISCOLORATION FROM MEDICATIONS

Epinephrine used while wearing contact lenses can cause a dark brown or black discoloration (Sugar, 1974; Miller *et al.*, 1976).

Topical vasoconstrictors such as tetrahydrozaline, when used with hydrogel lenses, have been reported to cause lens discoloration (Kleist, 1979b).

Topically applied drops containing phenylephrine, adrenaline and berberine have been reported to cause discoloration (Krezanoski, 1981).

It has also been reported that pyridium, tetracyline, phenolphthalein, rifamycin and nitrofurantoin are drugs that can discolor lenses (Aucamp, 1980). These drugs are taken

internally and excreted into the tears and stain the lenses. Rifampicin is a drug used systemically for treatment of tuberculosis or meningitis. It is secreted into the tears and will give the lenses an orange color (sometimes pink or red) (Lyons, 1979; Fraunfelder, 1980).

Sodium fluorescein used on the eye to evaluate corneal integrity can remain in the tears and get into the lens when the lens is placed on the eye. This will give a yellow-greenish discoloration that will fluoresce under ultraviolet light. With time the fluorescein will diffuse out and will not cause a problem. If large amounts of fluorescein get into lens it can be removed by repeatedly heat disinfecting the lens in distilled water changing water after each cycle or by just soaking the lens in distilled water or saline with several changes of solution over 12–24 hours.

47.20   DEPOSITS ON RIGID CONTACT LENSES

A majority of rigid gas permeable lenses used today are polymers containing silicone, acrylate and methylacrylic acid, HEMA or some other wetting agent. The addition of silicone increases the oxygen permeability but also increases the hydrophobicity of the lens surface creating spots or areas of relative nonwetting. Hydrophobic spots on the lens surface attract and hold nonaqueous compounds such as lipid (Fig. 47.39). Methylacrylic acid, HEMA or other compounds added to increase wettability helps the surface hold a tear film by adding a charge to the surface. In addition to holding water, the charged surface also attracts proteins and other tear film components. This coating or filming is the typical hazing seen on the lens surface when viewed under the biomicroscope (Fig. 47.40). Figure 47.41 shows both the surface hazing and spots of apparent lipid coating.

A number of methods can be used to

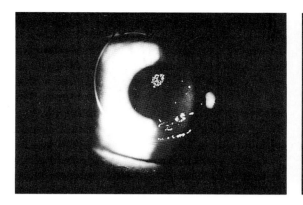

Figure 47.39 Lipid material deposited on the surface of a silicone/acrylate (rigid) lens.

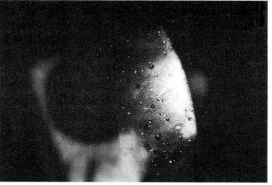

Figure 47.41 A protein type deposit (general hazy area) and a lipid deposit (spots) on a silicone/acrylate lens.

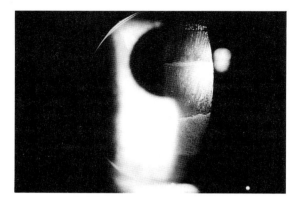

Figure 47.40 Deposit of protein type deposit on the surface of a silicone/acrylate (rigid) lens.

remove protein deposits from the lens surface. One is the daily use of surfactant cleaners. By rubbing the lens surface in the palm of the hand or between the fingers with the cleaner the majority of the deposits are removed. Deposits on the inside of the lens (base curve) are more difficult to remove because the patient tends not to rub the inside of the lens. If deposits are allowed to build up on the inside curve discomfort and corneal staining can occur. The inside of the lens should be cleaned at least once a week by placing a drop of the surfactant cleaner inside the lens and then rubbing the inside

curve with a cotton tipped applicator.

A number of surfactant cleaners clean the lenses well. Ones containing abrasive particles, usually either a polymer or aluminium oxide, work quite well. The patient must be sure to adequately rinse the cleaner off to prevent discomfort on lens placement. There has been concern that these particles might scratch the lens surface but clinically this does not seem presently to be a problem.

Enzymatic cleaners do a good job breaking down protein on rigid lenses as they do on hydrogel lenses. All present enzymes used on hydrogel lenses can also be used on rigid lenses. A schedule of once a week cleaning with the enzyme is usually sufficient. Many patients do fine without using enzyme, however, it should be recommended for any patient with protein coating problems.

Lipid deposits can often be more difficult to remove than protein deposits. The surfactants, particularly those with the abrasives, help. In some cases using a cleaner with some alcohol content will quickly remove these deposits. The alcohol is a good solvent for nonaqueous compounds. One must be careful not to allow the lenses to soak in the alcohol solution as it will be absorbed by the lens and distort it. If used to clean the lens and immediately rinsed off there is no apparent problem.

Foreign material from the hands, such as hand creams, cosmetics and oils, can coat the surfaces of gas permeable lenses (Fig. 47.42). Such material can often be difficult to remove. Using a good surfactant, particularly one containing alcohol, will often remove the foreign material. Preventing the deposit in the first place by proper hand washing with a soap not containing creams or lotions is best.

For especially tenanous deposits the lens surface can be polished using a soft polishing pad with a polish formulated for use on gas permeable lenses. The polish should not contain any solvents that might damage the material. In addition, one must be careful not to allow excessive heat to be generated during the polishing process as most gas permeable lenses are easily distorted.

47.21   SOFT SILICONE LENSES

Soft silicone lenses are finding only limited use because of surface deterioration and coating as well as due to fitting problems. These lenses must be surface treated in order to obtain a wettable surface. The surface

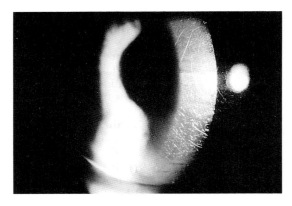

Figure 47.43 A deposit of tear film material on a soft silicone lens. The deposit has cracked.

coats easily with tear film components and can be very difficult to remove. The surface coating tends to crack (Fig. 47.43), probably due to the fact the lens material is elastic, and therefore stretches while the coating does not. Surfactants are used to help keep the surface clean but even with diligent use many lenses will still eventually coat. Enzymatic cleaning is helpful with some patients but not universally so. With any of the cleaning procedures deposits return quickly. The lenses can not be polished as this will result in a hydrophobic surface and a useless lens.

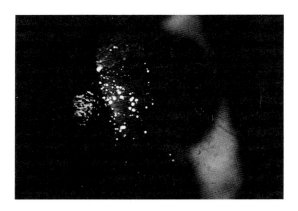

Figure 47.42 A heavy lipid deposit from hand cream on the surface of a silicone/acrylate (rigid) lens.

REFERENCES

Allen, J. (1978) Deposits on contact lenses. *The Optician*, **175**(4517), 8–9.
Antignani, A. *et al.* (1985) A determination of total protein and total lipid on individual worn contact lenses. Presented at the Am. Acad. Optom. Mtg. Atlanta, December 1985.
Aucamp, A. (1980) Drug excretion in human tears and its meaning for contact lens wearers. *The South African Optom.*, **39**, 128–36..
Bailey, N.J. (1976) Wrong solutions to the cleaning problem. *CLF*, **1**(8), 10–15.
Bier, N. and Lowther, G.E. (1977) *Contact Lens Correction*. Butterworths, London, pp.422–3.
Caroline, *et al.* (1985) Microscopic and elemental analysis of deposits on extended wear soft contact lenses. *The CLAO J.*, **11**(4), 311–16.

Dohlman, C.H. *et al.* (1973) Complications in use of soft contact lenses in corneal disease. *Arch. Ophth.*, **90**, 367–71.

Doughman, D.J. *et al.* (1975) The nature of 'spots' on soft lenses. *Ann. Ophth.*, **7**(3), 345–53.

Filippi, J.A. *et al.* (1973) Penetration of hydrophilic contact lenses by *Aspergillus fumagatus. Am. J. Optom*, **50**(7), 553–7.

Filippi, J.A., Pfister, G.E., Lowther, G.E. and Hill, R.M. (1973) Factors limiting hydrophilic lens life. *J. Am. Optom. Assoc.*, **44** (7), 722–5.

Fowler, S. *et al.* (1985) Deposits on soft contact lenses of various water contents. *The CLAO J.*, **11** (2), 124–7.

Fraunfelder, F.T. (1980) Orange tears. *Am. J. Ophth.*, **89**(5), 752.

Freiberg, J. (1977) Deposition of calcium carbonate and calcium phosphate on hydrophilic contact lenses. *ICLC*, **3**, 63.

Ganju, S.N. and Cordrey, P. (1977) A study of deposits on extended wear soft contact lenses made from Sauflon 85. *The Optician*, **173**(4466), 8–16.

Gudmundsson, O.F. *et al.* (1985) Identification of proteins in contact lens surface deposits by immunofluorescence microscopy. *Arch. Ophth.*, **103** (2), 196–7.

Hart, D. (1984) Lipid deposits which form on extended wear contact lenses. *ICLC*, **11**(6), 348–60.

Hathway, R.A. and Lowther, G.E. (1976) Appearance of hydrophilic lens deposits as related to chemical etiology. *ICLC*, **3**, 27–35.

Hathaway, R.A. and Lowther, G.E. (1978) Factors influencing the rate of deposit formation on hydrophilic lenses. *Aust. J. Optom.*, **61**, 92–6.

Hilbert, J., Lowther, G. and King, J. (1976) Deposition of substances within hydrophilic lenses. *Am. J. Optom.*, **53** (2), 51–4.

Holly, F.J. (1978) Preocular tear film. *Contact Intraocular Lens Med. J.*, **4**, 134.

Karageozian, H.L. (1974a) *Chemical Identity of Opaque Deposits on Human Worn Hydrophilic Lenses.* Allergan Report Series no. 92.

Karageozian, H.L. (1974b) *Laboratory Simulation Model for the Production of Opaque Deposits on Hydrophilic Lenses.* Allergan Report Series no. 93.

Keotting, R.A. (1976) Predicting soft lens surface problems. *CLF*, 1, 18–27.

Kimmerer, R.W. and Szabocsik J.M. (1978) Consideration of fungal invasion of hydrophilic contact lenses. In *Developments in Industrial Microbiology*, Proceedings of the 34th General Meeting of the Society for Industrial Microbiology, August 21–26, 1977, Society for Industrial Microbiology, Arlington, VA, pp. 237–44.

Kleist, F.D. (1979a) Appearance and nature of hydrophilic contact lens deposits. *ICLC*, **6**(3), 120–30.

Kleist, F.D. (1979b) Appearance and nature of hydrophilic contact lens deposits – Part 2: inorganic deposits. *ICLC*, **6**(4), 177–86.

Klintworth, G.K. *et al.* (1977) Calcification of soft contact lenses in patients with dry eye and elevated calcium concentrations in tears. *Invest. Ophth. Vis. Sci.*, **16**, 158.

Krezanoski, J. (1972) The significance of cleaning hydrophilic contact lenses. *J. Am. Optom. Assoc.*, **43** (3), 305–7.

Krezanoski, J. (1981) Topical medications. *Int. Ophth. Clin.*, **21**(2), 173–6..

Lamb, V.R. (1979) Rejuvenating discolored soft lenses. *CLF*, **4**(5), 33–5.

Liotet, S. *et al.* (1983) The genesis of organic deposits on soft contact lenses. *The CLAO J.*, **9** (1), 49–56.

Lowther, G.E. (1975) The relationship between the chemistry of the tear film and hydrophilic lens deposits. In *Proceedings of the 2nd National Research Symposium on Soft Contact Lenses*, Excerpta Medica, Princeton, NJ.

Lowther, G.E. and Hilbert, J.A. (1975) Deposits on hydrophilic lenses: differential appearance and clinical causes. *AJO*, **52** (10), 687–92.

Lowther, G.E., Hilbert J.A. and King, J.E. (1975) Appearance and location of hydrophilic lens deposits, *ICLC*, **2**, 30–4.

Lyons, R.W. (1979) Orange contact lenses from rifampin. *N. Eng. J. Med.*, **300**, 372.

Miller, D. *et al.* (1976) Adrenochrome staining of soft contact lenses. *Ann. Ophth.*, **8**, 65–7.

Morgan, J.F. *et al.* (1976) Blood constituents and hydrophilic lens coating. In *Proceedings of the 2nd International Medical Symposium* (ed. S. Mishima), Bausch & Lomb, Rochester, NY.

Phillips, A.J. (1979) Extended-wear hydrogel lenses in the United Kingdom. *ICLC*, **6**, 54–65.

Refojo, M.F. (1984) Binding of proteins and foreign materials. *J. Am. Optom. Assoc.*, **55**(3), 194.

Refojo, M.F. and Holly, G.J. (1977) Tear protein adsorption on hydrogel: a possible cause of contact lens allergy. *The Contact Lens*, **January/March** 23.

Ruben, M. *et al.* (1975) Calcium deposits as a cause of spoilation of hydrophilic soft contact lenses. *Br. J. Ophth.*, **59**, 141.

Ruben, M. (1976) Biochemical aspects of soft lenses. *Contact Intraoc Lens Med. J.*, **2**(4), 39–51.

Rudko, P. and Gregg, T.H. (1975) *A Study of the Safety of an Enzyme Preparation for Cleaning Hydrophilic Lenses*. Allergan Report Series #97.

Sack, R.A. (1985) Specificity and biological activity of lens bound protein layer to hydrogel structure. Presented at the Am. Acad. of Optom. Mtg., Atlanta, December 1985.

Sagan, W. (1976) Fungal invasion of a soft contact lens. *Arch. Ophth.*, **94**, 168.

Shapiro, I. (1974) Penicillium species fungus growth on a bionite hydrophilic contact lens. *Minn. Med.*, **57**(12), 943–4.

Sibley, M.J. and Chu, V. (1984) Understanding sorbic acid-preserved contact lens solutions. *ICLC*, **11**(9), 531–9.

Stone, R.P. *et al.* (1984) Protein: a source of lens discoloration. *CLF*, **9**, 33–41.

Sugar, J. (1974) Adrenochrome pigmentation of hydrophilic lenses. *Arch. Ophth.*, **91**(1), 11–12.

Trager, S.Y. (1972) Solutions for soft lenses. *Manufacturing Optics Intern.*, **May,** 403–5.

Tripathi, R.C. *et al.* (1980) The pathology of soft contact lens spoilage. *Am. J. Ophth.*, **87**(5), 365–80.

Uotila, M.H. and Gasset, A.R. (1972) Fitting Manual for Bausch and Lomb and Griffin Lenses. In *Soft Contact Lens* (ed. A.R. Gasset and H. Kaufman), C.V. Mosby Co., St Louis.

Wedler, F.C. (1977) Analysis of biomaterials deposited on soft contact lenses. *J. Biomed. Mater. Res.*, **11**, 525–35.

Wedler, F.C. and Riedhammer, T.M. (1982) Soft contact lenses: formation of deposits. *Biocompatibility in Clinical Practice*, **11**.

INDEX

Page numbers in **bold** refer to figures and page numbers in *italic* refer to tables.